NEPHROLOGY

SECRETS

T0195358

FOURTH EDITION

EDGAR V. LERMA, MD, FACP, FASN, FNKF, FPSN (Hon)
Clinical Professor of Medicine
Section of Nephrology
University of Illinois at Chicago College of Medicine/Advocate Christ
  Medical Center
Oak Lawn, Illinois

MATTHEW A. SPARKS, MD, FASN, FNKF
Assistant Professor of Medicine
Associate Program Director, Nephrology Fellowship
Duke University Medical Center;
Staff Physician
Durham VA Medical Center
Durham, North Carolina

JOEL M. TOPF, MD, FACP
Assistant Clinical Professor
Department of Medicine
Oakland University William Beaumont School of Medicine
Auburn Hills, Michigan

ELSEVIER

ELSEVIER

1600 John F. Kennedy Blvd.
Ste 1800
Philadelphia, PA 19103-2899

NEPHROLOGY SECRETS, FOURTH EDITION

ISBN: 978-0-323-47871-7

Notices

Previous editions copyrighted 2012, 2003, and 1999.

Library of Congress Cataloging-in-Publication Data

Names: Lerma, Edgar V., editor. | Sparks, Matthew A., editor. | Topf, Joel M., editor.
Title: Nephrology secrets / [edited by] Edgar V. Lerma, Matthew A. Sparks, Joel M. Topf.
Description: Fourth edition. | Philadelphia, PA : Elsevier, [2019] | Includes
    bibliographical references and index.
Identifiers: LCCN 2017060071 | ISBN 9780323478717 (hardcover : alk. paper)
Subjects: | MESH: Kidney Diseases
Classification: LCC RC903 | NLM WJ 300 | DDC 616.6/1--dc23
LC record available at https://lccn.loc.gov/2017060071

International Standard Book Number: 978-0-323-47871-7

Content Strategist: James Merritt
Content Development Specialist: Meghan Andress
Publishing Services Manager: Catherine Jackson
Senior Project Manager: Rachel E. McMullen
Design Direction: Bridget Hoette

Printed in India

Last digit is the print number: 9 8 7 6

Working together to grow libraries in developing countries

www.elsevier.com • www.bookaid.org

*To all my mentors, and friends, at the University of Santo Tomas
Faculty of Medicine and Surgery in Manila, Philippines, and
Northwestern University Feinberg School of Medicine in Chicago, IL,
who have in one way or another influenced and guided me to
become the physician that I am . . .
To all the medical students, interns, and residents at Advocate Christ
Medical Center whom I have taught or learned from, especially those
who eventually decided to pursue nephrology as a career . . .
To my parents and my brothers, without whose unwavering love
and support through the good and challenging times I would not have
persevered and reached my goals in life . . .
Most especially, to my two lovely and precious daughters, Anastasia
Zofia and Isabella Ann, whose smiles and laughter constantly
provide me with unparalleled joy and happiness; and my very loving
and understanding wife, Michelle, who has always been supportive
of my endeavors both personally and professionally, and who sacrificed
a lot of time and exhibited unwavering patience as I devoted a
significant amount of time and effort to this project. Truly,
they always provide me with motivation and inspiration.*
Edgar V. Lerma, MD, FACP, FASN, FNKF, FPSN (Hon)

*Editing the fourth edition of Nephrology Secrets has been both
rewarding and educational. Thanks to Edgar and Joel for embarking
on this journey with me. I could not ask for a better editorial team.
Thanks to each of the chapter authors for taking time to research
and write excellent chapters. Thanks to all of my mentors, especially
Tom Andreoli, Bob Safirstein, and Tom Coffman. Thanks to the many
undergraduates, medical students, residents, fellows, and my
colleagues I have had the privilege to work with both at Duke
University Medical Center and the University of Arkansas for Medical
Sciences. You have all played an important role in my life and continue
to inspire and motivate me. Thanks to my family, my siblings Jeff,
Shannon, and my parents for their encouragement and support.
Especially thanks to my wife, Neha, and the twins, Meera and Ishan,
for their unequivocal support and love throughout this project.
Thank you to the many patients and family members I have had
the privilege to care for over the years. I sincerely hope this book
helps others on their journey in medicine.*
Matthew A. Sparks, MD, FASN, FNKF

My hike through medicine and nephrology has been filled with teachers and mentors. It has been a rich and rewarding journey in ways that I could never have imagined. During this journey there have been particular people who have believed in me and have been willing to trust me on this somewhat unconventional path. Ernest Yoder at Wayne State School of Medicine, Mary Ciccarelli at Indiana University Med-Peds, and Patrick Murray at the University of Chicago Nephrology Fellowship immediately come to mind. After my formal education, Robert Provenzano has been a tireless cheerleader and more importantly, he built St Clair Specialty Physicians into the type of nephrology company where a physician who saw private practice a bit differently could thrive.

I probably owe the most to the online nephrology community that has blossomed in the last few years to be an always-on, all-hours, cocktail party, with interesting conversation and intelligent answers to the questions that bombard us all in clinical nephrology. #NephTwitter, you are the future of nephrology education. Don't slow down; keep going full speed ahead.

I want to thank my wife, Cathy. Without her I wouldn't be able to do any of this. She is understanding, helpful, and patient. She has excellent instincts and continues to be an awesome partner. She is better than I deserve. Thanks for everything. Cathy is a wonderful mother to our twins, Simon and Laura, who are great kids and always put a smile on my face. It has been a delight watching you mature into thoughtful and kind adults. Keep doing what you are doing, you are going to be the people this planet needs.

Finally, I am left with the impossible task of trying to express the amount of gratitude I have for my parents and how much they have given me. Nobody could have received a better childhood than my parents gave me and my sister. My mom and dad have always helped guide and support me. So many times they could have tried to block an unconventional decision, but instead, they understood what I was trying to do and supported and helped me along. Thanks.

Joel M. Topf, MD, FACP

CONTRIBUTORS

Rajiv Agarwal, MD
Professor of Medicine
Division of Nephrology
Indiana University School of Medicine
Indianapolis, Indiana

Talal Alfaadhel, MBBS, FRCPC
Assistant Professor
Department of Medicine
King Saud University Medical City
King Saud University
Riyadh, Saudi Arabia

Martin J. Andersen, DO
Assistant Professor of Clinical Medicine
Division of Nephrology
Indiana University School of Medicine
Indianapolis, Indiana

John Robert Asplin, MD
Medical Director
Litholink Corp, Laboratory Corporation of Americ
    Holdings
Chicago, Illinois

Rupali S. Avasare MD
Assistant Professor of Medicine
Department of Medicine
Oregon Health and Science University
Portland, Oregon

George L. Bakris, MD
Professor and Director, ASH Comprehensive
    Hypertension Center
Department of Medicine
The University of Chicago Medicine
Chicago, Illinois

Amar D. Bansal, MD
Division of Renal-Electrolyte
Section of Palliative Care and Medical Ethics
University of Pennsylvania
Philadelphia, Pennsylvania

Pravir V. Baxi, MD
Assistant Professor of Medicine
Division of Nephrology
Department of Internal Medicine
Rush University Medical Center
Chicago, Illinois

Michael Berkoben, MD, FACP
Associate Professor of Medicine
Division of Nephrology
Duke University Medical Center
Durham, North Carolina

Scott D. Bieber, DO
Clinical Associate Professor of Medicine
University of Washington
Seattle, Washington

Florian Buchkremer, MD
Division of Nephrology, Dialysis & Transplantation
Kantonsspital Aarau
Aarau, Switzerland

Anna Marie Burgner, MD, MEHP
Assistant Professor
Department of Nephrology and Hypertension
Vanderbilt University Medical Center
Nashville, Tennessee

James Brian Byrd, MD, MS
Assistant Professor
Department of Medicine
University of Michigan
Ann Arbor, Michigan

Daniel Cattran, MD
Professor of Medicine
Department of Medicine
University Health Network;
Senior Scientist
Toronto General Research Institute
University Health Network
Toronto, Ontario, Canada

Devasmita Choudhury, MD
Chief Renal Section
Salem Veterans Affairs Medical Center
Salem, Virginia;
Associate Professor Medicine
University of Virginia
Charlottesville Virginia;
Virginia Tech Carilion School of Medicine
Roanoke Virginia

Rolando Claure-Del Granado, MD, FASN
Professor of Medicine
Head Division of Nephrology
Hospital Obrero #2 - C.N.S.,
Universidad Mayor de San Simon School of Medicine
Cochabamba, Bolivia

Bradley M. Denker, MD
Associate Professor of Medicine
Harvard Medical School;
Clinical Chief
Renal Division
Beth Israel Deaconess Medical Center;
Chief of Nephrology
Harvard Vanguard Medical Associates
Boston, Massachusetts

Vimal K. Derebail, MD
Assistant Professor of Medicine
UNC Kidney Center
University of North Carolina
Chapel Hill, North Carolina

Robert J. Desnick, PhD, MD
Dean for Genetics and Genomic Medicine
Department of Genetics and Genomic Sciences
Icahn School of Medicine at Mount Sinai
New York, New York

Luca di Lullo, MD
Department of Nephrology and Dialysis
L. Parodi–Delfino Hospital
Colleferro, Italy

John V. Duronville, MD
Medical Instructor
Division of Nephrology
Duke University Medical Center
Durham, North Carolina

Garabed Eknoyan, MD
Selzman Institute of Kidney Health
Section of Nephrology
Department of Medicine
Baylor College of Medicine
Houston, Texas

Mina El Kateb, MD
Transplant Nephrology Fellow
St John Hospital and Medical Center
Detroit, Michigan

William J. Elliott, MD, PhD
Professor of Preventive Medicine, Internal Medicine
and Pharmacology
Chair
Department of Biomedical Sciences;
Chief
Division of Pharmacology
Pacific Northwest University of Health Sciences
Yakima, Washington

Jennifer L. Ennis, MD, FACP
Medical Director
Litholink Corporation, a LabCorp Company;
Clinical Assistant Professor of Medicine
Medicine, Division of Nephrology
University of Illinois at Chicago
Chicago, Illinois

Fernando G. Fervenza, MD, PhD
Professor of Medicine
Department of Nephrology and Hypertension
Mayo Clinic
Rochester, Minnesota

Robert A. Figlin, MD, FACP
Steven Spielberg Family Chair in Hematology
Oncology;
Professor of Medicine and Biomedical Sciences,
Director
Division of Hematology Oncology;
Deputy Director
Integrated Oncology Service Line;
Deputy Director
Samuel Oschin Comprehensive Cancer Institute
Cedars-Sinai Medical Center
Saperstein Critical Care Tower
Los Angeles, California

Zita Galvin, MD
Liver Transplant Unit
Toronto General Hospital
University Health Network
Toronto, Ontario, Canada

Pranav S. Garimella, MD
Division of Nephrology-Hypertension
University of California San Diego
San Diego, California

Debbie S. Gipson, MS, MD
Professor of Pediatrics
Department of Pediatrics
University of Michigan
Ann Arbor, Michigan

Patrick E. Gipson, MD
Professor of Pediatrics
University of Michigan
Ann Arbor, Michigan

David S. Goldfarb, MD, FACP, FASN, FNKF
Professor of Medicine and Physiology
NYU School of Medicine;
Interim Division Chief
Department of Nephrology
NYU Langone Medical Center
New York, New York

Arthur Greenberg, MD
Professor of Medicine, Emeritus
Division of Nephrology
Department of Medicine
Duke University Medical Center
Durham, North Carolina

Hermann Haller, MD
Professor,
Director
Department of Nephrology and Hypertension
Hannover Medical School
Hannover, Germany

Swapnil Hiremath, MD, MPH
Assistant Professor
Department of Medicine
University of Ottawa;
Senior Clinical Investigator
Clinical Epidemiology
Ottawa Hospital Research Institute
Ottawa, Ontario, Canada

Edward J. Horwitz, MD
Metrohealth Medical Center
Case Western Reserve University School of Medicine
Cleveland, Ohio

Susan Hou, MD
Professor of Medicine
Department of Medicine
Division of Nephrology and Hypertension
Loyola University Medical Center
Maywood, Illinois

Lesley A. Inker, MD, MS
Associate Professor of Medicine
Department of Medicine
Tufts University School of Medicine
Boston, Massachusetts

Maria V. Irazabal, MD
Assistant Professor of Medicine
Division of Nephrology
Department of Internal Medicine
Mayo Clinic
Rochester, Minnesota

Ashley Bruce Irish, MBBS, FRACP
Consultant Nephrologist
Department of Nephrology and Transplantation
Fiona Stanley Hospital;
Clinical Professor
Department of Medicine
University of Western Australia
Perth, Western Australia, Australia

Kenar D. Jhaveri, MD
Professor of Medicine
Division of Nephrology
Zucker School of Medicine at Hofstra/Northwell
Hempstead, New York

Jonathan Ashley Jefferson, MD, FRCP
Professor of Medicine
Division of Nephrology
University of Washington
Seattle, Washington

Kamyar Kalantar-Zadeh, MD, MPH, PhD
Professor and Chief
Division of Nephrology and Hypertension
University of California Irvine Medical Center
Orange, California

Elaine S. Kamil, MD
Health Sciences Clinical Professor of Pediatrics
David Geffen School of Medicine at UCLA;
Department of Pediatric Nephrology
Cedars-Sinai Medical Center
Los Angeles, California

Jon-Emile S. Kenny, MD
Assistant Professor of Medicine
Department of Internal Medicine
Icahn School of Medicine at Mount Sinai
New York, New York;
Masters Candidate
Department of Learning, Informatics, Management and Ethics
Karolinska Institutet
Stockholm, Sweden

Charbel C. Khoury, MD
Fellow
Department of Nephrology
Brigham and Women's Hospital;
Fellow
Department of Nephrology
Massachusetts General Hospital
Boston, Massachusetts

Jatinder Kohli, MD
University of Pennsylvania School of Medicine
Hospital of the University of Pennsylvania
Philadelphia Pennsylvania

Eugene C. Kovalik, MD, CM, FRCP(C), FACP, FASN
Associate Profesor of Medicine
Department of Medicine/Nephrology
Duke University Medical Center
Durham, North Carolina

Csaba P. Kovesdy, MD
Fred Hatch Professor of Medicine
Department of Medicine
University of Tennessee Health Science Center;
Nephrology Section Chief
Memphis VA Medical Center
Memphis, Tennessee

Warren Kupin, MD
Professor of Medicine
Miami Transplant Institute
Katz Family Division of Nephrology
University of Miami
Miami, Florida

Ruediger W. Lehrich, MD
Associate Professor of Medicine,
Program Director
Nephrology Fellowship,
Director of Home-Suitable Dialysis
Duke University Medical Center
Durham, North Carolina

Edgar V. Lerma, MD, FACP, FASN, FNKF, FPSN (Hon)
Clinical Professor of Medicine
Section of Nephrology
University of Illinois at Chicago College of Medicine/
  Advocate Christ Medical Center
Oak Lawn, Illinois

Moshe Levi, MD
Professor of Biochemistry and Molecular & Cellular
  Biology
Georgetown University Medical Center
Aurora, Colorado

Joseph L. Lockridge, MD
Medical Director
Kidney Transplant Program
Portland VA Health Care System;
Director of Transplant Nephrology
Fellowship Training Program,
Assistant Professor of Medicine
Oregon Health & Science University
Portland, Oregon

Jennifer Lopez, BS
Division of Pediatric Nephrology
NYU Langone Health
New York, New York

Etienne Macedo, MD, PhD
Assistant Adjunct Professor
University of California San Diego, School of
  Medicine
San Diego, California

Rajnish Mehrotra, MBBS, MD, MS
Professor of Medicine
Department of Medicine
University of Washington;
Section Head Nephrology
Department of Medicine
Harborview Medical Center
Seattle, Washington

Ravindra L. Mehta, MBBS, MD, DM, FACP, FASN
Professor of Clinical Medicine,
Associate Chair of Clinical Research,
Director CREST and MAS in Clinical Research
  Program
Department of Medicine
University of California San Diego
San Diego, California

Patrick H. Nachman, MD
Marion Stedman Covington Distinguished Professor
  of Medicine
UNC Kidney Center
University of North Carolina
Chapel Hill, North Carolina

Carol Nadai, MD
Medical Oncologist Instituto de Oncologia do Parana
Curitibia, Brazil

Lavinia Aura Negrea, MD
Associate Professor of Medicine
Department of Medicine
University Hospitals Case Medical Center
Cleveland, Ohio

Lindsay E. Nicolle, MD
University of Manitoba
Winnipeg, Manitoba, Canada

Keith C. Norris, MD, PhD
Professor
Department of Medicine
David Geffen School of Medicine, UCLA
Los Angeles, California

Alexander Novakovic, MD
Research Associate
Division of Genitourinary
Malignancies Department of Medical Oncology &
  Therapeutics Research
City of Hope Comprehensive Cancer Center
Duarte, California

Ali J. Olyaei, PharmD
Professor
Medicine and Pharmacy Practice
Division of Nephrology and Hypertension
OSU/OHSU
Portland, Oregon

Sumanta Kumar Pal, MD
Associate Professor
Department of Medical Oncology and Experimental
  Therapeutics
Division of Genitourinary Malignancies
City of Hope Comprehensive Cancer Center
Duarte, California

Paul M. Palevsky MD
Chief, Renal Section
VA Pittsburgh Healthcare System;
Professor of Medicine and Clinical & Translational
 Science
Department of Medicine
University of Pittsburgh
Pittsburgh, Pennsylvania

Ami M. Patel, MD
Assistant Professor of Medicine
University of Maryland School of Medicine,
Baltimore VA Medical Center
Baltimore, Maryland

Vikram Patney, MD
Nephrology and Hypertension Specialists, LLC
St. Louis, Missouri

Mark A. Perazella, MD
Professor of Medicine
Section of Nephrology
Yale University School of Medicine;
Director, Acute Dialysis Unit,
Medical Director, Yale Physician Associate
 Program,
Medical Director, Yale PA Online Program
New Haven, Connecticut

Phuong-Chi T. Pham, MD
Olive View-UCLA Medical Center
Los Angeles, California

Phuong-Thu T. Pham, MD
David Geffen School of Medicine at UCLA
Ronald Reagan UCLA Medical Center
Los Angeles, California

Joseph B. Pryor, BS
School of Medicine
Oregon Health & Sciences University
Portland, Oregon

C. Venkata S. Ram
Director
Apollo Heart Institute for Blood Pressure Management
 and Apollo Blood Pressure Clinics
Hyderabad, India

Mahboob Rahman, MD
University Hospitals Cleveland Medical Center
Case Western Reserve University School of Medicine
Cleveland, Ohio

Nathaniel Reisinger, MD
Instructor and Clinical Ultrasound Fellow
Department of Emergency Medicine
Penn Medicine;
Moonlighting Nephrologist
Division of Renal, Electrolyte, and Hypertension
Penn Medicine
Philadelphia, Pennsylvania

Michael V. Rocco, MD, MSCE
Vardaman M. Buckalew Jr. Professor of Internal
 Medicine/Nephrology
Internal Medicine, Section on Nephrology
Wake Forest School of Medicine
Winston-Salem, North Carolina

Claudio Ronco, MD
Director
Department of Nephrology
San Bortolo Hospital;
Director
International Renal Research Institute
San Bortolo Hospital
Vicenza, Italy

Mark E. Rosenberg, MD, FASN
Vice Dean for Education and Academic Affairs
University of Minnesota Medical School
Lino Lakes, Minnesota

Mitchell H. Rosner, MD
Professor of Medicine
Department of Medicine
University of Virginia Health System
Charlottesville, Virginia

Michael R. Rudnick, MD, FACP, FASN
Associate Professor of Medicine
University of Pennsylvania School of Medicine;
Chief
Nephrology Division
Penn Presbyterian Medical Center
Philadelphia, Pennsylvania

Ernesto Sabath, MD
Hospital General de Queretaro
Universidad Autonomo de Queretaro
Santiade Queretaro, Mexico

Mark J. Sarnak MD, MS
Tufts Medical Center
Boston, Massachusetts

Jane O. Schell, MD, MHS
Assistant Professor of Medicine
Division of Renal-Electrolyte
University of Pittsburgh Medical Center
Pittsburgh, Pennsylvania

N. Winn Seay, MD
Fellow, Division of Nephrology
Department of Medicine
Duke University Medical Center
Durham, North Carolina

John R. Sedor, MD
Professor Molecular Medicine
Cleveland Clinic Lerner College of Medicine
Case Western Reserve University;
Staff
Glickman Urology & Kidney Institute;
Staff
Department of Pathobiology
Lerner Research Institute
Cleveland, Ohio

Akash Nair Sethi, DO
Fellow
Renal, Electrolyte, and Hypertension Division
Hosptial of the University of Pennsylvania
Philadelphia, Pennsylvania

Anuja Shah, MD
Department of Medicine
Division of Nephrology
Harbor-UCLA Medical Center
Torrance, California;
David Geffen School of Medicine at UCLA
Los Angeles, California

Lori Shah, DO
Nephrology Fellow
Vanderbilt University Medical Center
Nashville, Tennessee

Benjamin A. Sherer
Clinical Fellow
Department of Urologic Surgery,
   Laparoscopy/Endourology
University of California San Francisco
San Francisco, California

Harpreet Singh, MD
Medical Instructor
Duke University Medical Center
Durham, North Carolina

**Rajalingam Sinniah, DSc, MD, PhD, FRCPI, FRCPA,
FRCPath**
Clinical Professor of Pathology
School of Pathology and Laboratory Medicine
The University of Western Australia;
Consultant Pathologist,
Anatomic Pathology
Pathwest Laboratory Medicine
Fiona Stanley Hospital
Western Australia, Australia

James A. Sloand, MD, FACP, FASN
Senior Medical Director, Global Therapeutic Area
   Lead, Peritoneal Dialysis
Renal Franchise
Baxter Healthcare Corporation
Deerfield, Illinois

Matthew A. Sparks, MD, FASN, FNKF
Assistant Professor of Medicine
Associate Program Director, Nephrology Fellowship
Duke University Medical Center;
Staff Physician
Durham VA Medical Center
Durham, North Carolina

Stuart M. Sprague, DO
NorthShore University HealthSystem
Evanston, Illinois;
Clincal Professor of Medicine
University of Chicago Pritzker School of Medicine
Chicago, Illinois

Susan Patricia Steigerwalt, MD
Clinical Associate Professor
Cardiovascular Medicine
University of Michigan
Ann Arbor, Michigan

Hillel Sternlicht, MD
Assistant Professor of Medicine
Hofstra University School of Medicine
Department of Medicine
Lenox Hill Hospital-Northwell Health
New York, New York

Marshall L. Stoller, MD
San Francisco, California

Beje Thomas, MD
Assistant Professor of Medicine
Division of Nephrology
University of Maryland School of Medicine
Baltimore, Maryland

Hakan R. Toka, MD, PhD, FASN
Manatee Memorial Hospital
Graduate Medical Education
Bradenton, Florida

Joel M. Topf, MD, FACP
Assistant Clinical Professor
Department of Medicine
Oakland University William Beaumont School of
   Medicine
Auburn Hills, Michigan

Vicente E. Torres, MD, PhD
Professor of Medicine
Department of Nephrology and Hypertension
Mayo Clinic
Rochester, Minnesota

Howard Trachtman, MD
Chief, Division of Pediatric Nephrology and
   Hypertension,
Professor of Pediatrics
Division of Nephrology
NYU Langone Medical Center
New York, New York

Carol Traynor, MB, BCh, BAO, BMedSci
Medical Instructor
Division of Nephrology
Duke University Medical Center
Durham, North Carolina

Bryan M. Tucker, DO, MS
Assistant Professor of Medicine
Department of Internal Medicine, Section
   of Nephrology
Wake Forest University School of Medicine
Winston-Salem, North Carolina

Beth A. Vogt, MD
Associate Professor
Department of Pediatrics
Case Western Reserve University;
Attending Physician
Division of Nephrology
Rainbow Babies and Children's Hospital
Cleveland, Ohio

Rimda Wanchoo, MD
Associate Professor of Medicine
Division of Nephrology
Zucker School of Medicine at Hofstra/Northwell
Hempstead, New York

Matthew R. Weir, MD
Professor of Medicine
Department of Medicine,
Director, Division of Nephrology
University of Maryland School of Medicine
Baltimore, Maryland

Adam Whaley-Connell, DO
Associate Professor of Medicine
Department of Medicine
Division of Nephrology and Hypertension
University of Missouri-Columbia School of Medicine;
Division of Endocrinology and Metabolism, and the
   Research Service
Harry S. Truman Memorial Veterans Hospital
Columbia, Missouri

William L. Whittier, MD, FASN
Associate Professor of Medicine
Division of Nephrology
Department of Internal Medicine
Rush University Medical Center
Chicago, Illinois

Jay B. Wish, MD
Professor of Clinical Medicine
Department of Medicine
Indiana University School of Medicine
Indianapolis, Indiana

Florence Wong, MB, BS, MD, FRACP, FRCPC
Professor
Department of Medicine, Division of
   Gastroenterology
University of Toronto
Toronto, Ontario, Canada

David C. Wymer, MD, FACR, FACNM
Associate Chair
Radiology
University of Florida;
Chief of Service, Imaging
Department of Radiology
Malcom Randall VAMC
Gainesville, Florida

David T.G. Wymer, MD
Resident
Department of Radiology
Mount Sinai Medical Center
Miami Beach, Florida

Ladan Zand, MD
Assistant Professor
Department of Nephrology and Hypertension
Mayo Clinic
Rochester, Minnesota

PREFACE

"Questions you will be asked on rounds, in the clinic, and on oral exams."

This was the subtitle to the first *Medical Secrets* textbook by Anthony Zollo from 1991. This was click bait before there was click bait. No medical student could resist a title like that. And it also is strangely compelling for attendings and teachers. Doctors don't get to peer inside the bedside teaching of other attendings, and the chance to see the questions that others are asking is hard to resist.

The book in your hand is the fourth edition of *Nephrology Secrets*. It has been nearly a decade since Lerma and Nissenson edited the third edition. All aspects of nephrology have evolved, and some topics have been completely revolutionized. Since the third edition was published, the cause of idiopathic membranous nephropathy has been elucidated, a genetic mutation explaining the high rate of kidney disease in African Americans has been discovered. We have an effective therapy for hepatitis C and its downstream kidney effects. Home dialysis modalities have recovered from being on the ropes and are now resurgent in both peritoneal and hemodialysis. The biomedical revolution in oncology has uncovered novel kidney diseases. The molecular mechanism of preeclampsia, the most common glomerular disease on the planet, has been elucidated. Nephrology is no longer the slow, methodical specialty of yore; it is fast moving and constantly changing.

Parallel to the changes in the science there has been a revolution in how nephrology educators teach and are recognized. More and more teaching is shifting from the classroom and bedside to the smartphone and internet. Therefore the current edition includes contributions from several individuals who have honed their skills teaching in that space.

In keeping with the design of the original *Medical Secrets*, we have included questions on everyday topics in addition to some "zebras" of particular academic interest. We hope that this book will be used not only by nephrologists and nephrology fellows, medical residents and interns, and medical students but also by primary care providers with particular interest in the art of homeostasis.

From personal experience, we know that very few people read a textbook from cover to cover. For a variety of reasons, people skim through books as patient encounters and interests guide them. To accommodate this reality, we tried to ensure that each chapter would be complete in itself. As a consequence, there is unavoidable overlap among some of the information provided in many chapters. Indulge this luxury; paper is cheap, and this makes the book a better information retrieval appliance.

Though only three names are on the cover, this book could not have been produced without a battalion of contributors. First, and most obviously, we are in debt to all of the contributing authors who have spent hours in producing high-quality, up-to-the-last-minute information that was rewarded with telephone, e-mail and Twitter direct messages with suggestions, rewrites, and "spirited discussions." The ISBN says fourth edition, but if you ask the authors, they will tell you it was closer to a clean-sheet rewrite. We express our sincere gratitude for all the authors' openness to this collaboration. Namaste. Additionally, we would need to express the highest gratitude to all the staff of Elsevier, most especially Meghan Andress, our Developmental Editor, Rachel McMullen, our Senior Project Manager; and James Merritt, our Senior Acquisitions Editor, all of whom have been very patient with our procrastinations and stubbornness.

Lastly, and philosophically, we thank our own teachers and our mentors, who devoted their time to train and form us to become nephrologists and teachers. We thank the undergraduates, medical students, residents, and fellows who have taught us how to teach. Lastly, we recognize and thank the patients, who are the reason we are here. Knowledge without application is an empty vessel. Every page contains information gleaned off the backs of patients. Their illness created this book, and on behalf of all the contributors to this book, we fervently hope that the efforts may help alleviate their suffering, prevent others from becoming similarly ill, and perhaps lead to their recovery.

Edgar V. Lerma, MD, FACP, FASN, FNKF, FPSN (Hon)
@EdgarVLermaMD

Matthew A. Sparks, MD, FASN, FNKF
@Nephro_Sparks

Joel M. Topf, MD, FACP
@Kidney_Boy

CONTENTS

XIII Acid-Base and Electrolyte Disorders

XIV Palliative Care in Nephrology

XV Nephrology Beginnings

TOP 100 SECRETS

These secrets are 100 of the top board alerts. They summarize the concepts, principles, and most salient details of nephrology.

1. The urine protein to creatinine (using a random urine specimen) ratio has been shown to have a good correlation with the 24-hour urine protein determination.

2. The most common complication associated with a kidney biopsy is bleeding, though it is usually self-limited and rarely life threatening.

3. The differential diagnosis of AKI includes prerenal azotemia, obstructive nephropathy, and intrinsic forms of AKI.

4. Hepatorenal Syndrome (HRS) is a functional kidney failure that occurs in end-stage liver cirrhosis with ascites.

5. The pharmacological treatment for HRS is a combination of albumin and vasoconstrictors, but the definitive treatment is liver transplantation.

6. Due to the high incidence of drug-induced AKI, a thorough review of the medication list should be performed in a patient at risk for AKI.

7. Sepsis is an important cause of AKI in critically ill patients and is associated with high mortality rates.

8. Rapid (<3 hours after presentation) administration of appropriate antibiotics is associated with improved outcomes and fewer cases of sepsis-associated AKI.

9. Early and vigorous volume resuscitation of patients with rhabdomyolysis (even before extrication in crush syndrome) is important for preventing AKI.

10. AKI secondary to rhabdomyolysis usually occurs with creatine kinase levels greater than 10,000 U/L.

11. Acute glomerulonephritis is a kidney injury syndrome characterized by the sudden onset of edema, new or worsening hypertension, and an active urinary sediment.

12. Rapidly progressive glomerulonephritis is a clinical syndrome characterized by rapid loss of kidney function that often results in ESKD.

13. Primary nephrotic syndrome is caused by one of the following four diseases—minimal change disease, focal segmental glomerulosclerosis, membranous nephropathy, or membranoproliferative glomerulonephritis—and the diagnosis is made based on a combination of clinical features, kidney biopsy findings, laboratory findings, and genetic testing.

14. Diuresis after relief of urinary obstruction may result from a physiologic excretion of water and urea, but can become pathologic. Patients should have electrolytes checked and replaced regularly, with free access to oral fluids. If necessary, the type and amount of intravenous fluids should be determined by serum and urinary electrolyte levels.

15. Struvite stones are due to infection with bacteria that contain the enzyme urease; *Proteus mirabilis* often has urease, *Escherichia coli* almost never has urease activity.

16. Uric acid stones are radiolucent on routine x-ray but are easily visualized by computed tomography scan.

17. Uric acid stones are almost always due to overly acidic urine and therefore the treatment of choice is alkali salts, not allopurinol.

18. Enteric hyperoxaluria requires that the patient have an intact colon because it is the sight of pathologic oxalate overabsorption.

19. Low calcium diets are not recommended in the treatment of patients with hypercalciuria, because a low calcium diet may contribute to bone demineralization.

20. The leading causes of CKD are diabetes, hypertension, glomerulonephritis, and cystic kidney disease, with about 40% of all cases due to diabetes.

21. The target hemoglobin level for patients receiving erythropoiesis-stimulating agent (ESA) therapy should be individualized based on transfusion avoidance, quality of life, physical activity, and ESA responsiveness, and should not exceed 12 g/dL.

22. Most patients receiving ESAs will require iron supplementation; however, oral iron supplements are often ineffective because of poor absorption and the magnitude of iron requirements.

23. Decreased kidney function is associated with abnormalities of mineral metabolism that results in decreased skeletal strength, bone pain, and abnormal calcification of the blood vessels and soft tissues.

24. Cardiovascular disease is the primary cause of death in patients with CKD, and is dramatically accelerated in CKD. Unfortunately, much of what is known about CVD may not apply to patients with CKD, so physicians should prioritize evidence performed in this special population.

25. Dyslipidemia is nearly universal in CKD and transplant. Kidney Disease Improving Global Outcomes (KDIGO) guidelines recommend that patients with CKD over the age of 50 and patients with a kidney transplant be treated with a statin.

26. Patients with progressive CKD opting for hemodialysis should have a timely evaluation for vascular access to ensure it is ready when dialysis starts. An arteriovenous fistula requires several months to mature.

27. Minimal change disease (MCD) is the cause of nephrotic syndrome in approximately 90% of children younger than 6 years of age, in approximately 65% of older children, and in approximately 20% to 30% of adolescents. In adults, only approximately 10% to 25% of nephrotic syndrome results from MCD, but it represents the third most common cause of primary nephrotic syndrome in adults after membranous nephropathy and FSGS.

28. Categorizing focal segmental glomerulosclerosis (FSGS) as genetic, secondary, or primary may inform type of treatment offered and influence posttransplant disease recurrence.

29. Patients with FSGS and high-risk *APOL1* are at greater risk of ESKD than patients with a low-risk *APOL2* genotype.

30. Membranous nephropathy is a cause of nephrotic syndrome that can be either primary or secondary to other diseases (malignancy, hepatitis B, lupus). Eighty percent of idiopathic (primary) membranous has increased anti-PLA_2R antibody levels.

31. IgA nephropathy is the most common primary glomerulonephritis. It is a nephritic syndrome that classically presents with hematuria. There is wide variability in kidney outcomes, from benign microscopic hematuria to rapidly progressive crescentic glomerular nephritis.

32. MPGN develops secondary to immune complex deposition or abnormalities in the alternate pathway of complement; it can progress to ESKD over 10 to 15 years.

33. There is no proven therapy for MPGN. It can recur in up to 30% of kidney transplant recipients.

34. Diabetic retinopathy is present in almost all patients with type 1 diabetes mellitus and diabetic nephropathy.

35. Early diagnosis of lupus nephritis is imperative because kidney function at the time of biopsy correlates with remission.

36. Anti-neutrophil cytoplasmic autoantibodies (ANCAs) are present in 90% of pauci-immune glomerulonephritis and are pathogenic for these diseases.

37. Induction therapy for ANCA vasculitis rests on the use of corticosteroids in combination with cyclophosphamide or rituximab. Plasma exchange should be considered in patients with severe pulmonary hemorrhage, advanced kidney disease, or concomitant anti glomerular basement membrane disease.

38. Postinfectious streptococcal glomerulonephritis occurs 7 to 21 days after a streptococcal infection (shorter for pharyngitis, longer for skin infections). It presents with acute nephritis and is generally self-limiting, without a defined role for immunomodulation.

39. The presence or absence of hepatitis B e antigen (HbeAg) is important with regard to the type of glomerular disease that may develop. Patients positive for both HbeAg and hepatitis B surface antigen are highly infectious and have a greater risk of kidney disease.

40. Hepatitis C–related glomerulonephritis is associated with type 2 cryoglobulinemia, resulting in activation of the classical complement pathway (low C3 and C4) with MPGN.

41. HIV-associated nephropathy (HIVAN) occurs almost exclusively in patients of black race who have high-risk *APOL1* genotypes.

42. HAART is the primary treatment for HIVAN and may lead to complete histologic reversal, but HAART is not as successful in HIV immune complex disease of the kidney (HIVICK).

43. Both rhabdomyolysis and tumor lysis syndrome can cause profound electrolyte abnormalities (hyperkalemia, hyperphosphatemia, hypocalcemia, and hyperuricemia) as a result of the release of intracellular constituents.

44. Rasburicase, a recombinant uric oxidase, rapidly lowers uric acid levels and is commonly used in the prevention of AKI secondary to tumor lysis syndrome.

45. Myeloma cast nephropathy is a medical emergency and requires immediate diagnosis and early institution of therapy in order to prevent irreversible kidney failure.

46. Kidney injury in myeloma is principally related to the light chain component of immunoglobulin because, unlike heavy chains, light chains are freely filtered at the glomerulus and reabsorbed in the proximal tubule.

47. Bortezomib-based chemotherapy regimens are recommended as the optimal management of AKI and myeloma

48. The measurement of serum-free light chains is the preferred study if suspecting myeloma and kidney disease due to light chain excess.

49. Patients with amyloidosis usually present with edema and nephrotic syndrome.

50. Treatments for metastatic renal cell carcinoma can be nephrotoxic—VEGF inhibitors can cause proteinuria, and programmed death-1 inhibitors can cause an autoimmune nephritis.

51. Thrombotic microangiopathies (TMAs) present with microangiopathic hemolytic anemia, thrombocytopenia, and altering degrees of kidney failure and neurologic dysfunction. The major causes of TMA are Shiga toxin–associated hemolytic uremia syndrome (ST-HUS), atypical hemolytic uremia syndrome (aHUS), and thrombotic thrombocytopenic purpura (TTP).

52. Fabry disease is an X-linked lysosomal storage disease that is unrecognized in 0.2% of patients with ESKD that can be detected in males by their marked decrease or absent plasma α-galactosidase-A activity.

53. Alport syndrome is associated with microscopic hematuria, proteinuria, sensorineural hearing loss, and progressive loss of kidney function.

54. Thin basement membrane nephropathy (TBMN) is a benign autosomal-dominant condition associated with microscopic hematuria without proteinuria, hearing loss, or progressive kidney failure.

55. The classical triad of fever, maculopapular rash, and peripheral eosinophilia is seen in only a minority of cases (<10%) of acute tubulointerstitial nephritis (ATIN).

56. Drug-induced ATIN is not dose dependent. A repeat exposure to the same drug can potentially lead to a recurrence of the disease process.

57. Asymptomatic bacteriuria should be treated only when present in pregnant women, or patients undergoing traumatic genitourinary procedures.

58. The major physiologic change in the kidney during pregnancy is a 50% increase in GFR.

59. The most important predictor of maternal and fetal problems when pregnancy occurs in women with preexisting kidney disease including prematurity, fetal loss, and loss of kidney function is prepregnancy kidney function.

60. Patients with sickle cell nephropathy may be particularly vulnerable to develop AKI as a result of hemodynamic insults, toxins, acute pyelonephritis, and urinary tract obstruction.

61. The rate of uremic toxin removal is determined by the time on dialysis, the blood and dialysate flow rates, and the efficiency of the dialyzer.

62. For patients receiving hemodialysis three times per week, it is recommended that the minimum delivered single pool Kt/V dose of dialysis is 1.2 and that the minimum treatment time of time should be 3 hours if residual kidney function is less than 2 mL/min.

63. Home hemodialysis provides a number of clinical benefits when compared with in-center hemodialysis, including decreased left ventricular mass, better volume control, improved serum phosphorous levels, less antihypertensive medication use, and improved quality of life.

64. Initiating incident patients on peritoneal dialysis (PD; i.e., "PD First") offers survival and other clinical benefits, particularly in situations where renal replacement is unplanned or a central venous catheter would otherwise be used.

65. In patients with ESKD achieving recommended renal replacement therapy parameters a high serum creatinine represents higher muscle mass and is associated with significantly better outcomes.

66. A team-based, multifaceted approach to continuous quality improvement with regular audit of infection rates and outcomes is essential to improving peritonitis rates in patients undergoing PD. Training and re-training of both patients and nurse patient-educators is a cornerstone of this effort.

67. In ANCA vasculitis, plasma exchange is presently recommended in addition to corticosteroids and cyclophosphamide for patients presenting with advanced kidney failure and/or pulmonary hemorrhage.

68. The new kidney transplant allocation system went into effect in December 2014. There were significant changes to allow for longevity matching between donors and recipients using the estimated posttransplant survival score and kidney donor profile index (KDPI) score to maximize graft survival. Another change was giving patients a time credit for time on renal replacement therapy.

69. The median time for waiting for a kidney transplant in the US is 3.6 years.

70. Living donor kidney transplantation offers the best long-term outcomes for patients with ESKD.

71. Calcineurin inhibitors remain a cornerstone of immunosuppressive regiments in kidney transplantation. They work by blocking calcineurin, an intricate protein in the signal transduction pathway that activates signal 3. The two prototypes are tacrolimus and cyclosporine, with tacrolimus being the primary drug of choice today.

72. Chronic rejection, better defined as chronic antibody-mediated rejection, is the main cause of late allograft loss and is histologically defined as transplant glomerulopathy.

73. Epstein-Barr virus is found in two-thirds of patients with posttransplant lymphoproliferative disorder.

74. Quantification of BK virus DNA in plasma by polymerase chain reaction has a sensitivity and specificity of 100% and 88%, respectively; a kidney transplant biopsy is still needed to rule out other diagnoses and confirm the diagnosis of BK nephropathy.

75. In patients who have received a kidney transplant, proteinuria is associated with cardiovascular events and mortality.

76. The traditional blood pressure target of <140/90 mm Hg is now <130/80 mm Hg for everyone except those with a <10% 10-year risk for cardiovascular events, where it is still <140/90.

77. No randomized trials to date have demonstrated a clear benefit for revascularization over medical management alone in the treatment of atherosclerotic renal artery stenosis.

78. Although endocrine and secondary forms of hypertension are uncommon, about 20% of patients with resistant hypertension can have their blood pressure controlled and occasionally "cured" with specific forms of treatment. This cannot occur if secondary forms of hypertension are not considered.

79. The most common form of secondary hypertension (~20% in some series) is associated with obstructive sleep apnea, the treatment of which improves blood pressure and quality of life.

80. Hypertensive emergencies occur when elevated blood pressure causes acute target-organ damage and requires blood pressure to be reduced gradually within minutes to hours.

81. Initial antihypertensive drug therapy can be with a thiazide or thiazide-like diuretic, an ACE inhibitor, an ARB, or a calcium channel blockers.

82. Spironolactone has emerged as the treatment of choice for treatment-resistant high blood pressure, but requires careful monitoring of serum potassium and kidney function.

83. Salt restriction is effective in reducing cardiovascular risk: reducing sodium consumption to approximately 1000 mg daily can reduce cardiovascular events by 25%, and every 1000 mg increase in daily dietary sodium can increase the relative risk of nonfatal stoke, myocardial infarction, and heart failure by 10%.

84. The Dietary Approaches to Stop Hypertension (DASH) diet, combined with sodium restriction of 1.5 g daily, can improve systolic blood pressure by approximately 9 mm Hg.

85. Diuresis of patients with chronic obstructive pulmonary disease and cor pulmonale can cause contraction alkalosis. Correction of contraction alkalosis with acetazolamide can lead to improved ventilation.

86. In patients with volume contraction and metabolic alkalosis, the urine sodium concentration may not be low. In this circumstance the urine chloride will typically be less than 15 mEq/L.

87. Abnormalities of serum potassium or bicarbonate, in the absence of diuretics, in patients with difficult-to-treat hypertension should trigger an evaluation for monogenic causes of hypertension.

88. Hypotonic hyponatremia arises from inadequate solute intake, excess electrolyte-free water intake, or reduced excretion of electrolyte-free water. Urine osmolality can distinguish the latter mechanism from the first two.

89. While acute hypotonic hyponatremia can be rapidly corrected, the rate of correction of chronic hyponatremia should be limited to prevent the osmotic demyelination syndrome.

90. In patients with severely symptomatic hyponatremia, raising the serum sodium concentration by just 3 to 4 mEq/L by administering one to three 100 mL boluses of 3% saline completely abrogates the risk of seizures, tentorial herniation, non-cardiogenic pulmonary edema, and other life-threatening complications.

91. Prediction equations for rate of rise of serum sodium concentration in response to hypertonic saline infusions do not account for ongoing urinary water loss. Measuring the serum sodium concentration change frequently when hypertonic saline is given is essential to be certain that the response meets the anticipated target rate.

92. Hyponatremia should be presumed to be chronic unless its time of onset is definitely known. This is especially true for hyponatremia developing prior to hospital presentation.

93. Definitive interventions to remove potassium from the body include hemodialysis or increasing fecal excretion by using potassium binders.

94. Intravenous calcium prevents life-threatening consequences of cardiac arrhythmias due to severe hyperkalemia by stabilizing the myocardial and conducting tissue cell membranes. This effect is rapid but short-lived and hence should be followed by definitive measures to lower serum potassium levels.

95. Hyperphosphatemia in the setting of normal kidney function: think excessive intake, cellular breakdown, or hypoparathyroidism.

96. Always ensure magnesium is replete in patients with hypokalemia.

97. The current "Surviving Sepsis" guidelines recommend against administration of sodium bicarbonate for arterial pH of 7.15 or more, and express uncertainty about whether giving it when pH is lower has any utility.

98. Measuring the concentration of Cl^- in the urine is an excellent first step in the clinical approach to patients with metabolic acidosis.

99. Hypokalemia plays a central role in the pathophysiology of metabolic alkalosis and must be corrected to successfully correct metabolic alkalosis.

100. Palliative care can be provided at any time during the course of a serious illness and is not synonymous with hospice, which is a Medicare benefit for patients with a terminal illness or a prognosis less than 6 months.

I

PATIENT
ASSESSMENT

HISTORY AND PHYSICAL DIAGNOSIS

Swapnil Hiremath and Edgar V. Lerma

CHAPTER 1

1. **How do patients with kidney disease typically present?**
   Patients with kidney disease typically present in several ways:
   - Abnormal blood laboratory studies (e.g., elevated blood urea nitrogen [BUN] and serum creatinine, decreased estimated glomerular filtration rate, or abnormal serum electrolyte values)
   - Asymptomatic urinary abnormalities (e.g., microscopic hematuria, proteinuria, microalbuminuria)
   - Changes in urinary frequency or problems with urination (e.g., polyuria, hematuria, nocturia, urgency)
   - New-onset hypertension
   - Worsening edema in dependent areas
   - Nonspecific symptomatologies (e.g., nausea, vomiting, malaise)
   - At times, symptoms can be specific (e.g., ipsilateral flank pain in those with obstructing nephrolithiasis)
   - Incidental discovery of anatomic kidney abnormalities on routine imaging studies (e.g., horseshoe kidney, congenitally absent or ptotic kidney, asymmetric kidneys, angiomyolipoma, kidney mass, polycystic kidneys)
   - Symptoms related to underlying systemic disease (e.g., skin changes and/or rash with scleroderma, vasculitis, systemic lupus erythematosus [SLE], arthritis due to gout, SLE, etc.)

2. **What important features need to be elicited in the history of patients referred for kidney disease evaluation?**
   - Previous diagnosis of kidney disease (e.g., previous documentation of BUN and serum creatinine values)
   - History of asymptomatic urinary abnormalities (e.g., hematuria, proteinuria)
   - History of alterations in urinary frequency or urgency, etc.
   - Change in the urinary character or appearance (e.g., smell, color, frothy appearance)
   - History of diabetes (duration, severity, end-organ damage)
   - History of hypertension (including cardiac history)
   - Previous exposure to nephrotoxic medications (e.g., nonsteroidal antiinflammatory drugs [NSAIDs], antibiotics such as aminoglycosides)
   - Previous adverse reactions to renin-angiotensin-aldosterone system blocking agents (e.g., angiotensin-converting enzyme inhibitors, angiotensin receptor antagonists)
   - Recent gastrointestinal endoscopic procedures requiring bowel cleansing (risk of acute phosphate nephropathy in those who use phosphate-containing enema)
   - Recent exposure to contrast-requiring procedures (risk of contrast-induced acute kidney injury)
   - Recent systemic infections or intercurrent illnesses
   - Family history of kidney disease or any relative requiring some form of renal replacement therapy (e.g., polycystic kidney disease [PKD], Alport syndrome)
   - History of autoimmune diseases
   - Recent changes in dose of a medication, or any new medication recently started
   - Any over-the-counter medications used (e.g., NSAIDs) and/or herbal, natural supplements

3. **Why is smoking history important in patients with kidney disease?**
   Chronic kidney disease has been shown to be closely related to cardiovascular disease and smoking. The concept of smoking as an "independent" progression factor in kidney disease has been a subject of interest in numerous investigations. Since 2003 several publications of clinical and experimental data concerning the adverse kidney effects of smoking have drawn interest, including large, prospective, population-based, observational studies. These studies clearly demonstrate that smoking is a relevant risk factor, and it does confer a significant increase in the risk for progression of kidney dysfunction (i.e., elevation of serum creatinine) regardless of the underlying cause of the kidney disease.

3

It has been suggested that urinary cotinine, a metabolite of nicotine, can potentially be used as an objective measure of smoking exposure. Its use has not been studied in the population with chronic kidney disease.

4. **What familial diseases are characterized by kidney involvement?**
   - Autosomal dominant PKD (ADPKD) (chromosomes 4 and 16)
   - Autosomal recessive PKD (linked to chromosome 6)
   - Autosomal dominant tubulointerstitial kidney disease (previously known as familial juvenile hyperuricemic nephropathy type 1, medullary cystic kidney disease type 2, and or uromodulin-associated kidney disease, linked to chromosomes 1, 16, 17)
   - Focal segmental glomerulosclerosis (linked to chromosomes 1, 9, 10, 11, 19)
   - Hypertension
   - Diabetes mellitus
   - Fabry disease
   - Alport syndrome
   - Sickle cell nephropathy
   - Familial hypercalcemic hypocalciuria
   - Cystinuria
   - HDR syndrome (syndrome of hypoparathyroidism, sensorineural hearing loss, and kidney disease; also called Barakat syndrome; mapped to chromosome 10p)
   - Liddle syndromes of apparent mineralocorticoid excess and other monogenic hypertension
   - Bartter and Gitelman syndromes
   - Congenital nephrotic syndrome (Finish and other variants, mapped to chromosomes 1, 3, 11, 19)

5. **What are the common symptoms and signs that are seen in patients with advanced kidney disease?**
   Chronic kidney disease is usually characterized by nonspecific signs and symptoms in the earlier stages and can be detected only by an increase in serum creatinine.

   Symptoms
   - Loss or decreased appetite (protein aversion)
   - Easy fatigability
   - Generalized weakness
   - Involuntary weight loss (resulting from cachexia) or gain (resulting from fluid retention)
   - Alterations in mentation (e.g., lethargy, coma, difficulty concentrating)
   - Nausea and vomiting; dyspepsia
   - Metallic taste
   - Generalized itching or pruritus
   - Seizures
   - Difficulty breathing
   - Edema
   - Intractable hiccups
   - Frothy" appearance of urine (usually results from proteinuria)
   - Decreased sexual interest (e.g., erectile dysfunction)
   - Restless legs

   Signs
   - Elevated blood pressure (BP)
   - Pallor (from anemia)
   - Volume overload (jugular venous distention, peripheral edema, pulmonary edema, anasarca)
   - Friction rub (pericarditis)
   - Asterixis and myoclonus (uremic encephalopathy)

6. **What is a bedside diagnostic test that will suggest the presence of underlying diabetic nephropathy.**
   Funduscopy. It is believed that the similarities in the vascularization between the retina and the kidneys account for the correlation of the typical microvascular complications commonly seen in patients with diabetes mellitus.

   Patients with type 2 diabetes with proliferative retinopathy often present with kidney involvement, manifested by either microalbuminuria (in the earlier stages) or overt proteinuria. Therefore it is recommended that all patients with diabetes and proliferative retinopathy undergo an evaluation of kidney function including testing for microalbuminuria.

   It must be remembered that although the presence of retinopathy does support a diabetic source of proteinuria, the lack of diabetic retinopathy does not rule out diabetic nephropathy.

7. **What are the common extrarenal manifestations associated with kidney diseases?**
   Dermatologic
   - See Question 8

   Arthritis and/or Musculoskeletal Symptoms
   - Lupus nephritis
   - Rheumatoid arthritis
   - Henoch-Schönlein purpura
   - Cryoglobulinemia
   - Sarcoidosis

- Amyloidosis
- Multiple myeloma
- Gouty nephropathy

Hemoptysis
- Acute kidney injury with community acquired pneumonia
- Pulmonary renal syndrome
  Goodpasture syndrome (also called anti-GBM disease)
  Henoch-Schönlein purpura and immuno-globulin A nephropathy
  Anti-Neutrophil Cytoplasmic Antibody (ANCA)-related vasculitides: Granulo-matosis with polyangiitis (previously called Wegener granulomatosis); eosinophilic granulomatosis with polyangiitis (previously called Churg-Strauss syndrome); microscopic polyangiitis; and pauci-immune crescentic glomerulonephritis
  Cryoglobulinemia
- Lupus nephritis with pneumonitis
- Pulmonary thromboembolism/infarction related to hypercoagulability (membranous

nephropathy and antiphospholipid syndrome)
- Volume overload (congestive heart failure, mitral stenosis)

Hearing loss
- Hearing loss from aminoglycosides or loop diuretics in someone with kidney disease
- Alport syndrome
- Charcot-Marie-Tooth syndrome
- HDR syndrome (hypoparathyroidism, sensorineural hearing loss, and kidney disease; also called Barakat syndrome)
- Wolfram syndrome (diabetes insipidus, diabetes mellitus, optic atrophy)
- Bartter syndrome (type IV)

Abdominal discomfort
- Henoch-Schönlein purpura
- Cryoglobulinemia
- Microscopic polyangiitis
- ADPKD

Cervicocranial aneurysms:
- ADPKD (also with mitral valve prolapse)
- Fibromuscular dysplasia

8. **What is importance of itching in kidney diseases, and how do you treat it?**
   Pruritus or itching is among the most common symptom of ESKD. In severe cases, it can be unrelenting. Although mostly benign in etiology (see xerosis, previous), it can lead to secondary complications, such as excoriations and lichen simplex chronicus, which may be disfiguring in extreme cases.
   The use of emollients, moisturizing lotions, keratolytic agents, and hydration have been commonly recommended as conservative treatment.
   In some cases, phototherapy (ultraviolet B radiation [UVB] administered as total body irradiation 3 times a week for a total of 8 to 10 sessions) has been shown to be helpful. It has been suggested that UVB (wavelength 280 to 315 nm) inactivates certain pruritogenic chemicals and induces the formation of metabolites with antipruritic effects. The risk of malignancy is fairly significant, especially in fair-skinned individuals.
   Topical capsaicin (0.025%), by reducing the levels of substance P in cutaneous type C sensory nerve endings, has been useful for localized pruritus.
   Topical tacrolimus (0.03% for 3 weeks, followed by 0.01% for another 3 weeks) may be beneficial but can predispose to dermatologic malignancies, so it is not recommended as a first line therapy or for prolonged use.
   Gabapentin (100 to 300 mg after each dialysis treatment) also has antipruritic effects. Prominent side effects include depression of the central nervous system.
   μ-opioid receptor antagonists, such as per os (PO) naltrexone, has antipruritic properties. In the same family, intranasal butorphanol (a F06BF06B-opioid receptor agonist and μ-opioid receptor antagonist) is another option.
   Other treatment options include PO-activated charcoal, selective serotonin antagonists (ondansetron and granisetron), oral cromolyn, cholestyramine, thalidomide, erythropoietin, and intravenous lidocaine.

9. **What is calciphylaxis?**
   Calcific uremic arteriolopathy (CUA), also known as calciphylaxis, is characterized by painful, subcutaneous purpuric plaques and nodules. These nodules may necrose in advanced disease. Although the skin manifestations are dramatic, it is useful to think of it as a systemic disease, and treat aggressively, given its high fatality rate. When the extremities are involved, the lesions tend to be bilateral and symmetric in distribution and often are described as a mottled or violaceous discoloration with a reticular pattern, similar to livedo reticularis (seen in atheroembolic kidney disease, antiphospholipid syndrome, and cryoglobulinemia). Of note, those with proximal lesions (trunk, buttocks, and thighs) tend to have a worse prognosis compared with those with more distal lesions (forearms and fingers; calves and toes).

Several known risk factors predispose to CUA—namely, poorly controlled secondary hyperparathyroidism, uncontrolled diabetes mellitus, obesity, female sex, duration of renal replacement therapy, history of skin trauma, and use of warfarin.

The increased expression of osteopontin and bone morphogenic protein 4 suggests the pivotal role that inducers of vascular calcification play in its pathogenesis.

Suspicion is the key to early diagnosis. When identified in its earlier stages (nonulcerative), initiation of therapeutic measures has been shown to improve prognosis.

Prevention is the key to management of CUA. Aggressive control of secondary hyperparathyroidism (see Chapter 21) is pivotal.

Sodium thiosulfate is one of the therapies for established CUA. It is believed to work by two mechanisms of action.
1. Chelates calcium from soft tissues
2. Antioxidant, inducing endothelial nitric oxide synthesis, thereby improving local blood flow and soft tissue oxygenation.

A commonly used regimen is 5 to 25 g of intravenous (IV) Na thiosulfate administered toward the end of dialysis for several weeks to months.

Bisphosphonates (IV pamidronate and ibandronate and PO etidronate) may be effective in altering ectopic deposition of calcium phosphate and directly inhibiting calcification via the nuclear factor F06BF06BB cascade, although there are limited data.

Hyperbaric oxygen therapy improves oxygen delivery to damaged tissues by increasing the partial pressure of oxygen; it also promotes wound healing by supporting phagocytosis and angiogenesis while decreasing tissue edema.

10. **What is nephrogenic systemic fibrosis (NSF)?**
NSF, previously known as nephrogenic fibrosing dermopathy, is characterized by progressive fibrosis and thickening of the skin (similar to scleroderma), which is particularly painful, and also fibrosis in other organs (e.g., pleura, diaphragm). The skin lesions appear as plaques, papules, or nodules distributed in an asymmetric fashion over the distal extremities. The pathogenesis is deposition of gadolinium (contrast material used in magnetic resonance imaging), which does not get cleared in the presence of severe chronic kidney disease or acute kidney injury. The interval between exposure to gadolinium and the early manifestations of NSF can range from 2 days to 18 months. This variability is attributed to mobilization of gadolinium from bone over time. The risk of NSF appears to be higher with the linear molecules (e.g., gadodiamide) compared with macro cyclic gadolinium molecules.

NSF has no effective treatment and a high fatality rate, so the primary focus is on prevention. Gadolinium-enhanced scans should be avoided in patients with severe chronic kidney disease or acute kidney injury. When gadolinium-enhanced scans are necessary, prophylactic measures that have been described include the use of hemodialysis (HD; eliminates 92% of gadolinium after two HD sessions; 99% after three HD sessions) in patients with advanced chronic kidney disease. Similarly, an intensified regimen of peritoneal dialysis (PD) can remove gadolinium (90% of the gadolinium in 2 days with a regimen of 10 to 15 exchanges per day of PD). The effectiveness of these measures is not clear.

11. **What are the other common dermatologic manifestations of kidney disease?**
Xerosis or dryness of the skin, especially on the extensor surfaces of the extremities, is common among patients receiving dialysis. It can lead to generalized pruritus and can be uncomfortable.

Changes in pigmentation—in particular, hyperpigmentation—have been attributed to the increased levels of melanocyte-stimulating hormone and the subsequent deposition of melanin in the basal layer of the epidermis.

Some patients may have a "sallow" discoloration of the skin believed to be caused by deposition of lipochrome pigment and carotenoids in the dermis and subcutaneous tissues.

Pallor is commonly associated with varying degrees of anemia as a result of chronic kidney disease.

Uremic frost refers to the deposition of crystallized urea that is excreted from sweat in the epidermis, seen in cases of untreated and advanced kidney disease.

Ecchymoses are commonly associated with uremic platelet dysfunction.

Lindsay nails, also known as "half and half nails," refer to the whitish discoloration of the proximal half of fingernails, believed to be a result of edema of the nail bed and underlying capillary network.

Acquired perforating dermatosis (Kyrle disease) is predominantly seen in African Americans with diabetes mellitus. It is usually characterized by a linear confluence of papules with a central, oyster shell–like keratotic plug, distributed on the trunk, proximal extremities, scalp, and face, and the lesions are pruritic. Possible etiologies include an inflammatory skin reaction secondary to the presence of uremic toxins, uric-acid deposits, or scratching-induced trauma.

Porphyria cutanea tarda (PCT) commonly presents as a vesiculobullous disease commonly involving the dorsum of both hands and feet but can affect any sun-exposed areas. It is commonly accompanied by sclerodermoid plaques (facial hyperpigmentation) and hypertrichosis. It is usually secondary to increased levels of uroporphyrins.

Avoidance of sun exposure is the cornerstone of management. Other measures to decrease uroporphyrin levels include the use of high-flux dialysis membranes (to improve dialysis efficacy) and small-volume weekly phlebotomies in extreme, rare cases.

Common precipitating factors are alcohol intake, use of estrogen and iron supplementations, and chronic infections (e.g., hepatitis B or C virus, human immunodeficiency virus).

One common differential diagnosis is pseudoporphyria, which is clinically similar to PCT with the exception of normal uroporphyrin levels.

12. **What are the causes of palpable kidneys?**
    Palpation for the kidneys is best performed bimanually, with one hand behind the patient in the costovertebral angle and the other anteriorly just below the costal margin. They may be normally palpable in very thin individuals. Pathologic causes include:
    - ADPKD (both kidneys will be palpable)
    - Large kidney tumors
    - Obstruction of the urinary tract with severe hydronephrosis
    - Very large kidney cyst(s)

13. **What are the causes and significance of an abdominal bruit?**
    - Normal: Approximately 5%–25% of normal individuals may have a midsystolic bruit audible, with the prevalence being higher in younger individuals.
    - Renovascular disease: The characteristic bruit seen in renovascular hypertension, due to renal artery stenosis, is an epigastric systodiastolic bruit. Although it has a low sensitivity, it has a high specificity in the patient in whom one is suspecting renovascular hypertension. Renovascular hypertension can be due to either atherosclerotic disease or fibromuscular dysplasia (typically seen in young or middle-aged women). In fibromuscular dysplasia, extrarenal disease is common, with cervicocranial and other abdominal arteries being involved in particular.
    - Nonrenal causes of abdominal bruit include portal hypertension (periumbilical venous hum), pancreatic neoplasia (epigastric bruit), splenic arteriovenous malformation (left upper quadrant), hepatic carcinoma (right upper quadrant), and abdominal aortic aneurysms.

14. **What are the other important aspects of physical examination in kidney disease?**
    - BP measurement is a keystone of assessment of kidney disease. High BP can be a cause or a consequence of kidney disease. Proper measurement, with adequate resting, measurement of both arms, and assessment of change with posture should be a part of BP measurement.
    - Assessment of volume: This is important for any case of acute kidney injury to make decisions about volume resuscitation, as well for advanced kidney disease to assess for volume overload. Typical components include jugular venous pressure, orthostatic BP measurements, skin turgor, and mucus membranes.
    - Chest examination: Signs of volume overload (pulmonary edema); pericardial friction rub (in uremic pericarditis)
    - Musculoskeletal system: See "Arthritis" section earlier.
    - Skin: Many diseases, especially autoimmune diseases, can be accompanied by a skin rash, such as SLE and Henoch-Schönlein purpura. Kidney disease can also have skin manifestations (see Question 11 for more details).

KEY POINTS

1. The similarities in the vascularization between the retina and the kidneys account for the correlation of the typical microvascular complications commonly seen in patients with diabetes mellitus.
2. Tobacco abuse confers a significant increase in the risk for progression of kidney dysfunction, regardless of the underlying cause of the kidney disease.
3. In patients with calciphylaxis, those with proximal lesions (trunk, buttocks, and thighs) tend to have worse prognosis compared with those with more distal lesions (forearms and fingers; calves and toes).

Commonly Used Terms for Signs and Symptoms of Kidney Disease and their Meaning and Significance

Term	Meaning	Significance
Oliguria	Decreased urine output (<0.5 mL/kghour in children, <400 mL/day in adults)	Volume depletion; kidney failure
Anuria	Severely decreased urine output (<100 mL/day)	Kidney failure
Absolute anuria	No (0 mL) urine output	Blocked/kinked catheter, urinary obstruction
Dysuria	Pain or burning while passing urine	Urinary tract infections, stones, sexually transmitted infections, interstitial cystitis
Hematuria	Presence of blood in urine; Gross: visible with naked eye Microscopic: only seen with dipstick/urinanalysis	Source of blood can be urinary tract or glomerulus
Proteinuria	Presence of protein in urine, by dipstick (trace or more) or quantitation	Usually suggests intrinsic kidney disease
Microalbuminuria	Very small amounts of albumin in urine, usually missed by urine dipstick	Sign of early diabetic kidney damage; in nondiabetic conditions suggests endothelial dysfunction
Polyuria	Increased amount of urine (opposite of oliguria)	Increased water intake; diabetes
Nocturia	Increased frequency of urine at night	Usually accompanies polyuria; also with chronic kidney disease (decreased urinary concentrating ability)
Pollakiuria	Frequent urination in the daytime	Benign condition in children; accompanies polyuria; neurogenic bladder; drugs (e.g., tolvaptan)

BIBLIOGRAPHY

Abu-Alfa, A. (2008). The impact of NSF on the care of patients with kidney disease. *Journal of the American College of Radiology, 5*, 42–52.

Glynne, P., Deacon, A., Goldsmith, D., Pusey, C., & Clutterbuck, E. (1999). Bullous dermatoses in end-stage renal failure: Porphyria or pseudoporphyria? *American Journal of Kidney Diseases, 34*, 155–160.

Jones-Burton, C., Vessal, G., Brown, J., Dowling, T. C., & Fink, J. C. (2007). Urinary cotinine as an objective measure of cigarette smoking in chronic kidney disease. *Nephrology, Dialysis, Transplantation, 22*(7), 1950–1954.

Kuypers, D. R. (2009). Skin problems in chronic kidney disease. *Nature Clinical Practice Nephrology, 5*, 157–170.

National Kidney Foundation. (2002). K/DOQI clinical practice guidelines for chronic kidney disease: evaluation, classification, and stratification. *American Journal of Kidney Diseases, 39*(2 Suppl. 1), S1–S266.

Orth, S. R., & Hallan, S. I. (2008). Smoking: A risk factor for progression of chronic kidney disease and for cardiovascular morbidity and mortality in renal patients—Absence of evidence or evidence of absence? *Clinical Journal of the American Society of Nephrology, 3*, 226–236.

Penfield, J. G., & Reilly, R. F., Jr. (2007). What nephrologists need to know about gadolinium. *Nature Clinical Practice Nephrology, 3*, 654–668.

CHAPTER 2

URINALYSIS

Swapnil Hiremath, Florian Buchkremer, and Edgar V. Lerma

1. **What is uroscopy?**
   Uroscopy comes from the word "uroscopia," meaning scientific examination of the urine. It is derived from the Greek words *ouron* meaning urine and *skopeo* meaning to behold, contemplate, examine, or inspect. Such analysis of the urine was historically termed uroscopy until the 17th century and is now called "urinalysis."

2. **What is the proper way of collecting and handling a urine specimen for analysis?**
   When collecting the urine specimen, the first 200 mL of early-morning voided urine should be discarded. In men a simple midstream urine collection should suffice, whereas in women the external genitalia should be cleaned first, to avoid contamination with secretions, before collecting a midstream specimen. The specimen should be collected in a clean but not necessarily sterile container.

   Urine should be analyzed within 30 to 60 minutes of voiding; the initially uncentrifuged specimen is analyzed for color, pH, specific gravity, blood, protein, and glucose. Subsequently, it is centrifuged at 3000 rpm for 3 to 5 minutes. The sediment is then examined under the microscope for various elements, such as red blood cells (RBCs) and RBC casts, white blood cells (WBCs) and WBC casts, squamous epithelial cells, hyaline, and granular casts.

3. **What are the typical elements in a urine dipstick?**
   See Table 2.1.
   - **Color:** Normal urine color can vary from pale or light yellow to deep amber or dark yellow. The color is due to the pigment urochrome. Two important characteristics influence the color: its chemical composition and concentration. In an individual who is volume depleted, urine concentration tends to be elevated, giving rise to a darker-yellow urine. However, in a patient with diabetes insipidus, the urinary concentrating ability is impaired, making the urine dilute and lighter yellow in color even in the presence of volume depletion. Certain medications and foods alter the urine color (Table 2.2). In porphyria cutanea tarda, the urine turns the color of port wine.
   - **Clarity or turbidity:** The degree of turbidity or cloudiness is usually influenced by excess amounts of cellular debris and casts but can also be secondary to proteinuria, crystals, or contamination with vaginal discharge.
   - **pH:** Normal urine pH ranges between 4.5 and 8.0. In a normal individual on a Western diet, the average endogenous acid production is 1 mEq/kg per day, and the kidneys are responsible for clearing this acid load, so urine is typically quite acidic, usually with a pH of 5 to 6. Urine pH is useful in differentiating the different types of renal tubular acidosis (RTA), which is characterized by the inability to acidify urine to a pH less than 5.5 (i.e., despite an overnight fast and acid loading). Similarly, it also provides a clue to the causes and therapies for certain disease states (e.g., nephrolithiasis). Alkaline urine is usually seen in urinary tract infection (UTI) caused by urea-splitting organisms *(Proteus mirabilis)*, associated with magnesium–ammonium phosphate crystals and staghorn calculi, whereas acidic urine is seen with uric acid calculi. Urine may also be deliberately (but cautiously, to avoid metabolic alkalemia and hypocalcemia) alkalinized, to a pH greater than 6.5, for therapeutic reasons, to aid in elimination of certain toxins (e.g., salicylates, barbiturates) or to prevent the crystallization of uric acid in tumor lysis syndrome or myoglobin in rhabdomyolysis.
   - **Specific gravity:** The urine specific gravity (1.005 to 1.025) reflects the ability of the kidneys to concentrate urine. In patients with impaired urinary-concentrating ability (acute tubular necrosis, sickle cell nephropathy, diabetes insipidus), the specific gravity tends to be low. Although imprecise at times, it can reflect a person's volume status.
   - **Blood:** The urinary dipstick test for blood detects the peroxidase activity of RBCs; however, myoglobin and hemoglobin also catalyze this reaction, so a positive dip stick may indicate hematuria, hemoglobinuria (paroxysmal nocturnal hemoglobinuria, transfusion-related reactions, infection with *Plasmodium falciparum,* infection with *Clostridium welchii*), or myoglobinuria (rhabdomyolysis). In the presence of positive blood on dipstick analysis, the presence of RBCs on urine microscopy confirms the diagnosis of hematuria (see Question 4 for more on this topic).

Table 2.1. Urine Dipstick Testing

MEASURED	CLINICAL SIGNIFICANCE	CAVEATS
Specific gravity	Expected value: 1.002–1.030 <1.005: inability to concentrate urine (e.g., diabetes insipidus, acute tubular necrosis) >1.030: SIAD, adrenal insufficiency, hypovolemia	Increased values in the presence of protein >1 g/L, ketoacids, iodinated contrast media, dextran *Urine osmolality is a more exact measure of urinary solutes*
pH	Expected value: 5.5–6.5 Alkaline: Diet (e.g., vegetarian), renal tubular acidosis (type I or II), salicylate overdose, acetazolamide, alkali therapy Acidic: diabetic ketoacidosis, diarrhea, furosemide, systemic acidosis	Increased values when urine left standing (increased ammonia synthesis)
Hemoglobin	Expected value: Negative Positive due to presence of erythrocytes, or free hemoglobin (e.g., with intravascular hemolysis)	False negative: Presence of ascorbic acid or formaldehyde, high nitrite concentration, delayed examination, high density of urine False positive: Myoglobin, microbial peroxidases, oxidizing detergents, hydrochloric acid
Glucose	Expected value: negative Positive in presence of glucose, typical diabetes mellitus, or with reduced renal threshold for glucose (e.g., proximal RTA, pregnancy, use of sodium-glucose transporter inhibitors, i.e., gliflozins)	False negative: Presence of ascorbic acid, urinary tract infection False positive: Presence of oxidizing detergents, hydrochloric acid
Albumin	Expected value: Negative Positive (+ or more): Proteinuria (glomerular disease)	False negative: Immunoglobulin light chains, hydrochloric acid, tubular proteins, other globulins, colored urine False positive: Alkaline urine (pH > 7.5), quaternary ammonium detergents, chlorhexidine, polyvinylpyrrolidone
Leukocyte esterase	Expected value: Negative Positive indicates pyuria, which would indicate a urinary tract infection, or other causes of sterile pyuria (as discussed previously)	False negative: Presence of ascorbic acid, recent treatment with gentamicin, tetracycline, cephalosporins, nitrofurantoin; proteinuria, glycosuria False positive: Oxidizing detergents, formaldehyde (0.4 g/L), sodium azide, colored urine from beet ingestion, or bilirubin
Nitrites	Expected value: Negative Positive in presence of bacteria that convert nitrates in urine to nitrites (typically gram-negative bacilli such as *E. coli, Klebsiella*)	False negative: Short bladder incubation time, presence of ascorbic acid, gram-positive bacteria False positive: colored urine
Ketones	Expected value: Negative Positive with ketonuria (e.g., ketoacidosis due to diabetes, starvation; may also occur in pregnancy, low-carbohydrate diets)	False negative: Test does not detect presence of β-hydroxybutyrate False positive: Free sulfhydryl groups (e.g., captopril), L-dopa, salicylates, phenothiazines, pigments in urine

Table 2.1. Urine Dipstick Testing *(Continued)*

MEASURED	CLINICAL SIGNIFICANCE	CAVEATS
Bilirubin	Expected value: Negative Positive in the presence of jaundice (hepatic or cholestatic disease) Negative in the presence of hyperbilirubinemia due to hemolysis	False negative: Presence of ascorbic acid, delayed examination, rifampin, exposure of urine to ultraviolet (UV) light False positive: Phenothiazines
Urobilinogen	Expected value: Negative Positive in presence of hyperbilirubinemia due to hepatic disease or hemolysis; negative in cholestatic disease	

RTA, Renal tubular acidosis; *SIAD*, syndrome of inappropriate diuresis.

Table 2.2. Possible Causes of Altered Urine Color

URINE COLOR	POSSIBLE CAUSES
Red	Foods: beets, blackberries, rhubarb Medications: laxatives, antipsychotics (chlorpromazine, thioridazine), anesthetics (propofol) Toxins: lead, mercury Conditions: urinary tract infections, nephrolithiasis, porphyria, hemoglobinuria (rhabdomyolysis); see Question 10
Orange	Foods: vitamin C, carrots Medications: rifampin, phenazopyridine
Green	Foods: asparagus Medications: vitamin B, propofol Conditions: *Pseudomonas* urinary tract infection
Blue	Medications: amitriptyline, indomethacin, IV cimetidine, IV promethazine, triamterene, methylene blue Conditions: blue diaper syndrome (see Question 6)
Brown	Foods: fava beans Medications: antimalarials (chloroquine, primaquine), antimicrobials (metronidazole, nitrofurantoin), laxatives (senna), methocarbamol, levodopa Conditions: hepatobiliary diseases (obstructive and nonobstructive), tyrosinemia, Gilbert syndrome
Pink	Uric acid crystals
Purple	See Question 5
Black	Conditions: malignant melanoma, porphyria, alkaptonuria (ochronosis)

IV, Intravenous.

- **Protein:** Normal urinary protein excretion should not exceed 150 mg/day. Among these urinary proteins are filtered albumin and the tubular Tamm-Horsfall mucoproteins (also called uromodulin). Urinary dipsticks detect only the presence of albumin, and hence they are notorious for being poor indicators of the presence of nonalbumin proteins, especially Bence Jones proteins (immunoglobulin [Ig] light chains, commonly seen in multiple myeloma). It is also important to recognize that the dipstick measurement of urine protein is dependent on the concentration of the urine specimen so that a patient with concentrated urine may test 2+ for protein, but when a 24-hour urine collection is obtained, the actual amount of protein excreted could be modest. Conversely, a patient with dilute urine may test only trace positive for protein but may have a larger amount of protein on a 24-hour collection. Thus it is important to quantify the amount of proteinuria found on dipstick testing. This can be done either with a 24-hour collection or with a random protein-to-creatinine ratio (PCR). A more reliable test for the presence of overall (including nonalbumin) proteins is called the sulfosalicylic acid test. It detects the presence of both albumin and nonalbumin proteins (including light chains) in the urine, even in low amounts. See Questions 16 to 19 for more on proteinuria.

- **Glucose:** Normal urinary glucose should not exceed 130 mg/day. Glucosuria (also termed glycosuria) commonly indicates the presence of diabetes mellitus. Other causes include the Fanconi syndrome (i.e., renal glycosuria accompanying proximal RTA) and the use of sodium-glucose cotransporter inhibitors. Urinary dipsticks (which use the glucose oxidase reaction) detect only the presence of glucose. For pediatric patients with suspected inborn errors of metabolism, other semiqualitative tests are used, such as Clinitest and Benedict test.
- **Ketones:** The presence of ketones in the urine is abnormal. There are three ketones found in diabetic ketoacidosis (acetone, acetoacetic acid, and bb-hydroxybutyric acid), but the urine dipstick detects only acetoacetate. Conditions whereby ketonuria may be present include poorly controlled diabetes, pregnancy, and starvation.
- **Nitrite:** Urinary nitrates are converted into nitrite by certain, commonly pathogenic bacterial species *(Escherichia coli, Klebsiella, Proteus, Pseudomonas, Enterobacter, Citrobacter)*. Therefore a positive nitrite is an indication of the presence of such bacteria. Other bacteria *(Haemophilus, Staphylococcus, Streptococcus)* do not have the ability to convert nitrate to nitrite. Therefore this test is considered specific but not very sensitive, whereas a positive nitrite may be suggestive of an active UTI; a negative result does not necessarily rule it out.
- **Leukocyte esterase:** When WBCs in the urine undergo lysis, esterases are released. Therefore a positive leukocyte esterase test implies pyuria and a UTI. If the urine culture is negative (i.e., sterile pyuria), this could indicate an infection that is not easily cultured (e.g., bacterial infections such as *Chlamydia, Ureaplasma urealyticum, Mycobacterium tuberculosis*, viral, fungal, or parasitic infections) or noninfectious causes of pyuria, such as urinary tract stones, interstitial nephritis, or acute glomerulonephritis.
- **Bacteria:** In the appropriate clinical scenario, with positive tests for nitrite and leukocyte esterase, the presence of bacteria further strengthens the diagnosis of an underlying UTI. However, despite this, one has to also consider the presence of squamous epithelial cells, which if abundant (≥15 to 20/high power field [hpf]) indicate a contaminated specimen.
- **Bilirubin and urobilinogen:** Normally, bilirubin in the urine should be undetectable. Conjugated bilirubin is secreted in bile and metabolized to urobilinogen, which is reabsorbed via the portal circulation, with a small amount being filtered by the glomerulus. The presence of significant amounts of water-soluble, conjugated bilirubin in the urine may be a clue to underlying liver disease or obstructive hepatobiliary conditions and gives the urine the dark characteristic color seen in jaundice. Increased levels of urobilinogen are seen in conditions characterized by excessive hemolysis and liver disease.

4. What are the important aspects of urine microscopy?
Casts: Urinary casts are cylindrical structures that are formed from coagulated protein (Tamm-Horsfall protein) secreted by tubular cells. As their name implies, they are usually formed in the long, thin, hollow renal tubules and take their shape. They develop in the distal convoluted tubule or the collecting duct. The proximal convoluted tubule and loop of Henle are not locations for cast formation. Low urine flow rate, high urinary salt concentration, and low urine pH all favor protein denaturation and precipitation of Tamm-Horsfall protein, the organic matrix that cements the casts together (Table 2.3; Fig. 2.1).
Cells: The presence of more than 15 to 20 squamous epithelial cells/low power field (lpf) is an indication that the urine specimen is contaminated (Fig. 2.2A). The presence of dysmorphic RBCs (also called acanthocytes, see Fig. 2.2G) and/or RBC casts (see Fig. 2.1E and F) is the sine qua non of glomerulonephritis. The presence of no more than two to five WBCs/hpf is considered normal. WBCs (see Fig. 2.2D) in the urine (pyuria) may be indicative of a UTI. If the urine culture is negative (i.e., sterile pyuria), this could indicate either an infection that is not easily cultured or noninfectious causes such as urinary tract stones, interstitial nephritis, or acute glomerulonephritis. However, when associated with other cellular elements or debris, pyuria may have limited diagnostic value. See also Fig. 2.2.
Crystals: See Table 2.4 and Fig. 2.3.
Bacteria: Because of the abundance of normal microbial flora in the vagina and/or external urethral meatus, it is not uncommon to see bacteria in urine specimens. Similarly, if the urine

Table 2.3. Casts

URINARY CASTS	DISEASE ASSOCIATIONS
Hyaline	May be nonspecific; seen in normal individuals or during severe intravascular volume depletion (after strenuous exercise or with diuretic use), first morning specimens, acidic and concentrated urine
Granular	May be nonspecific, result from the breakdown of cellular casts "Muddy-brown" heme-granular casts are seen in acute tubular necrosis
Waxy and broad	Advanced kidney disease
Red blood cell	Glomerulonephritis
White blood cell	Urinary tract infections (pyelonephritis, cystitis), tubulointerstitial nephritis, renal tuberculosis
Fatty	Nephrotic syndrome ("Maltese cross" appearance under polarized light)

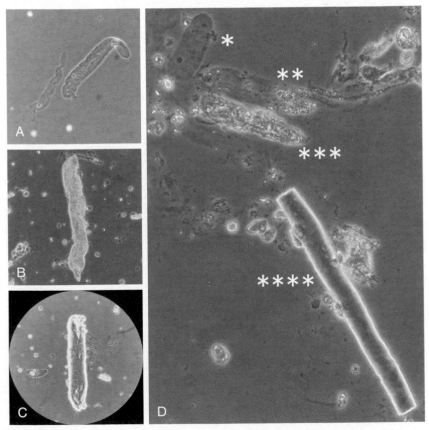

Figure 2.1. Casts. **A,** Two hyaline casts. **B,** Granular cast, signifying tubular injury. **C,** Huge waxy cast typical of severe kidney impairment. **D,** Aggregation of casts, *hyaline, **hyaline with granules, ***granular, ****waxy.

Continued

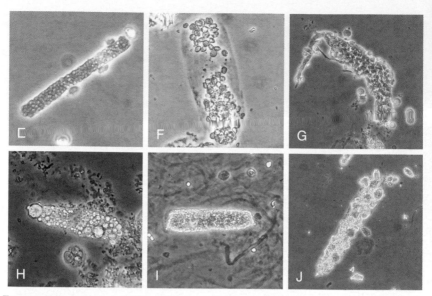

Figure 2.1. cont'd **E,** Red blood cell (RBC) cast with densely packed erythrocytes. **F,** RBC cast with easily discernable erythrocytes. **G,** White blood cell cast. **H** and **I,** Fatty or lipid casts. **J,** Tubular epithelial cell cast, typically found in patients with acute kidney injury (AKI).

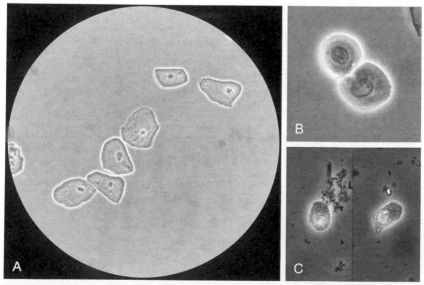

Figure 2.2. Cellular elements. **A,** Squamous epithelial cells. **B,** Urothelial cells. **C,** Tubular epithelial cells, suggesting acute tubular damage.

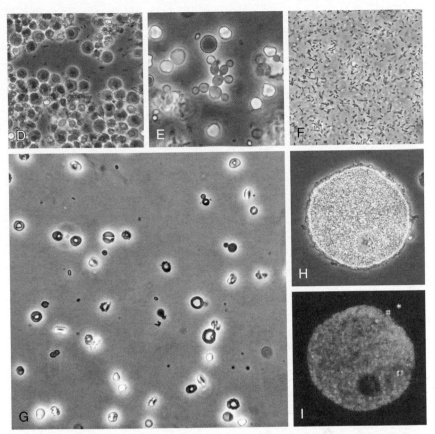

Figure 2.2. cont'd D, Abundant white blood cells. **E,** Budding yeasts (center), surrounded by normal red blood cells (RBCs). **F,** Countless bacteria. **G,** Dysmorphic RBCs, hallmark of glomerulonephritis. **H** and **I,** So-called oval fat body, a macrophage (or tubular epithelial cell) filled with lipid droplets, usually found in higher grade proteinuria. Note typical "Maltese cross" appearance *(*)* of singular lipid droplets in polarized light (I).

Table 2.4. Crystals

URINARY CRYSTALS	DESCRIPTION	DISEASE ASSOCIATION
Calcium oxalate dihydrate	Envelope shaped	Ethylene glycol toxicity
Calcium oxalate monohydrate	Dumbbell shaped	Ethylene glycol toxicity
Uric acid	Diamond or barrel shaped	Hyperuricosuria
Triple phosphate (also called struvite) or magnesium ammonium phosphate	Coffin lid	Urinary tract infection caused by urea-splitting organisms *(Proteus, Klebsiella)*
Cystine	Hexagonal	Cystinuria
Indinavir	Flat rectangular plates, fan shaped, or starburst in appearance	Indinavir therapy

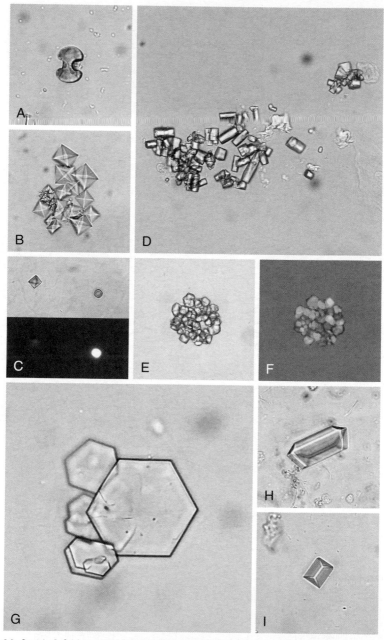

Figure 2.3. Crystals. **A,** Calcium oxalate monohydrate (dumbbell shaped). **B,** Calcium oxalate dihydrate (envelope shaped). **C,** Calcium oxalate dihydrate *(left)* and monohydrate *(right)*. Note intense birefringence of monohydrate crystal in polarized light *(bottom)*. **D–F,** Uric acid crystals show remarkable morphological variability. They exhibit strong and oftentimes colorful birefringence in polarized light **(F)**. **G,** Cystine crystals with classic hexagonal colorless plate. **H** and **I,** Triple phosphate crystals with typical coffin-lid appearance **(I)**.

specimen is left standing at room temperature for a considerable period, bacteria can multiply rapidly (see Fig. 2.2F). Therefore the identification of various microbial organisms (on Gram staining) in any urine specimen should be interpreted cautiously. (See Chapter 46 for discussion regarding asymptomatic bacteriuria.) The diagnosis of bacteriuria in those with suspected UTI should be followed by a urine culture. In general, the presence of more than 100,000 colony forming units (CFUs)/mL of a single organism reflects significant bacteriuria. The presence of multiple organisms usually reflects polymicrobial contamination. However, the presence of any organism obtained in a specimen via a catheter or suprapubic aspiration should be considered significant.

Yeasts: The presence of yeast cells (see Fig. 2.2E) usually represents contamination or can indicate a true infection. They are often difficult to distinguish from red cells and amorphous crystals but can be identified by their tendency to bud. Most often they are *Candida,* which may colonize the bladder, urethra, or vagina.

5. What is the purple urine bag syndrome (PUBS)?
   Initially described in medical literature in 1978, PUBS is a rare condition associated with alkaline urine and UTIs caused by sulfatase- and phosphatase-producing bacteria *(Providencia, E. coli, Proteus, Pseudomonas, Klebsiella).* It is commonly observed in institutionalized elderly females with chronic indwelling catheters, who are also constipated. The etiology remains unclear, although it is believed that indigo and indirubin pigments (which are metabolites of tryptophan) react with the synthetic material of the urinary catheter and bag and produce the purple urine.
   Of interest, from a historical perspective, England's "Mad" King George III was described by his physicians in 1812 to have a blue-tinged urine.

6. What is the blue diaper syndrome?
   This is another name for familial hypercalcemia with nephrocalcinosis and indicanuria, a rare, autosomal recessive disease caused by a metabolic defect in the reabsorption of tryptophan in the basolateral membrane of the proximal tubule. Bacterial degradation of tryptophan in the intestine leads to an excessive production of indole, thereby leading to indicanuria, which, during oxidation to indigo blue, causes a peculiar bluish discoloration of the urine. Symptoms generally involve the alimentary tract and include vision problems and fevers.

7. What is red diaper syndrome?
   It is seen in infants and is caused by prodigiosin, which is a red pigment produced by many strains of the gram-negative bacillus *Serratia marcescens.*

8. What is black urine disease?
   Also called alkaptonuria or homogentisuria, it is a rare, autosomal recessive condition, secondary to a defect in the enzyme homogentisate 1,2-dioxygenase, which is involved in the degradation of tyrosine. As a result, homogentisic acid is formed and excreted in the urine in excessive amounts. Excessive homogentisic acid causes ochronosis, pigmented sclerae, aortic and mitral regurgitation, and formation of kidney stones and prostatic stones. Of interest, most cases in the literature are in patients who are either from Slovakia or the Dominican Republic.

9. Does the odor of the urine have any diagnostic significance?
   The ammonia odor of normal urine is usually a result of bacterial (normal flora) breakdown of urea. The odor of urine is influenced by consumption of certain foods and medications. For instance, consumption of certain vegetables (commonly asparagus, Brussels sprouts) and certain curry spices (cumin, coriander, chili pepper) can cause a strong odor to urine.

10. Is red urine the same as hematuria?
    Gross hematuria is the presence of red or brown urine. The degree of discoloration has limited value because as little as 1 mL of blood per liter of urine can cause visible discoloration. In the initial evaluation of a patient with gross hematuria, it must be determined whether the urine discoloration is truly due to urinary tract bleeding. This can be difficult for patients who are menstruating or postpartum. Conditions in which the urine may appear red, in the absence of bleeding, include use of rifampin, phenothiazine, or phenazopyridine (analgesic) and dietary ingestion of beets in predisposed individuals. In these cases the urine dipstick will be negative for blood, and the microscopy will also not show any RBCs. It is also important to differentiate hematuria from other causes of red urine, such as hemoglobinuria (following intravascular hemolysis) and myoglobinuria (following acute rhabdomyolysis). In these cases the urine dipstick will be positive for blood, but the urine microscopy will not show many RBCs.

11. Can there be hematuria in the absence of red/brown urine?
    Yes, hematuria can be either gross or microscopic. Microscopic hematuria is defined as the presence of three or more RBCs/hpf in two of three urine samples. Often, it is detected incidentally by urine dipstick examination.

12. What should be your approach for a patient with hematuria?
    Careful history taking is central in the evaluation of hematuria and provides diagnostic clues. For instance, the occurrence of concomitant flank pain with radiation to the ipsilateral testicle or labia suggests underlying urinary tract stones; burning on urination or dysuria may point to possible UTI; a recent bout of upper respiratory tract infection may suggest either postinfectious glomerulonephritis or IgA nephropathy. A family history of hematuria is also helpful, because certain diseases tend to run in families, such as polycystic kidney disease or sickle cell nephropathy. Likewise, thin basement membrane nephropathy (TBMN; also known as benign familial hematuria) occurs in families and is notable for having a benign course. Exercise-induced hematuria is a benign condition seen in adolescents who exercise vigorously (e.g., long-distance runners).
    In elderly individuals (those older than age 50) the finding of gross or microscopic (even transient) hematuria should trigger an evaluation to rule out malignancy involving the genitourinary tract. The incidence of bladder cancer and other malignancies involving the kidneys and the ureters is significantly elevated, particularly in those with a history of smoking or analgesic use. Increased urgency and frequency with hematuria is suggestive of urinary tract obstruction secondary to either prostatic disease or cervical cancer.
    Asymptomatic hyperuricosuria or hypercalciuria (spot urine calcium to urine creatinine ratio >0.20 mg/mg) can also cause hematuria. These are more common causes of microscopic hematuria in children, although they have also been reported in adults.
    An important aspect of the evaluation of patients with hematuria is to differentiate glomerular from nonglomerular bleeding (Table 2.5). For those with glomerular bleeding, especially in the presence of other features such as proteinuria or progressive decline in kidney function, a percutaneous kidney biopsy may be necessary.

13. What is the "three tube test" for hematuria?
    The three tube test (also called three container method) is performed to determine the location of bleeding in the urinary tract. Three consecutive samples of the urine stream are collected: the first 10 to 15 mL, midstream 30 to 40 mL, and the last 5 to 10 mL. Hematuria (or predominance of RBCs on urine microscopy) primarily in the first sample (initial hematuria) is suggestive of an anterior urethral

Table 2.5. Glomerular Versus Nonglomerular Bleeding

GLOMERULAR	NONGLOMERULAR
Associated with:	Associated with:
Proteinuria >500 mg/day	Proteinuria <500 mg/day
Red blood cell (RBC) casts	Absent RBC casts
Dysmorphic RBCs	Absent dysmorphic RBCs
Usually seen in acute	Renal Causes:
glomerulonephritis, thin basement	Tubulointerstitial nephritis
membrane nephropathy (TBMN)	Polycystic kidney disease
	Sickle cell disease or trait
	Renovascular disease (atheroembolic renal disease, renal vein thrombosis, arteriovenous malformations, nutcracker syndrome)
	Urologic Causes:
	Tumors or malignancies
	Stones
	Infections (urethritis, prostatitis, cystitis, pyelonephritis)
	Medications:
	Chemotherapeutic agents (cyclophosphamide, ifosfamide, mitotane)
	Anticoagulants

source of bleeding, whereas hematuria primarily at the end of the urine stream (terminal hematuria) points to a lesion at the bladder trigone (bladder neck) or a posterior urethra. Hematuria in all three samples is seen in lesions that may be anywhere above the bladder neck (bladder, ureters, or kidneys).

14. **What is cyclic hematuria?**
Cyclic hematuria may be reported by women during menstruation where hematuria correlates with menstrual periods, suggesting the possibility of endometriosis involving the urinary tract. It is also seen with vesicouteral fistulae that usually arise as a complication of a previous cesarean section, Youssef syndrome.

15. **What is the loin pain hematuria syndrome (LPHS)?**
Considered a diagnosis of exclusion in patients with hematuria, LPHS is characterized by the presence of recurrent or persistent, severe, unilateral or bilateral flank pain accompanied by gross or microscopic hematuria. Commonly seen in young, white females, it has been associated with chronic pelvic pain and with TBMN.

16. **What is the nutcracker syndrome?**
Nutcracker syndrome is also known as left kidney vein entrapment syndrome. It is believed to be secondary to compression of the left kidney vein as it passes through the angle between the abdominal aorta and the superior mesenteric artery. Common presentations include hematuria (resulting from varices within the kidney pelvis and ureter), left-sided varicocele, and left flank discomfort. Diagnosis is established by performing a left kidney venography or a magnetic resonance angiography. In cases of recurrent or persistent pain, surgical treatment is considered (e.g., endovascular stenting, kidney vein reimplantation, and gonadal vein embolization).

17. **What is the significance of proteinuria?**
Proteinuria usually implies that there is a defect in glomerular permeability. In general, proteinuria can be classified into persistent or transient. Among the causes of persistent proteinuria there are three types: (1) glomerular, (2) tubular, or (3) overflow.
- Glomerular proteinuria includes diabetic nephropathy and other common glomerular disorders. It is caused by increased filtration of albumin and other proteins across the glomerular capillary wall. Other causes of glomerular proteinuria have a rather benign course, such as orthostatic and exercise-induced proteinuria. These latter causes are usually transient and characterized by significantly less proteinuria, usually less than 1 g a day.
- Tubular proteinuria is due to tubulointerstitial disease. Patients have decreased ability for the proximal tubules to reabsorb proteins that are normally filtered by the glomerulus. The amount of proteinuria is typically small (<2 g/day). Unlike the large macromolecules lost with glomerular proteinuria (albuminuria), in tubular proteinuria it is mostly low-molecular-weight proteins, such as β_2-microglobulin, that are lost in the urine. These will test negative by urinary dipstick.
- Overflow proteinuria (also called overproduction proteinuria) is exemplified by multiple myeloma, in which there is an overabundance of Ig light chains in circulation secondary to overproduction. These excess Igs get filtered by the glomerulus and exceed the tubular capacity for reabsorption, resulting in proteins appearing in the urine.

Although both glomerular and tubular proteinuria are secondary to abnormalities involving the glomerular capillary and tubular walls, respectively, in overflow proteinuria, the problem lies in overproduction of certain proteins.

Quantification of proteinuria is best accomplished by performing a 24-hour urine collection. However, this can be cumbersome, especially in the elderly, children, or those with urinary incontinence. The urine protein to urine creatinine ratio (urine PCR), using a random urine specimen, has good correlation with the 24-hour urine protein determination. The 24-hour urine protein in grams is approximately equivalent to the urine PCR in g/g (for SI units, multiply PCR in g/mmol by approximately 9 to estimate g/day). See Question 18 for more details.

In transient proteinuria conditions, there is a transient change in glomerular hemodynamics, causing increased excretion of urinary protein. These are usually benign and self-limited. Examples include congestive heart failure, fevers, strenuous exercise, seizure disorders, and even extremes of stress. Orthostatic proteinuria (see Question 17) falls under this category.

18. **What is the significance of a negative urine dipstick for protein along with an elevated urine PCR?**
The urine dipstick reacts to albumin and not to other nonalbumin proteins. The most important condition that one can miss here is overflow proteinuria, due to Ig light chains (Bence Jones proteins) from

multiple myeloma. It may also be seen with tubular proteinuria. In these cases, there is a discrepancy between the urine albumin-to-creatinine ratio, which may be low or normal, and the urine PCR, which will be elevated.

19. **What is orthostatic proteinuria?**

Orthostatic or postural proteinuria, by definition, is demonstration of increased urine protein excretion in the upright position and normal urine protein excretion in the supine position. It is a benign condition, typically seen in adolescents, whose mechanism is not clearly understood. The diagnosis is established by performing a split urine collection. The protocol for a split urine collection is as follows: (1) The first morning void is discarded. (2) A 16-hour upright collection is obtained between 7 AM and 11 PM, with the patient performing normal activities and finishing the collection by voiding just before 11 PM. (The times can be adjusted according to the normal sleep/wake times.) (3) The patient should assume the recumbent position 2 hours before the upright collection is finished to avoid contamination of the supine collection with urine formed when in the upright position. (4) A separate overnight 8-hour collection is obtained between 11 PM and 7 AM. Orthostatic proteinuria is diagnosed if the urinary protein excretion rate is normal for the nighttime collection (for children <4 mg/m^2 per hour and for adults <50 mg over an 8-hour period) and the daytime collection exceeds the normal protein excretion rate.

Orthostatic proteinuria has a benign course and does not progress to end-stage kidney disease; in fact, proteinuria resolves spontaneously in the majority of affected patients.

20. **What is the difference between a 24-hour protein excretion and a PCR on a random urine sample?**

The 24-hour urine protein excretion represents the reference (gold standard) method. It is used universally, averages the variation in proteinuria caused by circadian rhythm, and is the most accurate for monitoring proteinuria during treatment. However, it requires detailed instructions for urine collection and can be impractical in some circumstances (e.g., outpatient setting, infants, elderly, and incontinent patients). In practice, collection errors are common, compromising the accuracy of this "gold standard."

The PCR on a random urine sample is the recommended alternative to the 24-hour urine collection. It is easy to obtain, is not influenced by variation in water intake, and is not subject to collection errors, and the same sample can be used for microscopic investigation.

A normal PCR is sufficient to rule out the presence of pathologic proteinuria (which decreases the number of unnecessary 24-hour urine collections). Hence a random urine PCR serves as a useful screening tool. In general, the 24-hour urine protein in grams is approximately equivalent to the urine PCR in g/g (for SI units, multiply PCR in g/mmol by ~9 to estimate g/day). However, the correlation between the random PCR and a 24-hour collection is poorer at higher levels of proteinuria (>1g/L or >0.1 g/dL), and in such cases confirmation by a 24-hour collection should be considered. The validity of a random PCR in following response to treatment in patients with glomerular disorders is also unproven. In these settings, for intraindividual comparison of trends over time (e.g., for assessment of progression or response to treatment), it is important to use the same measure, either PCR or 24-hour collection, rather than use them interchangeably.

KEY POINTS

1. Normal urine color can vary from pale or light yellow to deep amber or dark yellow and is the result of the presence of a pigment called urochrome.
2. Urinary dipsticks detect only the presence of albumin; however, they are notorious for being poor indicators of the presence of nonalbumin proteins, especially light chains.
3. The presence of ketones in the urine is abnormal.
4. Careful history taking is important in the evaluation of hematuria.
5. The urine protein-to-creatinine (using a random urine specimen) ratio has been shown to have a good correlation with the 24-hour urine protein determination.

Bibliography

Armstrong, J. A. (2007). Urinalysis in western culture: A brief history. *Kidney International, 71*, 384.

Lerma, E. V. (2008). Approach to the patient with renal disease. In E. V. Lerma, J. R. Berns, & A. R. Nissenson (Eds.), *Current diagnosis and treatment in nephrology and hypertension.* New York: McGraw-Hill.

Pillai, B. P., Chong, V. H., & Yong, A. M. L. (2009). Purple urine bag syndrome. *Singapore Medical Journal, 50*(5), e193–194.

Simerville, J. A., Maxted, W. C., & Pahira, J. J. (2005). Urinalysis: A comprehensive review. *American Family Physician, 71*(6), 1153–1162.

Simonson, M. S. (2003). Measurement of urinary protein. In D. Hricik, T. R. Miller, & J. R. Sedor (Eds.), *Nephrology secrets* (2nd ed., pp. 11–14). Philadelphia: Hanley & Belfus.

CHAPTER 3

MEASUREMENT OF GLOMERULAR FILTRATION RATE

Joel M. Topf and Lesley A. Inker

1. **What is the glomerular filtration rate (GFR)?**
   The production of urine and the removal of waste products by the kidneys begin by filtering blood across the glomerular membrane. Blood enters the glomerulus and then can exit either through the efferent arteriole or by becoming filtrate by passing through the glomerular membrane into Bowman space and the tubules of the nephron. The GFR quantifies how fast fluid is crossing the glomerular membrane.

2. **What is the difference between single nephron GFR and total GFR?**
   Single nephron glomerular filtration rate (SNGFR), an experimentally derived value typically performed in animal models, refers to the filtration of a single nephron. SNGFR can be affected by hemodynamic alterations or structural damage. As part of the adaptation of the kidney to injury, uninjured nephrons undergo hypertrophy and hyperfiltration to compensate for the loss of functioning nephrons (compensatory hyperfiltration). Thus the total GFR that is measured or estimated) might remain relatively normal despite a decrease in functioning nephrons (see questions 5 and 8 for how to measure or estimate GFR). As such, the GFR is dependent on the number of nephrons (N) and the SNGFR, as described as follows:

   $$GFR = N \times SNGFR$$

   A change in measured or estimated GFR could reflect either a change in nephron number or SNGFR.

3. **What is the clinical significance of the GFR?**
   The GFR is the generally accepted, best index of kidney function. Chronic kidney disease (CKD) is defined as GFR less than 60 mL/min per 1.73 m^2 as well as markers of kidney damage. In the United States the most common marker of kidney damage is urine albumin. Other markers are kidney cysts or pathologic changes in the kidney, for example. The severity of CKD is also determined by the level of GFR (Table 3.1).
   Decreases in GFR are associated with increasing symptoms and metabolic abnormalities. These abnormalities include anemia, acidosis, malnutrition, and bone and mineral disorders. In addition, medications that are metabolized or excreted by the kidney need to be dose adjusted (or avoided

Table 3.1. The Six Stages of Chronic Kidney Disease Use GFR to DefineSeverity[a]

CKD STAGE	DEFINITION	DESCRIPTION
1	GFR $\geq$ 90 mL/min per 1.73 m^2 with other signs of kidney disease (usually an abnormal ultrasound or urinalysis)	Normal or high GFR
2	Slightly decreased GFR (60–89 mL/min per 1.73 m^2 with other signs of kidney disease	Mildly decreased GFR
3a	GFR of 45–59 mL/min per 1.73 m^2	Mildly to moderately decreased GFR
3b	GFR of 30–44 mL/min per 1.73 m^2	Moderately to severely decreased GFR
4	GFR 15–29 mL/min per 1.73 m^2	Severely decreased GFR
5	GFR < 15 mL/min per 1.73 m^2	Kidney failure

[a]Once the GFR falls below 60 mL/min the GFR alone is enough to define CKD. in the most recent KDIGO guidelines, CKD stages have been replaced with GFR categories, albuminuria categories, and assessment of the etiology of CKD.

CKD, Chronic kidney disease; *GFR*, glomerular filtration rate

completely) in patients with decreased GFR. Even drugs that are not excreted by the kidneys can have altered pharmacodynamics and pharmacokinetics in the presence of decreased GFR. Most importantly, a GFR less than 60 mL/min per 1.73 m^2 is associated with complications of CKD, including risk for kidney failure and increased total and cardiovascular disease mortality. For these reasons the GFR is the single number that best expresses kidney function.

4. **What are normal values for GFR in adults?**
Normal GFR varies according to age, sex, and body size; in young adults, it is approximately 120 to 130 mL/min per 1.73 m^2 and declines with age.

5. **How is GFR measured?**
GFR is measured as the clearance of an ideal filtration marker. Clearance refers to the amount of plasma that is completely cleared of a substance over a set amount of time. For example, if a person has substance X in his blood at a concentration of 2 g X per liter and he excretes 1 g of X in the urine, he will have theoretically removed all the X from half a liter of blood. If the person took 1 day to produce enough urine to get rid of 1 g of X, then his clearance will be 0.5 L (of plasma cleared of X) per day. The equation for calculating clearance is as follows:

$$Cl_x = \frac{Ur_x \times V}{P_x}$$

where Cl_x is the clearance of substance x, Ur_x is the urine concentration of X, and V is the urine flow rate.
   Plasma clearance is an alternative to urinary clearance for measurement of GFR. Plasma clearance is performed by measurement timed plasma levels following a bolus intravenous injection of an exogenous filtration marker computed from the following:

$$Cl_x = A_x/P_x$$

where A_x is the amount of the marker administered and P_x is the plasma concentration computed from the entire area under the disappearance curve.
   An ideal filtration marker is one that is freely filtered at the glomerulus but not reabsorbed, secreted, or metabolized by the kidney. Clearance of an ideal filtration marker can therefore be used to measure GFR. Inulin is the ideal filtration marker. Inulin is freely filtered by the glomerulus but is neither secreted nor reabsorbed by the tubules. However, inulin is rarely used, and alterative markers include iohexol and iothalamate and are more commonly used. In addition to exogenous substances, endogenous molecules that are filtered by the glomerulus can be measured to assess GFR. In particular, creatinine clearance assessed using timed urine collections is often used to estimate GFR.

6. **Why are units of GFR in milliliters/minute per 1.73 m^2?**
The clearance of substances is computed in units of milliliters/minutes. However, because kidney size (and therefore amount that can be cleared) varies by a person's body size, to determine whether a person has normal GFR, the clearance in units of mL/min is then adjusted for normal body surface area (BSA) by multiplying by 1.73 and dividing by the individual's BSA.

7. **How is measured creatinine clearance calculated?**
Creatinine clearance is calculated using timed urine collection. The time is often 24 hours but can be as short as 4 or 6 hours. The clearance formula and an example is as follows.

A. $Cl_{cr} = \dfrac{Ur_{cr} \times V}{P_{cr}}$

B. $Cl_{cr} = \dfrac{90\,mg/dL \times 2000\,ml/24\,hr}{2.3\,mg/dL \times 1{,}440\,min/24\,hr}$

C. $Cl_{cr} = \dfrac{90\,mg/dL \times 2000\,ml/24\,hr}{2.3\,mg/dL \times 1{,}440\,min/24\,hr} = 54.3\,ml/min$

where A is the generic clearance formula. B substitutes some typical values. C. Shows that the units all cancel out except mL/min.

Note: to convert the 24-hour measurement to the conventional units of mL/min, one needs to convert 24 hours to minutes, by dividing by the number of minutes in a day, 1440. All the units cancel each other out except mL/min.

8. **What are limitations to use of measured creatinine clearance?**

Several problems can compromise the utility of creatinine clearance. Firstly, accurate measurements of creatinine clearance require complete and carefully timed urine collections; inadequate urine collections yield spurious results. Secondly, because creatinine is secreted by the kidney tubules, the creatinine clearance systematically overestimates GFR. Between 10% and 20% of urinary creatinine is secreted rather than filtered, so the creatinine clearance will overestimate the GFR by a similar percentage. Cimetidine, the over-the-counter H2-blocker, competitively inhibits creatinine secretion. Thus a 24-hour urine creatinine clearance while a patient is on cimetidine is theoretically closer to the actual GFR. However, there the extent to which cimetidine blocks secretion occurs variable among individuals. Drugs that block creatinine secretion will also cause a slight elevation in serum creatinine that does not reflect a change in GFR, just a loss of tubular creatinine secretion.

Drugs that block creatinine secretion in the proximal tubule
- Cimetidine
- Trimethoprim
- Ranolazone
- Pyrimethamine
- Dronedarone
- Tenofovir

9. **How is GFR estimated in routine clinical practice?**

GFR is usually estimated using the serum creatinine and an estimating equation. Serum creatinine is the most common endogenous filtration marker. Endogenous filtration markers are markers produced by the body but are filtered by the glomerulus. All endogenous filtration markers are not perfect filtration markers in that there are non-GFR determinants of their levels in the blood, in particular, variation in generation (i.e., production) among people, secretion, or reabsorption by the tubule or extrarenal elimination.

Estimating equations combine endogenous filtration marker(s), such as creatinine and cystatin C, with other variables, such as age, sex, race, and body size, as surrogates for non-GFR determinants of the filtration markers, and therefore can overcome some of the limitations of the filtration marker alone. An estimating equation is derived using regression techniques to model the observed relationship between the serum level of the marker and measured GFR in a study population.

10. **What is the most accurate creatinine-based estimating equations?**

Kidney Disease International Global Outcomes (KDIGO) Guideline on Chronic Kidney Disease currently recommends using the Chronic Kidney Disease Epidemiology (CKD-EPI) 2009 creatinine equation:

$$\text{eGFR} = 141 \times \min(\text{SCr}/x,1)^{\alpha} \times \max(\text{SCr}/x,1)^{-1.209} \times 0.993^{age} \times 1.018 \text{ (if female)} \times 1.519 \text{ (if black)}$$

where x is 0.7 for females and 0.9 for males
where α is 0.329 for females and 0.411 for males
where min indicates the minimum of SCr/x or 1
where max indicates the maximum of SCr/x or 1

Several online calculators are also available that can easily compute estimated GFR (eGFR) values from creatinine (http://ckdepi.org/equations/gfr-calculator/). The CKD-EPI equation estimates GFR from serum creatinine, age, sex, and race. It was developed in a cohort of 8254 subjects pooled together from 10 research studies and clinical populations with diverse characteristics, including people with and without kidney diseases, and across a range of GFRs (2 to 198 mL/min per 1.73 m^2) and ages (18 to 97 years). The equation was validated in a separate cohort of 3896 people from 16 separate studies, GFR range (2 to 200 mL/min per 1.73 m^2) and age range (18 to 93 years).

11. **What are the major limitations of serum creatinine as a clinical index of kidney disease?**

Creatinine is generated from the breakdown of creatine in muscle, distributed throughout total body water, and excreted by the kidneys primarily by glomerular filtration. Although the serum level is affected primarily by the level of GFR, it is also affected by other physiologic processes, such as tubular secretion, generation, and extrarenal excretion of creatinine. Table 3.2 lists the factors that limit use of creatinine as estimated GFR. Due to variation in these processes among individuals and over time within individuals, especially creatinine generation, the cutoff for normal versus abnormal serum creatinine concentration differs among groups. In addition, assays for serum creatinine vary across clinical laboratories, leading to differences in GFR estimates for the same patient when creatinine is measured in different labs.

12. **What is cystatin C?**
Cystatin C is an alternative endogenous filtration marker to creatinine. It is a 13-kDa protein produced by all nucleated cells. It is freely filtered by the glomerulus and then catabolized by the proximal tubule cells but does undergo extrarenal elimination (see Table 3.2). Because cystatin C is filtered and destroyed, only small amounts of cystatin C are excreted in the urine and its urinary clearance cannot be measured. Although the generation of cystatin C is less variable and less affected by age and sex than serum creatinine, it is now recognized that there are non-GFR determinants of cystatin C (listed in Table 3.2). Several studies have shown that eGFRcys is more strongly associated with long term adverse events such as death and cardiovascular disease (Fig. 3.1). It is possible that this stronger association is due to the presence of these nonGFR determinants.

13. **What are the estimating equations that use cystatin C?**
The serum level of cystatin C can be used to estimate GFR (CKD-EPI 2012 Cystatin C equation):

$$eGFR = 133 \times \min(SCysC/0.8,1)^{-0.499} \times \max(SCysC/0.8,1)^{-1.328} \times 0.996^{Age} \times 0.932 \text{ [if female]}$$

Table 3.2. Factors That Limit Use of Estimated Glomerular Filtration Rate from Creatinine and Cystatin C

	CREATININE	CYSTATIN C
Factors affecting generation	Decreased eGFR from: • large muscle mass • high-protein diet • ingestion of cooked meat • creatine supplements Increased eGFR by: • small muscle mass • amputation • muscle wasting diseases	Decreased eGFR in hyperthyroidism Increased eGFR in: • hypothyroidism • obesity • glucocorticoid use • inflammation (higher CRP, lower serum albumin, higher WBC) • smoking Older age Male gender Elevated urine protein Malignancies
Factors affecting tubular reabsorption and secretion	Decreased eGFR by drug-induced inhibition of secretion (See list in the text)	Not known
Factors affecting extrarenal elimination	Decreased eGFR by inhibition of gut creatininase by antibiotics. Increased eGFR by: • dialysis • large losses of extracellular fluid (e.g., drainage of pleural fluid or ascites)	Increased eGFR by large losses of extracellular fluid (e.g., drainage of pleural fluid or ascites)
Interference with assays	Spectral interferences • bilirubin • some drugs Chemical interference • glucose • ketones • bilirubin • some drugs	Not known

CRP, C-reactive protein; *eGFR*, estimated glomerular filtration rate; WBC, white blood cell.
Sources of Error in Interpretation of Estimated GFR from creatinine and cystatin C.

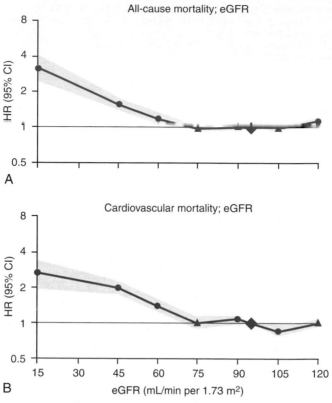

Figure 3.1. Relationship of eGFR With Mortality. HRs and 95% Cis for all-cause (A) and cardiovascular mortality (B) according to spline eGFR. HRs and 95% Cis *(shaded areas)* are adjusted for ACR, age, sex, ethnic origin, history of CVD, systolic BP, diabetes, smoking, and total cholesterol. The reference *(diamond)* was eGFR 95 mL/min per 1.73 m² and ACR 5 mg/g (0.6 mg/mmol), respectively. *Circles* represent statistically significant, and *triangles* represent not significant. *ACR,* Albumin-to-creatine ratio; *BP,* blood pressure; *CI,* confidence interval; *CVD,* cardiovascular disease; *eGFR,* estimated glomerular filtration rate; *HR,* hazard ratio. *(Reprinted with permission from Elsevier. Matshushita, K., van de Celde, M., Astor, B.C., et al. (2010). Association of estimated glomerular filtration rate and albuminuria with all-cause and cardiovascular mortality in general population cohorts: a collaborative meta-analysis,* Lancet, *vol 375, p 2073–2081.)*

where SCysC is serum cystatin C
min indicates the minimum of SCysC/0.8 or 1
max indicates the maximum of SCysC/0.8 or 1
   Cystatin C is less influenced than creatinine by race, so GFR estimates based on cystatin C alone (eGFRcys) include only age and sex, and not race. This allows GFR to be estimated without specification of race. This can be quite helpful in mixed-race populations. However, eGFRcys is not more accurate than creatinine-based estimating equations (eGFRcr); rather, it is the combination of the two markers (eGFRcr-cys) that results in the most accurate eGFR.
   The CKD-EPI 2012 creatinine-cystatin and cystatin C equations were developed using cystatin C measured using assays traceable to the international reference standard in a large database of subjects with diverse characteristics. KDIGO recommends using the CKD-EPI cystatin 2012 and creatinine-cystatin 2012 estimating equations:

$$eGFR = 135 \times min(SCr/x,1)^{\alpha} \times max(SCr/x,1)^{-0.601} \times min(SCysC/0.8,1)^{-0.375} \times max(SCysC/0.8,1)^{-0.711} \times 0.995^{Age} \times 0.969 \text{ [if female]} \times 1.08 \text{ [if black]}$$

where SCr is serum creatinine
SCysC is serum cystatin C

x is 0.7 for females and 0.9 for males
α is -0.248 for females and -0.207 for males
min(SCr/k,1) indicates the minimum of SCr/k or 1
max (SCr/k,1) indicates the maximum of SCr/k or 1
min(SCysC/0.8,1) indicates the minimum of SCysC/0.8 or 1
max(SCysC/0.8,1) indicates the maximum of SCysC/0.8 or 1
All eGFR equations are available online at http://ckdepi.org/equations/gfr-calculator/.

14. How should creatinine and cystatin C be used together?
The KDIGO CKD 2013 guidelines recommended using eGFRcr as an initial test, followed by a confirmatory test for situations in which eGFRcr is thought to be inaccurate (Box 3.1). Confirmation of the level of GFR may also be appropriate for clinical decisions regarding medications toxicity, initiation of dialysis, or candidacy for kidney donation. Confirmatory tests could include eGFRcr-cys or eGFRcys or a clearance measurement using either an exogenous filtration marker or a timed urine collection for creatinine clearance. In general, eGFRcr-cys is more accurate than eGFRcys and should be used as the confirmatory test. However, in certain populations (e.g., patients with neuromuscular diseases, limb amputation, eating disorders), eGFRcys has been hypothesized to be more accurate than eGFRcr. In states of pregnancy or rapidly changing kidney function, estimated GFR from cystatin C cannot be used and clearance measurements would be required.

15. What are other creatinine-based GFR estimating equations?
Prior to the CKD-EPI equation, there were two main creatinine equations in use: the Cockcroft-Gault and the Modification of Diet in Renal Diseases (MDRD) Study equation.
The Cockcroft-Gault formula was developed in 1973 using data from 249 hospitalized, veteran men. The multiplier of 0.85 for females was not based on any empiric data because the initial cohort was all men, and was suggested by the author as a reasonable decrease in creatinine generation in women compared with men. The Cockcroft-Gault formula estimates creatinine clearance rather than GFR, so it systematically overestimates GFR because of creatinine secretion. It was derived prior to creatinine standardization, which has led to lower serum values, hence it also systematically overestimates creatinine clearance. In addition, inclusion of a term for weight in the numerator leads to systematic overestimation of creatinine clearance in patients who are edematous or obese and underestimation in those who are thin or frail, and because of the form of the function of age, it systematically underestimates creatinine clearance in the elderly. The Cockcroft-Gault formula is less accurate than newer equations and should no longer be used.
The four-variable MDRD Study equation was developed in 1999 using data from 1628 patients with CKD with GFR from approximately 5 to 90 mL/min per 1.73 m^2. It estimates GFR adjusted for BSA. The equation was reexpressed in 2005 for use with a standardized serum creatinine assay (the four-variable MDRD Study equation):

$$eGFR = 175.6 \times SCr^{-1.154} \times Age^{-0.203} \times 1.212\,[black] \times 0.742\,[female]$$

The CKD-EPI equation was as accurate as the MDRD Study equation in the subgroup with estimated GFR less than 60 mL/min per 1.73 m^2 and substantially more accurate in the subgroup with estimated GFR greater than 60 mL/min per 1.73 m^2. Thus the MDRD Study equation is no longer recommended.
More recently, other creatinine-based equations have been developed in white Europeans—the Berlin Initiative Study and the CAPA (Caucasian, Asian, pediatric, and adult) equation—and both have been shown to be equivalent to CKD-EPI in elderly whites and more biased in blacks.

Box 3.1. Lists the Indications for an eGFRcrcys or Clearance Measurement Because eGFRcr May Be Inaccurate

Extremes of age and body size
Severe malnutrition or obesity
Disease of skeletal muscle
Paraplegia or quadriplegia
Vegetarian diet

eGFRcrcys, Estimated GFR from creatinine and cystatin; *eGFRcr,* estimated GFR from creatniine.

Several modifications to the MDRD or CKD-EPI equations have been developed for use in regions outside of North America, Europe, and Australia.

16. Can measurements of blood urea nitrogen (BUN) serve as an index of GFR?
BUN is not a reliable index of GFR. The kidney tubules reabsorb urea in quantities that vary depending on the state of hydration, thus rendering BUN an inaccurate marker for GFR. BUN concentration is also strongly affected by changes in catabolism and protein intake. Because urea is reabsorbed in the proximal tubule, urea clearance underestimates GFR. Some people advocate using the mean of the creatinine clearance (overestimates GFR due to tubular secretion of creatinine) and urea clearance (underestimates GFR due to tubular reabsorption) to get a better estimate of GFR.

17. How should GFR be assessed for drug dosing?
In its guidance to industry, the Food and Drug Administration (FDA) states that the method for assessment of kidney function that is most widely used in clinical practice ought to be the method used for adjustment of drug dosages. At the time, the Cockcroft-Gault equation was widely used, and the FDA provided this equation as an example of an estimate that could be used. Since then, more accurate equations are now available and widely reported (i.e., CKD-EPI equation and MDRD Study equation). The KDIGO 2011 clinical update on drug dosing in patients with acute and chronic kidney diseases recommended using the most accurate method for GFR evaluation for each patient rather than limiting the evaluation to the Cockcroft-Gault formula. Because larger people have larger kidneys which are able to clear more drug compared with smaller people, it is recommended to express GFR as mL/min, without indexing for BSA, for dosing adjustment based on GFR. Converting eGFR from mL/min per 1.73 m^2 to mL/min requires multiplication by BSA/1.73 m^2.

18. Can estimated GFR be used in patients with rapidly changing kidney function?
GFR-estimating equation assumes that GFR is in steady state. In acute kidney injury, GFR is not in steady state, and the endogenous filtration markers serum creatinine and cystatin C will rise more slowly than the change in GFR. In patients with rapidly changing kidney function, the rate and direction of change in the filtration marker reflects the magnitude and direction of the change in GFR.
• If the creatinine is increasing, the eGFR will overestimate the GFR.
• If the creatinine is decreasing, the eGFR will underestimate the GFR.
  A kinetic equation for change in GFR was developed, which allows one to estimate the GFR by using the rate of change in eGFR and an assumed creatinine generation rate.

19. How do we estimate GFR in pediatrics?
KDIGO recommends using an eGFR equation that incorporates height. Schwartz et al. produced an updated formula that does this. The data were from 349 children with CKD. GFR was measured using iohexol clearance (updated Schwartz formula):

$$eGFR = 39.1(height/SCr)^{0.516} \times (1.8/cystatin\ C)^{0.294} \times (30/BUN)^{0.169} \times 1.099(male) \times (height/1.4)^{0.188}$$

where eGFR is mL/min per 1.73 m2. Height is in meters. SCr is in mg/dL. Cystatin C is in mg/L. BUN is in mg/dL.
  All eGFR equations are available at https://www.kidney.org/professionals/KDOQI/gfr_calculatorPed.

KEY POINTS

1. The GFR is the generally accepted, best index of kidney function. CKD is defined as a GFR less than 60 mL/min per 1.73 m^2, as well as markers of kidney damage. In the United States the most common marker of kidney damage is urine albumin. The level of GFR is associated with metabolic complications of CKD, risk of death, risk of progression of CKD, and cardiovascular disease.
2. Normal GFR varies according to age, sex, and body size; in young adults, it is approximately 120 to 130 mL/min per 1.73 m^2 and declines with age.
3. The most common method used to assess GFR is serum creatinine combined with an estimating equation. The equation includes other variables, such as age, sex, race, and body size, as surrogates for non-GFR determinants of creatinine. The CKD-EPI equation is currently the most accurate way to estimate GFR from serum creatinine.
4. The two important limitations of serum creatinine are its generation from muscle mass and its presence in diet. Cystatin C is an alternative filtration marker that appears not to be generated

by muscle mass. The CKD-EPI creatinine-cystatin 2012 equation provides the most precise estimate of GFR.
5. Online calculators are available that easily allow eGFR to be computed.
6. KDIGO recommends that eGFRcr be used as an initial test with confirmatory tests used if eGFRcr is suspected to be inaccurate or for important clinical decisions.
7. For patients with rapidly changing kidney function, the estimated GFR is inaccurate. The equation depends on a stable creatinine. If the creatinine is increasing, the eGFR will overestimate the GFR. In contrast, if the creatinine is decreasing, the eGFR will underestimate the true GFR.

BIBLIOGRAPHY

Chen, S. (2013). Retooling the creatinine clearance equation to estimate kinetic GFR when the plasma creatinine is changing acutely. *Journal of the American Society of Nephrology, 24*(6), 877–888.

Fan, L., Inker, L. A., Rossert, J., Froissart, M., Rossing, P., Mauer, M., & Levey, A. S. (2014). Glomerular filtration rate estimation using cystatin C alone or combined with creatinine as a confirmatory test. *Nephrology, Dialysis, Transplantation, 29*(6), 1195–1203.

Inker, L. A., Lafayette, L. A., Upadhyay, A., & Levey, A.S. (2012). Laboratory evaluation of kidney disease. In T. M. Coffman, R. J. Falk, B. A. Molitoris, et al. (Eds.), *Schrier's diseases of the kidney* (9th ed., pp. 295–345). Philadelphia: Lippincott Williams and Wilkins.

Inker, L. A., Schmid, C. H., Tighiouart, H., Eckfeldt, J. H., Feldman, H. I., Greene, T, . . . CKD-EPI Investigators. (2012). Estimating glomerular filtration rate from serum creatinine and cystatin C. *New England Journal of Medicine, 367*(1), 20–29.

Levey, A. S., Inker, L. A., & Coresh, J. (2014). GFR estimation: From physiology to public health. *American Journal of Kidney Diseases, 63*(5), 820–834.

Levey, A. S., Stevens, L. A., Schmid, C. H., Zhang, Y. L., Castro, A. F., 3rd, Feldman, H. I., . . . , CKD-EPI (Chronic Kidney Disease Epidemiology Collaboration). (2009). A new equation to estimate glomerular filtration rate. *Annals of Internal Medicine, 150*(9), 604–612.

Kidney Disease Improving Global Outcomes. (2013). KDIGO 2012 clinical practice guideline for the evaluation and management of chronic kidney disease. *Kidney International Supplements, 3*(1), 1–150.

Matzke, G. R., Aronoff, G. R., Atkinson, A. J., Jr., Bennett, W. M., Decker, B. S., Eckardt, K. U., . . . Murray, P. (2011). Drug dosing consideration in patients with acute and chronic kidney disease—a clinical update from Kidney Disease: Improving Global Outcomes (KDIGO). *Kidney International, 80*(11), 1122–1137.

Schwartz, G. J., Muñoz, A., Schneider, M. F., Mak, R. H., Kaskel, F., Warady, B. A., & Furth, S. L. (2009). New equations to estimate GFR in children with CKD. *Journal of the American Society of Nephrology, 20*(3), 629–637.

Shlipak, M. G., Matsushita, K., Ärnlöv, J., Inker, L. A., Katz, R., Polkinghorne, K. R., . . . CKD Prognosis Consortium. (2013). Cystatin C versus creatinine in determining risk based on kidney function. *New England Journal of Medicine, 369*(10), 932–943.

Stevens, L. A., Coresh, J., Greene, T., & Levey, A. S. (2006). Assessing kidney function—measured and estimated glomerular filtration rate. *New England Journal of Medicine, 354*(23), 2473–2483.

Stevens, L. A., & Levey, A. S. (2009). Measured GFR as a confirmatory test for estimated GFR. *Journal of the American Society of Nephrology, 20*(11), 2305–2313.

CHAPTER 4

KIDNEY IMAGING TECHNIQUES

David C. Wymer and David T. Wymer

1. **List the most commonly used imaging modalities for the kidneys.**
   - Radiography (plain film, excretory urography [EU], retrograde pyelography, cystography)
   - Ultrasonography (US)
   - Computed tomography (CT) scan
   - Magnetic resonance imaging (MRI) and magnetic resonance angiography (MRA)
   - Radionuclide imaging
   - Kidney angiography

2. **Describe the information that can be provided about the urinary tract on the plain abdominal radiograph.**
   The plain abdominal radiograph, also called kidneys, ureters, bladder, can show the following:
   - Calcifications: kidney calculus, calcified neoplasm, sloughed papilla, medullary or cortical nephro-calcinosis, ureteric or bladder calculus/tumor
   - Air: air within or adjacent to the kidneys from severe infection
   - Soft tissue changes: obliteration of the psoas or kidney outline may indicate inflammation or tumor
   - Bone: changes of renal osteodystrophy and either lytic or blastic metastasis

3. **What is the current role of excretory urography (EU)?**
   - EU is also known as an intravenous pyelogram
   - The EU used to be the initial modality for upper tract imaging in patients with hematuria, flank pain, and other urologic disease
   - Now replaced by ultrasound, CT urography, and MR urography in most medical centers
   - Less sensitive than US, CT, or MRI for detecting kidney masses
   - EU does not allow reliable differentiation of solid masses from cysts

4. **What is retrograde pyelography?**
   The injection of contrast material directly into the distal ureter or the ureteral orifice of the bladder for visualization of the collecting system and ureter, without relying on the ability of the kidneys to excrete contrast media. The primary use of retrograde pyelography is to evaluate suspected ureteral obstruction or ureteral urothelial cancer in a patient whose ability to excrete contrast material is significantly impaired.

   This is an adjunctive technique when conventional imaging studies fail to adequately demonstrate the suspected pathology. Retrograde pyelography does not evaluate the kidney parenchyma and requires cystoscopy to place the catheters. This procedure is usually performed by a urologist.

   An alternative to the retrograde pyelography is antegrade pyelography, usually performed by an interventional radiologist. A percutaneous needle is placed into the kidney collecting system, and contrast is injected.

5. **What are the components of a CT urogram?**
   Comprehensive upper tract imaging includes the following:
   - Unenhanced axial CT of the kidneys—detection of calcification and baseline density measurement to determine enhancement of masses
   - Enhanced CT of the abdomen and pelvis with corticomedullary phase (early enhancement of the cortical tissue) and nephrographic phase (delayed imaging to view opacification of the medullary pyramids before calyceal excretion) for detection of enhancement of kidney masses
   - Excretory phase imaging of the abdomen and pelvis obtained with delayed imaging once contrast is in the collecting system essential for assessing subtle urothelial abnormalities including urothelial tumors; papillary necrosis; calyceal deformity; ureteral stricture; and inflammatory changes of the kidney collecting systems, ureters, and bladder
   - CT images may be reviewed as two-dimensional and three-dimensional reformatted images

6. **What is the diagnostic utility of ultrasound?**
   - Estimating kidney size
   - Assessing the echogenicity of the kidney (increased echogenicity may indicate chronic kidney disease but is nonspecific)
   - Preferred screening modality for suspected obstruction because it is very sensitive to dilatation of the collecting system, such as from obstruction in kidney failure, pelvic neoplasm, in kidney transplant, and in acute urinary tract infection with pyonephrosis
   - Complete ureteral obstruction can be excluded by documenting the presence of a ureteral jet (color flow seen on Doppler ultrasound as urine passes into the bladder from the ureteral orifice)
   - Can detect kidney calculi as echogenic foci with shadowing
   - Can differentiate solid from cystic mass
   - Diagnosing adult polycystic kidney disease and screening involved families
   - Guiding interventional procedures such as kidney biopsy and cyst aspiration
   - Detecting perinephric fluid collections
   - Evaluating kidney transplant allograft

7. **What is the diagnostic utility of ultrasound in the evaluation of a kidney transplant?**
   - Evaluating parenchymal echogenicity and masses
   - Detecting perinephric fluid collections (seroma, hematoma, urinoma, lymphocele)
   - Looking for hydronephrosis
   - Diagnosing ureteral obstruction/stenosis
   - Using Doppler to look for vascular compromise/complications
   - Used to guide for biopsies, aspiration, and drainage
   - Using resistive index to look for rejection.

8. **List the strengths of US in the evaluation of kidney disease.**
   - Sensitive for detection of perirenal fluid collections, pelvicalyceal dilatation, and cysts
   - Differentiates cortex and medulla
   - Differentiates cystic and solid masses
   - Shows the kidney contour and perinephric space
   - Demonstrates kidney blood flow by Doppler technique
   - Provides good kidney imaging irrespective of kidney function; may be used in patients with elevated serum creatinine
   - Can evaluate resistive indices to monitor chronic kidney disease and kidney transplants
   - Can be used portably at the bedside in the intensive care unit
   - Safe: no ionizing radiation or nephrotoxic contrast medium
   - Low cost

9. **List the weaknesses of US in the evaluation of kidney disease.**
   - Does not show fine pelvicalyceal detail
   - Does not show the entire normal ureter, although it may occasionally see proximal or distal ureters
   - Sometimes there is a limited acoustic window for seeing kidneys, especially on the left
   - Does not show the entire retroperitoneum
   - Can miss small kidney calculi and most ureteral calculi
   - Gives no functional information
   - Operator dependent

10. **When is CT scan superior to ultrasound for evaluation of kidney disease?**
    - For evaluation of an indeterminate mass on US or a solid mass when neoplasm is suspected
    - CT can define the extent of a neoplasm, evaluate for lymph node involvement, give a more comprehensive view of the perirenal, pararenal spaces, and Gerota fascia, evaluate vasculature (renal vein/inferior vena cava involvement), and stage neoplasms.
    - CT is the imaging method of choice in the evaluation of suspected kidney trauma.
    - CT provides information on the retroperitoneum and adrenal glands.
    - Complications of obstruction, such as infection, calyceal rupture, and kidney cortical atrophy, are readily seen.

11. **What is the Bosniak classification?**
    In 1986 Bosniak proposed a classification to characterize cystic kidney masses detected by CT scan as "nonsurgical" (i.e., benign) or "surgical" (i.e., requiring surgery). In his original classification, there were four categories:
    - Category I: simple benign cysts (fluid-filled, no perceptible wall)

- Category II: benign cystic lesions that are minimally complicated (mural calcifications, few thin septations)
  - Category IIF—added in 1993 (F = follow-up): more numerous thin septations, slight cyst wall thickening, totally intrarenal, nonenhancing, high-density lesions (i.e., hyperdense cysts)
- Category III: more complicated cystic lesions (calcifications, thickened or numerous septations, enhancement of the septations, mural nodules, thickened, irregular wall)
- Category IV: lesions that are clearly malignant cystic carcinomas (mural nodules with vascularization, enhancement of solid components)
  Categories I and II are considered nonsurgical, whereas categories III and IV are surgical. The risk that a category III or IV lesion is malignant is approximately 50% (range, 25% to 100%). The risk of malignancy in a Bosniak IIF cystic lesion is approximately 5%.

12. What are some clinical applications of magnetic resonance angiography?
    - Accurately evaluating patients suspected to have renal artery stenosis without the risks associated with nephrotoxic contrast agents, ionizing radiation, or arterial catheterization
    - Mapping the vascular anatomy for renal revascularization and abdominal aortic aneurysms
    - Assessing renal artery bypass grafts and kidney transplant anastomoses
    - Evaluating vascular involvement of kidney tumors

13. What are the limitations of magnetic resonance urography?
    - Relative insensitivity for kidney calculi
    - Relatively long imaging times—so they can be degraded by motion artifacts
    - More expensive and not universally available
    - Some people are claustrophobic.

14. Can MRI be done in patients with pacemakers?
    - Yes, unless the patient is pacemaker dependent
    - Newer generation of pacemakers are MRI compatible.
    - Coordination of the study with cardiology is required prior to scanning.

15. What are the clinical indications for radionuclide kidney imaging?
    - Estimation of glomerular filtration rate and effective renal plasma flow
    - Measurement of "split" kidney function to determine the relative contribution of the right and left kidneys to total kidney function. This can be important prior to a nephrectomy.
    - Differentiation of acute tubular necrosis (ATN) from rejection in cases of kidney transplant, where early blood flow images are normal in ATN with decreased delayed functioning as opposed to rejection where both are abnormal
    - Evaluation for urinary extravasation (leak)
    - Diuretic renogram is useful in differentiating functionally insignificant urinary tract dilatation from obstruction.
    - Diagnosis of acute pyelonephritis

16. What are the categories of radiotracers used in kidney imaging?
    Glomerular filtration agents to measure glomerular filtration rate:
    - Technetium 99 diethylenetriamine pentaacetic acid (99mTc-DTPA)
    - Technetium 99 mercaptoacetyl triglycine (99mTc-MAG3)
    - Iodine 131 o-iodohippurate (131I-OIH; mainly historical)
    - 99mTc-MAG3 is superior to 99mTc-DTPA in patient with poor kidney function

    Tubular secretion agents to estimate effective renal plasma flow:
    - 99mTc-MAG3
    - 131I-OIH

    Tubular retention agents used for cortical imaging (has some utility particularly in pediatrics for pyelonephritis evaluation):
    - Technetium 99 dimercaptosuccinate
    - Technetium 99 glucoheptonate (not often used anymore)
    - 99mTc-DTPA and 99mTc-MAG3 can both be used to evaluate transplant dysfunction

17. List the indications for kidney angiography.
    - Evaluation of cystic renal artery diseases
    - Preoperative evaluation of a complicated donor kidney
    - Evaluation and treatment of kidney transplant for renal artery occlusion or stenosis

- Evaluation and treatment of renal vein thrombosis
- Complex kidney masses or complications of polycystic disease or trauma
- Evaluation and treatment of bleeding involving the kidney vasculature (e.g., ruptured angiomyolipoma or following kidney trauma or procedure)
- The use of kidney angiography in the treatment of renovascular hypertension is controversial, especially in light of recent publication of the Cardiovascular Outcomes in Renal Atherosclerotic Lesions (CORAL) study (NEJM. January 2, 2014, vol. 370, no. 1), which suggests medical therapy is similarly efficacious

18. **What is an inexpensive first step in evaluating a patient with suspected ureteral stone?**
Radiography is often used as an inexpensive first step in examining a patient suspected of having urolithiasis, because the majority (approximately 90%) of urinary calculi are radiopaque. Large calculi can easily be seen; however, confounding factors such as overlying bowel gas, gallstones, or fecal material and osseous structures such as transverse processes or the sacrum can easily hide small calculi. In addition, distal ureteral stones can be confused with phleboliths in the pelvis.

19. **What is the test of choice for the examination of patient with acute flank pain?**
Unenhanced CT scan of the abdomen and pelvis is the preferred imaging modality, because virtually all stones are of sufficient attenuation to be detected on CT. The principle exception are stones consisting solely of indinavir sulfate (Crixivan, Merck, Rahway, New Jersey). In addition to direct visualization of a ureteral stone, secondary signs of obstruction on CT are commonly present. Unenhanced CT can also reveal many other causes of acute flank pain unrelated to the urinary system, such as pelvic masses, appendicitis, and diverticulitis.
   Ureteral dilatation has a sensitivity of approximately 90% for use in making a diagnosis of acute ureteral obstruction. Stranding of the perinephric fat and stranding of the periureteral fat both have sensitivities of approximately 85% but low specificity.

20. **Which is the study of choice for evaluating kidney trauma?**
The primary role of imaging in renal trauma:
- Accurately assess the severity and extent of injury
- Evaluate the injured kidney for underlying disorders
- Evaluate the anatomy and function of the opposite kidney
- Assess for other associated injuries
   Contrast-enhanced CT scan is the imaging technique of choice to evaluate the entire urinary tract, including the kidney vasculature, parenchyma, and collecting system.
   When a kidney laceration is detected on CT, a 10-minute delayed scan (excretory phase) should be obtained to assess the collecting system and evaluate for urinary extravasation. Delayed images are also helpful for characterizing the nature of a perinephric fluid collection and for distinguishing a hematoma from a urinoma.
   In patients with blunt trauma and suspected ureteropelvic junction injury, CT with excretory phase imaging is a reliable tool for evaluation.

21. **What is the role of radiology in kidney mass imaging?**
- Diagnosis of benign versus malignant
- Preoperative planning (surgery versus focused ablation)
- Renal artery embolization prior to surgery
- Split kidney function prior to nephrectomy

22. **What is the imaging work-up for hypertension?**
Imaging needs are defined by the possible etiology of the hypertension. For renovascular hypertension, per the American College of Radiology (ACR) Appropriateness Criteria (http://www.acr.org/quality-safety/appropriateness-criteria), MRI and CTA with and without contrast rank the highest tier.
- MRA without contrast
   - US Doppler and angiotensin converting enzyme I (ACE-I) renography are second tier.
- All other studies are **not** recommended.
- For patients with reduced kidney function, only MRA without contrast and ultrasound are recommended. If coarctation is suspected, then a chest x-ray along with either chest CT or chest MRI would be indicated. For suspected adrenal lesions, abdominal CT or abdominal MRI are the best modalities. For pheochromocytoma, nuclear studies with ^{131}I-metaiodobenzylguanidine (MIBG) is diagnostic.
- Echocardiography can be used prognostically looking for morphologic changes to the atria and ventricles as a result of hypertension.

23. What are the advantages and disadvantages of the various imaging methods used to diagnose renal artery stenosis?
    See Table 4.1.

24. What are the relative contraindications to intravenous (IV) contrast administration?
    - Previous allergic reaction to contrast media
    - Concern about contrast-induced nephrotoxicity
    - Asthma
    - Multiple allergies
    - Volume depletion
    - Pregnancy

25. What are the criteria for diagnosing contrast nephropathy?
    Although there is no universally accepted definition, an increase in serum creatinine level of 0.5 to 1.0 mg/dL or 25% to 50% from baseline is used after iodinated contrast administration. There is debate as to whether or not IV iodinated contrast induces nephropathy. The original studies showing harm were in patients receiving intra-arterial contrast for cardiac angiography. Recent studies have repeatedly failed to find contrast to be a risk factor for acute kidney injury.

26. What are risk factors for contrast nephropathy?
    - Preexisting CKD (creatinine level >1.5 mg/dL)
    - Diabetes
    - Age >75 years
    - Concurrent use of nonsteroidal anti-inflammatory drugs (NSAIDs), diuretics, ACE inhibitors, and angiotensin II receptor blockers (ARBs)
    - Large contrast volume

Table 4.1. Imaging Methods for the Diagnosis of Renal Artery Stenosis

METHOD	ADVANTAGES	DISADVANTAGES
Doppler ultrasound	• No ionizing radiation • Low cost	• Operator dependent • Bowel often obscures visualization of entire artery • Can be limited by body habitus • Low sensitivity for detection of accessory renal arteries
Computed tomography angiography	• Sensitivity and specificity near 100% • Accurate depiction of accessory renal arteries • Rapid acquisition	• Ionizing radiation • Only anatomic evaluation, cannot assess significance of any renal artery stenosis seen • Requires contrast administration
Magnetic resonance angiography	• 95% sensitivity • Lack of radiation	• Can miss small accessory arteries • Lower spatial resolution than computed tomography angiography • Risk of nephrogenic systemic fibrosis with contrast-enhanced techniques
Digital subtraction angiography	• Allows for interventional treatment	• Ionizing radiation • Requires contrast administration • Potential complication of groin puncture/vascular access
Nuclear Medicine— ACE inhibition renography	• Noninvasive	• Ionizing radiation • Time consuming with scans before and after ACE inhibition

- Hyperuricemia
- Use of ionic, high osmolar contrast media

27. **Is Myeloma a contraindication to IV contrast?**
No. Historically there has been a concern for precipitation of proteins in the collecting system; however, more recent studies have shown minimal or no risk if kidney function is otherwise normal.

28. **What is the typical time course of kidney impairment in a patient with contrast nephropathy?**
Serum creatinine level rises over 1 to 2 days after contrast administration, peaks at 4 to 7 days, and usually returns to normal by day 10 to 14.

29. **What are the issues of using contrast in patients on metformin?**
- None for MRI contrast.
- For IV iodinated contrast:

    Metformin in isolation is not considered a risk factor for contrast-induced nephropathy. However, patients who develop acute kidney injury (AKI) while taking metformin may be susceptible to the development of lactic acidosis.

    Per the Metformin package insert (perhaps overly cautious), metformin should be stopped at the time of contrast injection and withheld for 48 hours.

    Per ACR contrast guidelines:
- In patients with no evidence of AKI and with estimated glomerular filtration rate (eGFR) [33] 30 mL/min per 1.73 m^2, there is no need to discontinue metformin either prior to or following the IV administration of iodinated contrast media, nor is there an obligatory need to reassess the patient's kidney function following the test or procedure. http://www.acr.org/~/media/37D84428BF1D4E1B9A3A2918DA9E27A3.pdf

30. **What is nephrogenic systemic fibrosis (NSF)?**
A rare but debilitating or fatal fibrosing condition that most often affects the skin but may involve multiple organs. NSF occurs in the presence of kidney failure following the administration of gadolinium-based MR contrast agents. It was first described in 1997 and was called nephrogenic fibrosing dermopathy; the nomenclature was changed to NSF in 2005.

31. **What are the risk factors for developing NSF?**
- High doses of gadolinium-based contrast agents
- Decreased glomerular filtration rate (below 30 mL/min, although almost all documented cases have been dialysis dependent)
- Vascular injury
- Venous thrombosis
- Coagulopathy

    In patients with acute kidney injury, the use of gadolinium-based contrast agent should be avoided. For patients with chronic kidney disease, the Federal Drug Administration (FDA) has determined that the risk is greatest when the eGFR is less than 30 mL/min per 1.73 m^2. In this setting, it should be determined whether use of a gadolinium-based contrast agent is essential for diagnosis, and alternative imaging techniques and tests should be considered.

    For patients receiving hemodialysis when MRI is essential, it is recommended that hemodialysis be performed immediately after gadolinium-based contrast agent administration and again 24 hours later. However, the efficacy of dialysis is debated.

    Peritoneal dialysis clears gadolinium very slowly so gadolinium-based contrast agents should be avoided in these patients.

32. **Can contrast-enhanced MRI be done in patients with CKD?**
- Yes. Early-generation, linear gadolinium agents are the only ones in which NSF was reported. The newer cyclical agents bind gadolinium more tightly and are approved down to an eGFR of 30 mL/min per 1.73m^2. Most of these new agents have no documented cases of NSF, even in patients with eGFR below 30 mL/min per 1.73 m^2 or with dialysis (per some studies).
- See Table 4.2 for a current list of MRI contrast agents.

33. **What other potential risks are there with gadolinium contrast agents?**
- Recent studies have shown deposition of this heavy metal in the nervous system, even in patients with normal kidney function. Although no long-term adverse effects of this have been discovered, gadolinium should be used judiciously.

Table 4.2. Gadolinium-Based MRI Contrast Agents

NAME	TRADE NAME	MOLECULAR STRUCTURE	TYPE	NSF REPORTED
Gadotate	Dotarem	Macrocyclic ionic	Extracellular[a]	No
Gadodiamide	Omniscan	Linear ionic	Extracellular	Yes
Gadopentetate	Magnevist	Linear ionic	Extracellular	Yes
Gadobenate	Multihance	Linear ionic	Extracellular	No
Gadoteridol	Prohance	Macrocyclic nonionic	Extracellular	No
Gadoversetamide	Optimark	Linear nonionic	Extracellular	Yes
Gadobutrol	Gadavist	Macrocyclic nonionic	Extracellular	No
Gad oxetate	Eovist	Linear ionic	Hepatobiliary[b]	No
Gadofosveset	Ablavar	Macrocyclic albumin bound	Bloodpool[c]	No

[a]Gives general tissue enhanceement.
[b]Evaluate liver masses.
[c]Evaluates vasculature.
MRI, Magnetic resonance imaging; NSF, nephrogenic systemic fibrosis.

KEY POINTS

1. CT urography has replaced EU for evaluation of hematuria in most medical centers.
2. US provides adequate kidney imaging irrespective of kidney function.
3. Unenhanced CT scan is the preferred imaging modality for a patient with acute flank pain.
4. Gadolinium use with MRI has been associated with NSF in patients with kidney failure, although it is much rarer with newer cyclical agents; and gadolinium deposition is being seen in the central nervous system even in patients with normal kidney function.
5. Radionuclide renal imaging provides both functional and anatomic information about the kidneys.

BIBLIOGRAPHY

Brenner, B. M. (Ed.), (2008). *Brenner and Rector's the kidney* (8th ed.). Philadelphia: Saunders.
Dunnick, N. R., Sandler, C. M., Amis, E. S., & Newhouse, J. H. (Eds.), (2001). *Textbook of uroradiology* (3rd ed.). Philadelphia: Lippincott, Williams & Wilkins.
Hartman, D. S., Choyke, P. L., & Hartman, M. S. (2004). From the RSNA Refresher Course: A practical approach to cystic renal mass. *Radiographics*, 24(Suppl. 1), S101–S115.
Johnson, R. J., Floege, J., & Feehaly, J. (Eds.), (2003). *Comprehensive clinical nephrology* (3rd ed.). Philadelphia: Mosby.
Kawashima, A., Vrtiska, T. J., LeRoy, A. J., Hartman, R. P., McCollough, C. H., & King, B. F., Jr. (2004). CT urography. *Radiographics*, 24(Suppl. 1), S35–S54.
Pahade, J. K., LeBedis, C. A., Raptopoulos, V. D., Avigan, D. E., Yam, C. S., Kruskal, J. B., & Pedrosa, I. (2011). Incidence of contrast-induced nephropathy in patients with multiple myeloma undergoing contrast-enhanced CT. *American Journal of Roentgenology*, 196(5), 1094–1101.
Semelka, R. C., Ramalho, M., AlObaidy, M., & Ramalho, J. (2016). Gadolinium in humans: A family of disorders. *American Journal of Roentgenology*, 207(2), 229–233.

CHAPTER 5

KIDNEY BIOPSY

Pravir V. Baxi and William L. Whittier

1. **What are the major clinical uses for a kidney biopsy?**
   A kidney biopsy is performed to help establish a diagnosis and aid in the selection of an appropriate therapy when clinical and laboratory tests are unrevealing. The degree of active and chronic changes helps generate valuable information regarding the prognosis and likelihood of a treatment response. A kidney biopsy is routinely used to differentiate causes of transplant allograft dysfunction.

2. **In which clinical settings is a kidney biopsy most useful as an aid in the evaluation and management of a patient with undiagnosed kidney disease?**
   - **Acute Kidney Injury (AKI)**: A kidney biopsy is recommended when a patient has unexplained AKI that does not improve with supportive therapy. Prerenal disease, acute tubular necrosis, and obstruction must be ruled out, as these can be diagnosed based on clinical history.
   - **Nephrotic Syndrome:** Adults with evidence of nephrotic syndrome with no apparent underlying cause should undergo a kidney biopsy. Children with nephrotic syndrome are presumed to have minimal change disease and are treated empirically with steroids. A kidney biopsy is reserved for children with atypical features, including steroid resistance, hematuria, or kidney impairment.
   - **Systemic Disease:** Patients with vasculitis, systemic lupus erythematous, and viral infection-related nephropathy often require a kidney biopsy. Information is important in not only confirming a diagnosis but also in dictating further therapy based on the extent of active or chronic changes. In patients diagnosed with diabetes mellitus with kidney dysfunction, a kidney biopsy is sometimes suggested in the presence of features inconsistent with diabetic nephropathy, such as rapid progression or persistent hematuria. Additionally, a kidney biopsy is often recommended in the setting of various dysproteinemias when information would change the management strategy.
   - **Hematuria:** In patients with isolated microscopic hematuria, urologic causes must first be excluded. Patients with persistent non-urologic microscopic hematuria with proteinuria and/or kidney insufficiency often require a kidney biopsy for diagnostic and therapeutic purposes. In contrast, a kidney biopsy is usually not required in isolated microscopic non-urologic hematuria without kidney insufficiency, hypertension, or proteinuria. One may consider a kidney biopsy with microscopic hematuria and unique circumstances, such as in the evaluation of potential living kidney donors, life insurance, or employment purposes.
   - **Transplant Allograft:** Kidney biopsy is used in transplant kidney recipients who develop hematuria, proteinuria, or kidney transplant dysfunction to differentiate between the various forms of rejection versus other causes of kidney failure.
   - **Chronic Kidney Disease**: A kidney biopsy may be useful in prognostication for patients with unexplained chronic kidney disease and normal-sized kidneys on imaging.

3. **What are some clinical scenarios when a kidney biopsy may not be necessary?**
   - Acute kidney injury in which a clinical diagnosis of pre-renal disease, acute tubular necrosis, or obstruction is evident
   - Isolated glomerular hematuria without evidence of kidney dysfunction or proteinuria
   - Isolated non-nephrotic proteinuria with the absence of kidney insufficiency or glomerular hematuria
   - Patients with an insidious onset of proteinuria with a known diagnosis of long-standing diabetes mellitus (with slow progression of kidney disease) or massive obesity with presumed secondary focal segmental glomerulosclerosis
   - Patients with chronic kidney disease with small, hyperechoic kidneys. These patients are at higher risk of biopsy complications and are unlikely to have reversible disease.

4. **What are the clinical components of the pre-biopsy evaluation?**
   A complete history, physical examination, and selected laboratory tests are performed prior to a kidney biopsy. Current medications need to be reviewed with particular attention to antiplatelet agents,

aspirin, nonsteroidal anti-inflammatory drugs, and anticoagulants. Ideally, patients should be alert, cooperative, and able to follow simple directions. The skin overlying the planned biopsy site needs to be free from infection.

5. **What laboratory data should be obtained before undertaking a kidney biopsy?**
Routine laboratory tests that are obtained before biopsy include a complete biochemical profile, complete blood count, platelet count, prothrombin time, partial thromboplastin time, blood type, antibody screen for cross-matching, and a urinalysis. The practice of obtaining bleeding times prior to a percutaneous kidney biopsy is debated among different medical centers due to the lack of randomized, prospective studies, availability, and consistency. In a large prospective study of more than 1000 percutaneous kidney biopsies using real-time ultrasound guidance, patients with a bleeding time greater than 7.5 minutes had higher rates of biopsy-related complications. About 50% of these patients had a serum creatinine greater than 1.5 mg/dL. However, other studies have reported no increased risk. The use of bleeding times prior to a percutaneous kidney biopsy thus remains center dependent.

6. **What are the contraindications to percutaneous kidney biopsy?**
The absolute contraindications for performing a percutaneous kidney biopsy, as defined by the Health and Public Policy Committee of the American College of Physicians in 1988, include:
- Uncooperative patient
- Solitary native kidney
- Uncontrolled severe hypertension
- Uncontrolled bleeding diathesis
   With the exception of an uncontrolled bleeding diathesis, many consider these to be relative contraindications, which may be overridden in specific clinical circumstances. Percutaneous kidney biopsy of a solitary kidney has been performed successfully in small studies with technological advances of real-time ultrasound guidance and the use of automated needles. Other relative contraindications include:
- Active pyelonephritis
- Perinephric abscess
- Skin infection over the biopsy site
- Hydronephrosis
- Multiple cysts
- Kidney tumor
- Small hyperechoic kidneys
- Uncontrolled hypertension
- Hypotension

7. **What are non-percutaneous methods of kidney biopsy?**
A non-percutaneous kidney biopsy is performed when contraindications to the percutaneous method exist but tissue is required for diagnosis and treatment.
- **Transvenous Kidney Biopsy**: The transvenous, usually transjugular, kidney biopsy is performed by an interventional radiologist. The major indication for this technique is in patients with a bleeding diathesis. The reason that the transvenous approach is preferred for patients with bleeding diathesis is not that bleeding complications are less compared to the percutaneous approach, it is that an immediate bleeding complication can be treated quickly with the use of interventional techniques. A transvenous biopsy is also preferred in patients with morbid obesity, requiring multiple organ biopsies, and following unsuccessful attempts via the percutaneous route. Contraindications include bilateral internal jugular vein thrombosis and allergies to contrast material. The cost, the risk of contrast induced nephropathy, the variable operator experience, and the obtaining of an inadequate sample to establish a diagnosis are limitations of this technique.
- **Open Kidney Biopsy**: The open, or surgical, kidney biopsy is a safe and effective technique to obtain kidney tissue. The indications are similar to those outlined for the transvenous kidney biopsy, and it is performed in intensive care patients who are being mechanically ventilated. The risk of bleeding is low and mortality is rare. However, disadvantages of this technique include the risk of general anesthesia, fever, atelectasis, and a longer recovery time compared to the percutaneous approach.
- **Laparoscopic Kidney Biopsy**: Experience thus far suggests that the laparoscopic route is a safe, reliable, and accurate procedure to obtain kidney tissue.

8. **What factors are associated with an increased risk for bleeding following a kidney biopsy?**
Patients with a history of a bleeding diathesis are at increased risk for bleeding complications. Prolonged bleeding times are associated with increased bleeding in both retrospective and prospective studies, but

this test is not universally available. Advanced age, female gender, hypertension, and reduced glomerular filtration rate are all associated with increased risk of bleeding. Anemia was classically considered a risk factor for bleeding; however, patients with lower baseline hemoglobin pre-procedure are more likely to receive a blood transfusion based on the severity of the anemia as opposed to actual bleeding complications.

9. **How should patients on antiplatelet, antithrombotic, and/or nonsteroidal anti-inflammatory agents be managed in the setting of a kidney biopsy?**

A discussion regarding the absolute requirement of the biopsy for diagnosis and/or management, risk of thrombosis off medications, and risk of bleeding post-biopsy is necessary in patients on nonsteroidal anti-inflammatory, anti-platelet, and/or antithrombotic agents. Consultation with hematology and/or cardiology is often required in evaluating the risks and benefits.

Stopping the use of antiplatelet and nonsteroidal anti-inflammatory agents 5 days prior to a kidney biopsy has been shown to reduce the risk of minor complications. We recommend that patients stop these medications 1 to 2 weeks prior to and following a kidney biopsy. For patients on warfarin or heparin, there are no definitive guidelines for the management of anticoagulation specific to a kidney biopsy. The recommendations are generalized from studies of open surgical procedures.

- Warfarin should be held prior to the biopsy with a goal international normalized ratio less than 1.5
- Heparin should be stopped at least 4 to 6 hours (preferably up to 24 hours) prior to the biopsy
- Low-molecular-weight heparin should be held 24 hours prior to the procedure
- Anticoagulation medications should be held for 1 week following an uncomplicated biopsy

10. **What does the percutaneous biopsy procedure involve?**

The percutaneous kidney biopsy is usually performed on the right kidney under real-time ultrasonic guidance, but a computed tomography scan also offers adequate visualization. Local anesthesia is typically used, but mild sedation may be used. The patient is placed in the prone position, although the biopsy may rarely be performed in the seated, lateral decubitus, or supine anterolateral position in certain clinical situations. The lower pole is preferred to help reduce the risk of puncturing a major vessel while accessing the glomeruli of the kidney cortex. There are a variety of different biopsy needles available, but most operators prefer to use the automated spring-loaded biopsy needle. Two cores of kidney tissue are recommended for an adequate sample in most patients.

11. **What size needle should be used in kidney biopsies?**

There remains controversy regarding the ideal needle size to use in kidney biopsies. Most operators prefer the use of automated needles; however, there is no difference in the complication rates between an automatic needle and a manual needle of the same size. Several studies have shown no difference in the number of glomeruli obtained between automated needles of 14 gauge compared to 16 gauge. However, a recent meta-analysis found the rate of blood transfusion was significantly greater in patients biopsied using a 14-gauge needle as compared to a 16-gauge needle. There are also less asymptomatic perinephric hematomas demonstrated by routine screening ultrasound at 1 hour post-percutaneous kidney biopsy using 16-gauge needles compared to 14-gauge needles, suggesting a lower complication rate. In a prospective study undertaken in Norway, which included 9288 biopsies, there was a higher rate of complications with the use of 18-gauge needles as compared to 14-gauge or 16-gauge needles. Furthermore, the median number of glomeruli was significantly higher in both the 14-gauge and the 16-gauge needles compared to the 18-gauge needles. Based on these data, we recommend the use of the 16-gauge automated needle with real-time ultrasound sound guidance as our standard approach.

12. **What are the potential complications of a kidney biopsy?**

Due to the vascular nature of the kidney, the primary complications associated with a kidney biopsy are related to bleeding. Table 5.1 reviews the incidence of the various bleeding complications. Microscopic hematuria is the most common consequence of the procedure, but is asymptomatic and resolves spontaneously. Similarly, mild drops in hemoglobin concentration and silent perinephric hematomas (detected by routine screening imaging) are common but are not considered to be complications. Arteriovenous fistulas can be found in up to 18% of patients; however, most are clinically asymptomatic and resolve spontaneously within 2 years. Symptomatic fistulas can result in hematuria, hypertension, high-output cardiac failure, and kidney impairment, which can require arterial embolization or surgical ligation. Outside of bleeding, other complications of kidney biopsy are rare. They include Page Kidney (renin-mediated hypertension from pressure-induced ischemia from a perinephric hematoma), puncture of nearby organs (typically liver, pancreas, or spleen), pneumothorax, hemothorax, and perirenal soft tissue infection.

Table 5.1. Incidence of Percutaneous Kidney Biopsy (with Ultrasound Guidance) Bleeding Complications

COMPLICATION	APPROXIMATE INCIDENCE
Macroscopic hematuria	3.5%
Perinephric hematoma	2.5%–17%
Requirement of blood transfusion	0.9%–17%
Requirement of angiographic intervention	0.6%
Bladder obstruction from hemorrhage	0.3%
Requirement of nephrectomy	0.01%
Death	0.02%–0.1%

13. **What is the recommended post–kidney biopsy care?**
    Immediately after the kidney biopsy, the patient is placed on bedrest. The vital signs are closely monitored, and repeat labs are obtained at various points post-biopsy to monitor for bleeding and other complications. Urine is monitored for gross hematuria. In carefully selected patients, percutaneous biopsy of the kidney is being performed with increased frequency as an outpatient procedure. Individuals who are free of pain at the biopsy site have clear urine, stable hematocrit, and no hematoma on 1 hour post-ultrasound imaging could be discharged safely the same day. In a prospective study of over 1000 percutaneous kidney biopsies with real-time ultrasound guidance, post-biopsy observation of less than 8 hours was shown to miss 28% of complications, while 89% of major complications were identified by 24 hours. Although the timing of discharge post-kidney biopsy remains center- and nephrologist-dependent, an observation period of at least 6 hours and ideally 12 to 24 hours is recommended. Patients are instructed to avoid heavy exercise and any blood thinners (including nonsteroidal anti-inflammatory agents) for 10 to 14 days after the kidney biopsy.

KEY POINTS

1. The kidney biopsy is an effective, valuable, and safe procedure that provides insight into the diagnosis, prognosis, and treatment of patients with kidney disease.
2. A complete history, physical examination, and selected laboratory tests are important components of the pre–kidney biopsy evaluation.
3. The most common complication associated with a kidney biopsy is bleeding, though it is usually self-limited and rarely life threatening.
4. In patients with contraindications to the percutaneous approach, non-percutaneous methods should be considered when tissue is still required for diagnosis and treatment decisions.

BIBLIOGRAPHY

Chunduri, S., Whittier, W. L., & Korbet, S. M. (2015). Adequacy and complication rates with 14- vs. 16-gauge automated needles in percutaneous renal biopsy of native kidneys. *Seminars in Dialysis, 28*, E11–E14.

Corapi, K. M., Chen, J. L., Balk, E. M., & Gordon, C. E. (2012). Bleeding complications in native kidney biopsy: A systematic review and meta-analysis. *American Journal of Kidney Diseases, 60*, 62–73.

Fine, D. M., Arepally, A., Hofmann, L. V., Mankowitz, S. G., & Atta, M. G. (2004). Diagnostic utility and safety of transjugular kidney biopsy in the obese patient. *Nephrology, Dialysis, Transplantation, 19*, 1798–1802.

Khajehdehi, P., Junaid, S. M., Salinas-Madrigal, L., Schmitz, P. G., & Bastani, B. (1999). Percutaneous renal biopsy in the 1990s: Safety, value, and implications for early hospital discharge. *American Journal of Kidney Diseases, 34*, 92–97.

Korbet, S. M., Volpini, K. C., & Whittier, W. L. (2014). Percutaneous renal biopsy of native kidneys: A single-center experience of 1,055 biopsies. *American Journal of Nephrology, 39*, 153–162.

Mackinnon, B., Fraser, E., Simpson, K., Fox, J. G., & Geddes, C. (2008). Is it necessary to stop antiplatelet agents before a native renal biopsy? *Nephrology, Dialysis, Transplantation, 23*, 3566–3570.

Manno, C., Strippoli, G. F., Arnesano, L., Bonifati, C., Campobasso, N., Gesualdo, L., & Schena, F. P. (2004). Predictors of bleeding complications in percutaneous ultrasound-guided renal biopsy. *Kidney International, 66*, 1570–1577.

Simard-Meilleur, M. C., Troyanov, S., Roy, L., Dalaire, E., & Brachemi, S. (2014). Risk factors and timing of native kidney biopsy complications. *Nephron Extra, 4*, 42–49.

Stiles, K. P., Hill, C., LeBrun, C. J., Reinmuth, B., Yuan, C. M., & Abbott, K. C. (2001). The impact of bleeding times on major complication rates after percutaneous real-time ultrasound-guided renal biopsies. *Journal of Nephrology*, *14*, 275–279.

Thompson, B. C., Kingdon, E., Johnston, M., Tibballs, J., Watkinson, A., Jarmulowicz, M., . . . Wheeler, D. C. (2004). Transjugular kidney biopsy. *American Journal of Kidney Diseases*, *43*, 651–662.

Tøndel, C., Vikse, B. E., Bostad, L., & Svarstad, E. (2012). Safety and complications of percutaneous kidney biopsies in 715 children and 8573 adults in Norway 1988–2010. *Clinical Journal of the American Society of Nephrology*, *7*, 1591–1597.

Topham, P. S., & Chen, Y. (2015). Renal biopsy. In R. J. Johnson, J. Feehally, & J. Floege. (Eds.), *Comprehensive clinical nephrology* (5th ed., pp. 71–78). Philadelphia: Saunders.

Waldo, B., Korbet, S. M., Freimanis, M. G., & Lewis, E. J. (2009). The value of post-biopsy ultrasound in predicting complications after percutaneous renal biopsy of native kidneys. *Nephrology, Dialysis, Transplantation*, *24*, 2433–2439.

Whittier, W. L. (2012). Complications of the percutaneous kidney biopsy. *Advances in Chronic Kidney Disease*, *19*, 179–187.

Whittier, W. L., & Korbet, S. M. (2004). Timing of complications in percutaneous renal biopsy. *Journal of the American Society of Nephrology*, *15*, 142–147.

Whittier, W. L., & Korbet, S. M. (2014). Indications for and complications of renal biopsy. In T. Post (Ed.), *UpToDate*. Waltham, MA: UpToDate. http://www.uptodate.com. Accessed July 1, 2016.

II

ACUTE KIDNEY INJURY

EPIDEMIOLOGY, ETIOLOGY, PATHOPHYSIOLOGY, AND DIAGNOSIS

Paul M. Palevsky

CHAPTER 6

1. **What is acute kidney injury (AKI)?**

   AKI is a sudden decrease in kidney function occurring over a period of hours to days. The acute decrease in glomerular filtration rate (GFR) is usually manifested by the accumulation of waste products including, but not limited to, urea and creatinine in the blood (azotemia), and is sometimes accompanied by oliguria.

2. **What is the difference between AKI and acute renal failure (ARF)?**

   Although the terms AKI and ARF both described the sudden decrease in kidney function, the term AKI is now the preferred term, as it reflects the importance of smaller decrements in kidney function that do not result in complete loss of kidney function. The terms ARF or acute kidney failure now are generally used to describe AKI resulting in severe organ failure with the need for acute renal replacement therapy.

3. **What is oliguria?**

   Oliguria (literally, scanty urine) is a reduction in urine volume to a volume that is insufficient to excrete the necessary solute load. Oliguria is generally defined as a urine volume:
   - Less than 0.5 mL/kg per hour in children
   - Less than 20 mL/h in adults or
   - Less than 400 to 500 mL/day in adults
     Anuria (literally, the absence of urine) is defined as a urine output of <100 mL/day.

4. **How is AKI defined?**

   Although the concept of AKI is easily defined, multiple operational definitions have been used over the course of years, and coming up with a universal operational definition has been more of a challenge. Over the past 10 to 15 years, several consensus criteria for the operational definition of AKI have been developed, including the RIFLE (Risk, Injury, Failure, Loss, and End-stage) criteria developed by the Acute Dialysis Quality Initiative (ADQI) in 2004; the AKIN definition developed by the Acute Kidney Injury Network in 2007; and the Kidney Disease Improving Global Outcomes (KDIGO) definition developed by the Kidney Disease: Improving Global Outcomes Acute Kidney Injury Clinical Practice Guideline Workgroup in 2012. All three of these consensus definitions (Table 6.1) define AKI based either on changes in serum creatinine concentration or on the presence of oliguria. In the RIFLE criteria, AKI is defined based on at least a 50% increase in the serum creatinine concentration developing over a period of not more than 7 days or on the basis of a urine output of <0.5 mL/kg per hour for more than 6 hours. The AKIN definition added an absolute increase in serum creatinine of at least 0.3 mg/dL to the ≥50% increase in serum creatinine, and shortened the time frame for the change in serum creatinine to 48 hours. The KDIGO definition of AKI kept the ≥ 0.3 mg/dL increase in serum creatinine over 48 hours from the AKIN definition, but restored the time frame for the 50% relative increase in serum creatinine to 7 days, as was originally proposed in the RIFLE criteria. Both the AKIN and KDIGO definitions retained the same urine output criteria as proposed in the original RIFLE criteria.

5. **How is the severity of AKI staged?**

   In addition to standardizing the definitions of AKI, the RIFLE, AKIN, and KDIGO criteria stage the severity of AKI by the magnitude of change in creatinine or the duration of oliguria (see Table 6.1). The RIFLE criteria stratified AKI into three strata of severity (Risk, Injury, and Failure) on the basis of either change in serum creatinine (≥50%, ≥100%, or ≥200% increase) or the duration of oliguria (≥6 hours, ≥12 hours, or ≥24 hours) and two outcome stages based on the duration of kidney failure (see Table 6.1). The subsequent AKIN and KDIGO criteria kept the initial three strata of severity

Table 6.1. RIFLE, AKIN, and KDIGO Definition Staging Systems for Acute Kidney Injury

DEFINITION/ STAGING SYSTEM		INCREASE IN SERUM CREATININEa			URINE OUTPUT CRITERIAA
RIFLE	AKIN/ KDIGO	RIFLE	AKIN	KDIGO	
Risk	Stage 1	≥150% of baseline over 7 days	≥0.3 mg/dL over baseline over 48 h; or ≥150% of baseline over 48 h	≥0.3 mg/dL over baseline over 48 h; or ≥150% of baseline over 7 days	<0.5 mL/kg per hour for >6 h
Injury	Stage 2	≥200% of baseline	≥200% baseline	≥200% of baseline	<0.5 mL/kg per hour for >12 h
Failure	Stage 3	≥300% of baseline; or ≥0.5 mg/dL to a level >4.0 mg/dL	≥300% of baseline; or ≥0.5 mg/dL to a level >4.0 mg/dL	≥300% of baseline; or ≥0.5 mg/dL to a level >4.0 mg/dL	<0.3 mL/kg per hour for >24 h; or Anuria for >12 h
Loss		Need for RRT due to AKI for >4 weeks			
End Stage		Need for RRT due to AKI for >3 months			

aDefinition of AKI met by either increase in serum creatinine or urine output criteria; stage determined by highest severity of increase in serum creatinine or urine output criteria.

AKI, Acute kidney injury; AKIN, Acute Kidney Injury Network; KDIGO, Kidney Disease: Improving Global Outcomes; RIFLE, Risk, Injury, Failure, Loss, End-stage; RRT, renal replacement therapy.

(now called Stage 1, Stage 2, and Stage 3) but dropped the two outcome stages. In all three classification systems, the increasing severity of AKI is associated with the increasing risk of death and intensive care unit and hospital length of stay. The duration of AKI, which is not included in these staging criteria, is also associated with mortality risk. While these classification systems are important for epidemiologic studies and clinical trials, there remains uncertainty regarding the utility of AKI staging when applied prospectively in clinical practice.

6. What is acute kidney disease (AKD)?

With AKI defined as kidney dysfunction developing over less than 7 days, and chronic kidney disease (CKD) defined based on structural or functional damage to the kidney present for more than 3 months, a gap exists in patients who develop kidney dysfunction over more than 7 days but for less than 3 months. The KDIGO AKI workgroup proposed that AKD be defined as kidney disease that is present for less than 3 months, defined based on a GFR of <60 mL/min per 1.73 m², a decrease in GFR of ≥35% or an increase in serum creatinine of >50%. AKI is a subset of AKD.

7. How common is AKI?

Estimates of the incidence of AKI depend on the definition used for case finding and the population studied. It is estimated that 5% to 10% of hospitalized patients develop AKI. AKI is much more common in critically ill patients; 35% to 60% of critically ill patients will develop AKI based on the RIFLE, AKIN, or KDIGO criteria, and 5% will develop severe AKI requiring renal replacement therapy. Epidemiologic studies have demonstrated that AKI has become progressively more common, with an almost 20-fold increase in incidence over 25 years. Currently, more patients initiate renal replacement therapy for AKI than for CKD, progressing to end-stage kidney disease.

8. What are the causes of AKI?
   AKI encompasses any process that causes an abrupt decrease in kidney function. The differential diagnosis includes prerenal azotemia (approximately 50% to 70% of cases), obstructive nephropathy (approximately 5% of cases, see Chapter 17), and intrinsic forms of AKI.

9. Is acute tubular necrosis (ATN) the same as AKI?
   ATN is the most common form of intrinsic AKI. However, there are many other etiologies of AKI as described above, and the two terms are not synonymous.

10. Which patients are at risk for the development of AKI?
    The most important risk factor for the development of AKI is the presence of preexisting CKD. Elderly patients are at increased risk for the development of AKI, as they often have unrecognized diminished kidney function. Other risk factors include diabetes mellitus and volume depletion. Medications that cause intrarenal vasoconstriction, such as nonsteroidal anti-inflammatory drugs (NSAIDs), also predispose to the development of AKI.

11. What is prerenal azotemia?
    Prerenal azotemia is a functional form of AKI that results from diminished kidney perfusion. As there is no parenchymal injury, the hallmark of prerenal azotemia is the rapid normalization of kidney function when kidney perfusion is restored. Common etiologies of prerenal azotemia include intravascular volume depletion, congestive heart failure (cardiorenal syndrome, see Chapter 9), and advanced liver disease. The hepatorenal syndrome (see Chapter 8) is a severe form of prerenal azotemia in patients with cirrhosis of the liver and severe portal hypertension. Patients with prerenal azotemia are often (although not always) oliguric and generally manifest increased sodium reabsorption if they are not being treated with diuretics.

12. How can prerenal azotemia be differentiated from ATN?
    It is important to differentiate between prerenal azotemia and intrinsic forms of AKI, as prerenal azotemia will generally improve with the correction of the underlying hemodynamic disturbance. In contradistinction, the volume loading of patients with ATN or other forms of intrinsic AKI will not result in improved kidney function and may exacerbate volume overload. Characteristic laboratory findings that help differentiate between prerenal azotemia and ATN reflect the preservation of tubular function with increased sodium reabsorption and urinary concentration in prerenal azotemia (Table 6.2). Preexisting CKD or diuretic use may limit the usefulness of these indices. Novel biomarkers of tubular injury, such as neutrophil gelatinase-associated lipocalin (NGAL) and kidney injury molecule-1 (KIM-1), have been proposed as candidates for differentiating between prerenal azotemia and intrinsic tubular damage, but are not yet validated for clinical use.

13. What are the fractional excretion of sodium and urea and how are they calculated?
    The fractional excretion of sodium and urea are indices of tubular function that are useful in differentiating between prerenal azotemia and ATN, particularly in patients with oliguric AKI. In

Table 6.2. Laboratory Differentiation Between Prerenal Azotemia and Acute Tubular Necrosis

	PRERENAL AZOTEMIA	ACUTE TUBULAR NECROSIS
Serum BUN:creatinine ratio	>20:1	10:1
Urine specific gravity	>1.015	~1.010
Urine sodium	<20 mmol/L	>40 mmol/L
Fractional excretion of sodium	<1%	>2%
Fractional excretion of urea	<35%	>50%
Urine osmolality	>500 mOsm/kg	~300 mOsm/kg
Urine sediment	Normal, or hyaline casts	Kidney tubular cells and "muddy brown" granular casts
Biomarkers of tubular injury	Negative	Positive

BUN, blood, urea, nitrogen.

$$\text{Fractional Excretion of Na} = \frac{\text{Excreted Na} = \text{Ur}_{Na} \times V}{\text{Filtered Na} = P_{Na} \times \text{GFR}}$$

$$\text{GFR} = \text{Cl}_{Cr} = \frac{\text{Ur}_{Cr} \times V}{P_{Cr}}$$

$$\text{Fractional Excretion of Na} = \frac{\text{Ur}_{Na} \times V}{P_{Na} \times \dfrac{\text{Ur}_{Cr} \times V}{P_{Cr}}}$$

$$\text{Fractional Excretion of Na} = \frac{\text{Ur}_{Na} \times P_{Cr}}{P_{Na} \times \text{Ur}_{Cr}}$$

Figure 6.1. Fractional excretion of sodium calculation.

prerenal states, the tubular response of the kidney to decreased effective perfusion is to increase tubular sodium reabsorption. The fractional excretion of sodium (FE_{Na}), which is the percentage of the sodium filtered at the glomerulus that is excreted in the urine, will decrease from a normal value of slightly less than 1% and will be significantly less than 1%. In contrast, in many forms of ATN, impaired tubular function will result in elevated values of FE_{Na} ($>3\%$).

As shown in Fig. 6.1, FE_{Na} is calculated by dividing the urine sodium excretion by the filtered sodium load:
- The excreted $Na^+ = U_{Na} \times V$, where U_{Na} is the urine sodium concentration and V is the urine volume
- The filtered $Na^+ = P_{Na} \times \text{GFR}$, where P_{Na} is the plasma sodium concentration and GFR is the glomerular filtration rate
- The GFR can be estimated as the creatinine clearance, $U_{creat} \times V / P_{creat}$, where U_{creat} and P_{creat} are the urine and plasma creatinine concentrations, respectively.

Although the FE_{Na} is helpful in differentiating between prerenal azotemia and ATN, it is not completely reliable. Patients who develop ATN in the setting of true or effective volume depletion, such as with concurrent heart failure, cirrhosis, burn injury or sepsis, or as the result of contrast-induced nephropathy or rhabdomyolysis, may have a FE_{Na} $<1\%$. Conversely, the FE_{Na} may be $>1\%$ in patients with prerenal azotemia who are on diuretics or who have underlying CKD. In these patients, the fractional excretion of urea (FE_{urea}) may be helpful in differentiating between prerenal azotemia and ATN. The FE_{urea} is calculated in a fashion analogous to the FE_{Na} as:

$$FE_{urea} = (U_{urea} / P_{urea}) / (U_{creat} / P_{creat})$$

In prerenal azotemia FE_{urea} is usually $<35\%$; in ATN, values are typically $>50\%$. Fractional excretion of urea may be artificially lowered in the setting of infections with urea-splitting organisms. It should also be recognized that the while these diagnostic indices are guides in the differentiation between prerenal and intrinsic AKI, their diagnostic performance is imperfect and they should not be used as the sole criteria for establishing the etiology of AKI.

14. What is abdominal compartment syndrome?
Abdominal compartment syndrome is caused by an increase in intra-abdominal pressure resulting in the dysfunction of multiple organ systems including decreased cardiac output and hypotension, increased thoracic pressure, decreased pulmonary compliance and increased airway pressures leading to impaired ventilation, and decreased visceral perfusion, which in turn may lead to intestinal ischemia, and infarction and oliguric AKI. It is thought that increased renal venous pressure rather than increased intra-parenchymal pressure is the primary cause of AKI in the abdominal compartment syndrome. Common causes of abdominal compartment syndrome include trauma with intra-abdominal hemorrhage, abdominal surgery, retroperitoneal hemorrhage, peritonitis, pancreatitis, massive fluid resuscitation, abdominal banding, repair of large incisional hernia, laparoscopy and pneumoperitoneum, and ileus. It has been suggested that abdominal compartment syndrome may

contribute to as many as 30% of cases of AKI in critically ill patients. The treatment of abdominal compartment syndrome is abdominal decompression. In patients with massive ascites, paracentesis may be sufficient; however, the definitive therapy most commonly requires surgical decompression, often leaving the abdomen open until inflammation and edema subside.

15. **How is the abdominal compartment syndrome diagnosed?**
The hallmark of abdominal compartment syndrome is an intra-abdominal pressure over 20 mm Hg associated with a single or multiple organ system failure that was not previously present. Intra-abdominal pressure may be assessed by the transduction of urinary bladder pressure.

16. **What is obstructive (post-renal) AKI?**
Obstructive (post-renal) AKI results from blocked urine flow at the level of the ureters (upper tract) or the bladder outlet or urethra (see Chapter 16). For upper tract obstruction to cause AKI, the obstruction must either be bilateral, or be unilateral with an absent or nonfunctional contralateral kidney.

17. **What are the causes of intrinsic AKI?**
A variety of kidney parenchymal diseases can cause AKI:
- Acute and rapidly progressive forms of glomerulonephritis (see Chapter 14)
- Acute interstitial nephritis (AIN)
- ATN
- Acute vascular diseases (e.g., renal artery thromboembolism, atheroembolic disease)
- Intratubular deposition of crystals
  - Calcium oxalate in ethylene glycol positioning
  - Uric acid in tumor lysis syndrome
  - Acyclovir
  - Indinavir)
- Intratubular deposition of paraproteins (myeloma cast nephropathy)
  ATN is the most common etiology of intrinsic AKI

18. **How can the different causes of intrinsic AKI be differentiated?**
Although there are no specific therapies for the treatment of ATN, specific therapies are available for many of the other forms of intrinsic AKI. Diagnostic clues may be apparent from the history and physical examination, paying careful attention to (1) the history of medication use; (2) medical procedures; and (3) careful examination of the skin for evidence of vasculitis, drug eruption, and atheroembolism. Examination of the urine often provides key findings for differentiating between the etiologies of intrinsic AKI (Table 6.3). A definitive diagnosis may result in the requirement of a kidney biopsy.

19. **What is AIN?**
AIN is a form of AKI that results from immunologically mediated lymphocytic infiltration of the renal parenchymal interstitium, often with accompanying eosinophils. Although the classic presentation consists of AKI accompanied by the triad of fever, rash, and eosinophilia, the complete triad is observed in only a small minority of patients.

20. **What are the causes of AIN?**
Although AIN may develop as the result of infections, malignancy, and immunologically mediated systemic disease, it is most often associated with medication use (Box 6.1). The most common

Table 6.3. Urine Findings in Intrinsic Acute Kidney Injury (see Chapter 2)

AGN/RPGN	AIN	ATN	CRYSTAL NEPHROPATHIES	MYELOMA KIDNEY
Dysmorphic RBCs RBC Casts	RBCs WBCs WBC casts eosinophiluria	Tubular epithelial cells Coarse granular casts ("muddy brown" casts)	Crystaluria Oxalate—ethylene glycol Urate—tumor lysis syndrome Drug—acyclovir, indinavir	Bence-Jones proteinuria Free urinary light chains

AIN, Acute interstitial nephritis; *AGN,* acute glomerulonephritis; *ATN,* acute tubular necrosis; *RBC,* red blood cell; *RPGN,* rapidly progressive glomerulonephritis; *WBC,* white blood cell.

Box 6.1. Common Etiologies of Acute Interstitial Nephritis

Medications
  Penicillins
  Cephalosporins
  Sulfonamides
  Rifampin
  Proton pump inhibitors
  Phenytoin
  Furosemide
  Nonsteroidal antiinflammatory drugs
Infections
  Bacterial

Viral
Rickettsial
Tuberculosis
Systemic diseases
  Systemic lupus erythematosus
  Sarcoidosis
  Sjögren syndrome
  Tubulointerstitial nephritis and uveitis
Malignancy
Idiopathic

medications include antibiotics, particularly penicillins, cephalosporins, sulfonamides, rifampin, and proton pump inhibitors. Nonsteroidal antiinflammatory medications are associated with an atypical form of interstitial nephritis, which is usually not associated with fever, rash, or eosinophilia, and is often associated with nephrotic proteinuria.

21. **Does the presence of eosinophiluria mean a patient has AIN?**
Although eosinophiluria has been considered a hallmark finding, it is neither sensitive nor specific. It may be seen in many other conditions including pyelonephritis, prostatitis, cystitis, and atheroembolic disease. Routine assessment for eosinophiluria in patients with AKI is not appropriate.

22. **What are the causes of ATN?**
ATN may develop as the result of hypotension and kidney ischemia in the setting of sepsis with or without overt hypotension, or as the result of nephrotoxin exposure. Ischemia contributes to approximately 60% to 70% of cases of ATN, 50% to 60% of sepsis, and 30% to 40% of nephrotoxins. The nephrotoxins commonly associated with the development of ATN are listed in Box 6.2.

23. **What is the pathophysiology of ATN?**
Although ATN is characterized by a profound decrease in GFR, the connection between the tubular injury and the loss of glomerular function is not entirely understood. Three major mechanisms are thought to underlie the loss of kidney function in ATN:
1. *Intratubular obstruction:* Following an ischemic or nephrotoxic injury, tubular epithelial cells and cellular debris are sloughed from the tubular epithelium and occlude the tubular lumen distally. These sloughed cells and debris form the granular casts seen in the urine sediment.
2. *Tubular back leak:* The sloughing of apoptotic and necrotic tubular epithelial cells results in denuding of the tubular basement membrane and unregulated back leak of glomerular filtrate. The combination of tubular obstruction and back leak results in decreased urine flow through the tubular lumen.
3. *Vasoconstriction and microvascular injury:* Although the pathognomonic injury in ATN is damage to the tubular epithelium, there is both reactive vasoconstriction and endothelial injury in

Box 6.2. Common Etiologies of Acute Tubular Necrosis

Nephrotoxic
Exogenous
  Radiocontrast agents
  Aminoglycosides
  Vancomycin
  Amphotericin B
  Cisplatinum
Acetaminophen
Endogenous
  Hemoglobin
  myoglobin

Ischemic
  prolonged prerenal azotemia
  hypotension
  hypovolemic shock
  cardiopulmonary arrest
  cardiopulmonary bypass
  aortic surgery
Sepsis

the microvasculature that results in decreased glomerular perfusion, directly reducing the GFR and contributing to the extension of the initial injury.

24. **What is the clinical course of ATN?**
Clinically, four phases of ATN can be described. In the *initiation phase*, exposure to the nephrotoxic agent, ischemia, or sepsis initiates the injury to the kidney. In clinical practice, often there are multiple exposures whose cumulative effect results in the initiation of ATN. The initiation phase is then followed by an *extension phase*, during which there is continued cellular injury mediated by continued microvascular injury and the activation of inflammatory mediators despite the fact that the triggering exposure has resolved. This is then followed by a *maintenance phase*, which may last from days to 6 weeks or longer. During the maintenance phase, the GFR remains markedly depressed and is often accompanied by oliguria. During this phase, patients are often dependent on some form of renal replacement therapy (dialysis or continuous hemofiltration). With time, the patient may enter the *recovery phase*, during which time there is regeneration of the tubular epithelium and an improvement in kidney function. This phase is often characterized by a brisk increase in urine output, and is often referred to as the *diuretic phase*. Although the GFR may recover to near-normal levels, there is often residual kidney injury manifested by a decrease in GFR from the baseline, a loss of functional reserve of the kidneys or evidence of tubular dysfunction that may persist for months or years.

25. **What are the risk factors for the development of ATN?**
Preexisting kidney disease with a decrease in GFR is the most significant risk factor for the development of ATN. Patients with diabetic nephropathy are at increased risk as compared to patients with nondiabetic kidney disease of equal severity. Other factors that predispose to the development of ATN include volume depletion and the use of pharmacologic agents that decrease kidney perfusion, particularly nonselective NSAIDs and selective cyclooxygenase-2 (COX-2) inhibitors.

26. **Can AKI be prevented?**
Unfortunately, other than good medical care with the avoidance of volume contraction, the prevention of hypotension and the avoidance of nephrotoxic agents, there are no specific interventions that have been reliably demonstrated to prevent the development of AKI. The best model is the prevention of contrast-induced nephropathy following the administration of iodinated contrast agents for angiography and computed tomography. Although multiple agents, such *N*-acetylcysteine and sodium bicarbonate, have been evaluated, the efficacy of these agents beyond volume expansion with isotonic saline remains controversial (see Chapter 13).

27. **What is the treatment of AKI?**
The treatment of AKI depends on the specific cause. Prerenal states need to be treated with the correction of intravascular volume depletion and the optimization of cardiac function. AKI from urinary tract obstruction needs to be treated with decompression of the urinary tract. AIN is treated with discontinuation of the offending agent; however, the role of glucocorticoids therapy remains controversial. Acute glomerular syndromes need to be treated based on the specific etiology. Abdominal compartment syndrome is treated with abdominal decompression to reduce intra-abdominal pressure. Depending on the clinical setting, this may be accomplished with nasogastric drainage or paracentesis, but it may require surgical laparotomy, often leaving the abdomen open until edema and inflammation resolve. The management of ATN is entirely supportive. There are no effective pharmacologic agents. Renal replacement therapy is used to support patients while anticipating the recovery of kidney function.

28. **What is the role of novel biomarkers for the diagnosis of intrinsic AKI**
A number of potential novel urine and serum biomarkers have been investigated for the diagnosis and classification of AKI, including cystatin C, NGAL, KIM-1, liver fatty acid binding protein (L-FABP), interleukin-18, insulin-like growth factor binding protein 7 (IGFBP-7), and tissue inhibitor of metalloproteinase-2 (TIMP-2). Cystatin C is a marker of glomerular filtration that has a shorter serum half-life than creatinine and therefore increases more rapidly in the setting of AKI than creatinine does. Cystatin C is normally completely reabsorbed in the urine so there is no urinary excretion; in the setting of AKI, urinary cystatin C is increased as a result of tubular dysfunction. NGAL, KIM-1, L-FABP, and interleukin-18 are markers of tubular injury, and plasma and urine levels increase with intrinsic AKI. However, none of these markers are available for clinical use. IGFBP-7 and TIMP-2 are markers of cell cycle arrest; urine levels of these markers have been found to increase in patients at increased risk for AKI. A urine test incorporating these markers is clinically available; however, the optimal use of this technology remains uncertain.

29. **What are the outcomes of AKI?**
    AKI is associated with high rates of morbidity and mortality. In critically ill patients with severe ATN requiring dialytic support, hospital mortality rates are in the range of 40% to 70%. Even prerenal azotemia is associated with increased mortality, with mortality rates as high as 30% in some series. The recovery of kidney function in survivors is often incomplete, and there is a markedly increased risk of progressive CKD and the development of dialysis-requiring end-stage kidney disease after an episode of AKI.

KEY POINTS

1. Acute kidney injury (AKI) describes a sudden decrease in kidney function occurring over a period of hours to days.
2. The differential diagnosis of AKI includes prerenal azotemia, obstructive nephropathy, and intrinsic forms of AKI.
3. Prerenal azotemia is a functional form of AKI, which results from diminished kidney perfusion. As there is no parenchymal injury, the hallmark of prerenal azotemia is the rapid normalization of kidney function when kidney perfusion is restored.
4. A variety of renal parenchymal diseases can cause intrinsic AKI, including ATN, AIN, acute and rapidly progressive forms of glomerulonephritis, acute vascular diseases, and intratubular deposition of crystals or paraproteins. ATN is the most common etiology of intrinsic AKI.
5. The most important risk factor for the development of AKI is the presence of preexisting chronic kidney disease.
6. Other than good medical care with the avoidance of volume contraction, the prevention of hypotension, and the avoidance of nephrotoxic agents, there are no specific interventions that have been reliably demonstrated to prevent the development of AKI.

BIBLIOGRAPHY

Abdel-Kader, K., & Palevsky, P. M. (2009). Acute kidney injury in the elderly. *Clinics in Geriatric Medicine, 25*, 331–358.
Bellomo, R., Ronco, C., Kellum, J. A., Mehta, R. L., Palevsky, P., & Acute Dialysis Quality Initiative Workgroup. (2004). Acute renal failure—definition, outcome measures, animal models, fluid therapy and information technology needs: The Second International Consensus Conference of the Acute Dialysis Quality Initiative (ADQI) Group. *Critical Care, 8*, R204–R212.
Hoste, E. A., Bagshaw, S. M., Bellomo, R., Cely, C. M., Colman, R., Cruz, D. N., . . . Kellum, J. A. (2015). Epidemiology of acute kidney injury in critically ill patients: The multinational AKI-EPI study. *Intensive Care Medicine, 41*, 1411–1423.
Hsu, R. K., McCulloch, C. E., Dudley, R. A., Lo, L. J., & Hsu, C. Y. (2013). Temporal change in incidence of dialysis-requiring AKI. *Journal of the American Society of Nephrology, 24*, 37–42.
Hsu, C. Y., McCulloch, C. E., Fan, D., Ordoñez, J. D., Chertow, G. M., & Go, A. S. (2007). Community-based incidence of acute renal failure. *Kidney International, 72*, 208–212.
Kidney Disease Improving Global Outcomes (KDIGO), Acute Kidney Injury Work Group. (2012). KDIGO clinical practice guideline for acute kidney injury. *Kidney International Supplements, 2*, 1–138.
Mehta, R. L., Kellum, J. A., Shah, S. V., Molitoris, B. A., Ronco, C., Warnock, D. G., . . . Acute Kidney Injury Network. (2007). Acute Kidney Injury Network: Report of an initiative to improve outcomes in acute kidney injury. *Critical Care, 11*, R31.
Nash, K., Hafeez, A., & Hou, S. (2002). Hospital-acquired renal insufficiency. *American Journal of Kidney Diseases, 39*, 930–936.
Thadhani, R., Pascual, M., & Bonventre, J. V. (1996). Acute renal failure. *New England Journal of Medicine, 334*, 1448–1460.
Wald, R., Quinn, R. R., Luo, J., Li, P., Scales, D. C., Mamdani, M. M., . . . University of Toronto Acute Kidney Injury Research Group. (2009). Chronic dialysis and death among survivors of acute kidney injury requiring dialysis. *Journal of the American Medical Association, 302*, 1179–1185.

CHAPTER 7

MANAGEMENT OPTIONS: CONTINUOUS RENAL REPLACEMENT THERAPY

Rolando Claure-Del Granado, Etienne Macedo, and Ravindra L. Mehta

1. When should renal replacement therapy (RRT) be initiated?

There are accepted urgent indications for RRT in patients with acute kidney injury (AKI) and generally include: refractory fluid overload, hyperkalemia .6 mEq/L or rapidly rising potassium levels, signs of uremia, severe metabolic acidosis, and certain alcohol and drug intoxications. Although the maintenance of serum creatinine and blood urea nitrogen (BUN) concentrations below arbitrarily set levels is usually a reference for starting dialysis treatment, neither creatinine nor BUN should be used to absolutely determine when to initiate dialysis. BUN reflects factors not directly associated with kidney function, such as catabolic rate and volume status. Serum creatinine is influenced by age, race, muscle mass, and catabolic rate, and its volume of distribution varies in fluid overloaded patients. Other factors such as fluid balance control, nutrition needs, severity of the underlying disease, and acid base and electrolyte balance should guide the decision to start dialysis, as has been suggested by KDIGO AKI guidelines. We favor RRT initiation prior to the development of severe electrolyte disturbances in patients with severe metabolic acidosis (pH , 7.2) despite optimal medical management and with no signs that kidney function or metabolic acidosis is improving; and in patients with positive fluid balance despite aggressive use of diuretics, predominantly if they have increasing oxygen requirements. Therefore it is better to use RRT as a supportive therapy rather than a rescue therapy for late manifestations of AKI.

Since the optimal timing of RRT initiation is controversial, any presumed benefit from early dialysis needs to be balanced by the safety concerns from dialysis including:

- Risk for infection from an indwelling dialysis catheter
- Hypotension
- Potential for delayed kidney recovery
- Leukocyte activation from contact with dialysis membranes

Randomized, controlled trials that have compared strategies of early versus delayed initiation of RRT (in the absence of absolute indications) have yielded conflicting results. In fact, three of the largest trials have not demonstrated a benefit with earlier initiation of RRT. The best evidence comes from a randomized, controlled trial, which included 620 critically ill patients that had severe AKI (KDIGO stage 3) and required either or both mechanical ventilation and vasopressors (AKIKI Study). Patients were assigned to early RRT (within 6 hours after AKI was identified) or to delayed RRT; the delayed strategy required RRT initiation after the onset of severe hyperkalemia, metabolic acidosis, pulmonary edema, increase in BUN levels >112 mg/dL, or the development of oliguria for more than 72 hours after allocation. The choice of the method of RRT (intermittent or continuous technique, duration and interval between sessions, device setting, and anticoagulation method) was left to the discretion of each study site. The study showed no difference in terms of mortality between patients who received early RRT with a median time of initiation of 2 hours (patients with AKI stage 3 KDIGO without BUN levels >112 mmol/L, pH < 7.15, K levels > 6 mmol/L, and pulmonary edema due to fluid overload) and patients who received late RRT with a median time of initiation of 57 hours. An interesting finding in this study was that kidney recovery marked by increased diuresis was more rapid, and catheter-related infections were lower in the delayed-strategy RRT.

Another study was the ELAIN study: a single center, randomized, controlled trial that enrolled 231 critically ill patients with AKI KDIGO stage 2. All patients had severe sepsis, required vasopressors or catecholamines, or had refractory volume overload. In this study, early RRT (continuous venovenous hemodialfiltration) was started within 8 hours of diagnosis of AKI KDIGO stage 2, and delayed RRT was started within 12 hours of stage 3 AKI, or developed an absolute indication for RRT initiation (serum urea level >100 mg/dL, potassium >6 mEq/L, serum magnesium

>8 mEq/L, urine output 200 mL over 12 hours, or diuretic-resistant edema). Compared with delayed or no initiation, early RRT initiation reduced 90-day mortality. In addition, more patients recovered kidney function in the early versus delayed group by 90 days, and both the duration of RRT and the hospital stay were shorter in the early initiation group.

The timing of RRT, a modifiable factor, might exert an important influence on patient survival. We favor utilizing an approach that recognizes that the strategy in treating AKI is to minimize and avoid uremic and volume overload complications. Thus, it is not necessary to wait for progressive uremia to initiate dialytic support; it is better to use RRT as a supportive therapy in the presence of progressive azotemia and oliguria, rather than a rescue therapy for the late manifestation of AKI. Our recommendations to initiate RRT with worsening AKI are listed below:

- In patients with K >5.8 to 6.0 mEq/L or severe metabolic acidosis despite optimal medical management in patients that demonstrate no sign that kidney function or metabolic acidosis is improving
- In patients with positive fluid balance despite aggressive attempts of increasing diuresis, particularly if they have increasing oxygen support requirements

    Careful surveillance is mandatory when deciding to wait for RRT initiation in patients with severe AKI, so that any complication will be adequately detected and RRT will be started without delay.

2. **Which modalities of RRT are available for treating AKI patients?**
The modalities that could be used in the treatment of patients with AKI include:
a. Conventional intermittent hemodialysis (IHD)
b. Various types of continuous renal replacement therapies (CRRT) such as:
- Continuous venovenous hemofiltration (CVVH)
- Continuous venovenous hemodialysis (CVVHD)
- Continuous venovenous hemodiafiltration (CVVHDF)
c. Prolonged intermittent renal replacement therapies (PIRRT) that combine aspects of both IHD and CRRT, such as slow low-efficiency dialysis (SLED), slow continuous ultrafiltration (SCUF), or extended daily diafiltration.
d. Peritoneal dialysis (PD).

    The removal of solutes can be achieved by convection (hemofiltration), diffusion (hemodialysis), or the combination of the two methods (hemodiafiltration). The amount of solute transported per unit of time (clearance) depends on the molecular weight of the solute, the characteristics of the membrane, and both the dialysate and blood flows. IHD has been used widely for the last four decades to treat end-stage kidney disease (ESKD) and AKI.

- Diffusive clearance is more effective for small-molecular-weight solutes such as potassium, urea, and creatinine.
- Solutes with higher molecular weight (between 500 and 60,000 Da)—so-called middle molecules— are better removed by convection, where hydrostatic pressure forces plasma across a membrane. To provide effective solute clearance, the volume of plasma that must be removed by ultrafiltration is greater than the volume that can be tolerated, so it is replaced partially or completely with a hemofiltration solution. The solution can be infused pre- or post-filter. Intermittent ultrafiltration—in contrast to intermittent hemodiafiltration—can be done with the same machines as IHD, but is used specifically for volume removal. Most nephrologists use isolated ultrafiltration as a method of rapid fluid removal when the major indication for renal replacement or support is pulmonary edema or refractory congestive cardiomyopathy.

    Extended daily dialysis (EDD), or SLED, differs from IHD in that dialysate and blood flow are intentionally kept low, but the duration of the treatment is extended. These hybrid modalities can be performed at night for 8 to 12 hours, using intensive care unit (ICU) staff, thereby eliminating an interruption of therapy, reducing staff requirements, and avoiding scheduling conflicts. Studies comparing hybrid modalities to CRRT have revealed favorable hemodynamic tolerance in critically ill patients while achieving dialysis adequacy and ultrafiltration targets, since the fluid removal as well as the solute clearance is more gradual.

    There are few studies that have compared PD with other RRT modalities for treating patients with AKI. A single-center randomized trial found that there were no differences in the mortality rate and the recovery of kidney function when PD was compared to daily IHD, although PD was associated with a shorter duration of need for dialysis. Another study, a meta-analysis of eight observational cohorts and four randomized, controlled trials, found no difference in mortality comparing PD to extracorporeal modalities of RRT.

Since RRT can be provided in various forms as shown above, one should consider the use of continuous and intermittent RRT as complementary therapies in AKI patients. CRRT should be used, rather than standard intermittent RRT, for hemodynamically unstable patients. The choice of a specific type of RRT should be based also on the availability of resources, the needs of the patient, and the expertise of the staff.

3. What type of vascular access should be employed?
Guidelines recommend that for acute hemodialysis, access should be obtained by percutaneous placement using the ultrasound guidance of a double lumen catheter in the (order of preferences):
1. Right internal jugular
2. Femoral
3. Left internal jugular
4. Subclavian vein

If RRT is expected to extend beyond several days (>7 days), consideration should be given to early placement of a tunneled catheter in the internal jugular vein. Tunneled catheters have a larger diameter than do non-tunneled catheters, providing higher blood flows, and have a lower incidence of catheter-related bloodstream infections.

Catheter malfunction has a significant impact on the delivered dialysis dose as observed by the investigators of the ATN study; interestingly, one study showed that twin-tunneled catheters in the femoral vein provide better function than a conventional femoral vein catheter. The femoral vein is technically the easiest access to place; nevertheless, concern for infection by this type of access has limited its use. One randomized controlled trial showed that femoral catheters were not associated with an increased risk of infections compared with jugular catheters, except in patients with high body mass indexes. Jugular catheters could be used for prolonged periods of time (usually 3 weeks), with a low risk of bacteremia; on the other hand, femoral catheters—especially in obese and bed-bound patients—should not be used for more than 1 week. Thoracic catheters have the advantage of lower recirculation. However, it should be kept in mind that subclavian vein cannulation is associated with higher rates of both short-term and long-term complications, such as pneumothorax and hemorrhage, and central venous stenosis. Subclavian catheters should be placed only if all the other options are not viable. The use of portable ultrasound machines has improved the success rate of cannulation and decreased the rate of complications, and they should be used if available.

4. Which factors could affect the modality selection of RRT?
There is debate whether continuous modalities are better than intermittent modalities in the treatment of AKI patients. IHD has several advantages:
• Short duration of therapy
• Rapid correction of electrolyte and acid-base disturbances
• Rapid fluid removal
• Availability of the machines
• Availability of trained nurses

Often the machines and nurses available to deploy continuous therapies are not available. However, in intermittent dialysis, the duration of the procedure, 3 to 5 hours, limits the control of fluid regulation and acid-base and electrolyte balance. Patients with hemodynamic instability may not tolerate the high ultrafiltration rates necessary to achieve a fluid balance. CRRT can offer advantages over IHD:
• Slower fluid removal, which promotes hemodynamic stability
• Better solute clearance
• Better correction of acid-base and electrolyte abnormalities
• Better metabolic control

Some data have suggested that intradialytic hypotensive episodes during IHD could decrease the rate of recovery of kidney function. Still, CRRT can also have some limitations and disadvantages, such as the need for continuous anticoagulation, patient immobilization, and greater human resource requirement, including the need for ICU monitoring. Although there are many arguments that favor the use of CRRT in critically ill patients with AKI, current evidence has not shown any benefit to employing CRRT over IHD in this group of patients. The hybrid modalities, SLED and EDD, can provide the same adequate solute control as IHD can, but require less intensive monitoring and time, compared to CRRT.

It is now recognized that more than one therapy can be utilized for managing patients with AKI. Transitions in therapy are common and reflect the changing needs of patients during their hospital course. For instance, patients in the ICU may initially start on CRRT when they are hemodynamically unstable, then transition to SLED-EDD when they improve, and leave the ICU on IHD.

5. **Is there an ideal dose of dialysis?**

Since 2000, multiple studies in IHD as well as in CRRT have suggested that higher doses of RRT are associated with improved outcomes; however, two large multicenter, randomized, control trials (ATN study and RENAL study) do not support the hypothesis that a higher dose of RRT will improve outcomes. It appears that the relationship between the dose administered by RRT and survival has two regions: a dosage-dependent region where increases in the intensity of the dose are associated with improved survival; and a dosage-independent region after a threshold is reached. A further increase in the intensity of dose does not improve outcomes. These two studies suggest that dose should be measured, rather than implying that dose is not important in the treatment of critically ill patients with AKI. The influence on solute clearance of some operational characteristics of RRT, such as frequent filter clotting and protein fouling of the membrane, can translate into a lower dose of delivered dialysis; this explains why a simple prescription of a target dose, or adjusting for treatment interruptions, is not enough to find an ideal dose of dialysis. In order to ensure delivery of an effluent flow rate of 20 to 25 mL/kg per hour as recommended by 2012 KDIGO guidelines, we recommend prescribing an effluent flow rate of >25 mL/kg per hour in order to achieve the targeted dose of therapy.

For patients undergoing IHD, KDIGO recommend delivering a Kt/V of 3.9 per week. This recommendation is based on the results of the ATN study, and is just the arithmetic sum of the median dose in the less intensive arm that has been summed over the course of a week. We recommend that if IHD is provided three times per week, the targeted dose of therapy should be a Kt/V of ≥1.2 per treatment. The delivered dose of therapy should be monitored.

Besides a small solute clearance, other aspects of dosing should be considered (volume control, acid-base, nutritional status, etc.) in order to find an ideal dose of dialysis during AKI.

6. **How should dialysis dose be measured?**

Since the establishment of a link between dialysis dose measured by urea clearance and clinical outcomes in patients with ESRD, the clearance of urea adjusted for the volume of distribution of water has been used as an index of dialysis adequacy (Kt/V). Although widely used for chronic patients, the use of this dose assessment parameter in AKI is not clear. In AKI, the changes in body water volumes and urea generation rates result in inaccuracy of these formulas. The calculated Kt/V in AKI patients has been shown to be 30% higher than the measured clearance in the dialysate because of episodes of hypotension, dialyzer clotting, and vascular access recirculation. In CRRT, we also overestimate the true solute clearance by using the effluent volume as a surrogate marker of the delivered dose. Treatment interruptions, progressive decreased filter efficacy, and, consequently, reduced clearance over time result in a gap between the prescribed and the delivered dialysis dose. The use of dialysate-side measurements provides more accurate dose information (actual solute removal), as it accounts for the loss of filter efficacy. Thus, measuring the actual solute removal in the effluent, and calculating the clearance based on the mass extract, could dramatically improve the way we assess the effect of dose on outcomes in critically ill patients.

7. **What are the advantages of CRRT in a septic patient with AKI?**

The use of hemofiltration in CRRT techniques may have an immunomodulatory effect. Some of the inflammatory mediators are water-soluble cytokines (interleukin [IL]-6, IL-8, IL-1) and the tumor necrosis factor, and can be removed by convection according to their molecular weight and degree of plasma protein binding. Membrane characteristics such as molecular weight cut-off, structure, and charge also affect the ability of a solute to be cleared by RRT either by convection or by absorption.

In spite of some encouraging results, the clinical benefit of conventional CRRT in sepsis has been disappointing. Consequently, efforts have been made to improve the efficiency of soluble mediator removal by increasing the ultrafiltration rates and enlarging the pore size of the membranes.

8. **How can clotting of the dialyzer be prevented?**

The contact of blood with the extracorporeal circuit, lines, and membrane activates platelets and the production of a variety of inflammatory and prothrombotic mediators. The result is the induction of fibrin deposition and filter clotting. Clotting of the dialyzer reduces its longevity, and, more importantly, reduces the efficiency of solute clearance. Inefficient anticoagulation reduces the dialyzer performance by diminishing the surface of the membrane available for diffusion or convection.

The anticoagulation for RRT can be systemic or regional, when only the dialysis circuit is anticoagulated. Systemic anticoagulation with unfractionated heparin is the most commonly used method. Heparin is usually administrated as a bolus, followed by a continuous infusion into the arterial line. The optimal dose for AKI patients is not established. The target is to maintain a partial thromboplastin time of 1.5 to 2 times the normal level. The use of low-molecular-weight heparin (LMWH) requires the monitoring of factor Xa levels. In patients at high risk of bleeding, systemic anticoagulation should be avoided. Although IHD can often be performed without anticoagulation, using intermittent saline flushes (100 cc) every 15 to 30 minutes in the arterial line could improve the circuit and filter life. In CRRT, regional anticoagulation with citrate is the alternative method. Citrate is infused continuously in the arterial line and chelates the free calcium in the circuit, inhibiting the coagulation cascade. Part of the complex calcium citrate is removed by dialysis clearance and part is metabolized in the liver. Serum calcium concentrations (preferably ionized) should be monitored, and continuous or intermittent calcium infusion performed as necessary. The use of regional citrate anticoagulation (RCA) increases the buffer load during the treatment as citrate is converted to bicarbonate in the liver. The possibility of metabolic alkalosis requires modifications in the hemofiltration solution or dialysate.

9. **What complications should be expected when using CRRT?**
   The most common complications of CRRT are:
   - Hypotension
   - Bleeding
   - Electrolyte imbalances
   - Infection
   - Hypothermia

   Hypotension is the most common complication of dialysis, occurring in around 30% of treatments. Several factors associated with the dialysis treatment can cause hypotension (partial list):
   - Cardiac events
   - Electrolyte imbalances
   - Elevated dialysate temperature
   - Bacterial contamination of system
   - Low dialysate sodium concentration
   - Clearance of vasoactive drugs
   - Use of antihypertensive medications prior to treatment

   However, hypotension is most often related to the imbalance between fluid removal and fluid replacement by the extravascular compartment. A large amount of fluid removal is a major risk factor for hypotension, especially in patients with compromised refilling capacity, as in diabetic neuropathy, low cardiac ejection fraction, diastolic dysfunction, and sepsis. Although CRRT has been demonstrated to reduce episodes of hypotension and to allow better acid-base and electrolyte control, the prolonged time of therapy increases the risk of volume and electrolytes depletion. In spite of the expected safety of obtaining fluid removal over a longer period of time with CRRT, careful monitoring is mandatory. Hypotension and hemodynamic instability are still frequent in CRRT. In intensive and/or prolonged treatment, CRRT results in overcorrection of electrolyte imbalances, especially when non-physiologic solutions are used, such as dialysate or replacement fluids. Hypocalcemia, hypophosphatemia, and hypokalemia are common complications associated with higher doses of CRRT, requiring careful electrolyte monitoring during the procedure. The use of peritoneal dialysate fluids used for CRRT can cause hyperglycemia, demanding special attention with potassium imbalance. Patients receiving CRRT are at increased risk for hypothermia as blood circulates in the extracorporeal circulation for a prolonged time. Dialysate and replacement fluids should be warmed prior to administration, and the patient's body temperature should be frequently monitored. Because CRRT requires anticoagulation for a prolonged time, the risk of bleeding is also increased. The monitoring of hemoglobin and hematocrit is important to detect hidden bleeding. Patients on RRT are vulnerable to catheter-related infections, including systemic infections and those local to the vascular access site. The cooling effect of prolonged extracorporeal circulation in CRRT may mask fever; special monitoring for other signs of infection is mandatory.

10. **When you should stop CRRT?**
    CRRT is usually stopped when evidence of kidney function recovery is seen in patients; most often, recovery is assessed by an improvement in urine output, a progressive decline in serum creatinine levels, and an improvement in measured creatinine clearance. The precise level of kidney function required to allow the discontinuation of renal support has not been established; however, a creatinine clearance <12 mL/min could be inadequate to allow the discontinuation of renal replacement therapies. In the ATN study, investigators discontinued renal support when the measured creatinine clearance was >20 mL/min, and it was left to the discretion of the treating physicians when the range fell between 12 and 20 mL/min.

KEY POINTS

1. Urgent indications for CRRT in patients with AKI include volume overload refractory to diuretics, hyperkalemia, metabolic acidosis, uremia, and toxic overdose of a dialyzable drug. It is preferable that CRRT be electively initiated prior to the development of urgent indications.
2. CRRT should be used for hemodynamically unstable patients rather that standard intermittent hemodialysis. Also, it should be used for AKI patients with acute brain injury or other causes of increased intracranial pressure or generalized brain edema.
3. For anticoagulation in CRRT, regional citrate anticoagulation is preferable to heparin
4. CRRT should be provided with a delivered effluent flow rate of ≥20 mL/kg per hour, and in order to ensure delivery of this flow rate, the prescribed flow rate should be ≥25 mL/kg per hour. The CRRT delivered dose should be measured.
5. CRRT should be discontinued when it is no longer required because kidney function has recovered to the point that is adequate to meet the patient's needs; a measured creatinine clearance >20 mL/min should allow the discontinuation of CRRT.

BIBLIOGRAPHY

Bagshaw, S. M., Chakravarthi, M. R., Ricci, Z., et al. (2016). Precision continuous renal replacement therapy and solute control. *Blood Purif, 42*(3), 238–247.

Bagshaw, S. M., Uchino, S., Bellomo, R., et al. (2009). Timing of renal replacement therapy and clinical outcomes in critically ill patients with severe acute kidney injury. J *Crit Care, 24*(1), 129–140.

Baldwin, I., Bellomo, R., Naka, T., et al. (2007). A pilot randomized controlled comparison of extended daily dialysis with filtration and continuous veno-venous hemofiltration: Fluid removal and hemodynamics. *Int J Artif Organs, 30*(12), 1083–1089.

Berbece, A. N., & Richardson, R. M. A. (2006). Sustained low-efficiency dialysis in the ICU: Cost, anticoagulation, and solute removal. *Kidney Int. 70*(5), 963–968.

Cerdá, J., Baldwin, I., Honore, P. M., et al. (2016). Role of technology for the management of AKI in critically Ill patients: from adoptive technology to precision continuous renal replacement therapy. *Blood Purif, 42*(3), 248–265.

Elseviers, M. M., Lins, R. L., Van der Niepen, P., et al. (2010). Renal replacement therapy is an independent risk factor for mortality in critically ill patients with acute kidney injury. *Crit Care, 14*(6), R221.

Gaudry, S., Hajage, D., Schortgen, F., et al. (2016). Initiation strategies for renal-replacement therapy in the intensive care unit. *N Engl J Med, 375*(2), 122–133.

Gibney, N., Hoste, E., Burdmann, E. A., et al. (2008). Timing of initiation and discontinuation of renal replacement therapy in AKI: Unanswered key questions. *Clin J Am Soc Nephrol, 3*(3), 876–880.

Himmelfarb, J. (2007a). Continuous dialysis is not superior to intermittent dialysis in acute kidney injury of the critically ill patient. *Nat Clin Pract, 3*(3), 120–121.

Himmelfarb, J. (2007b). Continuous renal replacement therapy in the treatment of acute renal failure: Critical assessment is required. *Clin J Am Soc Nephrol, 2*(2), 385–389.

Holt, B. G., White, J. J., Kuthiala, A., et al. (2008). Sustained low-efficiency daily dialysis with hemofiltration for acute kidney injury in the presence of sepsis. *Clin Nephrol, 69*(1), 40–46.

Liao, Z., Zhang, W., Hardy, P. A., et al. (2003). Kinetic comparison of different acute dialysis therapies. *Artif Organs, 27*(9), 802–807.

Murugan, R., Hoste, E., Mehta, R. L., et al. (2016). Precision fluid management in continuous renal replacement therapy. *Blood Purif, 42*(3), 266–278.

Ostermann, M., Joannidis, M., Pani, A., et al. (2016). Patient selection and timing of continuous renal replacement therapy. *Blood Purif, 42*(3), 224–237.

Palevsky, P. M. (2009). Renal support in acute kidney injury—how much is enough? *N Engl J Med, 361*(17), 1699–1701.

Palevsky, P. M., O'Connor, T., Zhang, J. H., et al. (2005). Design of the VA/NIH Acute Renal Failure Trial Network (ATN) study: Intensive versus conventional renal support in acute renal failure. *Clin Trials, 2*(5), 423–435.

Pannu, N., & Gibney, R. T. N. (2005). Renal replacement therapy in the intensive care unit. *Ther Clin Risk Manag, 1*(2), 141–150.

Parienti, J. J., Thirion, M., Megarbane, B., et al. (2008). Femoral vs jugular venous catheterization and risk of nosocomial events in adults requiring acute renal replacement therapy: A randomized controlled trial. *JAMA, 299*(20), 2413–2422.

Payen, D., Mateo, J., Cavaillon, J. M., et al. (2009). Impact of continuous venovenous hemofiltration on organ failure during the early phase of severe sepsis: A randomized controlled trial. *Crit Care Med, 37*(3), 803–810.

Ronco, C. (2007). Continuous dialysis is superior to intermittent dialysis in acute kidney injury of the critically ill patient. *Nat Clin Pract, 3*(3), 118–119.

Schneider, A. G., Uchino, S., & Bellomo, R. (2012). Severe acute kidney injury not treated with renal replacement therapy: Characteristics and outcome. *Nephrol Dial Transplant, 27*(3), 947–952.

Seabra, V. F., Balk, E. M., Liangos, O., et al. (2008). Timing of renal replacement therapy initiation in acute renal failure: A meta-analysis. *Am J Kidney Dis, 52*(2), 272–284.

Kellum, J.A., Lameire, N., et al. Section 5. (2012). Dialysis interventions for treatment of AKI. *Kidney Int Suppl (2011), 2*(1), 89–115.

Vaara, S. T., Reinikainen, M., Wald, R., et al. (2014). Timing of RRT based on the presence of conventional indications. *Clin J Am Soc Nephrol, 9*(9), 1577–1585.

CHAPTER 8

HEPATORENAL SYNDROME

Zita Galvin and Florence Wong

1. **What is hepatorenal syndrome?**

   The current definition of hepatorenal syndrome (HRS) updated in 2007 by the International Ascites Club (IAC) states that it is "a potentially reversible syndrome that occurs in patients with cirrhosis, ascites and liver failure, consisting of impaired kidney function, marked abnormalities in cardiovascular function, and intense over-activity of the endogenous vasoactive systems." It can appear spontaneously or follow a precipitating event. It is important to emphasize that HRS is a form of prerenal acute kidney injury (AKI) not associated with structural changes; a kidney biopsy usually reveals normal histology.

2. **What is the incidence and prevalence of HRS?**

   In 1993, the annual incidence of HRS in patients with cirrhosis and ascites was reported as 8% and the probability of developing HRS was 18% at 1 year and 39% at 5 years. However, in 2006 a similar study showed a significantly lower prevalence of disease, with only 7.6% of cirrhotic patients developing HRS during the study period (40 $\pm$ 3 months) and a 5-year probability of developing HRS of 11.4%. These reductions are largely due to the increased recognition of the condition, the advances in the medical management of cirrhosis, and the availability of prophylactic antibiotics for spontaneous bacterial peritonitis (SBP).

3. **What is the pathophysiology of HRS? (Fig. 8.1)**
   - **Reduction in the effective arterial blood volume**: Hemodynamic changes of significant arterial vasodilatation occur in advanced cirrhosis, which preferentially localizes in the splanchnic circulation. The pooling of blood in the splanchnic circulation, *splanchnic steal syndrome*, results in insufficient blood volume in other vascular compartments, including the systemic circulation, *reducing the effective arterial blood volume*.
   - **Excess renal vasoconstriction**: The reduction in effective arterial blood volume activates the renin-angiotensin-aldosterone system (RAAS) and the sympathetic nervous system, and stimulates the nonosmostically induced release of vasopressin. The vasoconstrictors decrease renal blood flow and, consequently, the glomerular filtration rate (GFR).
   - **Abnormal renal autoregulation in advanced cirrhosis**: In cirrhosis, the renal autoregulation curve, which describes the relationship of mean arterial pressure and renal blood flow, is shifted to the right. This means that for any given arterial pressure, there is less renal blood flow than in a healthy individual. The decreased renal blood flow may be due to excess sympathetic drive seen in cirrhosis. The decreased renal blood flow makes patients with advanced cirrhosis more susceptible to AKI.
   - **Portal hypertension**: Independent of splanchnic vasodilatation and systemic hemodynamic changes, increased portal pressure reduces renal blood flow. This is mediated by increased sympathetic nervous activity and is called the hepatorenal reflex. Insertion of a transjugular intrahepatic portosystemic shunt (TIPS) eliminates portal hypertension and increases renal blood flow.
   - **Abnormal cardiac function in cirrhosis**: The presence of systemic arterial vasodilatation in advanced cirrhosis leads to a hyperdynamic circulation with tachycardia, high cardiac output, and low systemic vascular resistance. The presence of cirrhotic cardiomyopathy, consisting of myocardial thickening, diastolic dysfunction at rest, and systolic dysfunction under conditions of stress, means that the heart is unable to further increase cardiac output in periods of stress (e.g., sepsis). This lack of a cardiac reserve predisposes to the development of HRS.

4. **What is the clinical presentation of HRS?**

   HRS is a form of kidney injury, so patients present with increased serum creatinine and low urine output. Clinically, there are two types of HRS.
   1. Acute or type 1 HRS is characterized by a rapidly progressive kidney failure in a cirrhotic patient with ascites. It usually develops following a precipitating event but can occur spontaneously. Patients are usually very ill, with severe jaundice, coagulopathy, and liver failure. Type 1 HRS is now renamed as AKI-HRS.

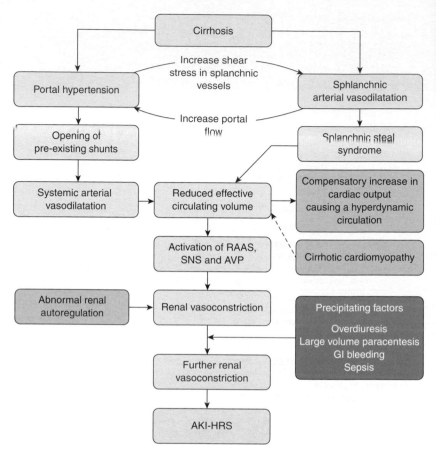

Figure 8.1. Pathophysiology of hepatorenal syndrome. *AKI*, Acute kidney injury; *AVP*, arginine vasopressin; *GI*, gastrointestinal; *HRS*, hepatorenal syndrome; *RAAS*, renin angiotensin aldosterone system; *SNS*, sympathetic nervous system.

2. Chronic or type 2 HRS is characterized by moderate kidney failure, with a serum creatinine between 1.5 and 2.5 mg/dL. It evolves slowly over weeks to months in patients with ascites refractory to diuretics. Patients with type 2 HRS are usually less ill than those with type 1 HRS, with a milder degree of jaundice and coagulopathy.

5. **What factors can precipitate the development of HRS?**
   Any condition that causes a further reduction of the effective arterial blood volume can precipitate HRS (see Fig. 8.1). These include over-diuresis, large-volume paracentesis (≥5 liters) without intravascular colloid replacement in patients with refractory ascites, and gastrointestinal bleeding. Other triggers are conditions that worsen the arterial vasodilatation, such as sepsis (especially SBP) or jaundice due to obstruction in the biliary tree (bile acids are vasodilators).

6. **How is HRS diagnosed?**
   The diagnostic criteria for HRS were updated by the IAC in 2015. This followed the adaptation of a set of uniform nomenclature and diagnostic criteria for AKI. Table 8.1 outlines the diagnosis, staging, and definitions of progression/regression of AKI as proposed by the IAC. Using these criteria, AKI is defined as an increase in serum creatinine by 0.3 mg/dL in less than 48 hours, or a 50% increase in serum creatinine presumed to have occurred in the past 7 days from baseline. Type 1 HRS or AKI-HRS is a special type of AKI that is not responsive to volume replacement. The new diagnostic criteria of AKI-HRS as set out in 2015 modified the previous criteria set by the IAC in 2007. There has to be at least a doubling of serum

Table 8.1. Diagnosis, Staging and Assessing Response to Treatment of Acute Kidney Injury in Patients With Cirrhosis According to International Ascites Club

PARAMETER	DEFINITION
Baseline SCr	Stable SCr in ≤ 3 months If not available, a stable SCr closest to the current one If no previous SCr at all, use admission SCr
Definition of AKI	↑ in SCr ≥ 0.3 mg/dL (26.4 μmol/L) ≤ 48 h, or ↑ 50% from baseline
Staging	Stage 1: ↑ SCr ≥ 0.3 mg/dL (26.4 μmol/L) or ↑ SCr ≥ 1.5–2.0 X from baseline Stage 2: ↑ SCr > 2.0–3.0 X from baseline Stage 3: ↑ SCr > 3.0 X from baseline, or SCr ≥ 4.0 mg/dL (352 μmol/L) with an acute ↑ of ≥ 0.3 mg/dL (26.4 μmol/L), or initiation of renal replacement therapy
Progression	Progression of AKI to a higher stage, or need for renal replacement therapy
Regression	Regression of AKI to lower stage
Response to treatment	None: No regression of AKI Partial: Regression of AKI stage with a ↓ in SCr to a value ≥ 0.3 mg/ dL (26.4 μmol/L) above baseline Complete: ↓ SCr < 0.3 mg/dL (26.4 μmol/L) from baseline

AKI, Acute kidney injury; *IAC,* International Ascites Club; *SCr,* serum creatinine.
From Angeli, P., Gines, P., Wong, F., et al. (2015). Diagnosis and management of acute kidney injury in patients with cirrhosis: revised consensus recommendations of the International Club of Ascites. *Gut*, 64(4):531–537.

creatinine without setting an absolute creatinine level (i.e., 2.5 mg/dL) for the diagnosis. The current proposed diagnostic criteria for AKI-HRS are:

- Cirrhosis and ascites
- Diagnosis of AKI according to the IAC-AKI criteria
- No reduction in serum creatinine after at least 48 hours of diuretic withdrawal and volume expansion with albumin. The recommended dose of albumin is 1 g/kg body weight/day up to a maximum of 100 g/day.
- Absence of shock
- No current or recent treatment with nephrotoxic drugs
- No evidence of structural kidney injury defined as:
  - Absence of proteinuria (>500 mg/day)
  - Absence of hematuria (>50 red blood cells/high power field)
  - Normal kidney ultrasonography

It is possible that patients who fulfill these criteria may still have structural damage, such as acute tubular necrosis (ATN). Urine biomarkers will become an important element in making a more accurate differential diagnosis between HRS and ATN.

Urinary electrolyte criteria are not required for the diagnosis of AKI-HRS, and the presence of infection does not preclude its diagnosis.

7. **Why was an absolute creatinine level removed from the diagnostic criteria for AKI-HRS?**
The current diagnostic criteria for AKI-HRS do not specify an absolute creatinine level. Serum creatinine is not an accurate measurement in patients with cirrhosis. In cirrhosis, low protein intake, loss of muscle mass, diminished hepatic synthesis of creatine, and an enlarged volume of distribution, all lower the serum creatinine irrespective of kidney function. This can delay the recognition of kidney dysfunction and have a negative impact on patient outcomes. Using a change in serum creatinine allows an earlier diagnosis of AKI and more timely intervention. This may lead to improved outcomes.

8. **What is the diagnostic work-up and initial management of the patient with cirrhosis and AKI?**
A trial of diuretic withdrawal, together with intravascular volume replacement should be done, as this can replenish the effective arterial blood volume. The intravascular volume replacement can be blood if the patient is anemic or albumin at the dose of 1 g/kg of body weight up to a maximum of 100 g/day.

The work-up should consist of a full work-up, including blood cultures, chest x-ray, urine and sputum cultures, a diagnostic paracentesis to exclude SBP, and the swabbing of any possible skin sources of infection. The threshold for starting antibiotics should be low. In order to exclude parenchymal kidney disease, the urine should be examined for the presence of protein, blood, and casts. An abdominal ultrasound should be performed to exclude small kidneys—indicative of parenchymal kidney disease—or structural abnormalities in the kidneys. Postrenal obstruction is an extremely uncommon cause of AKI in cirrhosis, and bladder catheterization is usually not done to avoid instrumentation-induced infections.

9. **What is the differential diagnosis of acute kidney injury in the patient with cirrhosis?**
   1. Prerenal azotemia is the most common cause of AKI in hospitalized patients with cirrhosis (approximately one-third of cases). Common causes are over-diuresis, large-volume paracentesis without colloid replacement, or gastrointestinal bleeding. AKI-HRS can be considered a form of prerenal azotemia which is not responsive to volume replacement in advanced cirrhosis with liver dysfunction and ascites.
   2. Intrinsic kidney failure occurs in approximately one-third of patients with cirrhosis; most commonly ATN, although systemic conditions, such as glomerulonephritis, also may be present.
   3. Postrenal failure occurs in <1% of patients in cirrhosis and results from obstruction to the passage of urine, as seen in a bladder neck obstruction.

10. **Can biomarkers assist in the diagnosis of AKI-HRS?**
    See Fig. 8.2A and B
    Biomarkers of kidney tubular injury may help with the differential diagnosis of AKI (prerenal azotemia ATN or AKI-HRS). Multiple biomarkers, including neutrophil gelatinase-associated lipocalin (NGAL), interleukin-18 (IL-18), liver type fatty acid binding protein (I-FABP), and kidney injury molecule-1 (KIM-1), have been shown to distinguish structural from functional causes of AKI in numerous clinical settings. NGAL performs well in the cirrhotic population, especially in distinguishing between prerenal azotemia, non-HRS cases of AKI, AKI-HRS, and ATN with an area under the receiver operating characteristic curve of 0.957. A study suggests that combining a panel of these biomarkers is the most accurate way to separate structural from functional causes of AKI. These biomarkers are still not readily commercially available worldwide. The commercially available biomarker strip, Nephrocheck, has never been tested in cirrhosis, and therefore cannot be recommended. In the future, clinicians should be able to diagnose ATN versus AKI-HRS early using biomarkers that differentiate these two conditions. Biomarkers may also be used to track transition from one type of AKI, such as prerenal azotemia, as it evolves into AKI-HRS over time, or to follow the response of the kidneys to treatment.

11. **What is the rationale for the various treatment options for HRS?**
    Treatments for HRS (mostly for AKI-HRS) are based on correcting the different aspects of pathophysiology of HRS.
    • Improving the effective arterial blood volume: Volume expanders
    • Reducing arterial vasodilatation: Vasoconstrictors
    • Eliminating portal hypertension: TIPS shunt
    • Correcting liver dysfunction and portal hypertension: Liver transplantation

12. **What are some general treatment measures for AKI in patients with cirrhosis?**
    See Fig. 8.3
    • Treat infection
    • Discontinue nephrotoxic medications, including nonsteroidal anti-inflammatory drugs
    • Discontinue angiotensin-converting enzyme inhibitors and angiotensin receptor blockers. In patients with decompensated cirrhosis, the RAAS is vital to maintaining arterial pressure and GFR in the face of marked splanchnic and systemic vasodilatation. Inhibition of the RAAS may precipitate hypotension and deterioration of kidney function.
    • Assess and correct effective circulating volume: While excess total body water is present in decompensated cirrhosis, it usually extravasates intra-abdominally or into peripheral tissue, and patients are still intravascularly deplete.

13. **How is volume expansion used in the treatment of AKI-HRS?**
    Hypoalbuminemia is common in cirrhosis secondary to reduced synthesis, dilution from plasma volume expansion, and increased transcapillary escape into extravascular space. In AKI-HRS, albumin infusions suppress sympathetic activity; specifically, it causes a decrease in plasma norepinephrine, reversing one of the primary abnormalities of cirrhotic pathophysiology.

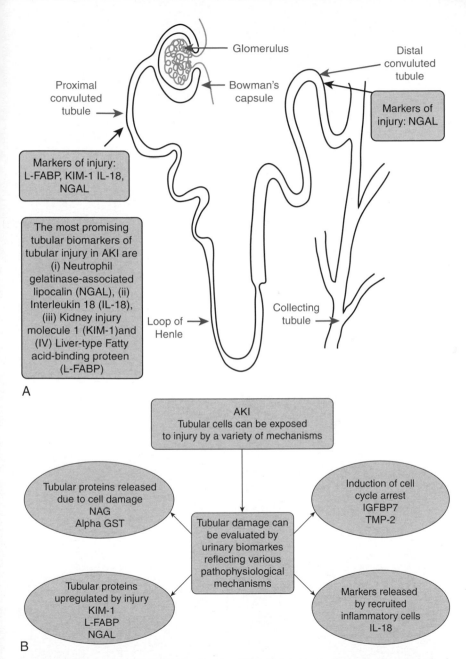

Figure 8.2. (A) Nephron localization of kidney injury biomarkers. (B) Tubular damage can be evaluated by urinary biomarkers reflecting various pathophysiological mechanisms. *AKI*, acute kidney injury; *alpha GST*, Alpha glutathione-s-transferase; *IGFBP 7*, insulin-like growth factor binding protein-7; *IL-18*, interleukin-18; *KIM-1*, kidney injury molecule-1; *L-FABP*, liver type fatty acid binding protein; *NAG*, N-acetyl-beta-glucosamide; *NGAL*, neutrophil gelatinase-associated lipocalin; *TIMP-2*, tissue inhibitor of metalloproteinase-2. *(From Francoz, C., Nadim, M.K., Durand, F. (2016). Kidney biomarkers in cirrhosis. J Hepatol, 65(4):809–24.)*

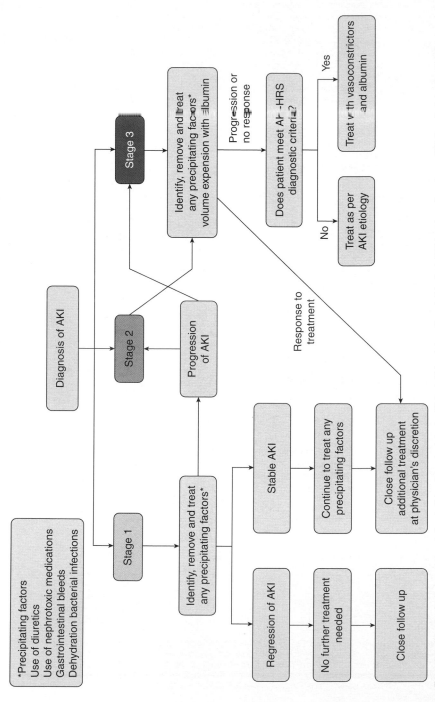

Figure 8.3. Algorithm for the management of acute kidney injury in cirrhosis. *AKI,* Acute kidney injury; *GI,* gastrointestinal; *HRS,* hepatorenal syndrome; *NAG,* N-acetyl-beta-glucosamide.

Albumin alone has been shown to be ineffective in the treatment of AKI-HRS. The use of albumin plus vasoconstrictor was superior in lowering serum creatinine and reversing AKI-HRS when compared to albumin alone or vasoconstrictor alone. However, there was no change in overall patient survival. A recent meta-analysis showed that within the group of patients who received vasoconstrictor plus albumin, a higher cumulative dose of albumin was associated with a significantly improved 6-month survival.

In AKI-HRS, albumin should be given with vasoconstrictors at the dose of 1 g/kg on day 1 followed by 20 to 40 g/day until vasoconstrictors are withdrawn. Where possible, the albumin dose should be titrated according to the level of the central venous pressure of up to 10 cm of water. Alternatively, albumin should be reduced or stopped in the presence of intravascular volume overload and/or pulmonary edema.

14. Should renal vasodilators be used in the treatment of AKI-HRS?
There is no proven efficacy for renal vasodilators such as low-dose dopamine, prostaglandin E1 analogues (e.g., misoprostol), or endothelin receptor antagonists in the treatment of AKI-HRS.

15. How are systemic vasoconstrictors used in the treatment of AKI-HRS?
See Fig. 8.3 and Table 8.2. Vasoconstrictors are the mainstay of treatment for patients with AKI-HRS.
• Terlipressin
Terlipressin is a vasopressin analogue, which causes vasoconstriction of the splanchnic vessels, thereby correcting one of the fundamental disease processes of cirrhotic pathophysiology. This improves the central circulation and reduces renal vasoconstriction. A continuous infusion is better tolerated and more effective at lower doses than intravenous boluses.
There are three randomized, controlled trials with 354 patients comparing the effects of
• terlipressin plus albumin versus albumin alone, or
• terlipressin versus placebo with or without albumin in both arms, or
• terlipressin versus placebo with albumin in both arms.

Table 8.2. Pharmacological Treatment of Hepatorenal Syndrome

MEDICATION	MECHANISM	DOSAGE	COMMENTS
Midodrine	Alpha agonist ↑ blood pressure ↑ renal perfusion pressure	Start with 5 mg tid and titrate to maintain a mean arterial pressure > 70 mm Hg	Used in combination with octreotide. Combination is inferior to continuous infusion of terlipressin.
Octreotide	Long-acting analogue of somatostatin ↓ splanchnic vasodilatation	Continuous intravenous infusion of 25 μg stat followed by 25 μg/h; or 100 μg tid subcutaneously	Octreotide alone has been shown to be ineffective as a treatment for HRS.
Vasopressin	V1 receptor agonist. Vasoconstriction of systemic and splanchnic circulations		Not commonly used because of ischemic side effects
Terlipressin	Vasopressin analogue	0.5–2 mg q4–6 h IV; or continuous intravenous infusion at 2–12 mg/day	Less ischemic side effects than vasopressin. Continuous infusion is better tolerated and more effective at lower doses than IV boluses.
Norepinephrine	Alpha, beta-adrenergic agonist. Systemic vasoconstriction	0.5–3 mg/h	Reversal of HRS. No significant ischemic side effects. Equally efficacious as terlipressin.

HRS, Hepatorenal syndrome; *IV,* intravenous.

Reversal of AKI-HRS was observed in 24% to 44% without overall survival benefit. The AKI-HRS reversal rate was low, which was partly related to patients stopping treatment early due to significant ischemic side effects or non-reversal of their AKI-HRS. The lack of overall survival benefit may be related to the fact that many of patients still had end-stage liver disease, which was one of the determinants of their survival. However, the use of terlipressin was able to sufficiently prolong patient survival to allow for liver transplant.

A post hoc analysis of the results of one of these studies found that patients with AKI-HRS and systemic inflammatory response syndrome (SIRS) at enrolment were more likely to respond to terlipressin with reversal of their AKI-HRS. This improved response was noted when compared with patients who received terlipressin without SIRS, and those who received albumin plus placebo with or without SIRS. Patients who received terlipressin and responded by reversing their AKI-HRS also survived better. Terlipressin is used as a first-line agent in AKI-HRS everywhere in the world except North America, where it is used only in the context of clinical trials.

- Norepinephrine and midodrine

  These are systemic vasoconstrictors that raise systemic arterial blood pressure and improve renal perfusion pressure. This leads to decreased renal vasoconstriction and increased GFR. Several randomized, controlled trials and a meta-analysis have shown that norepinephrine is as equally efficacious as terlipressin. Midodrine in combination with octreotide was inferior to terlipressin in reversing AKI-HRS in a randomized, controlled trial. It is popular in North America because terlipressin is not commercially available.

- Octreotide

  Octreotide is an analogue of somatostatin, a hormone involved in regulation of blood vessel tone in the gastrointestinal tract. Octreotide inhibits splanchnic vasodilatation and is used in combination with midodrine to treat AKI-HRS. Octreotide alone has not been shown to be effective in the treatment of AKI-HRS.

- N-acetylcysteine

  Isolated case reports have suggested the use of N-acetylcysteine (NAC) in combination with systemic vasoconstrictors or endothelin-receptor antagonists. This is based on a small case study of 12 patients with AKI-HRS who showed an improvement in serum creatinine after intravenous infusion of NAC, but it is not standard clinical practice at this time.

16. How is transjugular intrahepatic portosystemic stent shunt used in the treatment of AKI-HRS?
    TIPS is a prosthesis that can effectively reduce portal pressure. In addition, it returns a significant part of the splanchnic vascular volume into the systemic circulation, decreasing the activity of various vasoconstrictor systems.

    The use of TIPS in the management of AKI-HRS has been shown to lead to an improvement, but not normalization, of GFR. The use of vasoconstrictor therapy followed by TIPS insertion in AKI-HRS patients was able to normalize kidney function over the course of 12 months with an overall survival rate of 50%. The use of TIPS as a treatment for AKI-HRS is falling out of favor, as patients with AKI-HRS have advanced liver disease and there are valid concerns about precipitating liver failure if TIPS is inserted. Therefore TIPS is of limited use in AKI-HRS and can only be recommended in a very select group of patients with AKI-HRS, such as those with significant portal hypertension but minimal liver dysfunction.

17. How is extracorporeal albumin dialysis used in the treatment of AKI-HRS?
    Albumin dialysis removes albumin-bound substances, such as cytokines and bile acids, which are also systemic vasodilators. Albumin dialysis can filter out creatinine, and artificially reduces the serum creatinine without changing the GFR. Clinicians can be lured into a false sense of improvement when there is no recovery of kidney function. There are not enough data to accept it as a standard of care for AKI-HRS.

18. How is liver transplantation used in the treatment of HRS?
    Liver transplant is the definitive treatment for both AKI-HRS and chronic type 2 HRS. It corrects liver dysfunction and eliminates portal hypertension—the two pivotal pathogenetic mechanisms for the development of HRS. However, only 50% to 75% of patients with pre-transplant AKI-HRS will achieve normal kidney function following transplant, and this reversal to normal kidney function is independent of pre-transplant pharmacotherapy and dialysis. Dialysis is frequently started to deal with the electrolyte abnormalities and volume overload issues pre–liver transplant. Many studies have shown that the longer a patient is on dialysis pre-transplant, the less likely they are to reverse kidney dysfunction. Most guidelines suggest that patients should be considered for a combined liver and kidney transplant if they have spent a prolonged period on dialysis pre-transplant (≥8 weeks); however, there is no consensus on how long "a prolonged period" is. Liver transplantation reverses

chronic type 2 HRS in the majority of patients with survival outcomes comparable to matched controls.

For patients with AKI-HRS, overall survival is significantly better for those who recover kidney function post-transplant; therefore it is imperative that these patients are offered a timely liver transplant. The use of living donor liver transplants appears to provide similar results to cadaveric liver transplant donation.

19. Should dialysis be used for the treatment of HRS?
Intermittent hemodialysis has been used as a short-term bridge to liver transplantation. However, there is no evidence that it increases long-term survival without transplantation. It is not recommended unless there is a reversible component to the liver disease or the patient is listed for liver transplant.

20. What is the prognosis of HRS?
AKI-HRS is associated with a poor prognosis. Studies show a 2-week mortality of up to 80% in untreated AKI-HRS. In chronic type 2 HRS, the kidney function decline is more gradual, but it is also associated with a poor prognosis, with a median survival of 3 to 6 months.

21. Are there any scenarios in which AKI-HRS can be prevented?
- SBP: One-third of patients with SBP will develop kidney impairment despite appropriate antibiotic therapy. Patients who receive albumin in addition to antibiotics have been shown to have a lower incidence of kidney impairment and death compared to those treated with antibiotics alone. The benefit was particularly marked in patients with an elevated baseline creatinine >1 mg/dL (88 μmol/L) and/or bilirubin >4 mg/dL (68 μmol/L). Patients in this study received intravenous albumin at a dose of 1.5 g/kg body weight on day 1, then 1 g/kg body weight on day 3.
- Although antibiotics alone have not been shown to directly reduce the incidence of AKI-HRS, primary prophylaxis of SBP with norfloxacin reduces the incidence of SBP, which is a risk factor for AKI-HRS.
- Large-volume paracentesis: Removal of large (≥5 liters) amounts of ascites may precipitate post-paracentesis circulatory dysfunction, which can induce kidney failure in up to 20% of patients. Giving albumin at a dose of 6 to 8 g/L of ascitic fluid removed has been shown to reduce the incidence of kidney failure but not mortality.
- Gastrointestinal bleeds: Prophylactic antibiotics given to patients with gastrointestinal bleeds for a duration of 7 days have been shown to reduce the incidence of SBP, which is a recognized risk factor for AKI-HRS, especially in Child-Pugh Classes B and C patients.

KEY POINTS

1. Hepatorenal syndrome (HRS) is a form of functional acute kidney injury (AKI), which occurs in patients with end-stage liver cirrhosis and circulatory dysfunction.
2. The circulatory dysfunction of end-stage cirrhosis leads to a reduction in effective arterial blood volume, which stimulates renal vasoconstriction via the various systemic vasoconstrictor systems, predisposing patients to kidney failure.
3. Any condition that causes a further reduction of the effective arterial blood volume can potentially precipitate AKI-HRS. These include sepsis, over-diuresis, large-volume paracentesis (≥5 liters) without intravascular volume replacement, and gastrointestinal bleeding.
4. In hospitalized patients with cirrhosis, prerenal azotemia is the most common cause of acute kidney injury. HRS can be considered a form of prerenal azotemia, which is not volume responsive and which is seen exclusively in patients with severe liver dysfunction.
5. Type 1 HRS has been renamed AKI-HRS.
6. Pharmacologic treatment (e.g., midodrine and octreotide, terlipressin, norepinephrine) increases survival, but the only definitive treatment is liver transplantation.

BIBLIOGRAPHY
Angeli, P., Gines, P., Wong, F., Bernardi, M., Boyer, T. D., Gerbes, A., . . . Garcia-Tsao, G. (2015). Diagnosis and management of acute kidney injury in patients with cirrhosis: revised consensus recommendations of the International Club of Ascites. *Gut, 64*(4), 531–537.
Belcher, J. M., Sanyal, A. J., Peixoto, A. J., Perazella, M. A., Lim, J., Thiessen-Philbrook, H., . . . Parikh, C. R. (2014, August). Kidney biomarkers and differential diagnosis of patients with cirrhosis and acute kidney injury. *Hepatology, 60*(2), 622–632.

Cavallin, M., Kamath, P. S., Merli, M., Fasolato, S., Toniutto, P., Salerno, F., . . . Angeli, P. (2015). Terlipressin plus albumin versus midodrine and octreotide plus albumin in the treatment of hepatorenal syndrome: A randomized trial. *Hepatology, 62*(2), 567–574.

Cavallin, M., Piano, S., Romano, A., Fasolato, S., Frigo, A. C., Benetti, G., . . . Angeli, P. (2016). Terlipressin given by continuous intravenous infusion versus intravenous boluses in the treatment of hepatorenal syndrome: A randomized controlled study. *Hepatology, 63*(3), 983–992.

Nassar Junior, A. P., Farias, A. Q., D' Albuquerque, L. A., Carrilho, F. J., & Malbouisson, L. M. (2014). Terlipressin versus norepinephrine in the treatment of hepatorenal syndrome: a systematic review and meta-analysis. *PLoS One, 9*(9), e107466.

Salerno, F., Gerbes, A., Ginès, P., Wong, F., & Arroyo, V. (2007). Diagnosis, prevention and treatment of hepatorenal syndrome in cirrhosis. *Gut, 56*(9), 1310–1318.

Salerno, F., Navickis, R. J., & Wilkes, M. M. (2015). Albumin treatment regimen for type 1 hepatorenal syndrome: a dose–response meta-analysis. *BMC Gastroenterol, 15*, 167.

Wong, F., & Angeli, P. (2017). New diagnostic criteria and management of acute kidney injury. *J Hepatol, 66*(4), 860–861.

Wong, F., Nadim, M. K., Kellum, J. A., Salerno, F., Bellomo, R., Gerbes, A., . . . Arroyo, V. (2011). Working Party proposal for a revised classification system of renal dysfunction in patients with cirrhosis. *Gut, 60*(5), 702–709.

CARDIORENAL SYNDROME

Claudio Ronco and Luca di Lullo

CHAPTER 9

BACKGROUND

1. What does cardiorenal syndrome (CRS) mean?
   The term CRS has been used to define different clinical conditions in which heart and kidney dysfunction overlap. A consensus classification of CRS is outlined in Table 9.1.

2. What is CRS type 1?
   CRS type 1 (CRS-1) is when patients have acute worsening of cardiac function that leads to acute kidney injury (AKI). This is usually seen with acute decompensated heart failure (ADHF) that follow ischemic (acute coronary syndrome, cardiac surgery complications) or non-ischemic (valvular disease, pulmonary embolism) heart disease.

3. Which pathophysiologic pathways are involved in the development of CRS-1?
   Hemodynamic mechanisms probably play a major role. With ADHF, decreases in kidney artery blood flow result in decreased glomerular filtration rate (GFR). Two patterns have been described for CRS-1: *cold* and *warm* patients.
   1. In cold patients, severe vasoconstriction from activation of the renin angiotensin-aldosterone system (RAAS) and the systemic nervous system, or reduced effective circulating volume compromise kidney artery blood flow.
   2. In warm (also described as "wet") patients, marked increases in central venous pressure (CVP) decreases perfusion pressure throughout the kidney. Increased CVP also increases interstitial pressure, collapsing the tubules and further lowering GFR.
      Patients with a warm hemodynamic profile have pulmonary and/or systemic congestion. The warm profile is the most frequent profile in acute and chronic advanced heart failure (HF). The cold hemodynamic profile may also have an increased CVP, but kidney perfusion pressure is better maintained due to higher arterial blood pressures.

4. Are there any non-hemodynamic mechanisms for CRS-1?
   Non-hemodynamic mechanisms may also be involved in CRS-1, specifically increased reactive oxygen species and impaired of nitric oxide production.

Table 9.1. Classification of Cardiorenal Syndrome

TYPE	NAME	DESCRIPTION	EXAMPLE
1	Acute cardiorenal	Heart failure leading to acute kidney injury (AKI)	Acute coronary syndrome leading to acute heart and kidney failure
2	Chronic cardiorenal	Chronic heart failure leading to kidney failure	Chronic heart failure
3	Acute nephrocardiac	AKI leading to acute heart failure	Uremic cardiomyopathy AKI-related
4	Chronic nephrocardiac	Chronic kidney disease leading to heart failure	Left ventricular hypertrophy and diastolic heart failure due to kidney failure
5	Secondary	Systemic disease leading to heart and kidney failure	Sepsis, vasculitis, diabetes mellitus

5. **What is the prevalence of CRS-1?**
   Type 1 CRS occurs in about 25% of patients hospitalized for ADHF; among these patients, chronic kidney disease (CKD) is quite common and contributes to AKI in 60% of cases. Developing AKI is an independent risk factor for death in ADHF.

6. **Could biomarkers be helpful in type 1CRS diagnosis?**
   Many biomarkers have been proposed for the early diagnosis of kidney injury in CRS-1. Cystatin C represents a valid surrogate to test kidney function and it has been recognized as more predictive of long-term mortality and rehospitalization for ADHF than serum creatinine or serum brain natriutetic peptide (BNP). Neutrophil gelatinase-associated lipocalin (NGAL) correlates with kidney function markers, adverse cardiovascular outcomes, or death in ADHF patients. Type 1 CRS also can be diagnosed by bioimpedance electrical devices that track total body water. The use of bioimpedance has demonstrated an association between increased body fluid volume and rehospitalization and death.

7. **Is there a diagnostic role for ultrasound?**
   Echocardiography could show abnormal heart function including:
   - Abnormal myocardial kinetics (indicating an ischemic condition)
   - Left ventricular hypertrophy
   - Valvular stenosis
   - Valvular regurgitation
   - Pericardial effusions
   - Aortic aneurysm
   - Aortic dissection

   The echocardiogram should show normal inspiratory collapse of the inferior vena cava to exclude severe hypervolemia. Kidney ultrasound usually shows normal or slightly increased kidney size and increased cortical-to-medullary ratio, and Doppler evaluation will show regular intraparenchymal blood flow, often with an increased resistance index (>0.8 cm/s)

8. **What are the main treatment approaches in CRS-1 patients?**
   Diuretics, beta blockers, angiotensin-converting enzyme inhibitors, or angiotensin receptor blockers should be started or maximized in the setting of ADHF. The management of patients with cardiogenic shock can be challenging because of the limited effectiveness of pharmacological therapy. Among patients requiring emergency coronary artery bypass graft (CABG) surgery, the in-hospital mortality rate in Europe and the United States is about 20%, with a high incidence of stroke (8%), kidney failure requiring dialysis (8.3%), and bleeding (63.3%). Inotropic support remains the central therapy for depressed myocardium, and correction of the underlying cause, such as ischemia, will improve outcomes and produce less kidney injury.

9. **How is type 2 cardiorenal syndrome (CRS-2) defined?**
   CRS-2 is characterized by chronic abnormalities in cardiac function leading to kidney injury or dysfunction. CKD has been observed in 45% to 63% of congestive heart failure (CHF) patients.

10. **What are the main pathophysiologic pathways involved in CRS-2?**
    Intrinsic to its definition, CRS-2 is characterized by CKD onset or progression in HF patients, but two fundamental features are proposed: CHF and CKD are found simultaneously, and CHF is the cause of the CKD or responsible for its progression. Examples of CRS-2 include cyanotic nephropathy occurring in patients with congenital heart disease, when heart disease clearly precedes kidney involvement or acute coronary syndrome leading to left ventricular dysfunction and the onset or progression of coexisting CKD. The pathophysiological mechanisms of CRS-2 include:
    - Neurohormonal activation
    - Kidney hypoperfusion
    - Venous congestion
    - Inflammation
    - Atherosclerosis
    - Oxidative stress

    These mechanisms are operative in recurrent episodes of acute heart and kidney decompensation associated with HF and CKD progression.

11. **Is there a pathophysiological role for the RAAS?**
    Patients with decompensated HF and venous congestion often have significant RAAS activation without decreased circulating volume. Kidneys of HF patients release renin, which

increases angiotensin II production. Persistent RAAS and sympathetic nervous system (SNS) activation could contribute to CKD progression.

Angiotensin II production and aldosterone release increase sodium reabsorption leading to increased blood pressure and volume overload. Increased aldosterone levels also contribute to glomerular fibrosis due to the up-regulation of transforming growth factor-β (TGF-β) and increased fibronectin.

Persistent inflammation triggered by cardiac decompensation also promotes CKD progression in CHF.

12. What about new biomarkers for the diagnosis of type 2 CRS?

Assessment of kidney injury in chronic HF patients previously has been limited to creatinine, estimated glomerular filtration rate (eGFR), and urinary protein excretion. Recently, novel kidney biomarkers (cystatin C, NGAL, kidney injury molecule-1 and N-acetylbeta-glucosaminidase) have been evaluated in CHF patients, and may eventually become effective prognostic markers for CKD and cardiovascular outcomes.

13. Is there a diagnostic role for ultrasound?

In CRS-2, the kidney ultrasound shows a reduction of cortical thickness, reduced cortico-medullary ratio, and increased parenchymal echogenicity. Echocardiography may show:

- High atrial volumes and areas as indices of volume overload
- Normal or decreased ejection fraction (EF)
- Right chamber dilation
- Increased pulmonary arterial pressure
- Pericardial effusion
- Valvular disease (calcific disease)

MANAGEMENT

PHARMACOLOGICAL TREATMENT APPROACH

In the treatment of CRS-2, the main issues are:

- Preventing new-onset kidney dysfunction, emerging in a setting of CHF
- Counteract kidney dysfunction once it has developed

Special attention should be paid to several CHF drugs that may worsen kidney function. Diuresis-associated hypovolemia, the early introduction of RAAS blockade, and drug-induced hypotension may all contribute to the genesis or aggravation of CRS-2. In patients with a poor response to oral loop diuretics, a number of strategies can be employed to improve urine output. Loop diuretics can be switched to intravenous (IV) infusions. This removes the problem of erratic bioavalability found in furosemide. Often HF patients require nearly continuous exposure to a diuretic in order to achieve adequate diuresis. This can be achieved through increased frequency or a continuous infusion. Adding thiazide diuretics to block distal sodium resorption can enhance loop diuretic activity. High doses of IV loop diuretics in patients with signs and symptoms of HF adequately controlled should be lowered because of the side effects:

- Hypokalemia
- Hypotension
- Dysnatremia
- Marked neurohormonal activation
- Kidney impairment

These iatrogenic influences may often account for kidney damage as much as the congestive nephropathy itself.

ULTRAFILTRATION FOR CARDIORENAL SYNDROME TYPE 2

Isolated ultrafiltration (IUF) in the setting of CRS-2 allows rapid correction of fluid overload when standard management (high-dose IV diuretics with or without inotrope support) has failed. Current American Heart Association/American College of Cardiology and the European Society of Cardiology treatment guidelines establish that IUF is an option (class IIa, level of evidence B and C) if all diuretic strategies have failed. IUF does not affect electrolytes or significantly reduce urea levels like dialysis or hemofiltration.

14. How is type 3 cardiokidney syndrome (CRS-3) defined?

CRS-3 is characterized by acute worsening of kidney function leading to heart disease (Box 9.1). AKI represents an independent cardiovascular risk factor for mortality in hospitalized patients, especially in those on renal replacement therapy (RRT).

Box 9.1. Potential Biomarkers in Acute Kidney Injury

Biomarkers of Acute Kidney Injury, Acute Cardiac Dysfunction and Type 3 Cardiorenal Syndrome

Potential Biomarkers for Early Detection of Acute Kidney Injury
NGAL
KIM-1
Cystatin C
IL-18
NAG
L-FABP
Netrin-1
Klotho
Midkine
TIMP-2
IGFBP-7

Potential Biomarkers for Differential Diagnosis of Acute Kidney Injury
KIM-1
IL-18

Potential for Prognosis of AKI
NGAL
Cystatin C
NAG

Potential Biomarkers for Inflammation and Immune Response
Urinary IL-18
TNFR-1
VCAM-1
CP-1

Early Detection of Acute Cardiac Dysfunction
BNP/NT-proBNP
cTnT, cTnI
Myoglobin
MPO
CRP
H-FABP

BNP/NT-proBNP, Brain natriuretic peptide/N-terminal (NT)-proBNP; *CRP*, C-reactive protein; *H-FABP*, human heart fatty acid binding protein; *IGFBP-7*, insulin-like growth factor-7; *IL-18*, interleukin-18; *KIM-1*, kidney injury molecule-1; *L-FABP*, liver-type fatty acid-binding protein; *MCP-1*, monocyte chemoattractant protein-1; *MPO*, myeloperoxidase; *NAG*, N-acetyl-(D)-glucosaminidase; *NGAL*, neutrophil gelatinase-associated lipocalin; *TIMP-2*, tissue inhibitor of metalloproteinase-2; *TNFR-1*, tumor necrosis factor receptor-1; *VCAM-1*, urinary vascular cell adhesion molecules-1.

AKI can occur in all hospitalized patients but is especially prevalent in:
- Patients over age 65
- Patients with infections
- Underlying cardiovascular disease
- Hepatic cirrhosis
- Respiratory distress
- Chronic HF
- Hematologic neoplasia
- Intensive care unit (ICU) patients (mainly due to sepsis, major surgery, hypovolemic status with low cardiac output, HF).

15. What's the epidemiology of CRS-3?
AKI may occur in 70% of ICU patients. From 5% to 25% of ICU patients develop severe AKI with mortality rates ranging from 50% to 80%.

ADHF, defined as new-onset, gradual or rapid worsening of preexisting HF with signs and symptoms requiring immediate therapy, represents the most common etiology of acute cardiac dysfunction syndrome.

Cardiac valvular disease, atrial fibrillation, arterial hypertension as well as noncardiac comorbidities (kidney dysfunction, diabetes, anemia) and medications (especially nonsteroidal anti-inflammatory drugs and glitazones) can contribute to ADHF development. According to the Acute Decompensated Heart Failure National Registry database, kidney dysfunction increases mortality in ADHF patients from 1.9% in those with mild kidney disease to 7.6% in those with severe kidney dysfunction. Other adverse prognostic factors are a low EF, low systolic blood pressure, hyponatremia, older age, and elevated C-reactive protein (CRP) levels. AKI leads to heart dysfunction, which then decreases perfusion of the kidney, which further compromises cardiac function in a self-perpetuating cycle of cardiac and kidney failure.

16. How can AKI directly affect heart function?
Pathophysiological interactions between kidney and heart in AKI are called "cardiorenal connectors," which include immune modulation (both pro- and antiinflammatory cytokines and chemokines), sympathetic nervous system, RAAS activity, and activation of the coagulation cascade.

Circulating levels of tumor necrosis factor-alpha (TNFα), interleukin-1 (IL-1) and interleukin-6 (IL-6), increase immediately after experimental kidney ischemia and, together with other cytokines as well as interferon-alfa (IFN-α), have direct cardiodepressant effects, such as a reduction in the left ventricular EF and elevation of the left ventricular end diastolic and systolic volumes and areas. Cytokines can decrease myocardial contractility directly or by interacting with the extracellular matrix to cause negative inotropic effects. Cellular mechanisms involve secondary mediators, such as sphingolipids, arachidonic acid, and alterations in intracellular calcium.

Hyperactivity of the SNS with abnormal secretion of norepinephrine is found in AKI and impairs myocardial activity in several ways:
- Direct norepinephrine effect
- Impairment in Ca2+ metabolism
- Increased myocardial oxygen demand with potential evolution to myocardial ischemia
- β1-adrenergic mediated apoptosis of myocardial cells
- Stimulation of α1 receptors
- Activation of RAAS
- Angiotensin II promotion of cellular hypertrophy and apoptosis.

Increased RAAS activity could be accountable for diminished coronary response to adenosine, bradykinin, and L-arginine. Other animal models exemplify how the inflammatory cascade of AKI can contribute to altered permeability of lung vessels, resulting in interstitial edema and microhemorrhage mediated by inflammatory mediators and altered expression of epithelial sodium channel and aquaporin-5.

17. **How can AKI indirectly decrease heart function?**
As kidney function declines, it can result in significant pathophysiological derangement, leading to cardiac injury. AKI can lead to fluid overload causing hypertension, pulmonary edema, and myocardial injury. Electrolyte imbalances, primarily hyperkalemia, can cause arrhythmias and sudden death. Acidemia can worsen pulmonary vasoconstriction, increased right ventricular afterload, and contribute to a negative inotropic effect. Uremia itself can directly decrease myocardial contractility and promote pericardial effusions and pericarditis.

In response to systemic and kidney hemodynamic changements, baroceptor and intrarenal chemoceptors lead to SNS and RAAS activation.

18. **What is the role for ultrasound in the diagnosis of CRS-3?**
Kidney size and echogenicity are the primary features that distinguish acute from chronic kidney damage. Of note, enlarged kidneys can be seen in some forms of CKD (e.g., early stages of diabetic nephropathy, HIV-related glomerulonephritis, or cast nephropathy). A hyperechogenic kidney cortex with low corticomedullary ratio is predictive of CKD.

The echocardiographic pattern is not diagnostic of CRS-3. It may show increased atrial volumes or areas as indices of volume overload, pleural or pericardial effusions.

19. **How do you manage type-3 CRS?**
The strategy to manage these patients depends on the stage of AKI.

Patients at high risk of developing AKI. Special care should be taken to avoid AKI. This should include avoiding or minimizing nephrotoxic medications and procedures. Preventing hypoperfusion, volume depletion, or volume overload is a cornerstone of avoiding AKI. This is especially important in patients with higher filling pressures and signs of right heart dysfunction due to increased preload.

Stage 1 (risk). In addition to the above recommendations, these patients should get a urine analysis, routine blood tests, biomarkers, and a kidney ultrasound to investigate the etiology and to correct problems. Close monitoring and supportive care should also be provided.[1]

Stage 2 (injury). Stage 2 patients are characterized by high risk of morbidity/mortality due to kidney injury. In addition to conservative therapy, these patients should receive functional hemodynamic monitoring to guide resuscitation, especially pulse pressure variation in ventilated patients. Attention should be paid to the maintenance of electrolytes and acid-base homeostasis. Drug dosing may need to be altered due to the decreased renal clearance.

Stage 3 (failure). At this stage patient are at a high risk of death and have a high probability of extrarenal complications, including CRS. RRT may be needed to provide clearance or to avoid life-threatening complications. The prevention of left ventricular volume overload is critical to maintain adequate cardiac output and systemic perfusion. Continuous infusion of furosemide may be needed to establish and maintain diuresis. Combining loop diuretics with thiazide diuretics will also increase efficacy.

RENAL REPLACEMENT THERAPY

Once pharmacological treatment fails in AKI patients and oligo-anuric kidney failure is established, RRT should be started. The timing of RRT initiation is a point of debate, with some arguing for a survival advantage from starting dialysis early. The largest randomized controlled trials (RCT) to date was unable to demonstrate a survival advantage. RRT may be initiated in response to electrolyte and acid-base imbalance, hypercreatininemia, and severe fluid overload that is unresponsive to pharmacological treatment.

RRT can be stopped when improvement in kidney function is clear as pointed out by increased urine output or decreased serum creatinine levels in patients with constant continuous renal replacement therapy (CRRT) dose. A urine output of more than 400 ml /day or a creatinine clearance of 15 to 20 ml /min could allow CRRT withdrawal.

CRRT and intermittent hemodialysis (IHD) both present pros and cons; when correctly applied, both CRRT and IHD can achieve good metabolic control. In randomized, controlled trials and meta-analyses, CRRT seems to be associated with more frequent kidney recovery in critically ill patients.

Together with CRRT and IHD therapies, some "hybrid therapies" have been proposed, such as sustained low-efficiency (daily) dialysis (SLED) and extended daily dialysis in which IHD techniques are adapted to provide longer dialysis sessions.

Some clinical trials have not found any difference between SLED and continuous veno-venous hemofiltration in terms of cardiovascular stability and mortality rates, but SLED seems to be associated with a shorter duration of mechanical ventilation.

Concerning the RRT dose, large multicenter, randomized, controlled trials have found no advantage to doses higher than 20 to 30 mL of effluent/kg per hour. Clinicians should tailor RRT therapy of critically ill patients to provide the ideal blood purification treatment.

20. What is the definition of type-4 cardiorenal syndrome (CRS-4)?

    CRS-4, also called chronic renocardiac disease, is characterized by cardiovascular involvement in patients affected by CKD at any stage. Kidney dysfunction is an independent risk factor for cardiovascular disease with higher mortality for myocardial infarction and sudden death in CKD.

21. What is the incidence and prevalence of CRS-4?

    All patients with CKD are at increased risk of cardiovascular outcomes. This was shown in a meta-analysis by Tonelli et al that looked at 1.4 million patients and found higher mortality rates as eGFR declined, with the odds ratio going from 1.9 to 2.6 to 4.4 for eGFRs of 80, 60, and 40 mL/min, respectively. The single largest epidemiological study to look at this was done by Go et al. on over 1 million people. They found elevated cardiovascular risk in patients with K/DOQI stage IIIb–IV CKD, as well as patients undergoing RRT (hemodialysis, peritoneal dialysis, and transplant).

    The Chronic Renal Insufficiency Cohort (CRIC) Study investigators focused their attention on 190 patients with stage III to end-stage kidney disease (ESKD) and performed serial echocardiograms. Over the 2-year evaluation period, during which patients shifted from stage 5 to ESKD, EF dropped from 53% to 50%, and the fraction of patents with an EF less than 50% increased by a fifth.

22. Pathophysiology of CRS-4 role of risk factors and CKD comorbidities

    CRS-4 shows close interactions between CKD and cardiovascular involvement. CKD can indirectly (exacerbating ischemic heart disease) and directly (pressure and volume overload leading to left ventricular hypertrophy) contribute to heart disease.[2] Left ventricular hypertrophy is highly prevalent in patients starting hemodialysis and is associated with subsequent hospitalizations for HF. Left ventricular hypertrophy results from comorbid conditions, such as hypertension and calcific valvular disease, which are particularly prevalent in hemodialysis and pre-dialysis patients. Hyperphosphatemia and secondary hyperparathyroidism can cause calcification of coronary vessels and valves due to osteoblastic transformation of vascular smooth muscle cells. Hypertension itself can contribute to vascular calcification. CKD patients, especially those undergoing dialysis, are prone to arrhythmias, especially atrial fibrillation and ventricular tachyarrhythmias.

    Almost half of cardiovascular deaths in ESKD are related to cardiac arrhythmia or sudden death. An increased risk for sudden death is associated with prolonged dialytic intervals in subjects undergoing thrice-weekly hemodialysis treatment. This may be due to large shifts of electrolytes and fluids.

    In the CRIC study, atrial fibrillation had a prevalence of 18%.

    Volume overload is common in CKD due to anemia plus sodium and water retention, and it can be exacerbated by hemodialysis vascular access.

    Chronic inflammation, insulin resistance, and lipid abnormalities also contribute to cardiovascular disease in CKD patients.

23. **What are the main available diagnostic tools in CRS-4?**

Cardiac function is widely assessed by N-terminal (NT)-proBNP serum levels, while eGFR represents the primary biochemical test to evaluate kidney function.

Kidney ultrasound shows features of CKD, such as thin and hyperechogenic cortex with the reduced corticomedullary ratio.

Echocardiography reveals signs of volume overload, and left and right ventricular dysfunction, especially in ESKD and hemodialysis patients. Increased atrial volumes and pleural or pericardial effusion suggest volume overload. It is quite common to describe valvular calcifications (related to secondary hyperparathyroidism) and signs of right heart dysfunction, such as high pulmonary artery pressure, low tricuspid annulus plane systolic excursion, or right chamber dilation.

24. **How should CRS-4 patients be managed?**

The Irbesartan Diabetic Nephropathy Trial study was designed to evaluate renoprotective effects of irbesartan versus amlodipine or placebo in type 2 diabetes. The results showed that the irbesartan group had a lower incidence of HF compared to the amlodipine or placebo groups. The use of carvedilol together with ACE inhibitors or ARBs is associated with better cardiovascular and kidney outcomes in dialysis patients with dilated cardiomyopathy. Although the Evaluation of Cinacalcet Hydrochloride Therapy to Lower Cardiovascular Events study did not meet its primary end-point, the investigators did note a reduction in the first HF episode with cinacalcet in ESKD patients.

Di Lullo et al. found that treating pre-dialysis patients with sevelamer chloridrate (1600 mg/day), a calcium-free phosphate binder, reduced cardiac valve calcifications and delayed kidney function decline was observed. However, Bellasi et al. found an increase in cardiac calcification and no change in CKD progression with the use of phosphorus binders in pre-dialysis patients. (54.5)

Dyslipidemia represents another potential target in managing cardiovascular complications in CKD patients. The Study of Heart and Renal Protection (SHARP) trial was the largest trial on statin use in CKD patients and showed a significant benefit with the combination of simvastatin and ezetimibe on major atherosclerotic events, although all-cause mortality was not improved.

25. **What is type-5 CRS?**

CRS-5 occurs when cardiac and kidney injury occur simultaneously. This can be seen in sepsis, where heart and kidney are involved secondary to a common underlying pathological trigger.

26. **What is the pathophysiology of CRS-5?**

The pathophysiology of CRS-5 depends on the underlying disease. Acute CRS-5 results from systemic processes: for example, sepsis, infections, drugs, toxins, and connective tissue disorders, such as lupus, granulomatosis with polyangiitis, and sarcoidosis. The temporal course of the development of CRS-5 is variable. For example, in sepsis-induced acute CRS-5, there is a fulminant disease process with an acute impact on both the kidney and heart. On the other hand, in cirrhosis, CRS-5 has a more insidious onset, and the kidney and cardiac dysfunction may develop slowly until a crucial point is reached and full decompensation occurs.

The development of CRS-5 can be divided into four categories:
1. Hyper-acute, 0 to 72 hours after diagnosis
2. Acute, 3 to 7 days
3. Sub-acute, 7 to 30 days
4. Chronic, over 30 days

Pathophysiological changes in sepsis-related CRS-5 depend on the systemic effects of sepsis, and from cross-talk between the damaged heart and kidney. In early stages of sepsis microcirculatory perfusion derangements are found despite normal systemic hemodynamics, and they strongly correlate with morbidity and mortality rates.

Sepsis-associated cardiomyopathy represents one of the main predictors of mortality in septic patients. Both the left and right ventricles can be injured with dilation and decreased EF, and are often unresponsive to fluid and catecholamine therapy. Septic cardiomyopathy, when severe, can mimic cardiogenic shock, but it is usually reversible. Myocardial blood flow and oxygen consumption do not seem involved in the pathophysiology of septic cardiomyopathy. Proinflammatory mediators and complement factors have been proposed as crucial actors in the development of cardiac involvement during sepsis.

In sepsis-associated AKI, there are clear signs of intraparenchymal blood flow compromise independent of systemic hemodynamic changes linked to the septic process. Recent experimental animal data have demonstrated increased kidney vascular resistance and early rises in pro-inflammatory cytokines (IL-6) and oxidative stress markers in animals that later went on to AKI.

Sepsis affects the autonomic nervous system (ANS), RAAS, and hypothalamus-pituitary-adrenal axis independently, each of which can impact cardiac and kidney function. The severity of ANS dysfunction correlates with morbidity and mortality. Autonomic dysfunction can be assessed by observing decreased heart rate variability, often associated with the release of inflammatory biomarkers such as IL-6, IL-10, and CRP.

During combined heart and kidney dysfunction, as in sepsis, several cellular and molecular changes occur in both tissues. The activation and induction of cytokines (TNF-α and IL-6) and leukocytes (macrophages, neutrophils, and lymphocytes) are well documented in both the heart and kidney. Myocardial contractility is decreased due to altered muscle protein expression. Increased secretion of lipopolysaccharide during sepsis alters bicarbonate transport, leading to abnormalities in urine acidification. Lipopolysaccharide also modifies megalin, a glomerular protein leading to increased albuminuria and intrarenal inflammation.

27. Are there CRS-5 specific biomarkers?

A recent review has pointed out some characteristic biomarkers whose elevation is typical during the septic process: lipopolysaccharide binding protein, pro-calcitonin, CRP, and proinflammatory cytokines (IL-6, TGF-β).

The assessment of cardiac function in CRS-5 is similar to other clinical situations with myocardial dysfunction. Natriuretic peptides and troponins provide information about cardiac chambers (especially the left cardiac chambers) and myocardial cells damage. In early stages of the septic process there is a low-output myocardial involvement; after starting fluid therapy, the clinical picture shifts to stereotypical distributive shock, which is characterized by increased cardiac output and systemic vasodilatation.

The diagnosis of kidney involvement in sepsis-related CRS-5 overlaps with other forms of AKI, relying primarily on acute changes in serum creatinine as defined by Risk, Injury, Failure, Loss and End stage (RIFLE), Acute Kidney Injury Network (AKIN), and Kidney Disease: Improving Global Outcomes (KDIGO) criteria.

28. How should CRS-5 patients be managed?

The primary goal of managing type-5 CRS is maintaining hemodynamic stability and tissue perfusion. Fluid therapy must be carefully managed to avoid fluid overload and other iatrogenic complications.

Since inflammation and immune disorders play an important role in the pathogenesis of sepsis, the removal of cytokines and immunomodulation can be obtained with high permeability membranes, although it is yet to be determined if this translates into better patient outcomes. To manage heart complications, IV fluids, together with vasopressors, vasodilators, and inotropes, may be required to maintain filling pressures. Vasopressors must be carefully administered because of the depressive effects on cardiac output. Levosimendan is a novel inotrope with some benefits in decompensated HF: for example, increasing stroke volume, heart rate, and coronary blood flow, while decreasing systemic vascular resistance, systolic blood pressure, wedge pressure, pulmonary artery pressure, and myocardial oxygen consumption. It has been shown to improve symptoms and BNP, although its efficacy is still unproven in CRS-5. Renal support includes the removal and avoidance of nephrotoxins, the maintenance of adequate perfusion, and, if indicated, early intervention with RRT. There is no role for dopamine for improving kidney hemodynamics. Likewise, fenoldopam has not shown improved outcomes in AKI. Norepinephrine decreases kidney perfusion in normal conditions but increases systemic blood pressure in septic patients, while vasopressin increases diuresis and GFR in septic patients.

RRT with CRRT should be started, when indicated, to control metabolite concentrations and fluid status.

KEY POINTS

1. CRS-1 usually presents in the setting of an acute cardiac disease such as ADHF and it can follow an ischemic (acute coronary syndrome, cardiac surgery complications) or non-ischemic (valvular disease, pulmonary embolism) heart disease.
2. Cystatin C represents a valid surrogate to test kidney function and it has been recognized as being more predictive of long-term mortality and re-hospitalization for ADHF than serum creatinine or serum BNP.
3. Diuretic resistance can be suspected when the urine output is relatively poor (e.g., <1000 mL/ day), in spite of the maximal tolerated oral dose of a loop diuretic (for example, 250 mg of furosemide per day), and in the presence of signs and symptoms of refractory hydrosaline retention.

4. BNP/NT proBNP ratio is the best diagnostic and prognostic marker in patients with acute kidney injury.
5. Increased risks of sudden death appear to be particularly related to longer dialytic intervals in subjects undergoing thrice-weekly hemodialysis treatment because of extreme shifts of electrolytes and fluids.

BIBLIOGRAPHY

Bellasi, A., Ferramoscam E., Rattim, C., et al. (2012). Cardiac valve calcification is a marker of vascular disease in prevalent hemodialysis patients. *J Nephrol. 25*(2):211–218.

Bellomo, R., Kellum, J. A., & Ronco, C. (2012). Acute kidney injury. *Lancet, 380*, 756–766.

Bongartz, L. G., Cramer, M. J., Doevendans, P. A., Joles, J. A., & Braam, B. (2005). The severe cardiorenal syndrome: "Guyton revisited." *European Heart Journal, 26*(1), 11–17.

Celes, M. R., Prado, C. M., & Rossi, M. A. (2013). Sepsis: Going to the heart of the matter. *Pathobiology*, 80(2), 70–86.

Cruz, D. N., Fard, A., Clementi, A., Ronco, C., & Maisel, A. (2012). Role of biomarkers in the diagnosis and management of cardio-renal syndromes. *Seminars in Nephrology, 32*(1), 79–92.

Di Lullo, L., Floccari, F., Granata, A., D'Amelio, A., Rivera, R., Fiorini, F., . . . Timio, M. (2012). Ultrasonography: Ariadne's thread in the diagnosis of cardiorenal syndrome. *Cardiorenal Medicine, 2*(1), 11–17. doi:10.1159/000334268.

Di Lullo, L., Floccari, F., Rivera, R., Barbera, V., Granata, A., Otranto, G., . . . Ronco, C. (2013). Pulmonary hypertension and right heart failure in chronic kidney disease: New challenge for 21st-century cardionephrologists. *Cardiorenal Medicine, 3*, 96–103.

Di Lullo, L., Floccari, F., Santoboni, A., Barbera, V., Rivera, R. F., Granata, A., . . . Russo, D. (2013). Progression of cardiac valve calcification and decline of renal function in CKD patients. *Journal of Nephrology, 26*(4), 739–744.

Di Lullo, L., Rivera, R., Barbera, V., Bellasi, A., Cozzolino, M., Russo, D., . . . Ronco, C. (2016). Sudden cardiac death and chronic kidney disease: From pathophysiology to treatment strategies. *International Journal of Cardiology, 217*, 16–27.

Go, A.S., Chertow, G.M., Fan, D., et al. (2004). Chronic kidney disease and the risks of death, cardiovascular events, and hospitalization. *N Engl J Med. 351*(13), 1296–1305.

Kajstura, J., Cigola, E., Malhotra, A., Li, P., Cheng, W., Meggs, L. G., & Anversa, P. (1997). Angiotensin II induces apoptosis of adult ventricular myocytes in vitro. *Journal of Molecular and Cellular Cardiology, 29*(3), 859–870.

Lassus, J. P., Nieminen, M. S., Peuhkurinen, K., Pulkki, K., Siirilä-Waris, K., Sund, R., Harjola, V. P.; FINN-AKVA study group. (2010). Markers of renal function and acute kidney injury in acute heart failure: Definitions and impact on outcomes of the cardiorenal syndrome. *European Heart Journal, 31*, 2791–2798.

Lemm, H., Dietz, S., Janusch, M., & Buerke, M. (2017). Use of vasopressors and inotropics in cardiogenic shock. *Herz, 42*(1), 3–10.

Lewis, E. J., Hunsicker, L. G., Clarke, W. R., Berl, T., Pohl, M. A., Lewis, J. B., . . . Collaborative Study Group. (2001). Renoprotective effect of the angiotensin-receptor antagonist irbesartan in patients with nephropathy due to type 2 diabetes. *New England Journal of Medicine, 345*(12), 851–860.

Palmer, S.C., Mavridis, D., Navarese, E., et al. (2015). Comparative efficacy and safety of blood pressure-lowering agents in adults with diabetes and kidney disease: a network meta-analysis. *Lancet, 385*(9982), 2047–2056.

Prabhu, S. D. (2004). Cytokine-induced modulation of cardiac function. *Circulation Research, 95*(12), 1140–1153.

Remuzzi, G., Cattaneo, D., & Perico, N. (2008). The aggravating mechanisms of aldosterone on kidney fibrosis. *Journal of the American Society of Nephrology, 19*(8), 1459–1462.

RENAL Replacement Therapy Study Investigators, Bellomo, R., Cass, A., Cole, L., Finfer, S., Gallagher, M., . . . Su, S. (2009). Intensity of continuous renal-replacement therapy in critically ill patients. *New England Journal of Medicine, 361*, 1627–1638.

Schmidt, H., Hoyer, D., Hennen, R., Heinroth, K., Rauchhaus, M., Prondzinsky, R., . . . Werdan, K. (2008). Autonomic dysfunction predicts both 1- and 2-month mortality in middle-aged patients with multiple organ dysfunction syndrome. *Critical Care Medicine, 36*(3), 967–970.

Uchino, S., Kellum, J. A., Bellomo, R., Doig, G. S., Morimatsu, H., Morgera, S., . . . Beginning and Ending Supportive Therapy for the Kidney (BEST Kidney) investigators. (2005). Acute renal failure in critically ill patients: A multinational, multicenter study. *Journal of the American Medical Association, 294*, 813–818.

Wu, V. C., Wang, C. H., Wang, W. J., Lin, Y. F., Hu, F. C., Chen, Y. W., . . . NSARF Study Group. (2010). Sustained low-efficiency dialysis versus continuous veno-venous hemofiltration for postsurgical acute renal failure. *American Journal of Surgery, 199*, 466–474.

CHAPTER 10

MEDICATIONS

Bryan M. Tucker and Mark A. Perazella

DRUGS COVERED

1. Nonsteroidal antiinflammatory drugs (NSAIDs)
2. Angiotensin-converting enzyme (ACE) and angiotensin-receptor blocker (ARB)
3. Sodium phosphate
4. Pamidronate and zoledronate
5. Proton pump inhibitors (PPIs)
6. Checkpoint inhibitors (CPI) chemotherapy
7. Antiangiogenesis drugs
8. Cisplatin
9. Braf inhibitors
10. Intravenous immune globulin (IVIG)
11. Tenofovir
12. Vancomycin + piperacillin/tazobactam
13. Ciprofloxacin
14. Topiramate
15. Crystalline nephropathy
16. Metformin
17. Bath salts
18. Dialyzability
19. Contrast

1. **What classic syndromes involving the kidneys are associated with NSAIDs?**
   NSAIDs are well described to cause a number of clinical syndromes involving the kidneys many which are related to decrease in prostaglandin production by the kidneys. Whereas others are idiosyncratic, those associated with NSAIDs include:
   - Acute kidney injury (AKI)
   - Hyponatremia
   - Hyperkalemia
   - Hypertension
   - Edema/congestive heart failure (CHF)
   - Acute interstitial nephritis (AIN)
   - Minimal change/membranous nephropathy
   - Acute papillary necrosis
   - Uroepithelial malignancies

   The following factors increase the risk for APN:
   - Preexisting CKD
   - Concomittant diuretic or ACE-I use
   - Older age
   - Female sex
   - Volume depletion

2. **What are the clinical scenarios where ACE inhibitors and ARBs are likely to cause AKI?**
   Any clinical circumstance where perfusion to the kidney is impaired will cause a decline in glomerular filtration rate (GFR) and AKI by inducing efferent arteriolar vasodilatation through blockade of angiotensin II production or receptor binding. Clinical scenarios include:
   - Disease states associated with hypotension
   - Decreased blood volume (i.e., diuretics, diarrhea, vomiting, etc.)
   - Decreased effective circulating blood volume (i.e., CHF, cirrhosis, nephrotic syndrome, etc.)
   - Critical renal artery stenosis
   - Treatment with medications such as NSAIDs, calcineurin inhibitors (CNIs), and vasoconstrictors
     The typical scenario is that the GFR continues to decline with ACE inhibitor/ARB therapy and does not stabilize until drug withdrawal or correction of the underlying disease process. Stabilization of kidney function, without hyperkalemia or hypotension, with continued ACEi/ARB therapy is likely associated with beneficial effects on both the heart and the kidneys.

3. **What are the major adverse effects on the kidney of ACE inhibitors and ARBs?**
   ACE inhibitors and ARBs are associated with AKI and hyperkalemia. These effects are due to inhibition of angiotensin II production by ACE inhibitors or competitive antagonism of the angiotensin II receptor by ARBs. This results in loss of angiotensin II–induced efferent arteriolar tone, leading to a drop in glomerular filtration fraction and GFR. The efferent arteriolar vasodilation reduces intraglomerular hypertension (and pressure-related injury) and maintains perfusion (and oxygenation) of the peritubular capillaries. Hyperkalemia occurs due to reduced adrenal aldosterone synthesis from decreased angiotensin II production/receptor binding. AIN is a rare complication of ACE inhibitors.

4. What are risk factors for the development of acute phosphate nephropathy (APN)?

Oral sodium phosphate-containing purgatives used for colonoscopy preparation can cause both acute and chronic kidney disease (CKD). The acute form is called APN. The following factors increase risk for development of APN. It is notable that two-thirds of patients that developed APN had three or more of these risk factors. APN may resolve or progress to CKD.

5. What are the histopathologic lesions associated with APN?

The hallmark of APN is abundant tubular and less prominent interstitial calcium phosphate deposits. Greater than 30 calcifications and sometimes greater than 100 calcifications per tubular profile may be seen. The calcifications form basophilic rounded concretions, are mainly confined to the distal tubules and collecting ducts, and are prominent in the kidney cortex. The calcifications do not polarize and have a strong histochemical reaction with the von Kossa stain, indicating that they are composed of calcium phosphate. Acute tubular degenerative changes and interstitial edema are seen with early lesions. Biopsies performed more than 3 weeks after exposure to sodium phosphate exhibit chronicity (tubular atrophy/interstitial fibrosis). Acute and/or chronic tubulointerstitial nephropathy, reminiscent of changes seen in nonresolving acute tubular necrosis (ATN), may be present. There may also be an association between PPI's and hyponatremia via SIADH. But due to the paucity of data and the many confounding variables, causation has not been demonstrated.

6. What lesions in the kidneys can be caused by pamidronate and zoledronate?

The bisphosphonates have been described to cause a couple of lesions involving the kidneys. High-dose pamidronate causes collapsing focal and segmental glomerulosclerosis (FSGS) and minimal change lesion, along with some tubular injury. In contrast, high-dose zoledronate causes a pure tubular injury pattern with severe ATN. These agents target epithelial cells, visceral epithelial cells with pamidronate, and tubular epithelial cells with zoledronate.

7. What syndromes involving the kidneys are associated with PPIs?

PPIs, regardless of class, can cause AIN. Hyponatremia, likely the result of SIADH, is less common. Most PPIs are metabolized predominantly by hepatic CYP450 enzymes, in particular CYP3A4 and CYP2C19. PPIs can cause CNI toxicity due to their effects to reduce CNI metabolism by these 2 CYP450 enzymes. Hypomagnesemia is another complication of PPIs. This is due to reduced GI absorption rather than magnesium loss via the kidneys. A reduction in TRPM-6/7 function, which are magnesium pores in apical membranes of gastrointestinal (GI) epithelial cells, lead to this effect. Discontinuation of the PPI generally reverses GI magnesium wasting.

8. Are PPIs associated with CKD?

PPIs are widely used and maintain a fairly good safety profile; however, recent observational evidence has described an association of PPI use with a variety of risks, including hip fractures, cardiovascular events, pneumonia, Clostridium difficile infection, and most recently CKD and end-stage kidney disease (ESKD). Higher-dose PPI use was associated with a greater incident risk of CKD, an association that remained significant with a time-varying model. The duration of PPI use was also significantly associated with incident CKD and ESKD. One can hypothesize that CKD and ESKD occurring in the setting of chronic PPI use is due to unrecognized (and untreated) AIN, which then transitions into chronic interstitial nephritis. However, little is known beyond the epidemiological observation of association. Therefore the precise mechanism as well as whether PPI therapy itself is causative is unclear.

9. Are CPIs associated with AKI?

The immune system has the capacity to differentiate self from foreign invaders by the use of "checkpoints," which allow cellular communication via cell surface receptors on T cells. Cancer cells use tumor products acting via checkpoints to deactivate T cells. Ipilimumab, a CTLA-4 antibody, was the first CPI approved by the Food and Drug Administration (FDA). Thereafter, immune-related adverse events were observed in many organ systems. Kidney toxicity from ipilimumab is rare but has been associated with granulomatous AIN. This was attributed to a steroid responsive autoimmune mechanism. The CPIs, nivolumab and pembrolizumab, which are antiprogrammed cell death protein 1 (PD1) antibodies, have also been associated with AIN. Nephritogenic drugs (NSAIDs, PPIs) may prime drug-specific effector T-cells and then the drug-induced inhibition of the PD-1 pathway, resulting in a loss of tolerance and AIN. An alternate hypothesis is that PD-1 inhibition causes a loss of T-cell self-tolerance, resulting in a general autoimmune disease in the kidney.

10. What adverse effects on the kidneys can be caused by antiangiogenesis drugs such as bevacizumab, sorafenib, and sunitinib?

Drugs that target the angiogenesis pathway are important in treatment of certain malignancies. However, a number of adverse effects involving the kidneys have been described. The two most common are hypertension and proteinuria, which appear to be the result of vascular endothelial growth factor (VEGF) deficiency. In the vasculature, VEGF maintains vasodilatation through the nitric oxide pathway. Hypertension results when the antiangiogenesis drugs disrupt this pathway. VEGF has a role in maintaining healthy glomerular endothelial cell function as well. Thus a common adverse event is the development of proteinuria. Rarely, if microvascular injury is significant and is not repaired, thrombotic microangiopathy (TMA) can develop. AIN have also been described with sorafenib and sunitinib. Tyrosine kinase inhibitors (sorafenib, sunitinib, axitinib, etc.) have been associated with direct podocyte toxicity, leading to minimal change disease/collapsing FSGS lesions, which contrasts the TMA lesion observed with anti-VEGF drugs (bevacizumab, aflibercept). This direct podocyte injury is thought to result from an upregulation of c-mip (c-maf-inducing protein), which disrupts intracellular signaling in podocytes.

11. **How does cisplatin cause AKI and proximal tubule injury?**
Cisplatin is a platinum-based agent whose nephrotoxicity is thought related to the chloride in the *cis* position. Cisplatin gains entry into tubular cells via uptake by the OCT-2 system on the basolateral membrane of proximal tubular cells.
- Cellular apoptosis/necrosis develops due to endoplasmic reticulum-induced stress, mitochondrial injury pathways, and a death receptor pathway.
- Normal cell-cycle regulation is disrupted by cisplatin, leading to tubular apoptosis and kidney injury.
- Cisplatin-induced DNA damage activates p53, which through various intracellular signals promotes cell apoptosis.
- Cisplatin stimulates production of reactive oxygen species and oxidative stress by depleting and inactivating glutathione and other related antioxidants.
- Cisplatin induces both inflammation and vascular injury, which further promotes kidney injury.
    In addition to AKI, cisplatin causes proximal tubulopathy, salt wasting, loss of urinary concentrating ability, and magnesium wasting.

12. **Do BRAF (v-Raf murine sarcoma viral oncogene homolog B) inhibitors cause AKI?**
BRAF is a protooncogene involved in cell signaling that, when mutated, has been associated with development of a number of other malignancies. Vemurafenib is associated with ATN, which can be associated with proteinuria (~500 g/day), and usually resolves with drug discontinuation. Reintroduction with dose reduction may cause recurrent AKI. Vemurafenib-induced nephrotoxicity may also include Fanconi syndrome and Sweet syndrome (also called acute febrile neutrophilic dermatosis; it is an uncommon skin condition characterized by fever and inflamed or blistered skin and mucosal lesions). Dabrafenib is associated with a lower incidence of AKI, although when combined with trametinib, an mitogen-activated protein kinase kinase (MEK) inhibitor, AKI incidence increases. The manifestations involving the kidneys are more commonly seen with dabrafenib are hyponatremia, hypokalemia, and hypophosphatemia. BRAF inhibitor–induced AKI causes both tubular and interstitial damage.

13. **How do IVIG and intravenous (IV) hydroxyethyl starch (HES) cause AKI?**
IVIG preparations are stabilized with sucrose (vs. maltose and glucose), which can cause "osmotic nephropathy." Similarly, the plasma expander HES also causes "osmotic nephropathy." In fact, large prospective sepsis trials comparing HES with other plasma expanders demonstrate that HES use was associated with excess AKI, increased renal replacement therapy, and mortality. Sucrose and HES are both filtered by the glomerulus and then endocytosed by proximal tubular cells. Once inside the cells, they are transported to lysosomes and can not be degraded. The cells become swollen with enlarged lysosomes, which can cause tubular obstruction. Also, as the cells are injured, they detach from the basement membrane and are released into the tubular lumens. Risk factors include kidney impairment and high doses.

14. **How is tenofovir (TDF) excreted by the kidneys, and how is it related to the drug's nephrotoxicity?**
TDF causes AKI and Fanconi syndrome. TDF damages the proximal tubule. It enters the proximal tubular cells via the basolateral circulation and is then transported into the intracellular space via the human organic anion transporter (OAT). It is subsequently secreted into the urinary space via efflux transporters such as multidrug-resistant protein-2 (MRP-2). Endogenous substances and drugs compete for the MRP-2 efflux transporter, impairing TDF excretion and leading to higher intracellular concentrations. A single nucleotide polymorphism of the MRP-2 gene (loss-of-function mutation) increases the risk for Fanconi syndrome. Mitochondrial injury is the major cause of the proximal tubulopathy associated with high intracellular TDF concentrations.

15. Do vancomycin and piperacillin-tazobactam cause AKI?

Vancomycin is an antibiotic that inhibits cell wall synthesis in gram-positive bacteria. The incidence of vancomycin-induced nephrotoxicity is highly variable, ranging from <1% to >40%, depending on the population studied, dosing regimens, event under/overreporting, and the definitions employed. Risk factors for vancomycin-induced AKI include increased exposure of the kidneys to vancomycin from higher doses or higher trough levels (>20 mg/L) and underlying CKD. Piperacillin-tazobactam is an antibiotic combination containing an extended-spectrum beta lactam with β-lactamase inhibitor. Retrospective studies demonstrate a significant increase in serum creatinine (incidence ~30%), with the combination of vancomycin and piperacillin-tazobactam. This may reflect pseudo-nephrotoxicity, a situation where piperacillin competes with creatinine for uptake by the OAT in the proximal tubule. This effect would raise serum creatinine and lead to a diagnosis of AKI. True AKI may also result from either AKI or AIN.

16. What are risk factors for ciprofloxacin-associated crystalline nephropathy?

While AIN is the most common cause of AKI with ciprofloxacin, crystalluria does occur. The drug is insoluble at alkaline pH. Ciprofloxacin causes crystalluria when the urine pH is greater than 7.3, especially with higher drug doses. AKI develops within 2 days to 2 weeks of exposure and urinalysis reveals crystals, which are strongly birefringent and show a wide array of appearances, including needles, sheaves, stars, fans, butterflies, and other unusual shapes. Needle-shaped birefringent crystals are seen within the tubules on biopsy. Ciprofloxacin crystalline nephropathy should be considered as a cause of AKI in elderly patients with impaired kidney function, volume depletion, and urine pH > 6.0. Prevention includes dose adjustment for GFR and volume repletion.

17. What is the adverse effect of topiramate on the kidney and what is the underlying pathomechanism?

Topiramate is an antiseizure drug that is also used to prevent migraine headaches. Nephrolithiasis was noted at a higher-than-expected rate in patients treated with this medication, raising the possibility of a drug-related complication. It was subsequently shown that topiramate acts as a carbonic anhydrase inhibitor and causes a defect in hydrogen secretion in both the proximal tubule and collecting duct. This is a drug-induced type 1 and type 2 renal tubular acidosis (RTA). These abnormalities produce an alkaline urine and promotes the formation of calcium phosphate stones.

18. What other drugs cause crystalline-induced nephropathy?

AKI from drug-induced crystalline nephropathy requires the presence of a significant amount of drug crystal within tubular lumens that favor crystal insolubility in a low urinary flow state. This is accomplished by supersaturation of constituent molecules, low or high urine pH (depending on the drug), volume depletion, and the absence of urinary inhibitors of crystallization. Sulfadiazine causes crystalline nephropathy or nephroliths in the setting of hypoalbuminemia, volume depletion, acid urine, and high drug doses. Prevention and/or treatment are directed at correcting hypovolemia and alkalizing the urine. Acyclovir can precipitate in the setting of hypovolemia, rapid IV bolus administration, and with excessive dosing. IV fluids and slower IV administration are employed to prevent/reduce the occurrence. IV methotrexate and its metabolites can precipitate within the tubules when given in high doses, with acid urine, and in the setting of hypovolemia. Prevention includes aggressive alkaline IV fluids and induction of high urine flow rates. When AKI develops, in addition to leucovorin rescue, drug removal can be achieved with prolonged high-flux hemodialysis (HD) or drug metabolism with carboxypeptidase G.

19. What is the risk of lactic acidosis with metformin therapy in patients with acute or CKD?

Metformin can be rarely associated with lactic acidosis, with an incidence of 3 to 10 per 100,000 person-years. Metformin binds to complex I of the mitochondrial respiratory chain, inhibiting oxidative phosphorylation and thereby increasing the proportion of uncoupled respirations. This leads to increased glycolysis and glucose uptake and shuts off gluconeogenesis in the liver. Because oxidative phosphorylation is inhibited, pyruvate is shunted to lactate instead of acetyl CoA in order to restore the NAD+ needed for glycolysis. If metformin levels get too high, the lactate can increase to clinically significant levels and cause metformin associated lactic acidosis (MALA). The greatest risk factor for MALA is impaired kidney function. The FDA recently relaxed use in certain patients with diminished kidney function based on its favorable safety profile. The prior contraindication of a serum creatinine ≥1.5mg/dL in males and ≥1.4mg/dL in females was updated to a genderless, GFR-based definition of <30mL/min. The FDA does not recommend starting metformin in patients with an eGFR of 30 to 45 mL/min, but does support continuing metformin if drug was started at an eGFR >45 mL/min and the patient's kidney function gradually declines to an eGFR 30 to 45 mL/min. However, kidney function should be monitored frequently. MALA is reversible with drug discontinuation and improvement of kidney function, but has been associated with fatalities. In cases of overdose, HD should be considered to remove metformin and correct the underlying acidosis.

20. **Are bath salts and spice associated with AKI?**
Bath salts, which are cathinones, contain 3,4-methylenedioxypyrovalerone and 4-methylcathinone (mephedrone), which give users a feeling of euphoria, alertness, and increased sexual arousal. AKI is reported with bath salts, most often due to pigment-associated ATN in the setting of rhabdomyolysis. It is unclear whether AKI results from a direct nephrotoxic drug effect, pigment-related tubular injury, or an ischemic tubular insult. Spice is a synthetic cannabinoid with clinical presentations ranging from euphoria to psychosis. The active ingredient, δ^9THC, binds to the cannabinoid receptor 1 in the central nervous system, modulating GABAergic and glutaminergic transmission. While there is variability in the type of AKI syndromes, the majority is due to ATN. Nearly 25% of AKI patients may need temporary dialysis. Urine metabolites may damage kidney tubules and cause AKI.

21. **What factors determine if a drug is effectively removed by extracorporeal therapies?**
There are clinical situations where an overdose or intoxication with certain drugs warrants removal with an extracorporeal therapy such as hemodialysis (HD) or continuous venovenous hemofiltration (CVH). Efficient drug removal by extracorporeal therapies is determined primarily by:
- Drug characteristics associated with efficient removal
  Small molecular weight ($<$10,000 Da)
  Limited protein binding ($<$50%)
  Small volume of distribution ($<$1.0 L/kg, which suggests the drug is limited to the plasma space or extracellular space)
  Water versus lipid solubility
- Dialyzer characteristics associated with efficient clearance
  Large surface membrane
  Large pore size
  High blood flow rates
  High dialysate flow rates

Examples of drugs efficiently removed by HD include the toxic alcohols, lithium, metformin, theophylline, and salicylates. CVVH is inferior to HD due to its low drug clearance, which is primarily determined by the lower blood flow rates and dialysate flow rates employed with this extracorporeal modality. CVVH does have a role to treat drug rebound following HD for drugs such as lithium, metformin, and methotrexate.

22. **What is the risk for development of AKI following exposure to IV and intraarterial contrast agents?**
Refer to Chapter 14 on Contrast-Induced Nephropathy

KEY POINTS

- Hypertension and proteinuria are the most common adverse effects on the kidneys of the antiangiogenesis inhibitors (bevacizumab, sorafenib, sunitinib), which target the vascular endothelial growth factor signaling pathway.
- The proton pump inhibitors are associated primarily with acute interstitial nephritis (AIN); however, less common adverse effects involving the kidneys include hyponatremia, impaired calcineurin inhibitor metabolism, and hypomagnesemia, and may increase the risk of incident chronic kidney disease.
- Checkpoint inhibitors (ipilimumab, nivolumab, pembrolizumab) are a group of antineoplastic agents aimed at activating a person's immune system to remove cancerous cells that can cause immune-mediated interstitial nephritis.
- Synthetic cannabinoids, also known as *spice*, is a drug of abuse that is associated with severe acute kidney injury related to acute tubular necrosis (ATN), AIN, and acute oxalate nephropathy.
- Bath salts, also called synthetic cathinones, are associated with ATN usually in the setting of rhabdomyolysis, although an exact mechanism of tubular injury has not been elucidated.
- BRAF (v-Raf murine sarcoma viral oncogene homolog B) is a protooncogene that, when mutated, leads to a variety of malignancies; hence BRAF inhibitors, vemurafenib and dabrafenib, are effective cancer treatment options but associated with AKI from ATN and electrolyte abnormalities, respectively.
- Crystalline-induced nephropathy can occur with a variety of medications (ciprofloxacin, sulfadiazine, acyclovir, methotrexate), and the management is primarily aimed at correcting volume deficits and creating a more soluble environment to prevent precipitation.

BIBLIOGRAPHY

American Diabetes Association. (2016). Standards of medical care in diabetes. *Diabetes Care*, *39*(suppl. 1), S1–S106.

Brewster, U. C., & Perazella, M. A. (2007). Proton pump inhibitors and the kidney: Critical review. *Clin Nephrol*, *68*, 65–72.

FDA Drug Safety Communication. (2017). FDA revises warnings regarding use of the diabetes medicine metformin in certain patients with reduced kidney function. https://www.fda.gov/Drugs/DrugSafety/ucm493244.htm. Accessed October 2, 2017.

Flory, J. H., & Hennessy, S. (2015). Metformin use reduction in mild to moderate renal impairment: Possible inappropriate curbing of use based on Food and Drug Administration contraindications. *JAMA Intern Med*, *175*(3), 458–459.

Gambaro, G., & Perazella, M. A. (2003). Adverse renal effects of anti-inflammatory agents: Evaluation of selective and nonselective cyclooxygenase inhibitors. *J Intern Med*, *253*, 643–652.

Ghannoum, M., Roberts, D. M., Hoffman, R. S., et al. (2014). A stepwise approach for the management of poisoning with extracorporeal treatments. *Semin Dial*, *27*(4), 362–370.

Gupta, A., Biyani, M., & Khaira, A. (2011). Vancomycin nephrotoxicity: Myths and facts. *Neth J Med*, *69*(9), 379–383.

Gurevich, F., & Perazella, M. A. (2009). Renal effects of anti-angiogenesis therapy: Update for the internist. *Am J Med*, *122*, 322–328.

Hayashi, T., Watanabe, Y., Kumano, K., et al. (1989). Protective effect of piperacillin against the nephrotoxicity of cisplatin in rats. *Antimicrob Agents Chemother*, *33*(4), 513–518.

Inzucchi, S. E., Lipska, K. J., Mayo, H., et al. (2014). Metformin in patients with type 2 diabetes and kidney disease, A systematic review. *JAMA*, *312*(24), 2668–2675.

Izzedine, H., Gueutin, V., Gharbi, C., et al. (2014). Kidney injuries related to ipilimumab. *Invest New Drugs*, *32*(4), 769–773.

Jensen, J. U. S., Hein, L., Lundgren, B., et al. (2012). The Procalcitonin and Survival Study (PASS) Group. Kidney failure related to broad-spectrum antibiotics in critically ill patients: Secondary end point results from a 1200 patients randomised trial. *BMJ Open*, *2*(2), e000635.

Kamel, M., & Thajudeen, B. A. (2015). Case of acute kidney injury and calcium oxalate deposition associated with synthetic cannabiniods. *Saudi J Kidney Dis Transpl*, *26*(4), 802–803.

Kazory, A., & Aiyer, R. (2013). Synthetic marijuana and acute kidney injury: An unforeseen association. *Clin Kidney J*, *6*, 330–333.

Komuro, M., Maeda, T., Kakuo, H., et al. (1994). Inhibition of renal excretion of tazobactam by piperacillin. *J Antimicrob Chemother*, *34*(4), 555–564.

Lalau, J. D. (2010). Lactic acidosis induced by metformin: Incidence, management and prevention. *Drug Saf*, *33*(9), 727–740.

Lazarus, B., Chen, Y., Wilson, F. P., et al. (2016). Proton pump inhibitor use and the risk of chronic kidney disease. *JAMA Intern Med*, *176*(2), 238–246.

Lee, L., Gupta, M., & Sahasranaman, S. (2016). Immune checkpoint inhibitors: An introduction to the next-generation cancer immunotherapy. *J Clin Pharmacol*, *56*(4), 157–169.

Luciano, R. L., & Perazella, M. A. (2014). Nephrotoxic effects of designer drugs: Synthetic is not better! *Nat Rev Nephrol*, *10*, 314–324.

Markowitz, G. S., & Perazella, M. A. (2005). Drug-induced renal failure: A focus on tubulointerstitial disease. *Clin Chim Acta*, *351*, 31–47.

Markowitz, G. S., & Perazella, M. A. (2009). Acute phosphate nephropathy. *Kidney Int*, *76*, 1027–1034. doi:10.1038/ki.2009.308.

Moledina, D. G., & Perazella, M. A. (2016). Proton pump inhibitors and CKD. *J Am Soc Nephrol*, *27*(10), 2926–2928.

Perazella, M. A. (2009). Renal vulnerability to drug toxicity. *Clin J Am Soc Nephrol*, *4*, 1275–1283.

Perazella, M. A., & Markowitz, G. S. (2008). Bisphosphonate nephrotoxicity. *Kidney Int*, *74*(11), 1385–1393.

Shirali, A. C., Perazella, M. A., & Gettinger, S. (2016). Association of acute interstitial nephritis with programmed cell death (PD)-1 inhibitor therapy in lung cancer patients. *AJKD*, *68*(2), 287–291.

van Hal, S. J., Paterson, D. L., & Lodise, T. P. (2013). Systemic review and meta-analysis of vancomycin-induced nephrotoxicity associated with dosing schedules that maintain troughs between 15 and 20 milligrams per liter. *Antimicrob Agents Chemother*, *57*(2), 734–744.

Wanchoo, R., Jhaveri, K. D., Deray, G., et al. (2016). Renal effects of BRAF inhibitors: A systematic review by the Cancer and the Kidney International Network. *Clin Kidney J*, *9*(2), 245–251.

Wyman, J. F., Lavins, E. S., Engelhart, D., et al. (2013). Postmortem tissue distribution of MDPV following lethal intoxication by "bath salts." *J Anal Toxicol*, *37*(3), 182–185.

Xie, Y., Bowe, B., Li, T., et al. (2016). Proton pump inhibitors and risk of incident CKD and progression to ESRD. *J Am Soc Nephrol*, *27*, 1–11.

Yarlagadda, S. G., & Perazella, M. A. (2008). Drug-induced crystal nephropathy: An update. *Expert Opin Drug Saf*, *7*(2), 147–158.

CHAPTER 11

SEPSIS

Mitchell H. Rosner

1. How is sepsin associated acute kidney injury (SA-AKI) defined?

   SA-AKI is characterized by the simultaneous presence of AKI (based on a nonconsensus definition such as the Acute Kidney Injury Network [AKIN] or Kidney Disease Improving Global Outcomes [KDIGO] criteria; see Chapter 10) and the 2016 consensus criteria for sepsis (defined as life-threatening organ dysfunction caused by a dysregulated response to infection). Causes of AKI not related to sepsis (e.g., nephrotoxic drugs or rhabdomyolysis) should be ruled out. However, there is no standardized method for distinguishing SA-AKI from other causes of AKI, and in many cases the cause of AKI may be multifactorial and thus difficult to attribute to sepsis.

2. What are the key epidemiologic aspects of AKI in the setting of sepsis?

   Sepsis is common among intensive care unit (ICU) patients with a prevalence ranging from 8.2% to 35.3% of all ICU patients. Sepsis is becoming more common. A recent large study in the United States showed an increase of 8.7% of sepsis as the primary diagnosis from the previous year. However, the overall sepsis-associated mortality rate appears to be decreasing (between 18% and 25%). Sepsis is associated with significant deleterious effects on outcomes:
   • Extended mechanical ventilation
   • Prolonged hospitalization
   • Secondary infections
   • Increased long-term mortality

   Although the etiology of AKI in patients who are critically ill is often multifactorial, sepsis has consistently been found to be an important, if not the most important, contributing factor. Several studies have shown that approximately 40% to 50% of patients with AKI on presentation to an ICU have concomitant sepsis and that up to 64% of patients who are critically ill with a diagnosis of severe sepsis or septic shock have concomitant AKI.

3. Does the degree of sepsis determine the incidence and severity of AKI?

   In contrast to AKI, sepsis syndrome has benefited from the development of a consensus-driven standardized definition for more than 20 years. This definition was modified to reflect advances in the pathobiology, management, and epidemiology of sepsis. In this new schema, sepsis is defined as "life-threatening organ dysfunction caused by a dysregulated host response to infection." Organ dysfunction is best identified as an acute change in the total Sequential Organ Failure Assessment score ≥ 2 points, which reflects an overall mortality risk of approximately 10%. Septic shock is the most severe form of sepsis with profound cellular, metabolic, and hemodynamic abnormalities that include hypotension (requiring vasopressors), as well as elevated serum lactate levels. Septic shock is associated with mortality rates over 40%.

   While there are no studies assessing the incidence of AKI utilizing the new definition of sepsis, prior studies have shown that there is a stepwise increase in the severity of AKI in patients who are stratified by the severity of sepsis. For instance, in one study, the incidence and severity of AKI, defined by the AKIN criteria, increased markedly when stratified by sepsis severity. Furthermore, as patients progress from sepsis to severe sepsis to septic shock, the incidence of AKI that requires dialysis also increased. See Table 11.1.

   Definitions:
   • **Sepsis**: criteria for systemic inflammatory response syndrome (SIRS) with suspected or present source of infection. SIRS criteria:
     • Temperature $>38°C$ or $<36°C$
     • Heart rate $>90/min$
     • Respiratory rate $>20/min$ or $PaCO_2 < 32$ mm Hg
     • White blood cell count $>12,000/mm^3$, $<4000/mm^3$ or $>10\%$ bands
   • **Severe Sepsis**: sepsis plus organ dysfunction, hypotension, or hypoperfusion as defined by:
     • Lactic acidosis
     • Systolic blood pressure <90
     • Systolic blood pressure drop ≥ 40 mm Hg of normal
   • **Septic Shock**: severe sepsis with hypotension despite adequate fluid resuscitation

Table 11.1. Incidence of Acute Kidney Injury That Requires Dialysis

	INCIDENCE OF AKI	AKI REQUIRING DIALYSIS
Sepsis	4.2%	24%
Severe sepsis	22.7%	39%
Septic shock	52.8%	89%

AKI, Acute kidney injury.

4. **What is the timing of AKI resulting from sepsis?**
AKI in sepsis is usually evident at the time of ICU admission or develops early in the illness course. In a multicenter study of patients who were critically ill presenting with septic shock, investigators found 64% had AKI within 24 hours of developing shock.

5. **When should physiologic derangements in sepsis be corrected?**
In 2001, a seminal paper from Rivers et al. demonstrated that timely intervention, called "early goal-directed therapy" (EGDT), for the treatment of severe sepsis and septic shock improved outcomes. In particular, treatment goals for improving tissue oxygenation, such as central venous pressure (CVP), mean arterial blood pressure (MAP), central venous oxygen saturation (ScvO$_2$), and blood lactate concentration, were achieved as a protocolized bundle within 6 hours after presentation. These measures were codified as the surviving sepsis care bundles:
a. To be completed within 3 hours:
   i. Measure lactate level
   ii. Obtain blood cultures prior to administration of antibiotics
   iii. Administer broad-spectrum antibiotics
   iv. Administer 30 mL/kg crystalloid solutions for hypotension or serum lactate ≥4 mmol/L
b. To be completed within 6 hours:
   i. Add vasopressors (for hypotension refractory to initial fluid resuscitation) to maintain MAP ≥ 65 mm Hg
   ii. In the event of persistent arterial hypotension despite volume resuscitation (shock) or initial serum lactate ≥4 mmol/L:
      1. Measure CVP with goal of ≥8 mm Hg
      2. Measure ScvO$_2$ with a goal of ≥70%
   iii. Re-measure serum lactate if initial serum lactate was elevated (goal is normalization of lactate)
      Since the institution of this bundle, the prognosis for patients with sepsis has improved, and one study demonstrated a fall in in-hospital mortality of 59%. However, in 2014, two studies (the PROCESS and ARISE studies) raised uncertainties regarding the efficacy of protocol-based EGDT in contributing to improvements in mortality. In the ARISE study, in critically ill patients presenting to the emergency department with early septic shock, EGDT did not reduce all-cause mortality at 90 days. In the PROCESS study, protocol-based resuscitation of patients in whom septic shock was diagnosed in the emergency department did not improve outcomes as well. A third study in 2015 reached a similar conclusion that EGDT did not lead to improvements in outcome but was also associated with increased costs. Importantly, in all three of these studies, the majority of patients met the goals of the 3-hour bundle, highlighting the importance of rapid antibiotic administration and fluid resuscitation, and downgrading the benefits of hemodynamic targets, such as CVP and ScvO$_2$.

6. **What is the role of resuscitation strategies on the incidence of AKI in patients with septic shock?**
In the ProCESS trial, the development of AKI was common (approximately 38%) and was not influenced by protocolized resuscitation compared with usual care. Furthermore, the duration of AKI and the need for dialysis did not differ between the protocolized care and usual care groups. Of note, 60-day hospital mortality was 6.2% for patients without AKI, 16.8% for those with stage 1, and 27.7% for stages 2 to 3. Thus, while AKI is common in patients with septic shock and is associated with significant mortality, its rates and outcomes do not appear to be influenced by resuscitation protocols.

7. **Is there an optimal fluid management approach for patients with AKI and sepsis?**
Several studies have addressed whether various intravenous fluids are superior to one another in the treatment of patients with sepsis. These trials have compared albumin, normal (0.9%) saline, various starches, and a balanced pH solution (such as lactated ringers or in various combinations). The bottom

line from trials is that volume expansion with normal (0.9%) saline is either associated with similar if not better outcomes than other intravenous solutions. Of note, the various starch solutions have been associated with an increased incidence of AKI and poor outcomes, and should be avoided. Thus, a reasonable initial approach for volume resuscitation in the patient with sepsis is to initiate therapy with intravenous normal (0.9%) saline, and if the patient develops a metabolic acidosis associated with a high chloride load, then switch to a more balanced pH solution, such as Lactated Ringer's.

8. **What are the demographic characteristics of AKI resulting from sepsis?**
   Observational data have found SA-AKI occurs more commonly among elderly patients and females when compared with non-septic AKI. Patients with SA-AKI are also more likely to have a higher burden of preexisting comorbid disease when compared with patients with non-septic AKI. In particular, patients with SA-AKI have a higher prevalence of congestive heart failure, chronic obstructive pulmonary disease, chronic kidney disease (CKD), liver disease, diabetes mellitus, active malignancy, and immune system compromise. Positive blood cultures are associated with a significantly higher risk of developing AKI (37% vs. 29%) and delays in administering antibiotics further increase the risk of developing AKI.

   Patients with SA-AKI have been shown across a range of observational studies to have higher rates of oliguria, despite having received more fluid therapy and/or diuretic therapy when compared with patients with non-septic AKI or those with sepsis only. Consequently, these patients are more likely to accumulate fluid and develop a positive fluid balance early in their clinical course. Data have accumulated to suggest significant fluid accumulation is associated with worse clinical outcome in patients who are critically ill with AKI and should be avoided.

9. **What are the hemodynamic factors that play a role in the development of septic AKI?**
   - In SA-AKI, multiple and overlapping mechanisms lead to AKI. These include: alterations in systemic and kidney hemodynamics, cellular injury, and immune and inflammatory mediator-induced injury.
   - Hemodynamically, sepsis is associated with decreased peripheral vascular resistance, maldistribution of tissue blood flow, and profound abnormalities in the microcirculation. These abnormalities lead to a heterogeneous distribution of tubular cell injury that can be quite variable in severity. Mechanistically, several mechanisms contribute to alterations in regional renal blood flow: (1) increases in renal vascular resistance; (2) capillary (micro-circulatory) occlusion due to platelet activation, fibrin deposition, and leukocyte aggregation along with endothelial cell swelling; (3) increases in vascular permeability that within an encapsulated organ, such as the kidney, which lead to interstitial edema, venous congestion, and alterations in transmural pressures; (4) changes in nitric oxide production; and (5) imbalances between vasodilators and vasoconstrictors resulting in more pronounced vasoconstriction and redistribution of regional blood flow

10. **What are the non-hemodynamic factors that occur in sepsis that can lead to AKI?**
    a. Inflammatory mediators (cytokines [such as interleukin-6 and -10], vasoactive substances, arachidonic acid metabolites) are released during sepsis and may have a significant pathogenic role.
    b. Apoptosis (programmed cell death) occurs in response to immune-mediated cell injury. In contrast, tubular necrosis caused by ischemia also happens in sepsis. There is now good evidence to show that human kidney tubular cells die by apoptosis and necrosis in experimental models of acute ischemic and toxic kidney injury.
    c. Endothelial cell dysfunction may also lead to ischemia.
    d. Activation of coagulation pathways may impair renal microcirculatory blood flow.
    e. Reactive oxygen species, proteases, elastases, myeloperoxidase, and other enzymes are released from activated immune cells and damage tubular cells.

11. **What are the histopathologic findings associated with AKI resulting from sepsis?**
    There is no consistent or typical kidney histopathologic pattern, and the fall in glomerular filtration rate (GFR) is often much greater than would be anticipated from the bland histology observed. In part, this is a result of a lack of data, because kidney biopsies are not typically performed in these critically ill patients. Acute tubular necrosis may be seen in some cases and is simply the end-result of overlapping ischemic and immune-mediated injury to the tubules.

12. **What are the urinary findings in AKI resulting from sepsis?**
    The urinary findings are highly variable in this setting. Studies have shown either a high or low fractional excretion of sodium or urea and either high or low urinary osmolalities. This wide range of findings likely reflects the timing of the urine studies in relation to the amount of irreversible injury versus hemodynamic factors (i.e., the fractional excretion of sodium may be initially low when the mechanism of AKI results from vasoconstriction but may be elevated in the setting of tubular injury).

The most common findings on urine microscopic examination are granular ("muddy brown") casts that represent shedding and degradation of tubular cells. However, the absence of these casts does not exclude the diagnosis of AKI.

13. **What are the outcomes associated with sepsis-associated AKI?**
Patients with septic AKI have a mortality rate of approximately 70% compared to 20% for patients with severe sepsis, or 49% for patients with septic shock in the absence of AKI. In addition, septic AKI is an independent predictor of hospital death. AKI is associated with a doubling in the length of ICU stays.

14. **What are the clinical factors in patients with septic AKI associated with worse outcomes?**
    a. Older age
    b. Higher acuity of disease
    c. Greater burden of illness
    d. Longer stays in ICU and hospital
    e. AKI severity as defined by the RIFLE criteria
    f. Delay in the initiation of appropriate antimicrobial therapy
    g. Positive fluid balance

15. **What is the therapy of AKI resulting from sepsis?**
Currently, there are no specific therapies for either prevention or treatment of septic AKI. However, it is critically important that appropriate and timely supportive care be delivered. This includes the following:
    a. Rapid fluid resuscitation to ensure adequate blood pressure and organ perfusion
    b. Appropriate use of vasopressors to ensure adequate blood pressure and organ perfusion
    c. Timely administration of antimicrobials
    d. Avoidance of nephrotoxic exposures, such as intravenous contrast or nonsteroidal anti-inflammatory drugs
    e. Timely initiation of dialysis in patients with oliguria, positive fluid balance, and signs of irreversible kidney injury or with metabolic derangements (hyperkalemia and metabolic acidosis) that cannot be treated with non-dialysis therapies. The exact timing for the initiation of dialysis remains controversial.
    Novel therapies that target specific pathogenic pathways are being actively studied in animal models and offer promise for future human use.

16. **In patients who develop AKI from sepsis, what is the rate of recovery of kidney function?**
Recovery of kidney function is increasingly recognized as an important determinant of morbidity with long-term health resource implications. Data have suggested that kidney recovery and independence from dialysis may be greater in septic compared with nonseptic AKI. In the BEST Kidney study (a large multicenter study of patients with AKI), in survivors to hospital discharge with normal baseline kidney function, 5.7% of septic AKI compared with 7.8% of nonseptic AKI were dialysis dependent. However, in patients with preexisting CKD, recovery to dialysis independence trended lower in septic compared with non-septic AKI (16.7% vs. 24.7%, $P = .28$). Another study found 95.7% of patients with septic AKI had complete kidney function recovery occurring on average 10.1 ± 8 days after hospital discharge. It is important to note that patients with SA-AKI who do recover kidney function may be left with residual kidney damage and are at high risk of future CKD. Thus, SA-AKI patients should be closely followed by a nephrologist to monitor for CKD and partial recovery.

17. **What, if any, is the role of serum or urine biomarkers in detecting SA-AKI?**
A concern among nephrologists has been that rises in serum creatinine occur relatively late (at least 24 to 48 hours) after the kidney injury from sepsis or other causes. This late diagnosis may compromise the ability of clinicians to rapidly intervene with strategies that could protect the kidneys from further damage. Thus, a series of serum and urine biomarkers that can detect early stages of small degrees of kidney injury have been investigated. Only one panel of urine biomarkers has yet to meet Federal Drug Administration (FDA) approval criteria for risk stratification of patients for AKI: a combination of urinary tissue inhibitor of metalloproteinase-2 and insulin-like growth factor binding protein-7. A combination level of these two biomarkers has a relatively strong predictive ability to tell whether a patient will develop moderate to severe AKI within 12 hours. However, it is not yet known whether care protocols based upon this risk score will lead to improved outcomes, and the routine use of biomarkers for the detection of early AKI has not yet gained clinical acceptance.

KEY POINTS

1. Several studies have shown that approximately 40% to 50% of patients with acute kidney injury (AKI) on presentation to an intensive care unit have concomitant sepsis and that up to 64% of patients who are critically ill with a diagnosis of severe sepsis or septic shock have concomitant AKI (also known as sepsis-associated AKI [SA-AKI]).
2. AKI resulting from sepsis occurs early in the course of the disease. Of patients presenting with septic shock, investigators found 64% had evidence of AKI, defined by the RIFLE criteria, within 24 hours of the onset of sepsis.
3. Physiologic derangements resulting from sepsis need to be corrected as early as possible utilizing goal-directed therapy. Normal saline is a reasonable initial fluid choice and rapid administration of appropriate antibiotics is associated with improved outcomes.
4. Patients with septic AKI have a mortality rate of approximately 70% compared to 20% for patients with severe sepsis, or 49% for patients with septic shock in the absence of AKI.
5. Patients recovering from SA-AKI are at risk for long-term chronic kidney disease and should be followed by a nephrologist once discharged from the hospital.

BIBLIOGRAPHY

ARISE Investigators, ANZICS Clinical Trials Group, Peake, S. L., Delaney, A., Bailey, M., . . . Williams, P. (2014). Goal-directed resuscitation for patients with early septic shock. *New England Journal of Medicine, 371,* 1496–1506.

Bagshaw, S. M., Uchino, S., Bellomo, R., Morimatsu, H., Morgera, S., Schetz, M., . . . Beginning and Ending Supportive Therapy for the Kidney (BEST Kidney) Investigators. (2007). Septic acute kidney injury in critically ill patients: Clinical characteristics and outcomes. *Clinical Journal of the American Society of Nephrology, 2,* 431–439.

Hoste, E. A., Lameire, N. H., Vanholder, R. C., Benoit, D. D., Decruyenaere, J. M., & Colardyn, F. A. (2003). Acute renal failure in patients with sepsis in a surgical ICU: Predictive factors, incidence, comorbidity, and outcome. *Journal of the American Society of Nephrology, 14,* 1022–1030.

Jiang, L., Jiang, S., Zhang, M., Zheng, Z., & Ma, Y. (2017). Albumin versus other fluids for fluid resuscitation in patients with sepsis: A meta-analysis. *PLoS One, 9,* e114666. doi:10.1371/journal.pone.0114666.

Kashani, K., Al-Khafaji, A., Ardiles, T., Artigas, A., Bagshaw, S. M., Bell, M., . . . Kellum, J. A. (2013). Discovery and validation of cell cycle arrest biomarkers in human acute kidney injury. *Critical Care, 17,* R25.

Kellum, J. A., Chawla, L. S., Keener, C., Singbartl, K., Palevsky, P. M., Pike, F. L., . . . ProCESS and ProGReSS-AKI Investigators. (2016). The effects of alternative resuscitation strategies on acute kidney injury in patients with septic shock. *American Journal of Respiratory and Critical Care Medicine, 193,* 281–287.

Langenberg, C., Bagshaw, S. M., May, C. N., & Bellomo, R. (2008). The histopathology of septic acute kidney injury: A systematic review. *Critical Care, 12*(2), R38.

Lopes, J. A., Jorge, S., Resina, C., Santos, C., Pereira, A., Neves, J., . . . Prata, M. M. (2009). Acute kidney injury in patients with sepsis: A contemporary analysis. *International Journal of Infectious Diseases, 13,* 176–181.

Marik, P. E. (2014). Early management of severe sepsis: Concepts and controversies. *Chest, 145,* 1407–1418.

Marshall, J. C., Vincent, J. L., Fink, M. P., Cook, D. J., Rubenfeld, G., Foster, D., . . . Reinhart, K. (2003). Measures, markers, and mediators: Toward a staging system for clinical sepsis. A report of the Fifth Toronto Sepsis Roundtable, Toronto, Ontario, Canada, October 25–26, 2000. *Critical Care Medicine, 31,* 1560–1567.

McCullough, P. A., Shaw, A. D., Haase, M., Bouchard, J., Waikar, S. S., Siew, E. D., . . . Ronco, C. (2013). Diagnosis of acute kidney injury using functional and injury biomarkers: Workgroup statements from the tenth acute dialysis quality initiative consensus conference. *Contributions to Nephrology, 182,* 13–29.

Mouncey, P. R., Osborn, T. M., Power, G. S., Harrison, D. A., Sadique, M. Z., Grieve, R. D., . . . ProMISe Trial Investigators. (2015). Trial of early, goal-directed resuscitation for septic shock. *New England Journal of Medicine, 372,* 1301–1311.

ProCESS Investigators, Yealy, D. M., Kellum, J. A., Huang, D. T., Barnato, A. E., Weissfeld, L., . . . Angus, D. C. (2014). A randomized trial of protocol-based care for early septic shock. *New England Journal of Medicine, 370,* 1683–1693.

Ricci, Z., & Ronco C. (2009). Pathogenensis of acute kidney injury during sepsis. *Current Drug Targets, 10,* 1179–1183.

Rivers, E., Nguyen, B., Havstad, S., Ressler, J., Muzzin, A., Knoblich, B., . . . Early Goal-Directed Therapy Collaborative Group. (2001). Early goal-directed therapy in the treatment of severe sepsis and septic shock. *New England Journal of Medicine, 345,* 1368–1377.

Rochwerg, B., Alhazzani, W., Sindi, A., Heels-Ansdell, D., Thabane, L., Fox-Robichaud, A., . . . Fluids in Sepsis and Septic Shock Group. (2014). Fluid resuscitation in sepsis: a systematic review and network meta-analysis. *Annals of Internal Medicine, 161,* 347–355.

Singer, M., Deutschman, C. S., Seymour, C. W., Shankar-Hari, M., Annane, D., Bauer, M., . . . Angus, D. C. (2016). The third international consensus definitions for sepsis and septic shock (sepsis-3). *Journal of the American Medical Association, 315,* 801–810.

RHABDOMYOLYSIS

Scott D. Bieber and Jonathan Ashley Jefferson

CHAPTER 12

1. **What is rhabdomyolysis?**
   Rhabdomyolysis is a condition characterized by muscle injury leading to myocyte necrosis and the release of intracellular contents into the circulation. The term is usually applied when acute kidney injury (AKI) results from the muscle injury, but AKI does not always occur, even following severe muscle injury.

2. **How does rhabdomyolysis cause AKI?**
   Rhabdomyolysis causes AKI through a combination of kidney vasoconstriction, direct oxidant injury, and tubular obstruction.
   - **Kidney vasoconstriction:** Muscle damage causes interstitial edema at the site of injury. The fluid shift from the intravascular space leads to activation of the renin-angiotensin-aldosterone system (RAAS) and sympathetic nervous system. Vasoconstrictor mediators including endothelin-1, thromboxane-A2, tumor necrosis factor-α, and F2-isoprostanes are also upregulated. The binding of nitric oxide to myoglobin may further contribute to vasoconstriction. The net result is early and prolonged kidney vasoconstriction, which may manifest as oliguria with a low urine sodium concentration prior to progression to acute tubular injury.
   - **Oxidant injury:** Free iron released from myoglobin may lead to the formation of oxygen-free radicals as ferrous iron is converted to ferric iron (Fenton reaction). Myoglobin itself has been found to be directly toxic to tubular cells by causing lipid peroxidation of tubular cellular membranes.
   - **Tubular obstruction:** Under normal conditions, small amounts of myoglobin are filtered, then endocytosed and metabolized by proximal tubular cells. When myoglobin levels in the tubules exceed the absorptive capacity of the proximal tubular cells, myoglobin may complex with Tamm-Horsfall protein (THP) in the distal nephron to form casts leading to intra-tubular obstruction. An acidic environment (urine pH < 6.5) favors the formation of these complexes.

3. **What are some of the common causes of rhabdomyolysis?**
   Rhabdomyolysis may be caused by a wide range of conditions (Table 12.1). Trauma or direct muscle injury is the most common cause and should be considered in any patient who presents with multiple injuries/trauma.

4. **How does alcohol intoxication contribute to rhabdomyolysis?**
   Alcohol is directly toxic to myocytes (and also proximal tubular cells). Alcoholics are often phosphorus, magnesium, and potassium depleted:
   - Hypokalemia impairs the ability of muscle arterioles to vasodilate, promoting ischemic muscle injury.
   - Hypomagnesemia can worsen concurrent hypokalemia.
   - Phosphorus deficiency may result from poor diet, the use of phosphorus-binding medications used for gastrointestinal upset, and urinary phosphorus wasting. Phosphorus is critical in the production of adenosine triphosphate (ATP) and multiple cellular enzymes. Furthermore, alcohol intoxication leading to altered mental status may result in compressive injuries from trauma or to muscle injury from prolonged motionlessness in unconscious individuals.

5. **Do statins cause rhabdomyolysis?**
   Yes. 3-hydroxy-3-methylglutaryl-coenzyme A (HMG-CoA) reductase inhibitors (statins) are commonly associated with mild myositis and, rarely, can progress to severe rhabdomyolysis. This may be more common in those who have other risk factors or with drug–drug interactions that increase statin levels (e.g., calcineurin inhibitors, macrolide antibiotics, antifungals). It has been suggested that statins cause muscle cell damage by inhibiting coenzyme Q and the electron transport chain, interfering with ATP generation. Statin-induced myositis can occur within days of starting the drug but has been described years later. Muscle pain is a common reason to discontinue statin use.

6. **Can you get rhabdomyolysis from excessive exercise?**
   Yes. Exercise-induced muscle injury typically occurs in cases of vigorous exercise, such as in marathon runners or weight lifters. Strenuous exercise may cause thermal injury to the muscle cells combined

Table 12.1. Common Causes of Rhabdomyolysis

CAUSE	EXAMPLES
Trauma related/crush injury	Motor vehicle accidents, falls, workplace accidents, earthquakes
Vascular occlusion	Thrombosis, embolism, vessel clamping during surgery, malfunctioning endovascular stents
Muscular strain	Exercise induced, seizures, delirium tremens
Toxins/drugs	Alcohol, HMG-CoA reductase inhibitors, barbiturates, corticosteroids, colchicine, fibrates, isoniazid, zidovudine, amphotamines, ecstasy, opiates, cocaine, neuroleptic malignant syndrome
Infection	Viral: Influenza, human immunodeficiency virus, Epstein-Barr virus, legionella, polio, coxsackievirus Bacterial: Streptococcus, Staphylococcus, toxic shock syndrome
Electrolyte disorders	Hypokalemia, hypophosphatemia, hypocalcemia
Inherited disorders of metabolism	Carnitine palmitoyl transferase II deficiency, phosphofructokinase deficiency, myophosphorylase deficiency (McArdle), coenzyme Q10 deficiency, myoadenylate deaminase deficiency
Autoimmune	Polymyositis, dermatomyositis
Others	Hyperthermia, hypothermia, electrical injury

with ATP depletion. Hypokalemia and volume depletion may also play a role. High temperature and humidity conditions put athletes at increased risk for exercise-induced rhabdomyolysis. Inherited disorders of muscle metabolism may be present in those with recurrent episodes of exercise-induced rhabdomyolysis.

7. **Why do some people develop recurrent episodes of rhabdomyolysis?**
   Behavioral issues should be explored in patients with recurrent rhabdomyolysis. Often recurrent episodes of rhabdomyolysis are linked to alcohol and substance abuse. Toxicology screening can be useful to identify drug or alcohol ingestions as a cause of recurrent muscle injury. The athlete who is abusing diuretics or laxatives is another example. In the latter setting, the combination of strenuous exercise with concurrent diuretic- or laxative-induced hypokalemia can lead to muscle injury.
   Less frequently, patients with recurrent episodes of rhabdomyolysis have underlying inherited disorders of cell metabolism (see Table 12.1). These disorders impair cellular energetics as a result of abnormalities in carbohydrate or lipid metabolism. Usually, patients with inherited metabolic myopathies present in childhood, but adult presentation also occurs. The most common inherited disorder causing rhabdomyolysis is carnitine palmitoyltransferase deficiency. Often these inherited disorders of metabolism present with a concurrent precipitating factor, such as strenuous exercise or infection.

8. **Do the creatine kinase (CK) or myoglobin levels help with the diagnosis of rhabdomyolysis?**
   Creatine kinase (CK) or creatine phosphokinase (CPK) and myoglobin are present in muscle cells and are released into the circulation in large quantities in the presence of significant muscle injury. The main role of CK is to catalyze the formation of phosphocreatine from creatine. In muscle cells, phosphocreatine serves as a store for high-energy phosphates, which can be transferred to adenosine diphosphate (ADP) when extra adenosine triphosphate (ATP) is needed. Myoglobin is an iron- and oxygen-containing molecule found in muscle cells that is structurally similar to hemoglobin and functions to carry oxygen in muscle tissue.

9. **Should I check CK (CPK) levels or myoglobin levels when diagnosing and following patients with rhabdomyolysis?**
   CK levels are the most sensitive marker of muscle injury. Normal CK levels can go as high as 400 U/L. In muscle injury, CK levels tend to rise in the first 12 hours and peak in 1 to 3 days, with levels remaining elevated for up to 5 days after resolution of the muscle injury. CK levels correlate with the degree of muscle injury and may correlate with the risk of AKI. The risk of developing AKI is usually low when the CK level is below 10,000 U/L. Persons who develop AKI at lower levels of CK often have coexisting conditions predisposing them to AKI, such as sepsis, hypotension, or underlying chronic kidney disease.

Myoglobin levels rise rapidly (within 3 hours) and serum levels peak prior to serum CK levels. Myoglobin has a short half-life of 2 to 3 hours and is rapidly excreted by the kidneys. Rapid and unpredictable metabolism makes serum myoglobin a less useful marker of muscle injury than CK, and is rarely used in assessing the risk of AKI.

10. **What are the clinical features of rhabdomyolysis?**
The clinical features of rhabdomyolysis are variable depending on the underlying cause and extent of the muscle injury. Patients usually complain of myalgias and may have associated muscle weakness. Blood pressure in rhabdomyolysis is usually maintained secondary to vasoconstriction, in part because of the sequestration of nitric oxide by free myoglobin. Affected muscles may be tender, sometimes with marked stiffness and swelling. The large muscles of the leg and lower back are most commonly involved. Sometimes muscle swelling within a myofascial compartment may compress blood vessels, limiting local blood supply, leading to further muscle ischemia. This is known as compartment syndrome and requires urgent surgical intervention (fasciotomy) to prevent ongoing ischemic muscle damage. The measurement of intramuscular pressures can be used to help guide decisions regarding the need for surgical intervention. Note that less severe rhabdomyolysis may be asymptomatic and may be detected only on routine laboratory testing.

11. **How do I know when an intervention is necessary for compartment syndrome causing rhabdomyolysis?**
Compartment pressures greater than 30 mm Hg are usually associated with muscle ischemia and may require surgical intervention. Fasciotomy should be performed emergently if intramuscular pressures are greater than 50 mm Hg or remain above 30 mm Hg for 6 hours.

12. **What can I expect to happen to urine output in a patient with rhabdomyolysis?**
In severe rhabdomyolysis, the patient is typically oliguric and may demonstrate the classic "tea-colored" urine secondary to myoglobinuria.

13. **What is the differential diagnosis in a patient with reddish-brown urine?**
The differential diagnosis for red-brown urine is broad. Most cases involve the presence of heme pigment in the urine, or food or drugs that alter the color of the urine. Some of the more common causes of red-brown urine are as follows:
- Heme pigment: Gross hematuria, hemoglobinuria, myoglobinuria, bile pigments, porphyria
- Foods: Beets, rhubarb, food coloring, fava beans, blackberries
- Drugs: Rifampin, phenolphthalein, vitamin B_{12}, phenytoin, deferoxamine, doxorubicin, chloroquine, methyldopa, levodopa, metronidazole, nitrofurantoin, iron sorbitol

14. **How does the urinalysis help in the diagnosis of rhabdomyolysis?**
The urinalysis (dipstick) detects both heme pigments (free hemoglobin, myoglobin) and hemoglobin within red blood cells. In rhabdomyolysis, the urinalysis will be positive for heme (myoglobin) but urine microscopy will not show red blood cells.

15. **What laboratory abnormalities are commonly seen in patients with rhabdomyolysis?**
Common laboratory findings in rhabdomyolysis include an increase in muscle enzyme levels (e.g., creatinine kinase), hyperkalemia, hypocalcemia, hyperphosphatemia, hyperuricemia, and an anion gap acidosis. Potassium and phosphorus are released from damaged muscle cells into the circulation as muscle cells are lysed. If muscle injury is coupled with AKI, the excretion of potassium and phosphorus by the kidneys is further impaired.

By contrast, calcium levels in rhabdomyolysis are typically decreased as calcium precipitates in injured muscle and occasionally massive heterotropic calcification occurs. High phosphorus levels contribute to hypocalcemia by directly binding free calcium and inhibiting 1aa-hydroxylase (the enzyme that catalyzes the conversion of 25-hydroxycholecalciferol to 1,25-dihydroxycholecalciferol, the active form of vitamin D).

An anion gap metabolic acidosis is seen from the combination of anaerobic respiration in hypoxic muscles (lactic acidosis) and the accumulation of organic acids from AKI. Elevated uric acid levels are a direct result of the release of purine nucleosides from degrading muscle cells. It should be noted that a low urine pH promotes the formation of tubular myoglobin casts and uric acid crystals, both of which can lead to tubular obstruction in the development of AKI.

16. **How do we prevent kidney injury in patients with rhabdomyolysis?**
The treatment of rhabdomyolysis should be specific to the patient and to the underlying etiology of muscle injury. Reversal of the underlying cause of muscle injury is of paramount importance.

Volume resuscitation is the key initial therapy in patients with crush syndrome and trauma. Ideally, patients with crush syndrome should be started on intravenous fluids prior to extraction or relief of the compressive injury. Severe muscle injuries may also require surgical intervention, such as amputation or fasciotomy for compartment syndrome.

The amount of fluid administered should be tailored to the patient and take into account the underlying etiology of muscle injury. In traumatic crush injury cases, 1 to 2 L of isotonic saline should be given as a bolus prior to extraction. Caution should be utilized in giving excess IV fluid hydration if the patient is oliguric or anuric at presentation. Patients with traumatic muscle injury or large fluid losses may require 10 to 15 L per day of fluid resuscitation, titrating to a urine output of 200 to 300 mL/hr. The use of chloride-restrictive solutions (e.g., Lactated Ringer's solution) have been proposed but not studied in this setting. By comparison, it is inadvisable to administer large amounts of fluid to an elderly patient with heart failure and statin-related rhabdomyolysis.

17. **Should sodium bicarbonate or mannitol or diuretics be given to prevent kidney injury in rhabdomyolysis?**
Urinary alkalinization in animal models has been shown to increase the solubility of the myoglobin-THP complex and inhibit reduction-oxidation cycling of myoglobin and lipid peroxidation. Some experts advocate for the administration intravenous sodium bicarbonate (aiming for a urine pH greater than 6.5), in addition to volume expansion with normal saline. However, alkalinization may lower serum ionized calcium levels as a result of enhanced binding to albumin (but not change total calcium) in patients who are already hypocalcemic. Retrospective studies have shown that bicarbonate administration does not improve outcomes with regard to kidney failure, the need for dialysis, or mortality in most patients, although there may be benefit in the subgroup with severe rhabdomyolysis (CK level >30,000 U/L).

Loop diuretics may increase urinary flow but have not been shown to protect against AKI. Mannitol is an osmotic diuretic and a weak free-radical scavenger. Unfortunately, mannitol may worsen AKI by causing osmotic nephrosis and can accumulate if the urine output falls; it is now rarely used. Notably, any diuretic therapy should be limited to patients who have been resuscitated and are volume replete.

18. **How should electrolyte abnormalities be managed in rhabdomyolysis?**
Hyperkalemia in rhabdomyolysis should be managed in a similar fashion to hyperkalemia from other causes (see Chapter 77). However, the potassium load may be very large, and patients who receive dialysis for hyperkalemia may develop post-dialysis "rebound" hyperkalemia, so potassium should be monitored frequently, even after dialysis.

Serum calcium levels often decline early, but replacing calcium may exacerbate muscle calcium deposition and can lead to rebound hypercalcemia as the calcium leaves myocytes during the recovery period. Indications for calcium replacement include symptomatic hypocalcemia (e.g., seizures, tetany), ionized serum calcium <0.8 mmol/L, and severe hyperkalemia with electrocardiogram changes. High phosphorus levels in rhabdomyolysis are difficult to manage and usually respond poorly oral PO_4 binder medications. As muscle injury resolves and kidney injury improves, hyperphosphatemia usually resolves.

19. **When is dialysis indicated in the treatment of rhabdomyolysis?**
Indications for dialysis in AKI from rhabdomyolysis are similar to those in other forms of AKI. Life-threatening hyperkalemia, refractory acidosis, and volume overload are standard indications for renal replacement therapy in rhabdomyolysis. The clearance of myoglobin using conventional intermittent hemodialysis or continuous therapies, such as continuous venovenous hemofiltration, continuous venovenous hemodiafiltration, or slow extended daily dialysis, is low and currently does not have a role in the prevention of AKI in rhabdomyolysis. Super-high-flux dialyzers have increased myoglobin clearance; however, their role in the treatment or prevention of AKI remains unclear.

KEY POINTS

1. Early and vigorous volume resuscitation of patients with rhabdomyolysis (even prior to extrication in crush syndrome) is the key to preventing acute kidney injury (AKI).
2. Serum creatine kinase levels correlate with the degree of muscle injury and help predict the risk of AKI (less common if <10,000 U/L).
3. Blood pressure in rhabdomyolysis is often maintained, even in the setting of large amounts of fluid loss, secondary to vasoconstriction partly due to nitric oxide sequestration by free myoglobin.
4. Life-threatening hyperkalemia may be prominent as a result of the lysis of muscle cells and the release of intracellular potassium.

BIBLIOGRAPHY

Chavez, L. O., Leon, M., Einav, S., & Varon, J. (2016). Beyond muscle destruction: A systematic review of rhabdomyolysis for clinical practice. *Critical Care, 20*(1), 135.

Nance, J. R., & Mammen, A. L. (2015). Diagnostic evaluation of rhabdomyolysis. *Muscle Nerve, 51*(6), 793–810.

Panizo, N., Rubio-Navarro, A., Amaro-Villalobos, J. M., Egido, J., & Moreno, J. A. (2015). Molecular mechanisms and novel therapeutic approaches to rhabdomyolysis-induced acute kidney injury. *Kidney and Blood Pressure Research, 40*(5), 520–532.

Torres, P. A., Helmstetter, J. A., Kaye, A. M., & Kaye, A. D. (2015). Rhabdomyolysis: Pathogenesis, diagnosis, and treatment. *Ochsner Journal, 15*(1), 58–69.

CHAPTER 13

CONTRAST-INDUCED NEPHROPATHY

Akash Nair Sethi, Jatinder Kohli, Ami M. Patel, and Michael R. Rudnick

1. **What is contrast-induced nephropathy (CIN), and how does it occur?**
   Iodinated contrast media can lead to a usually reversible form of non-oliguric acute kidney injury (AKI) that occurs typically 24 to 48 hours after intravenous (IV) or intra-arterial administration of contrast. CIN does not occur with oral delivery of contrast media because contrast is not absorbed through the gut. Contrast media causes AKI through two major mechanisms: (1) renal vasoconstriction causing ischemia, and (2) direct tubular epithelial toxicity from the contrast. After contrast administration, there is an immediate transient increase in renal blood flow followed by a prolonged period of reduced flow resulting in renal ischemia. Contrast media stimulates the release of vasoconstrictive mediators, such as endothelin, while blocking the release of vasodilators, such as prostaglandins and nitric oxide, which causes hypoperfusion. The renal medulla, which is poorly oxygenated in normal conditions, is susceptible to injury from contrast-induced reductions in oxygen delivery. This ischemic injury generates reactive oxygen species, which causes tubular injury by affecting renal endothelial cells. Furthermore, contrast agents are directly toxic to renal epithelial cells, causing proximal tubular vacuolization, interstitial inflammation, and cellular necrosis.

2. **What is the typical clinical presentation of atheroembolic acute AKI? What is the differential diagnosis for kidney failure following cardiac catheterization?**
   The differential diagnoses of kidney failure following cardiac catheterization includes ischemic acute tubular necrosis, cardiorenal syndrome, renal atheroemboli/cholesterol emboli syndrome, and prerenal causes of AKI. The presence of diffuse atherosclerosis predisposes a patient to renal atheroemboli, which is characterized by a stair-step pattern to the increase in creatinine that occurs days to weeks after the procedure with little or no recovery of kidney function. Other distinguishing features of atheroembolic acute AKI are the presence of embolic lesions (as on the toes and fingers), livedo reticularis, transient eosinophilia, hypocomplementemia, vague abdominal pain (due to small vessel ischemic disease), and Hollenhorst plaques (cholesterol emboli to retinal vessels).

3. **What is the clinical significance of CIN?**
   CIN is defined as an increase in the pre-contrast baseline serum creatinine within 48 to 72 hours following contrast administration. Most studies have defined CIN as an elevation of serum creatinine of >0.5 mg/dL or >25% of baseline value. Some studies now define using the AKIN criteria of >0.3 mg/dL. CIN has been shown to be associated with an increase in hospital and long-term morbidity and mortality. It is noted as the third leading cause of AKI for inpatients with retrospective studies showing its incidence varying between 3% and 30% depending on contrast volume, concomitant risk factors, and whether the contrast is given intravenously or arterially. Lower incidences are seen with venous administration. The in-hospital mortality rates in a large retrospective analysis were 1.1% without CIN, 7.1% in CIN not requiring dialysis, and 35.7% for those with CIN requiring dialysis; fortunately, CIN requiring dialysis is rare (typically representing less than 2% of CIN). Although CIN is usually reversible and rarely requires renal replacement, studies have shown that CIN requiring dialysis has a 2-year survival rate of less than 40%. This high mortality rate is difficult to interpret and difficult to solely contribute to CIN, as these patients tend to have confounding comorbidities that also place them at higher mortality risk. CIN also has been shown to be an independent risk factor for subsequent chronic kidney disease (CKD), as noted in many retrospective studies. There has been an association between CIN and mortality, but a causal relationship has never been truly established. Several retrospective studies have shown that less than one-third of patients with CIN will have some permanent loss of kidney function following an episode of CIN.

4. **What are the risk factors for the development of CIN?**
   - CKD: The main predisposing risk factor is preexisting kidney disease with serum creatinine ≥1.5 mg/dL or estimated glomerular filtration rate below 60 mL/min/1.73 m2. Furthermore, the more severe the degree of CKD, the greater the risk of CIN.
   - Diabetes: The presence of diabetes further enhances this risk; however, diabetes itself without kidney disease has not been associated with CIN.
   - Contrast volume: High doses of contrast are associated with increased risk. Several studies in percutaneous coronary intervention (PCI) patients have shown that low-volume contrast (<50 mL) during coronary angiography can be adequate for coronary artery visualization and stent placement, but they have not directly looked at the decreased rates of CIN. However, it would be expected—with minimal contrast volumes—that the incidence of CIN post-PCI would be either eliminated or mitigated.
   - Intra-arterial administration carries a higher risk of injury than does IV administration.
   - Advanced age
   - Proteinuria
   - Hypotension
   - Volume depletion
   - Congestive heart failure
   - Multiple myeloma (historical risk factor; unlikely a risk factor with modern contrast agents)
   - Concurrent use of nonsteroidal anti-inflammatory agents
   - Renin-Angiotensin-Aldosterone System (RAAS) blockade*
   - Kidney transplant without CKD*
   - Cirrhosis*
   Although CIN has been described for years following IV contrast radiologic studies, large trials with propensity matching suggest that IV contrast media has had no statistically significant increase in AKI, dialysis, or mortality, compared to patients with similar procedures without contrast. Despite these findings, we still recommend that in high-risk patients (i.e., with impaired kidney function) scheduled for IV contrast radiologic studies, the usual prophylactic steps be followed (see later) to minimize risk and prophylactic techniques.

5. **What are the clinical features and how the diagnosis is made?**
   CIN usually manifests with AKI developing within 24 to 48 hours, with peak injury anywhere between 72 and 120 hours after insult. It may take 7 to 10 days before serum creatinine returns to baseline. The injury typically does not cause proteinuria, and the urinalysis resembles acute tubular necrosis with muddy brown casts and renal tubular epithelial cells. The fractional excretion of sodium is typically below 1%, which presumably is due to the severe vasoconstriction, although the significance of this is confounded in that CIN is almost always non-oliguric. Kidney biopsy is not indicated unless the presentation is atypical and the diagnosis is unclear.

6. **What prophylactic hydration measures are recommended?**
   Beyond supportive measures there are no treatments to reverse CIN once it is established, so prophylactic measures are the only intervention available. Prophylaxis should be used in high-risk individuals, primarily patients with impaired kidney function. Volume expansion is the only consistently effective prophylactic measure to reduce the risk for CIN. Volume expansion may work by:
   - Suppressing the renin-angiotensin system
   - Reducing vasoconstrictive mediators
   - Diluting the contrast media
   - Increasing the transit time of contrast media through the kidney
   Pre-procedure hydration has been done with a variety of fluids, including oral hydration, hypotonic solutions (0.45% Normal Saline), and isotonic crystalloids (normal saline, Ringer's lactate, and isotonic bicarbonate solutions). In a prospective trial, normal saline was superior to 0.45% saline. This is expected because the isotonic fluid provides more effective volume expansion. IV hydration is recommended over oral hydration for the same reason. Until recently, isotonic bicarbonate was suggested to be a better prophylactic solution than normal saline possibly by reducing reactive oxygen species formation. However a large study (4993 patients) comparing isotonic bicarbonate to normal saline has now been completed (PRESERVE Trial) and did not show any benefit of isotonic

---

* Synergistic risk factors; controversial data about true risk.

bicarbonate over normal saline. Thus, the former should not be used due to lack of benefit, increased cost, and risk of compounding errors.

Our recommended infusion rate is:

- Outpatient: 3 mL/kg/hr for 1 hour pre-contrast administration and 1 to 1.5 mL/kg/hr for 4 to 6 hours after contrast
- Inpatients: 1 mL/kg/hr for 6 to 12 hours pre-procedure and intra-procedure, and 6 to 12 hours post-procedure

Infusion rates may need to be reduced in patients at risk for heart failure. The safe administration of prophylactic fluids in these patients may be done by monitoring left ventricular and diastolic pressures, which was shown to be an effective measure in reducing CIN in the POSEIDON trial.

7. **What is the role of N-acetylcysteine?**

Another prophylactic treatment has been N-acetylcysteine (also known as Mucomyst), which has antioxidative properties by increasing intracellular glutathione levels. It is believed that N-acetylcysteine may exert its activity by negating some of the effects of the reactive oxygen species. In prospective studies, N-acetylcysteine is not consistently effective at reducing the risk of contrast nephropathy. The PRESERVE Trial referenced in the Prophylactic Hydration section also randomized patients at risk for CIN to N-acetylcysteine or placebo and found no prophylactic benefit of N-acetylcysteine. Based on these results, we do not recommend N-acetylcysteine prophylaxis.

8. **What are the historical prophylactic therapies that reduce CIN risk and how effective are they?**

Several classes of pharmacologic agents have been investigated to provide prophylaxis from contrast nephropathy. The following agents failed in prospective trials and are not recommended:

- Theophylline has been examined as a prophylactic treatment for CIN because of its effect on renal vasodilation through non-selective blockage of the adenosine receptor; however, it is not generally recommended because of its lack of evidence in large, randomized, controlled trials and potential drug-related toxicity when administered intravenously (such as ventricular arrhythmias, seizures, and shock)
- Mannitol
- Furosemide
- Dopamine
- Atrial natriuretic peptide
- Fenoldopam
- Endothelin receptor antagonist

9. **Does hemodialysis prevent CIN?**

The use of hemodialysis or hemofiltration for the prevention of CIN has been proposed to prevent CIN. Although dialysis can remove the majority of the contrast media, a recent meta-analysis has failed to show that periprocedural dialysis decreases the risk for CIN. One explanation for this finding is that hemodynamic changes in the renal vasculature occur within seconds of contrast administration, and subsequent histopathologic changes occur within 15 minutes. It is logistically difficult to arrange for dialysis within minutes of contrast delivery, and there is significant associated risk involved with dialysis. Therefore, we do not recommend dialysis as prophylaxis from CIN. Residual kidney function in dialysis patients still portends better outcomes in mortality; therefore, CIN can still have an adverse effect in dialysis patients. Multiple studies suggest that when contrast media needs to be given to dialysis patients, emergent dialysis post-contrast administration is not needed and patients do well when the post-contrast dialysis is delayed for 24 to 48 hours. The only exception may be in patients with severe volume overload or significantly reduced left ventricular function; in these patients, dialysis, shortly after contrast administration, may be advisable.

10. **Is there any benefit to discontinuing angiotensin-converting enzyme inhibitors and angiotensin receptor blockers (ACE-I/ARBs) prior to contrast exposure?**

There are two opposing theories concerning the effects of ACE-I/ARBs on the kidneys in the setting of contrast administration. First, ACE-I/ARBs increase the risk of CIN because these drugs are associated with a decrease in the glomerular filtration rate. The second theory is that ACE-I/ARBs are protective against CIN by counteracting the afferent arteriolar vasoconstriction and the subsequent medullary ischemia precipitated with contrast. Retrospective and prospective studies are mixed on the questions, with some studies showing a neutral effect and others demonstrating a deleterious effect of ACEi/ARB. We do not recommend holding these drugs unless there is concern for volume depletion, and we do not feel that there is sufficient evidence to recommend starting these agents before a contrast administration purely for prophylactic purposes. Volume depletion increases the risk for CIN; therefore, holding diuretics immediately before and after contrast administration is prudent.

11. **Is there a role for statin therapy in preventing contrast nephropathy?**
Statins have been shown to possess pleiotropic effects including antioxidant and anti-inflammatory properties. Because reactive oxygen species are involved in the pathogenesis of CIN, the administration of statins has been proposed to reduce the risk for CIN. However, several meta-analyses have not found a statistical reduction in CIN with statins. While there is no indication to add a statin prior to contrast, patients currently taking them should continue to receive them.

12. **Can remote ischemic preconditioning (RIPC) prevent contrast nephropathy?**
RIPC is a technique that uses brief episodes of non-injurious ischemia and reperfusion to reduce the risk of tissue injury after an ischemic event. The proposed mechanism involves the neuronal and humoral pathways that modulate the anti-inflammatory and anti-oxidant mediators to protect organs from injury. Several methods of RIPC have been explored, including the use of a sphygmomanometer inflated above systolic blood pressure or using a stent balloon. There have been conflicting results about efficacy, but RIPC seems to be an exciting new prospect that warrants further evaluation before it can be recommended as a prophylactic technique for CIN prevention.

13. **What different types of iodinated contrast are available? Is there one contrast agent that is more nephrotoxic than others?**
Clinical studies have suggested that the osmolality of contrast might have an impact on the development of CIN. Iodinated contrast media are either ionic or non-ionic, and they are further classified by their osmolality. The first-generation contrast media are ionic high-osmolal agents with an osmolar range of 1500 to 1800 mOsm/kg, compared to plasma osmolality of 290 mOsm/kg. These high-osmolal agents are no longer used for intravascular contrast administration. In the 1980s, second-generation contrast media replaced high osmolal ionic contrast media because they were less nephrotoxic and better tolerated by the patient. Second-generation contrast media are known as low-osmolal non-ionic agents, although they are still hyperosmolar at 600 to 700 mOsm/kg. Third-generation contrast media, referred to as iso-osmolol agents, such as iodixanol, typically have an osmolality around 290 mOsm/kg. Since low-osmolal contrast agents were shown to be less nephrotoxic than high-osmolal contrast agents, it was hoped that iso-osmolal contrast agents would be less nephrotoxic than low-osmolal contrast agents. While early studies did show a reduction in CIN, subsequent studies were unable to confirm the benefit of iso-osmolal contrast agents. The current recommendation by experts is to use either low-osmolal or iso-osmolal agents in high-risk patients.

14. **What is gadolinium, and what risks are associated with it?**
Gadolinium is a lanthanide metal with paramagnetic properties, making it a suitable contrast agent. Initially, it was assumed to be a safe alternative to iodinated contrast; however, subsequently, it was shown to cause nephrogenic systemic fibrosis (NSF) in patients on dialysis or with severe impairment of kidney function. NSF is a severe fibrosing disorder of the skin and other organs that can be debilitating and fatal. The majority of cases of NSF occur in patients with end-stage kidney disease who were receiving renal replacement therapy. No cases have been reported with stage 1 to 3 CKD, and only a few cases with CKD 4. If gadolinium must be administered in patients with advanced CKD, experts recommend:
- Using a macrocyclic ionic chelate-based gadolinium rather than linear nonionic type
- Administering the lowest dosage possible
- Avoiding repeated exposures
- Consider hemodialysis after gadolinium administration.
- Due to the risk of NSF in patients at high-risk for CIN, gadolinium contrast media cannot be recommended for the reduction of CIN risk.

KEY POINTS

1. Contrast media cause acute kidney injury through two major mechanisms: renal vasoconstriction and direct tubular epithelial toxicity.
2. In most cases, contrast-induced nephropathy (CIN) is characterized by an elevation (>0.5 mg/dL or 25%) of the baseline creatinine within 24 to 48 hours following exposure, reaching a peak within 3 to 5 days, usually followed by a return to baseline within 7 to 10 days. Most patients with CIN are

non-oliguric. Typically, the urinalysis is characterized by coarse granular casts and renal tubular epithelial cells along with a high specific gravity and fractional excretion of sodium <1%.

3. The main predisposing factor for CIN is preexisting kidney disease with serum creatinine ≥1.5 mg/dL or estimated glomerular filtration rate <60 mL/min/1.73 m². Other risk factors include diabetes only when coupled with CKD, high contrast load, advanced age, proteinuria, hypotension, volume depletion, congestive heart failure, and nonsteroidal anti-inflammatory drug (NSAID) use.

4. Volume expansion, using minimal contrast volumes, and removal of nephrotoxins, including NSAIDs, are the principal prophylactic measures to reduce the risk for CIN. The recent demonstration in the PRESERVE Trial of a lack of prophylactic advantage of isotonic bicarbonate over normal saline results in our recommendation that the former solution should not be used and prophylactic hydration should be with normal saline only. The recommended infusion rates are:

   • Outpatient: 3 mL/kg/hr for 1 hour pre-contrast administration and 1 to 1.5 mL/kg/hr for 4 to 6 hours after contrast

   • Inpatients: 1 mL/kg/hr for 6 to 12 hours pre-procedure and intra-procedure, and 6 to 12 hours post-procedure

5. The recent PRESERVE Trial has demonstrated no prophylactic benefit to N-acetylsteine and we no longer recommend it as a prophylaxis.

6. Statins should be continued, but not routinely started before contrast exposure. We do not recommend discontinuing drugs that block the renin-angiotensin-aldosterone system prior to contrast administration. Prophylactic use of hemodialysis or hemofiltration is not recommended. Remote ischemic preconditioning remains an exciting option, but is not yet proven for CIN prophylaxis.

BIBLIOGRAPHY

Brar, S., Aharonian, V., Mansukhani, P., Moore, N., Shen, A. Y., Jorgensen, . . . Kane, K. (2014). Hemodynamic-guided gluid administration for the prevention of contrast-induced acute kidney injury: The POSEIDON randomized controlled trial. *Lancet, 60*(5), 1394. doi:10.1016/j.jvs.2014.09.019.

Brar, S. S., Hiremath, S., Dangas, G., Mehran, R., Brar, S. K., & Leon, M. B. (2009). Sodium bicarbonate for the prevention of contrast induced-acute kidney injury: A systematic review and meta-analysis. *Clinical Journal of the American Society of Nephrology, 4*(10), 1584–1592.

Cruz, D. N., Perazella, M. A., Bellomo, R., Corradi, V., de Cal, M., Kuang, D., Ocampo, C., Nalesso, F., & Ronco, C. (2006). Extracorporeal blood purification therapies for prevention of radiocontrast-induced nephropathy: A systematic review. *American Journal of Kidney Diseases, 48*(3), 361–371.

Jefferson, J. A., & Schrier, R. W. (2007). Pathophysiology and etiology of acute renal failure. In J. Feehaly, J. Floege, & R. Johnson (Eds.), *Comprehensive clinical nephrology* (3rd ed., pp. 755–770). Philadelphia: Mosby Elsevier.

Jo, S. H., Koo, B. K., Park, J. S., Kang, H. J., Cho, Y. S., Kim, Y. J., . . . Kim, H. S. (2008). Prevention of radiocontrast medium-induced nephropathy using short-term high-dose simvastatin in patients with renal insufficiency undergoing coronary angiography (PROMISS) trial—A randomized controlled study. *American Heart Journal, 155*, 499.e1–e8.

Kiski, D., Stepper, W., Brand, E., Breithardt, G., & Reinecke, H. (2010). Impact of renin-angiotensin-aldosterone blockade by angiotensin-converting enzyme inhibitors or AT-1 blockers on frequency of contrast medium-induced nephropathy: A post-hoc analysis from the Dialysis-versus-Diuresis (DVD) trial. *Nephrology Dialysis Transplantation, 25*, 759–764.

Meier, P., Ko, D. T., Tamura, A., Tamhane, U., & Gurm, H. S. (2009). Sodium bicarbonate-based hydration prevents contrast-induced nephropathy: A meta-analysis. *BMC Medicine, 7*, 23.

Navaneethan, S. D., Singh, S., Appasamy, S., Wing, R. E., & Sehgal, A. R. (2009). Sodium bicarbonate therapy for prevention of contrast-induced nephropathy: A systematic review and meta-analysis. *American Journal of Kidney Diseases, 53*, 617–627.

Perazella, M. A. (2009). Current status of gadolinium toxicity in patients with kidney disease. *Clinical Journal of the American Society of Nephrology, 4*, 461–469.

Persson, P. B., & Tepel, M. (2006). Contrast medium-induced nephropathy: The pathophysiology. *Kidney International Supplement, 100*, S8–S10.

Rudnick, M., & Feldman, H. (2008). Contrast-induced nephropathy: What are the true clinical consequences? *Clinical Journal of the American Society of Nephrology, 3*, 263–272.

Tepel, M., & Zidek, W. (2004). N-Acetylcysteine in nephrology: Contrast nephropathy and beyond. *Current Opinion in Nephrology and Hypertension, 13*, 649–654.

Toso, A., Maioli, M., Leoncini, M., Gallopin, M., Tedeschi, D., Micheletti, C., . . . Bellandi, F. (2010). Usefulness of atorvastatin (80 mg) in prevention of contrast-induced nephropathy in patients with chronic renal disease. *American Journal of Cardiology, 105*, 288–292.

Trivedi, H., Daram, S., Szabo, A., Bartorelli, A. L., & Marenzi, G. (2009). High-dose N-acetylcysteine for the prevention of contrast-induced nephropathy. *American Journal of Medincine, 122*, 874.e9–e15.

Weisbord, S.D., Gallagher, M., Jneid, H., et al. for the PRESERVE Trial Group. (2017). Outcomes after angiography with sodium bicarbonate and acetylcysteine. *N Engl J Med*, November 12. [Epub ahead of print].

Wu, S., Shah, S., Sterling, K. (2009). Prevention of contrast-induced nephropathy. *US Nephrology, 4*, 35–38.

ACUTE GLOMERULONEPHRITIS AND RAPIDLY PROGRESSIVE GLOMERULONEPHRITIS

John R. Sedor

CHAPTER 14

1. **What is the syndrome of acute glomerulonephritis?**

   Acute glomerulonephritis is an acute kidney injury (AKI) syndrome characterized by the sudden onset of edema and new-onset or worsening hypertension. Urinalysis demonstrates an active sediment, including abnormal proteinuria (usually >30 mg/dL or 1+ on a semiquantitative scale), hematuria, and red cell casts. Patients with acute glomerulonephritis are often azotemic (i.e., they have elevated serum blood urea nitrogen and creatinine concentrations) and occasionally develop severe kidney injury requiring dialysis. Acute glomerulonephritis can be a primary kidney disease, which is usually classified on the basis of kidney histopathology, or can result from a number of systemic diseases. Although this chapter focuses on primary acute glomerulonephritis, the diagnostic and therapeutic approaches for kidney-limited glomerulonephritis and glomerulonephritides associated with systemic diseases are similar. The reader is referred to the sections on primary (Part IV) and secondary (Part V) glomerular disorders for additional information.

2. **What are the major causes of acute glomerulonephritis? What approaches should be used to develop an appropriate differential diagnosis?**

   The patient's history and a physical examination can provide clues to the diagnosis of acute glomerulonephritis. Looking for skin lesions and disease in other organ systems can help determine if the cause of the acute glomerulonephritis syndrome is a result of kidney-limited or systemic disease. A focused laboratory examination, including serologic studies, directed by the findings in the patient's history and physical examination, can also be useful in establishing a diagnosis. Hematuria with dysmorphic red cell morphology and red cell casts are usually detected on urinalysis. Moderate proteinuria, usually in the non-nephrotic range, is typical. Nephrotic-range proteinuria occurs in <30% of patients. Mild to severe azotemia is universally present.

   Table 14.1 presents major causes of acute glomerulonephritis stratified by their association with serum complement levels (low vs. normal or high). Complement levels can help a clinician focus on a differential diagnosis on the most likely causes of the acute glomerulonephritis syndrome. Measuring serum complement levels (C3, C4) and/or activity (CH50) is a somewhat arbitrary choice of initial tests, but they provide a practical approach to further testing and management of the patient with presumptive glomerulonephritis. A kidney biopsy is almost always indicated to establish a definitive diagnosis and direct treatment. The extent of acute inflammation and fibrosis present in the biopsy can provide important data on prognosis and can be used to project responsiveness to therapy. In order to optimize patient care, a standardized kidney biopsy classification system based on current concepts of glomerulonephritis etiology/pathogenesis has been proposed.

3. **What are dysmorphic red cells?**

   Phase-contrast morphology can be used to characterize urinary erythrocyte morphology. Glomerular bleeding, a characteristic of glomerulonephritis, causes red cells in the urine to have a non-uniform morphology with irregular outlines and small blebs projecting from their surfaces (i.e., the red cells are "dysmorphic"). Red cells in the urine from non-glomerular bleeding in the urinary tract are uniform in shape and similar in appearance to red cells in the circulation. Urine can be analyzed by the clinical laboratory for the presence of dysmorphic red cells. The sensitivity, specificity, and predicative values for this test are limited, and results need to be interpreted in the context of other clinical and diagnostic data. Clinical labs most often quantify numbers of dysmorphic red cells as a percentage of total red cells, and define the upper limit of normal to aid in the interpretation of the test.

Table 14.1. Some Causes of Acute Glomerulonephritis (Serologic and Other Tests that Provide Diagnostic Clues)

	LOW SERUM COMPLEMENT LEVEL	NORMAL SERUM COMPLEMENT LEVEL
Systemic diseases	Systemic lupus erythematosus (ANA+, anti-DNA antibody+) Cryoglobulinemia (cryoglobulin+) Henoch-Schönlein purpura Infectious endocarditis (positive blood cultures) "Shunt" nephritis (positive blood cultures) Infection-associated glomerulonephritis	Microscopic polyangiitis (ANCA+) Granulomatosis with polyangiitis (ANCA+) Goodpasture syndrome (anti-GBM Ab+) Hypersensitivity vasculitis Visceral abscess (positive blood cultures)
Primary kidney diseases	Post-infection glomerulonephritis (β-hemolytic streptococci) C3 glomerulopathy Dense deposit disease Membranoproliferative glomerulonephritis	IgA nephropathy Idiopathic RPGN Type I: Anti-GBM disease (Goodpasture disease; anti-GBM Ab+) Type II: Immune complex/immune deposit disease Type III: Pauci-immune (ANCA+)

ANA, Antinuclear antibody; ANCA, anti-neutrophil cytoplasmic antibodies; GBM, glomerular basement membrane; IgA, immunoglobulin-A; RPGN, rapidly progressive glomerulonephritis.
Modified from Manoharon, A., Schelling, J. R., Diamond, M., Chung-Park, M., Madaio, M., & Sedor, J. R. (2013). Immune and inflammatory glomerular diseases. In R. J. Alpern, M. J. Caplan, & O. W. Moe (Eds.), *Seldin and Giebisch's the kidney: Physiology and pathophysiology* (pp. 2763–2816). Amsterdam: Elsevier.

4. Describe glomerulonephritis in the setting of infection.
Glomerulonephritis associated with infection is varied. Post-infectious glomerulonephritis occurs after an infection and latent period in which the patient returns to her or his baseline health. Beta-hemolytic Streptococcus is almost exclusively the etiology of post-infectious glomerulonephritis. In contrast, infection-associated glomerulonephritis occurs concurrently with the infection. While an active staphylococcal infection is a classically recognized cause of infection-associated glomerulonephritis, it can be caused by many different viruses, bacteria, and fungi. Complement levels, especially C3, are often—but not always—depressed in infection-associated glomerulonephritis. Recognizing the distinction between these clinical presentations is necessary for appropriate clinical management. The management of post-streptococcal glomerulonephritis is supportive, primarily managing hypertension and volume overload. For infection-associated glomerulonephritis, the primary goal is to treat the infection.

5. Define the syndrome of rapidly progressive glomerulonephritis (RPGN).
Patients with RPGN have evidence of glomerular disease (proteinuria, hematuria, and red cell casts) accompanied by rapid loss of kidney function over days to weeks. If untreated, RPGN often results in kidney failure. The pathologic hallmark of RPGN is the presence of crescents on kidney biopsy, and RPGN is also described as crescentic nephritis (see later for further discussion). Fortunately, the disorders associated with this syndrome are rare, so that RPGN makes up only 2% to 4% of all cases of glomerulonephritis. Importantly, RPGN is not a specific diagnosis, and multiple different diseases can cause this syndrome. Diagnosis almost always requires a biopsy of the affected tissue if the presentation suggests systemic involvement, or of the kidney if it is kidney-limited.

6. What are crescents in kidney biopsies?
Crescent formation is a nonspecific response to severe injury of the glomerular capillary wall. As a result, fibrin leaks into Bowman's space, causing parietal epithelial cells to proliferate and mononuclear phagocytes to migrate into the glomerular tuft from the circulation. Large crescents can compress glomerular capillaries and impair filtration. Although crescent formation can resolve, some inflammatory chemotactic signals recruit fibroblasts into Bowman's space, which ultimately can cause both the crescents and glomeruli to scar. Extensive scarring results in end-stage kidney disease (ESKD). Similar to RPGN, crescentic nephritis is not a specific pathologic diagnosis. Crescents can be seen with a number of specific glomerular diseases (see question 9).

7. **Do crescentic nephritis and RPGN describe the same syndrome?**
Although the terms *crescentic nephritis* and *RPGN* are used interchangeably, these diagnoses are not synonymous. RPGN describes a *clinical* syndrome of rapid loss of kidney function over days to weeks in patients with evidence of glomerulonephritis. In contrast, crescentic nephritis is a *histopathologic* description of kidney biopsy specimens, which demonstrate the presence of crescents in more than 50% of glomeruli. Biopsies of patients with RPGN very commonly reveal crescentic nephritis. However, RPGN can occur in the absence of crescentic nephritis, and extensive glomerular crescent formation is rarely identified in kidney biopsy specimens from patients without the clinical syndrome of RPGN.

8. **How is primary RPGN classified?**
RPGN can occur as a primary disorder in the absence of other glomerular or systemic diseases. Crescentic nephritis, the pathologic correlate of RPGN, is classified into three types using immunofluorescence microscopy to describe the presence or absence of immune deposits and the character of their distribution within the glomerular basement membrane (GBM; Table 14.1 and Box 14.1):
1. Type I RPGN is characterized by linear deposition of antibodies directed against type IV collagen, a matrix protein that is a constituent of the GBM. These antibodies are commonly referred to as anti-GBM antibodies (discussed later). Type I RPGN comprises approximately 10% to 20% of patients with primary RPGN without pulmonary hemorrhage.
2. Type II RPGN is characterized by a granular pattern of immune complex deposition. This is found in 20% to 30% of patients with primary RPGN without pulmonary hemorrhage.
3. Type III RPGN has no immune deposits ("pauci-immune") in glomeruli using immunofluorescence or electron microscopy, and occurs in 50% to 60% of patients with crescentic glomerulonephritis on kidney biopsy.

9. **What glomerular diseases are associated with RPGN?**
RPGN can complicate the clinical course of some primary glomerular diseases, such as immunoglobulin A (IgA) nephropathy, membranous nephropathy, membranoproliferative glomerulonephritis, and hereditary nephritis (Alport syndrome). In addition, RPGN is associated with infectious and multisystem diseases, including systemic lupus erythematosus, cryoglobulinemia, and systemic vasculitides. Box 14.1 summarizes the kidney-limited and systemic causes of RPGN.

Box 14.1. Classification of RPGN

Primary	**Secondary to Systemic Disease**
Type I: Anti-GBM antibody disease (Goodpasture disease)	Superimposed on a primary glomerular disease
Type II: Granular glomerular immune complex association	Infection related
Type III: Pauci-immune glomerulonephritis	Post-streptococcal and rarely post-viral glomerulonephritis
	Visceral abscess and other infection-associated
	Vasculitides:
	Small Vessel (Pauci-Immune):
	Microscopic polyangiitis
	Granulomatosis with polyangiitis (Wegener's syndrome)
	Eosinophilic granulomatosis (Churg-Strauss syndrome)
	Small Vessel (Immune Complex):
	Systemic lupus erythematosus
	Henoch-Schönlein purpura
	Cryoglobulinemia
	Medium Vessel:
	Polyarteritis nodosa (rare)
	Goodpasture syndrome and disease
	Malignancy-related
	Medication-associated:
	ANCA-associated (hydralazine, propylthiouracil, minocycline)
	Drug-induce lupus

ANCA, Anti-neutrophil cytoplasmic antibodies; *GBM*, glomerular basement membrane; *RPGN*, rapidly progressive glomerulonephritis.

10. **Aside from urinalysis, which other laboratory tests are useful in determining the etiology of acute glomerulonephritis?**

    Certain serologic studies or other laboratory tests may be useful in narrowing the differential diagnosis, but ordering these labs should be guided by the patient's history and clinical presentation. Complement levels (C3, C4) are usually normal in patients with either primary RPGN or RPGN associated with systemic diseases (see Table 14.1). Lupus is an exception, as these patients usually have depressed C3 and C4 levels. In almost all patients, an antinuclear antibody level is a useful screen for lupus or other connective tissue diseases. Identification of anti-GBM antibodies and anti-neutrophil cytoplasmic antibodies (ANCA) can be useful in establishing a diagnosis in patients with RPGN. Patients who are ANCA antibody positive frequently have a primary small vessel vasculitis. The patient's clinical presentation determines the predictive value of ANCA testing. For example, the predictive value of a positive ANCA test is lower in a patient who presents with hematuria, proteinuria, and a normal creatinine than in a patient with similar urinalysis findings in the presence of azotemia. Laboratory testing to identify infections with *Streptococcus*, hepatitis, or HIV, or causes of autoimmune diseases in addition to lupus and ANCA vasculitis, may be indicated. Antibodies to phospholipase A2 receptor (PLA$_2$R) are found in 70% of cases of idiopathic membranous nephropathy. Testing for anti-PLA$_2$R antibodies is reasonable in selected patients with RPGN syndromes.

11. **What are anti-GBM antibodies?**

    Anti-GBM antibodies are targeted toward the noncollagenous domain 1 (NC1) domain of the α3 chain of type IV collagen, which is a component of the GBM. Formation of the type IV collagen network in normal GBM sequesters these epitopes from the immune system, preventing tolerance during fetal development. Anti-GBM-associated disease occurs after the kidney is injured in a manner that exposes these regions of the collagen molecule; the collagen is not recognized as "self" and generates an immune response. Anti-GBM antibodies are found in 90% to 95% of patients with Goodpasture disease and are deposited in the GBM. On kidney biopsy immunofluorescence, they form linear deposits of immunoglobulin along the basement membranes.

12. **Are Goodpasture syndrome and anti-GBM glomerulonephritis (Goodpasture disease) the same?**

    No. Although both disease entities result from circulating anti-GBM antibodies, *Goodpasture syndrome* describes a systemic disease with a clinical constellation of pulmonary hemorrhage, circulating anti-GBM antibodies, and glomerulonephritis. Anti-GBM glomerulonephritis, or *Goodpasture disease*, is kidney-limited and describes a proliferative glomerulonephritis, which results from the deposition of anti-GBM antibodies. Anti-GBM antibodies are the same in patients with Goodpasture syndrome and Goodpasture disease. Because alveolar basement membrane contains the epitope of type IV collagen that is recognized by anti-GBM antibodies, the variable presence of pulmonary disease seems to reflect whether alveolar basement membrane epitope is accessible to the circulating anti-GBM antibodies. Alveolar injury from infections, smoking, toxins, or other underlying lung disease may predispose the lungs to the deposition of anti-GBM antibodies.

13. **What are ANCA?**

    Kidney biopsies from patients with type III RPGN have no immune deposits, but type III RPGN usually results from small-vessel vasculitides associated with circulating ANCA. The ANCA-associated small vessel vasculitides are:
    - Granulomatosis with polyangiitis (GPA, formerly Wegener's granulomatosis)
    - Microscopic polyangiitis (MPA; systemic and kidney-limited)
    - Eosinophilic granulomatosis with polyangiitis (EGPA, formerly known as Churg-Strauss syndrome)

    These are usually systemic diseases but can be limited to the kidney. ANCA are directed against neutrophil proteinase 3 (PR3) or myeloperoxidase (MPO). Screening for ANCA uses an indirect immunofluorescence examination of normal neutrophils, which, if positive, demonstrates a staining pattern characteristic of the target antigen (cytoplasmic for PR3 [C-ANCA] against PR3 and perinuclear for anti-MPO ANCA [P-ANCA]). The P-ANCA screening test has low specificity because other anti-neutrophil antibodies give a similar pattern by indirect immunofluorescence. A screening test that is positive for either C-ANCA or P-ANCA needs confirmation with an antigen-specific technique. C-ANCA positivity is associated with active GPA, and P-ANCA positivity is associated with active MPA and less so EGPA. However, ANCA testing results have to be interpreted in the context of the clinical presentation, and the diagnosis of a vasculitis or glomerulonephritis often requires a tissue biopsy. ANCA antibodies can be present in patients with non-vasculitic rheumatologic diseases, infections, and autoimmune gastrointestinal diseases, and can co-occur with other types of acute glomerulonephritis (e.g., anti-GBM disease).

14. **What is the treatment for acute glomerulonephritis?**

    The treatment for acute glomerulonephritis is primarily supportive: diuretics to reduce the edema and antihypertensive drugs to reduce elevated blood pressure. Anti-inflammatory therapy with corticosteroids, cytotoxic agents, and other classes of immunosuppressive agents is used for some etiologies of acute glomerulonephritis. Therapeutic approaches for acute glomerulonephritis due to systemic lupus nephritis and the pauci-immune vasculitides have been extensively studied, and reasonable evidence from multicenter trials is available to guide treatment for these diseases. Treatment strategies for other etiologies of acute glomerulonephritis are often based on observational studies of small numbers of patients. Approaches to therapy in children and adults with the same etiology of acute glomerulonephritis are not always identical.

15. **What are the treatment options for patients with RPGN?**
RPGN needs to be treated aggressively and early in its course to reduce the likelihood of ESKD. Glucocorticoid and immunosuppressive regimens are the mainstay of RPGN treatment. The benefit of these agents is greatest in patients with ANCA-associated vasculitis. The most common complications of therapy are infections. Hemorrhagic cystitis, a complication of cyclophosphamide therapy, occurs less commonly with use of aggressive intravenous saline infusions to promote the excretion of metabolites toxic to bladder epithelial cells. In addition, 2-mercaptoethanesulfonate (MESNA), an agent that binds and sequesters the metabolite responsible for injury to the uroepithelia, is often given with cyclophosphamide. Malignancies, especially bladder cancers and leukemias, can occur decades after treatment of GPA with cyclophosphamide. Randomized, clinical trials continue to be performed in order to determine optimal therapy for patients with either ANCA-associated vasculitis or lupus nephritis. The reader is encouraged to review the most current literature and expert opinion to develop treatment regimens for patients with these diseases. The most current immunosuppressive protocols include several different immunosuppressive agents directed at different molecular targets to induce and maintain a remission. Therapy with these agents is often prolonged, lasting months to more than 1 year, necessitating the need for expert diagnosis and almost always biopsy confirmation. Of course, all treatment protocols have significant risk for adverse events, and patients require close monitoring and drug dose adjustments to reduce drug toxicity. Consultation with an expert in the treatment of these patients is highly recommended.

16. **Should treatment for RPGN be initiated prior to definitive diagnosis?**
Yes. Data obtained in experimental animal models of acute glomerulonephritis/crescentic nephritis show that fibrosis begins within days after disease initiation. Because patients usually present with evidence of active kidney inflammation and are often azotemic, significant kidney scarring has likely occurred by the time patients receive medical attention. Starting treatment should be viewed as urgent. Patients can be treated with corticosteroids until kidney biopsy results are available and treatment can be directed by the results (see next question). While some experts do treat patients based on clinical diagnosis alone, the toxicities and duration of the immunosuppressive therapies used to treat RPGN make a compelling rationale for biopsy confirmation of the diagnosis. Before initiating any immunosuppressive therapies, the treating physician must rule out infection.

17. **What is appropriate empiric therapy for patients with acute glomerulonephritis or RPGN?**
Kidney biopsy should be performed expeditiously and appropriate laboratory studies should be sent when the patient presents. While waiting for these results, the initiation of steroid therapy—the mainstay inductive anti-inflammatory therapy for most acute inflammatory glomerular diseases—is reasonable. Toxicities from high-dose steroid therapy are minimal and manageable during this short "window" between patient presentation and obtaining diagnostic test results. The initiation of cytotoxic or other immuno-suppressive treatments, which consolidate treatment response to steroids, or plasma exchange, should wait until a definitive diagnosis is established. Analysis of clinical trial outcomes for some glomerular diseases suggests that benefit from cytotoxic drugs occurs well after disease onset, and most experts feel that the use of these agents can be delayed until diagnosis is established. Dosing for cyclophosphamide must be adjusted in the patient with altered kidney function to avoid leukopenia. The spectrum of agents used in modern protocols has expanded greatly to include biologics as well as additional classes of nonspecific immunosuppressive drugs, such as calcineurin inhibitors and mycophenolate.

18. **Is there any role for plasma exchange in the therapy for RPGN?**
Plasma exchange is thought to remove circulating pathogenic autoantibodies from the circulation. Trials evaluating efficacy of plasma exchange for all causes of RPGN have included only small numbers of patients. However, plasma exchange is a safe procedure in experienced centers and may be an appropriate therapeutic modality for subsets of patients with RPGN, in view of the high risk of kidney failure with this syndrome. The European Vasculitis Study Group published a randomized trial that demonstrated that adjunctive plasma exchange improved kidney outcomes in patients with severe kidney failure (serum creatinine >2.3 mg/dL) and active ANCA vasculitis. In addition, the prompt initiation of plasma exchange and aggressive immunosuppression with corticosteroids and

cyclophosphamide can be lifesaving in patients with ANCA vasculitis and diffuse alveolar hemorrhage. Patients who are dialysis-dependent with ANCA vasculitis can respond to treatment (see question 19).

Plasma exchange and immunosuppressive therapy are standard treatments for patients with anti-GBM antibody disease. Most evidence supporting the use of plasma exchange in anti-GBM-associated diseases is from case reports, although one small, randomized, controlled trial demonstrated a non-significant trend toward improved outcome in patients treated with plasma exchange. Patients who are dialysis-dependent with anti-GBM disease are unlikely to respond to aggressive treatment, and the potential benefit of treatment does not outweigh the risk in these individuals (see question 19).

19. What is the prognosis of RPGN?

The prognosis and response to treatment in patients with anti-GBM antibody or Goodpasture disease have not been studied in large trials. Data from a number of small case series with similar, but not identical, treatment strategies suggest that patient survivals are high (70% to 90%). Overall, only 40% of patients remain off dialysis 1 year after presentation. However, patients who do not require dialysis and who are treated with immunosuppression and plasma exchange have 1-year kidney survivals of approximately 70% to 75%, even if kidney failure is severe. In contrast, kidney survival is poor in patients with anti-GBM antibody-associated disease, who require dialysis within 72 hours of presentation. Aggressive therapy with immunosuppressive drugs and plasma exchange may not be appropriate in this subgroup of anti-GBM antibody patients, unless significant acute tubular necrosis, in addition to crescentic nephritis, is demonstrated on kidney biopsy. Clinical, laboratory, and pathologic parameters do not have sufficient predictive value for kidney outcomes to be used in an individual patient.

Although data on patients with kidney-limited, ANCA-positive RPGN are limited, treatment responses have been recently reported in several cohorts of patients with ANCA-associated necrotizing glomerulonephritis and either GPA or MPA. Many patients (approximately 75%) achieve remission after induction therapy, but only 40% to 50% remain in long-term remission after 4 to 10 years. Serum creatinine at presentation is the strongest predictor of kidney survival in patients who are ANCA positive. In contrast to patients with anti-GBM glomerulonephritis, patients with ANCA-associated glomerulonephritis can respond to therapy even if they have already required the initiation of dialysis.

KEY POINTS

1. Acute glomerulonephritis is a kidney injury syndrome characterized by the sudden onset of edema, new or worsening hypertension, and an active urinary sediment.
2. Rapidly progressive glomerulonephritis is a clinical syndrome characterized by rapid loss of kidney function that often results in ESKD.
3. Acute glomerulonephritis and rapidly progressive glomerulonephritis (RPGN) are not specific diagnoses. Kidney biopsy is almost always required for definitive diagnosis and patient management.
4. If you think a patient has either acute glomerulonephritis or RPGN, expeditious diagnosis and initiation of therapy is vital because early intervention is associated with better outcomes.
5. Optimal patient management often requires referral to an expert in the care of patients with these diseases.

BIBLIOGRAPHY

Beck, L. H., Jr., & Salant, D. J. (2014). Membranous nephropathy: From models to man. *Journal of Clinical Investigation, 124*(6), 2307–2314.

Cattran, D. C., & Brenchley, P. E. (2017). Membranous nephropathy: Integrating basic science into improved clinical management. *Kidney International, 91*(3), 566–574.

Glassock, R. J., Alvarado, A., Prosek, J., Hebert, C., Parikh, S., Satoskar, A., . . . Hebert, L. A. (2015). Staphylococcus-related glomerulonephritis and poststreptococcal glomerulonephritis: Why defining "post" is important in understanding and treating infection-related glomerulonephritis. *American Journal of Kidney Diseases, 65*(6), 826–832.

Glassock, R. J., & Rovin, B. H. (2016). Primary and secondary glomerular diseases. *Nephrology Self-Assessment Program, 15*(3), 1–346.

Manoharon, A., Schelling, J. R., Diamond, M., Chung-Park, M., Madaio, M., & Sedor, J. R. (2013). Immune and inflammatory glomerular diseases. In R. J. Alpern, M. J. Caplan, & O. W. Moe (Eds.), *Seldin and Giebisch's the kidney: Physiology and pathophysiology* (pp. 2763–2816). Amsterdam: Elsevier.

Nasr, S. H., Radhakrishnan, J., & D'Agati, V. D. (2013). Bacterial infection-related glomerulonephritis in adults. *Kidney International, 83*(5), 792–803.

Sethi, S., Haas, M., Markowitz, G. S., D'Agati, V. D., Rennke, H. G., Jennette, J. C., . . . Fervenza, F. C. (2016). Mayo clinic/renal pathology society consensus report on pathologic classification, diagnosis, and reporting of GN. *Journal of the American Society of Nephrology, 27*(5), 1278–1287.

CHAPTER 15

NEPHROTIC SYNDROME

Jennifer Lopez and Howard Trachtman

1. What is nephrotic syndrome?

Nephrotic syndrome is one of the most rigidly defined entities in clinical medicine. The term is not a specific diagnosis, but instead represents a cluster of abnormal findings. Specifically, it is comprised of four distinct elements: one physical sign, edema; and three laboratory test abnormalities, massive proteinuria, hypoalbuminemia, and hypercholesterolemia. A hypercoagulable state is an optional fifth feature, especially in adults, who have a 10-fold higher risk of thromboembolic complications compared to pediatric patients. The hypercoagulable state in the nephrotic syndrome is due to many factors including urinary loss of antithrombin III, increased platelet aggregation, and endothelial dysfunction. It is important to note that reduced glomerular filtration rate or azotemia is not a defining feature of the nephrotic syndrome in any age group.

Edema is a key feature in patients with nephrotic syndrome. Studies suggest that it can develop by two distinct mechanisms. According to the underfill hypothesis, the hypoalbuminemia leads to decreased plasma oncotic pressure, reduction in the effective intravascular compartment size, activation of the renin–angiotensin axis, and stimulation of renal sodium reabsorption. In contrast, the overfill hypothesis posits that sodium retention in nephrotic syndrome is a primary abnormality in the kidney due to corin-mediated activation of the epithelial sodium channel. It is likely most patients have a component of each mechanism operating in the formation of edema. In most cases, the edema is controlled with modest dietary salt restriction and the administration of diuretics. In cases with severe underfilling, infusions of albumin and furosemide may be required to control edema.

2. How does one make the diagnosis of nephrotic syndrome?

The diagnosis is made in a patient with edema and massive proteinuria; that is, a urine protein:creatinine ratio greater than 2 (mg:mg) in a first morning sample in children or >3.5 g/24 hours in adults. Quantitation of urine protein excretion is mandatory to confirm the diagnosis of new-onset nephrotic syndrome. However, subsequent monitoring can be accomplished using qualitative dipstick urine testing. It is important to exclude cirrhosis, congestive heart failure, or gastrointestinal disease (protein-losing enteropathy or malabsorption) before conclusively attributing edema to kidney disease.

3. What are the causes of nephrotic syndrome?

Nephrotic syndrome is classified into primary (or idiopathic) and secondary causes. There are four principal primary etiologies of nephrotic syndrome:
1. Minimal change nephrotic syndrome (MCNS)
2. Focal segmental glomerulosclerosis (FSGS)
3. Membranous nephropathy (MN)
4. Membranoproliferative glomerulonephritis (MPGN)

There are variants of MCNS characterized by subtle changes in mesangial cell hypercellularity or the deposition of specific immunoglobulins such as IgM. However, the clinical significance of these entities is unclear. In adults, IgA nephropathy, fibrillary, and immunotactoid glomerulonephritis can present with nephrotic syndrome.

The secondary causes of nephrotic syndrome include:
• Post-infectious glomerulonephritis
• Systemic lupus erythematosus
• Henoch-Schoenlein purpura
• Medications
• Infections (e.g., hepatitis B, hepatitis C, HIV)
• Malignancies (Hodgkin's diseases)
• Amyloidosis
• Diabetes

This chapter will focus on primary nephrotic syndrome as a group, because the secondary causes are detailed in specific chapters for each entity.

4. What is the incidence and prevalence of nephrotic syndrome and has it changed in recent years?
The incidence of nephrotic syndrome is approximately 2 to 4 new cases per 100,000 population per year. There are data suggesting that the incidence of nephrotic syndrome is rising in certain populations around the world, such as Indians and Southeast Asians. However, the overall figure has been fairly steady and is applicable around the world and in most racial and ethnic groups.
      There may be a difference in the incidence of specific types of primary nephrotic disease in children and adults. The prevalence of nephrotic syndrome as a cause of chronic kidney disease varies from country to country depending on the practice patterns for disease detection and treatment. Nonetheless, primary nephrotic syndrome is an uncommon illness and qualifies for designation as a rare disease.

5. What is the clinical presentation of patients with nephrotic syndrome?
The most common presenting complaint for patients with nephrotic syndrome is edema. It usually involves the lower extremities in adults because they are more sedentary. While children also have pedal edema, it tends to be less severe because of increased physical activity. Periorbital edema and ascites occur in all age groups. The edema is symmetric and painless.

6. Are there extra-renal manifestations of nephrotic syndrome?
Less common presentations include peritonitis. This can even occur before the implementation of immunosuppressive therapy. In addition, thromboembolic events can complicate the course of nephrotic syndrome. The latter complaint is much more common, at least ten fold higher, in adults. Patients with nephrotic syndrome can present with acute kidney injury, attributable either to intra-renal edema and tubular obstruction or severe contraction of the effective intravascular compartment. In addition, patients with unremitting nephrotic syndrome and persistent hypercholesterolemia are at risk of premature atherosclerosis and cardiovascular disease.

7. What is the natural history of nephrotic syndrome?
The natural history of the primary nephrotic syndrome depends on the underlying cause.
   • MCNS: Patients have an excellent long-term prognosis. Most patients are responsive to therapy, and while the majority will follow a relapsing course, eventually most patients outgrow the disease without permanent kidney injury. However, there are some children with MCNS who continue to have relapsing disease well into adulthood.
   • FSGS: Nearly half of patients with primary FSGS progress to end-stage kidney disease (ESKD) over 5 to 10 years. Additionally, there is recurrent disease in 25% to 30% following a kidney transplant.
   • MPGN: Nearly 50% of patients with MPGN will progress to ESKD over 10 to 15 years and 20% to 25% of these patients develop recurrent disease in a transplanted kidney.
   • Membranous nephropathy: The long-term course of MN is more variable. Approximately one-third will go into remission, another third have persistent proteinuria with stable kidney function, and the remaining patients will experience a steady decline in kidney function. Recent findings suggest that monitoring the level of antibody to M-type phospholipase A(2) receptor (PLA(2)R) can be useful to predict prognosis and response to therapy.

8. Are there any patient groups at special risk of developing nephrotic syndrome or adverse long-term outcomes?
Primary nephrotic syndrome occurs in all racial ethnic groups. It affects boys more commonly than girls; however, the outcomes are similar irrespective of the patient's gender.

9. What is the appropriate work-up for patients with nephrotic syndrome?
   • Patients with primary nephrotic syndrome require **quantitation of urine protein** excretion to demonstrate nephrotic-range proteinuria. This can be accomplished by measuring the protein:creatinine ratio in the first morning urine specimen where a value >2 (mg:mg) in children is indicative of nephrotic syndrome. Alternatively, in adults, a 24-hour urine collection can be performed, and a level of protein in excess of 3.5 g is diagnostic of nephrotic-range proteinuria. While assessment of the first morning urine specimen is the standard of care in pediatric patients, there is greater diversity of practice in adult patient, with use of first morning urine samples, spot urine specimens, and 24-hour urine collections to monitor disease activity.
   • A **complete metabolic profile** is obtained to demonstrate hypoalbuminemia and hypercholesterolemia. The blood urea nitrogen and creatinine are generally normal. Total serum calcium level is low secondary to the low hypoalbuminemia. Serum sodium concentration may be low if there is water reabsorption in excess of sodium. Pseudohyponatremia secondary to hyperlipidemia is no longer a concern with the widespread use of ion selective electrodes in clinical chemistry analyzers.

- The **C3 level** is measured in all patients to exclude MPGN.
- A **complete blood count** is part of the routine evaluation even though it usually has little information value about the cause of nephrotic syndrome. In select cases in which the nephrotic syndrome is secondary to a systemic illness or malignancy, the complete blood count may provide useful data.

10. Are there any unique laboratory tests that are relevant to patients with nephrotic syndrome?
    - Anti-streptolysin O
    - ANA, and double stranded DNA titers
    - HIV testing
    - Hepatitis B and C testing
    - Assays for C3 nephritic factor with MPGN
    - Antibodies to M-type phospholipase A_2 receptor PLA$_2$R is useful in idiopathic MN
    - thrombospondin type-1 domain-containing 7A may be useful in idiopathic MN
    - Venography is often performed in adults with new-onset primary nephrotic syndrome to detect renal vein thrombosis, especially in patients with MN.

11. What is the role of a kidney biopsy in the assessment of patients with nephrotic syndrome?
    A kidney biopsy is necessary to definitively distinguish between the four causes of primary nephrotic syndrome. There are differences in the application of kidney biopsy in pediatric and adult patients.
    - In children, the criteria for performing a kidney biopsy prior to treatment are:
      - Age below 6 months
      - Onset in adolescence; that is, Tanner stage 3 or greater
      - Low C3 level
      - Any unusual clinical feature
    - Otherwise, most pediatric nephrologists defer a kidney biopsy until after completion and resistance to steroids. The rationale for this approach is the high frequency of MCNS in children with new-onset nephrotic syndrome. Importantly, a standard course of steroids will not modify the underlying renal histopathology if there is a lesion other than MCNS.
    - In adults with nephrotic syndrome, a kidney biopsy is done prior to therapy because of diverse potential pathology and reduced tolerance of corticosteroids. The tissue sample should be processed for light microscopy, immunofluorescence, and electron microscopy to establish the diagnosis.
    - Special stains for glomerular proteins, such as synaptopodin and dystroglycan, may help discriminate among the causes of primary nephrotic syndrome. These are podocyte-associated proteins whose expression has been shown to be different in patients with MCNS versus FSGS.

12. What is the cause of nephrotic syndrome?
    The cause of primary nephrotic syndrome is generally unknown. In MCNS, an immune-mediated mechanism has been proposed based on the association of the disease with atopy, various malignancies, and the response to immunosuppressive medications. In addition, a variety of permeability factors, including vascular endothelial growth factor and interleukin-8, presumably derived from immunoeffector cells, have been linked to proteinuria. Genetic mutations (see below) are increasingly recognized as the cause of primary MCNS and FSGS. The pathogenesis of idiopathic MN is linked to the development of antibodies to M-type phospholipase A2 receptor and thrombospondin type-1 domain-containing 7A. Infants and young children may develop MN because of antibodies to bovine albumin. Types I and III MPGN are immune-complex disorders, while type II disease (DDD, dense deposit disease) is associated with abnormal regulation of the alternative pathway of complement.

13. Is there a genetic contribution to nephrotic syndrome?
    Approximately 5% of cases of MCNS occur in a familial pattern with parent-child or sibling-sibling clusters. However, there are little data about the frequency of causative genetic mutations in steroid-responsive disease. In nearly 30% to 40% of cases of primary FSGS, genetic mutations in podocyte proteins have been identified. The most commonly affected protein is podocin, detected in up to 20% of sporadic and familial cases. Other proteins linked to FSGS include α-actinin-4, CD2AP, Wilms tumor-1 (Denys-Drash syndrome), phospholipase C epsilon1, TRPC6, and the inverse formin gene INF2. Defects in the nephrin gene and laminin β2 (Pierson syndrome) are associated with congenital nephrotic syndrome and disease in the first year of life. Recently, mutations in mitochondrial and nuclear transport proteins have been associated with FSGS. The list of genetic causes of nephrotic syndrome, and FSGS in particular, is likely to grow over time. However, the exact frequency remains to be determined as methods to distinguish disease-causing genetic mutations from normal variants

are refined. MN has been linked to various HLA polymorphisms. MPGN type II (DDD) is associated with a variety of genetic mutations in proteins involved in the alternative pathway of complement.

Currently, the role of genetic testing in patients with new-onset nephrotic syndrome that is resistant to corticosteroids is subject to ongoing debate. Patients with nephrotic syndrome who have a genetic basis for the disease may have not only a lower response rate to immunosuppressive therapy but also a lower risk of recurrent disease following transplantation.

14. What is the first-line treatment for nephrotic syndrome?

Corticosteroids are generally considered the first agent used in an attempt to reduce proteinuria in all patients with nephrotic syndrome caused by MCNS or FSGS, unless there is a clinical contraindication to their use. The dose and duration of therapy is highly contingent on the age of the patient, and the likelihood of response varies from greater than 90% in children with MCNS to less than 20% to 30% in patients with FSGS. In patients with MN, current recommendations suggest using conservative therapy with agents that block the renin–angiotensin axis, and resorting to corticosteroids if the proteinuria does improve or if the patients are symptomatic. The therapy of MPGN and the role of corticosteroids is determined by the specific disease subtype.

15. What are the second-line therapies for nephrotic syndrome?

The choice of therapy in patients with steroid-resistant nephrotic syndrome is a highly contentious topic because of a lack of sufficiently powered clinical trials. Alternative therapies are applied in MCNS in children who are suffering intolerable side effects from steroids. These patients respond well to mycophenolate mofetil, cyclophosphamide, or calcineurin inhibitors, such as cyclosporine or tacrolimus. Cyclosporine is the only agent that has been proven to be superior to placebo in patients with FSGS. In those with MN, combined therapy with steroids and an alkylating agent is effective in patients at high risk of progressive deterioration in kidney function. There are ongoing trials to assess the efficacy of calcineurin inhibitors (CNIs) and rituximab in the treatment of MN. In those with MPGN, a regimen involving steroids, antiplatelet drugs and an alkylating agent has been utilized with uncertain efficacy. The role of inhibitors of the alternative pathway of complement, such as eculizumab in patients with type II MPGN, remains to be determined.

16. What is the appropriate supportive care for patients with nephrotic syndrome?

Patients who have edema from nephrotic syndrome require dietary sodium restriction and judicious use of diuretics. These agents are often needed in combination (site of action in the loop of Henle and distal tubule), and careful monitoring for hyponatremia, hypokalemia, and metabolic alkalosis is mandatory. Angiotensin-converting enzyme inhibitors and angiotensin receptor blockers can be used to lower blood pressure and reduce urinary protein excretion. Hypercholesterolemia can be treated with an HMG-CoA reductase inhibitor. Immunization against *Streptococcus pneumoniae* should be administered to prevent bacterial infections, such as peritonitis. In select cases, prophylactic antibiotics may be necessary. Careful surveillance for thromboembolic complications and the administration of anticoagulants may be needed in adult patients. There are tools that can be used to identify patients at higher risk of thromboembolism and in whom prophylactic interventions are warranted. The use of lipid-lowering drugs is usually not needed in patients with treatment-responsive nephrotic syndrome. In those with refractory disease, statins may reduce but will not normalize the hyperlipidemia.

17. What is the role of kidney transplantation in the treatment of patients with nephrotic syndrome?

Kidney transplantation is a viable option in all patients with nephrotic syndrome who progress to ESKD. However, there is a substantial risk of recurrent disease that is in the range of 20% to 40% for patients with FSGS and MPGN. Thus, patients who have lost more than one kidney allograft to recurrent glomerular disease are often considered ineligible for subsequent transplant procedures.

18. Are there novel therapies for nephrotic syndrome that are under development?

Dietary interventions, such as a gluten-free diet, may be useful in a subset of children with MCNS. Rituximab, a monoclonal antibody to CD20 on B-cells, is being tested in the full array of causes of nephrotic syndrome. Abatacept, a monoclonal antibody to B7.1, has been shown to be effective in inducing remission of proteinuria in the open-label treatment of patients with FSGS and is being evaluated in an ongoing randomized clinical trial. Strategies to prevent kidney fibrosis using thiazolidinediones (rosiglitazone) and monoclonal anti-tumor necrosis factor antibodies (adalimumab) are under evaluation to protect the kidney in resistant forms of nephrotic syndrome. The identification of a subgroup of patients with a specific disease mechanism may improve the likelihood of achieving a favorable response to therapeutic interventions targeted at the underlying pathophysiological cause.

KEY POINTS

1. The nephrotic syndrome is comprised of four distinct elements
   a. edema
   b. massive proteinuria, defined as a urine protein:creatinine ratio >2 (mg:mg) in children and >3.5 g/24 hours in adults
   c. hypoalbuminemia
   d. hypercholesterolemia
   e. with an optional fifth feature, a hypercoagulable state
2. Nephrotic syndrome is classified as primary (or idiopathic) and secondary causes. There are four principal primary etiologies:
   a. Minimal change nephrotic syndrome (MCNS)
   b. Focal segmental glomerulosclerosis (FSGS)
   c. Membranous nephropathy (MN)
   d. Membranoproliferative glomerulonephritis (MPGN)
3. A kidney biopsy is necessary to definitively distinguish among the four causes of primary nephrotic syndrome or confirm a secondary cause. Genetic testing may be an alternative diagnostic test in infants in the first year of life or in those with a family history of disease.
4. The natural history of primary nephrotic syndrome depends on the underlying cause. Patients with MCNS have an excellent long-term prognosis. Half of patients with primary FSGS will progress to end-stage kidney disease over 5 to 10 years. Additionally, 25% to 30% of primary FSGS patients develop recurrent disease following a kidney transplant.
5. Corticosteroids are generally considered the first agent to be tried to reduce proteinuria in all patients with nephrotic syndrome, unless there is a clinical contraindication to their use. Calcineurin inhibitors are the most widely accepted second-line therapeutic option in patients with nephrotic syndrome who are unresponsive to corticosteroids or who are experiencing significant side effects.

BIBLIOGRAPHY

Banh, T. H. M., Hussain-Shamsy, N., Patel, V., Vasilevska-Ristovska, J., Borges, K., Sibbald, C., . . . Parekh, R. S. (2016). Ethnic differences in incidence and outcomes of childhood nephrotic syndrome. *Clinical Journal of the American Society of Nephrology*, *11*(10), 1760–1768.

Beck, L. H., Jr., Bonegio, R. G., Lambeau, G., Beck, D. M., Powell, D. W., Cummins, T. D., . . . Salant, D. J. (2009). M-type phospholipase A2 receptor as a target antigen in idiopathic membranous nephropathy. *New England Journal of Medicine*, *361*, 11–21.

Hahn, D., Hodson, E. M., Willis, N. S., & Craig, J. C. (2015). Corticosteroid therapy for nephrotic syndrome in children. *Cochrane Database of Systematic Reviews*, (3), CD001533.

Iijima, K., Sako, M., & Nozu, K. (2017). Rituximab for nephrotic syndrome in children. *Clinical and Experimental Nephrology*, *21*(2), 193–202. http://doi:org/10.1007/s10157-016-1313-5.

Jahan, A., Prabha, R., Chaturvedi, S., Mathew, B., Fleming, D., & Agarwal, I. (2015). Clinical efficacy and pharmacokinetics of tacrolimus in children with steroid-resistant nephrotic syndrome. *Pediatric Nephrology*, *30*, 1961–1967.

Karp, A. M., & Gbadegesin, R. A. (2016). Genetics of childhood steroid-sensitive nephrotic syndrome. *Pediatric Nephrology*. http://doi:org/10.1007/s00467-016-3456-8.

Lemley, K. V., Faul, C., Schramm, K., Meyers, K., Kaskel, F., Dell, K. M., . . . Trachtman, H. (2016). The effect of a gluten-free diet in children with difficult-to-manage nephrotic syndrome. *Pediatrics*, *138*(1), e20154528. http://doi:org/10.1542/peds.2015-4528.

Lombel, R. M., Gipson, D. S., & Hodson, E. M. (2013). Treatment of steroid sensitive nephrotic syndrome: New guidelines from KDIGO. *Pediatric Nephrology*, *28*, 415–426.

McCaffrey, J., Lennon, R., & Webb, N. J. (2016). The non-immunosuppressive management of childhood nephrotic syndrome. *Pediatric Nephrology*, *31*, 1383–1402. http://doi:org/10.1007/s00467-015-3241-0.

Rüth, E. M., Landolt, M. A., Neuhaus, T. J., & Kemper, M. J. (2004). Health-related quality of life and psychosocial adjustment in steroid-sensitive nephrotic syndrome. *Journal of Pediatrics*, *145*, 778–783.

CHAPTER 16

OBSTRUCTIVE UROPATHY

Benjamin A. Sherer and Marshall L. Stoller

1. **What is obstructive uropathy?**
   Obstructive uropathy is structural or functional interference of normal urine flow anywhere along the urinary tract. Obstructive uropathy can be acute or chronic, partial, or complete, and unilateral or bilateral.

2. **What is obstructive nephropathy?**
   Long-standing obstructive uropathy may ultimately lead to kidney damage. Obstructive nephropathy is typically caused by elevated pressures in the renal pelvis and calyces due to hydronephrosis and can lead to dilation and ischemia of the distal tubules of nephrons and subsequent interstitial fibrosis and kidney atrophy.

3. **What are the most common causes of obstructive uropathy?**
   The causes of obstructive uropathy vary with age and gender. In older men, benign prostatic hyperplasia (BPH) and prostate cancer are the most common causes. In older women, gynecologic malignancies can cause extrinsic compression on the urinary tract and ureteral obstruction. In younger patients, nephrolithiasis is the most common cause of ureteral obstruction. In children, obstruction is most often a result of congenital anomalies such as ureteropelvic junction obstruction and posterior urethral valves in newborn boys.

4. **What is the role of ultrasound in the evaluation of obstructive uropathy?**
   Ultrasound is the primary modality used for detection and characterization of obstructive uropathy. Hydronephrosis is the most common finding in unilateral upper urinary tract obstruction involving the ureteropelvic junction or ureter. In early obstruction (first 1 to 3 days) or in an anuric or dehydrated state, hydronephrosis may be mild or absent in the setting of obstruction. Duplex Doppler ultrasonography can be used to calculate renal arterial resistive indices, which can improve the sensitivity and specificity in detecting obstruction. In acute obstruction, a resistive index of >0.70 is often indicative of obstruction. In chronic obstruction, there is often a progressive loss of the echo-rich fat in the plane of Gil Vernet. Ultrasonography may also identify a distended urinary bladder in the setting of bladder outlet obstruction.

5. **Does hydronephrosis always indicate obstruction?**
   Mild hydronephrosis found on ultrasound can be a normal physiologic variant; kidney ultrasonography is therefore associated with a high false-positive rate (~24%) in detecting obstruction. Another common "false positive" ultrasonographic finding is hydronephrosis of pregnancy, which is physiologic and rarely clinically significant. This is hypothesized to result from both hormonal changes (elevated progesterone) influencing the ureter and mechanical extrinsic compression on the ureter from the uterus. Hydronephrosis of pregnancy is more common in the right kidney because the sigmoid colon occupies space within the left pelvis and pushes the uterus toward the right ureter.

6. **What other imaging modalities are helpful in the evaluation of obstructive uropathy?**
   A computed tomography (CT) scan can provide a more detailed evaluation of hydronephrosis, hydroureter, and/or bladder distension from outlet obstruction. The noncontrast phase of a CT scan is best for identifying obstruction from stones. If kidney function permits the use of contrast, a delayed contrast phase can show contrast draining from the kidneys to the bladder and identify the cause and location of intrinsic (inside the ureter) and extrinsic (compression of ureter from the outside) forms of ureteral obstruction. A MAG-3 (mercaptoacetyltriglycine) nuclear medicine renal scan can evaluate differential kidney function (kidney uptake) and can quantify drainage times for each kidney unit after administration of a diuretic.

7. **What procedures can aid in the diagnosis and treatment of urinary obstruction?**
   Cystourethroscopy (endoscopic visualization of the urethra and bladder) can identify urethral strictures and/or prostatic hyperplasia that may be causing bladder outlet obstruction. If other imaging studies are equivocal or patients are unable to receive intravenous contrast administered (due to severe chronic kidney disease (CKD) or allergy), a retrograde pyelography (injection of contrast up the ureters during cystoscopy) may be necessary. Retrograde pyelography provides excellent delineation of filling

defects within the ureter, renal pelvis, or renal calyces. Collection of urinary cytology is possible during retrograde pyelography. Cystoscopy also allows for intervention to relieve ureteral obstruction in the same setting, such as placement of a ureteral stent. If a ureteral stent is unable to bypass a ureteral obstruction or does not provide adequate drainage of the kidney collecting system, a percutaneous nephrostomy tube may be necessary to optimize kidney decompression.

8. **How can urinary retention lead to obstructive uropathy?**
   Normal patients should have the ability to void at least 80% of their bladder volume, with a postvoid residual of less than 50 mL. In the setting of bladder outlet obstruction (BOO) or poor bladder contractility, the efficiency of bladder emptying may decrease and residual urine may increase. An elevated postvoid residual is associated with increased risk of infection and can lead to a distended and a hypotonic bladder. If high (typically >40 cm H_2O) intravesical pressures develop due to excessive bladder volumes and/or poor bladder compliance, urine can reflux up the ureters and cause hydroureteronephrosis and obstructive nephropathy.

9. **What are common causes of urinary retention?**
   The most common cause of anatomic cause of urinary retention in men is BOO due to BPH. Urethral strictures can also cause BOO. In females, urinary retention can be caused by the presence of a cystocele or pelvic organ prolapse. Common nonanatomic causes of urinary retention include diabetes, neurologic deficits (spinal cord injury, multiple sclerosis, Parkinson disease), urinary tract infections, and medications (especially anticholinergics).

10. **What are common signs/symptoms of urinary retention?**
    Common symptoms of subacute and chronic urinary retention include urinary frequency, urgency, decreased urinary flow, intermittent urinary stream, and bothersome nocturia. In severe acute urinary retention (inability to urinate in the setting of a full bladder), patients often develop pelvic pain and anxiety. In contrast, patients with progressive chronic retention, large bladders, hypotonic bladders, neurogenic bladders, or decreased bladder sensation may not have any symptoms in the presence of significant underlying urinary retention. Some patients develop incontinence due to unexpected detrusor contractions or overflow of urine in the setting of a full bladder. On physical exam, a full bladder may be palpable between the pubic bone and the umbilicus.

11. **Is pain always present in patients with hydronephrosis?**
    The pain in obstruction of the upper urinary tract is a result of distention of the renal collecting system. If obstruction and distention occur acutely, then pain can be excruciating and is often associated with nausea and vomiting. However, if obstruction is slowly progressive, then the process can be painless (a.k.a. "silent" obstruction).

12. **Describe the three hemodynamic phases of acute unilateral upper tract urinary obstruction.**
    In the first phase of unilateral upper tract obstruction (first 1 to 2 hours), intrarenal pressure rises due to obstruction. In response, tubuloglomerular feedback mechanisms allow for afferent arteriolar vasodilation (mediated by prostaglandin E_2 and nitric oxide), which increases kidney blood flow to maintain glomerular filtration rate (GFR). In the second phase (lasting 3 to 4 hours), intrarenal pressures remain elevated, but elevated renin released during phase one results in angiotensin II mediated preglomerular vasoconstriction and decreased kidney blood flow. A third phase (beginning ~5 hours after obstruction) is marked by a further decline in kidney blood flow and GFR mediated by a number of vasoconstrictors (including angiotensin II, thromboxane A_2, endothelin).

13. **How does the physiologic response to bilateral obstruction differ from unilateral obstruction?**
    In unilateral ureteral obstruction, the renin release from the obstructed kidney causes a compensatory increase in kidney blood flow and GFR in the contralateral kidney. Because the contralateral kidney provides compensatory function, there is little change to total GFR, urine output, electrolyte levels, or serum creatinine. In bilateral ureteral obstruction, there is no compensation by the contralateral kidney. Thus there can be dramatic decreases in GFR, which is often associated with oliguria, electrolyte abnormalities, creatinine elevation, and fluid retention. Bilateral obstruction can also result in hypertension. In acute bilateral obstruction, hypertension is caused by elevated renin levels. In chronic bilateral obstruction, hypertension is secondary to fluid overload.

14. **What electrolyte abnormalities are seen in bilateral obstructive nephropathy?**
    Bilateral kidney obstruction is often associated with hyperkalemia and metabolic acidosis resulting from defects in the excretion of potassium and hydrogen in the distal convoluted tubules and cortical collecting ducts in the setting of relative aldosterone resistance.

15. Can obstructive uropathy be associated with infection?

Urinary tract infection is a common complication of urinary tract obstruction and results from stasis of urine. Infection in the setting of hydronephrosis can lead to pyonephrosis, pyelonephritis, bacteremia, and sepsis. Infection associated with hydronephrosis typically warrants urgent decompression with ureteral stent placement or nephrostomy tube placement. Elimination of infection is difficult until the obstruction is relieved.

16. What is postobstructive diuresis?

After obstruction is relieved, a physiologic diuresis occurs with the excretion of excess total body water, along with an osmotic diuresis stimulated by the excretion of urea. This process can lead to a pathologic diuresis, with negative fluid balance and electrolyte deficiencies. Pathologic postobstructive diuresis is caused by decreased expression of aquaporin channels in the collecting duct, excessive presence of atrial natriuretic peptide, and concentrating defects in the corticomedullary gradient. Patients should have electrolytes checked and replaced regularly with free access to oral fluids. If intravenous fluids are required, their type and amount should be determined by serum and urinary electrolyte levels. Postobstructive diuresis is most likely to occur after relief of obstruction in patients with severe urinary retention, high serum creatinine, and elevated serum bicarbonate.

KEY POINTS

1. Acute urinary tract obstruction can cause acute kidney injury. Chronic obstruction can lead to end-stage kidney disease.
2. Acute urinary obstruction is often associated with pain, whereas chronic urinary obstruction may be asymptomatic.
3. Ultimate recovery of kidney function after relief of obstruction is based on severity of obstruction, duration of obstruction, patient age, and baseline kidney function.
4. Hypertension from bilateral urinary obstruction is initially a result of the release of renin and later a result of retention of fluid.
5. Diuresis after obstruction may result from a physiologic excretion of water and urea, but can become pathologic. Patients should have electrolytes checked and replaced regularly, with free access to oral fluids. If necessary, the type and amount of intravenous fluids should be determined by serum and urinary electrolyte levels.
6. Infection is a common complication of urinary tract obstruction and is a result of urinary stasis. Hydronephrosis with infection warrants urgent urologic intervention for decompression.

BIBLIOGRAPHY

Hamdi, A., Hajage, D., Van Glabeke, E., Belenfant, X., Vincent, F., Gonzalez, F., . . . Das V. (2012). Severe post-renal acute kidney injury, post-obstructive diuresis and renal recovery. *BJU International, 110,* E1027–E1034.

Harris, R. H., & Yarger, W. E. (1974). Renal function after release of unilateral ureteral obstruction in rats. *American Journal of Physiology, 227,* 806–815.

Kamholtz, R. G., Cronan, J. J., & Dorfman, G. S. (1989). Obstruction and the minimally dilated renal collecting system: US evaluation. *Radiology, 170,* 51–53.

Kerr, W. S., Jr. (1954). Effect of complete ureteral obstruction for one week on kidney function. *Journal of Applied Physiology, 6,* 762–772.

Kim, S. W., Lee, J., Park, J. W., Hong, J. H., Kook, H., Choi, C., & Choi, K. C. (2001). Increased expression of atrial natriuretic peptide in the kidney of rats with bilateral ureteral obstruction. *Kidney International, 59,* 1274–1282.

Klahr, S., & Morrissey, J. (2002). Obstructive nephropathy and renal fibrosis. *American Journal of Physiology. Renal Physiology, 283,* F861–F875.

Lameire, N., Van Biesen, W., & Vanholder, R. (2005). Acute renal failure. *Lancet, 365,* 417–430.

Rokaw, M. D., Sarac, E., Lechman, E., West, M., Angeski, J., Johnson, J. P., & Zeidel, M. L. (1996). Chronic regulation of transepithelial Na+ transport by the rate of apical Na+ entry. *American Journal of Physiology, 270,* C600–C607.

Schlossberg, S. M., & Vaughan, E. D., Jr. (1984). The mechanism of unilateral post-obstructive diuresis. *Journal of Urology, 131,* 534–536.

Vaughan, E. D., Jr., & Gillenwater, J. Y. (1971). Recovery following complete chronic unilateral ureteral occlusion: Functional, radiographic, and pathologic alterations. *Journal of Urology, 106,* 27–35.

Wein, A. J., Kavoussi, L. R., Novick, A. C., Partin, A. W., & Peters, C. A. (2011). *Campbell-Walsh urology* (10th ed., 4 v., xlii, 4320, cxv). Philadelphia: W.B. Saunders.

CHAPTER 17

NEPHROLITHIASIS

John Robert Asplin and Jennifer L. Ennis

1. How common are kidney stones?

   In industrialized countries, approximately 12% of men and 7% of women will form at least one kidney stone in their life, and the prevalence of nephrolithiasis is increasing. Historically men were much more likely to form kidney stones than women, but recent data show the prevalence in women is approaching that of men. After presenting with their initial stone, about 50% of patients will have at least one more stone within 8 years.

2. What are kidney stones made of?

   Approximately 80% of kidney stones are predominantly calcium salts. Calcium oxalate is the major component in 85% to 90% of calcium stones, the rest being calcium phosphate, in the form of apatite or brushite. It is common for small amounts of apatite to be found in calcium oxalate stones. About 10% of stones are uric acid and 5% to 10% are struvite (magnesium ammonium phosphate). Cystine accounts for about 1% of all stones. Stones may be a single pure substance or may be a mix of crystal types, such as calcium oxalate and uric acid.

3. What is the best radiologic test to diagnose kidney stones?

   Noncontrast computed tomography (CT) scan or ultrasound are the tests of choice for imaging patients with suspected kidney stones. Advantages of CT include much greater sensitivity for small stones, no intravenous contrast, ability to detect uric acid stones (which are radiolucent on standard x-rays), and the potential to diagnose other causes of flank/abdominal pain if no stones are found. The main drawback with CT scans is the radiation exposure. If a patient requires serial radiologic evaluation, a KUB (kidneys, ureters, and bladder) x-ray is preferred, but only if the stone of interest can be adequately visualized.

   Ultrasound can identify hydronephrosis and document stones, but it is not as sensitive or specific as CT. Ultrasound is clearly the preferred imaging method in pregnant women, and many clinicians prefer to use it in children to avoid excessive radiation.

4. Do all patients with renal colic require urologic intervention to remove the stone?

   Most patients with renal colic will pass the stone without surgical intervention. Stones <5 mm will pass without intervention 80% to 90% of the time; stones >6 mm pass only 25% of the time. Pharmaceuticals, such as the alpha blocker tamsulosin or calcium channel blockers, which act as ureteral muscle relaxants, can be used to promote stone passage. Corticosteroids may be used to reduce swelling and inflammation. Indications for emergent removal of an obstructing stone include fever, intractable pain, persistent nausea and vomiting, obstruction of a unilateral kidney, or a stone deemed unlikely to pass because of its size.

5. What is extracorporeal shock-wave lithotripsy (ESWL)?

   ESWL is a noninvasive method to remove urolithiasis in the renal pelvis or in the ureter. Shock waves are conducted through water to the patient's flank. The shock waves are focused on the stone, pulverizing it into multiple small pieces. ESWL is an outpatient procedure that requires only mild anesthesia. Disadvantages include the requirement for the patient to pass the fragments, which may cause renal colic, and the potential for some stone fragments to remain in the kidney, particularly stones in the lower pole of the kidney. Some stones, such as cystine and brushite, are difficult to fragment by ESWL.

6. Is open surgery still used for kidney stones?

   Open surgery has been replaced by percutaneous nephrolithotomy (PCNL) and ureteroscopy. PCNL is performed by placing a nephroscope through the patient's flank into the renal pelvis. Stones can be directly visualized and fragmented, and fragments removed through the scope. PCNL most often is used for large stones (>2 cm), stones in a lower pole of the kidney, or stones that have been resistant to ESWL. Ureteroscopy is used for stones in the ureter and some stones in the renal pelvis. The ureteroscope is introduced through the urethra, into the bladder, and then the ureter. Stones may

113

be removed using a basket or destroyed using a laser. The choice of surgical approach depends on the type of stone, location of the stone, and expertise of the urologist.

7. Is it worthwhile having kidney stone composition analyzed?
Whenever stone material is available, crystallographic analysis should be performed. Although 70% of stones will be composed of calcium oxalate, it is the finding of noncalcium stones that provides the most benefit. Struvite and cystine stones are uncommon but cause serious stone diseases; their diagnosis via stone analysis leads to specific and intensive therapy. Uric acid stones are always treated with alkalinization. Crystallization of medications such as indinavir, guaifenesin, and triamterene in the urinary tract can lead to stones, which can only be diagnosed by the analysis of stone material.

8. If an initial stone has been analyzed, do subsequent stones need to be analyzed?
Yes. Analysis of stones as they recur may reveal that stone composition has changed, which could require revision of the stone prevention protocol. In fact, a change in stone type may be a result of preventive therapy, such as calcium phosphate stones forming because of excessive alkalinization in a patient with cystinuria.

9. How much of a workup should a patient with a single kidney stone have?
When adults present with their initial stone episode, they should have a limited workup to identify the more serious issues related to nephrolithiasis. Serum chemistries will reveal hypokalemia and/or acidosis that would indicate distal renal tubular acidosis (RTA), hypercalcemia to identify patients who should be evaluated for hyperparathyroidism, and serum creatinine to estimate kidney function. Stone analysis should always be performed. Urinalysis and/or urine culture should be done to identify infection and microscopy for stone-related crystals. Radiographic evaluation should be performed to quantify stone burden. If multiple stones are seen on CT scan or x-ray, the patient should be considered a recurrent stone former.

10. Who should have 24-hour urine chemistries measured as part of their evaluation?
Adults with recurrent stone disease should have 24-hour urine chemistries measured. Some adults with a single stone event will require full evaluation as dictated by their career, such as airline pilots. Recent AUA guidelines suggest performing 24-hour urine studies in first-time stone formers if they are highly motivated to prevent future stones. In addition, all children with kidney stones should have urine chemistries performed, because they have a higher likelihood of having a severe inherited form of nephrolithiasis such as cystinuria or primary hyperoxaluria.

11. What chemistries should be ordered on a 24-hour urine collection?
Urine chemistries should include:
- Calcium
- Oxalate
- Uric acid
- Phosphorus
- Urine volume: All patients should try to maintain a urine volume of at least 2.5 liters/day.
- Citrate forms a complex with calcium in the urine; thus low urine citrate is a commonly found risk factor for calcium stone formation.
- pH should be measured in a 24-hour urine sample; low pH is a risk factor for uric acid stones, and high pH is a risk factor for calcium phosphate stones.
- Creatinine should be measured in all timed urine specimens to ensure that the urine specimen was collected properly.

12. Is a random urine pH an adequate replacement for a 24-hour urine pH?
A random urine pH should not be used to assess stone risk, because pH is too variable for a single measurement to provide meaningful information. Urine pH in a normal subject varies from 5.0 to 7.0, depending on diet and time of day. A 24-hour sample gives the time-averaged urine pH; normal range is 5.7 to 6.3 for a 24-hour collection.

13. Is a single 24-hour urine collection adequate when evaluating a patient with nephrolithiasis?
Urine chemistries vary much more than serum chemistries, because urine excretions are dependent on lifestyle, diet, and each patient's particular physiology. As such, it is wise to perform at least two 24-hour urine collections during the initial evaluation. Optimally, one collection would be on a weekend and the other on a weekday to assess both the home and work environment, because diet, fluid intake, and levels of exertion can vary tremendously.

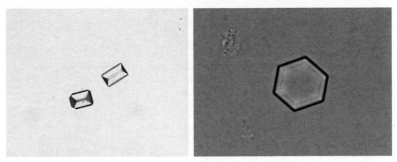

Figure 17.1. Struvite crystals (left panel) are rectangular prisms with the appearance of coffin lids. Cystine crystals (right panel) are hexagonal plates.

14. Are crystals seen during urine microscopy helpful in the diagnosis of stone disease?

Cystine crystals and struvite crystals are always abnormal and diagnostic of an underlying disorder (Fig. 17.1). Cystine crystals are only present in people with cystinuria, an uncommon genetic disorder in which cystine is not reabsorbed normally by the kidney. Struvite crystals only form in humans when there is urinary infection with bacteria that possess urease activity. Uric acid and calcium crystals may be more frequent in the urine of stone formers, but they are not diagnostic of disease because they also may be found in healthy people. One situation in which the finding of calcium or uric acid crystals may be helpful is in patients with renal colic without a documented stone, where transient bursts of crystalluria may be causing symptoms.

15. Is it really true that drinking water prevents kidney stones?

Creating dilute urine will reduce the concentration of lithogenic substances and thus the driving force for crystallization. A prospective randomized trial proved the effectiveness of high fluid intake; the urine volume in the treated group averaged 2.5 L/day, providing a reasonable goal for patients with nephrolithiasis. Generally it is better to prescribe a specified urine flow rather than an absolute amount of fluid intake because patients' fluid needs vary. Although physicians usually recommend water as the preferred fluid, other beverages seem to provide equal benefit.

16. Why do uric acid stones form?

Urate is an end product of purine metabolism. Urate solubility is pH dependent; as urine pH falls below 5.5, uric acid becomes the predominant form of urate. Uric acid is poorly soluble such that even at normal rates of urate excretion, uric acid can crystallize when urine pH is low. In fact, most patients with uric acid stones do not over-excrete uric acid, but have an abnormally low urine pH as the cause of stone formation. Low urine pH may be the result of high dietary intake of animal protein, chronic kidney disease (CKD), metabolic syndrome, or gastrointestinal (GI) alkali loss, as may be seen with chronic diarrhea.

17. How does metabolic syndrome lead to kidney stones?

Metabolic syndrome is a constellation of abnormalities (hypertension, glucose intolerance, dyslipidemia, and increased waist size) associated with an increased risk of cardiovascular disease. Recent studies also have shown an increased risk of uric acid stone formation. Patients with metabolic syndrome have a lower urine pH because they excrete more of their daily net acid production as titratable acid and less as ammonium, with the net effect being a lower urine pH. The lower ammonia production by the proximal tubule results from insulin resistance. As might be expected, patients with diabetes appear to develop uric acid stones more frequently than nondiabetics.

18. What is the best treatment for uric acid stones?

Lowering dietary intake of animal protein will reduce the dietary acid load, raising urine pH. Because most dietary purine comes from animal tissue, lowering animal protein intake will also lower uric acid excretion. The mainstay of therapy to prevent uric acid stone formation is to raise urine pH with alkali. Potassium citrate is generally preferred. If a patient cannot tolerate potassium salts because of GI side effects or hyperkalemia, then sodium alkali may be used. The goal of therapy is a 24-hour urine pH of 6.0 to 6.5; raising urine pH to higher levels will not provide additional benefit. Allopurinol is a second-line drug for uric acid stones, used when the patient also has gout or when the patient is unable to take sufficient alkali to raise urine pH higher than 6.0. Allopurinol should be used in diseases with massive urate overproduction such as Lesch-Nyhan syndrome.

19. **What is idiopathic hypercalciuria?**
    Idiopathic hypercalciuria is generally defined as a urine calcium excretion higher than 300 mg/day in a man or 250 mg/day in a woman, with normal serum calcium in the absence of any systemic disorder known to affect mineral metabolism, such as sarcoidosis or primary hyperparathyroidism.

20. **How much calcium should a patient with calcium stones have in their diet?**
    For many years, low-calcium diets (400 mg/day) were standard for patients with calcium stones and hypercalciuria. Although low-calcium diets clearly reduce urine calcium, there is not a clinical trial proving that low-calcium diets reduce stone formation. Epidemiologic studies challenged this approach by showing people with low-calcium diets were more likely to form kidney stones than those on high-calcium diets. A subsequent study showed that a low-sodium, low-protein diet with normal calcium intake was more effective in preventing stones than a standard low-calcium diet. In general, patients should be encouraged to avoid calcium gluttony but should maintain a calcium intake of 1000 to 1200 mg/day.

21. **What treatments are available to prevent recurrent nephrolithiasis?**
    Treatments vary, depending on the type of stone and the underlying metabolic abnormality that has caused the stone to form. Table 17.1 lists possible treatments to prevent stone recurrence.

22. **Can thiazide diuretics be used in patients with a sulfa allergy?**
    Sulfonamide antibiotics are one of the most common causes of drug allergies. However, there is minimal evidence of cross-reactivity between sulfonamide antibiotics and nonantibiotics, such as thiazide diuretics. Available data suggest that cross-reactivity may be due to a susceptibility to allergic drug reactions in general, rather than a specific sulfa allergy. Considerations before prescribing a thiazide in patients with a sulfa allergy include the nature and severity of the initial reaction, the type of medication implicated (antibiotic vs. nonantibiotic), and whether alternative treatments are available. Loop diuretics are not alternatives to thiazide diuretics because they increase calcium excretion.

23. **Do patients with nephrolithiasis get bone disease from renal calcium losses?**
    Multiple studies have documented reduced bone mineral density in calcium stone formers, particularly those with idiopathic hypercalciuria. Patients with hypercalciuria are likely to go into negative calcium balance when placed on a low-calcium diet. Because many patients avoid dairy products after a stone episode, they may be contributing to their bone loss. Higher fracture rates have been noted in stone

Table 17.1. Medical Therapy for Recurrent Nephrolithiasis

STONE TYPE	METABOLIC ABNORMALITY	POTENTIAL TREATMENT
Calcium oxalate (therapy for calcium phosphate stone focuses on hypercalciuria and hypocitraturia)	Hyperparathyroidism	Parathyroidectomy
	Hypercalciuria	Low-sodium, low-protein diet
		Thiazide diuretic
	Dietary hyperoxaluria	Low-oxalate, normal-calcium diet
	Enteric hyperoxaluria	Low-oxalate, low-fat diet
		Calcium supplements with meals
	Primary hyperoxaluria	Pyridoxine
		Neutral phosphate
		Potassium citrate
	Hypocitraturia	Potassium citrate
		Sodium bicarbonate if potassium salts not tolerated
	Hyperuricosuria	Low-purine diet
		Allopurinol
Uric acid	Low urine pH	Alkali salts, potassium citrate preferred
	Severe hyperuricosuria	Allopurinol
Cystine	Cystinuria	Alkali salts, potassium citrate preferred
		Tiopronin, D-penicillamine

formers. To treat bone loss, diet calcium should be 1000 to 1200 mg/day and diet sodium should be 2300 to 3000 mg/day. Thiazide diuretics can improve bone mineral level and reduce stone risk.

24. **How does distal RTA cause kidney stones?**
In distal RTA, stone formation is common, and most stones are calcium phosphate. The systemic metabolic acidosis leads to increased proximal tubule reabsorption of citrate, lowering urine citrate excretion. Because there is less citrate available to complex calcium, there is more calcium available to combine with phosphate or oxalate. Acidosis increases renal calcium excretion, further increasing the risk of stones. Finally, the inability to acidify urine leads to a persistent alkaline urine, which increases the amount of divalent phosphate (pK $= 6.8$) and thus the risk of calcium phosphate crystallization. Carbonic anhydrase inhibitors, such as topiramate and acetazolamide, can cause kidney stones by creating an RTA.

25. **Why do patients with bowel disease have a higher risk of kidney stone formation?**
Diarrheal states cause low urine flow, as patients lose excess water from the GI tract, and patients may restrict fluid intake to lower GI output. In addition, chronic diarrhea leads to GI bicarbonate loss, causing metabolic acidosis. The acidosis leads to low urine pH, a risk factor for uric acid stones, and low urine citrate, a risk factor for calcium stones. These abnormalities are commonly found in patients who have colectomy, with or without ileostomy. If a patient has fat malabsorption from Crohn disease or small bowel surgery, they can develop enteric hyperoxaluria, as steatorrhea leads to increased oxalate absorption in the colon. Note that enteric hyperoxaluria does not occur in patients who have had a colectomy.

26. **Does bariatric surgery lead to kidney stones?**
Only the malabsorptive bariatric procedures, roux-en-Y gastric bypass and biliopancreatic diversion, have been linked to an increased risk of kidney stones. The purely restrictive procedures such as gastric banding are not associated with stones. Stone risk from the malabsorptive procedures is mainly a result of hyperoxaluria. The hyperoxaluria can be severe, not only causing stone formation but at times loss of kidney function from oxalate nephropathy.

27. **What are infection stones?**
Infection stones are composed of struvite. Struvite stones only form in the presence of urinary infection with bacteria that possesses the enzyme urease, which converts urea to ammonium and bicarbonate, leading to the unique condition of high urine ammonium concentration with a high urine pH. The bacteria most likely to possess urease are the *Proteus* species, although many other bacterial species may also possess urease. *Escherichia coli,* the most common urinary tract pathogen, does not possess urease. Struvite stones can grow to fill the entire renal pelvis (staghorn stones) and may lead to recurrent infection and loss of kidney function. Treatment of struvite stones requires complete surgical removal of the stone and a prolonged course of antibiotics.

28. **Do kidney stones cause damage and lead to CKD?**
Cystine and struvite stones have long been recognized as causing kidney damage and even loss of a kidney. These stones can form large staghorn calculi and recur frequently, which leads to kidney damage. Patients with kidney stones do have slightly lower estimated glomerular filtration rate (eGFR) than a healthy population. Whether the CKD is a result of recurrent surgical procedures, lithotripsy, or intermittent obstruction during stone passage is not known.

29. **How should symptomatic stone disease be managed during pregnancy?**
Ultrasound is the radiologic procedure of choice, although it may be difficult to interpret because ureters become dilated during pregnancy, making the diagnosis of hydronephrosis difficult. If a patient has a symptomatic stone, hydration and observation to let the stone pass spontaneously are the preferred approaches. If the stone does not pass and pain persists, infection/pyelonephritis is present, or there is complete unilateral obstruction, then the stone should be removed ureteroscopically. If the stone cannot be removed, then placement of a stent may be needed to relieve the obstruction. ESWL is not recommended during pregnancy. Final surgical removal of a stone may be delayed until after delivery, if necessary. Medical evaluation for the cause of the stone should be delayed until after pregnancy and nursing are over, because urine calcium excretion will be markedly different than the non-pregnant state.

30. **Are magnesium salts or pyridoxine (vitamin B$_6$) effective therapies for calcium nephrolithiasis?**
Both of these agents have been proposed as ways to lower urine oxalate excretion—magnesium because it can bind dietary oxalate and lower intestinal absorption, and pyridoxine because it is a

cofactor for a key enzyme that can lower endogenous oxalate production. There are no controlled trials to prove that these therapies are effective in lowering urine oxalate or preventing calcium stone recurrence. However, a subset of patients with primary hyperoxaluria, an autosomal recessive disorder characterized by severe hyperoxaluria, nephrolithiasis, and CKD, may significantly lower urine oxalate excretion when treated with pyridoxine.

31. **Does the intestinal microbiome play a role in kidney stone risk?**
Of the numerous organisms comprising the intestinal microbiome, oxalate-degrading bacteria, particularly *Oxalobacter formigenes*, are the most interesting in relation to stone disease. *O. formigenes* is an anaerobic bacterium that is a common component of colonic flora. *O. formigenes* metabolizes oxalate and presumably lowers the amount of oxalate available for intestinal absorption. It appears *O. formigenes* can stimulate colonic secretion of oxalate, which should reduce urine oxalate as well. Some observational studies have found lower rates of *O. formigenes* colonization in patients with kidney stones, suggesting a role in stone formation. Though animal models of hyperoxaluria have shown reduced urinary oxalate excretion when treated with *O. formigenes*, there are no controlled trials demonstrating a convincing effect in humans to date.

KEY POINTS: FEATURES OF CYSTINURIA

1. Cystinuria is a stone disease in which the clinical phenotype follows an autosomal recessive pattern.
2. Reduced proximal tubule reabsorption of cystine and dibasic amino acids is present.
3. Hexagonal crystals may be seen in the urine.
4. First presentation is usually in childhood.
5. The mainstays of therapy are very high fluid intake, alkalinization of the urine, and the use of thiol-binding drugs such as tiopronin or D-penicillamine.

KEY POINTS: MEDICATIONS THAT CAN LEAD TO STONE FORMATION

1. Protease inhibitors
2. Carbonic anhydrase inhibitors (such as topiramate)
3. Calcium supplements
4. Triamterene
5. Guaifenesin/ephedrine

BIBLIOGRAPHY

Asplin, J. R. (2016). The management of patients with enteric hyperoxaluria. *Urolithiasis, 44,* 33–43.
Campschroer, T., Zhu, Y., Duijvesz, D., Grobbee, D. E., & Lock, M. T. (2014). Alpha-blockers as medical expulsive therapy for ureteral stones. *Cochrane Database of Systematic Review,* (4), CD008509. doi:10.1002/14651858.CD008509.pub2.
Hernandez, J. D., Ellison, J. S., & Lendvay, T. S. (2015). Current trends, evaluation, and management of pediatric nephrolithiasis. *JAMA Pediatrics, 169,* 964–970.
Pearle, M. S., Goldfarb, D. S., Assimos, D. G., Curhan, G., Denu-Ciocca, C. J., Matlaga, B. R., . . . American Urological Assocation. (2014). Medical management of kidney stones: AUA guideline. *Journal of Urology, 192,* 316–324.
Rodríguez, D., & Sacco, D. E. (2015). Minimally invasive surgical treatment for kidney stone disease. *Advances in Chronic Kidney Diseases, 22,* 266–272.
Sakhaee, K. (2014). Epidemiology and clinical pathophysiology of uric acid kidney stones. *Journal of Nephrology, 27,* 241–245.
Shoag, J., Tasian, G. E., Goldfarb, D. S., & Eisner, B. H. (2015). The new epidemiology of nephrolithiasis. *Advances in Chronic Kidney Diseases, 22,* 273–278.
Smith-Bindman, R., Aubin, C., Bailitz, J., Bengiamin, R. N., Camargo, C. A., Jr., Corbo J., . . . Cummings, S. R. (2014). Ultrasonography versus computed tomography for suspected nephrolithiasis. *New England Journal Medicine, 371,* 1100–1110.
Sumorok, N., & Goldfarb, D. S. (2013). Update on cystinuria. *Current Opinion in Nephrology and Hypertension, 22,* 427–431.

III
CHRONIC KIDNEY DISEASE

CHAPTER 18

EPIDEMIOLOGY, ETIOLOGY, PATHOPHYSIOLOGY, AND STAGING OF CHRONIC KIDNEY DISEASE

Mark E. Rosenberg

1. **What is the definition of chronic kidney disease (CKD)?**
   CKD is defined as the presence of kidney damage or decreased kidney function (defined as estimated glomerular filtration rate [eGFR] <60 mL/min per 1.73 m^2) for 3 or more months, irrespective of the cause. The persistence for at least 3 months is necessary to distinguish CKD from acute kidney injury (AKI). Markers of kidney damage include:
   - Albuminuria with albumin to creatinine ratio (ACR) ≥30 mg/g
   - Urine sediment abnormalities
   - Electrolyte abnormalities due to tubular disorders
   - Abnormalities detected by histology
   - Structural abnormalities detected by imaging
   - History of kidney transplantation

2. **How is this definition of CKD derived?**
   This definition is derived from the Kidney Disease: Improving Global Outcomes (KDIGO) 2012 Clinical Practice Guideline for the Evaluation and Management of Chronic Kidney Disease. For this definition, eGFR is calculated from serum creatinine using the Chronic Kidney Disease Epidemiology Collaboration (CKD-EPI) equation. Those with eGFR <60 mL/min per 1.73m^2 are considered to have reduced kidney function. Urinary albumin is assessed from the ACR, with four levels of ACR considered: <10 mg/g, 10 to <30 mg/g (normal to slightly elevated), 30 to 300 mg/g (moderately increased), and >300 mg/g (severely increased).

3. **What is the staging system for CKD?**
   Among patients who are diagnosed using the criteria described previously, staging of CKD should be done according to Table 18.1 and based on:
   - Cause of disease
   - Six categories of eGFR (G stages)
   - Three levels of albuminuria (A stages)
   eGFR is used clinically to evaluate the degree of kidney impairment, to follow the course of the disease, and to assess the response to therapy.

4. **Why should there be a staging system for CKD?**
   Staging patients with CKD according to cause, eGFR, and albuminuria enhances risk stratification for the major complications of CKD. As seen in Fig. 18.1, increasing albuminuria is associated with a higher risk of adverse events at every level of eGFR. These complications include kidney outcomes and mortality. Risk stratification is used to inform appropriate treatments, determine the intensity of monitoring, and facilitate patient education. In addition, the definition and staging of CKD has been useful in providing a common terminology for CKD to facilitate the study of the epidemiology, natural history, and prognosis of CKD.

5. **Why is it important to identify CKD at an early stage?**
   The main reasons for identifying CKD at an early stage are:
   - To make a definitive diagnosis in case there are specific therapies that can be started
   - To institute treatment to prevent progression of kidney disease such as inhibition of the renin-angiotensin system
   - To manage the complications of CKD, including anemia, mineral and bone disorders, acidosis, and most importantly cardiovascular disease

Table 18.1. Chronic Kidney Disease Classification Based on Glomerular Filtration Rate and Albuminuria

GFR STAGES	eGFR (mL/min/1.73m2)	TERMS
G1	>90	Normal or high
G2	60–89	Mildly decreased
G3a	45–59	Mildly to moderately decreased
G3b	30–44	Moderately to severely decreased
G4	15–29	Severely decreased
G5	<15	Kidney failure (add D if treated by dialysis)
ALBUMINURIA STAGES	**ALBUMIN/CREATININE RATIO (mg/g)**	**TERMS**
A1	<30	Normal to mildly increased
A2	30–300	Moderately increased
A3	>300	Severely increased

The cause of chronic kidney disease is also included in the Kidney Disease: Improving Global Outcomes classification.

eGFR, Estimated glomerular filtration rate; GFR, glomerular filtration rate.

				Persistent albuminuria categories description and range		
				A1	A2	A3
Prognosis of CKD by GFR and albuminuria categories: KDIGO 2012				Normal to mildly increased	Moderately increased	Severely increased
				<30 mg/g <3 mg/mmol	30–300 mg/g 3–30 mg/mmol	>300 mg/g >30 mg/mmol
GFR categories (ml/min/1.73 m²) description and range	G1	Normal or high	≥90			
	G2	Mildly decreased	60–89			
	G3a	Mildly to moderately decreased	45–59			
	G3b	Moderately to severely decreased	30–44			
	G4	Severely decreased	15–29			
	G5	Kidney failure	<15			

☐ Low risk (if no other markers of kidney disease, no CKD   ☐ High risk

■ Moderately increased risk   ■ Very high risk

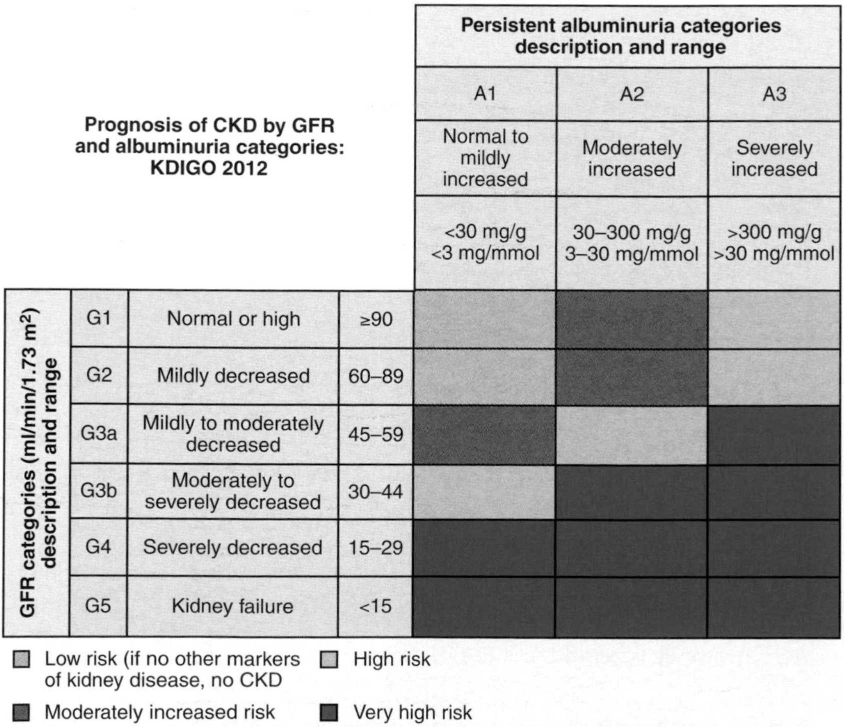

Figure 18.1. Prognosis of chronic kidney disease (CKD) by glomerular filtration rate (GFR) and albuminuria categories. The colors represent different risks. (Obtained with permission from Kidney Disease: Improving Global Outcomes (KDIGO) CKD Work Group. (2013). KDIGO 2012 clinical practice guideline for the evaluation and management of chronic kidney disease. *Kidney International Supplement, 3*(1), 1–150.)

- To enhance measures to prevent and detect AKI, given CKD is associated with a higher incidence of AKI
- To plan for renal replacement therapy, whether it be initiating a transplant evaluation or planning for vascular or peritoneal access for initiation of dialysis

Not recognizing CKD results in patients presenting at or near end-stage, often requiring the emergency initiation of dialysis, which is associated with worse outcomes.

6. **Why use eGFR and not just serum creatinine to assess kidney function?**
Serum creatinine alone is an imperfect marker of kidney function, since creatinine level can be influenced by such factors as muscle mass, protein intake, and drugs that affect tubular creatinine secretion such as trimethoprim or fenofibrate. The estimating equations have been derived using regression analysis of studies where GFR and serum creatinine have been directly measured, and the equations include a combination of other demographic and clinical variables.

7. **Why is it important to include urinary albumin excretion in the definition of CKD?**
Urinary albumin measurement is the most abundant protein lost in the urine, and its measurement is more standardized than that of urinary total protein. Albuminuria is a risk factor for the development of end-stage kidney disease (ESKD) in the general population, and a powerful predictor of kidney outcomes in CKD patients (see Fig. 18.1), with prognosis being worse with higher levels of albuminuria. Nephrotic range proteinuria (ACR > 2200 mg/g) is associated with even higher risks. Reduction of proteinuria in clinical trials is usually, but not always, associated with improved kidney outcomes.

8. **Should elderly patients be classified as CKD even though there is an expected decline in GFR with aging?**
The normal GFR in young adults is approximately 125 mL/min per 1.73 m^2. GFR declines with age, with the mean GFR being 65 mL/min per m^2 at ages 80 to 89 years. Other studies have demonstrated a decline in GFR ranging from 6 to 12 mL/min per 1.73 m^2 per decade of age. Increased ACR also occurs with aging. There has been controversy as to whether a decreased eGFR or increased ACR is a disease or part of normal aging. Since these abnormalities are associated with adverse outcomes, these people should be classified as having CKD.

9. **What are the causes of CKD?**
The leading causes of CKD are:
- Diabetes
- Hypertension
- Glomerulonephritis
- Cystic kidney disease.

The current prevalence of each of these causes in the U.S. population from 1996 to 2013 is displayed in Fig. 18.2. As can be seen, diabetes is the most common cause, with almost half of all people with CKD having diabetes. All four of these leading causes have been increasing over time.

10. **How do you make the diagnosis of the cause for CKD?**
An attempt should be made to obtain a specific kidney diagnosis. The first step in this process is a careful urinalysis, looking for proteinuria, hematuria, and cellular casts. Further evaluation may include quantification of proteinuria, kidney ultrasound, referral to a nephrologist, and a kidney biopsy. The biopsy can be done as an outpatient and has a relatively low complication rate. The kidney tissue is examined by light, immunofluorescent, and electron microscopy. Serum and urine electrolytes may be used to assess for renal tubular disorders, and serum and urine immunofixation can be performed to rule out a monoclonal protein. If glomerulonephritis is suspected, further evaluation could include hepatitis serology, ANCA, anti-GBM antibodies, antinuclear antibodies, and anti–double-stranded DNA.

11. **How do you further classify kidney disease?**
CKD can be classified into glomerular diseases, tubulointerstitial diseases, vascular diseases, and cystic and congenital diseases (Table 18.2). These can be due to systemic diseases (e.g., systemic lupus erythematosus causing glomerulonephritis) or be a primary kidney disease (e.g., idiopathic focal and segmental glomerulosclerosis). CKD is not one unifying diagnosis but a term encompassing multiple diseases with unique pathophysiology and treatment.

12. **Do all diabetic patients develop CKD?**
Only 30 to 40% of type 1 or type 2 diabetics develop kidney disease. In diabetic patients with albuminuria and the presence of other diabetic complications, the cause of the underlying kidney

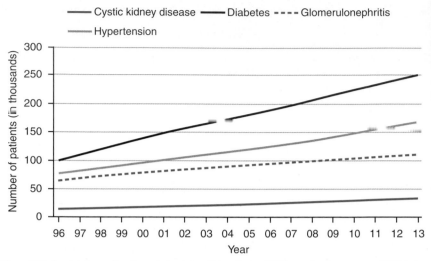

Figure 18.2. Trends in the number of prevalent end-stage kidney disease (ESKD) cases by primary cause of ESKD in the U.S. population, 1996 to 2013. (In public domain from United States Renal Data System. (2015). *2015 USRDS annual data report: Epidemiology of Kidney Disease in the United States.* Bethesda, MD: National Institutes of Health, National Institute of Diabetes and Digestive and Kidney Diseases.)

Table 18.2. Causes of Chronic Kidney Disease

LOCATION	EXAMPLES
Glomerular	Focal and segmental glomerulosclerosis, IgA nephropathy, membranous nephropathy, diffuse proliferative glomerulonephritis, minimal change disease
Tubulointerstitial	Urinary tract infection, autoimmune disease, stones, obstruction
Vascular	Anti-neutrophil cytoplasmic antibody-associated kidney limited vasculitis, fibromuscular dysplasia
Cystic and congenital	Kidney dysplasia, medullary cystic disease

disease is often presumed to be diabetic nephropathy and a kidney biopsy is not performed. If there are unusual features to the kidney disease such as red blood cell casts, nephropathy early in the course of diabetes, or rapid progression of kidney disease, then a biopsy may be warranted. In some studies, half of type 2 diabetic patients have kidney disease due to diseases other than diabetes.

13. Why do African American patients have a higher incidence of CKD?
    The incidence of CKD is higher in African Americans compared with other populations, and there is marked familial aggregation of ESKD in African American families.
    In patients of African ancestry, diseases such as idiopathic focal and segmental glomerulosclerosis, human immunodeficiency virus–associated nephropathy (HIVAN), and hypertensive nephropathy are associated with coding variants in the apolipoprotein L1 (APOL1) gene on chromosome 22q13. The risk of these kidney diseases is greatly increased if two APOL1 nephropathy risk variants are inherited. These risk variants confer an advantage in the ability to kill *Trypanosoma brucei rhodesiense*, the parasite causing African sleeping sickness, providing a survival advantage in patients with these APOL1 alleles in endemic areas.

14. How common is CKD?
    The overall prevalence of all stages of CKD in the US general population is about 14% and has remained stable over the past decade. In contrast, there has been an increase in Stage 3 CKD, with prevalence of 6%. There were 661,648 prevalent cases of ESKD at the end of 2013, and the unadjusted prevalence was 2034 per million in the US population. Fig. 18.3 shows the trends in ESKD prevalence and annual

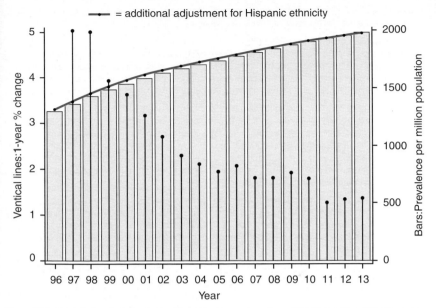

Figure 18.3. Trends in the adjusted end-stage kidney disease prevalence (per million) (bars; scale on left) and annual change (%) (lines; scale on right) in the U.S. population, 1996 to 2013. The data are adjusted for age, sex, and race. (In public domain from United States Renal Data System. (2015). *2015 USRDS annual data report: Epidemiology of Kidney Disease in the United States*. Bethesda, MD: National Institutes of Health, National Institute of Diabetes and Digestive and Kidney Diseases.)

change from 1996 to 2013. The number of incident (newly reported) ESKD cases in 2013 was 117,162. The adjusted incidence rate of ESKD in the United States rose sharply in the 1980s and 1990s, leveled off in the early 2000s, and has declined slightly since its peak in 2006.

15. What are the risk factors for developing CKD?
    Risk factors for CKD include:
    - Diabetes
    - Hypertension
    - Cardiovascular disease
    - Multisystem diseases with potential kidney involvement such as systemic lupus erythematosus (SLE)
    - Family history of kidney failure
    - Smoking
    - History of and recovery from AKI
    - Obesity
    - Metabolic syndrome
    - Frequent urinary tract infections
    - Kidney stones
    - Lower urinary tract obstruction
    - Reduction in kidney mass
    - Low birth weight
    - Exposure to nephrotoxic drugs
        Socioeconomic risk factors associated with CKD are age, U.S. ethnic minorities (African Americans, American Indian, Hispanics), and exposure to certain chemicals or environmental conditions.

16. Should there be routine screening for CKD?
    Guidelines recommend targeted screening versus mass screening for CKD. The American College of Physicians recommends against screening low-risk patients. High-risk groups, as defined in question 15, should be screened on a regular basis especially those with hypertension, diabetes, cardiovascular

disease, structural disorders of the urinary tract, a familial history of kidney failure, those recovering from AKI, and those with proteinuria or hematuria discovered serendipitously.

17. **How do you predict the prognosis of CKD?**
The prognosis of CKD varies depending on the underlying cause, the level of GFR, the amount of albuminuria, and the presence of other comorbidities such as cardiovascular disease or diabetes. The contributions of each of these factors vary, depending on the outcome of interest. For example, the development of ESKD is more dependent on the cause of CKD and GFR than on other factors.

18. **Do all patients with CKD progress to ESKD?**
No, not all patients with CKD progress to ESKD. More patients will die before they reach ESKD, predominantly of cardiovascular disease. These competing risks between ESKD and cardiovascular disease depend on the population of patients studied, with the general finding that older patients with milder CKD are more likely to die of cardiovascular disease, while younger patients with more severe CKD are more likely to progress to ESKD. Emphasis should be placed on both reducing cardiovascular risk and in slowing the progression of CKD.

19. **How often should eGFR and albuminuria be assessed in people with CKD?**
It is recommended to assess eGFR and albuminuria at least annually in people with CKD and more often in those at a higher risk for progression, or when measurement will impact therapeutic decisions. Both lower eGFR and greater albuminuria are associated with an increased rate of kidney disease progression.

KEY POINTS: CHRONIC KIDNEY DISEASE DEFINITION AND RISK FACTORS

1. CKD is defined as the presence of kidney damage or decreased kidney function (defined as eGFR $<$60 mL/min per 1.73 m^2) for 3 or more months, irrespective of the cause.
2. Albuminuria is a risk factor for the development of ESKD in the general population, and a powerful predictor of kidney outcomes in CKD patients, with prognosis being worse with higher levels of albuminuria.
3. The leading causes of CKD are diabetes, hypertension, glomerulonephritis, and cystic kidney disease, with about 40% of all CKD due to diabetes.
4. Risk factors for CKD include diabetes, hypertension, cardiovascular disease, structural kidney tract disease, multisystem diseases with potential kidney involvement such as SLE, family history of kidney failure, hereditary kidney disease, and smoking.

20. **How fast does CKD progress?**
Progression of CKD is variable, depending on the population being studied, underlying disease, adequacy of therapy, presence of risk factors, and unknown factors. To provide perspective on CKD progression, it is important to note the decline in kidney function in various populations. A decline in kidney function of 0.3 to 1.0 mL/min per 1.73 m^2 per year has been demonstrated in those without proteinuria or comorbidity. In patients with established CKD, rates of progression vary between 2.5 and 4.5 mL/min per 1.73 m^2 per year, with rapid progression defined as rates of more than 5 mL/min per 1.73 m^2 per year.

21. **What are the risk factors for progression of CKD?**
Progression of kidney disease is defined as a loss of GFR over time and includes the need to initiate renal replacement therapy. Factors that affect progression are GFR and albuminuria categories, absolute amounts of albuminuria, the cause for the underlying kidney disease, hypertension, age, race/ethnicity, obesity, exposure to nephrotoxic agents, episodes of AKI, and laboratory parameters such as hemoglobin, serum albumin, calcium, phosphate, and bicarbonate.

22. **Why does kidney disease progress?**
Common mechanisms underlie the progression of most kidney diseases. These mechanisms initially involve adaptive changes to loss of nephrons that eventually have maladaptive consequences. The best-described common mechanism of progression is glomerular hyperfiltration. Reductions in the nephron number cause increased filtration rate in residual nephrons—the greater the degree of nephron loss, the greater the compensatory increase in the function of the residual units. After these initially adaptive increases in function, pathologic changes appear, ultimately resulting in glomerular

sclerosis. Other mechanisms of progression include kidney fibrosis, loss of podocytes, activation of the renin-angiotensin-aldosterone system, and proteinuria.

23. **What are the most common symptoms of CKD?**
CKD is often asymptomatic in the early stages. In the late stages of kidney failure, symptoms include:
- Fatigue
- Weakness
- Anorexia
- Nausea and vomiting
- Volume overload with pulmonary edema
- Pericarditis
- Peripheral neuropathy
- Central nervous system abnormalities (ranging from loss of concentration and lethargy to seizures, coma, and death), which can occur when kidney function is severely impaired
    No direct correlation exists between the absolute serum levels of blood urea nitrogen or creatinine and the development of these symptoms.

24. **Why do diabetics develop CKD?**
Diabetic nephropathy is the leading cause of ESKD in the industrialized world, and its incidence continues to increase. Clinically it manifests as albuminuria and progressive loss of kidney function. The structural manifestations are:
- Glomerular basement membrane thickening
- Tubular basement membrane thickening
- Expansion of the mesangium at times forming nodules called Kimmelstiel-Wilson lesions
- Arteriolar hyalinosis
- Tubulointerstitial fibrosis
    The pathophysiology of CKD in diabetics is complex and involves a combination of glucose toxicity, glomerular hypertension, oxidative stress, toxic effects of other metabolites, cytokines, and growth factors including advanced glycation end-products and transforming growth factor-beta, combined with poorly defined genetic risk factors.

25. **What are the complications of CKD?**
Complications of CKD are discussed in subsequent chapters and include disorders of fluid and electrolyte balance such as volume overload, hyperkalemia, metabolic acidosis, and hyperphosphatemia. Other complications are hypertension, anemia, malnutrition, mineral and bone disorders, dyslipidemia, and sexual dysfunction. In more advanced CKD, complications include uremic bleeding, increased susceptibility to infection, pericarditis, uremic neuropathy, thyroid dysfunction, and infection. Most importantly, CKD is a risk factor for cardiovascular disease.

26. **Why do CKD patients have a high incidence of cardiovascular disease?**
Patients with CKD have a substantial increase in cardiovascular risk and disease (Fig. 18.4) that can be in part explained by an increase in traditional risk factors such as hypertension, diabetes, and metabolic syndrome. CKD alone is also an independent risk factor for cardiovascular disease. Among patients with CKD, the risk of death, particularly due to cardiovascular disease, is much higher than the risk of eventually requiring dialysis. CKD patients have worse outcomes from cardiovascular disease, including a higher mortality after acute myocardial infarction.

27. **Can the progression of CKD be slowed?**
The diagnosis of CKD and assessment of the tempo of progression set the stage for implementing therapies directed at slowing progression and preventing the development of ESKD. Therapy includes:
- Blood pressure control
- Inhibition of the renin-angiotensin-aldosterone system
- Dietary protein restriction (in certain populations and settings)
- Glycemic control in diabetics
- Bicarbonate supplementation when serum bicarbonate concentration is <22 mEq/L
    Other principles of therapy include avoidance of nephrotoxic drugs such as NSAIDs or aminoglycoside antibiotics, and avoidance of radiographic contrast agents. In addition, attention should be paid to reversible causes of progression, such as urinary obstruction.

28. **What drugs should be avoided in patients with CKD?**
Whenever possible, nephrotoxic medications should be avoided including NSAIDs, which should be stopped when eGFR is <30 mL/min per $1.73m^2$ and not prescribed long-term in patients with eGFR

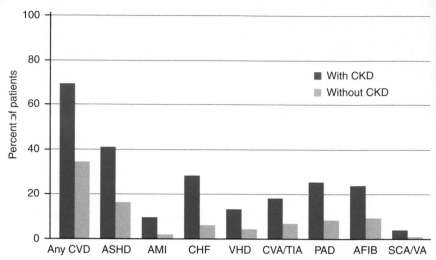

Figure 18.4. Cardiovascular disease in patients with or without CKD, 2013. Data Source: Special analyses, Medicare 5% sample. Patients aged 66 and older, alive, without end-stage kidney disease, and residing in the United States on 12/31/2013 with fee-for-service coverage for the entire calendar year. Totals of patients for the study cohort: N = 1,238,888; With CKD = 132,840; Without CKD = 1,106,048. *AFIB*, Atrial fibrillation; *AMI*, acute myocardial infarction; *ASHD*, atherosclerotic heart disease; *CHF*, congestive heart failure; *CKD*, chronic kidney disease; *CVA/TIA*, cerebrovascular accident/transient ischemic attack; *CVD*, cardiovascular disease; *PAD*, peripheral arterial disease; *SCA/VA*, sudden cardiac arrest and ventricular arrhythmias; *VHD*, valvular heart disease. (In public domain from United States Renal Data System. (2015). *2015 USRDS annual data report: Epidemiology of Kidney Disease in the United States.* Bethesda, MD: National Institutes of Health, National Institute of Diabetes and Digestive and Kidney Diseases.)

<60 mL/min per 1.73m². Other nephrotoxic medications are aminoglycosides, amphotericin, and cisplatin. The GFR level needs to be considered when dosing drugs that undergo kidney excretion, especially for such medications as lithium and digoxin. Caution should be used when nutritional supplements are being used. Metformin should be discontinued in people with eGFR < 30 mL/min per 1.73m². Oral phosphate-containing bowel preparations (used for colonoscopy prep) should be avoided in people with an eGFR <60 mL/min per 1.73m² because of the risk of phosphate nephropathy.

29. When should a CKD patient be referred to a nephrologist?
    Early referral to a nephrologist is associated with improved outcomes once patients initiate dialysis. Referral to a nephrologist is recommended when eGFR <30 mL/min per 1.73m² and/or urine albumin creatinine ratio is >300 mg/g, with earlier referral recommended in specific cases. Early referral has been associated with several beneficial effects, including decreased mortality, reduced hospitalization, and improvement in the appropriate use of fistulas and grafts as opposed to catheters at the initiation of hemodialysis.

KEY POINTS: CKD PROGRESSION AND CONSEQUENCES

1. In patients with established CKD, rates of progression vary between 2.5 and 4.5 mL/min per 1.73m² per year, with rapid progression defined as rates of more than 5 mL/min per 1.73 m² per year.
2. CKD is a risk factor for all forms of cardiovascular disease, and aggressive risk factor reduction should be standard therapy for patients with CKD.
3. Early referral to a nephrologist is associated with improved outcomes once patients initiate dialysis.

BIBLIOGRAPHY

Drawz, P., Hostetter, T. H., & Rosenberg, M. E. (2015). Slowing progression of chronic kidney disease. In P. L. Kimmel & M. E. Rosenberg (Eds.), *Chronic renal disease* (1st ed., pp. 598–612). San Diego, CA: Elsevier.

Kidney Disease: Improving Global Outcomes (KDIGO) CKD Work Group. (2013). KDIGO 2012 clinical practice guideline for the evaluation and management of chronic kidney disease. *Kidney International Supplement, 3*(1), 1–150.

Levey, A. S., Stevens, L. A., Schmid, C. H., Zhang, Y. L., Castro, A. F., 3rd, Feldman, H. I., ... CKD-EPI (Chronic Kidney Disease Epidemiology Collaboration). (2009). A new equation to estimate glomerular filtration rate. *Annals of Internal Medicine, 150,* 604–612.

National Kidney Foundation. (2002). K/DOQI Clinical practice guidelines for chronic kidney disease: evaluation, classification and stratification. *American Journal of Kidney Diseases, 39*(2 Suppl. 1), S1–S266.

United States Renal Data System. (2015). *2015 USRDS annual data report: Epidemiology of kidney disease in the United States.* Bethesda, MD: National Institutes of Health, National Institute of Diabetes and Digestive and Kidney Diseases.

CHAPTER 19

ANEMIA IN CHRONIC KIDNEY DISEASE

Jay B. Wish

1. **What causes anemia in patients with kidney disease?**

   The anemia of chronic kidney disease (CKD) is primarily caused by deficiency of erythropoietin (EPO). The kidneys are the major source of EPO, and as kidney function declines, production of EPO declines proportionately. Several other factors decrease red blood cell (RBC) life span from the normal 120 days to approximately 70–80 days in patients with CKD. These include:
   - RBC trauma due to microvascular disease from diabetes or hypertension
   - Blood loss from hemodialysis (HD)
   - Increased incidence of gastrointestinal bleeding from peptic ulcer disease and angiodysplasia of the bowel
   - Increased oxidative stress

2. **What are the adverse effects of anemia?**

   Anemia leads to decreased oxygen-carrying capacity of the blood and decreased delivery of oxygen to tissues. This results in fatigue (both with exercise and at rest), decreased cognitive function, loss of libido, and decreased sense of well-being. The increased workload on the heart may lead to left ventricular hypertrophy. Observational studies of dialysis patients in the 1990s demonstrated decreased hospitalizations and mortality among patients with higher hemoglobin (Hb) levels, but these may have been confounded by comorbidities that decreased Hb levels and also led to poorer outcomes. Randomized controlled trials (RCTs) of erythropoiesis-stimulating agents (ESAs) to raise Hb levels have not led to improved outcomes or consistently improved quality-of-life (QOF; Table 19.1 and question 17).

3. **How does one evaluate anemia in a patient with CKD?**

   EPO deficiency is a diagnosis of exclusion, and checking EPO levels in patients with CKD is generally not indicated. The routine evaluation of such patients should include:
   - Measurement of RBC indices
   - Reticulocyte count
   - Transferrin saturation (TSAT)
   - Serum ferritin
   - Stool for occult blood testing
     If these tests reveal no alternative cause of anemia, it can be presumed that the anemia is primarily due to EPO deficiency.

4. **How does one interpret TSAT?**

   TSAT is calculated by dividing the serum iron level by the total iron-binding capacity. The total iron-binding capacity reflects circulating transferrin, the major iron-binding protein in plasma. TSAT correlates with the amount of iron available for erythropoiesis, because only circulating iron is available to the bone marrow for incorporation into RBC. Patients with TSAT <20% have decreased iron delivery to the erythroid marrow, but supplemental iron can only correct this if the iron is effectively released from storage sites to the transferrin carrier protein.

5. **How does one interpret the serum ferritin?**

   The serum ferritin level correlates with storage iron, located primarily in the reticuloendothelial system. Interpretation of serum ferritin levels is confounded by ferritin being an acute-phase reactant and rising with acute or chronic inflammation. In patients with CKD, serum ferritin level <100 ng/mL correlates with a deficiency in storage iron; such patients almost invariably respond to supplemental iron therapy.

Table 19.1. Large Randomized Studies in Patients With Anemia and Chronic Kidney Disease Not Receiving Dialysis

	CHOIR	CREATE	TREAT
Location	United States	Europe	International
ESA	Epoetin alfa	Epoetin beta	Darbepoetin alfa
Number of patients	1432	603	4038, type 2 diabetics
High Hb target g/dL	13.5	13–15	13
Low Hb target g/dL	11.3	10.5–11.5	Placebo control, ESA rescue for Hb <9
Cardiovascular endpoints	Higher in high Hb group	No difference	No difference except higher stroke and lower coronary revascularization in high Hb group
Progression of CKD	No difference	More in high Hb group	No difference
Cancer deaths	Not noted	Not noted	Higher in high Hb group among patients with prior cancer
Quality of life	No difference	Better in high Hb group	No difference except less fatigue in high Hb group

CHOIR, Correction of Hemoglobin and Outcomes in Renal Insufficiency; CKD, chronic kidney disease; CREATE, Cardiovascular Risk Reduction of Early Anemia Treatment with Epoetin Beta; ESA, erythrocyte-stimulating agent; Hb, hemoglobin; TREAT, Trial to Reduce Cardiovascular Events with Aranesp Therapy.

6. **What is functional iron deficiency?**
   Functional iron deficiency is a bone marrow iron supply-demand mismatch in a patient with normal or elevated iron stores. It can occur in the setting of inflammation when elevated hepcidin levels impair the release of storage iron to circulating transferrin. It can also occur in patients treated with pharmacologic doses of ESAs when the bone marrow is stimulated to produce RBCs faster than the transferrin carrier protein can deliver adequate iron substrate. In such patients, TSAT tends to be low or low-normal, whereas serum ferritin level may be normal or even high. The operative definition of functional iron deficiency is based on a response to intravenous (IV) iron supplementation characterized by either an increase in Hb or a decrease in ESA requirements to achieve the same Hb.

7. **What is the role of IV iron?**
   Studies have demonstrated that functional iron deficiency is common in patients with end-stage kidney disease (ESKD) who are treated with ESAs and that IV iron supplementation decreases ESA requirements by 20% to 25%. In CKD patients with iron deficiency anemia not receiving ESAs, 1 gm IV iron generally raises the Hb 1 gm/dL. For iron-deficient, non-hemodialysis patients who fail oral iron therapy, IV iron can be given in larger doses over fewer treatments for patient convenience and vein sparing. In HD patients, IV iron is generally administered in smaller, more frequent doses through the dialysis circuit.

8. **What are the adverse effects of IV iron?**
   IV iron may be associated with acute reactions such as nausea/vomiting and hypotension, which are likely related to free iron in the preparation. IV iron may be associated with allergic or anaphylactic reactions to the carbohydrate that binds the iron. There have been concerns regarding the long-term effects of IV iron administration, including iron accumulation in tissues, oxidative damage to endothelial cells, and increased susceptibility to infection. Retrospective studies in HD patients have shown an association with adverse clinical outcomes and monthly IV iron doses over 400 mg, but it is impossible to exclude confounding by indication. In a prospective study comparing IV and oral iron in patients with nondialysis patients with iron deficiency anemia, patients receiving IV iron had a 2.51 higher incidence of cardiovascular events and a 2.12 increased risk of hospitalization due to infection over a 2-year follow-up period. This supports the Kidney Disease Improving Global Outcomes recommendation that in patients with nondialysis CKD and iron deficiency anemia, a 1- to 3-month trial of oral iron therapy be considered prior to initiating IV iron therapy.

9. **Why are oral iron supplements ineffective in treating the iron deficiency in patients receiving chronic HD?**

   Increasing the Hb from 8 g/dL to 11 g/dL in a 70-kg patient requires the incorporation of 600 mg elemental iron into newly synthesized RBC. Daily iron losses in HD patients are approximately 4 to 7 mg (averaged over dialysis and nondialysis days). Thus the 2 to 4 mg of oral iron absorbed daily from conventional oral supplements in dialysis patients with elevated hepcidin levels could barely keep pace with ongoing iron losses, and would not allow the patient to repair the accumulated deficit. Compounding this problem is the phenomenon of functional iron deficiency, which often results in the need for high levels of storage iron to facilitate the release of iron to transferrin and delivery of that iron to the erythroid marrow.

10. **Are there other options for iron supplementation in HD patients?**

    Oral ferric citrate, a phosphate binder, has absorbable iron that has been shown to increase serum ferritin and TSAT and decrease IV iron requirements in HD patients. Unlike other oral iron supplements, ferric citrate is associated more with diarrhea than with constipation. Sodium ferric pyrophosphate added to the hemodialysate solution can replace 5 to 7 mg iron per treatment, decreasing IV iron requirements by 48%. Dialysate sodium ferric pyrophosphate has a similar safety profile to placebo.

11. **What is hepcidin?**

    Hepcidin is a protein synthesized by the liver in the setting of inflammation, which is usually present in patients with CKD. Hepcidin decreases iron absorption from the gastrointestinal tract and movement of iron from the reticuloendothelial system to the circulation. Hepcidin causes an increase in serum ferritin levels, a decrease in TSAT, and contributes to functional iron deficiency. Investigational drugs that decrease hepcidin activity improve ESA responsiveness.

12. **How are ESAs administered?**

    Human recombinant erythropoietin (epoetin) is a polypeptide hormone that, like insulin, must be given through a subcutaneous or IV route. Subcutaneously administered epoetin, because of its slower absorption and longer half-life, is more effective than a comparable dose administered through IV. Epoetin dose can be reduced 20% to 30% by switching patients from IV to subcutaneous dosing while achieving the same Hb.

13. **What is the recommended dose of epoetin?**

    For patients receiving epoetin IV on HD, the recommended starting dose is 50 units/kg of body weight three times weekly. For patients receiving epoetin therapy subcutaneously, the recommended starting dose is 30 units/kg administered three times weekly (as is typically done in HD facilities) or 100 units/kg/week administered weekly or biweekly (which is typical for predialysis and peritoneal dialysis patients). Dose should be titrated at monthly intervals, depending on the Hb response.

14. **What is the recommended dose of darbepoietin?**

    Darbepoetin alfa is an analog of human EPO, with two extra carbohydrate side chains and a longer duration of action when compared with both native and recombinant hormone. The recommended starting dose for darbepoetin alfa is 0.45 mcg/kg administered weekly or 0.75 mcg/kg administered biweekly in dialysis and patients with CKD for both IV and subcutaneous administration, with subsequent titration based on the Hb concentration. Success with longer dosing intervals for both epoetin and darbepoetin has been reported.

15. **What is the target Hb for patients with CKD receiving ESA therapy?**

    After considering the results of several RCTs of higher versus lower Hb targets in patients with CKD receiving ESA therapy, the Food and Drug Administration (FDA) changed the product information for epoetin and darbepoetin in 2011. In these RCTs patients experienced greater risks for death, major adverse cardiovascular events, and stroke when administered ESAs to target Hb level >11 g/dL (per the FDA; see the next section). No trial has identified a Hb target level, ESA dose, or dosing strategy that does not increase these risks. Therefore it is recommended that the lowest ESA dose be used that is sufficient to reduce the need for RBC transfusions.

16. **What is the evidence on which the FDA based its recommendations regarding target Hb level?**

    The Normal Hematocrit Cardiovascular Trial, published in 1998, demonstrated a tendency toward more cardiovascular events among patients undergoing HD and receiving epoetin who were randomized to a target hematocrit of 42% versus 30%. Three additional studies comparing high versus low Hb targets for ESA therapy in patients with nondialysis CKD are summarized in Table 19.1.

Retrospective analyses of these studies suggest that the risk of adverse outcomes is correlated with the ESA dose received, rather than the Hb level achieved. A patient who achieves an Hb of 13 g/dL using a low dose of ESA is at lower risk than a patient who requires a large dose of ESA to increase the Hb level from 9 to 11 g/dL. It should be noted that the target Hb level in the high Hb arm of all the principal trials was at least 13 g/dL, and the FDA's statement that the risk for adverse outcomes occurred when ESAs were administered to a target Hb >11 g/dL is a very cautious, non-evidence-based interpretation of the studies' results.

17. Are ESAs toxic?

ESAs are administered to more than 95% of patients receiving dialysis in the United States. Like any other pharmacologic agent, ESAs have risks that must be weighed against their benefits. The most compelling benefit of ESA therapy is transfusion avoidance. A pre- versus posttreatment QOL benefit of ESA therapy was reported in patients receiving dialysis whose baseline Hb in the pre-ESA era was 7–8 g/dL, and the Hb level was increased with ESA to 10–11 g/dL; however, no significant QOL benefit has been shown in the RCTs comparing Hb targets of 9–11.5 and 13–15 g/dL. None of the randomized clinical trials of ESA therapy has ever shown a mortality benefit, and the three large trials in patients with CKD who are not receiving dialysis summarized in Table 19.1 suggest that caution must be used when treating patients with ESAs to minimize the risk of adverse outcomes. Data demonstrating an improvement in the rates of stroke, venous thromboembolism, and heart failure (but not mortality) among dialysis patients following a reduction in mean Hb levels from a change in ESA reimbursement also suggest that ESAs and/or higher Hb levels have adverse effects in this vulnerable population.

18. What is pure red cell aplasia (PRCA)?

PRCA is caused by antibodies produced against an exogenous ESA cross-reacting with endogenous EPO. This results in the complete loss of RBC precursors from the bone marrow and severe anemia. Most reported cases of PRCA have been associated with alterations of the ESA protein due to manufacturing, packaging, or distribution issues, and PRCA is almost exclusively associated with subcutaneous ESA administration. Most patients with PRCA recover after withdrawal of the ESA and the use of immunosuppressive agents. PRCA is very rare in industrialized countries with robust regulatory and pharmacovigilance systems.

19. Do ESAs promote cancer?

The increased number of cancer deaths noted in the high Hb arm of the TREAT study, coupled with data from the oncology literature demonstrating increased tumor progression or recurrence among patients treated with ESAs, suggests that ESAs should be used with caution in patients with CKD with existing malignancies. The recommendation is that ESA treatment and dosing should be individualized in the patient with CKD to weigh benefit versus risk and that very high doses of ESAs should be avoided.

20. Are there newer ESAs?

Methoxy-pegylated epoetin beta (Mircera) was approved by the FDA in 2008, but its introduction into the U.S. market was delayed until 2015 because of patent infringement issues. Methoxy-pegylated epoetin beta is effective when administered once monthly and has the same FDA recommendations regarding dosing and target Hb levels as epoetin and darbepoetin. Its long duration of action may make it attractive to non-hemodialysis patients who require subcutaneous ESA administration.

21. What are biosimilars?

Since ESAs are complex proteins with side chains, not every molecule is identical to each other, and therefore it is impossible to develop a "generic" version that is identical to the originator molecule. For biologic drugs whose patents have expired, the FDA has developed an approval pathway for biosimilar agents whose safety, efficacy, and potency is sufficiently similar to the originator molecule that it can be used as a therapeutic alternative. The advantage of biosimilar agents is that they are expected to be 20% to 30% less expensive than the originator molecule. Biosimilar ESAs have been used successfully in Europe since 2008, and at least two biosimilar ESAs are under development in the United States as of 2016.

22. What are hypoxia-inducible factor (HIF) prolyl hydroxylase inhibitors?

Several agents are under development that potentiate the activity of HIF, the substance in the kidney and other tissues that senses decreased delivery of oxygen (from hypoxemia or anemia) and stimulates the production of EPO. In the absence of hypoxia, HIF is rapidly degraded by an enzyme, prolyl hydroxylase (HIF-PH). By inhibiting HIF-PH, these agents increase HIF and endogenous EPO activity. These agents are orally active and effective, even in patients with ESRD, suggesting that significant EPO production can be induced in nonrenal tissues This is supported by the observation that HIF-PH inhibitors are effective in anephric patients with ESRD.

23. **Are there special considerations for patients with CKD and sickle cell disease?**
There are no evidence-based guidelines regarding whether the anemia of patients with CKD and sickle cell disease should be treated differently from other patients with anemia and CKD. Because of ongoing RBC destruction, patients with sickle cell disease have lower Hb levels and higher ESA requirements than their anemic CKD counterparts. Transfusions are more often required in patients with sickle cell disease than in other patients with anemia and CKD, so attention must be paid to the potential for iron overload and sensitization for future kidney transplantation. As in all patients, ESA and transfusion therapy in patients with sickle cell disease should carefully weigh risk versus benefit.

24. **What is the role of transfusions in the treatment of CKD-associated anemia?**
RBC transfusion therapy for the anemia of CKD in the pre-ESA era was associated with the transmission of bloodborne infections, iron overload, and sensitization for future kidney transplantation. Despite the controversies regarding the risk versus benefits of ESA therapy, there is no dispute that ESAs decrease RBC transfusion requirements, and far fewer patients receiving ESAs require RBC transfusions than patients not receiving ESAs. Nonetheless, RBC transfusions are occasionally required in patients with anemia and CKD, despite the use of ESA and iron therapy, especially in the setting of acute blood loss.

25. **What Hb level should trigger transfusion in a CKD patient?**
Because RBC transfusions carry the risk of sensitization for future kidney transplantation, they should be used judiciously in patients with CKD, especially those who are transplant candidates. There is no single Hb or Hb range that is considered a trigger for RBC transfusions in patients with CKD based on current practice guidelines, although most practitioners will transfuse patients with Hb <7 g/dL. It should be pointed out that the Hb target/trigger for transfusion is not the same as the Hb target range for ESA therapy.

KEY POINTS

1. The anemia of chronic kidney disease (CKD) is primarily caused by deficiency of erythropoietin.
2. Many patients with CKD not receiving hemodialysis and most patients receiving hemodialysis are iron deficient and require iron supplementation.
3. Because higher target hemoglobin levels and higher erythropoiesis-stimulating agent (ESA) doses have been associated with adverse outcomes, the FDA recommends using the smallest ESA dose sufficient to reduce the need for red blood cell transfusions.
4. Biosimilar ESAs and hypoxia-inducible factor prolyl hydroxylase inhibitors may be promising alternatives to anemia treatment with "originator" ESAs.

BIBLIOGRAPHY

Bailie, G. R., Larkina, M., Goodkin, D. A., Li, Y., Pisoni, R. L., Bieber, B., . . . Robinson, B. M. (2015). Data from the Dialysis Outcomes and Practice Patterns Study validate an association between high intravenous iron doses and mortality. *Kidney International, 87*(1), 162–168.

Chertow, G. M., Liu, J., Monda, K. L., Gilbertson, D. T., Brookhart, M. A., Beaubrun, A. C., . . . Collins, A. J. (2016). Epoetin alfa and outcomes in dialysis amid regulatory and payment reform. *Journal of the American Society of Nephrology, 27*(10), 3129–3138.

Epogen (epoetin alfa) for injection [prescribing information]. (2016). Thousand Oaks, CA: Amgen Inc; Available at: http://pi.amgen.com/united_states/epogen/epogen_pi_hcp_english.pdf. Accessed October 1, 2016.

Kidney Disease: Improving Global Outcomes. (2012). KDIGO Clinical Practice Guideline for Anemia in Chronic Kidney Disease. *Kidney International Supplement, 2*(4), 28–335. Available at: http://www.kdigo.org/clinical_practice_guidelines/pdf/KDIGO-Anemia%20GL.pdf. Accessed October 1, 2016.

Lewis, J. B., Sika, M., Koury, M. J., Chuang, P., Schulman, G., Smith, M. T., . . . Collaborative Study Group. (2015). Ferric citrate controls phosphorus and delivers iron in patients on dialysis. *Journal of the American Society of Nephrology, 26*(2), 493–503.

Macdougall, I. C., Bircher, A. J., Eckardt, K. U., Obrador, G. T., Pollock, C. A., Stenvinkel, P., . . . Conference Participants. (2016). Iron management in chronic kidney disease: Conclusions from a "Kidney Disease: Improving Global Outcomes" (KDIGO) controversies conference. *Kidney International, 89*(1), 28–39.

Pfeffer, M. A., Burdmann, E. A., Chen, C. Y., Cooper, M. E., de Zeeuw, D., Eckardt, K. U., . . . TREAT Investigators. (2009). A trial of darbepoetin alfa in type 2 diabetes and chronic kidney disease. *New England Journal of Medicine, 361*(21), 2019–2032.

Provenzano, R., Besarab, A., Sun, C. H., Diamond, S. A., Durham, J. H., Cangiano, J. L., . . . Neff, T. B. (2016). Oral hypoxia-inducible factor prolyl hydroxylase inhibitor roxadustat (FG-4592) for the treatment of anemia in patients with CKD. *Clinical Journal of the American Society of Nephrology, 11*(6), 982–991.

Vaziri, N. D., Kalantar-Zadeh, K., & Wish, J. B. (2016). New options for iron supplementation in maintenance hemodialysis patients. *American Journal of Kidney Diseases, 67*(3), 367–375.

Wish, J. B. (2014). The approval process for biosimilar erythropoiesis-stimulating agents. *Clinical Journal of the American Society of Nephrology, 9*(9), 1645–1651.

CHAPTER 20

BONE AND MINERAL METABOLISM

Stuart M. Sprague

1. **What is chronic kidney disease–mineral and bone disorder (CKD-MBD)?**
   CKD-MBD is a systemic disorder of mineral and bone metabolism resulting from CKD that may be manifested by either one or a combination of the following:
   - Laboratory abnormalities associated with disturbed mineral metabolism, including abnormalities of:
     - Calcium
     - Phosphorus,
     - Parathyroid hormone (PTH)
     - Vitamin D metabolites
   - Bone disease defined as renal osteodystrophy (ROD) including abnormalities in:
     - Bone turnover
     - Bone mineralization
     - Bone volume
     - Bone strength
     - Linear growth
   - Calcification of extraskeletal tissue, which would include the vasculature and other soft tissues

2. **How do we define ROD?**
   ROD is the term used to describe the bone lesions associated with CKD-MBD. ROD is an alteration of bone morphology in patients with CKD. It represents the skeletal component of the systemic disorder CKD-MBD. It is assessed by bone histomorphometry. There are three key histologic descriptors:
   - Bone turnover: normal, increased, or decreased
   - Bone mineralization: normal or abnormal
   - Bone volume: normal, increased, or decreased
        This is referred to as the TMV (turnover, mineralization, and volume) system—with any combination of each of the descriptors possible in each specimen. The TMV classification scheme provides a clinically relevant description of the underlying bone pathology.

3. **Name the factors contributing to secondary hyperparathyroidism and high-turnover bone disease.**
   The factors responsible for secondary hyperparathyroidism associated with CKD include:
   - Hyperphosphatemia from diminished kidney phosphorus excretion
   - Hypocalcemia, impaired kidney production of active 1,25-dihydroxyvitamin D (calcitriol)
   - Alterations in the control of PTH gene transcription
   - Skeletal resistance to the calcemic action of PTH
   - Fibroblastic growth factor 23 (FGF23), which may indirectly promote hyperparathyroidism by inhibiting production of 1,25-dihydroxyvitamin D

4. **Describe the bone lesion associated with hyperparathyroidism.**
   The primary histologic bone lesion associated with moderate to severe hyperparathyroidism is a high-turnover lesion, sometimes called *osteitis fibrosa cystica*. Clinically it is associated with nonspecific bone pain, proximal myopathy. The serum-intact PTH level is usually higher than 350 to 500 pg/mL. Radiologic features are subperiosteal resorption, Brown tumors, and a mottled and granular salt-and-pepper appearance to the skull. The histologic features include:
   - Increased turnover (T) as indicated by increased bone resorption and formation with increased numbers of osteoclasts and osteoblasts, and increased tetracycline uptake
   - Abnormal mineralization (M), as indicated by increase of woven bone, peritrabecular fibrosis and there may or may not be increased osteoid
   - Generally increased volume (V)

5. **How is high-turnover bone disease treated?**
   Treatment of this disorder entails prevention and correction of the factors leading to secondary hyperparathyroidism:
   • Phosphorus control: dietary restriction, phosphate binders, adequate dialysis
   • Prevention of hypocalcemia: oral calcium supplements, correction of vitamin D deficiency, dialysis
   • Suppression of PTH production and secretion: vitamin D receptor activators (VDRA), including calcitriol, paricalcitol, and doxercalciferol, and/or the use of calcimimetics (cinacalcet, elecalcetide; Table 20.1)
   • Surgical parathyroidectomy: in severe cases, parathyroidectomy may be required; however, bone biopsy should be considered prior to surgery

6. **What disorders are associated with low-turnover bone disease?**
   Low-turnover or adynamic bone disease is defined by the presence of low or absent bone formation as determined by decreased tetracycline uptake into bone, in conjunction with a paucity of bone-forming osteoblasts and bone-resorbing osteoclasts (decreased T). It may also be associated with a defect in mineralization (abnormal M), resulting in the histologic lesion referred to as osteomalacia. Bone volume (V) is variable. Clinically it may manifest with nonspecific bone pain and fractures. PTH concentrations are relatively low (less than 100 to 200 pg/mL), and hypercalcemia is a common feature. There may be a tendency for increased extraskeletal calcification. Low turnover is

Table 20.1. Impact and Challenges With Vitamin D to Treat Secondary Hyperparathyroidism in Patients With Chronic Kidney Disease

VITAMIN D COMPOUND	BIOLOGIC AND CLINICAL IMPACT	CHALLENGES
Ergocalciferol (D_2) Cholecalciferol (D_3)	Effective in repleting 25-D and 1,25-D in patients with early-stage CKD and adequate kidney function	Requires activation in the liver to generate 25-D Requires activation in the kidney to generate active 1,25-D Provides only partial suppression of PTH in patients with later-stage CKD
ER Calcifediol	Effective in repleting 25-D and 1,25-D in patients with CKD 3 and 4 Effectively suppresses SHPT	No data in CKD stage 5
Calcitriol	Biologically active VDR agonist Effectively suppresses SHPT Reduces abnormal high bone turnover	Hypercalcemia, hypercalciuria, and hyperphosphatemia evident at high doses
Doxercalciferol	Suppresses SHPT similar to or better than calcitriol Noted reduction in serum bone-specific alkaline phosphatase and osteocalcin	Requires activation in liver to generate active 1,25-D Induces significant elevation of serum P, elevating need for phosphate binder use
Alphacalcidol	Suppresses SHPT similar to or better than calcitriol	Requires activation in kidney to generate active 1,25-D Induces significant elevation of serum P, elevating need for phosphate binder use
Paricalcitol	Biologically active VDR agonist Effectively suppresses SHPT Noted reduction in serum bone-specific alkaline phosphatase and osteocalcin	Minimal elevation in Ca, P, and Ca × P product, requiring Ca and P monitoring

1,25-D, 1,25-Dihydroxyvitamin D; *25-D*, 25-hydroxyvitamin; *Ca*, calcium; *CKD*, chronic kidney disease; *ER*, extended release; *P*, phosphorus; *PTH*, parathyroid hormone; *SHPT*, Secondary hyperparathyroidism; *VDR*, vitamin D receptor.

characterized histologically by absence of cellular (osteoblast and osteoclast) activity, osteoid formation, and endosteal fibrosis. This is a disorder of decreased bone formation, accompanied by a secondary decrease in bone mineralization. Low turnover disease was initially described as a result of aluminum toxicity. Aluminum bone disease is diagnosed by special staining, which demonstrates the presence of aluminum deposits at the mineralization front. Outside of aluminum, the major risk factors for low turnover bone disease include diabetes, aging, and malnutrition. The other causes of low bone formation in CKD are multifactorial and include:

- Vitamin D deficiency
- High serum phosphate
- Metabolic acidosis
- Elevated circulating cytokine levels (interleukin [IL]-I, tumor necrosis factor [TNF])
- Low estrogen and testosterone levels

   Normal or mildly elevated serum PTH concentrations have been associated with adynamic bone disease, as there is a resistance to the bone stimulatory effect of PTH in CKD. PTH receptor downregulation is one potential mechanism to explain the bone resistance effect to PTH resulting, in part, from persistently elevated PTH.

7. What is osteomalacia?

Osteomalacia is an abnormality of mineralization (M) that is characterized by an excess of unmineralized osteoid, manifested as wide osteoid seams and a markedly decreased mineralization rate. The presence of increased unmineralized osteoid per se does not necessarily indicate a mineralizing defect, because increased quantities of osteoid appear in conditions associated with high rates of bone formation when mineralization lags behind the increased synthesis of matrix. Other features of osteomalacia include the absence of cell activity and the absence of endosteal fibrosis; there is normal or decreased osteoid volume and decreased mineralization. Frequently, aluminum disease is associated with osteomalacia. Serum PTH is, in general, normal or low, and hypercalcemia is common. Looser zones or pseudofractures are radiologic characteristics.

8. What is mixed uremic osteodystrophy (MUO)?

MUO is the term that has been used to describe bone biopsies that have features of secondary hyperparathyroidism together with evidence of a mineralization defect. There is extensive osteoclastic and osteoblastic activity and increased endosteal peritrabecular fibrosis, coupled with more osteoid than expected, and tetracycline labeling uncovers a concomitant mineralization defect. Unfortunately, MUO, in particular, and high- and low-turnover bone disease have been inconsistent and poorly defined. Thus it is best to describe bone histology or ROD according to the TMV system, as defined as part of CKD-MBD.

9. What is calcific uremic arteriolopathy (CUA)?

CUA, or calciphylaxis is a rare but life-threatening syndrome characteristically occurring in individuals with ESRD, but has been described in patients with normal kidney function and calcium/phosphate metabolism. CUA generally presents as excruciatingly painful eschars on the lower limbs but may affect other sites, including the abdominal wall, breasts, and penis, and only rarely the face or upper extremities. The syndrome typically begins with dysesthesia, followed by the development of erythema resembling livedo reticularis, and progression to frank ulceration. There may be palpable deposits of calcium subcutaneously. The lesions are intensely painful, and the surrounding tissue may be pruritic. The lesions have been proposed to occur at sites of adipose tissue where diminished blood flow contributes to hypoxia. Major risk factors for CUA include:

- Female gender
- Diabetes mellitus
- Obesity
- Malnutrition
- Elevated serum phosphate
- Warfarin

   The underlying pathology is vascular calcification. The calcification was historically assumed to be a passive event caused by deranged calcium and phosphate metabolism; however, this calcification is an actively regulated process. Elevated phosphate levels has been regarded as one of the most important factors in initiating CUA, with persistent hyperphosphatemia and hypercalcemia promoting vascular mineralization. Defects in a number of inhibitors of calcification, including matrix GLA protein and fetuin, play a causative role. Most patients with CUA die from complications of wound infections. Therapy should be focused on wound management and controlling serum phosphate levels. Parathyroidectomy is controversial and is generally not recommended unless PTH levels are markedly elevated (>900 ng/mL). Aggressive dialysis, nutrition, and non-calcium-containing phosphate binders are the mainstay of therapy. Some studies have demonstrated anecdotal response to sodium thiosulfate. It is unclear if calcimimetics or bisphosphonates are beneficial.

10. **How should treatment be approached for patients with CKD stages 3 to 4?**
    The earliest manifestations of CKD-MBD in the evolution of CKD are increases in FGF23, phosphate retention, decreases in calcitriol, then increases in PTH, and finally (in late stage 4, early stage 5 disease) hyperphosphatemia and eventually hypocalcemia. Most patients are also calcidiol (25-hydroxy vitamin D) deficient. Unfortunately, adequate studies demonstrating clinical outcome benefit to various therapies are lacking. Therefore treatment recommendations have been based on expert opinion and clinical judgment. The current approach to therapy should be aimed at reversing or preventing these perturbations in mineral metabolism. A reasonable approach would be to prevent phosphate retention either through moderate phosphate restriction or the introduction of phosphate binders (Table 20.2). To date, the use of phosphate binders has not been approved in CKD stages 3 and 4, nor are there adequate studies demonstrating that the use of phosphate binders results in improved patient outcome. Furthermore, there may be a risk of worsening coronary artery calcifications, especially with the use of calcium-containing phosphate binders. It is also reasonable to correct the calcidiol deficiency by replacing nutritional vitamin D, either with cholecalciferol (1200 to 2000 units/day) or ergocalciferol (50,000 units once monthly to once weekly). Cholecalciferol is vitamin D_3, which comes from animal sources, as opposed to ergocalciferol, vitamin D_2, which comes from plants. Although cholecalciferol is more readily orally absorbed, once absorbed, both D_2 and D_3 compounds are essentially equivalent. Extended-release (ER) calcifediol (25-hydroxycholecalciferol) may be more effective than nutritional vitamin D in correcting both the vitamin D deficiency and hyperparathyroidism. If PTH levels remain elevated after some degree of phosphate control and correction of vitamin D deficiency, then it would be reasonable to use a VDRA—calcitriol, paricalcitol, or doxercalciferol. There does not appear to be a role for calcimimetics in CKD stages 3 and 4. Although the National Kidney Foundation's Kidney Disease Outcomes Quality Initiative (K/DOQI) and Kidney Disease: Improving Global Outcomes (K/DIGO) have suggested therapeutic targets for PTH concentrations, unfortunately there are insufficient data to support those targets, and patients should be treated using clinical judgment (Table 20.3).

11. **How should treatment be approached for patients with CKD stage 5?**
    Patients with stage 5 CKD who have not been previously treated generally present with hyperphosphatemia, hyperparathyroidism, and very low calcitriol concentrations, and may have low, normal, or elevated serum calcium. Furthermore, most of these patients are also calcidiol deficient. Similar to patients with CKD stages 3 and 4, there is a lack of prospective clinical studies demonstrating that correction of mineral abnormalities improve hard clinical endpoints. However, expert consensus agrees that therapy should definitely be focused to control serum phosphate to at least 5.5 mg/dL, if not to normal values by the use of adequate dialysis, dietary phosphate restriction, and phosphate binders. The use of calcium-containing binders (calcium carbonate or calcium acetate) should be limited to less than 1500 mg of calcium a day. Calcium acetate is a more effective phosphate binder per mg of calcium compared with calcium carbonate. Thus the use of calcium carbonate may result in greater absorption of calcium relative to phosphate binding, compared with calcium acetate. If patients have evidence of vascular calcifications, calcium-containing binders should be avoided. The non-calcium-containing binders include either sevelamer, lanthanum, or iron-based compounds (see Table 20.2). Both sevelamer, as either sevelamer HCl or carbonate, and lanthanum carbonate have been available for many years and have proven to be effective with few side effects or long-term risks. However, the dose for sevelamer generally requires three to four times the number of pills than that required for lanthanum with comparable phosphate control. Two iron-based phosphate binders, ferric citrate and sucroferric oxyhydroxide, are effective, with few side effects. Ferric citrate increases iron loading and lowers erythropoietin stimulating agent (ESA) requirements. Succoferric oxyhydroxide is as effective as sevelamer carbonate, with about a third of the pill burden. Succoferric oxyhydroxide does not significantly affect iron balance or ESA dosing.
    If patients have extremely elevated serum phosphorus, a short course of aluminum-containing phosphate binder may be considered; however, its long-term use should be avoided because of the risk of aluminum toxicity.
    Hyperparathyroidism and calcitriol deficiency could be addressed with the use of VDRAs. Calcitriol is effective but carries a greater risk of causing hypercalcemia and/or hyperphosphatemia,

Table 20.2. Characteristics of Commonly Used Phosphate Binders

PHOSPHATE BINDER	BENEFITS	HAZARDS	BONE BIOPSY FINDINGS
Aluminum	Potent and effective Useful for short term in severe hyperphosphatemia	Dementia Low-turnover bone disease/osteomalacia Anemia Should not be used as maintenance therapy	Markedly decreases turnover, markedly impairs mineralization, and moderately decreases volume
Calcium salt based	Effective Inexpensive Treats hypocalcemia Antacid properties useful for reflux and peptic ulcer disease	High calcium load Hypercalcemia Development of adynamic bone disease Extraosseous/vascular calcifications	May slightly decrease bone turnover, no effect on mineralization or volume
Sevelamer	Effective No systemic absorption Lowers level of low-density lipoprotein cholesterol Lower risk of hypercalcemia Reduces aortic and coronary calcification versus calcium salts Lower risk of adynamic bone disease versus calcium salts	Expensive Binds bile acids May inhibit absorption of active vitamin D Not effective in acidic environment Gastrointestinal symptoms such as diarrhea/constipation High pill burden	May slightly increase bone turnover, no effect on mineralization, and may slightly increase bone volume
Lanthanum carbonate	Potent and effective over wide pH range Lack of hypercalcemia No evidence of increased risk of low bone turnover disease Reduced pill burden	Expensive Gastrointestinal symptoms such as dyspepsia	May increase bone turnover, no effect on mineralization, and increases in bone volume
Ferric citrate	Effective Significant absorption of iron that may decrease iron and ESA requirements Lack of hypercalcemia	Expensive Gastrointestinal symptoms such as diarrhea/dark stools High pill burden Potential for iron overload	Unknown
Sucroferric oxyhydroxide	Potent and effective over wide pH range Lack of hypercalcemia No significant systemic absorption Reduced pill burden	Expensive Gastrointestinal symptoms such as diarrhea/dark stools	Unknown

whereas paricalcitol appears to have the lowest risk for hypercalcemia and hyperphosphatemia. Doxercalciferol, a prohormone, is also effective at reducing PTH, but may have a higher incidence of hypercalcemia and/or hyperphosphatemia than paricalcitol. Only one study has directly compared VDRAs in patients receiving dialysis, and that was between calcitriol and paricalcitol, which demonstrated comparable reduction in PTH but greater incidence of hypercalcemia and increase in calcium $\times$ phosphate product in those receiving calcitriol. Unfortunately, no prospective studies have yet been performed that have demonstrated the use of VDRAs improve hard clinical outcomes, such as survival, fractures, and cardiovascular events.

Table 20.3. Comparison of Kidney Disease Outcomes Quality Initiative With Kidney Disease: Improving Global Outcomes Mineral Guidelines

	K/DIGO	K/DOQI
Monitoring of Ca, phos, PTH	Starting at CKD stage 3 CKD stage 5 Ca and phos monthly PTH quarterly Include alkaline phosphatase: high or low levels may predict bone turnover	Same, no comment on alkaline phosphatase
Goal calcium	Normal range CKD stages 3–5	Same, weighted to lower end of normal range (8.4–9.5 mg/dL)
Goal phosphorus	Normal range stages 3–5	Range 2.7–4.6 mg/dL stages 3–4, 3.0–5.5 mg/dL for stage 5
Goal PTH	Evaluate patients with PTH above upper limits of normal for correctable factors: low phos/ca, low vitamin D. Treat based on trends to achieve PTH between 2 and 9 times the upper limit of normal	Target ranges: CKD3 35–70 pg/mL CKD4 70–110 pg/mL CKD5 150–300 pg/mL
Bone biopsy	Reasonable in various settings and prior to bisphosphonate therapy in CKD-MBD	Should be considered

Ca, Calcium; *CKD*, chronic kidney disease; *CKD-MBD*, chronic kidney disease–mineral and bone disorder; *K/DIGO*, Kidney Disease: Improving Global Outcomes; *K/DOQI*, Kidney Disease Outcomes Quality Initiative; *phos*, phosphorus; *PTH*, parathyroid hormone.

The calcimimetic, cinacalcet lowers PTH, calcium, and phosphate concentrations in ESKD patients. The EVOLVE study, a 5-year prospective trial of cinacalcet, used in combination of VDRAs, did not reduce mortality, cardiovascular disease, or fractures, but was associated with decrease in parathyroidectomies, compared with VDRA use alone. In addition to cinacalcet, there is a parenteral calcimimetic, elecalcetide, which also appears to be similarly effective to cinacalcet.

There has been some controversy as to the optimal PTH concentration to achieve in patients with stage 5 CKD. K/DIGO has expanded the K/DOQI range (150 to 300 pg/mL) to two to nine times the upper limit of normal for the particular PTH assay being used. The problem is that it has not clearly been defined as to what PTH values are consistently associated with normal bone histology. Furthermore, it has been noted that there are great discrepancies between various PTH assays. Thus a reasonable approach is to manage patients with only one PTH assay, to follow trends in PTH levels (as suggested by K/DIGO), and to use appropriate clinical judgment in managing PTH levels. Whether it is reasonable to correct the calcidiol deficiency by replacing nutritional vitamin D with cholecalciferol or ergocalciferol remains open for debate. To date, there is no data on the use of ER calcifediol in patients with stage 5 CKD.

12. Can osteoporosis be diagnosed in patients with CKD?

Osteoporosis is a condition of decreased bone mass, leading to fragile bones, which are at an increased risk for fractures. The diagnosis of osteoporosis is generally based on measurements of bone mineral density (BMD). The World Health Organization (WHO) has established criteria for making the diagnosis of osteoporosis. These criteria are based on comparing the BMD of the patient with that of a typical healthy, young gender-matched adult. BMD values that fall well below the average for healthy young adults (stated statistically as 2.5 standard deviations below the average referred to as the T-score) are diagnosed as osteoporosis. Although these criteria are widely used, they were based and validated only on Caucasian females. Furthermore, underlying diseases, such as chronic kidney disease, were excluded from the analyses. In non-CKD populations, fracture risk increases approximately 1.6-fold for every SD decrement in BMD, irrespective of gender. Although CKD patients have decreased BMD, the degree of bone loss is not directly associated with the decrease in estimated GFR. Furthermore, BMD measurements are not able to discriminate between the histological or microarchitectural abnormalities seen in CKD and thus have not been able to consistently discriminate between CKD patients who fracture and those who do not fracture. It is important to remember that there are many potential causes for decreased bone density in CKD patients, including hypogonadism, sedentary lifestyle, smoking, use of steroids, poor protein intake, vitamin D deficiency, diabetes, and Ca deficiency. Thus in CKD patients, fractures are not necessarily related to osteoporosis, and the diagnosis could only be made after ruling out and correcting all underlying causes of CKD-MBD and generally requires a bone biopsy prior to proceeding with traditional anti-osteoporotic therapy.

13. **Is there a role for parathyroidectomy?**
    Ideally, parathyroidectomy should be avoided with the initiation of early therapy to prevent the development of severe hyperparathyroidism with monoclonal nodular transformation of the parathyroid gland. As the parathyroid glands develop monoclonal nodularity, there is loss of both the calcium-sensing receptor and the vitamin D receptor. Thus, as the parathyroid glands develop large nodules, they are no longer responsive to normal physiologic control and are resistant to pharmacologic therapy, which is a poor prognostic sign. An attempt should be made to treat patients early before severe hyperparathyroidism develops. In patients with severe hyperparathyroidism, treatment with high-dose VDRAs and cinacalcet may be necessary; however, if severe hyperparathyroidism persists and patients develop hypercalcemia and hyperphosphatemia, a parathyroidectomy may be required. There is much controversy as to the best approach for parathyroidectomy, whether a subtotal parathyroidectomy should be performed or a total parathyroidectomy with reimplantation of part of a gland into either the forearm or the sternocleidomastoid muscle. The problem of reimplantation is that frequently the implanted tissue becomes fibrotic and does not function, or the patient (rarely) could develop parathyroidomatosis, in which microscopic cells produce high levels of PTH. A relatively common complication following parathyroidectomy is the development of the hungry bone syndrome. This occurs in patients with long-standing, severe hyperparathyroidism. Following the rapid drop in PTH concentrations, the bones rapidly take up both calcium and phosphate as they remineralize, resulting in hypocalcemia and possibly hypophosphatemia. These patients require high doses of calcium and calcitriol to prevent symptomatic hypocalcemia. Depending on the severity of the preexisting hyperparathyroidism, this can last for weeks to even months. Experienced parathyroid surgeons may be able to perform partial parathyroidectomy, while trying to selectively remove nodular tissue, and leave behind normal-appearing gland. Surgery should be performed utilizing intraoperative PTH measurements. Although several studies have suggested improved survival in dialysis patients following parathyroidectomy, a cohort analysis of USRDS ESRD database demonstrated increased morbidity following parathyroidectomy.

14. **What are the biochemical changes in mineral metabolism following kidney transplantation?**
    Significant changes in mineral metabolism are observed following transplantation. PTH concentrations decrease significantly during the first 3 months but typically stabilize at elevated values after 1 year. It is common for PTH values to range from one to two times the upper limit of normal. Serum calcium tends to increase after transplant and then stabilize at the higher end of the normal range within 2 months. A small percentage of patients will have persistent hypercalcemia. Serum phosphorus generally decreases rapidly to within or below normal levels after surgery, and hypophosphatemia, if present, generally resolves within 2 to 4 months. However, a small group of patients will have persistent hypophosphatemia. Low levels of calcitriol typically do not normalize until almost 18 months after transplantation. If patients have persistent hypercalcemia with hyperparathyroidism, the practice is to wait at least 1 year prior to considering a parathyroidectomy. Lately it has become relatively common practice to treat patients with hypercalcemia and hyperparathyroidism with cinacalcet; however, data demonstrating a long-term benefit of this practice presently are lacking.

15. **What bone lesion is typical after kidney transplantation?**
    Fractures are very common following kidney transplantation associated with bone loss in the first 1 to 2 years. The use of corticosteroids for immunosuppression is considered to be the major contributor. The decreased use of corticosteroids has resulted in less fractures following transplantation. However, other factors such as persistent hyperparathyroidism, vitamin D deficiency, persistent and/or progressive CKD, and hypophosphatemia are contributing factors. Therapy should be focused on identifying the underlying metabolic disorder and appropriately managing it.

KEY POINTS

1. Chronic kidney disease–mineral and bone disorder (CKD-MBD) is a systemic disorder of mineral and bone metabolism resulting from CKD that may be manifested by at least one of the following:
   a. Laboratory abnormalities associated with disturbed mineral metabolism
   b. Bone disease, defined as ROD
   c. Calcification of extraskeletal tissue
2. The manifestations of CKD-MBD in the chronologic evolution of CKD are:
   a. Phosphate retention
   b. Increases in FGF23
   c. Decreases in calcitriol
   d. Increases in PTH
   e. Finally (in late stage 4, early stage 5 disease), hyperphosphatemia and eventually hypocalcemia. Most patients are also calcidiol (25-hydroxy vitamin D) deficient.
3. In stage 5 CKD, therapy is focused on maintaining the serum phosphate below 5.5 mg/dL by the use of adequate dialysis, dietary phosphate restriction, and phosphate binders.
4. Treatment of hyperparathyroidism in stage 5 CKD should be addressed with the use of vitamin D receptor activators (VDRAs) and calcimimetics.
5. The optimal PTH concentration in patients with stage 5 CKD has not been prospectively determined, and there are significant discrepancies between various PTH assays. Thus a reasonable approach is to manage patients with only one PTH assay, to follow trends in PTH levels (as suggested by K/DIGO), and to use appropriate clinical judgment in managing PTH levels. Kidney Disease: Improving Global Outcomes (K/DIGO) suggests a target of two to nine times the upper limit of normal for the particular PTH assay being used.

BIBLIOGRAPHY

Andress, D. L. (2008). Adynamic bone in patients with chronic kidney disease. *Kidney International, 73,* 1345–1354.

Andress, D. L., Coyne, D. W., Kalantar-Zadeh, K., Molitch, M. E., Zangeneh, F., & Sprague, S. M. (2008). Management of secondary hyperparathyroidism in stages 3 and 4 chronic kidney disease. *Endocrine Practice, 14*(1), 18–27.

Block, G. A., Wheeler, D. C., Persky, M. S., Kestenbaum, B., Ketteler, M., Spiegel, D. M., . . . Chertow, G. M. (2012). Effects of phosphate binders in moderate CKD. *Journal of the American Society of Nephrology, 23,* 1407–1415.

EVOLVE Trial Investigators, Chertow, G. M., Block, G. A., Correa-Rotter, R., Drüeke, T. B., Floege, J., . . . Parfrey, P. S. (2012). Effect of cinacalcet on cardiovascular disease in patients undergoing dialysis. *New England Journal of Medicine, 367,* 2482–2494.

Gal-Moscovici, A., & Sprague, S. M. (2008). Role of bone biopsy in stages 3 to 4 chronic kidney disease. *Clinical Journal of the American Society of Nephrology, 3*(Suppl. 3), S170–S174.

Lewis, J. B., Sika, M., Koury, M. J., Chuang, P., Schulman, G., Smith, M. T., . . . Collaborative Study Group. (2015). Ferric citrate controls phosphorus and delivers iron in patients on dialysis. *Journal of the American Society of Nephrology, 26,* 493–503.

Moe, S., Drüeke, T., Cunningham, J., Goodman, W., Martin, K., Olgaard, K., . . . Kidney Disease: Improving Global Outcomes (KDIGO). (2006). Definition, evaluation, and classification of renal osteodystrophy: A position statement from Kidney Disease: Improving Global Outcomes (KDIGO). *Kidney International, 69,* 1945–1953.

Rogers, N. M., Teubner, D. J., & Coates, P. T. (2007). Calcific uremic arteriolopathy: Advances in pathogenesis and treatment. *Seminars in Dialysis, 20,* 150–157.

Sprague, S. M., Bellorin-Font, E., Jorgetti, V., Carvalho, A. B., Malluche, H. H., Ferreira, A., . . . Moe, S. M. (2016). Diagnostic accuracy of bone turnover markers and bone histology in patients with chronic kidney disease treated by dialysis. *American Journal of Kidney Diseases, 67*(4), 559–566.

Sprague, S. M., Belozeroff, V., Danese, M. D., Martin, L. P., & Olgaard, K. (2008). Abnormal bone and mineral metabolism in kidney transplant patients—A review. *American Journal of Nephrology, 28,* 246–253.

Sprague, S. M., & Coyne, D. (2010). Control of secondary hyperparathyroidism by vitamin D receptor activators in chronic kidney disease. *Clinical Journal of the American Society Nephrology, 5,* 512–518.

Sprague, S. M., Crawford, P. W., Melnick, J. Z., Strugnell, S. A., Ali, S., Mangoo-Karim, R., . . . Bishop, C. W. (2016). Use of extended-release calcifediol to treat secondary hyperparathyroidism in stages 3 and 4 chronic kidney disease. *American Journal of Nephrology, 44*(4), 316–325.

CHAPTER 21

CARDIOVASCULAR DISEASE
Anuja Shah, Charbel C. Khoury, and Rajnish Mehrotra

1. What is the relationship between the decrease in the glomerular filtration rate and cardiovascular disease?
   Patients with chronic kidney disease (CKD) have a substantial increase in risk for death from cardiovascular disease. Even small decreases in kidney function, as measured by the estimated glomerular filtration rate (eGFR), are associated with this higher risk, and it increases progressively as kidney function declines. Patients with CKD are substantially more likely to die from heart disease than progress to dialysis. In patients with end-stage kidney disease (ESKD), the risk for death is 10- to 100-fold higher than age- and gender-matched individuals without kidney disease. Conversely, in patients with known heart disease (like coronary artery disease or heart failure), the greater the severity of kidney disease, the worse the patient outcome, including higher mortality and, in patients hospitalized for non-ST segment elevation myocardial infarction, a longer length of stay.

2. What is the relationship between albuminuria/proteinuria and cardiovascular disease?
   The presence of albuminuria is also associated with a higher risk of death from cardiovascular disease. This risk begins even when the amount of urine albumin is not enough to meet the criteria for the diagnosis of microalbuminuria. As the amount of urine albumin increases, so does the risk for death from heart disease—the risk is higher in individuals with microalbuminuria and even higher among those with overt proteinuria.

3. Why is the risk for cardiovascular disease increased in CKD?
   Both traditional and nontraditional risk factors are important contributors to cardiovascular disease. Diabetes mellitus and hypertension are the two most common causes of CKD—both are also known cardiovascular risk factors. Moreover, diseases like hypertension are more severe in the setting of CKD. However, traditional risk factors are insufficient to explain the high cardiovascular risk seen with CKD. A large number of nontraditional risk factors have been identified, such as systemic inflammation, high serum phosphorus, and oxidative stress (among others). However, at this time, it remains unclear if any of the traditional or nontraditional risk factors can be modified to reduce the risk of heart disease (Table 21.1).

4. What types of cardiovascular disease are seen in patients with CKD?
   There are two major overlapping categories of cardiovascular disease associated with CKD: disorders of cardiovascular perfusion, which includes atherosclerotic cardiovascular disease; and disorders of cardiac function, such as congestive heart failure and left ventricular hypertrophy. Disorders of vascular perfusion include coronary artery disease, cerebrovascular disease, peripheral vascular disease, and renovascular disease.

5. Are there other forms of cardiovascular disease seen in patients with CKD?
   Cardiovascular calcification is a frequent contributor to cardiovascular disease in CKD; it can occur either in heart valves, the tunica intima, or the tunica media of the blood vessels. Calcified blood vessels

Table 21.1. Nontraditional Risk Factors for Cardiovascular in Chronic Kidney Disease

Salt and volume overload	Anemia
Left ventricular hypertrophy	Metabolic acidosis
Uremic toxins	Use of immunosuppressants
Sympathetic overactivity	Oxidative stress
Altered mineral metabolism	Inflammation
Vascular calcification	Endothelial cell dysfunction
Protein-energy wasting	Albuminuria/proteinuria

can often be seen on plain x-rays in patients with CKD, particularly among the elderly or those being treated with dialysis. Though not fully understood, during vascular calcification, the smooth muscle cells of vessels express osteocytic phenotypes and the calcium phosphate deposition resembles hydroxyapatite seen in bone. The greater the severity of vascular calcification, the greater the risk of death. There are many reasons why patients with CKD develop vascular calcification; an increase in serum phosphorus is considered to be an important contributor, and this may be a potentially modifiable risk factor. Hence, the management of elevated phosphorus levels may reduce the risk for heart disease; however, this approach remains unproven.

Calciphylaxis, or cacificic uremic arteriolopathy, is an accelerated form of vascular calcification typically seen in patients with CKD stage 5. Risk factors include warfarin therapy, altered mineral metabolism, and obesity. The process can lead to nonhealing wounds and is often fatal. Parathyroidectomy and/or sodium thiosulfate therapy may be of benefit.

6. **What are the clinical manifestations of cardiovascular disease in CKD?**
   Manifestations of cardiovascular disease include angina pectoris, myocardial infarction, congestive heart failure, stroke, peripheral vascular disease, arrhythmias, and sudden cardiac death. In advanced CKD, cardiovascular disease is often manifested by left ventricular hypertrophy, diastolic dysfunction, and heart failure. The national registry for dialysis patients—the United States Renal Data System—reports that about 30% of patients with CKD over 66 years of age have congestive heart failure. Left ventricular hypertrophy may be accompanied by left ventricular remodeling and fibrosis, and these changes, with or without coronary artery disease (in addition to electrolyte shifts and volume expansion), may contribute to the high incidence of sudden cardiac death in this population. Indeed, sudden cardiac death is the most common cause of death in dialysis patients.

   The clinical manifestations of acute coronary syndrome are also atypical in patients with CKD, and the electrocardiographic findings may be obscured by the presence of left ventricular hypertrophy.

7. **What should be the goal blood pressure for the treatment of hypertension in patients with CKD?**
   Long-term follow-up of participants with nondiabetic CKD in the Modification of Diet in Renal Disease study showed that aggressive control of blood pressure was associated with slowing in the rate of loss of kidney function. However, the results of other studies examining the association of intensity of blood pressure control on the progression of kidney disease has not been consistent, and a recent meta-analyses of clinical trials in patients with nondiabetic kidney disease was not able to show the benefit as seen in the Modification of Diet in Renal Disease study. The results of the Systolic Blood Pressure Intervention Trial (SPRINT) trial have recently been published and show that targeting blood pressure <120 mm Hg systolic, measured using a standardized approach distinct from how measurements are made in clinical practice, was associated with a 25% lower risk for the composite primary outcome of myocardial infarction, other acute coronary syndromes, stroke, heart failure, or death from cardiovascular causes. The benefit was the same in patients with and without kidney disease; the results of the effect of aggressive control of blood pressure on the rate of loss of kidney function are awaited. Given the results of this landmark study, it seems prudent to target lower blood pressure in patients with CKD, which has not been the norm recently.

8. **Does reduction in proteinuria decrease cardiovascular risk?**
   The greater the proteinuria, the higher the cardiovascular risk. A reduction in urine protein excretion is associated with long-term slowing in the loss of kidney function. However, whether or not reduction in proteinuria will reduce cardiovascular risk is unclear at this time. Nevertheless, given the benefit of the slowing rate of decline of the GFR, attempts should be made to reduce urine protein excretion to at least <1.0 g/day.

   There are two broad strategies for reducing urine protein excretion:
   - Therapies specific to the underlying disease (like that for glomerular diseases)
   - Nonspecific therapies. Angiotensin-converting enzyme inhibitors or angiotensin receptor blockers are the most effective nonspecific anti-proteinuric therapies and should be the first-line antihypertensive therapies as long as there are no contraindications for their use. The combined use of angiotensin-converting enzyme inhibitors and angiotensin receptor blockers is no longer recommended, as it is associated with a higher risk for clinically meaningful acute worsening of kidney function.

9. **What is the role of lipid management in CKD?**
   The greater the amount of proteinuria, the worse the abnormalities in the lipid panel. Patients with proteinuria generally have elevated total cholesterol and low-density lipoprotein cholesterol, as well as low levels of high-density lipoprotein cholesterol. Patients with diabetes may have, in addition, elevated triglyceride levels.

Lipid-lowering therapies are as effective in lowering cholesterol levels in patients with CKD as in the general population. No dosage adjustments are required for statins, bile acid sequestrants, niacin, or ezetemibe. Fibrates do require a dosage adjustment for kidney function. However, the magnitude of effect of these drugs on reducing cardiovascular disease may not be as large as that seen in the general population. Two large, randomized, controlled trials have been unable to show any significant reduction in fatal and/or nonfatal cardiovascular events in dialysis patients. The Study of Heart and Renal Protection (SHARP) study demonstrated that treatment of patients with CKD with simvastatin/ezetimibe was associated with a significant reduction in cardiovascular events; however, there was no effect on cardiovascular or all-cause mortality. The results were the same whether or not the patients were undergoing dialysis. These data indicate that the benefit with lipid lowering in patients with CKD may not be as large as that seen in patients without kidney disease.

10. **What is the relationship between anemia and its management to the cardiovascular mortality in CKD?**
    Anemia is a cardinal manifestation of CKD and it generally is apparent when the eGFR is <30 mL/min per 1.73 m². Observational studies have shown that the greater the severity of anemia, the higher the risk for death. However, several randomized, controlled trials have failed to demonstrate a reduction in mortality risk with erythropoietin therapy, the cornerstone of anemia management in patients with CKD. In fact, some of these studies have shown a higher risk for stroke and/or death when the treatment was targeted to achieve a hemoglobin level of 13 g/dL. Hence, erythropoietin therapy should not be started unless the hemoglobin level decreases to between 9.0 and 10.0 g/dL, and care should be exercised to prevent it from increasing to above 12.0 g/dL.

11. **Can serum troponin be used in the diagnosis of myocardial infarction in patients with kidney disease?**
    The use of biomarkers for the diagnosis of myocardial infarction in patients with CKD can be problematic. Serum troponin has been found to be elevated in patients with CKD who have no clinical suspicion of acute myocardial injury. It is not absolutely clear why this is the case. This may have to do with subclinical myocardial ischemia or decreased clearance of troponin degradation products because of kidney disease.
    Baseline elevations in troponin are associated with the higher risk of cardiovascular death in these patients. Troponin I is a more specific marker of infarction that troponin T in these patients. Even so, whether or not an elevation in serum troponin in a given patient indicates acute myocardial injury, it is necessary to take into account the patient's clinical presentation and change in the blood levels of troponin over time. For example, a rising troponin level in a patient who presents with typical chest pain would be consistent with the diagnosis of acute myocardial infarction. On the other hand, small and unchanging elevations in an otherwise asymptomatic patient would portend a poor long-term prognosis but are unlikely to be of any immediate import.

12. **Are there special considerations for treatment of myocardial infarction in CKD?**
    Patients with CKD who present with acute myocardial infarction generally do not do as well as those without kidney disease. Furthermore, CKD patients do not do as well after percutaneous coronary intervention, with or without stenting or after coronary artery bypass grafting. The risk-benefit ratio of all these procedures should be carefully considered, and a decision should be made on a case-by-case basis.
    The treatment of an acute myocardial infarction with percutaneous coronary intervention also involves a risk for acute kidney injury, which may be secondary to contrast-induced nephropathy or cholesterol emboli. Patients at increased risk of contrast-induced nephropathy are those with a serum creatinine ≥1.5 mg/dL or an eGFR <60 mL/min per 1.73 m², patients with diabetes mellitus, those treated with biguanides, and the elderly.

13. **What are the clinical manifestations of cholesterol emboli?**
    Patients will have progressive and often irreversible loss of kidney function after an intra-arterial procedure (over days and weeks), which often does not improve. Livedo reticularis, low complement levels, peripheral and or urinary eosinophilia, and physical findings of distal emboli (in the digits or retina) may be seen.

14. **How reliable is the measurement of serum brain natriuretic peptide in patients with CKD?**
    Like serum troponin, serum levels of brain natriuretic peptide are elevated in patients with CKD; in many cases, marked elevations are noted. The magnitude of increase in serum brain natriuretic peptide depends on the degree of left ventricular hypertrophy and/or left ventricular systolic dysfunction. It is unclear if serum brain natriuretic peptide can be used to diagnose circulatory congestion in

patients with CKD or to serially monitor response to diuretics or ultrafiltration with dialysis. A fair bit of caution should be exercised before ordering and/or interpreting brain natriuretic peptide levels in patients with advanced CKD or those treated with dialysis.

15. **Is there an increased risk of atrial fibrillation and stroke in CKD?**
The risk of atrial fibrillation increases with the decline in the GFR. By the time patients have progressed to ESKD and are requiring dialysis, the prevalence of atrial fibrillation is at least 10-fold higher than in the general population, so around 1 in 8 dialysis patients suffer from atrial fibrillation. Previous and ongoing studies with arrhythmia-monitoring devices suggest that atrial fibrillation may be even more common and underdiagnosed in the dialysis population. It is thought that coronary artery disease, degenerative valvular disease, left ventricular hypertrophy, and fluctuating levels of electrolytes during hemodialysis likely promote the arrhythmia.
   Atrial fibrillation carries an increased risk of thromboembolic stroke in CKD patients. The US Renal Data System reported an annual incidence of 15% in hemodialysis patients compared with 10% in patients with CKD not undergoing dialysis, and 3% in individuals without CKD. The 2-year mortality rates after stroke in these subgroups were 74%, 55%, and 28%, respectively.

16. **What are the special considerations for the management of atrial fibrillation in CKD patients?**
Oral anticoagulation can be considered for the prevention of cardioembolic strokes from atrial fibrillation. This is supported by subgroup analyses from one single, randomized, controlled trial (Stroke Prevention in Atrial Fibrillation SPAF-3 trial), which found that warfarin reduced the risk of strokes in patients with CKD stages 3A to 3B. However, strong evidence is lacking in the advanced stages of CKD. There are no randomized trials assessing the benefits and risks of anticoagulation in patients with advanced stages of CKD or on dialysis, and the observational studies published so far have been split. Moreover, platelet dysfunction, anemia, endothelial, and vascular dysfunction, as well as other factors make the risk of intracranial hemorrhage or gastrointestinal bleeding significantly higher in people with advanced kidney disease. As such, the risk-benefit balance of anticoagulation in advanced CKD may be tilted by increased bleeding complications.
   Overall, in patients with CKD and not on dialysis, the risk of thromboembolism should be assessed using the CHA2DS2-VASc score. This scoring system accounts for congestive heart failure, hypertension, age ≥75 (doubled), diabetes, stroke or transient ischemic attack, or systemic embolism (doubled), vascular disease, age 65 to 74, and sex. Men with a CHA2DS2-VASc score ≥1 and women with a score ≥2 should be considered for anticoagulation. For patients on dialysis, the initiation of anticoagulation needs to be individualized. Careful monitoring of the degree of anticoagulation is necessary in these patients, and the risk of bleeding is further increased when oral anticoagulation is combined with aspirin therapy. The HAS-BLED (hypertension, abnormal kidney/liver function [1 point each], stroke, bleeding history or predisposition, labile INR, elderly [>65 years], drugs/alcohol concomitantly [1 point each]) is used in atrial fibrillation patients to determine those at a higher risk of bleeding. However, while it accounts for abnormal kidney function, its use has not been formally validated in patients with advanced CKD and dialysis.

17. **Which oral anticoagulants can be used in CKD patients with atrial fibrillation?**
When the decision is made to anticoagulate, the 2014 American Heart Association and the 2016 European Society of Cardiology guidelines recommend warfarin as the oral anticoagulant of choice in patients with atrial fibrillation and advanced CKD or ESKD. Warfarin has less than 1% kidney elimination, and should not accumulate with decreased kidney function or on dialysis. However, patients with advanced CKD and dialysis have alterations of their hepatic metabolism and tend to require lower doses of warfarin.
   Non–vitamin K oral anticoagulants (NOACs), also referred to as direct oral anticoagulants, are increasingly being used in non-valvular atrial fibrillation. They include the direct thrombin inhibitor (dabigatran) and factor Xa inhibitors (rivaroxaban, apixaban, edoxaban). These drugs are at least noninferior to warfarin in the prevention of thromboembolic complications of atrial fibrillation for the average patient. However, they have not been properly studied in advanced CKD and ESKD.
   All NOACs are, to some extent, renally cleared (Table 21.2), and may potentially accumulate in patients with a low GFR. This could lead to an increased risk for bleeding, especially since no clinically available coagulation parameter accurately estimates the level of anticoagulation. As such, dosage adjustments are recommended in patients with CKD using the Cockcroft-Gault creatinine clearance formula (Table 21.3). Using the body surface area standardized CKD-EPI GFR formula may lead to dosing error, as it is not in line with the randomized controlled trials used to make these suggestions.

Table 21.2. Non–Vitamin K Oral Anticoagulants

	WARFARIN	DABIGATRAN	APIXABAN	RIVAROXABAN	EDOXABAN
Renal clearance	<1%	80%	27%	36%	50%
Removal after 4 h of hemodialysis	<1%	50%–60%	7%	<1%	9%

Table 21.3. US Food and Drug Administration-Recommended Dosing of Non–Vitamin K Oral Anticoagulants by Creatinine Clearance

	Creatinine Clearance mL/min (Cockcroft-Gault Equation)				
	>90	51–90	31–50	15–30	<15 OR ON DIALYSIS
Dabigatran[a]	150 mg BID	150 mg BID	150 mg BID	75 mg BID	NR
Apixaban[b]	5 or 2.5 mg BID	5 or 2.5 mg BID	5 or 2.5 mg BID	5 or 2.5 mg BID	5 or 2.5 mg BID
Edoxaban[c]	60 mg QD	60 mg QD	30 mg QD	30 mg QD	NR
Rivaroxaban	20 mg QD	20 mg QD	15 mg QD	15 mg QD	NR

[a]Dabigatran is not approved in the rest of the world for CrCl 15 to 29 mL/min.
[b]Apixaban is only approved for CrCl <15 mL/min in the United States; 2.5 mg twice daily if the patient has any two of the following: serum creatinine ≥1.5 mg/dL, age ≥80 years, or body weight ≤60 kg.
[c]Not recommended in patients with eCrCl >95 mL/min due to high renal clerance.
BID, Twice daily; QD, daily; NR, not approved by the FDA.

Currently, the US Food and Drug Administration approved the use of apixaban for patients with a creatinine clearance <15 mL/min or on dialysis. Caution should still be exercised when using this medication, since these suggestions were based on small pharmacokinetic studies.

18. How do you manage major hemorrhage in patients on oral anticoagulants?
For warfarin, and all the NOACs, 4-factor prothrombin complex concentrate rather than fresh frozen plasma is recommended for reversing anticoagulation in acute life-threatening hemorrhages. Antifibrinolytic agents, such as tranexamic acid and epsilon-aminocaproic acid, may also be used.
For warfarin-associated bleeding, intravenous vitamin K can be used concomitantly. As for dabigatran, idarucizumab is a humanized anti-dabigatran monoclonal antibody fragment that is effective for emergency reversal. Hemodialysis has also been used to clear dabigatran, but it is not suitable for factor Xa inhibitors.

KEY POINTS

1. Even small changes in kidney function—either a decrease in the GFR or an increase in urine albumin excretion—are associated with a higher risk of death from cardiovascular causes.
2. Both traditional and nontraditional cardiovascular risk factors are more common and are often severe in patients with CKD, and they account for the high risk for heart disease.
3. The serum levels of biomarkers, such as troponin and brain natriuretic peptide, are sometimes increased in patients with CKD; their diagnostic value depends on the clinical setting and change over time.

BIBLIOGRAPHY

Abboud, H., & Henrich, W. L. (2010). Clinical practice. Stage IV chronic kidney disease. *N Engl J Med, 362*(1), 56–65.
Baigent, C., Landray, M. J., Reith, C., Emberson J, Wheeler, D. C., Tomson, C., . . . SHARP Investigators. (2011). The effects of lowering LDL cholesterol with simvastatin plus ezetimibe in patients with chronic kidney disease (Study of Heart and Renal Protection): a randomized placebo-controlled trial. *Lancet, 377*, 2181–2192.

Chan, K. E., Giugliano, R. P., Patel, M. R., Abramson, S., Jardine, M., Zhao, S., . . . Piccini, J. P. (2016). Non-vitamin K anti-coagulant agents in patients with advanced chronic kidney disease on dialysis with atrial fibrillation. *J Am Coll Cardiol, 67*, 2888–2899.

Cheung, A. K., Rahman, M., Reboussin, D. M., Craven, T. E., Greene, T., Kimmel, P. L., . . . SPRINT Research Group. (2017). Effects of intensive BP control in CKD. *J Am Soc Nephrol, 28*(9), 2812–2823.

Dukipatti, R., Adler, S. A., & Mehrotra, R. (2008). Cardiovascular implications of chronic kidney disease in older adults. *Drugs and Aging, 25*(3), 241–253.

Fellström, B. C., Jardine, A. G., Schmieder, R. E., Holdaas, H., Bannister, K., Beutler, J., . . . AURORA Study Group. (2009). Rosuvastatin and cardiovascular events in patients undergoing hemodialysis. *N Engl J Med, 360*, 1395–1407.

Go, A. S., Chertow, G. M., Fan, D., McCulloch, C. E., & Hsu, C. (2004). Chronic kidney disease and the risks of death, cardiovascular events, and hospitalization. *N Engl J Med, 351*, 1296–1305.

Hart, R. G., Pearce, L. A., Asinger, R. W., & Herzog, C. A. (2011). Warfarin in atrial fibrillation patients with moderate chronic kidney disease. *Clin J Am Soc Nephrol, 6*, 2599–2604.

Kanderian, A. S., & Francis, G. S. (2006). Cardiac troponin and chronic kidney disease. *Kidney Int, 69*(7), 1112–1114.

Mavrakanas, T. A., & Charytan, D. M. (2016). Cardiovascular complications in chronic dialysis patients. *Curr Opin Nephrol Hypertens, 25*(6), 536–544.

National Kidney Foundation. (2002). K/DOQI clinical practice guidelines for chronic kidney disease: Evaluation, classification and stratification. *Am J Kidney Dis, 39*(2 Suppl. 1), S1–S266.

Pfeffer, M. A., Burdmann, E. A., Chen. C. Y., Cooper, M. E., de Zeeuw, D., Eckardt, K. U., . . . TREAT Investigators. (2009). A trial of darbepoetin alfa in type 2 diabetes and chronic kidney disease. *N Engl J Med, 361*, 2019–2032.

Pun, P. H., Smarz, T. R., Honeycutt, E. F., Shaw, L. K., Al-Khatib, S. M., & Middleton, J. P. (2009). Chronic kidney disease is associated with increased risk of sudden cardiac death among patients with coronary artery disease. *Kidney Int, 76*, 652–658.

Reinecke, H., Brand, E., Mesters, R., Schäbitz, W. R., Pavenstädt, H., & Breithardt, G. (2009). Dilemmas in the management of atrial fibrillation in chronic kidney disease. *J Am Soc Nephrol, 20*(4), 705–711.

Rucker, D., & Tonelli, M. (2009). Cardiovascular risk and management in chronic kidney disease. *Nat Rev Nephrol, 5*, 287–296.

Sarma, A., & Giugliano R. P. (1995). Current and developing strategies for monitoring and reversing direct oral anticoagulants in patients with non-valvular atrial fibrillation. *Hosp Pract, 43*, 258–267.

Sarnak, M. J., Greene, T., Wang, X., Beck, G., Kusek, J. W., Collins, A. J., & Levey, A. S. (2015). The effect of a lower target blood pressure on the progression of kidney disease: Long-term follow-up of the modification of diet in renal disease study. *Ann Intern Med, 142*, 342–351.

Schlieper, G., Schurgers, L., Brandenburg, V., Reutelingsperger, C., & Floege, J. (2016). Vascular calcification in chronic kidney disease: An update. *Nephrol Dial Transplant, 31*, 31–39.

The SPRINT Research Group. (2015). A randomized trial of intensive versus standard blood pressure control. *N Engl J Med, 373*, 2103–2116.

Tsai, W. C., Wu, H. Y., Peng, Y. S., Yang, J. Y., Chen, H. Y., Chiu, Y. L., . . . Chien, K. L. (2017). Association of intensive blood pressure control and kidney disease progression in nondiabetic patients with chronic kidney disease: A systematic review and meta-analysis. *JAMA Intern Med, 177*, 792–799.

United States Renal Data System. (2015). *2015 USRDS annual data report: Epidemiology of kidney disease in the United States.* Bethesda, MD: National Institutes of Health, National Institute of Diabetes and Digestive and Kidney Diseases.

Zimmerman, D., Sood, M. M., Rigatto, C., Holden, R. M., Hiremath, S., & Clase, C. M. (2012). Systematic review and meta-analysis of incidence, prevalence and outcomes of atrial fibrillation in patients on dialysis. *Nephrol Dial Transplant, 27*(10), 3816–3822.

CHAPTER 22

DYSLIPIDEMIA

Pranav S. Garimella and Mark J. Sarnak

1. **What is the typical lipid profile in patients with chronic kidney disease (CKD)?**
   Dyslipidemias are common in patients with CKD, those on dialysis (both hemodialysis and peritoneal dialysis), and those who have undergone kidney transplantation. Dyslipidemia is also prevalent in over 60% of people who have received cardiac or liver transplantation, and this may be partially due to the long-term use of calcineurin inhibitors and/or steroids as immunosuppressants. Proteinuria, and particularly nephrotic syndrome, is associated with a greater elevation in total cholesterol, low-density lipoprotein (LDL) cholesterol, triglycerides, and lipoprotein(a) (Lp-a) than in persons with CKD without proteinuria. The concentration of high-density lipoprotein (HDL) cholesterol is also often reduced in nephrotic syndrome. Hemodialysis and peritoneal dialysis patients have increased levels of triglycerides and Lp-a compared to patients with milder degrees of CKD, with peritoneal dialysis patients having particularly atherogenic lipid profiles, perhaps due to constant dextrose absorption. LDL cholesterol is often normal or low in hemodialysis patients, perhaps due to poor nutrition and chronic inflammation. Table 22.1 depicts the most common lipid abnormalities seen across the spectrum of kidney disease.

2. **What are the unique characteristics of the pathophysiology of dyslipidemia in CKD?**
   A number of unique clinical features among patients with CKD and those on dialysis lead to changes in the structure and function of lipid molecules. Uremia and frequent heparinization in dialysis patients can decrease the activity of lipoprotein lipase and hepatic triglyceride lipase necessary to cleave triglycerides into free fatty acids. Incomplete triglyceride catabolism causes an accumulation of remnant particles (chylomicrons) that contribute to increased atherosclerosis. Although the concentration of LDL cholesterol is often no higher than that in the general population, there are differences in the qualitative nature of LDL cholesterol. Small dense LDL (sdLDL) and intermediate LDL (ILDL) fractions are increased in CKD. The decreased activity of lipases described above prevents the degradation of very-low-density LDL (VLDL) into LDL cholesterol, resulting in the accumulation of ILDL. The increased plasma residence time of these particles further results in structural changes in the apo(B) protein they carry, decreasing hepatic clearance. Decreased clearance by the liver results in uptake by macrophages, which may result in adherence to the vascular endothelium, leading to plaque formation.
   CKD is also associated with change in the distribution of HDL cholesterol fractions. Low apo-AI level and decreased lecithin:cholesterol acyltransferase (LCAT) activity result in reduced esterification of free cholesterol and a reduced cholesterol-carrying capacity of HDL molecules. Proteinuric kidney diseases, especially nephrotic syndrome, are characterized by elevations in plasma Lp(a) concentrations, LDL, and total cholesterol due to increased liver production. In addition, there is a reduction in the cardioprotective HDL2 component of HDL cholesterol. Proteinuria also leads to an elevated free fatty acid to albumin ratio. Angiopoietin-like 4 (angptl4) is a protein expressed primarily in the liver, and its levels are elevated in nephrotic syndrome in response to these free fatty acids. Angptl4 inhibits lipoprotein lipase, leading to hypertriglyceridemia in persons with nephrotic syndrome.

3. **When should patients with kidney disease be evaluated for dyslipidemia?**
   Recent guidelines from the Kidney Disease Improving Global Outcomes (KDIGO) have recommended that all adult patients with newly identified CKD, including those on dialysis or kidney transplant recipients, should be evaluated with a lipid profile. Although the evidence to suggest improved clinical outcomes after measuring lipids is lacking, the risks of testing are low, and the data may provide information on cardiovascular disease (CVD) prognosis and guide treatment.

4. **What tests should be used to evaluate dyslipidemia in patients with CKD?**
   As with the general population, a complete lipid profile including total, HDL, LDL cholesterol, and triglycerides should be obtained when evaluating dyslipidemia. While a lipid profile obtained after an

Table 22.1. Lipid Profiles Across the Spectrum of Kidney Disease as Compared to the General Population

	CKD NOT ON DIALYSIS	NEPHROTIC SYNDROME	HEMODIALYSIS	PERITONEAL DIALYSIS	POST-TRANSPLANT
Total cholesterol	↑ or ↔	↑ ↑	↓ or ↔	↑ or ↔	↑ or ↔
HDL cholesterol	↓ or ↔	↓	↓	↓	↓ or ↔
LDL cholesterol	↑	↑ ↑	↓	↑	↑
Triglycerides	↑	↑ ↑	↑	↑ ↑	↑ or ↔
Lp(a)	↑	↑ ↑	↑	↑ ↑	↑ or ↔

CKD, Chronic kidney disease; HDL, high-density lipoprotein; LDL, low-density lipoprotein; Lp(a), lipoprotein(a). Modified from Kwan, B.C., Kronenberg, F., Beddhu, S., et al. (2007). Lipoprotein metabolism and lipid management in chronic kidney disease. *J Am Soc Nephrol.* 18(4):1246–1261.

overnight fast is ideal, even nonfasting values can provide important information. Fasting lipid profiles should be considered when significant abnormalities, especially high triglycerides, are noted with non-fasting samples. The routine measurement of lipoprotein(a), apolipoprotein B, and other lipid markers is not recommended due their lack of utility in current clinical practice.

5. **How often should lipids be checked in persons with CKD and dyslipidemia?**
   There is no recognized clinical benefit of measuring lipids annually in most people with CKD, especially if they are already on a statin. Possible reasons for remeasuring lipids include:
   1. Assessing treatment adherence by ensuring an appropriate decrease in LDL cholesterol levels, although this can be achieved through questionnaires, pill counts, and verifying prescription refills.
   2. Reevaluating the 10-year CVD risk in persons younger than 50 years of age who are not being treated with a statin.
   3. Determining the need for a greater treatment intensity to achieve target lipid goals (at least 30% reduction in LDL cholesterol) after initial treatment is begun.

6. **Are the principles of testing different in children with CKD?**
   A number of organizations, including the American Academy of Pediatrics, American Heart Association, and KDIGO, recommend that all children older than 2 years of age with any CVD risk factors, including CKD, have a fasting lipid profile checked. In contrast to adults, despite an absence of high-quality evidence, it is recommended that children undergo annual fasting lipid profiles in order to detect secondary causes of dyslipidemia, and because growth and development can affect the lipid profile.

7. **What is the association of dyslipidemia with CVD and mortality in patients with CKD?**
   Unlike in the general population, the linear association between higher levels of cholesterol and CVD-related mortality is less evident in patients with CKD, especially those on dialysis. Instead, observational studies have demonstrated a "reverse epidemiology" between total cholesterol levels and mortality in dialysis patients; that is, increased risk at low cholesterol levels, with evidence that malnutrition and chronic inflammation may act as affect modifiers of this association. Hypercholesterolemia is an independent risk factor for cardiovascular and all-cause mortality in dialysis patients without evidence of malnutrition or inflammation. Observational data from non-dialysis CKD populations has been conflicting. Data from the Atherosclerosis Risk in Communities (ARIC) study suggested that higher total cholesterol and triglyceride levels were associated with a higher risk of CVD events in patients with CKD. However, the Cardiovascular Health Study (CHS) and the Modification of Diet in Renal Disease (MDRD) study reported that dyslipidemia was not associated with the increased risk of kidney failure and cause, or CVD mortality.

8. **Does treatment of dyslipidemia reduce the risk of CVD events and mortality in patients with CKD?**
   The 10-year cardiovascular risk for most adults over the age of 50 years with CKD is >10%, thereby meeting the general population requirements for statin therapy. Data supporting the use of statins in

the primary prevention of CVD comes primarily from post hoc analysis of trials of the general population. A meta-analysis of 50 such trials, which included 45,285 participants with stage 3 or 4 CKD, reported a significant reduction in all-cause and cardiovascular mortality and nonfatal CVD outcomes. The best randomized controlled trial (RCT) evidence in patients with CKD comes from the Study of Heart and Renal Protection (SHARP) trial, which is the only randomized trial to focus on statin therapy for the primary prevention of CVD events and mortality in patients with kidney disease. The SHARP trial included 9438 participants with CKD with a mean estimated glomerular filtration rate (eGFR) of 27 mL/min per 1.73 m². Participants were randomized to either simvastatin 20 mg, ezetimibe 10 mg, or placebo. Among 6247 SHARP participants with CKD not on dialysis, there was a reduced incidence of CVD mortality, nonfatal myocardial infarction, and stroke (9.5% vs. 11.9%) among patients treated with simvastatin and ezetimibe compared to placebo. Whether combination therapy with ezetimibe is superior to monotherapy with statins in CKD patients is yet unknown.

9. **Is dyslipidemia associated with a decline in kidney function?**
   A number of observational studies have demonstrated an association between dyslipidemia and a higher risk of kidney function decline. Post hoc analysis from the Reduction of Endpoints in NIDDM with the Angiotensin II Antagonist Losartan (RENAAL) trial showed that in persons with type 2 diabetes, proteinuria of at least 300 mg/day and at least CKD stage 3, higher total, and LDL cholesterol at baseline was associated with an increased risk of end-stage kidney disease (ESKD). Low HDL cholesterol and high triglyceride levels in the setting of even mild to moderate CKD were also associated with a decline in kidney function. In addition, among diabetics without kidney disease, the presence of high total cholesterol was associated with an increased risk of developing albuminuria.

10. **Does treatment of dyslipidemia prevent the progression of kidney disease?**
    The best trial evidence for this comes from a secondary analysis of the SHARP study, which randomized 6245 individuals with non-dialysis-requiring CKD, to either simvastatin/ezetimibe or placebo. There was no difference in the risk of ESKD, or the composite outcome of ESRD, or the doubling of serum creatinine between the two groups. A meta-analysis of 57 studies including 143,888 participants demonstrated that while therapy with statins did not decrease the risk of kidney failure events, the rate of decline in the estimated glomerular filtration rate (eGFR) and the change in proteinuria or albuminuria were lower for those receiving statin therapy. Therefore while dyslipidemia is a risk factor for progressive kidney disease, it remains unclear if treating dyslipidemia results in better kidney outcomes.

11. **Which CKD patients should receive pharmacological statin therapy for dyslipidemia?**
    The KDIGO guidelines recommend that all adults aged over 50 years with an eGFR less than 60 mL/min per 1.73 m² not treated with dialysis or kidney transplantation (GFR categories G3a-G5) should be treated with a statin or statin/ezetimibe combination. This recommendation is based on the results of the SHARP trial and the fact that most patients older than 50 years with at least CKD 3a would have a greater than 10% risk of coronary heart disease (CHD) at 10 years, thus warranting statin therapy. Therefore the level of LDL cholesterol would not be required to assess the CHD risk and initiate therapy in this population. The treatment of hypertriglyceridemia in CKD is limited by a lack of data. A subgroup analysis of nearly 1000 men from the Veterans Affairs High-Density Lipoprotein Intervention Trial (VA-HIT) did not demonstrate a mortality benefit with lowering triglycerides in participants with CKD. Currently, due to the increased risk of drug-related adverse events, co-administration of fibrates in patients receiving statin therapy is not recommended and is contraindicated in persons with advanced CKD. The exception to this may be the prevention of pancreatitis when levels are >500 mg/dL despite lifestyle modification therapy.

12. **Why should pharmacologic therapy not be initiated in patients receiving chronic dialysis but be continued if patients are already taking statins?**
    The KDIGO guidelines recommend against initiating statins in dialysis patients. Two trials—4D (Die Deutsche Diabetes Dialyse) study, in which hemodialysis patients with diabetes and high serum LDL were treated with atorvastatin or placebo; and AURORA (Use of Rosuvastatin in subjects On Regular hemodialysis: an Assessment of survival and cardiovascular events), in which dialysis patients were treated with rosuvastatin or placebo—failed to demonstrate a significant reduction in mortality or other CVD outcomes. The SHARP trial reported no interaction between dialysis and non-dialysis participants with regard to the simvastatin/ezetimibe benefit; however, an analysis limited to dialysis patients did not demonstrate a benefit. In the SHARP trial, 34% of CKD stage 3 to 5 patients progressed to ESKD during the course of the trial, and because an overall benefit in the non-dialysis patients was reported, the KDIGO guidelines recommend that statins be continued at the time of dialysis initiation. Importantly,

these guidelines in dialysis patients do not consider patients with recent acute coronary events, younger patients with longer life expectancies, and those who might receive a kidney transplant and therefore receive a yet unquantified benefit from the initiation of statin therapy.

13. **What is the evidence for statin therapy in patients with CKD and eGFR >60mL/min per 1.73 m²?**
The KDIGO guidelines recommend that all patients older than 50 years with CKD diagnosed with structural kidney abnormalities but with an eGFR greater than 60 mL/min per 1.73 m² (GFR categories G1-G2) be treated with a statin. However, given the lack of robust clinical evidence, this recommendation is weaker than recommendations for persons older than 50 years with an eGFR less than 60 mL/min per 1.73 m². Albuminuria is the most common non-GFR marker that identifies structural CKD. In people both with and without diabetes, albuminuria is associated with adverse CVD outcomes and mortality. However, there is a lack of RCT data on whether statins reduce CVD events in this particular population. The CARE (Cholesterol and Recurrent Events) Study and CARDS (Collaborative Atorvastatin Diabetes Study) included people with albuminuria who were at an increased risk of CVD events, and found a lower risk of CVD events with atorvastatin therapy. In contrast, the PRE-VEND IT (Prevention of Renal and Vascular Endstage Disease Intervention Trial), which was a 2 × 2 study of fosinopril/placebo and pravastatin/placebo, did not find a significantly lower risk of cardiovascular outcomes with pravastatin therapy.

14. **Should all patients who have received kidney transplants receive statin therapy?**
The KDIGO guidelines suggest that all kidney transplant recipients should receive therapy with a statin. The ALERT (Assessment of Lescol in Renal Transplant) trial was a large study that randomly assigned 2102 kidney transplant recipients aged 30 to 75 years to either fluvastatin, 40 mg (later 80 mg), or placebo. Over 5.7 years of follow-up, fluvastatin reduced the risk of cardiac deaths and nonfatal myocardial infarction but did not reduce the rates of coronary intervention cerebrovascular events, noncardiovascular death, all-cause mortality, and graft loss. In a subsequent 2-year open-label extension in which all participants of the trial were offered fluvastatin treatment, 1652 participants agreed to receive 80 mg of fluvastatin while 442 participants declined. An intention-to-treat analysis by original treatment group demonstrated that participants randomized to the drug had a borderline statistically significant lower risk of incident CVD events and mortality. A meta-analysis of 22 RCT studies further reported that statin treatment had uncertain effects on overall mortality, but that CVD outcomes may be reduced. Given the lack of robust data, KDIGO suggested, rather than recommended, the use of statins in these patients.

15. **What is the role of proprotein convertase subtilisin/kexin type 9 inhibitors in treating dyslipidemia in CKD?**
Proprotein convertase subtilisin/kexin type 9 (PCSK-9) is an enzyme that binds to the LDL receptor, reduces its cell surface density, and leads to hypercholesterolemia. In recent years, a number of studies of antibodies inhibiting PCSK-9 have been shown to effectively treat hypercholesterolemia and reduce CVD events in persons already being treated with maximal statin therapy. Data suggests that levels of PCSK-9 are elevated in kidney disease, are removed by dialysis, and are lowered after kidney transplantation. The recently completed Long-term Safety and Tolerability of Alirocumab in High Cardiovascular Risk Patients with Hypercholesterolemia Not Adequately Controlled with Their Lipid Modifying Therapy (ODYSSEY LONG TERM) trial enrolled 174 patients with an eGFR <60 mL/min per 1.73 m² at baseline. In this subgroup, treatment with aliroucumab was associated with 62% reduction in LDL cholesterol levels, compared to 8% elevation in the placebo arm (P value, .02). This study was not powered to evaluate the effect of the intervention on clinical outcomes, and further studies are needed that include a larger number of patients with CKD. Whether these drugs offer the same degree of lipid reduction and cardiovascular benefit in patients not taking statins, for instance those with statin intolerance, remains unknown.

16. **What is the role of LDL apheresis in persons with kidney disease?**
Persons who are homozygous for familial hypercholesterolemia, or those with an LDL cholesterol ≥200 mg/dL and documented coronary heart disease, or those with an LDL cholesterol ≥300 mg/dL despite medical therapy, or people intolerant of medical therapy are often candidates for LDL apheresis. Apheresis decreases LDL cholesterol by 50% to 75% per session and are usually performed on a weekly or biweekly basis. The above indications and results are based on small-scale studies done in the general population without specific recommendations for persons with kidney disease.

17. **Which patients should be monitored for statin-induced adverse events?**
Myopathy is the most common adverse event due to statin therapy and can occur in up to 10% of persons taking the drug. Of the statins, pravastatin, fluvastatin, and rosuvastatin are ones associated

with the lowest risk of myopathy, especially when concomitant drugs that inhibit cytochrome P450 3A4 cannot be avoided. In addition, fibrates have a synergistic effect on the occurrence of myopathy in patients already receiving statins, and this may be partially responsible for their limited use to treat hypertriglyceridemia in patients with advanced CKD. Certain patient populations, such as the elderly, (>80 years), frail persons, Asian populations, and those with underlying liver disease, may be at an increased risk of adverse events from statin therapy. Routine monitoring is not recommended. Decreasing the dose of the drug, switching to a statin with less myopathy risk, and vitamin-D repletion if deficient are some strategies that can be adopted to mitigate the risk of myopathy. Persons who develop statin-induced rhabdomyolysis should not be treated with statins in the future due to the risk of recurrence. Alternatives, such as PCSK9 inhibitors, may be considered.

KEY POINTS

1. Patients with CKD usually have high triglycerides and low HDL cholesterol concentrations, while total and LDL cholesterol are normal or low. In patients with nephrotic syndrome, all except HDL cholesterol are high.
2. All adult patients with newly identified CKD, including those on dialysis, or kidney transplant recipients, should be evaluated with a complete lipid profile.
3. Unlike the general population, dyslipidemia is not linearly associated with kidney function decline or mortality in patients with CKD, perhaps due to confounding from malnutrition or inflammation.
4. All adults older than 50 years with eGFR <60 mL/min per 1.73 m² not treated with dialysis or kidney transplantation should be treated with a statin or a statin/ezetimibe combination.
5. Most trial data do not suggest a benefit for statin treatment in dialysis patients.

BIBLIOGRAPHY

Fellström, B. C., Jardine, A. G., Schmieder, R. E., Holdaas, H., Bannister, K., Beutler, J., . . . AURORA Study Group. (2009). Rosuvastatin and cardiovascular events in patients undergoing hemodialysis. *N Engl J Med, 360*(14), 1395–1407.

Baigent, C., Landray, M. J., Reith, C., Emberson, J., Wheeler, D. C., Tomson, C., . . . SHARP Investigators. (2011). The effects of lowering LDL cholesterol with simvastatin plus ezetimibe in patients with chronic kidney disease (Study of Heart and Renal Protection): A randomized placebo-controlled trial. *Lancet, 377,* 2181–2192.

Chawla, V., Greene, T., Beck, G. J., Kusek, J. W., Collins, A. J., Sarnak, M. J., & Menon, V. (2010). Hyperlipidemia and long-term outcomes in nondiabetic chronic kidney disease. *Clin J Am Soc Nephrol, 5*(9), 1582–1587.

Clement, L. C., Macé, C., Avila-Casado, C., Joles, J. A., Kersten, S., & Chugh, S. S. (2014). Circulating angiopoietin-like 4 links proteinuria with hypertriglyceridemia in nephrotic syndrome. *Nat Med, 20*(1), 37–46. doi:10.1038/nm.3396.

German Diabetes and Dialysis Study Investigators. (2005). Atorvastatin in patients with type 2 diabetes mellitus undergoing hemodialysis. *N Engl J Med. 353*(3), 238–248.

Gerstein, H. C., Mann, J. F., Yi, Q., Zinman, B., Dinneen, S. F., Hoogwerf, B., . . . HOPE Study Investigators. (2001). HOPE Study Investigators. Albuminuria and risk of cardiovascular events, death, and heart failure in diabetic and nondiabetic individuals. *JAMA. 286*(4), 421–426.

Holdaas, H., Fellström, B., Jardine, A. G., Holme, I., Nyberg, G., Fauchald, P., . . . Assessment of LEscol in Renal Transplantation (ALERT) Study Investigators. (2003). Effect of fluvastatin on cardiac outcomes in renal transplant recipients: A multicentre, randomized, placebo-controlled trial. *Lancet, 361*(9374), 2024–2031.

IMPROVE-IT Investigators. (2015). Ezetimibe added to statin therapy after acute coronary syndromes. *N Engl J Med, 372*(25), 2387–2397.

Kasiske, B., Cosio, F. G., Beto, J., Bolton, K., Chavers, B. M., Grimm, R., Jr., . . . National Kidney Foundation. (2004). National Kidney Foundation. Clinical practice guidelines for managing dyslipidemias in kidney transplant patients: A report from the Managing Dyslipidemias in Chronic Kidney Disease Work Group of the National Kidney Foundation Kidney Disease Outcomes Quality Initiative. *Am J Transplant, 4*(Suppl. 7), 13–53.

Kidney Disease: Improving Global Outcomes (KDIGO) Lipid Work Group. (2013). KDIGO clinical practice guideline for lipid management in chronic kidney disease. *Kidney Int Suppl, 3,* 259–305.

Kidney Disease: Improving Global Outcomes (KDIGO) Lipid Work Group. (2013). KDIGO Clinical Practice Guideline for Lipid Management in Chronic Kidney Disease: Chapter 3: Assessment of lipid status in children with CKD. *Kidney Int Suppl, 3,* 280.

Konarzewski, M., Szolkiewicz, M., Sucajtys-Szulc, E., Blaszak, J., Lizakowski, S., Swierczynski, J., & Rutkowski, B. (2014). Elevated circulating PCSK-9 concentration in renal failure patients is corrected by renal replacement therapy. *Am J Nephrol, 40*(2), 157–163.

Kwan, B. C., Kronenberg, F., Beddhu, S., & Cheung, A. K. (2007). Lipoprotein metabolism and lipid management in chronic kidney disease. *J Am Soc Nephrol, 18*(4), 1246–1261.

Liu, Y., Coresh, J., Eustace, J. A., Longenecker, J. C., Jaar, B., Fink, N. E., . . . Klag, M. J. (2004). Association between cholesterol level and mortality in dialysis patients: Role of inflammation and malnutrition. *JAMA, 291,* 451–459.

Muntner, P., He, J., Astor, B. C., Folsom, A. R., & Coresh, J. (2005). Traditional and nontraditional risk factors predict coronary heart disease in chronic kidney disease: Results from the Atherosclerosis Risk in Communities study. *J Am Soc Nephrol, 16,* 529–538.

Robinson, J. G., Farnier, M., Krempf, M., & ODYSSEY LONG TERM Investigators. (2015). Efficacy and safety of alirocumab in reducing lipids and cardiovascular events. *N Engl J Med, 372*(16), 1489–1499. doi:10.1056/NEJMoa1501031.

Sabatine, M. S., Giugliano, R. P., Keech, A. C., Honarpour, N., Wiviott, S. D., Murphy, S. A., . . . FOURIER Steering Committee and Investigators. (2017). Evolocumab and Clinical Outcomes in Patients with Cardiovascular Disease. *N Engl J Med, 376*(18), 1713–1722. doi:10.1056/NEJMoa1615664.

Sarnak, M. J., Bloom, R., Muntner, P., Rahman, M., Saland, J. M., Wilson, P. W., & Fried, L. (2015). KDOQI US commentary on the 2013 KDIGO Clinical Practice Guideline for Lipid Management in CKD. *Am J Kidney Dis, 65*(3), 354–366.

Baigent, C., Landray, M. J., Reith, C., Emberson, J., Wheeler, D. C., Tomson, C., . . . SHARP Investigators. (2011). The effects of lowering LDL cholesterol with simvastatin plus ezetimibe in patients with chronic kidney disease (Study of Heart and Renal Protection): A randomised placebo-controlled trial. *Lancet, 377,* 2181–2192.

Shlipak, M. G., Fried, L. F., Cushman, M., Manolio, T. A., Peterson, D., Stehman-Breen, C., . . . Psaty, B. (2005). Cardiovascular mortality risk in chronic kidney disease: Comparison of traditional and novel risk factors. *JAMA, 293,* 1737–1745.

Wanner, C., Tonelli, M., & Kidney Disease: Improving Global Outcomes Lipid Guideline Development Work Group Members. (2014). KDIGO Clinical Practice Guideline for Lipid Management in CKD: Summary of recommendation statements and clinical approach to the patient. *Kidney Int, 85*(6), 1303–1309.

1. What is malnutrition?
To define malnutrition, an expert panel of the International Society of Renal Nutrition and Metabolism (ISRNM) has recommended the use of the term "protein-energy wasting" (PEW) to encompass states of undernutrition that could result from a complex interplay of decreased nutrient intake and/or increased catabolism.

2. How is nutritional status examined, and how is malnutrition diagnosed in patients with chronic kidney disease (CKD)?
   - There is no single way to assess nutritional status, which is a consequence of a complex interplay of nutrient intake and catabolism, with significant effect modification by comorbid conditions, especially inflammatory conditions.
   - PEW can be diagnosed in clinical practice using five different criteria:
     - Biochemical measures (serum albumin, prealbumin, transferrin, and cholesterol)
     - Measures of body mass (body mass index [BMI], unintentional weight loss, and total body fat)
     - Measures of muscle mass (total muscle mass, mid-arm muscle circumference, and creatinine appearance)
     - Measures of dietary intake (dietary protein and energy intake)
     - Integrative nutritional scoring systems (subjective global assessment of nutrition and malnutrition-inflammation score)
   - In addition to these readily available measures of PEW, a series of other markers have also been proposed, which could have applicability as research tools; these include measures of appetite, food intake and energy expenditure, other measures of body mass and composition (such as dual energy x-ray absorptiometry [DEXA], bioimpedance, near-infrared interactance, or computed tomography/magnetic resonance imaging of muscle mass) and laboratory measures (such as growth hormone levels, C-reactive protein, interleukin-1, interleukin-6, tumor necrosis factor alpha, serum amyloid-A or peripheral blood cell counts; Box 23.1).

3. Why is malnutrition associated with mortality in CKD?
Markers of PEW are some of the strongest independent predictors of adverse outcomes in patients with CKD and end-stage kidney disease. The link between PEW and mortality has been established almost exclusively in epidemiologic and observational studies. Thus only an association has been established. Causality needs to be verified in randomized controlled trials of nutritional interventions, even though the association is strong, robust, and consistent. Multiple pathophysiologic mechanisms have been invoked to explain the link between poor nutritional status and mortality in CKD:
   - Lower muscle and adipose mass decrease circulating lipoprotein that normally suppresses circulating endotoxin
   - Gastrointestinal, hematopoietic, and immune dysfunctions leading to more infections
   - Micronutrient deficiency leading to oxidative stress and endothelial dysfunction
   - Inadequate circulating gelsolin to oppose deleterious effects of circulating actin, including platelet activation leading to increased thromboembolic events
   - The maladaptive activation of the inflammatory and oxidative cascade can potentiate the effects of low nutrient intake by increasing catabolism
   - Novel factors such as proinflammatory high-density lipoprotein (HDL), myeloperoxidase, and pentraxin may also play important roles

4. What is the obesity paradox in patients with CKD?
Obesity has reached epidemic proportions in the general population and has been linked to increased morbidity and mortality. Several epidemiologic studies have suggested a link between obesity and higher risk of developing incident CKD; the link between obesity and adverse outcomes in the general population is evident from epidemiologic studies showing a linear increase in mortality associated with higher BMI, especially greater than 30 kg/m². Studies in patients with moderate to advanced CKD

Box 23.1. Criteria for the Clinical Diagnosis of Protein-Energy Wasting in Patients With Kidney Disease

Serum Chemistry and Other Laboratory Markers

Serum albumin <3.8 g/dL (Bromcresol Green)
Serum prealbumin (transthyretin) <30 mg/dL
Serum cholesterol <100 mg/dL
Serum biochemistry: transferrin, urea, triglyceride, bicarbonate
Hormones: leptin, ghrelin, growth hormones
Inflammatory markers: CrP, IL-6, TNF-α, IL-1, SAA
Peripheral blood cell count: lymphocyte count or percentage

Body Mass and Composition

Body mass index <22 kg/m^2 (<65 years) <23 kg/m^2 (>65 years)
Unintentional weight loss over time: 5% over 3 months or 10% over 6 months
Total body fat percentage <10%
Weight-based measures: weight for height
Total body nitrogen
Total body potassium
Energy-beam based methods: DEXA, BIA, NIR
Underwater weighing and air displacement weighing
14 K Dalton fragment of actomyosin
Microarrays
Muscle fiber size
Relative proportions of muscle fiber types

Muscle alkaline soluble protein
Computed tomography and/or magnetic resonance imaging of muscle mass

Muscle Mass

Muscle wasting: reduced muscle mass 5% over 3 months or 10% over 6 months
Reduced mid-arm muscle circumference area (>10% of reduction in relation to 50th percentile of reference population)
Urinary creatinine appearance

Dietary Intake

Unintentional low dietary protein intake: <0.80 g/kg per day for at least 2 months for dialysis patients or <0.6 g/kg per day for patients on CKD stages 2–5

Appetite, Food Intake, and Energy Expenditure

Appetite assessment questionnaires
Population based dietary assessments: food frequency questionnaires
Measuring energy expenditure by indirect or direct calorimetry

Nutritional Scoring Systems

SGA and its modifications
Malnutrition-Inflammation Score

BIA, bioelectrical impedance analysis; CRP, C-reactive protein; DEXA, dual energy x-ray absorptiometry; IGF-1, insulin-like growth factor 1; IL, interleukin (e.g., IL-1 and IL-6); NIR, near-infrared interactance; SAA, serum amyloid A; SGA, subjective global assessment of nutritional status; TNF-aa, tumor necrosis factor alpha.

have shown *a reversal* of this risk factor pattern, with a linear *decrease* in mortality in those with higher BMI. In fact, patients with BMI levels reaching morbid obesity have shown the best survival, questioning the validity of the obesity paradigm in this patient population. Similar reversals in risk factor patterns, also known as "obesity paradox" or "reverse epidemiology," have emerged in other patient populations characterized by chronic disease states and a high burden of comorbid conditions (such as those with advanced chronic obstructive pulmonary disease, congestive heart failure, rheumatoid arthritis, malignancies, and liver cirrhosis). The common thread in the populations displaying this phenomenon of reverse epidemiology is their extremely high short-term mortality rate, which probably explains the mechanism whereby obesity appears protective within short periods of time: in such patients the mechanisms responsible for the long-term deleterious effects seen in the general population (metabolic syndrome/insulin resistance/atherosclerosis) are likely overshadowed by the beneficial effects of higher overall nutritional reserves.

5. Can manipulations of weight improve outcomes in patients with CKD?
    Interventions aimed at alleviating obesity are advocated in the general population to prevent long-term deleterious consequences. Such interventions are based on robust evidence linking obesity to adverse outcomes. Because descriptive studies in patients on renal replacement therapy suggest that obesity may confer a survival benefit rather than a risk, it may be less likely that interventions validated in the general population can be extrapolated to these patients without critical appraisal of the consequences. There is currently no evidence from clinical trials that have tested the risks versus benefits of weight reduction interventions in dialysis patients. Due to the marked discrepancy between epidemiologic studies of obesity in the general population and in patients on dialysis, any weight loss–based intervention in the latter group would have to proceed with utmost care taken to ensure that no harm is done. There also has to be openness about the possibility that gain in dry (edema free) weight could in fact be beneficial in this patient population because the complex homeostatic

changes occurring in the process of increasing lean body mass end even adiposity may entail short-term benefits.

6. **What is known about weight reduction strategies in advanced CKD?**
Weight reduction strategies bring up even more complex questions in patients with non–dialysis-dependent CKD. Some, but not all, observational studies in this patient population have also indicated a salutary association between higher BMI and lower mortality, but at the same time obesity has also been linked to more severe loss of kidney function, and restriction of dietary protein intake may be beneficial in retarding progressive loss of kidney function. Due to such complex interplays, weight loss–based interventions could in fact have benefits on kidney function in these patients, but any attempt to induce weight loss through limiting nutrient intake in patients with non–dialysis-dependent CKD has to be coordinated by trained personnel to ensure no deleterious effects on broader nutritional status and consequently on survival.

7. **What is the effect of cholesterol-lowering interventions in CKD patients?**
Blood lipid (cholesterol) level is one of the biochemical markers linked to nutritional status and used to define PEW in CKD. However, in the general population, lowering blood cholesterol is the cornerstone of primary and secondary cardiovascular disease (CVD) prevention. Given the extremely high CVD morbidity and mortality observed in the CKD population, it appeared seemingly reasonable to use cholesterol-lowering therapies in patients on dialysis, especially because such pharmacologic interventions are not only antiinflammatory, but they are not burdened by worsening PEW. One issue that appeared to contradict the cholesterol-CVD paradigm in the CKD population was that high cholesterol was not associated with higher mortality in CKD. In fact, epidemiologic data showed that high lipids may in fact be protective. This is referred to as the "lipid paradox" and is another component of the "reverse epidemiology" phenomenon.
- Due to the uncertainty, two randomized controlled trials (Study to Evaluate the Use of Rosuvastatin in Subjects on Regular Hemodialysis: An Assessment of Survival and Cardiovascular Events [AURORA] and Die Deutsche Diabetes Dialyse Studie [4D Study]) were designed to test the hypothesis that lowering blood cholesterol by statin therapy can decrease CVD event rates and mortality in patients in dialysis. Both of these studies yielded negative results, corroborating the findings of epidemiologic studies, and again suggesting that the classical Framingham risk factor patterns cannot be automatically translated to patients with kidney disease.
- A third study (Study of Heart and Renal Protection, SHARP) enrolled patients with non–dialysis-dependent CKD (besides dialysis patients) found that cholesterol lowering resulted in lower risk of a composite CVD event rate. SHARP did not find improvement in all-cause mortality. The CVD benefit of cholesterol lowering was significant only in patients with CKD not on renal replacement therapy, but there was no statistically significant interaction with dialysis status, suggesting that the lack of statistically significant effect in patients on hemodialysis may have been the result of the lower number of patients on hemodialysis enrolled. The results of SHARP suggest that therapeutic cholesterol lowering has a modest CVD benefit in patients with kidney diseases, especially those with non–dialysis-dependent CKD.

8. **What is the role of nutritional counseling?**
Compared with the general population, nutritional interventions in patients with CKD and especially those undergoing maintenance hemodialysis therapy are more complex. The most basic intervention is dietary counseling, the goals of which are aimed on the one hand to provide the necessary amount of energy, protein, and other nutrients and on the other hand to avoid biochemical imbalances that are the result of the lack of kidney function. These two goals of dietary intervention are often in conflict with each other, as for example, adequate amounts of protein in diet will result in an obligatory intake of potassium and phosphorus and could lead to hyperkalemia and/or hyperphosphatemia. Dietary counseling is even more complex in patients with CKD, in whom protein restriction of 0.6 to 0.8 g/kg per day has been suggested as an intervention to retard progression of kidney disease, but in whom restrictions of this magnitude may result in unintended worsening in their nutritional status. Because of this complexity, nutritional management (including formal assessment of nutritional status and formal nutritional interventions) should be provided by trained nutritionists to ensure the adequacy of the nutritional value of any imposed restricted diets.

9. **Can meals consumed during dialysis improve nutritional status?**
Meals during hemodialysis are routine in many countries but not in the United States, although recent studies have popularized the concept of oral dietary supplements in dialysis clinics. A randomized controlled trial in 110 hemodialysis patients showed that high-protein meals during in-center hemodialysis improved serum albumin while serum phosphorus remained within target range by use of a potent phosphorus binder.

10. What types of nutritional interventions are there in dialysis patients?
    Due to the complex medical conditions that are common in CKD, nutritional interventions often extend far beyond dietary counseling in these patients.
    Nutritional interventions for malnourished CKD patients can be classified into three groups of oral/enteral, parenteral, and pharmacologic (Box 23.2). Among dialysis patients, the goal of nutritional interventions is to maintain serum albumin greater than 4.0 g/dL, and this may be achieved by maintaining oral supplements of 1 to 2 servings per day (Fig. 23.1).
    Artificial nutrition through feeding tubes, gastrostomy tubes, or parenteral nutrition (which is sometimes applied in the context of hemodialysis, called intradialytic parenteral nutrition) can be applied in certain conditions, usually over short periods of time.

11. Can pharmacologic interventions be used in patients on dialysis to improve nutritional status?
    Pharmacologic measures to improve nutrition include appetite stimulators (megestrol acetate) or interventions to improve biochemical measures of PEW, such as the use of anabolic hormones. These

Box 23.2. Nutritional Support and Therapy

Oral or Eternal Interventions
- Meals during dialysis treatment
- Intense/tailored protein-energy
  - Oral nutritional supplements
  - Tube feeding

Parenteral Interventions
- Intradialytic parenteral nutrition (IDPN)
- Total parenteral nutrition (TPN)

Pharmacologic Interventions
- Appetite stimulators
- Antidepressant
- Antiinflammatory and/or antioxidative
- Anabolic and/or muscle enhancing

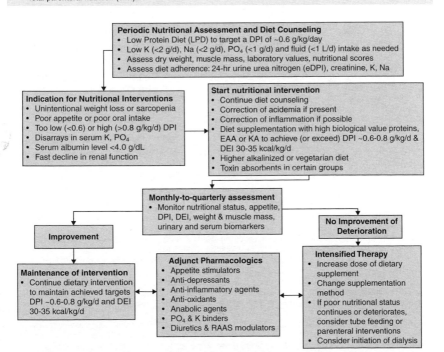

Figure 23.1. Proposed nutritional therapy algorithm for the entire range of chronic kidney disease. *Adapted from Kovesdy, C. P., Kopple, J. D., & Kalantar-Zadeh, K. (2013). Management of protein-energy wasting in non-dialysis-dependent chronic kidney disease: Reconciling low protein intake with nutritional therapy. American Journal of Clinical Nutrition, 97, 1163–1177.*

interventions have been tested in small clinical trials, but their use in clinical practice remains uncommon, due to their potential to cause adverse effects, and due to the lack of robust outcome studies supporting their application.

12. **Can nutritional interventions result in better outcomes in patients with CKD?**
PEW is the strongest predictor of increased mortality in patients with CKD of all stages. Based on the compelling results of epidemiologic studies, it is plausible to postulate that interventions aimed at improving nutritional status could be beneficial in these patients. Unfortunately, there are no clinical trial data to prove this hypothesis, and because of this, nutritional interventions cannot be advocated as a means to improve patient survival. Clinical trials have shown that various interventions can be successfully applied to improve biochemical measures of PEW (such as serum albumin) or to favorably change body composition, but it remains unclear if the application of such interventions (which include dietary and pharmacologic interventions) can result in better clinical outcomes. Well-conducted large observational studies have suggested that nutritional supplementation in dialysis patients is associated with favorable outcomes. The clinical benefit of such interventions would have to be proven in dedicated randomized controlled clinical trials.

KEY POINTS

1. PEW and its markers are among the strongest predictors of mortality in dialysis patients.
2. Obesity is associated with higher risk of incident CKD, but once CKD is established, obesity is paradoxically associated with survival advantages.
3. Oral nutritional supplements and other nutritional and dietary interventions should maintain serum albumin greater than 4.0 g/dL.

BIBLIOGRAPHY

KDIGO 2012 clinical practice guideline for the evaluation and management of chronic kidney disease. (2013). *Kidney International Supplement, 3,* 1–150.

Baigent, C., Landray, M. J., Reith, C., Emberson, J., Wheeler, D. C., Tomson, C., . . . SHARP Investigators. (2011). The effects of lowering LDL cholesterol with simvastatin plus ezetimibe in patients with chronic kidney disease (Study of Heart and Renal Protection): A randomised placebo-controlled trial. *Lancet, 377,* 2181–2192.

Cheu, C., Pearson, J., Dahlerus, C., Lantz, B., Chowdhury, T., Sauer, P. F., . . . Ramirez, S. P. (2013). Association between oral nutritional supplementation and clinical outcomes among patients with ESRD. *Clinical Journal of the American Society of Nephrology, 8,* 100–107.

Fellström, B. C., Jardine, A. G., Schmieder, R. E., Holdaas, H., Bannister, K., Beutler, J., . . . AURORA Study Group. (2009). Rosuvastatin and cardiovascular events in patients undergoing hemodialysis. *New England Journal of Medicine, 360,* 1395–1407.

Fouque, D., Kalantar-Zadeh, K., Kopple, J., Cano, N., Chauveau, P., Cuppari, L., . . . Wanner, C. (2008). A proposed nomenclature and diagnostic criteria for protein-energy wasting in acute and chronic kidney disease. *Kidney International, 73,* 391–398.

Hsu, C. Y., McCulloch, C. E., Iribarren, C., Darbinian, J., & Go, A. S. (2006). Body mass index and risk for end-stage renal disease. *Annals of Internal Medicine, 144,* 21–28.

Ikizler, T. A., Cano, N. J., Franch, H., Fouque, D., Himmelfarb, J., Kalantar-Zadeh, K., . . . International Society of Renal Nutrition and Metabolism. (2013). Prevention and treatment of protein energy wasting in chronic kidney disease patients: A consensus statement by the International Society of Renal Nutrition and Metabolism. *Kidney International, 84,* 1096–1107.

Kalantar-Zadeh, K., & Ikizler, T. A. (2013). Let them eat during dialysis: An overlooked opportunity to improve outcomes in maintenance hemodialysis patients. *Journal of Renal Nutrition, 23,* 157–163.

Kalantar-Zadeh, K., & Kopple, J. D. (2006). Obesity paradox in patients on maintenance dialysis. *Contributions to Nephrology, 151,* 57–69.

Kalantar-Zadeh, K., Tortorici, A. R., Chen, J. L., Kamgar, M., Lau, W. L., Moradi, H., . . . Kovesdy, C. P. (2015). Dietary restrictions in dialysis patients: Is there anything left to eat? *Seminars in Dialysis, 28,* 159–168.

Kovesdy, C. P. (2016). Malnutrition in dialysis patients—the need for intervention despite uncertain benefits. *Seminars in Dialysis, 29*(1), 28–34.

Kovesdy, C. P., Anderson, J. E., & Kalantar-Zadeh, K. (2007). Paradoxical association between body mass index and mortality in men with CKD not yet on dialysis. *American Journal of Kidney Diseases, 49,* 581–591.

Kovesdy, C. P., George, S. M., Anderson, J. E., & Kalantar-Zadeh, K. (2009). Outcome predictability of biomarkers of protein-energy wasting and inflammation in moderate and advanced chronic kidney disease. *American Journal of Clinical Nutrition, 90,* 407–414.

Kovesdy, C. P., & Kalantar-Zadeh, K. (2009). Why is protein-energy wasting associated with mortality in chronic kidney disease? *Seminars in Nephrology, 29,* 3–14.

Kovesdy, C. P., Kopple, J. D., & Kalantar-Zadeh, K. (2013). Management of protein-energy wasting in non-dialysis-dependent chronic kidney disease: Reconciling low protein intake with nutritional therapy. *American Journal of Clinical Nutrition, 97,* 1163–1177.

Lacson, E., Jr., Wang, W., Zebrowski, B., Wingard, R., & Hakim, R. M. (2012). Outcomes associated with intradialytic oral nutritional supplements in patients undergoing maintenance hemodialysis: A quality improvement report. *American Journal of Kidney Diseases, 60,* 591–600.

Lu, J. L., Kalantar-Zadeh, K., Ma, J. Z., Quarles, L. D., & Kovesdy, C. P. (2014). Association of body mass index with outcomes in patients with CKD. *Journal of the American Society of Nephrology, 25,* 2088–2096.

Lu, J. L., Molnar, M. Z., Naseer, A., Mikkelsen, M. K., Kalantar-Zadeh, K., & Kovesdy, C. P. (2015). Association of age and BMI with kidney function and mortality: A cohort study. *Lancet. Diabetes & Endocrinology, 3,* 704–714.

Rhee, C. M., You, A. S., Koontz Parsons, T., Tortorici, A. R., Bross, R., St-Jules, D. E., . . . Kalantar-Zadeh, K. (2017). Effect of high-protein meals during hemodialysis combined with lanthanum carbonate in hypoalbuminemic dialysis patients: Findings from the FrEDI randomized controlled trial [published online ahead of print]. *Ncphrology, Dialysis, Transplantation, 32*(7), 1233–1243.

Wanner, C., Krane, V., März, W., Olschewski, M., Mann, J. F., Ruf, G., . . . German Diabetes and Dialysis Study Investigators. (2005). Atorvastatin in patients with type 2 diabetes mellitus undergoing hemodialysis. *New England Journal of Medicine, 353,* 238–248.

CHAPTER 24

CLINICAL MANAGEMENT OF CHRONIC KIDNEY DISEASE

Carol Traynor and Eugene C. Kovalik

1. **How do you recognize progressive kidney failure?**

   Progressive kidney failure is recognized by an increasing serum creatinine over time. However, some patients may have a normal creatinine early in the course of their chronic kidney disease (CKD). Individuals with an abnormal urinary sediment (e.g., proteinuria or hematuria) or abnormal pathology on a kidney biopsy are at risk for progressive kidney failure.

   Because serum creatinine is a reflection of muscle mass, a person with low muscle mass can have CKD despite a creatinine in the normal range. Conversely, patients with larger muscle mass may have an abnormally elevated creatinine despite normal kidney function. For these reasons, calculating an estimated glomerular filtration rate (eGFR) is the recommended way to assess kidney function (see chapter on Glomerular Filtration Rate). These equations should not be used in acute kidney injury because the calculations assume a stable serum creatinine.

2. **How do you monitor the rate of loss of kidney function?**

   Kidney function is monitored with serum creatinine (or eGFR correlates as outlined previously) and urinalysis. A certain degree of fluctuation in serum creatinine can be expected and is usually related to changes in volume status, medications, and diet. Creatinine values should be viewed over time to judge progression of CKD.

   Creatinine-based GFR-estimating equations are less accurate in elderly patients and lead to overdiagnosis of CKD, particularly in those patients with higher eGFR. Directly measuring creatinine clearance or using creatinine in combination with cystatin C–based eGFR equations can be used to further assess kidney function in older patients if a definitive diagnosis of CKD is required (e.g., a potential kidney donor).

   A rise in urine protein excretion (or a failure to decrease urine protein excretion following treatment) is also an indicator of disease activity and progression of kidney disease. Therapy should be aimed at reducing proteinuria to slow the progression of kidney disease. This can be done by treating the underlying disease, if possible, or using inhibitors of the renin angiotensin system (such as angiotensin-converting enzyme [ACE] inhibitors or angiotensin receptor blockers [ARBs] but not in combination) to decrease proteinuria.

3. **What are the risk factors, diseases, and complications that should be considered in the management of patients with progressive kidney failure?**

   See Box 24.1.

4. **What is the blood pressure (BP) goal for a person with progressive kidney failure?**

   Although guidelines such as Joint National Committee (JNC) 8 relaxed BP goals compared with prior treatment recommendations, there has been evidence from studies published subsequent to these guidelines supporting a more aggressive approach to BP management.

   The Systolic Blood Pressure Intervention Trial (SPRINT) was a prospective randomized controlled trial that was enriched with CKD patients (although without significant proteinuria) that assigned patients to a systolic BP goal of less than 120 mm Hg (intensive treatment) or less than 140 mm Hg (standard treatment). BP was measured differently from typical office BPs, using a device that can average multiple consecutive readings with the patient resting alone in a room. A mean of three consecutive BPs was used as the visit BP.

   Overall, participants assigned to the intensive treatment group, as compared with those assigned to the standard treatment group, had a 25% lower relative risk (RR) of major cardiovascular events, with consistent results across subgroups defined according to age, sex, race, medical history, and baseline BP. In addition, the intensive treatment group had a 27% lower RR of death from any cause. SPRINT was the first randomized controlled trial (RCT) to demonstrate a benefit in lower BP goals (i.e., systolic <140). Of note, the method of BP assessment in the trial is rarely used in clinical practice.

Box 24.1. Factors to Consider in the Management of Patients With Progressive Kidney Failure (No Matter the Original Etiology)

Contributors to the Loss of Kidney Function

- Hypertension
- Diabetes mellitus
- Dietary salt intake
- Proteinuria
- Metabolic acidosis

Complications of Chronic Kidney Disease

- Anemia
- Platelet dysfunction
- Abnormal bone and mineral metabolism (e.g., secondary hyperparathyroidism)
- Lipid abnormalities (elevated cholesterol and triglycerides)
- Metabolic acidosis
- Volume overload
- Electrolyte disturbances (e.g., hyperkalemia)
- Cardiovascular disease

In an earlier RCT, the African American Study of Kidney Disease and Hypertension, African Americans with hypertension and CKD were randomly assigned one of two mean arterial pressure goals: 102 to 107 mm Hg or 92 mm Hg or less. Achieved BP averaged 128/78 mm Hg in the lower BP group and 141/85 mm Hg in the usual BP group. The mean change in GFR over the 4 years of the study did not differ significantly between arms (−2.21 vs. −1.95 mL/min per 1.73 m^2 per year, in the lower and usual BP arms, respectively; $P = .24$).

To address BP targets in diabetic patients, the Action to Control Cardiovascular Risk in Diabetes blood pressure (ACCORD BP) trial randomly assigned 4733 patients with type 2 diabetes who had cardiovascular disease or at least two additional risk factors for cardiovascular disease to either intensive therapy (goal systolic BP less than 120 mm Hg) or standard therapy (goal systolic BP less than 140 mm Hg). There was no significant difference in the annual rate of the primary composite outcome of nonfatal myocardial infarction, nonfatal stroke, or death from cardiovascular causes between the intensive versus standard therapy groups. There was an increase in drug side effects, including hypotension (2.4% vs. 1.4%), syncope (2.3% vs. 1.7%), and acute kidney injury (4.1% vs. 2.5%), in the intensive therapy group versus standard therapy group. Both SPRINT and ACCORD used the same BP targets, with different patient populations (ACCORD was diabetes only and SPRINT used patients at high cardiovascular disease (CVD) risk but excluded diabetes) and had different results. Of note, SPRINT had twice the number of patients as ACCORD did.

Given conflicting data, current treatment goals are systolic <130 and diastolic <80 for CKD with proteinuria. Kidney Disease: Improving Global Outcomes (KDIGO) currently recommends a goal BP of systolic <140 and diastolic <90 for nonproteinuric CKD patients.

5. What are the preferred antihypertensive medications for a patient with progressive kidney failure?
Multiple studies suggest that in CKD, particularly with increased urine protein excretion, an ACE inhibitor or ARB is the preferred antihypertensive medications (and perhaps direct renin inhibitors if ACE inhibitors or ARBs are not tolerated). For a patient with proteinuria, BP reduction and urine protein excretion should be goals of therapy and used to titrate doses of either of these medication classes upward. Studies of ACE inhibitors and ARBs in patients with diabetes, human immunodeficiency virus (HIV)-associated nephropathy, and multiple other glomerular diseases demonstrate a benefit from the use of these agents in slowing the progression of kidney disease *independent* of their BP effects.

Due to their effects on glomerular hemodynamics, patients treated with ACE inhibitors and ARBs should have their serum creatinine and potassium levels monitored. Side effects include hyperkalemia and acute kidney injury (AKI). Late-onset kidney failure from angiotensin blockade has been described. A study of older patients who had significant worsening of creatinine with angiotensin blockade (>25% increase in serum creatinine) found that once angiotensin blockade was stopped, most showed improvement or stabilization in kidney function. Whether these changes represent a transient hemodynamic effect or true progression of their underlying CKD needs further investigation.

6. What studies have demonstrated that BP control slows the progression of CKD?
Multiple observational studies show that individuals with lower BPs have better overall kidney outcomes and slower progression to ultimate kidney failure. However, it is important to demonstrate this effect through a randomized clinical trial looking at kidney end points with different BP goals. For instance, if patients are randomized to a higher versus lower BP, do the patients in the lower BP group have slower progression to kidney failure? The answer to this question is, No. In large studies

including the Modification of Diet in Renal Disease (MDRD) study, African American Study of Kidney Disease and Hypertension (AASK), Ramipril Efficacy in Nephropathy-2 (REIN-2) Study as well as in SPRINT, lower BP goals failed to slow the progression of kidney failure. This was confirmed in a 2016 meta-analysis of 613,815 patients and 123 studies.

Every 10-mm Hg reduction in systolic BP significantly reduced the risk of major cardiovascular disease events (RR 0.80, 95% CI 0.77 to 0.83), coronary heart disease (RR 0.83, 95% CI 0.78 to 0.88), stroke (RR 0.73, 95% CI 0.68 to 0.77), and heart failure (RR 0.72, 95% CI 0.67 to 0.78), which, in the populations studied, led to a significant 13% reduction in all-cause mortality (RR 0.87, 95% CI 0.84 to 0.91). However, the effect on kidney failure was not significant (RR 0.95, 95% CI 0.84 to 1.07).

At this time, we do not have compelling evidence that lowering BP preserves kidney function but given its powerful effect at modulating risk of stroke, heart disease, and total mortality, this should not dissuade from careful and thoughtful BP management.

7. **What is the goal hemoglobin A1c (HbA1c) in patients with progressive kidney failure?**
The goal HbA1c in patients with CKD with respect to its effect on hard clinical outcomes has not been clearly established and is beyond the scope of the chapter; from the kidney perspective, glucose control close to normal range is associated with the slowest rate of progression of kidney disease. The Diabetes Control and Complications Trial (DCCT) randomly assigned approximately 1400 patients with type I diabetes to intensive therapy aimed at maintaining glucose concentrations close to the normal range as compared with conventional therapy. Intensive therapy reduced the occurrence of microalbuminuria by 39% and albuminuria by 54%.

The Epidemiology of Diabetes Interventions and Complications (EDIC) Study is a long-term, observational study which follows the DCCT cohort of patients to determine the effects of prior DCCT treatment on diabetes complications, particularly nephropathy and macrovascular complications. It showed that the benefits of intensive diabetes controlled were sustained: after 16 years of follow-up in EDIC (22 years since the start of the DCCT trial), patients originally assigned to intensive glycemic control were significantly less likely to develop impaired kidney function (eGFR < 60 mL/min per 1.73 m^2) −3.9% versus 7.6% in the standard therapy group.

Thus a goal HbA1c of close to 7%, particularly in older patients, is a reasonable target and is consistent with the 2012 Kidney Disease Outcomes Quality Initiative and KDIGO guidelines for patients with CKD.

8. **Is hemoglobin A1c a good marker of blood sugar control in a person with progressive kidney failure?**
Although hemoglobin A1c is a sufficient marker of blood sugar control in a patient with earlier stages of kidney disease who does not yet require dialysis, this parameter has limited utility in patients with stage 5 disease. Studies suggest little correlation between average blood glucose level and hemoglobin A1c with clinical outcomes in late-stage CKD due to nonenzymatic glycosylation of hemoglobin in the uremic serum and shortened red blood cell survival. Multiple other potential markers have been studied, and glycosylated albumin may be a good alternative for assessment of glycemic control.

9. **Does the management of lipids affect the course of patients with progressive kidney failure?**
Current treatment guidelines recommend treatment of hyperlipidemia in patients with CKD. A meta-analysis published in 2009 included 26 studies with 25,017 participants with stage 3 or stage 4 CKD. Compared with placebo, statin therapy decreased the risk of all-cause mortality, cardiovascular death, and nonfatal cardiovascular events. There was no effect on rate of GFR decline. More evidence supporting the use of statins came from the SHARP trial (Study of Heart and Renal Protection). This randomized controlled trial evaluated the efficacy of simvastatin plus ezetimibe compared with placebo in lowering cardiovascular morbidity in patients with CKD, approximately one-third of whom were on maintenance dialysis. SHARP included 6247 patients with CKD who were not treated with maintenance dialysis. During a median follow-up of 4.9 years, simvastatin/ezetimibe lowered the incidence of the primary end points of coronary death, myocardial infarction, ischemic stroke, or any revascularization procedure (9.5% vs. 11.9% in the placebo group).

The evidence for the use of statins in patients who are on dialysis is discussed elsewhere in this book.

10. **How does diet (salt, protein, and fluids) affect the progress of kidney disease?**
Sodium restriction to less than 2 g/day in patients with CKD can facilitate better BP and volume control, as well as reducing albuminuria. Early studies of dietary protein restriction suggested that a lower-protein diet decreased hyperfiltration and glomerular pressure and may potentially benefit the progression of kidney disease. However, the large MDRD study failed to demonstrate a benefit in slowing kidney disease progression among people who reduced their protein intake, only delaying the onset of symptoms. KDIGO currently recommends that patients at risk of progressive CKD to avoid

high protein intake ($>$1.3 g/kg per day) and patients with CKD stage 4 should restrict protein intake to 0.8 g/kg per day.

11. How should proteinuria be used as a marker and a target of disease activity in the person with progressive kidney disease?
Proteinuria is an important surrogate outcome for disease activity in someone with progressive kidney disease. In a patient with glomerular kidney disease, the level of proteinuria correlates with disease activity and potential risk for progression. Therefore therapeutic decisions aimed at lowering protein excretion should be implemented in a paradigm similar to BP management; baseline protein excretion should be estimated using a urine test such as the urine protein-to-creatinine ratio. The urine protein-to-creatinine ratio roughly approximates the amount of protein a patient excretes in a single 24-hour period. A lower value of approximately 0.3 g or less is considered normal. A value $>$0.3 g is abnormal.
    In a patient with an abnormal level of proteinuria, therapy, such as ACE inhibitors or ARBs, should be initiated to lower urine protein excretion. The urine protein excretion should be rechecked to determine the effect of therapy. The therapeutic goal is to decrease the urine protein-to-creatinine ratio to the lowest value possible. If, after initiating the therapy, the desired urine protein-to-creatinine ratio is not reached, the medication chosen should be titrated up as tolerated. However, patients should not be treated with a combination of both ACE inhibitors and ARBs or a combination of ACEi and direct renin inhibitors because studies have shown that these drugs in combination are associated with an increased risk of adverse events and a more rapid decline in GFR, despite effectively lowering proteinuria.

12. When is anemia likely to occur in the person with progressive kidney disease?
Anemia is a common feature in patients with advanced CKD. It becomes increasingly common as the eGFR declines to less than 60 mL/min per 1.73 m^2. In a study of more than 15,000 participants in the National Health and Nutrition Examination Survey (NHANES), the prevalence of anemia (hemoglobin $<$12 g/dL in men and $<$11 g/dL in women) increased from 1% at an eGFR of 60 mL/min per 1.73 m^2 to 9% at an eGFR of 30 mL/min per 1.73 m^2 and to 33% in males and 67% in females at an eGFR of 15 mL/min per 1.73 m^2.

13. What are the mechanisms by which anemia develops in the patient with progressive kidney disease?
The mechanism for anemia is multifactorial in the person with CKD. An important contributor is decreased endogenous erythropoietin production related to decreased nephron mass; however, also contributing to anemia are factors including iron deficiency, both absolute and functional.

14. What are the therapeutic options in the treatment of anemia in the patient with progressive kidney disease?
Therapies available for the patient with anemia and kidney disease include iron supplementation and erythrocyte-stimulating agents (ESAs) once iron stores are replete. The initial evaluation in patients with anemia should include red cell indices, iron, ferritin, total iron-binding capacity, transferrin saturation, vitamin B12 and folate, reticulocyte count, and platelets. Patients with iron deficiency should be treated with iron. Iron stores may be supplemented through oral iron supplementation. When oral iron is not efficacious, intravenous iron is an alternative option.
    Patients whose hemoglobin falls to less than 10 g/dL despite adequate iron stores can be treated with ESAs such as epoetin-alfa or darbepoetin given subcutaneously.

15. What are the treatment goals for anemia in a patient with progressive kidney disease?
The treatment goals for anemia in a patient with progressive kidney disease are based on several clinical trials. Three clinical trials have been performed to evaluate the effect of anemia correction with ESAs on clinical outcomes such as death, congestive heart failure, myocardial infarction, and stroke. Two clinical trials enrolled a wide range of patients with CKD and anemia, randomly assigning them to treatment for correction of their anemia to hemoglobin of approximately 13 versus hemoglobin of approximately 11. Although one study failed to demonstrate any benefit or harm when the two arms were compared, the other demonstrated worse outcomes in the group randomized to the higher hemoglobin level. Finally, a trial randomly assigning patients to receive darbepoetin to achieve a target hemoglobin of 13 g/dL as compared with placebo (i.e., no anemia correction) failed to demonstrate a difference in cardiovascular outcomes or mortality between the two arms. However, it is noteworthy that this trial did demonstrate a significantly increased risk of stroke in the arm receiving active treatment with the ESA. In addition, there was an increase in cancer-related deaths in patients with a prior history of cancer.
    The treatment goal recommended by the US Food and Drug Administration (FDA) for ESAs is to consider starting ESA therapy when the hemoglobin is $<$10 g/dL if the rate of hemoglobin decline indicates the likelihood of requiring a red blood cell transfusion and a reduction in alloimmunization- and

transfusion-related risks is the goal. In addition, the previously mentioned trials have demonstrated an increased risk of adverse cardiovascular events when hemoglobin >11 g/dL, and the FDA now specifies that ESA dosing should be reduced or stopped if the Hb level exceeds 11 g/dL. The relative benefit to quality of life as compared with the increased risk of cardiovascular events, particularly stroke, should be considered on a case-by-case basis.

16. **What are the parameters that should be monitored in bone and mineral metabolism, and when are changes in these parameters likely to occur in the person with progressive kidney disease?**
The parameters that should be monitored in patients with progressive kidney disease with respect to bone and mineral metabolism include serum levels of calcium, phosphorous, 25-hydroxyvitamin D, and intact parathyroid hormone (PTH). Although phosphorous retention occurs early in CKD, a rise in PTH (particularly when GFR < 60) serves to maintain serum calcium and serum phosphorous within normal ranges in the vast majority of patients until late stages of progressive kidney disease.

17. **What is the mechanism by which bone and mineral metabolism changes in the person with progressive kidney disease?**
The earliest changes involve rising fibroblast growth factor (FGF)-23 levels, which increase phosphate excretion in the urine and suppress 1,25 vitamin D production. Increased phosphorous and low 1,25-vitamin D lead to hypocalcemia, which stimulates PTH production (secondary hyperparathyroidism) to normalize serum calcium.

18. **What are the therapeutic options to treat the changes in bone and mineral metabolism seen in progressive kidney disease?**
The therapeutic options available for a person with derangements in bone and mineral metabolism include normalizing 25 vitamin D levels and dietary counseling to decrease phosphorous intake. In the setting of persistent hyperphosphatemia, a phosphate binder can be used. These binders are taken with the patient's meal to bind the phosphorus in the food, preventing absorption. Phosphate binders include calcium carbonate, calcium acetate, sevelamer, lanthanum, and iron-based binders. Aluminum-containing binders are not recommended due to the increased risk of aluminum toxicity. It should be noted that no studies have demonstrated an improvement in clinical outcomes with the use of phosphate binders. Indeed, there is concern that the use of calcium-based binders can lead to an increase in vascular calcification. This was demonstrated in a study by Block et al., in which patients treated with binders had increased calcification of the coronary arteries and abdominal aorta compared with placebo.

In addition to treating 25 vitamin D deficiency, active 1,25 vitamin D (calcitriol) or active vitamin D analogues (paricalcitol, ergocalciferol) and the calcimimetic cinacalcet can be used to suppress secondary hyperparathyroidism. However, similar to phosphate binders, the evidence of the effectiveness of vitamin D analogues on clinical outcomes in CKD is lacking. The relative combination of these agents should be considered on a case-by-case basis following measurement of serum calcium, phosphorus, vitamin D and intact PTH levels.

19. **What are the treatment goals for changes in bone and mineral metabolism in the patient with progressive kidney disease?**
The treatment goals for a patient with derangements in bone and mineral metabolism are focused on maintaining serum calcium and phosphorous within the normal range. With regard to PTH, current treatment guidelines suggest initiating therapy when the serum PTH is progressively rising and remains persistently greater than the upper limit of normal for the assay.

20. **What are the potential benefits of treating metabolic acidosis and what is the target bicarbonate level?**
The prevalence of metabolic acidosis (serum $HCO_3^- < 22$) increases as CKD progresses. Chronic metabolic acidosis in CKD is associated with adverse consequences such as increased muscle catabolism, bone reabsorption, systemic inflammation, impaired myocardial contractility, and increased mortality. It is also associated with a higher risk of progressive loss of kidney function. Patients with metabolic acidosis can be treated with alkali therapy to maintain bicarbonate in the normal range (23 to 29 mEq/L). Options include sodium bicarbonate, sodium citrate, and alkali-rich diets (fruits and vegetables). Therapy with bicarbonate slowed progression of CKD in multiple single-center trials.

21. **What is the effect of smoking on progression of CKD?**
Smoking is associated with a higher incidence of cardiovascular- and cancer-related deaths in patients with CKD, similar to the general population. Some studies have also found an association between smoking cessation and a slower rate of progression of CKD.

22. In preparation for dialysis, when and what should patients be told to assist them in their decision regarding modality choice?
Patient education should begin early. The patients may wish to understand their options early in their disease progression; however, referral to a nephrologist and education with respect to options for kidney or placement therapy should begin no later than stage 4 CKD. Options such as conservative care, hemodialysis, peritoneal dialysis, home hemodialysis, and renal transplantation should be discussed and plans established.

23. In a person interested in hemodialysis, when and what should be done to facilitate the timely placement of a functional vascular access, and why is that important?
For a patient who is opting for hemodialysis, vascular access should be placed early enough so that the vascular access is usable when hemodialysis is initiated. Patients and their health care providers should be instructed to avoid venipuncture above the hands, particularly in the nondominant arm, to preserve the veins for arteriovenous fistula (AVF) formation. An AVF takes several months to mature and will fail to mature in approximately half the cases. Arteriovenous grafts will be able to be used 2 to 3 weeks after placement. Peritoneal dialysis requires sufficient time for not only catheter placement and healing (approximately 2 to 4 weeks) but also the training that will be required for the patient and his or her family prior to the full initiation of the therapy. Having a patient's vascular access or peritoneal access ready when it is necessary to initiate renal replacement therapy is important to avoid placement of an intravenous catheter and hospitalization to initiate hemodialysis. Catheters have increased risk of infection and mortality compared with AVF.

24. Can a person receive a kidney transplant without having been on dialysis?
Patients can be listed for kidney transplant when eGFR $\leq$ 20. Preemptive transplantation (i.e., prior to initiation of dialysis) has been shown to provide a patient and graft survival benefit over transplantation following the initiation of dialysis. In that regard, education and timely referral of a patient for kidney transplantation should be considered for those patients with progressive CKD who are appropriate candidates (Fig. 24.1).

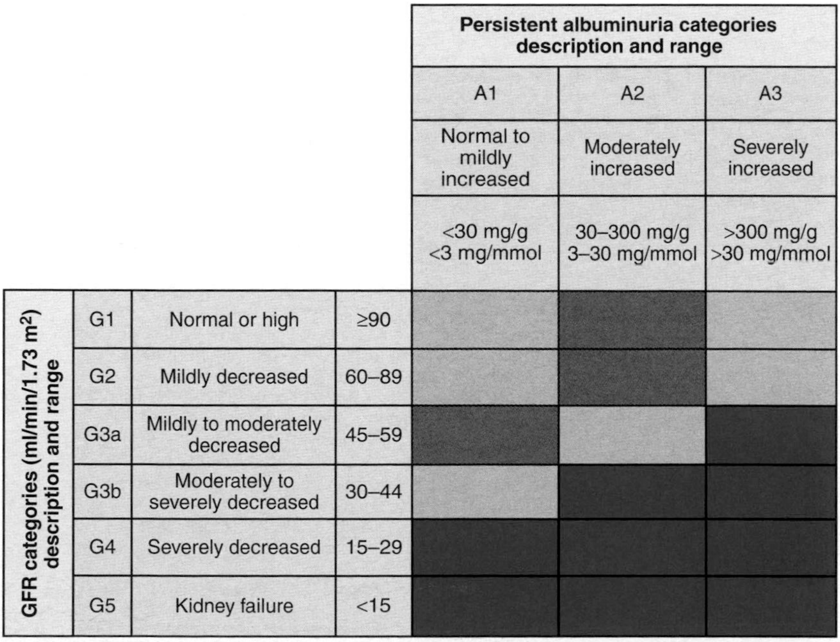

				Persistent albuminuria categories description and range		
				A1	A2	A3
				Normal to mildly increased	Moderately increased	Severely increased
				<30 mg/g <3 mg/mmol	30–300 mg/g 3–30 mg/mmol	>300 mg/g >30 mg/mmol
GFR categories (ml/min/1.73 m²) description and range	G1	Normal or high	≥90			
	G2	Mildly decreased	60–89			
	G3a	Mildly to moderately decreased	45–59			
	G3b	Moderately to severely decreased	30–44			
	G4	Severely decreased	15–29			
	G5	Kidney failure	<15			

Figure 24.1. Prognosis of chronic kidney disease (CKD) by glomerular filtration rate (GFR) and albuminuria categories: KDIGO 2012. *(Kidney Disease: Improving Global Outcomes (KDIGO) CKD Work Group. (2013). KDIGO 2012 clinical practice guideline for the evaluation and management of chronic kidney disease. Kidney International Supplements, 3, 1–150.)*

KEY POINTS

1. Chronic kidney disease (CKD) progression can be monitored using serum creatinine and urine protein excretion.
2. Proteinuria is an important surrogate outcome for disease activity in someone with progressive kidney disease. In a patient with glomerular kidney disease, the level of proteinuria correlates with disease activity and potential risk for progression. Proteinuria can be reduced with angiotensin-converting enzyme inhibitors or angiotensin receptor blockers; however, several studies have shown that these drugs should not be used in combination due to an increased risk of adverse events.
3. Although hemoglobin A1c is a sufficient marker of blood sugar control in a patient with early stages of kidney disease, it has limited utility in patients with stage 5 disease. Studies suggest little correlation between average blood glucose level and hemoglobin A1c in CKD stage 5 due to nonenzymatic glycosylation of hemoglobin and shortened red blood half-life.
4. Patients with progressive CKD should be educated about treatment options, including conservative care, hemodialysis, peritoneal dialysis, and transplantation.
5. In patients with metabolic acidosis, treatment with oral bicarbonate may slow progression of CKD, improve bone health, and nutritional status.

BIBLIOGRAPHY

ACCORD Study Group, Cushman, W. C., Evans, G. W., Byington, R. P., Goff, D. C., Jr., Grimm, R. H., Jr., . . . Ismail-Beigi, F. (2010). Effects of intensive blood-pressure control in type 2 diabetes mellitus. *New England Journal of Medicine, 362*(17), 1575.

Baigent, C., Landray, M. J., Reith, C., Emberson, J., Wheeler, D. C., Tomson, C., . . . SHARP Investigators. (2011). The effects of lowering LDL cholesterol with simvastatin plus ezetimibe in patients with chronic kidney disease (Study of Heart and Renal Protection): A randomized placebo-controlled trial. *Lancet, 377*(9784), 2181.

Block, G. A., Wheeler, D. C., Persky, M. S., Kestenbaum, B., Ketteler, M., Spiegel, D. M., . . . Chertow, G. M. (2012). Effects of phosphate binders in moderate CKD. *Journal of the American Society of Nephrology, 23*(8), 1407.

de Brito-Ashurst, I., Varagunam, M., Raftery, M. J., & Yaqoob, M. M. (2009). Bicarbonate supplementation slows progression of CKD and improves nutritional status. *Journal of the American Society of Nephrology, 20*(9), 2075.

The Diabetes Control and Complications Trial/Epidemiology of Diabetes Interventions and Complications Research Group, Lachin, J. M., Genuth, S., Cleary, P., Davis, M. D., & Nathan, D. M. (2000). Retinopathy and nephropathy in patients with type 1 diabetes four years after a trial of intensive therapy. *New England Journal of Medicine, 342,* 381–389.

Drüeke, T. B., Locatelli, F., Clyne, N., Eckardt, K. U., Macdougall, I. C., Tsakiris, D., . . . the CREATE Investigators. (2006). Normalization of hemoglobin level in patients with chronic kidney disease and anemia. *New England Journal of Medicine, 355,* 2071–2084.

Ettehad, D., Emdin, C. A., Kiran, A., Anderson, S. G., Callender, T., Emberson, J., . . . Rahimi, K. (2016). Blood pressure lowering for prevention of cardiovascular disease and death: A systematic review and meta-analysis. *Lancet, 387*(10022), 957–967.

Kidney Disease: Improving Global Outcomes (KDIGO) Anemia Work Group. (2012). KDIGO clinical practice guideline for anemia in chronic kidney disease. *Kidney International Supplements, 2,* 279–335.

Kidney Disease: Improving Global Outcomes (KDIGO) CKD-MBD Work Group. (2009). KDIGO clinical practice guideline for the diagnosis, evaluation, prevention, and treatment of chronic kidney disease–mineral and bone disorder (CKD–MBD). *Kidney International Supplements, 76*(Suppl. 113), S1–S130.

Klahr, S., Levey, A. S., Beck, G. J., Caggiula, A. W., Hunsicker, L., Kusek, J. W., & Striker, G. (1994). The effects of dietary protein restriction and blood-pressure control on the progression of renal disease. Modification of Diet in Renal Disease Study Group. *New England Journal of Medicine, 330,* 877–884.

ONTARGET Investigators, Yusuf, S., Teo, K. K., Pogue, J., Dyal, L., Copland, I., . . . Anderson, C. (2008). Telmisartan, ramipril, or both in patients at high risk for vascular events. *New England Journal of Medicine, 358*(15), 1547.

Onuigbo, M. A., & Onuigbo, N. T. (2008). Late-onset renal failure from angiotensin blockade (LORFFAB) in 100 CKD patients. *International Urology and Nephrology, 40,* 233–239.

The SPRINT Research Group. (2015). A randomized trial of intensive versus standard blood-pressure control. *New England Journal of Medicine, 373,* 2103–2116.

Staplin, N., Haynes, R., Herrington, W. G., Reith, C., Cass, A., Fellström, B., . . . SHARP Collaborative Group. (2016). Smoking and Adverse Outcomes in Patients with CKD: The Study of Heart and Renal Protection (SHARP). *American Journal of Kidney Diseases, 68*(3), 371–380.

Wright, J. T., Jr., Bakris, G., Greene, T., Agodoa, L. Y., Appel, L. J., Charleston, J., . . . for the African American Study of Kidney Disease and Hypertension Study Group. (2002). Effect of blood pressure lowering and antihypertensive drug class on progression of hypertensive kidney disease: results from the AASK trial. *Journal of the American Medical Association, 288,* 2421–2431.

DRUG DOSING IN PATIENTS WITH CHRONIC KIDNEY DISEASE

Joseph B. Pryor, Joseph L. Lockridge, and Ali J. Olyaei

CHAPTER 25

1. **How can chronic kidney disease (CKD) alter the pharmacokinetic behavior of most drugs?**
   CKD directly and indirectly affects the pharmacokinetic properties of most drugs. Alterations of drug pharmacokinetics in patients with kidney failure are based on changes in absorption, distribution, metabolism, and elimination.

2. **How can changes in absorption resulting from CKD alter the pharmacokinetic behavior of drugs?**
   - Alkaline saliva. As CKD progresses, saliva becomes more alkaline. This compromises absorption of drugs that need an acid milieu (e.g., iron supplements) and contributes to a higher gastric pH.
   - Nausea and vomiting may reduce drug ingestion and absorption.
   - Volume overload states: Edema of the gastrointestinal tract limits absorption.
   - Drug interactions: Many drugs used in the management of CKD limit drug absorption by forming nonabsorbable complexes (e.g., iron, phosphate-binding agents).
   - Gastrointestinal neuropathy: Uremia may delay gastric emptying time, particularly in patients with diabetes.

3. **How can changes in distribution from CKD alter the pharmacokinetic behavior of drugs?**
   The volume of distribution (V_D) represents the ratio of administered dose to the resulting plasma drug concentration. The calculated V_D is a theoretic representation of the size of the anatomic space occupied by the drug if it were present throughout the body in the same concentration as that in the plasma. Drugs with a large V_D, such as digoxin, are distributed widely throughout the tissues and are present in relatively small amounts in the blood. In patients with CKD, changes in drug distribution may arise from either fluid retention or reductions in the extent of protein binding in tissue and plasma. CKD has very limited effects on drugs with large volume distribution. Conversely, drugs that are less lipid soluble and highly protein bound will tend to have a lower V_D because they are more restricted to the vascular compartment. Kidney impairment and hemodialysis has a significant effect on drugs with small V_D. For example, in critically ill patients with CKD, for a drug like vancomycin with a small V_D, higher than recommended loading and daily doses are needed to rapidly achieve therapeutic serum concentrations.

   Malnutrition and proteinuria reduce the amount of protein available for protein binding, and uremic stage may alter the affinity of many drugs to albumin. Thus the concentration of free drug will increase in these settings, which can result in increased free fraction and potential adverse drug reactions. Therapeutic drug monitoring (TDM) for free or unbound drug concentrations in patients with kidney insufficiency or heavy proteinuria (e.g., free phenytoin levels) is an important consideration.

4. **How can changes in metabolism as a result of CKD alter the pharmacokinetic behavior of drugs?**
   Even drugs without or with only minimal kidney elimination can have altered pharmacokinetics in advanced CKD. CKD may increase, decrease, or have no effect on nonkidney clearance. Some drugs are metabolized to active metabolites that are insignificant with normal kidney function but accumulate in CKD. For example, morphine metabolizes to 6- and 3-morphine-gluconate with respiratory depression and seizure properties. In CKD the clearance of the parent compound (morphine) is not significantly affected; however, morphine metabolizes to 6- and 3-morphine-gluconate, which accumulate and place patients at risk for serious adverse drug reactions. Therefore it is recommended that morphine be used cautiously in patients with CKD or avoided completely if high doses or a prolonged use is indicated.

5. **How can changes in elimination as a result of CKD alter the pharmacokinetic behavior of drugs?**
   A reduction in the glomerular filtration rate (GFR) will generally lead to an increased half-life of a drug that is eliminated primarily by the kidney. Clearance is a measure of the efficiency of the kidney at

169

excreting a specific compound. The clearance of a drug is the amount of plasma from which the drug is completely removed from over unit time. For example, a furosemide clearance of 20 mL/min means that every minute enough furosemide is excreted in the urine to completely clear out all of the furosemide from 20 mL of plasma.

6. **What characteristics determine whether a drug is removed by dialysis?**
   - **Molecular weight.** As a general rule, smaller molecular weight substances pass through the dialyzer membrane much more easily than larger weight molecules. In general, free drug molecules with a molecular weight of less than 500 Daltons (D) are removed efficiently by hemodialysis.
   - **Protein binding.** Decreased protein binding may increase the amount of free drug available for removal during dialysis. In the setting of an overdose, the amount of ingested drug may exceed the normal protein-binding capacity. This would allow removal of the excess drug by hemodialysis, even though dialysis has a minimal effect when the drug is used at normal doses.
   - **V_D.** Drugs with large volumes of distribution are not removed effectively by dialysis. Lipid-soluble drugs usually have large volumes of distribution, making significant removal of the drug difficult because the plasma volume is rapidly replenished from other tissues (e.g., cyclosporine and digoxin).
   - **Water solubility.** Drugs with high water solubility will be dialyzed to a greater extent than those with high lipid solubility.
   - **Dialyzer membrane.** The pore size, surface area, and geometry are the primary factors in determining whether a dialysis membrane will clear a specific drug. Historically, standard dialysis membranes did not effectively remove vancomycin (molecular weight, 3300 D) given its size. Currently, high-flux membranes that remove larger-molecular-weight molecules have become standard of care in dialysis practice. Therefore vancomycin and many other antibiotics are removed by these membranes. Dosing of these medications should be held until after dialysis on those days.
   - **Blood and dialysate flow rates.** Increased flow rates during hemodialysis will increase drug clearance. Patients who cannot tolerate standard blood flow rates will require less replacement dosing of a drug after hemodialysis.

7. **How is kidney function assessed for drug dosing determination?**
   The best way is to estimate the GFR. The gold standard is measurement of the clearance of inulin; however, this is cumbersome and impractical for clinical use. Measurement of the 24-hour creatinine clearance (CrCl) is no longer recommended for similar reasoning. This has led to the development of equations to estimate GFR such as the Cockcroft-Gault (CG) and Modification of Diet in Renal Disease (MDRD) study. These equations use serum creatinine as one of the variables and both generally provide similar dosing recommendations. Adverse events such as drug accumulations are relatively uncommon when the GFR remains >50 mL/min.
   It is still important to consider potential analytic interferences in these calculations based on the concurrent drug therapy. Some drugs may artifactually increase or decrease the measured serum creatinine concentration without directly influencing GFR. Drugs that inhibit the tubular secretion of creatinine will raise the serum level (e.g., trimethoprim, cimetidine, and probenecid).

8. **What the best method to estimate kidney function for drug dosing in CKD?**
   Most approved drugs advice to use CG method by the way to estimated kidney function for medication dosage adjustment in patients with kidney disease. Recently, it has been questioned that other methods of estimating kidney function perhaps are more accurate than CG method for estimating kidney function. It is important to remember that CG formula, MDRD, and Chronic Kidney Disease-Epidemiology (CKD-EPI) Collaboration equation are only an "estimation" and "approximation" of kidney function. Neither of these methods provides accurate "measurement" or "calculation" of kidney function. In addition, there are many other changes in the kidney that might affect drug handling than just filtration rate such tubular function and organic acid accumulations. Health care providers should also consider drug safety and efficacy for dosage adjustment. In general, a number of recent studies comparing the equations for their influence on drug dosage adjustment have shown that the MDRD perhaps is a better method with a greater concordance with measured GFR compared with other methods.

9. **What commonly prescribed drugs cause hyperkalemia in patients with CKD and receiving dialysis?**
   Many drugs used as therapy for CKD and associated conditions, such as heart failure and hypertension, can cause or worse hyperkalemia. Often, it is combinations of these medications that lead to hyperkalemia. Potassium (K+) supplements are used frequently in combination with diuretic therapy. K+-sparing diuretics (spironolactone, amiloride) inhibit kidney elimination of K+. Angiotensin-converting enzyme

(ACE) inhibitors and angiotensin receptor blockers (ARBs) are common causes via alterations in the renin-angiotensin-aldosterone system (RAAS). Digoxin inhibits the basolateral Na-K ATPase in cardiac myocytes. Because of a narrow therapeutic window, overdose states are not uncommon and can result in elevated K+. Acute and/or chronic reductions in GFR in association with the previously mentioned medications can tip a patient into hyperkalemia by compromising K+ excretion by the kidneys. Nonsteroidal antiinflammatory drugs (NSAIDs) and beta blockers also impair kidney K+ excretion mainly through inhibition of RASS system leading to hyperkalemia. Digoxin inhibits the basolateral Na-K ATPase in cardiac myocytes. Penicillin infusion solutions contain a high amount of K+ for drug stability.

    Calcineurin inhibitors (CNIs) such as tacrolimus or cyclosporine are the backbone of immunosuppression in kidney transplant and are additionally used in the treatment of some glomerulonephritis. Both of these are associated with various electrolyte abnormalities including hyperkalemia.

10. **Which antimicrobials should be avoided prior to hemodialysis on scheduled dialysis days?**
    Many antibacterial agents are water-soluble, small molecules, and not highly protein bound; thus they are well dialyzed and will require supplementation post-dialysis. Many of these agents are already administered in a reduced dose or frequency given the reduced kidney clearance. Beta-Lactam agents such as penicillins, cephalosporins, carbapenems, and monobactams are examples of such compounds. Aminoglycosides also exhibit similar properties. Carbapenem and imipenem can lower the seizure threshold and should be avoided altogether in patients receiving dialysis; meropenem in a reduced dose is a therapeutic alternative. Antifungals such as fluconazole may require supplemental dosing; however, the echinocandins (caspofungin, micafungin) and the amphotericin family do not. Antiviral agents should receive individual consideration given their varying properties. Entecavir and telbivudine appear to be removed by hemodialysis, whereas lamivudine does not.

11. **When is re-dosing or a supplemental dose required following hemodialysis?**
    Dialysis clearance must increase total clearance by at least 30% to be considered clinically significant and to require a replacement dose after hemodialysis. The physicochemical characteristics as discussed previously determine the extent that a drug may be affected by dialysis.

12. **How does kidney failure effect drug metabolism?**
    Although the kidney is largely thought to be responsible for drug elimination, the kidney plays an important role in drug metabolism, thus contributing to need for dose adjustments. Current drug dosing guidelines are based on CKD, but both CKD and acute kidney injury (AKI) have been associated with decreased metabolism, specifically via cytochrome P450 (CYP) enzymes. The proposed mechanism is through increased circulating levels of urea, PTH, and cytokines, all of which are thought to downregulate both hepatic and intestinal CYP activity. In addition, individuals in kidney failure have been noted to have decreased drug transport (organic anion transporters and P-glycoprotein) capacity, further decreasing metabolism. Although the exact mechanism is not fully understood, improvement in drug metabolism has been noted in patients on dialysis.

13. **How should aminoglycosides be adjusted for hemodialysis?**
    First, the patient's dosing weight should be determined. Use ideal body weight (IBW) unless total body weight (TBW) is less.
    - Nonobese is: TBW < 130% of IBW
    - IBW (males) = 50 kg + (2.3 × height in inches >60 inches)
    - IBW (females) = 45 kg + (2.3 × height in inches >60 inches)
    - In patients who are obese, adjust IBW: ABW (kg) = IBW + 0.4 (TBW − IBW), where ABW is actual body weight.
      Second, select the appropriate loading and maintenance doses:
    - Loading dose should be considered in life-threatening infection (for gentamicin and tobramycin, give 2.5 mg/kg; for amikacin give 7.5 mg/kg as a loading dose).
    - Select appropriate maintenance dose according to indications (Table 25.1).

14. **What adjustments should be made for administering vancomycin to patients receiving hemodialysis?**
    It is important to load patients receiving dialysis with 15 to 20 mg/kg based on ABW. Maintenance doses will depend on the dialysis membrane used during hemodialysis (Table 25.2).

15. **What adjustments should be made for patients with diabetes?**
    The breakdown of insulin decreases as kidney function deteriorates. Patients with diabetes must be monitored for symptoms of hypoglycemia because their insulin requirement may decrease concurrently.

Table 25.1. Aminoglycoside Dosing in Patients Undergoing Dialysis

DRUG	Dose and Frequency in Patients Undergoing Dialysis		
	HEMODIALYSIS (DOSE POSTDIALYSIS)	PERITONEAL DIALYSIS (EVERY 48 H)*	CONTINUOUS RENAL REPLACEMENT THERAPY (EVERY 24 H)
Gentamicin	1.5–2 mg/kg	1.5–2 mg/kg	1.5–2 mg/kg
Serious infection	1 mg/kg	1 mg/kg	1 mg/kg
Urinary tract infection	1 mg/kg	1 mg/kg	1 mg/kg
Synergy			
Tobramycin	1.5–2 mg/kg	1.5–2 mg/kg	1.5–2 mg/kg
Urinary tract infection	1 mg/kg	1 mg/kg	1 mg/kg
Amikacin	7.5 mg/kg	7.5 mg/kg	7.5 mg/kg

Sulfonylureas that are excreted primarily by the kidneys can accumulate and result in a prolonged hypoglycemic effect. For example, glyburide is metabolized to active metabolites with hypoglycemic properties. A substitute to a drug with greater hepatic excretion, such as glipizide, should be considered when GFR is reduced to less than 50 mL/min. Sodium-glucose cotransporter-2 (SGLT-2) inhibitors are a new class of hypogluycemic agents that work by inhibiting glucose absorption from the kidney. The use of these agents should be avoided in patients with estimated glomerular filtration rate (eGFR) less than 40 mL/min. In addition, AKI has been reported with the use of SGLT2 inhibitors, most likely related to hypoxic injury from osmotic diuresis and dehydration or concomitant use of NSAIDs. Finally, metformin should be used with caution in patients with CKD (Table 25.3).

16. What is the new guideline for the appropriate use of metformin in patients with various degree of kidney disease?
Historically, metformin was contraindicated in patients with CKD. The U.S. Food and Drug Administration (FDA) required a labeling change for metformin. Dosing is now based off of eGFR rather than the previous serum creatinine. The eGFR should be calculated before patients begin treatment with metformin and at least annually thereafter. In patients with an eGFR ≥60 mL/min, no dose adjustments are required for the use of metformin with annual monitoring. However, patients with an eGFR between 30 and 60 mL/min require more frequent kidney function monitoring every 3 to 6 months and dosage to be adjusted to no more than 1000 mg per day. In patients with an eGFR less than 30 mL/min, metformin should be discontinued to avoid the risk of lactic acidosis.

17. How does narcotic pain management differ in patients with CKD?
Meperidine should be avoided in patients with kidney failure because of accumulation of its metabolite (normeperidine), which undergoes kidney elimination. Normeperidine also has an excitatory effect on the central nervous system and causes seizures if it accumulates.

Propoxyphene should also be avoided in patients with kidney failure because of the accumulation of a metabolite (norpropoxyphene). Both can cause ventricular arrhythmias as a result of class IA antiarrhythmic properties. Another complication, propoxyphene-induced hypoglycemia, can be seen in patients with CKD.

Morphine should be used with caution in patients with kidney failure. Morphine undergoes glucuronidation to morphine-6-glucuronide (M6G) and morphine-3-glucuronide. M6G accumulates in kidney failure and is a more potent analgesic than the parent compound. In patients with end-stage kidney disease, the half-life of M6G is estimated to be 38 to 103 hours.

Codeine is metabolized in the liver to codeine-6-glucuronide, norcodeine, and morphine. A dose reduction of 50% is generally recommended in kidney failure.

Hydromorphone is considered to be relatively safe and effective in patients with kidney failure. It is metabolized in the liver to hydromorphone-3-glucuronide followed by a reduction to 6-a-hydroxyhydromorphone and 6-b-hydroxyhydromorphone, both of which are less potent analgesics than the parent drug. Seizure activity and cognitive impairment have been reported in patients with kidney failure receiving high-dose hydromorphone therapy.

Fentanyl is another good option for pain management in patients with kidney failure, even though the kidneys eliminate both the parent drug and its metabolites.

Table 25.2. Vancomycin Administration in Patients Undergoing Dialysis

	HEMODIALYSIS (HD) (HIGH FLUX)	CONTINUOUS VENOVENOUS HEMOFILTRATION (HD, HEMODIAFILTRATION)	PERITONEAL
Loading dose	15–20 mg/kg dose based on actual body weight (ABW) Note: Not to exceed 1500 mg May consider 20 mg/kg in severe infections (i.e., meningitis, severe sepsis, endocarditis, osteomyelitis, and hospital-acquired pneumonia [HAP])	15–20 mg/kg dose based on ABW Note: Not to exceed 1500 mg May consider 20 mg/kg in severe infections (i.e., meningitis, severe sepsis, endocarditis, osteomyelitis, HAP)	Not necessary
Maintenance dose (postdialysis)	<75 kg: 500 mg after HD for predialysis level <20 >75 kg: 1000 mg after HD for predialysis level <20	10–15 mg/kg every 24 h Note: May consider higher doses in patients who are obese not to exceed 1500 mg Intravenous (IV) q24h	IP (intraperitoneal): 30 mg/kg loading dose 15 mg/kg every 3–5 days Note: Patients that are not anuric may need to adjust dosing frequency because there is residual kidney function IV: 15–20 mg/kg per dose
Serum level monitoring	Draw serum level prior to the second HD session, then get random levels with AM labs on HD days only (or q48 h) Note: Subsequent serum levels should be drawn prior to every or every other HD session	Draw serum level prior to the second or third dose (approximately 24 h after last dose) Note: May draw random daily levels with AM labs	IP: Draw serum trough level 72 h after loading dose IV: Draw serum trough level 48–72 h after initial dose
Dosing based on serum levels	If pre-HD level is: >20: hold dose 10–20: give dose after HD (based on weight) <10: administer another loading dose after HD	If serum level is: >20: hold dose 10–20: continue with q24h dosing <10: 15–20 mg/kg loading dose → consider more frequent dosing or increasing the dose	If level is: >20: hold dose <20: administer another dose

Table 25.3. Medication Adjustments for Patients With Diabetes

	NORMAL KIDNEY FUNCTION	CHRONIC KIDNEY DISEASE STAGES 3–5	HEMODIALYSIS
Metformin	500–2000 mg/day	Avoid	Avoid (lactic acidosis)
Rosiglitazone	4–8 mg/day	Caution	Caution (heart failure and fluid retention)
Pioglitazone	15–30 mg/day	Caution	Caution (heart failure and fluid retention)
Glyburide	2.5–10 mg bid	50%	Avoid
Glipizide	5–20 mg bid	100%	50%
Glimepiride	1–8 mg/day	50%	Avoid
Nateglinide	120–180 tid	100%	100%
Dapagliflozine	5-10 mg/day	Avoid	Fungal urinary tract infections, dehydration and AKI
Canaglifozine	100-300 mg/day	Avoid	Fungal urinary tract infections, dehydration and AKI
Rapaglinide	0.5–4 mg tid	100%	100%
Sitagliptin	100 mg/day	50 mg/day	25 mg/day

18. **How is dosage of anticonvulsants adjusted in patients with CKD?**
Phenytoin is a highly protein-bound drug. In patients receiving dialysis or in patients with CKD and significant proteinuria, the free fraction of phenytoin (free phenytoin) is elevated, although plasma phenytoin levels seem low. If not adjusted, total phenytoin levels are of little value. In patients receiving dialysis, the monitoring of free concentration is recommended for a target plasma concentration of 1 to 2 mcg/mL.
    If unable to obtain a free phenytoin level, the following equations can be used to adjust the serum concentrations based on either reduced albumin levels or presence of kidney failure (CrCl < 10 mL/min).
    • Hypoproteinemia: $C_{adjusted} = C_{measured}/[(0.2 \times albumin) + 0.1]$
    • AKI and dialysis: $C_{adjusted} = C_{measured}/[(0.1 \times albumin) + 0.1]$

19. **List the common drug interactions for cyclosporine and tacrolimus in kidney transplant recipients.**
Many drugs are known to interact with CNIs (cyclosporine and tacrolimus); some agents are more problematic than others. Antiepileptic medications such as phenytoin, carbamazepine, and phenobarbital; antituberculosis agents such as rifampin, rifabutin, and isoniazid (INH); and herbal supplements such as St. John's wort are well-known inducers of the cytochrome P-450 (CYP3A4) pathway and would decrease plasma concentrations of CNIs. Thus these drug-drug interactions may increase the risk of acute rejection following transplantation. The use of these agents in combination with CNIs requires dose escalation and careful TDM.
    Coadministration of CNIs with agents that strongly inhibit the CYP3A4 enzymatic system may conversely result in nephrotoxicity. Nefazodone, nondihydropyridine calcium channel blockers (verapamil, diltiazem), antibiotics (erythromycin, clarithromycin, telithromycin, but not azithromycin), antifungal agents (ketoconazole, fluconazole, itraconazole, voriconazole), and grapefruit are strong CYP3A4 inhibitors. Grapefruit and grapefruit juice are known inhibitors of the cytochrome P-450 pathway and should be avoided in transplant patients and patients with CKD taking statins and calcium channel blockers.

20. **What are the common risk factors for aminoglycoside kidney toxicity?**
Dose and duration of therapy, advanced age, use of other nephrotoxic agents (cyclosporine, tacrolimus, vancomycin), sepsis, hypotension, dehydration, and intravenous radiologic contrast medium have been reported as important risk factors in the development of aminoglycoside-induced nephrotoxicity. However, when confounding factors are adjusted using multivariate analysis, only dose, duration, advanced age, and baseline creatinine level have been associated with nephrotoxicity.

21. **What drugs have been associated with or precipitate nephrolithiasis?**
    Several agents can crystallize in the urine, such as indinavir, topirmate, acyclovir, sulfadiazine, and triamterene. Stones related to these drugs usually involve the crystalline structure. Topirmate is a carbonic anhydrase inhibitor and causes systemic metabolic acidosis, which leads to decreased urinary citrate excretion. Alternation of urinary pH may increase the risk of calcium phosphate stones. Nephrolithiasis also has been reported with prolonged use of ceftriaxone in children. Large amounts of vitamin C intake in men have been associated with an increased risk of calcium-based stone formation, presumably related to its metabolism to oxalate. Initiation of uricosuric therapy with probenecid can precipitate uric acid stone formation. Loop diuretics (e.g., furosemide) can also play a role as a result of increased urinary calcium excretion and volume contraction related to diuresis. Conversely, thiazide-type diuretics reduce urinary calcium excretion.

22. **How can ACE inhibitors and ARBs cause kidney dysfunction while being protective in diabetic nephropathy?**
    ACE inhibitors and ARBs exert their effects by blocking the RAAS pathway. The pharmacodynamic effects of these agents are achieved by inhibiting the vasoconstrictive effect of angiotensin II at the efferent arteriole in the glomerulus. RAAS blockade at the glomerular structure of the nephron reduces glomerular capillary pressure, which is associated with reduced proteinuria, an important surrogate outcome for kidney function. As a result of the reduced filtration fraction associated with this hemodynamic change, an increase in the baseline serum creatinine concentration prior to drug initiation of 30% is generally determined acceptable. However, this increased in the serum creatinine has been associated with an increased risk of adverse outcomes long term. Increases in creatinine beyond this are suggestive of atherosclerotic kidney artery stenosis and should be further evaluated.

23. **What is the association between proton pump inhibitors (PPIs) and acute interstitial nephritis (AIN)?**
    The PPIs (i.e., omeprazole and lansoprazole) are fast becoming one of the most common causes of drug-induced AIN. The first documented case was in 1992. Since then, numerous case series with biopsy-proven disease have been published. The interaction appears to be a class effect because all PPIs have been documented to cause AIN. The onset of disease is idiosyncratic in that the development of symptoms has ranged from 1 week to 18 months after drug initiation. PPI-induced AIN generally does not manifest as the typical hypersensitivity reaction. The PPI should be withdrawn upon suspicion of this diagnosis. However, although most patients do recover kidney function, many are left with some level of CKD.

24. **What are the dosing recommendations and indications for use of bisphosphonates in states of kidney injury?**
    In general, most of the data for the use of bisphosphonates in patients with varying degrees of AKI have come from trials looking at treatment of hypercalcemia associated with multiple myeloma and other malignancies. Metabolic changes in bone morphology associated with CKD complicate the definition of osteoporosis and thus the validity of the indication for these therapies in this population (Table 25.4).

Table 25.4. Dosing Recommendations for Bisphosphonates in Kidney Injury

	HYPERCALCEMIA IN ACUTE KIDNEY INJURY	CHRONIC KIDNEY DISEASE STAGES 3–5	HEMODIALYSIS
Pamidronate (Avedia)	OK	Avoid—associated with development of focal segmental glomerulosclerosis	OK—for 1 dose of 30 mg if failing other therapies
Alendronate (Fosamax)	—	Avoid in glomerular filtration rate <30–35	Avoid
Ibandronate (Boniva)	OK		Avoid
Risedronate (Actonel)	—		Avoid
Zoledronic acid (Zometa)	Use with caution	Avoid	Avoid

25. What are the dosing recommendations for enoxaparin and other low-molecular-weight heparin in CKD?
    Enoxaparin dose should be adjusted for the treatment of the most common thrombotic disorders in patient with CKD. For patients with stable estimated GFR less than 30 mL/min, the dose should be adjusted to 1 mg/kg per day and Xa activities should be monitored twice a week initially, then weekly after 2 weeks of treatment. The heparin level should be drawn 4 hours after the dose and the dose should be adjusted to heparin level of 0.7 to 1.1. Unfractionated heparin should be considered the alternative of choice for patients with unstable kidney function or undergoing dialysis (Table 25.5).

26. Discuss the dosing of antigout drugs in adults with CKD.
    Gout is a common inflammatory arthritis disorder in patients with CKD. Although NSAIDs are the drugs of choice for the treatment of acute attack in patients with normal kidney function, NSAIDs should be avoided or used with caution in patients with CKD. Corticosteroids orally, intravenously,

Table 25.5. Dosage Recommendations for Anticoagulations in Chronic Kidney Disease

DRUGS	NORMAL DOSAGE	CKD STAGE 3-5	HD
Alteplase	60 mg over 1 h, then 20 mg/h for 2 h	100%	100%
Anistreplase	30 U over 2–5 min	100%	100%
Apixaban	5 mg po bid	100%	50%
Aspirin	81–325 mg/day	100%	100%
Clopidogrel	75 mg/day	100%	100%
Dabigatran	150 mg po bid	100%	AVOID
Dalteparin	100 U/kg	100%	Avoid Check anti–factor Xa activity 4 h after second dose in patients with kidney dysfunction
Dipyridamole	50 mg tid	100%	100%
Enoxaparin	1 mg/kg q12h	100%	50%
Fondaparinux	2.5–10 mg Subq	100%	Avoid
Heparin	75 U/kg load then 15 U/kg/h	100%	100%
Iloprost	0.5–2.0 ng/kg/min for 5–12 h	100%	100%
Prasugrel	10 mg	100%	100%
Rivaroxaban	20 mg/day	50%–75%	Avoid
Streptokinase	250,000-U load, then 100,000 U/h	100%	100%
Sulfinpyrazone	200 mg bid	100%	100%
Ticlopidine	250 mg bid	100%	100%
Tinzaparin	175 U/kg	100%	Avoid
Tranexamic acid	25 mg/kg tid–qid	50%	25%
Urokinase	4,400-U/kg load, then 4,400 U/kg qh	100%	100%
Warfarin	5 mg per day then adjust per INR	100%	50%–100%

CKD, Chronic kidney disease; HD, hemodialysis; INR, international normalized ratio; U, units.

Table 25.6. Dosage Recommendations for Antigout Drugs in Chronic Kidney Disease

	NORMAL KIDNEY FUNCTION	CKD STAGES 3–5	HEMODIALYSIS
Allopurinol	300–400 mg	25%–50%	25%
Colchicine	1 mg, then 0.5 mg q8h	25%	Avoid
Corticosteroids	40 mg	100%	100%
Febuxostat	40–80 mg/day	100%	NA
Rasburicase	0.15–0.2 mg/kg	100%	100%

CKD, Chronic kidney disease; NA, not applicable.

intra-articularly, or indirectly via adrenocorticotropic hormone can be given safely in this setting. Colchicine also can be used for the treatment of gout flare-up; however, the dose should be adjusted to 0.5 mg orally 2 to 3 times per day for patients with eGFR between 10 and 50 mL/min. Intravenous colchicines is contraindicated in CKD because of the associated risk for multiorgan failure. Recombinant urate oxidase (rasburicase) can be used in patients with hyperuricemia and have failed other standard oral antihyperuricemic drug therapy. No dosage adjustment is required in this setting (Table 25.6).

KEY POINTS

1. Kidney disease alters pharmacokinetic and pharmacodynamic of most commonly used drugs.
2. Pharmacologic agents that could cause hyperkalemia in patients with CKD and undergoing dialysis should be used with caution.
3. Consider a loading dose of antibiotic in the treatment of serious infection and adjust dosage according to kidney function to avoid toxicities.
4. Drug-induced kidney injury should be differentiated from other form of kidney impairment.

BIBLIOGRAPHY

Bakris, G. L. (2012). Lipid disorders in uremia and dialysis. *Contributions to Nephrology, 178,* 100–105.
Bansal, A. D., Hill, C. E., & Berns, J. S. (2015). Use of antiepileptic drugs in patients with chronic kidney disease and end stage renal disease. *Seminar in Dialysis, 28*(4), 404–412.
Corsonello, A., Onder, G., Bustacchini, S., Provinciali, M., Garasto, S., Gareri, P., & Lattanzio, F. (2012). Estimating renal function to reduce the risk of adverse drug reactions. *Drug Safety, 35*(Suppl. 1), 47–54.
Helou, R. (2010). Should we continue to use the Cockcroft-Gault formula? Nephron. *Clinical Practice, 116*(3), c172–c185.
Hudson, J. Q., & Nyman, H. A. (2011). Use of estimated glomerular filtration rate for drug dosing in the chronic kidney disease patient. *Current Opinion in Nephrology and Hypertension, 20*(5), 482–491.
Judd, E., & Calhoun, D. A. (2015). Management of hypertension in CKD: Beyond the guidelines. *Advances in Chronic Kidney Disease, 22*(2), 116–122.
Khanal, A., Peterson, G. M., Jose, M. D., & Castelino, R. L. (2017). Comparison of equations for dosing of medications in renal impairment. *Nephrology (Carlton), 22*(6), 470–477.
Levey, A. S., & Inker, L. A. (2017). Assessment of glomerular filtration rate in health and disease: A state of the art review. *Clinical Pharmacology and Therapeutics, 102*(3), 405–419.
Lutz, J., Jurk, K., & Schinzel, H. (2017). Direct oral anticoagulants in patients with chronic kidney disease: Patient selection and special considerations. *International Journal of Nephrology and Renovascular Disease, 10,* 135–143.
MacCallum, L. (2014). Optimal medication dosing in patients with diabetes mellitus and chronic kidney disease. *Canadian Journal of Diabetes, 38*(5), 334–343.
Miller, K., & Miller, E. M. (2015). Hot topics in primary care: Role of the kidney and SGLT-2 inhibition in type 2 diabetes mellitus. *Journal of Family Practice, 64*(Suppl. 12), S54–S58.
Momper, J. D., Venkataramanan, R., & Nolin, T. D. (2010). Nonrenal drug clearance in CKD: Searching for the path less traveled. *Advances in Chronic Kidney Disease, 17*(5), 384–391.
Nolin, T. D. (2015). A synopsis of clinical pharmacokinetic alterations in advanced CKD. *Seminars in Dialysis, 28*(4), 325–329.

Offurum, A., Wagner, L. A., & Gooden T. (2016). Adverse safety events in patients with Chronic Kidney Disease (CKD). *Expert Opinion on Drug Safety, 15*(12), 1597–1607.

Philips, B. J., Lane, K., Dixon, J., & Macphee, I. (2014). The effects of acute renal failure on drug metabolism. *Expert Opinion on Drug Metabolism and Toxicology, 10*(1), 11–23.

Saltiel, M. (2010). Dosing low molecular weight heparins in kidney disease. *Journal of Pharmacy Practice, 23*(3), 205–209.

Tortorici, M. A., Cutler, D. L., Hazra, A., Nolin, T. D., Rowland-Yeo, K., & Venkatakrishnan, K. (2015). Emerging areas of research in the assessment of pharmacokinetics in patients with chronic kidney disease. *Journal of Clinical Pharmacology, 55*(3), 241–250.

Vellanki, K., & Bansal, V. K. (2015). Neurologic complications of chronic kidney disease. *Current Neurology and Neuroscience Reports, 15*(8), 50.

IV
PRIMARY GLOMERULAR DISORDERS

CHAPTER 26

MINIMAL CHANGE DISEASE

Elaine S. Kamil

1. **What are the diagnostic criteria for nephrotic syndrome?**
   Nephrotic syndrome is a syndrome that results from severe proteinuria. Heavy glomerular protein losses (≥ 3.5 g in an adult or >40 mg/m^2 per hour in a child) lead to the other three criteria for nephrotic syndrome: hypoalbuminemia, hyperlipidemia, and edema. From a practical standpoint, measuring a urine total protein-to-creatinine ratio is preferable to collecting a 24-hour urine for protein. A ratio of ≥ 3.5 correlates with nephrotic-range proteinuria.

2. **What is minimal change disease (MCD; minimal change nephrotic syndrome)?**
   MCD is a disorder of glomeruli that leads to heavy proteinuria. Kidney biopsy shows normal glomeruli by light microscopy but shows effacement of the podocyte foot processes on electron microscopy. Immunofluorescent microscopy typically is negative, although some patients may show staining for immunoglobulin M (IgM) in the mesangial regions of the glomeruli. Technically, a patient cannot be said to have MCD with certainty without a kidney biopsy. However, so many young children with nephrotic syndrome have MCD that kidney biopsies are performed only in children with atypical findings or after failure of a trial of glucocorticoids. Older adolescents and adults are diagnosed with MCD after a kidney biopsy is performed.

3. **How likely is MCD to be the cause of nephrotic syndrome in any individual?**
   MCD is the cause of nephrotic syndrome in approximately 90% of children younger than age 6, in approximately 65% of older children, and in approximately 20% to 30% of adolescents. In adults with primary glomerular diseases, only 10% to 25% of nephrotic syndrome results from MCD, which puts it third after membranous nephropathy and focal, segmental glomerulosclerosis.

4. **What causes MCD?**
   MCD is an immune-mediated disease, thought to be due to a circulating factor capable of inducing proteinuria. Presumably the circulating factor is secreted by lymphoid cells and functions as a vascular permeability factor and directly affects podocyte function. Although most cases are idiopathic, MCD, particularly in adults, may be associated with neoplastic disease such as lymphoma, toxic or allergic reactions to drugs, certain infections, allergies, or other autoimmune disorders.

5. **How common is MCD?**
   The prevalence of MCD in children is approximately 16 per 100,000, but it is much less prevalent in adults.

6. **What is the typical clinical presentation of MCD?**
   Patients with MCD typically present with mild to severe edema. Because the onset with periorbital edema commonly follows an upper respiratory infection in young children, nephrotic syndrome may sometimes be confused with an allergic reaction until a more thorough evaluation is performed. In the youngest children, there is a 2:1 male to female prevalence, but by adolescence and beyond males and females are equally affected. Other symptoms can include abdominal pain, diarrhea, poor appetite, and decreased urine output. Rarely, a patient may present with sepsis.

7. **How is MCD diagnosed?**
   MCD presents with nephrotic syndrome. However, the child who presents with typical features (see question 1) of nephrotic syndrome is presumed to have MCD and does not undergo a kidney biopsy unless there are unusual factors such as resistance to prednisone therapy, hypertension, decreased kidney function, or hypocomplementemia.

8. **What is the standard initial therapy for MCD in children?**
   The cornerstone of therapy of typical nephrotic syndrome in young children is high-dose glucocorticoids. Children treated with a longer initial course of prednisone may be less likely to experience frequent relapses than those children treated with a more abbreviated course of steroid therapy. Children older than 4 years of age are treated with 60 mg/m^2 daily given early in the morning for 6 weeks followed by

40 mg/m^2 every other morning for an additional 6 weeks. Children younger than age 4 receive the same initial 6-week course of daily prednisone but then should receive a slower taper of 60 mg/m^2 every other morning for 4 weeks, tapering further by 10 mg/m^2 every 4 weeks for an additional 20 weeks. Approximately 95% of young children will experience a complete remission of the nephrotic syndrome within 4 weeks; 75% will respond within 2 weeks.

9. What is the standard initial therapy for MCD in adults?

   Prednisone is also the standard initial therapy for adults with MCD. Adults with MCD tend to require a longer course of prednisone before remission is attained. The optimal initial prednisone regimen varies somewhat among nephrologists, but typically a single morning dose of 1 mg/kg per day, maximum of 80 mg, is continued for a minimum of 8 weeks. For patients not in remission at 8 weeks, daily prednisone may be continued for another 2 months until remission is attained. A gradual taper is then recommended on an every-other-day schedule until the patient is tapered off over many months. The slow taper is recommended to sustain the remission and to reduce the likelihood of problems with adrenal insufficiency.

10. How do you define remission in nephrotic syndrome?

    Typically, patients with nephrotic syndrome are taught to monitor their urine protein at home using dipsticks. A complete remission is defined in children as a urine dipstick of trace to negative or a urine protein/creatinine ratio of <0.2. In adults, a complete remission is defined as a reduction of proteinuria to ≤300 mg of urinary protein in a 24-hour period; however, a urine protein-to-creatinine ratio of <0.2 is also an appropriate benchmark for adults. A partial remission is defined as a ≥50% reduction in 24-hour protein or a 24-hour urine protein of <3.5 g with a normal serum albumin. Patients with MCD almost always experience a complete, as opposed to a partial, remission. Normalization of serum albumin quickly follows the reduction in proteinuria, but hyperlipidemia may take several months to resolve.

11. What other supportive therapies are useful for MCD?

    A no-added-salt diet is always recommended for patients with MCD—it will reduce edema and the tendency to develop hypertension. In addition, angiotensin-converting enzyme (ACE) inhibitors and/or angiotensin receptor blockers (ARBs) are useful in ameliorating proteinuria and are the first choice for the treatment of hypertension in these patients. Oral diuretics may be used with caution in patients with moderate edema. For those patients with severe edema accompanied by ascites, scrotal or labial edema, and/or pleural effusions, intravenous infusions of 25% salt-poor albumin may be helpful. A dose of 1 g/kg, up to a maximum of 50 g, is infused over 2 to 4 hours once or twice a day, followed by intravenous furosemide at a dose of 1 mg/kg. Caution must be observed in the patient with oliguria because that patient could have acute kidney injury, making him or her unresponsive to the diuretic and susceptible to mobilization of peripheral edema, leading to the risk of pulmonary edema with respiratory compromise.

12. What is the typical course for a patient with MCD?

    Most children (60% to 75%) with MCD experience relapses of the disease, and sometimes they are frequent—three or more relapses per year. Relapses tend to be precipitated by infections, particularly upper respiratory infections, or allergies. Approximately 50% to 75% of adults who respond to steroids will have a relapse, and 10% to 25% become frequent relapsers. A minority of patients develop steroid dependence of variable severity where the patient cannot be tapered off the prednisone. The steroid dependence can vary from being maintained in remission on low-dose, alternate-day steroids to requiring high-dose, daily steroids to maintain a remission.

13. How are relapses of MCD treated?

    Relapses of MCD are treated with the same initial doses of corticosteroids as the initial episode of nephrotic syndrome but for a more abbreviated course, at least in children. Children are treated with daily steroids until the urine is negative for protein for 3 days. The prednisone dose is then lowered to 40 mg/m^2 every other morning for 4 weeks with either a rapid taper over 2 months or a slow taper over 6 to 12 months. The rapidity of the taper is usually based on the patient's prior response to tapering. Adults who relapse are also re-treated with a regimen similar to the initial corticosteroid protocol outlined previously.

14. If the patient responds to steroids but develops steroid toxicity or steroid dependence, what other treatment options are there?

    Several treatment options are available for the child or adult with steroid toxicity or steroid dependence, each with its own unique risk-benefit profile. The goal of therapy for these patients is to avoid the complications of nephrotic syndrome (see question 16) by maintaining remission while minimizing the toxicities of therapy. The first therapy used for these patients is alternate-day prednisone therapy, tapered slowly to the lowest dose that will maintain a remission. If that fails, other options include 12-week courses of oral cyclophosphamide (or chlorambucil), longer courses (1 to 2 years) of cyclosporine, mycophenolate mofetil, azathioprine, tacrolimus, or levamisole. These medications should only be prescribed by physicians who are familiar with their toxicities.

15. **If the patient is steroid resistant, what are the treatment options?**
The patient who is steroid resistant should have a kidney biopsy if one has not yet been performed. The biopsy may show focal, segmental glomerulosclerosis; MCD; or membranous nephropathy. Treatment options include a course of high-dose intravenous methylprednisolone, oral cyclosporine, or tacrolimus. Mycophenolate mofetil may also be tried. Some newer reports have shown some promise with rituximab, a CD20 monoclonal antibody, but those reports are still preliminary.

16. **What are the complications of MCD?**
The complications of MCD are those of nephrotic syndrome or are related to the toxicities of the treatments used. For the patient with frequent relapses, there is a delicate trade-off between the complications of the disease and the side effects of the medications. MCD may have life-threatening complications. These include the risks of overwhelming infection, thromboembolic phenomenon, and the cardiovascular complications related to hyperlipidemia. The cause of the increased risk of infection is multifactorial but is in part related to loss of opsonizing factors in the urine. Opsonizing factors are particularly important in defense against encapsulated bacteria such as *Pneumococcus* and *Haemophilus influenzae*. Another risk factor for infection in the patient with MCD is the frequent occurrence of hypogammaglobulinemia in these patients, especially during episodes of relapse. There is an increased risk of serious bacterial infections when the plasma IgG levels fall to less than 400 mg/dL and a very increased risk when levels fall to less than 200 mg/dL. In a patient with low IgG levels and sepsis, or in those patients with chronic hypogammaglobulinemia, intravenous gamma globulin may be used.

Thromboembolism may be seen in patients with MCD, more commonly in the adult with MCD than in the child with MCD. Children are more prone to sagittal sinus thrombosis, pulmonary artery thrombosis, or inferior vena caval thrombosis, whereas adults with MCD are more prone to deep vein or renal vein thrombosis. The hypercoagulable state in MCD results from several factors, including increased clotting factor synthesis (fibrinogen, II, V, VII, IX, X, XIII), urinary losses of anticoagulants (antithrombin III), platelet abnormalities (thrombocytosis, increased aggregability), hyperviscosity, and hyperlipidemia.

Patients in a severe relapse have an increased risk of developing acute kidney injury secondary to decreased kidney perfusion and edema of the kidney interstitium. Acute kidney injury is usually reversible in this setting. Intravenous albumin therapy should not be given during an episode of acute kidney injury because of the risk of pulmonary edema.

Chronic hyperlipidemia in the patient with MCD can lead to the accelerated development of arteriosclerosis.

17. **What steps can be taken to reduce the complications of MCD?**
The complications of nephrotic syndrome can be avoided by keeping the patient in remission whenever possible. The risk of some of the infectious complications can be avoided by making sure that patients receive vaccines against all infectious agents that can cause life-threatening infections. All adults and children older than 2 years of age should receive the 23-valent pneumococcal vaccine. All patients with MCD should receive yearly influenza vaccines. Children should receive their childhood vaccines with deferral of live virus vaccines (measles, mumps, and rubella; varicella) until they are in remission off of immunosuppressive medications. The administration of live virus vaccine may be associated with a relapse, but that risk is minimal when compared with the risk of vaccine-preventable disease. Adults and children with MCD should also have the status of their immunity against varicella determined by checking a varicella-zoster IgG titer. Varicella infections in individuals who are immune compromised, including those individuals taking prednisone, may be fatal. If the patient does not have a protective titer against varicella, vaccine should be given if possible. If the patient cannot receive vaccine because of continued immunosuppression, varicella-zoster immune globulin should be administered as soon as possible after exposure to an individual with chicken pox. If a patient who is immunosuppressed develops chicken pox or zoster, he or she should receive immediate treatment with intravenous acyclovir.

A reduction in thromboembolic complications can be attempted by being vigilant for situations in which thromboembolism is more of a risk, particularly protecting the intravascular volume of a critically ill patient in relapse. Central venous catheters should be avoided whenever possible in this patient population. If a patient experiences a thromboembolic event, treatment should include heparin or low-molecular-weight heparin, followed by warfarin for 6 months. Prophylactic anticoagulation therapy should be administered for future relapses in these patients.

Chronic hyperlipidemia, if present, warrants therapy in adults; there are little data on its use in children at this point and should only be considered in children who are chronically hyperlipidemic. Hypertension is best treated initially with an ACE inhibitor and/or an ARB, which should help reduce the risk of cardiovascular complications later.

18. **What is the prognosis for a patient with MCD?**
The vast majority of children with MCD have a favorable prognosis. In children, a prompt remission within 7 to 9 days of steroid therapy, the absence of microhematuria, and age greater than 4 years at presentation predict fewer relapses. By 10 years from diagnosis, only 16% of children with MCD are still experiencing relapses. Many children will "outgrow" their disease by or during adolescence, although some continue to experience relapses into adulthood. The long-term cardiovascular risk in children with MCD who have experienced long periods of steroid therapy and periods of hyperlipidemia and hypertension is largely unknown. In adults with MCD the most important prognostic factor is the patient's initial response to steroid therapy and whether he or she can experience extended periods of time off steroids, which carry a more serious toxicity profile in adults.

KEY POINTS

1. Minimal change disease (MCD) is the cause of nephrotic syndrome in approximately 90% of children younger than age 6, in approximately 65% of older children, and in approximately 20% to 30% of adolescents. In adults, only approximately 10% to 25% of nephrotic syndrome results from MCD, but it represents the third most common cause of nephrotic syndrome in adults after membranous nephropathy and focal, segmental glomerulosclerosis.
2. MCD is an immune-mediated disease, thought to be mediated by a circulating factor capable of inducing proteinuria. Presumably the circulating factor is secreted by lymphoid cells and functions as a vascular permeability factor that directly affects the function of the podocytes.
3. Patients with MCD typically present with mild to severe edema. Because the onset with periorbital edema commonly follows an upper respiratory infection in young children, nephrotic syndrome may sometimes be confused with an allergic reaction until a more thorough evaluation is performed.
4. The cornerstone of therapy of typical nephrotic syndrome in young children is high-dose glucocorticoids. Children treated with a longer initial course of prednisone are less likely to experience frequent relapses than those children treated with a more abbreviated course of steroid therapy. Prednisone is also the standard initial therapy for adults with MCD. Adults with MCD tend to require a longer course of prednisone before remission is attained.
5. The vast majority of children with MCD have a very favorable prognosis. In children a prompt remission within 7 to 9 days of steroid therapy, the absence of microhematuria, and age greater than 4 years at presentation predict fewer relapses.

BIBLIOGRAPHY

Brenchley, P. E. (2003). Vascular permeability factors in steroid-sensitive nephrotic syndrome and focal segmental glomerulosclerosis. *Nephrology, Dialysis, Transplantation, 18*(Suppl. 6), vi21–vi25.

Filler, G. (2003). Treatment of nephrotic syndrome in children and controlled trials. *Nephrology, Dialysis, Transplantation, 18*(Suppl. 6), vi75–vi78.

Gipson, D. S., Massengill, S. F., Yao, L., Nagaraj, S., Smoyer, W. E., Mahan, J. D., . . . Greenbaum, L. A. (2009). Management of childhood onset nephrotic syndrome. *Pediatrics, 124*(2), 747–757.

Glassock, R. J. (2003). Secondary minimal change disease. *Nephrology, Dialysis, Transplantation, 18*(Suppl. 6), vi52–vi58.

Hodson, E. M., Habashy, D., & Craig, J. C. (2006). Interventions for idiopathic steroid-resistant nephrotic syndrome in children. *Cochrane Database of Systematic Reviews*, (2), CD003594.

Hodson, E. M., Willis, N. S., & Craig, J. C. (2007). Corticosteroid therapy for nephrotic syndrome in children. *Cochrane Database of Systematic Reviews*, (4), CD001533.

Hogg, R. J., Portman, R. J., Milliner, D., Lemley, K. V., Eddy, A., & Ingelfinger, J. (2000). Evaluation and management of proteinuria and nephrotic syndrome in children: Recommendations from a pediatric nephrology panel established at the National Kidney Foundation Conference on Proteinuria, Albuminuria, Risk Assessment, Detection, and Elimination (PARADE). *Pediatrics, 105*, 1242–1249.

Kamil, E. S. (2009). Minimal change disease. In E. V. Lerma, J. S. Berns, & A. R. Nissenson (Eds.), *Current diagnosis and treatment nephrology and hypertension* (pp. 217–221). New York: McGraw-Hill Company.

Kyrieleis, H. A., Löwik, M. M., Pronk, I., Cruysberg, H. R., Kremer, J. A., Oyen, W. J., . . . Levtchenko, E. N. (2009). Long-term outcome of biopsy-proven, frequently relapsing minimal change nephrotic syndrome in children. *Clinical Journal of the American Society of Nephrology, 4*(10), 1593–1600.

Mathieson, P. W. (2003). Immune dysregulation in minimal change nephropathy. *Nephrology, Dialysis, Transplantation, 18*(Suppl. 6), vi26–vi29.

Nakayama, M., Katafuchi, R., Yanase, T., Ikeda, K., Tanaka, H., & Fujimi, S. (2002). Steroid responsiveness and frequency of relapse in adult-onset minimal change nephrotic syndrome. *American Journal of Kidney Diseases, 39*, 503–512.

Palmer, S. C., Nand, K., & Strippoli, G. F. (2008). Interventions for minimal change disease in adults with nephrotic syndrome. *Cochrane Database of Systematic Reviews*, (1), CD001537.

Tse, K. C., Lam, M. F., Yip, P. S., Li, F. K., Choy, B. Y., Lai, K. N., & Chan, T. M. (2003). Idiopathic minimal change nephrotic syndrome in older adults: Steroid responsiveness and pattern of relapses. *Nephrology, Dialysis, Transplantation, 18*, 1316.

Vivarelli, M., Massella, L., Ruggiero, B., et al. (2017). Minimal change disease. *Clin J Am Soc Nephrol 12*(2), 332–345.

CHAPTER 27

FOCAL SEGMENTAL GLOMERULOSCLEROSIS

Patrick E. Gipson and Debbie S. Gipson

1. **What is focal segmental glomerulosclerosis?**

   Focal segmental glomerulosclerosis (FSGS) is a class of glomerular diseases defined by focal and segmental patterns of scar in the kidney glomeruli. This disease spectrum includes primary, genetic, and secondary diseases. Primary FSGS is diagnosed in patients without a known cause. There are a number of genetic mutations that disrupt the structure and function of the glomerular podocyte and slit diaphragm that manifest as FSGS. Secondary FSGS may arise from various kidney insults that lead to a common end point of glomerular damage. These secondary insults include:

   - Viral infection: HIV, parvovirus
   - Drugs: heroin, pamidronate
   - Postinflammatory conditions: autoimmune diseases
   - Vascular issues: atheroembolic disease, hypertension, sickle cell disease
   - Reflux nephropathy

     The sclerosing type of C1q nephropathy may be grouped with primary or secondary FSGS with the distinguishing factor of C1q in the glomeruli revealed on kidney biopsy immunofluorescence staining and electron dense deposits with electron microscopy. The etiology of C1q nephropathy is unknown. Obesity-related glomerulopathy is also often considered a secondary FSGS that manifests with glomerular hypertrophy in addition to the sclerosis of FSGS. The common factor in these conditions is damage to the glomerular structure.

2. **How common is FSGS?**

   FSGS is a rare condition with an estimated incidence of 1.8/100,000 per year. The lifetime risk is estimated to be more than four times higher for African Americans compared with other races. FSGS is the underlying cause of approximately 4% of patients with end-stage kidney disease (ESKD) in the United States and up to 10.8% of those younger than 24 years. In adults, FSGS is the fourth most common cause of ESKD, following diabetes, hypertension, and glomerulonephritis not otherwise specified. Among children, FSGS is the second leading cause of ESKD, following congenital kidney anomalies.

3. **What is the clinical presentation of FSGS?**

   FSGS may present as nephrotic syndrome with edema, hypoalbuminemia, and hypercholesterolemia, or it may present in a patient with isolated proteinuria. Microscopic hematuria is found in approximately half of patients at diagnosis. However, gross hematuria is rare. Children are more likely to present with nephrotic syndrome, but the entire phenotypic spectrum of FSGS occurs in both children and adults. Kidney function as assessed by glomerular filtration rate may be normal but is impaired in up to 60% at presentation. ESKD at presentation is rare.

   Clinical clues may help distinguish whether a patient has primary or secondary FSGS. Patients with primary FSGS more often have low serum albumin levels (<3 g/dL) and edema, whereas patients with secondary FSGS more often present with albumin levels >3.5 g/dL, without edema, and with some historical evidence of a predisposing primary condition or exposure.

4. **What is the cause of primary FSGS?**

   There are likely several causes of primary FSGS. Research has focused on possible immune defects, such as T-cell dysregulation, and the presence of a circulating permeability factor, such as cardiotrophin-like cytokine 1, that induces changes in the glomerular filtration barrier with resultant proteinuria. Genetic and gene expression studies have identified structural abnormalities in the podocyte cytoskeleton and slit diaphragms, as well as signaling and inflammatory pathways that contribute to the cause of FSGS.

5. **What genetic defects lead to sporadic and familial FSGS?**

   Over the past decade, much of the biology of the glomerular filtration barrier has been explained and defects in multiple structural and functional components of this barrier have been implicated in FSGS.

There are more than 50 genetic mutations associated with FSGS. Mutations may occur in podocyte structural components from genes such as NPHS2 (podocin), NPHS1 (nephrin), ACTN4 (alpha-actinin 4), TRPC6, alpha-5, beta-4 integrins, CD2AP may present as kidney-limited structural anomalies. Mutations in WT1, LAMB2, COQ2, and LMX1B have been identified as causative of syndromic conditions in which FSGS in only one of the multiple anomaly manifestations within an individual. Autosomal dominant inheritance patterns are documented in familial FSGS with ACTN4, TRPC6, and INF2, which were first implicated in adult-onset disease. Familial FSGS of childhood with NPHS1, NPHS2, and PLCE1 mutations are transmitted in an autosomal recessive pattern. Autosomal recessive and dominant inheritance patterns have been documented with child- and adult-onset FSGS (Table 27.1).

The prevalence of specific gene mutations in patients with FSGS depends on the ancestry of the cohort being studied. For example, NPHS2 mutations are found in 26% of children from families of Eastern European and Middle Eastern descent with familial FSGS and 19% of sporadic cases in that population. These mutations are rare causes of FSGS in Asian, African-American, and European-American populations of the United States. Apolipoprotein L1 (APOL1) has alleles that increase the risk of FSGS. These risk alleles are found in African Americans of west African descent. APOL1 polymorphisms convey protection against *Trypanosoma brucei*.

Table 27.1. List of Genes Implicated in Familial Focal Segmental Glomerulosclerosis

GENE	PHENOTYPE
Autosomal Recessive	
NPHS1 (Nephrin)	FSGS; Congenital Nephrotic Syndrome
NPHS2 (Podocin)	FSGS; Congenital Nephrotic Syndrome
NPHS3 (PLCE1)	FSGS; Diffuse Mesangial Sclerosis
LAMB2	FSGS; Pierson Syndrome
MYH9	FSGS; Sensorineural Deafness; Macrothrombocytopenia; Epstein, Fechtner & Sebastian Syndromes
MYOE1	FSGS
ADCK4	FSGS
SGPL1	FSGS; Adrenal Insufficiency; Ichthyosis; Acanthosis; Immunodeficiency
COQ6	FSGS; Diffuse Mesangial Sclerosis; Sensorineural Deafness; Neurologic abnormalities
WDR73	FSGS; Galloway-Mowat Syndrome
NUP93	FSGS
NUP205	FSGS
Autosomal Dominant	
ACTN4	FSGS
ANLN	FSGS
ARHGAP24	FSGS
CD2AP	FSGS
TRPC6	FSGS
INF2	FSGS; Charcot-Marie-Tooth Disease
LMX1B	FSGS; Nail-Patella Syndrome
PAX2	FSGS; Papillorenal Syndrome
WT1	FSGS; Denys–Drash, WAGR & Frasier Syndrome

FSGS, Focal segmental glomerulosclerosis.

Genotype/phenotype correlations are still being investigated and have not yet reached the point of guiding clinical care with a few notable exceptions:
- Genetic testing of patients with FSGS may be considered during the assessment of infantile FSGS
- FSGS that is part of a multiple congenital anomaly syndrome
- Familial FSGS, in regions with a high prevalence of consanguinity
- In some cases, prior to kidney transplantation to assess the risk of FSGS recurrence

6. How is FSGS diagnosed?

A kidney biopsy is required to establish the diagnosis of FSGS. Patients presenting with sustained proteinuria, whether nephrotic (>3 g/day) or subnephrotic, will typically be evaluated for secondary forms of glomerular disease, including screens for systemic illnesses that may have a kidney component. Hepatitis B and C and HIV should be excluded by serology. Antinuclear antibody level should be obtained to screen for systemic lupus erythematosus (SLE). Complement C3 levels may be low in membranoproliferative glomerulonephritis, SLE, and postinfectious glomerulonephritis. In appropriate-age adults, urine and protein electrophoresis and/or serum free light-chain measurements should be obtained to evaluate for paraproteinemias.

Unfortunately, urine or blood biomarkers have not yet been developed and validated to support the diagnosis or prognosis of FSGS in clinical contexts. Biomarkers are being evaluated, but they must survive validation and independent replication, steps that have repeatedly flummoxed previous promising candidates.

7. What are the pathologic findings in FSGS?

As noted by its descriptive name, FSGS initially is characterized by sclerotic lesions restricted to a segment of a subset (focal) of the glomeruli. Electron microscopy may confirm these changes and show widespread foot process effacement. There are some pathology clues that suggest the FSGS is secondary rather than primary:
- Less diffuse foot process effacement
- Foot process width may be normal
- Glomeruli may be enlarged (glomerulomegaly)

However, pathology alone cannot distinguish between the three categories of FSGS: primary, genetic, or secondary. There are a few exceptions:
- Immunoglobulin A (IgA) nephropathy as a secondary cause of FSGS has IgA deposits identifiable by immunofluorescence
- Obesity-related glomerulopathy and FSGS secondary to cyanotic congenital heart disease often have enlarged glomeruli in addition to the typical glomerular fibrosis

As the disease progresses, involvement of more glomeruli and sclerosis of entire glomeruli may occur. Interstitial fibrosis with tubular atrophy is a frequent finding. No significant immunoglobulin deposits are found in cases of primary FSGS, and their presence suggests an alternative etiology or, at low amounts, trapping of immunoglobulin that is not pathogenic.

8. Does histopathology predict prognosis?

FSGS is diagnosed through findings on the kidney biopsy. The glomerular scarring pattern has been classified as five variants of FSGS based solely on histologic description:
- Collapsing
- Tip
- Cellular
- Perihilar
- FSGS not otherwise specified.

These variants are defined by the location and type of glomerular scars. Unfortunately, FSGS variant assignment can be inconsistent between pathologists, and patient response to therapy is variable within groups of patients defined by FSGS pathology variants. Collapsing FSGS appears to represent a particularly virulent form of FSGS, and overall progression to ESKD is more rapid when compared with groups of FSGS patients with other variants. Increased tubular atrophy and interstitial scarring portend worse prognosis.

9. What is the clinical course of FSGS?

Primary FSGS has a variable course. Clinical factors such as the degree of proteinuria at disease presentation, the amount of interstitial fibrosis and tubular atrophy noted on kidney biopsy, proteinuria reduction in response to therapy, and collapsing histologic variant are considered prognostic factors for kidney survival. Spontaneous remission is reported in less than 5% of patients with primary FSGS. Therapy may result in complete proteinuria remission (normal urinary protein excretion), partial remission, or resistance to therapy. Patients with complete remission have an expected 90% 10-year kidney survival. For patients with proteinuria in the nephrotic range that is resistant to treatment, the 10-year kidney survival is approximately 50%. Patients with partial proteinuria remission have intermediate 10-year kidney survival. Patients with high-risk APOL1 genotype have a poorer kidney survival relative to low-risk genotype. As in many kidney diseases, patients who present with an elevated serum creatinine have a poorer prognosis.

10. **What therapies are indicated for primary FSGS?**
Angiotensin-converting enzyme (ACE) inhibitor/angiotensin receptor blocker (ARB) therapy has been shown to be beneficial in reducing proteinuria and slowing the decline in kidney function in proteinuric kidney diseases. There is only one randomized controlled trial of ACE therapy in adults with FSGS and one in children with steroid-resistant nephrotic syndrome. These studies document a reduction in urinary protein excretion by approximately 30%. Long-term data to assess a benefit in preventing a decline in kidney function are not available. Regardless, ACE inhibitor/ARB therapy is considered standard care for proteinuria control and hypertension management.
    Therapy targeted at a presumed immunologic basis of FSGS has been used clinically and in controlled and uncontrolled trials. Corticosteroids induce remission in 20% to 30% of patients. Treatment may begin with daily dosing and then progress to alternate-day therapy for primary FSGS. The duration of treatment may affect response to therapy with a typical initial course up to 3 months in children and 6 months in adults. A summary of common therapies is presented in the Fig. 27.1.
    Cyclosporine, tacrolimus, and mycophenolate mofetil have been reported to be effective in case reports. In a few small, randomized trials, calcineurin inhibitors, cyclosporine and tacrolimus, show combined complete and partial remission rates of 50% to 60% in primary FSGS. Mycophenolate appears to be less effective, with a combined complete and partial remission rate of approximately 33%. However, mycophenolate has less kidney toxicity than calcineurin inhibitors.
    There are several case reports and small case series of other therapeutic agents. Rituximab, a CD20 monoclonal antibody, adalimumab, a tumor necrosis factor (TNF) inhibitor, adrenocorticotropin hormone with potential action through corticosteroid-associated avenues, as well as melanocortin receptor agonism, and perfenidone as an antifibrotic agent have all been used in the treatment of FSGS.
    Plasmapheresis can be used to treat FSGS recurrence after kidney transplant. The mechanism of action is postulated to be removal of circulating factors that increase glomerular permeability.
    Therapy for dyslipidemia is also a component of standard therapy in patients with nephrotic syndrome, with a goal to improve nephrotic syndrome–associated dyslipidemia.
    Diuretics are indicated for control of edema in patients with nephrotic syndrome. Intravenous albumin infusion with diuretic therapy may be beneficial to control severe edema in select patients with nephrotic syndrome, but it has not been shown to have significant additive benefit in controlled trials and carries with it the risk of pulmonary edema and hypertensive crisis.

11. **What are the therapeutic options for secondary forms of FSGS?**
Treatment of the secondary forms of FSGS is directed at the underlying disease. Resolution of FSGS manifestations can occur with weight loss in obesity-related glomerulopathy and following heart transplantation in cyanotic heart disease–associated FSGS. Mitochondrial dysfunction in animal models of obesity-related glomerulopathy is modifiable by mitochondrial-targeted antioxidants. Human investigations are needed to assess whether these findings can be translated to humans safely and effectively. In addition, therapies such as ACE inhibitors, ARBs, and lipid-lowering agents may be prescribed with a goal of reducing proteinuria, controlling blood pressure, and minimizing further cardiovascular or kidney insults.

12. **Should those with FSGS be on a special diet?**
Low-protein diets may reduce proteinuria and slow the progression of proteinuric kidney disease. This was studied and failed in multiple, large, randomized controlled trials. If this is going to be attempted, special concern should be given to children, especially if they have profound proteinuria, to avoid protein malnutrition. All patients should be on low-salt diets to help with hypertension and edema and maximize the effectiveness of angiotensin converting enzyme inhibitor (ACEi) and angiotensin receptor blocker (ARB).

13. **What is the role of the primary care physician in a patient with FSGS?**
Primary care physicians have an important role monitoring and maintaining therapy for hypertension, hyperlipidemia, and edema. They also should be aware of and monitor for other complications of

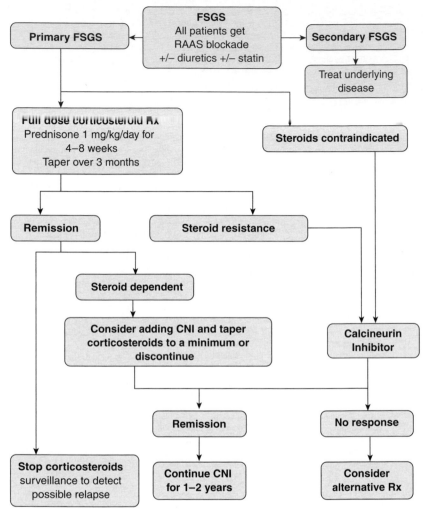

Figure 27.1.   Treatment algorithm for primary focal segmental glomerulosclerosis (FSGS). *CNI,* Calcineurin inhibitor; *RAAS,* renin angiotensin aldosterone system.

FSGS, including peritonitis, thromboembolism, and side effects of immunosuppressive therapy. Maintenance of appropriate immunizations is important, especially 23-valent pneumococcal and influenza. Before using live virus vaccines, doctors should consult the national vaccination guidelines for special populations.

14. Are there special issues in patients with FSGS with respect to kidney transplantation?
    Primary FSGS recurs in 10% of initial kidney allografts. Proteinuria may develop within minutes of allograft implantation. In this setting, circulating factors in the recipient cause acute glomerular capillary permeability, podocyte foot process effacement, and subsequent glomerulosclerosis. If uncontrolled, recurrent FSGS reduces allograft survival. Patients with a history of rapid FSGS recurrence have a very high risk for FSGS recurrence in subsequent kidney transplants.
        Patients with FSGS may receive an allograft from either deceased donors or living related donors. Concerns about using that living related donors may have increased risk of recurrence have not born out.

Plasmapheresis can be used in the immediate pretransplant and posttransplant period in an attempt to remove the substances responsible for inducing proteinuria and recurrent FSGS. Rituximab has been used in the setting of posttransplant FSGS recurrence. These approaches have not been evaluated in randomized studies, but case series suggest they may be helpful in preventing and treating early FSGS recurrence. However, the addition of these therapies to standard kidney transplant induction immunosuppression leads to profound immunocompromised state increasing the risk for life-threatening infections.

KEY POINTS

1. FSGS represents a spectrum of primary, genetic, and secondary diseases that manifest with characteristic glomerular scaring and proteinuria.
2. FSGS is more common in African Americans, mostly due to a high-risk APOL1 genotype in individuals of African ancestry.
3. Proteinuria is the common clinical laboratory manifestation of FSGS and may be accompanied by edema, reduced glomerular filtration rate, and hypertension.
4. Mutations in multiple genes that direct the structure and function of the podocyte and slit diaphragm have been implicated in familial and sporadic FSGS.
5. Primary FSGS recurs in 10% of initial kidney allografts and increases the risk for allograft failure.

BIBLIOGRAPHY

Bierzynska, A., McCarthy, H. J., Soderquest, K., Sen, E. S., Colby, E., Ding, W. Y., . . . Saleem, M. A. (2017). Genomic and clinical profiling of a national nephrotic syndrome cohort advocates a precision medicine approach to disease management. *Kidney International, 91*(4), 937–947.
D'Agati, V. D., Kaskel, F. J., & Falk, R. J. (2011). Focal segmental glomerulosclerosis. *New England Journal of Medicine, 365*(25), 2398–2411. doi:10.1056/NEJMra1106556. Review. PMID:22187987.
Francis, A., Trnka, P., & McTaggart, S. J. (2016). Long-term outcome of kidney transplantation in recipients with focal segmental glomerulsclerosis. *Clinical Journal of the American Society of Nephrology, 11*(11), 2041–2046. PMID:27797890.
Hickson, L. J., Gera, M., Amer, H., Iqbal, C. W., Moore, T. B, Milliner, D. S., . . . Griffin, M. D. (2009). Kidney transplantation for primary focal segmental glomerulosclerosis: Outcomes and response to therapy for recurrence. *Transplantation, 87,* 1232–1239.
Kidney Disease: Improving Global Outcomes (KDIGO) Glomerulonephritis Work Group. (2012). KDIGO clinical practice guideline for glomerulonephritis. *Kidney International Supplement, 2,* 139–274.
Kitiyakara, C., Eggers, P., & Kopp, J. B. (2004). Twenty-one-year trend in ESRD due to focal segmental glomerulosclerosis in the United States. *American Journal of Kidney Disease, 44*(5), 815–825.
Laurin, L. P., Gasim, A. M., Derebail, V. K., McGregor, J. G., Kidd, J. M., Hogan, S. L., . . . Nachman, P. H. (2016). Renal survival in patients with collapsing compared with not otherwise specified FSGS. *Clinical Journal of American Society of Nephrology, 11*(10), 1752–1759.
Rubin, L. G., Levin, M. J., Ljungman, P., Davies, E. G., Avery, R., Tomblyn, M., . . . Infectious Diseases Society of America. (2014). 2013 IDSA clinical practice guideline for vaccination of the immunocompromised host. *Clinical Infectious Diseases, 58*(3), 309–318. doi:10.1093/cid/cit816. Erratum in: *Clinical Infectious Diseases*, 59(1), 144. PMID: 24421306.
Swaminathan, S., Leung, N., Lager, D. J., Melton, L. J., 3rd, Bergstralh, E. J., Rohlinger, A., & Fervenza, F. C. (2006). Changing incidence of glomerular disease in Olmsted County, Minnesota: A 30-year renal biopsy study. *Clinical Journal of the American Society of Nephrology, 1,* 483–487.
Thomas, D. B., Franceschini, N., Hogan, S. L., Ten Holder, S., Jennette, C. E., Falk, R. J., & Jennette, J. C. (2006). Clinical and pathologic characteristics of focal segmental glomerulosclerosis pathologic variants. *Kidney International, 69,* 920–926.
Troyanov, S., Wall, C. A., Miller, J. A., Scholey, J. W., Cattran, D. C; Toronto Glomerulonephritis Registry Group. (2005). Focal and segmental glomerulosclerosis: Definition and relevance of a partial remission. *Journal of the American Society of Nephrology, 16,* 1061–1068.
United States Renal Data System. (2010). *USRDS 2010 Annual Data Report: Atlas of chronic kidney disease and end-stage renal disease in the United States.* Bethesda, MD: National Institutes of Health, National Institute of Diabetes and Digestive and Kidney Diseases.
Yu, H., Artomov, M., Brähler, S., Stander, M. C., Shamsan, G., Sampson, M. G., . . . Shaw, A. S. (2016). A role for genetic susceptibility in sporadic focal segmental glomerulosclerosis. *Journal of Clinical Investigation, 126*(3), 1067–1078. doi:10.1172/JCI82592. Erratum in, 126(4), 1603. PMID: 26901816.

CHAPTER 28

MEMBRANOUS NEPHROPATHY

Ladan Zand and Fernando C. Fervenza

1. What is membranous nephropathy (MN)?

   MN is a common immune-mediated glomerular disease that remains the leading cause of nephrotic syndrome in white adults. It is a histologic diagnosis based on the presence of immunoglobulins (Ig; usually IgG and C3) deposition along the capillary walls on immunofluorescence microscopy and subepithelial deposits along the glomerular basement membrane (GBM) on electron microscopy (EM). MN can be either a primary or secondary disease. Secondary MN is caused by:
   - Autoimmune diseases
     - Systemic lupus erythematosus
     - Autoimmune thyroiditis
     - Rheumatoid arthritis
     - Sjögren syndrome
   - Infections
     - Hepatitis B
     - Hepatitis C
     - Malaria
     - Schistosomiasis
     - Tuberculosis
     - Leprosy
   - Drugs
     - Penicillamine
     - Gold
     - Nonsteroidal antiinflammatory drugs
     - Captopril
   - Malignancies
     - Prostate cancer
     - Lung cancer
     - Colon cancer
     - Stomach cancer
     - Breast cancer
     - Cervical cancer
     - Lymphoma
     - Leukemia

2. What are the kidney biopsy findings of MN?

   The diagnosis of MN is based on the following findings:
   - Thickened GBM, often showing pinholes or spikes on silver and periodic acid–Schiff stains, and occasionally subepithelial fuchsinophilic deposits on trichrome stains
   - Immunofluorescence microscopy showing granular Ig (usually IgG and C3) along the capillary walls
   - Subepithelial deposits on EM.

   However, in the early stages of the disease, light microscopy may be completely normal. Based on the location of the deposits on EM, MN has been divided into four stages:
   - Stage I, sparse small deposits without thickening of the GBM
   - Stage II, more extensive subepithelial deposits with formation of basement membrane spikes between the deposits and thickening of the GBM
   - Stage III, combination of stage II along with deposits completely surrounded by basement membrane (intramembranous deposits)
   - Stage IV, incorporation of deposits in the GBM and irregular thickening of the GBM
   - However, these stages have no correlation with clinical outcome.

3. What are the clinical manifestations of MN?

At presentation, 60% to 70% of patients have nephrotic syndrome, with the remaining 30% to 40% of patients presenting with proteinuria <3.5 g/24 hours in an otherwise asymptomatic patient. Although more than 90% of patients have no evidence of impaired kidney function at the time of presentation, hypertension at onset is found in 10% to 20% of patients. The presence of microscopic hematuria is common (30% to 40%), but macroscopic hematuria and red cells casts are rare and these findings should suggest an alternative diagnosis. Findings of physical examination may vary from mild peripheral edema to full-blown nephrotic syndrome, including ascites and pericardial and pleural effusions.

4. What is the cause of primary MN?

M-type phospholipase A2 receptor (PLA2R) on the human podocytes is the target antigen in at least 70% of patients with primary MN, and anti-PLA$_2$R autoantibodies have been detected in the sera of these patients. Thrombospondin type-1 domain containing 7A (THSD-7A) is another podocyte antigen that accounts for an additional 10% of patients with primary MN that are negative for anti-PLA$_2$R antibody. As a rule, patients with positive anti-THSD-7A autoantibodies have negative sera for anti-PLA$_2$R antibodies, although rare cases of dual positivity have been reported. Taken together, autoantibodies to these podocyte-specific antigens are the cause of primary MN in almost 80% of patients. Although these findings do not explain the cause in all cases of MN, they suggest that additional antibodies against podocyte proteins are likely to be identified.

5. Can kidney biopsy findings be helpful in identifying secondary causes of MN?

Although it is often difficult to determine whether the MN is primary or secondary based on kidney pathology, certain features are helpful in identifying a primary versus secondary cause. Commercial tests are available that allow for staining of kidney tissue for anti-PLA$_2$R and THSD-7A, which aids in identifying primary forms of MN. Features in favor of a secondary cause, in particular an autoimmune disease, include the following:

- Proliferative features (mesangial or endocapillary)
- Full-house pattern of Ig staining including staining for C1q on immunofluorescence microscopy
- Glomerular deposits predominantly containing Ig other than IgG4 on immunofluorescence microscopy
- Electron-dense deposits in the subendothelial location of the capillary wall and mesangium or along the tubular basement membrane and vessel walls
- Endothelial tubuloreticular inclusions on EM (EM showing only few superficial scattered subepithelial deposits may suggest a drug-associated secondary MN)

6. What is the clinical course of MN?

MN is a chronic disease, with spontaneous remission and relapses clearly documented. The clinical course is characterized by great variability in the rate of disease progression, and the natural course is difficult to assess in part because of the selection criteria, geographic variability, and genetic characteristics of the subjects presented in different studies. Although in most patients the disease progresses relatively slowly, approximately 40% of patients eventually develop ESKD after focal segmental glomerulosclerosis and lupus nephritis.

7. What evaluation should be considered if there is rapid loss of kidney function?

When progressive loss of kidney function occurs faster than usual, patient should be evaluated for other causes of worsening kidney function, such as acute tubular necrosis, acute interstitial nephritis, kidney vein thrombosis, or urinary tract obstruction. A superimposed crescentic glomerulonephritis should also be considered in the differential, anti-neutrophil cytoplasmic antibody (ANCA)-associated vasculitis and anti-GBM disease in particular. A repeat kidney biopsy may be indicated in these patients.

8. What factors are associated with poor outcomes in MN?

Several factors are associated with worse outcome in patients with MN including:

- Advanced age (>50)
- Male sex
- Elevated blood pressure
- CKD (low estimated glomerular filtration rat at presentation)
- Severity of initial proteinuria
- Persistent proteinuria

   Persistent proteinuria of >4 g/24 hours is the strongest predictor of progressive kidney disease. Histologic changes such as tubular atrophy, interstitial fibrosis, and glomerulosclerosis have also been associated with poor prognosis. Elevated β$_2$-microglobulin urinary excretion rate has been shown to predict poor outcome, but accurate measurement of urinary β_2-microglobulin can be challenging. Increasing evidence suggests that high anti-PLA$_2$R autoantibody levels may be used in diagnosis and management of MN and to predict long-term outcomes.

9. **Can one predict who would progress to ESKD in patients with MN?**
   Finding useful markers that predict this group is difficult. The best model for identifying patients at risk was developed from the Toronto Glomerulonephritis Registry. This model takes into consideration the initial creatinine clearance (CrCl), the slope of the CrCl, and the lowest level of proteinuria during a 6-month observation period.
   • Patients who present with a normal CrCl, proteinuria ≤4 g/24 hours, and stable kidney function over 6 months have an excellent long-term prognosis and are classified as low risk for progression.
   • Patients with normal kidney function and whose CrCl remains unchanged during 6 months of observation but continue to have proteinuria >4 g but <8 g/24 hours have a 55% probability of developing CKD and are classified as medium risk for progression.
   • Patients with persistent proteinuria >8 g/24 hours, independent of the degree of kidney dysfunction, have a 66% to 88% probability of progression to ESKD within 10 years and are classified as high risk of progression.
   The discovery of anti-PLA$_2$R autoantibodies and its potential role in the pathogenesis of the disease, its correlation with disease activity and long-term remission is changing the approach to patients with MN. Therefore anti-PLA$_2$R positivity and antibody levels should be evaluated and taken into account when making decisions regarding treatment.

10. **What are the complications of MN?**
    The main complications of MN are related to presence of nephrotic syndrome including hypogammaglobulinemia and increased risk of infection, hypovitaminosis D due to loss of vitamin D binding protein, and most importantly increased risk of thromboembolic event, with an incidence as high as 50% in patients with severe proteinuria. An increased risk of cardiovascular events in particular in the first 2 years in the setting of severe nephrosis is well documented in this population.

11. **Is anticoagulation recommended for patients with MN?**
    Patients with severe nephrotic syndrome are at increased risk for thromboembolic complications, and this risk tends to be higher in patients with MN for unclear reasons. Although no consensus has emerged regarding whether prophylactic anticoagulation should be used, a decision analysis tool is now available (www.gntools.com) that helps estimate the benefit from prophylactic anticoagulation based on serum albumin and taking into account the risk of bleeding. Some recommend anticoagulation in patients with MN who are severely nephrotic (proteinuria >10 g/day and serum albumin <2.5 g/day) unless there are contraindications.

12. **What is the conservative treatment in MN?**
    Conservative therapy for MN consists of low sodium diet (<2.3 grams/day), lowering lipids and controlling blood pressure (target blood pressure ≤125/75 mm Hg). Inhibition of the renin-angiotensin-aldosterone system (RAAS) with angiotensin-converting enzyme (ACE) inhibitors or angiotensin receptor blockers (ARBs) are effective antihypertensive agents that can reduce proteinuria and slow progression of kidney disease in patients with nephropathy with or without diabetes, and for these reasons they are the preferred agents to treat hypertension in MN. However, the antiproteinuric effect of ACE inhibitors or ARB is modest (<30% decrease) and is more significant in patients with lower levels of proteinuria.

13. **Is there a role for dual RAAS inhibition in MN?**
    Another approach to reducing proteinuria in MN is the use of dual RAAS inhibition with ACE inhibitors and ARBs (or addition of aliskiren [renin inhibitor]). This approach will necessitate close monitoring secondary to the increased risk of hyperkalemia and AKI. Symptomatic hypotension on dual RAAS blockade can be an insuperable barrier in patients with normal or low baseline blood pressures, and therefore close monitoring of blood pressure is paramount. The goal of dual blockade is to ameliorate glomerular sieving function, reduce proteinuria, and increase serum albumin levels with consequent improvement in hypercholesterolemia and other components of the nephrotic syndrome. The risk of adverse events in patients on dual RAAS therapy with MN is primarily derived from patients with cardiovascular disease and proteinuria. It should be noted that long-term outcome studies examining dual RAAS inhibition in MN have not been conducted, but only short-term studies looking at albuminuria reduction. Therefore we recommend a cautious approach when considering dual RAAS blockade.

14. **Is there a role for dietary protein restriction in MN?**
Restricting dietary protein has been shown to reduce proteinuria in a variety of proteinuric kidney diseases including MN. Thus restricting dietary protein intake to 0.8 g/kg of ideal body weight per day of high-quality protein may be attempted in patients with refractory proteinuria. However, long-term studies with clinical end points are lacking that compare protein restriction to control diet.

15. **How effective are lipid-lowering drugs in patients with MN?**
Lipid abnormalities associated with proteinuria are likely important players in the high cardiovascular risk seen in patients with MN and thus provide an important target for treatment. Statins can improve the lipid profile and reduce cardiovascular morbidity and mortality in patients with chronic kidney disease. Statins have a synergistic antiproteinuric effect when combined with ACE inhibitors, but this effect is small and mainly observed in patients with proteinuria <3 g/24 hours.

16. **What is the role of immunosuppressive agents in the treatment of MN?**
The ideal treatment option in patients with primary MN remains unclear, and use of immunosuppression is controversial. This is partly due to the variable natural history of the disease and the risks associated with drug toxicity. Immunosuppression is generally reserved for those patients with deteriorating kidney function or heavy proteinuria that persists despite conservative treatment or those with high anti-PLA$_2$R antibody titers. Various agents have been used including corticosteroids, cyclophosphamide, chlorambucil, mycophenolate mofetil, calcineurin inhibitors (e.g., cyclosporine, tacrolimus), rituximab, and adrenocorticotropic hormone (ACTH) with variable success.

17. **What are the traditional treatment options in patients with MN?**
Corticosteroids have been examined extensively in treatment of patients with MN with inconsistent outcomes. In meta-analysis and a secondary pooled analysis, corticosteroid therapy alone was not associated with an increased rate of remission or preservation of kidney function. Therefore corticosteroid therapy alone is not recommended for treatment of patients with MN.
   Cytotoxic agents (cyclophosphamide, chlorambucil) in combination with corticosteroids have been studied in multiple trials and increase the rate of complete and partial remission and result in preservation of kidney function short term. In the largest meta-analysis of 36 clinical trials, cytotoxic agents combined with corticosteroids were associated with a lower rate of mortality and ESRD and higher rate of complete and partial remissions but also led to a higher rate of adverse events. Kidney Disease: Improving Global Outcomes currently recommends initial therapy to consist of a 6-month course of alternating monthly cycles of oral and intravenous corticosteroids and oral cyclophosphamide (grade 1B).
   Calcineurin inhibitors (cyclosporin and tacrolimus) with or without corticosteroids have also been used in treatment of patients with primary MN and are associated with high rate of complete and partial remission; however, risk of relapse after discontinuation of the drug is similarly high. If calcineurin inhibitors are used as first line therapy, we recommend treatment for at least 12 months, with a slow taper afterwards. However, lack of reduction in proteinuria $>30\%$ after 6 months of therapy with calcineurin inhibitor suggests resistance.
   Several studies have evaluated the use of mycophenolate mofetil in patients with primary MN, but the outcomes have been disappointing and we do not recommend use of Mycophenolate Mofetil (MMF) monotherapy in this population.

18. **What other therapies are available for treatment of MN?**
Rituximab, an anti-CD20 monoclonal antibody, has become a popular choice for treating patients with primary MN after small, prospective but uncontrolled cohorts suggested that it can be effective in inducing remission in approximately 60% of patients. A randomized controlled study of 75 patients with primary MN and proteinuria ≥3.5 g/24 hours compared rituximab therapy plus nonimmunosuppressive treatment with nonimmunosuppressive treatment alone and showed that those treated with rituximab have a remission rate of 65% compared with 34% in the control group at 12 months. A randomized controlled study comparing rituximab to cyclosporin is currently being conducted. It should be noted that rituximab has been linked to unusual infections, such as progressive multifocal leukoencephalopathy, and caution should be taken prior to its widespread use until results from larger randomized studies become available.
   Both synthetic and natural ACTH have been studied as treatment options for treating patients with MN. Synthetic ACTH administered for 1 year was compared with corticosteroid plus cyclophosphamide or chlorambucil in a randomized study, and synthetic ACTH resulted in equal reduction in proteinuria. Natural ACTH (Acthar Gel) has also been studied as a treatment option at a dose of 80 units twice weekly for at least 12 weeks and was associated with more than 50%

reduction in proteinuria. ACTH is overall well tolerated. Adverse effects include glucose intolerance, swelling, and development of bronze-colored skin, which resolve after the end of the therapy. ACTH may be a potential therapy in treatment of patients with MN but requires further evaluation to define its role.

19. What are the follow-up strategies regarding cancer in patients with MN?

   Patients with MN have an increased incidence of malignancy. Therefore patients with MN should be regularly screened for the development of cancer. Age, smoking, and the presence of glomerular leukocytic infiltrates increase the likelihood of malignancy in these patients. In patients with secondary MN due to malignancy, clinical remission of cancer is usually associated with a reduction of proteinuria. Studies suggest an association between cancer-associated MN and presence of anti-THSDA-7a antibodies. In the largest cohort of 25 patients with positive anti-THSDA-7a antibodies, 7 were found to have a malignant tumor. This supports the hypothesis of molecular mimicry in which antibodies produced by the tumor cells recognize the related antigen expressed on podocytes. Patients with MN and positive serology for anti-THSDA-7a antibody should be carefully screened for malignancy.

20. What percentage of patients relapse after complete or partial remission is achieved?

   Approximately 40% of MN cases will relapse after a complete remission. Many will relapse only to subnephrotic-range proteinuria and will have stable function long term. These patients can be retreated with immunosuppressive therapy.

21. Does MN recur after kidney transplantation?

   MN can recur after kidney transplantation in close to 50% of the patients and can result in proteinuria, allograft dysfunction, and graft loss. Patients with positive anti-PLA2R antibodies prior to kidney transplantation who continue to have persistently positive titers despite standard immunosuppression post transplant are at increased risk of clinically relevant recurrent MN and should be considered for treatment with rituximab post transplantation.

KEY POINTS

1. Membranous nephropathy (MN) remains the leading cause of nephrotic syndrome in white adults. Patients who remain nephrotic are likely to progress to ESKD and are also at an increased risk for thromboembolic and cardiovascular events.
2. Antibodies against podocyte proteins such as M-type phospholipase A2 receptor (PLA2R) and thrombospondin type-1 domain containing 7A are responsible for approximately 80% of cases of primary MN.
3. Secondary causes of MN include autoimmune diseases, infection, and malignancies.
4. Up to 70% of patients with MN will have nephrotic syndrome at the time of presentation. MN is a chronic disease, with spontaneous remission and relapses clearly documented.
5. The standard model for the identification of patients at risk for progression to ESKD was developed by the Toronto Glomerulonephritis Registry. This model considers the initial creatinine clearance (CrCl), the slope of the CrCl, and the lowest level of proteinuria during a 6-month observation period, but new models incorporating PLA2R titers are being developed.
6. Conservative therapy consists of restricting dietary protein intake and controlling blood pressure, hyperlipidemia, and edema. Angiotensin-converting enzyme inhibitors and angiotensin receptor blockers are effective antihypertensive medication. However, their antiproteinuric effect is poor (average proteinuria reduction approximately 30%), and they work best in patients with lower degrees of proteinuria.
7. The use of immunosuppression in the setting of primary MN should be reserved for those patients with deteriorating kidney function and/or heavy proteinuria that persist despite conservative therapy, and/or have high anti-PLA2R antibody levels.
8. Current data suggest that new therapeutic agents such as rituximab and synthetic adrenocorticotropic hormone are effective in reducing proteinuria while having few adverse effects.
9. Membranous nephropathy can recur after kidney transplantation in close to 50% of patients and can result in proteinuria, allograft dysfunction, and graft loss. Recurrence most often occurs during the first year.
10. The relationship between anti-PLA2R antibody levels in patients with MN and clinical response to different treatment modalities needs to be evaluated further.

Bibliography

Bech, A. P., Hofstra, J. M., Brenchley, P. E., & Wetzels, J. F. (2014). Association of anti-PLA2R antibodies with outcomes after immunosuppressive therapy in idiopathic membranous nephropathy. *Clinical Journal of the American Society of Nephrology, 9,* 1386–1392.

Beck, L. H., Jr., Bonegio, R. G., Lambeau, G., Beck, D. M., Powell, D. W., Cummins, T. D., . . . Salant, D. J. (2009). M-type phospholipase A2 receptor as target antigen in idiopathic membranous nephropathy. *New England Journal of Medicine, 361*(1), 11–21.

Cattran, D. C., Pei, Y., & Greenwood, C. (1992). Predicting progression in membranous glomerulonephritis. *Nephrology Dialysis Transplantation, 7*(Suppl. 1), 48–52.

De Vriese, A.S., Glassockm R., Nathm K., et al. (2017). A proposal for serology-based approach to membranous nephropathy. *Journal of the American Society of Nephrology, 28*(2), 421–430.

Dussol, B., Morange, S., Burtey, S., Indreies, M., Cassuto, E., Mourad, G., . . . Berland, Y. (2008). Mycophenolate mofetil monotherapy in membranous nephropathy: A 1-year randomized controlled trial. *American Journal of Kidney Diseases, 52*(4), 699–705.

Hladunewich, M. A., Cattran, D., Beck, L. H., Odutayo, A., Sethi, S., Ayalon, R., . . . Fervenza, F. C. (2014). A pilot study to determine the dose and effectiveness of adrenocorticotrophic hormone (H.P. Acthar® Gel) in nephrotic syndrome due to idiopathic membranous nephropathy. *Nephrology Dialysis Transplantation, 29,* 1570–1577.

Kattah, A., Ayalon, R., Beck, L. H., Jr., Sethi, S., Sandor, D. G., Cosio, F. G., . . . Fervenza, F. C. (2015). Anti-phospholipase A2 receptor antibodies in recurrent membranous nephropathy. *American Society of Transplantation, 15*(5), 1349–1359.

Ponticelli, C., Altieri, P., Scolari, F., Passerini, P., Roccatello, D., Cesana, B., . . . Bellazzi, R. (1998). A randomized study comparing methylprednisolone plus chlorambucil versus methylprednisolone plus cyclophosphamide in idiopathic membranous nephropathy. *Journal of the American Society of Nephrology, 9,* 444–450.

Praga, M., Barrio, V., Juárez, G. F., Luño, J., & Grupo Español de Estudio de la Nefropatía Membranosa. (2007). Tacrolimus monotherapy in membranous nephropathy: A randomized controlled trial. *Kidney International, 71*(9), 924–930.

Ruggenenti, P., Cravedi, P., Chianca, A., Perna, A., Ruggiero, B., Gaspari, F., . . . Remuzzi, G. (2012). Rituximab in idiopathic membranous nephropathy. *Journal of the American Society of Nephrology, 23*(8), 1416–1425.

Thomas, N. M., Beck, L. H., Jr., Meyer-Schwesinger, C., Seitz-Polski, B., Ma, H., Zahner, G., . . . Lambeau, G. (2014). Thrombospondin Type-1 Domain-containing 7A in idiopathic membranous nephropathy. *New England Journal of Medicine, 371,* 2277–2287.

CHAPTER 29

IMMUNOGLOBULIN A NEPHROPATHY AND HENOCH–SCHÖNLEIN DISEASE

Daniel Oattran and Talal Alfaadhol

1. **What is immunoglobulin A nephropathy (IgAN)?**
   IgAN is a glomerular disease characterized by the deposition of type A immunoglobulin in the mesangial areas of the glomerulus. This leads to inflammation and damage to the glomerulus and the surrounding structures. Originally known as Berger disease, IgAN is the most common biopsy-proven primary glomerular disease.

2. **What are the typical biopsy findings in IgAN?**
   On light microscopy (LM), mesangial cellular proliferation and matrix expansion are the classic findings. In cases with rapid deterioration in kidney function, diffuse proliferation of both the mesangial and endocapillary cells can be appreciated, in association with segmental necrosis and crescents. Nonspecific pathologic features associated with advanced glomerular diseases in general can be seen in IgAN, including glomerulosclerosis, tubular atrophy, and interstitial fibrosis.

   On immunofluorescence (IF), the defining feature of IgAN is the presence of prominent IgA deposits within the mesangium in a dominant or codominant intensity with IgG and more rarely IgM.

   On electron microscopy (EM), electron-dense mesangial deposits are the typical finding. Paramesangial and subendothelial extension of the deposits may be present but are less common.

3. **What is the pathogenesis of IgAN?**
   A unifying theory of the pathogenesis has not been fully elucidated. The available data suggest that tissue injury can be initiated by the deposition of abnormally underglycosylated IgA subclass 1 (IgA1) immune complexes in the mesangium. These complexes somehow trigger mesangial cell activation, which in turn releases proinflammatory cytokines and profibrotic mediators, affecting nearby glomerular structures. It is also suggested that IgA deposits activate the local complement system. The higher C3 deposition compared with C1q suggests that the lectin and alternative complement pathways are implicated.

4. **What is the etiology of IgAN?**
   The etiology of IgAN is unknown in the majority of cases. There appears to be a dysregulation of the mucosal-type IgA immune response that results in the production of the aberrant IgA1. The aberrant IgA1 forms immune complexes that deposit in the glomerulus, although the specific relationship between the complexes glomerular deposition and injury remain incompletely understood. It is likely that there are contributions from both genetic and environmental factors that cause the production of aberrant IgA1.

   In familial IgAN, genetic linkage studies have suggested some specific genetic abnormalities. Most of the reported kindreds with IgAN are inherited in an autosomal-dominant pattern with incomplete penetrance. Genomewide association studies that include populations of IgAN from across the world have identified associated variants in the HLA gene family. Associations have described abnormalities within 1q32 that contains multiple complement regulatory genes as a possible IgAN susceptibility locus. In most cases, especially the more common sporadic variants, additional environmental factors are necessary to produce the clinical phenotype.

5. **Is IgAN associated with any other conditions?**
   Yes. Although IgAN is most commonly a primary (idiopathic) disorder, there are some well-established associations. The most common are
   - Liver cirrhosis (both alcohol- and virus-induced)
   - Celiac disease

- HIV infection
- Inflammatory bowel disease
- Some rheumatic conditions
  IgAN has also been described in association with
- Minimal change disease (MCD)
- Membranous nephropathy
- Antineutrophil cytoplasmic antibody-positive vasculitis
  There is increased recognition of IgA deposition with *Staphylococcus*-related glomerulonephritis (GN). However, unlike primary IgAN, the presence of the active infection and typical large subepithelial deposits (humps) on microscopy can help distinguish between these two entities.

6. **How does IgAN present?**
   About 20% to 30% of patients present with recurrent gross hematuria, typically within a few days of an upper respiratory infection. Classically known as "synpharyngetic hematuria," this presentation is much more common in children and young adults than in the older population. Dull flank pain and low-grade fever may be present, and this pattern can mimic both urinary tract infection and urolithiasis.
   The majority of the remaining patients with IgAN are asymptomatic at presentation and are detected on routine examination of the urine (positive for microscopic hematuria with or without mild proteinuria [<500 mg/day]). Systemic hypertension may also be found. Nephrotic-range proteinuria or lesser degrees of proteinuria without hematuria are unusual but also occur. In less than 5% of patients, IgAN can present with acute kidney injury. It is felt that the kidney injury is most commonly secondary to tubular obstruction and/or damage by red cell casts, which form in the course of the gross hematuria. Crescentic GN in IgAN can also produce a similar clinical phenotype and should be considered whenever an acute deterioration of kidney function occurs. Because this is a relatively rare clinical presentation, a kidney biopsy should be obtained to differentiate acute tubular damage from crescentic GN. This is particularly important given that their outcome and management are so distinctly different.
   At least 20% of patients with IgAN present with chronic kidney disease as a result of long-standing but undiagnosed disease. The clinical phenotype usually includes hypertension, mild to moderate proteinuria, and hematuria of undetermined duration in combination with varying degrees of chronic kidney disease.

7. **What is the differential diagnosis of synpharyngitic hematuria?**
   The onset of hematuria shortly after a respiratory infection is common to both IgAN and poststreptococcal GN. However, the latent period from infection to gross hematuria averages 1 to 3 days in IgAN versus 10 to 14 days in poststreptococcal GN. Poststreptococcal GN can also be distinguished from IgAN by the presence of hypocomplementemia, which is rarely seen in IgAN, and the elevation of antistreptococcal antibodies in the early phase of infection.

8. **How is the IgAN diagnosis established?**
   Even if IgAN is suspected on the basis of the clinical and laboratory findings, the diagnosis can be confirmed only by the findings on kidney biopsy. The presence of mesangial proliferation and matrix expansion on LM with dominant or codominant deposition of IgA and complement on IF microscopy confirms the diagnosis.

9. **Are there any biomarkers to diagnose IgAN or monitor the activity of the disease?**
   Not yet. Although increased levels of serum IgA can be found in up to 50% of cases, this finding is not specific and has no diagnostic or prognostic value. Alternative biomarkers have been identified, including serum galactose-deficient IgA1 (GD IgA1) and GD IgA1 antibodies and immune complexes, but their utility in routine clinical practice has not been established.

10. **Should a kidney biopsy always be performed?**
    No. Asymptomatic patients with isolated hematuria or mild proteinuria (<500 mg/day) usually follow a benign course. General interventions known to slow progression that are used in other cases of chronic kidney disease should be implemented. Given that histologic findings at this stage of disease are not likely to alter therapy and considering the risk, a kidney biopsy is not warranted. The decision to perform a biopsy in these cases even when IgAN is highly suspected is a matter of debate. Although biopsy can at least confirm the diagnosis, this decision varies widely among nephrologists and the affected patients as well as by geographic region.
    Regardless of whether a kidney biopsy is performed, ongoing follow-up of these patients is imperative, because a more concerning phenotype may evolve at any time and is unpredictable. Kidney biopsy is generally recommended in patients with an unexplained serum creatinine above normal for age and sex and/or proteinuria > 500 to 1000 mg/day.

11. What is the prognosis of IgAN?

Most patients who present with isolated hematuria and no proteinuria have a low risk of progression provided these laboratory features do not change. Among patients who develop significant persistent proteinuria > 500 to 1000 mg/day, approximately 25% to 30% will require renal replacement therapy (RRT) within 20 to 25 years of presentation. A higher percentage will require RRT if they have persistent higher-grade proteinuria of more than 2000-3000 mg/day with or without hypertension. This is particularly true if the proteinuria cannot be reduced with therapy.

Spontaneous improvement in laboratory findings in those with isolated hematuria (without significant proteinuria or impairment of glomerular filtration rate [GFR]) has been reported. It appears to be more common in children and has been estimated to occur in between 5% and 30% of such cases.

There is a geographic variability in IgAN prognosis that is in large part explained by lead time bias related to differing clinical thresholds for performing a kidney biopsy. Calculating the influence of other factors such as genetics, diet, ethnicity, or treatment is relevant but currently impossible to quantitate.

12. Do any kidney biopsy findings predict outcome?

Yes. Several variables have been found to correlate with a poor renal outcome. The Oxford classification (Table 29.1) shows that histopathology has a predictive value—independent of the clinical parameters of hypertension, proteinuria, and GFR—related to the degree of mesangial proliferation, presence of endocapillary proliferation, segmental glomerulosclerosis, the degree of tubular atrophy/interstitial fibrosis, and the percentage of crescents. This classification has been validated in many different countries and in cohorts comprising a wider variety of presentations and degrees of progression than the original studies. Although uncommon and not part of the original MEST classification, crescent formation also points to a poor renal prognosis. Extension of the IgA deposits into the subendothelial location of the capillary wall has also been associated with a worse prognosis, but this has been somewhat inconsistent.

13. Are there clinical features predictive of outcome?

Yes. In fact, they have been known to have a stronger predictive value than the histologic ones, particularly because they can be measured serially. The level of sustained proteinuria over time (usually after 2 years of follow-up) has been shown to be the strongest predictor of progression. Regardless of the level of proteinuria at presentation, achieving a complete (proteinuria <300 mg/day) or partial remission (proteinuria <1000 mg/day) is associated with a significant reduction in the rate of progression of the kidney disease. Mean arterial pressure over time and level of impairment of kidney function have also been identified as important predictors. Combining clinical factors with the pathologic variables of the Oxford classification can improve risk stratification and management decisions at the time of presentation. Whether isolated hematuria or recurrent macroscopic hematuria are prognostic indicators is still debated. It seems likely that recurrent gross hematuria may leave subclinical kidney damage that will eventually result in tubular interstitial scarring and a worse long-term outcome, but currently there is little evidence to support that theory.

Table 29.1. The Oxford Classification MEST Criteria

PATHOLOGIC FEATURE	Score		
	0	**1**	**2**
Mesangial hypercellularity (M)	<50% of the glomeruli showing hypercellularity	>50% of the glomeruli showing hypercellularity	Not applicable
Endocapillary hypercellularity (E)	No endocapillary hypercellularity	Any glomeruli showing endocapillary hypercellularity	Not applicable
Segmental sclerosis (S)	No segmental sclerosis	Any glomeruli showing segmental sclerosis	Not applicable
Tubular atrophy/interstitial fibrosis (T)	≤25% tubular atrophy/interstitial fibrosis	>25%–50% tubular atrophy/interstitial fibrosis	>50% tubular atrophy/interstitial fibrosis
Crescents (C)[a]	No cellular/fibrocellular crescents	10%–25% of glomeruli having cellular/fibrocellular crescents	>25% of glomeruli having cellular/fibrocellular crescents

[a]Crescents were studied in addition to the MEST score in 2016 and were validated.

14. **Is there a specific treatment for IgAN?**
There is no known treatment that specifically modifies the presumed pathogenesis of IgAN. Nonimmune-modulating treatment with renin-angiotensin system blockade is still the best evidence-based intervention for slowing IgAN progression. The blood pressure target should be <125/75 to 130/80 mm Hg in adults and similar targets adjusted appropriately for body size and age in the pediatric population. The aim should be to reduce the proteinuria to less than 500 to 1000 mg/day.

Angiotensin-converting enzyme inhibitors (ACEIs) or, alternatively, angiotensin receptor blockers (ARBs) should be initiated and titrated up to maximum doses as tolerated. There is an increased risk of adverse events with combined use of these agents; thus it is generally inadvisable to combine them, especially with the limited evidence of benefit in the literature.

15. **Should all patients with IgAN receive treatment?**
No. The approach to therapy in individual patients should take into account their relative risk of progression and their clinical and pathologic findings as well as a careful assessment of the potential risks and benefits of therapy.
    * Patients with isolated hematuria, no proteinuria, and a normal GFR do not require treatment; however, monitoring every 6 to 12 months for potential indicators of worsening disease (such as increasing proteinuria, blood pressure, and/or serum creatinine) is warranted.
    * For patients with persistent proteinuria >500–1000 mg/day, angiotensin inhibition is recommended with ACEI and/or ARB therapy, aiming for reduction in proteinuria to <500 to 1000 mg/d.
    * Many physicians advocate the use of fish oil supplements because of their lack of toxicity and because they may provide a nonspecific anti-inflammatory/vasoprotective effect. However, it must be noted that randomized trials using fish oil have yielded conflicting results.

16. **When should immunosuppressive therapy be considered?**
    * **Persistent proteinuria:** In patients with persistent proteinuria (>1000 mg/day) despite optimal conservative therapy (ACEI or ARB) with preserved kidney function, earlier studies have shown benefit of a 6-month course of steroid therapy in patients, with a lower risk of side effects. However, a randomized controlled trial (STOP-IgA) has cast doubt on the short-term benefit of preserving GFR, even when steroid treatment showed significant improvement in proteinuria. Steroid side effects associated with such courses include glucose intolerance and a higher risk of infection.
    * **Nephrotic syndrome:** In patients presenting with nephrotic syndrome and clinical/pathologic features suggestive of concurrent MCD, corticosteroids prescribed in a manner similar to that used in the treatment of MCD alone will commonly induce a complete remission of proteinuria.
    * **Accelerated decline in GFR:** In patients with a rapidly declining GFR (to less than 50 mL/min per 1.73 m^2), a biopsy can be helpful in risk stratification. If advanced sclerosis and fibrosis is found, the risk of immunosuppression usually outweighs the benefit. However, if significant inflammatory activity is seen with less sclerosis and fibrosis, immunosuppression can halt or substantially reduce the rate of decline of kidney function. The evidence to guide treatment in this group of patients is scarce and limited. With higher grades of activity, additional treatment beyond a course of prednisone—such as cyclophosphamide (typically for 3 months)—has been used, especially when glomerular crescents are found. Further maintenance treatment and/or steroid-sparing agents in the form of azathioprine or mycophenolate mofetil have been used, but no randomized controlled trials have confirmed their value.
    * **Resistant and relapsed disease:** In some patients, first-line immunosuppression (steroid monotherapy or in combination with cyclophosphamide) may fail to diminish proteinuria. In other patients, relapse after the achievement of remission may occur shortly after an immunosuppressive course is completed or after many years. In such situations, additional courses of immunotherapy increase their risk, and a kidney biopsy may be needed to define the activity versus chronicity of the disease and help guide treatment.
    * **Advanced disease:** Advanced glomerular sclerosis and interstitial fibrosis usually follow chronic unremitting IgAN or acute/subacute aggressive variants of the disease. Such irreversible findings on biopsy will be reflected in the declining GFR. The level of sclerosis/fibrosis and GFR at which the risk of therapy outweighs the benefit is unclear and remains a subject of debate. The Kidney Disease: Improving Global Outcomes (KDIGO) guidelines suggest to withhold immunosuppressive treatment if the GFR is less than 30 mL/min per 1.73 m^2 unless active crescentric IgAN is found. Although these recommendations are not based on strong evidence, they are reflective of general practice.

17. **Is tonsillectomy recommended?**
No. Although tonsillectomy has been performed as a treatment for IgAN, particularly in the Japanese population, it is not a risk-free procedure, and the evidence of its usefulness is weak.

18. Does IgAN recur after transplantation?

Yes, but the spectrum of recurrence is wide. This ranges from histologic recurrence (the presence of IgA on IF staining without features of active disease) to the full-blown clinical phenotype with manifestations similar to those present in the pretransplant IgAN course. The rate of recurrence in the literature is variable and has been reported from 10% to greater than 50% with extended follow-up. However, graft loss from recurrent IgAN is rare, typically less than 5% to 10%, at least within a decade of transplantation. Because of this, transplantation, when feasible, remains the optimal form of RRT for patients with IgAN.

19. What is Henoch-Schönlein purpura (HSP)?

HSP is a systemic leukocytoclastic vasculitis affecting small vessels, characterized by IgA immune deposits. The incidence increases in the fall and winter, possibly due to increased infectious or allergic triggers. The classic presentation is a tetrad of skin rash, abdominal pain, arthralgias, and hematuria/proteinuria. HSP has a peak incidence at ages 4 to 6 and shows a 2:1 male-to-female predilection. It is the most common cause of vasculitis in children. The four classic clinical features are as follows:

- **Skin:** Palpable purpura affecting mainly the forearms, lower limbs, and buttocks. Skin manifestations usually predominate in children.
- **Gastrointestinal:** Bowel vasculitis causing colicky abdominal pain. Gastrointestinal bleeding may occur.
- **Joints:** Symmetric polyarthralgia typically limited to the knees and ankles.
- **Kidney:** This may be clinically and pathologically indistinguishable from IgAN. Kidney involvement is more commonly seen and more severe in older children and adults than in young children.

20. What is the prognosis of HSP nephritis?

Most patients have a self-limiting course and a good prognosis. A minority of patients have persistent hematuria or proteinuria that may eventually lead to end-stage kidney disease. In these patients, the evolution and prognosis of the nephritis is comparable to that of patients with IgAN; thus the follow-up and approach to treatment should be similar. There is limited evidence to guide treatment, but steroids with or without other immunosuppressive agents may be a reasonable option for severe and progressive kidney disease.

Recurrent/relapsing episodes can occur but may not predict a worse long-term outcome. Disease behavior after transplantation is similar to that of IgAN but occasionally can be severe, with features of rapidly progressive GN and crescentic disease.

KEY POINTS

1. Immunoglobulin A nephropathy (IgAN) is the most common biopsy-proven primary glomerulonephritis.
2. The classic presentation is painless gross hematuria 1 to 3 days after an upper respiratory infection.
3. When accompanied only by microscopic hematuria, the long-term prognosis of IgAN is excellent.
4. Persistent proteinuria greater than 1 g/day with/without hypertension is associated with up to a 50% likelihood of developing end-stage kidney disease within 10 years.
5. Renin-angiotensin system blockade with angiotensin-converting enzyme inhibition or angiotensin receptor blockade has been proven in randomized controlled trials in both children and adults to improve prognosis.
6. Of the available immunosuppressive treatments, only steroids have shown reasonable evidence of benefit. However, trials have indicated a significant risk of toxicity, and careful assessment of the risk/benefit ratio is needed before embarking on therapy.

BIBLIOGRAPHY

Ballardie, F. W., & Roberts, I. S. (2002). Controlled prospective trial of prednisolone and cytotoxics in progressive IgA nephropathy. *Journal of the American Society of Nephrology, 13*, 142–148.

Cattran, D. C., Coppo, R., Cook, H. T., A Working Group of the International IgA Nephropathy Network and the Renal Pathology Society, Feehally, J., Roberts, I. S., . . . Zhang, H. (2009). The Oxford classification of IgA nephropathy: Rationale, clinicopathological correlations, and classification. *Kidney International, 76*, 534–545.

Coppo, R., Andrulli, S., Amore, A., Gianoglio, B., Conti, G., Peruzzi, L., . . . Cagnoli L. (2006). Predictors of outcome in Henoch-Schönlein nephritis in children and adults. *American Journal of Kidney Diseases, 47*, 993–1003.

Kidney Disease: Improving Global Outcomes (KDIGO) Glomerulonephritis Work Group. (2012). KDIGO clinical practice guideline for glomerulonephritis. *Kidney International Supplements, 2*, 139–274.

Kiryluk, K., Julian, B. A., Wyatt, R. J., Scolari, F., Zhang, H., Novak, J., & Gharavi, A. G. (2010). Genetic studies of IgA nephropathy: Past, present, and future. *Pediatric Nephrology, 25*(11), 2257–2268.

Pozzi, C., Andrulli, S., Del Vecchio, L., Melis, P., Fogazzi, G. B., Altieri, P., . . . Locatelli, F. (2004). Corticosteroids effectiveness in IgA nephropathy: Long-term results of a randomized controlled trial. *Journal of the American Society of Nephrology, 15*, 157–163.

Praga, M., Gutiérrez, E., González, E., Morales, E., & Hernández, E. (2003). Treatment of IgA nephropathy with ACE inhibitors: A randomized and controlled trial. *Journal of the American Society of Nephrology, 14*, 1578–1583.

Rauen, T., Eitner, F., Fitzner, C., Sommerer, C., Zeier, M., Otte, B., . . . STOP-IgAN Investigators. (2015). Intensive supportive care plus immunosuppression in IgA nephropathy. *New England Journal of Medicine, 373*(23), 2225–2236.

Reich, H. N., Troyanov, S., Scholey, J. W., Cattran, D. C., & Toronto Glomerulonephritis Registry. (2007). Remission of proteinuria improves prognosis in IgA nephropathy. *Journal of the American Society of Nephrology, 18*, 3177–3183.

Wyatt, R. J., & Julian, B. A. (2013). IgA nephropathy. *New England Journal of Medicine, 368*(25), 2402–2414.

CHAPTER 30

MEMBRANOPROLIFERATIVE GLOMERULONEPHRITIS

Jennifer Lopez and Howard Trachtman

1. What is membranoproliferative glomerulonephritis (MPGN)?
   (MPGN) is a rare form of glomerular disease that occurs in both children and adults. It is characterized by a unique histopathologic feature, namely splitting of the glomerular basement membrane (GBM) with interposition of mesangial cells and extracellular matrix material. It is associated with variable degrees of endothelial and mesangial hypercellularity. Together with postinfectious glomerulonephritis, systemic lupus erythematosus (SLE), and cholesterol embolic disease, it is one of the glomerulopathies that is marked by hypocomplementemia (i.e., a low level of serum C3).

2. How is MPGN diagnosed and classified?
   Although the disease may be suspected in a patient with hematuria and/or proteinuria and a reduced level of C3, a kidney biopsy is required to confirm the diagnosis. Examination of the kidney histopathology demonstrates a lobular appearance of the glomerular tuft, mesangial expansion, hypercellularity, and the characteristic "tram track" finding with a double contour of the GBM. Immunofluorescence staining is usually positive for C3, IgG, and IgM in a capillary wall distribution. Classic complement cascade components are seen in type I but not types II and III MPGN.
   Primary MPGN is divided into three subtypes based on the nature and location of electron-dense deposits in addition to the expected changes in the GBM: type I, subendothelial deposits; type II, large, ribbon-like intramembranous deposits, so-called dense deposit disease (DDD); and type III, subendothelial and subepithelial deposits. The deposits can be numerous or sparse. They are homogeneous in density and have no defining ultrastructural appearance. The presence of C4d on immunofluorescence staining has been utilized to distinguish type I (positive) from type II (negative) MPGN.
   Recently the term *C3 glomerulopathy* has been introduced to define cases of MPGN. It corresponds to type II MPGN (DDD) as opposed to the immune-complex–mediated forms of the disease, types I and III.
   The diagnostic label MPGN is focused mainly on the light microscopy appearance (hypercellular, lobulated glomerular tuft) and the ultrastructural changes in the GBM (splitting of the GBM with mesangial cell interposition) as well as the specific location of the electron-dense deposits (subepithelial, intramembranous, or subendothelial). In contrast, the term, C3 glomerulopathy, highlights the presence of C3 as the dominant or codominant molecule detected by immunofluorescence examination of the kidney tissue. In this way the diagnosis sheds light on the underlying cause of the disease—activation of the alternative pathway of complement in the pathogenesis of the glomerulopathy. Moreover, it points the way to a new therapeutic approach to MPGN and C3 glomerulopathy that reduces kidney injury by inhibiting the activity of the alternative pathway of complement (see Question 16).

3. What is the cause of MPGN?
   MPGN can be primary (idiopathic) in nature. Alternatively, it can be secondary to a wide variety of medical conditions including infections (hepatitis B, hepatitis C, and bacterial endocarditis), autoimmune diseases (e.g., SLE), chronic liver disease (e.g., α1-antitrypsin deficiency), malignancies, lymphoproliferative disorders, plasma cell dyscrasias leading to monoclonal gammopathy, and essential cryoglobulinemia. MPGN has been associated rarely with Lyme disease, autoimmune thyroiditis, and type I diabetes mellitus. Some newer medications have been linked to type I MPGN, such as granulocyte colony-stimulating factor. Because MPGN is a rare condition that requires a kidney biopsy for diagnosis, there is no systematic information about the relative incidence of primary versus secondary MPGN.
   Postinfectious glomerulonephritis and MPGN likely represent a spectrum of the same disease. They share common histopathologic features. Long-term follow-up and detailed assessment of the alternative pathway of complement are required to distinguish these two entities. Type II MPGN has

been linked to genetic mutations in proteins involved in the regulation of the alternative pathway of complement. These include alterations in factor H, factor H–related proteins, and complement receptor 1.

4. What are the incidence and prevalence of MPGN?

Primary MPGN is one of the least common causes of primary nephrotic syndrome, accounting at most for 5% to 10% of cases. Therefore the incidence is probably in the range of 1 to 2 per million population per year; as such, it qualifies for the federal designation of a rare disease. The incidence of MPGN may have been declining over the last two decades. The secondary causes of MPGN have a less clear-cut epidemiology because of varying patterns of performing a kidney biopsy in patients with urinary abnormalities and subtle changes in glomerular filtration rate (GFR). In addition, clinical practice may differ in those with primary versus secondary disease. In primary disease, where extrarenal symptoms are limited, a kidney biopsy is essential to make a diagnosis. In contrast, the presence of a defined secondary cause may be viewed as sufficient to make a clinical diagnosis. The net result may underestimate the incidence of this complication in patients with MPGN. Nonetheless, MPGN is a rare cause of end-stage kidney disease (ESKD) in children and adults, accounting for less than 5% of patients on dialysis or receiving a kidney transplant.

5. What is the clinical presentation of patients with MPGN?

MPGN can be present with the full spectrum of glomerular disease.
- Hematuria can be the sole manifestation in rare cases.
- Glomerular hematuria (including gross hematuria) and proteinuria with normal kidney function may be the presenting finding in 10% to 30%.
- New-onset nephrotic syndrome may be seen in 40% to 70%.
- Nephritic syndrome occurs, with hypertension, azotemia, hematuria, and proteinuria.
- There may be anemia that is out of proportion to the degree of kidney dysfunction.

6. Are there extrarenal manifestations of MPGN?

Patients with primary MPGN generally have primarily kidney manifestations. However, in nearly 25% of cases, patients with type II disease, which is more common in children, manifest partial lipodystrophy (gradual loss of subcutaneous fat tissue in the face and upper body). There may be other associated findings in patients with MPGN, such as macular degeneration and mild visual field and color defects. Retinal angiography demonstrates the presence of choroidal neovascularization.

Patients with secondary MPGN may have extrarenal abnormalities related to the underlying disease. For example, patients with MPGN in association with cryoglobulinemia may have ulcerative skin lesions, Raynaud phenomenon, peripheral neuropathy, hepatomegaly, and signs of cirrhosis.

7. What is the natural history of MPGN?

Although spontaneous remission has been described in children and adolescents with MPGN, nearly 50% progress to ESKD over 10 to 15 years. Similar outcomes are found in adults, with 50% progressing to ESKD within 5 years and 64% after 10 years of follow-up. Indicators of poor outcome include
- Elevated serum creatinine at presentation
- Nephrotic-range proteinuria
- Severe hypertension
- Crescents in more than 50% of glomeruli
- Diffuse interstitial fibrosis and tubular atrophy
- A reduced calculated GFR after 1 year of treatment
- Primary versus secondary forms of MPGN
- Type II MPGN compared as opposed to types I and III

8. Are there any patient groups at special risk of developing MPGN or adverse long-term outcomes?

MPGN appears to involve children and adults of both genders and all ethnic groups, and the prognosis is comparable in all patient groups.

9. What is the appropriate workup for patients with MPGN?

The critical laboratory test that suggests the diagnosis of MPGN is hypocomplementemia—namely, reduced C3 and CH50 levels, which are confirmed in 80% to 90% of cases. The C4 and factor B levels are also low in approximately 40% of those with type I MPGN. This is less common in those with type II or III MPGN. Molecular markers of activation of the alternative pathway of complement, such as Bb and C3d, are elevated in patients with type II MPGN. Measurement of all components of the complement cascade to distinguish between the different types of MPGN is usually not performed in clinical chemistry laboratories and currently is available only in select research facilities. Activity of C3 nephritic factor, an IgM autoantibody that stabilizes C3 convertase, should be assayed in all forms of primary and secondary MPGN. In adults with cryoglobulinemia, testing should be performed for hepatitis B and C infection. Hepatitis serology should be evaluated in pediatric patients with MPGN even in the absence of mixed cryoglobulinemia. Other laboratory abnormalities will be present depending on the underlying disease. The confirmatory test in patients with hypocomplementemia or a suggestive history is a kidney biopsy demonstrating the characteristic histopathological findings.

10. **Are there any unique laboratory tests that are relevant to patients with MPGN?**
Mutations in the alternative pathway of complement proteins or detectable levels of the activity of C3 nephritic factor, an IgM autoantibody to the alternate pathway C3 convertase (C3bBb), are more common in type II disease—that is, in up to 80% of patients, compared with 20% to 25% of patients with types I or III disease. C3 nephritic factor can be measured in a hemolytic or solid-phase assay. This autoantibody is also detectable in up to 50% of patients with secondary forms of MPGN. Patients with type III MPGN may have a nephritic factor of the terminal complement pathway that stabilizes properdin-dependent C5 convertase.

11. **What is the pathogenesis of MPGN?**
In primary forms of MPGN, the mechanism of disease centers on abnormal activation of the complement cascade. There are three distinct patterns of complement activation in the three types of MPGN.
- In type I disease, the process is initiated by immune complex deposition within the kidney and involvement of the classic pathway. The source of the immune complexes is unknown in the idiopathic form of the disease. Patients have low levels of C3, C4, C6, C7, and/or C9.
- In the type II variant, continuous overactivity of the complement cascade involves an amplification loop in the alternative pathway, characterized mainly by markedly depressed C3 levels. An IgG or IgM autoantibody, termed C3 nephritic factor, is present in the majority of patients with DDD.
- Type III MPGN appears to have features in common with type I disease as well as evidence of activation of the terminal complement pathway, with low levels of C3, C5, and properdin. In the secondary forms of MPGN, it is presumed that there is immune complex–mediated activation of the complement cascade.

12. **Is there a genetic contribution to MPGN?**
Abnormal complement activation in MPGN can occur as a consequence of genetic mutations with reduced endogenous inhibitors of the alternate pathway, such as factor H, or because of the presence of a circulating autoantibody that stabilizes C3 convertase. MPGN occurs in patients who carry homozygous mutations in factor H. Other genetic causes of MPGN include isolated C4 deficiency.

13. **What is the first-line treatment for MPGN?**
Children who are clinically well and free of symptoms or only have minor urinary abnormalities generally do not require aggressive therapy. These patients may be treated with antihypertensive agents, specifically an angiotensin-converting enzyme inhibitor (ACEI) or angiotensin receptor blocker (ARB), to reduce proteinuria and prevent progressive kidney damage. Those with more severe disease are treated with prolonged alternate-day therapy with oral steroids, prednisone 40 to 60 mg/m^2, or 2 to 2.5 mg/kg every other day for an average period of 6.5 years, leading to an improved outcome compared with historic controls or patients treated at other centers. Repeat biopsies performed after 2 years of therapy have shown an increase in open capillary loops and a reduction in mesangial matrix expansion, suggesting that there may be an increase in glomerulosclerosis despite clinical improvement. The efficacy of therapy was greater in patients who began treatment within 1 year of disease onset and in those whose GFR was well preserved (i.e., >70 mL/min per 1.73 m^2).

In adults, there is widespread concern about the risks of prolonged steroid therapy. Therefore the current evidence-based medicine recommendation is to prescribe steroids only for adults with nephrotic syndrome or impaired kidney function. Treatment is maintained for 6 months. Patients with asymptomatic urinary findings or who fail to respond to steroids should be treated conservatively. ACEIs have been demonstrated to be effective in reducing proteinuria in patients with MPGN. Combined therapy with dipyridamole, cyclophosphamide, and warfarin does not appear to be beneficial, and this treatment is no longer recommended.

In patients with hepatitis C infection and MPGN, several new antiviral agents (e.g., boceprevir, telaprevir, simeprevir, sofosbuvir, and the ledipasvir-sofosbuvir combination) have been introduced into clinical practice. They have led to dramatically improved viral clearance and outcomes. However, the impact of these agents on the incidence of hepatitis C–related MPGN has not been assessed.

14. **What are the second-line therapies for MPGN?**
There is a compelling argument in favor of optimal control of blood pressure, preferably with an ACEI or ARB. Plasmapheresis has been reported to be useful in small numbers of patients with severe idiopathic MPGN and acute kidney failure or rapidly deteriorating disease. Mycophenolate mofetil has been tried in patients with cryoglobulinemic MPGN related to hepatitis B infection. Although treatment resulted in reduced proteinuria, viral replication was induced by the drug. Therefore caution is advisable when considering this immunosuppressive agent for the treatment of MPGN. Mycophenolate mofetil has also been utilized in open-label studies of patients with type II MPGN and C3 glomerulopathy. Cyclosporine is another alternative form of immunosuppressive therapy that may be beneficial in patients with refractory MPGN; however, it has not been studied systematically in a large case series.

15. **What is the role of kidney transplantation in the treatment of patients with MPGN?**
Kidney transplantation is a viable treatment for patients with MPGN who progress to ESKD. However, there is a variable risk of recurrent disease in both primary and secondary categories of disease. In patients with primary MPGN, the recurrence rate is approximately 20% to 40% in those with type I and III disease and up to 80% to 90% in those with type II (DDD). In those with secondary disease, the recurrence is directly linked to control of the underlying illness. The risk of recurrent disease may be marginally higher in recipients of living-donor kidneys. Recurrent disease usually leads to allograft loss.

16. **Are there novel therapies in development for MPGN?**
Agents to block the abnormal activation of the alternate pathway of complement, including eculizumab, a monoclonal antibody to C5a and recombinant factor H, are being considered as potential treatments for primary MPGN, especially type II disease. Initial studies suggest that this treatment may be most effective in patients with evidence of activation of the alternative pathway of complement (e.g., elevated circulating levels of the soluble membrane attack complex). However, this observation requires confirmation in larger randomized clinical trials. Newer anticomplement therapies are under development and will also require testing in patients with MPGN. In secondary disease, removal of cryoglobulins with cryofiltration is an experimental modality.

KEY POINTS

1. Membranoproliferative glomerulonephritis (MPGN) is diagnosed based on a kidney biopsy with renal kidney histopathology demonstrating a lobular appearance of the glomerular tuft, mesangial expansion, and hypercellularity, the characteristic "tram track" finding with a double contour of the glomerular basement membrane, and immunofluorescence staining that is usually positive for C3, IgG, and IgM in a capillary wall distribution.
2. There are three subtypes:
    a. Type I—subendothelial deposits
    b. Type II—large, ribbon-like intramembranous deposits, so-called dense deposit disease
    c. Type III—subendothelial and subepithelial deposits
3. A new term, *C3 glomerulopathy*, which highlights the presence of C3 as the dominant or codominant immunoreactant in the glomerulus and the role of the alternative pathway of complement activation, has been introduced to describe subtypes II and III of MPGN.
4. MPGN can be primary or idiopathic. A substantial proportion of these primary conditions are due to genetic mutations in proteins involved in the alternative complement pathway. Secondary causes of MPGN may be due to:
    a. Infections
    b. Autoimmune diseases
    c. Chronic liver disease
    d. Malignancies
    e. Lymphoproliferative disorders
    f. Plasma cell dyscrasias
    g. Essential cryoglobulinemia
5. Primary MPGN is one of the least common causes of idiopathic nephrotic syndrome, accounting for at most 5% to 10% of cases and an incidence in the range of 1 to 2 per million population per year.

6. Together with postinfectious glomerulonephritis, systemic lupus erythematosus, and cholesterol embolic disease, MPGN is one of the glomerulopathies characterized by hypocomplementemia (i.e., a low serum C3 level).

7. Spontaneous remission is rare and nearly 50% of patients with MPGN progress to end-stage kidney disease over 10 to 15 years.

8. Children with severe disease are treated with prolonged alternate daily therapy with oral steroids, prednisone 40 to 60 mg/m², or 2 to 2.5 mg/kg every other day for an average period of 6.5 years, with an improved outcome compared to historic controls or patients treated at other centers. The role of immunosuppressive therapy is less clear in adults. Further study is needed to clarify the role of anticomplement therapies in patients with MPGN.

BIBLIOGRAPHY

Alchi, B., & Jayne, D. (2010). Membranoproliferative glomerulonephritis. *Pediatr Nephrol, 25*(8), 1409–1418. doi:10.1007/s00467-009-1322-7.

Alexander, M. P., Fervenza, F. C., De Vriese, A. S., Smith, R. J. H., Nasr, S. H., Cornell, L. D., . . . Sethi, S. (2016). C3 glomerulonephritis and autoimmune disease: More than a fortuitous association? *J Nephrol, 29*(2), 203–209. doi.org/10.1007/s40620-015-0218-9.

Appel, G. B., Cook, H. T., Hageman, G., Jennette, J. C., Kashgarian, M., Kirschfink, M., . . . Zipfel, P. F. (2005). Membranoproliferative glomerulonephritis type II (Dense deposit disease): An update. *J Am Soc Nephrol, 16,* 1392–1403.

Bomback, A. S., Smith, R. J., Barile, G. R., Zhang, Y., Heher, E. C., Herlitz, L., . . . Appel, G. B. (2012). Eculizumab for dense deposit disease and C3 glomerulonephritis. *Clin J Am Soc Nephrol, 7,* 748–756.

Cansick, J. C., Lennon, R., Cummins, C. L., Howie, A. J., McGraw, M. E., Saleem, M. A., . . . Taylor, C. M. (2004). Prognosis, treatment and outcome of childhood mesangiocapillary (membranoproliferative) glomerulonephritis. *Nephrol Dial Transplant, 19,* 2769–2777.

Green, H., Rahamimov, R., Rozen-Zvi, B., Pertzov, B., Tobar, A., Lichtenberg, S., . . . Mor, E. (2015). Recurrent membranoproliferative glomerulonephritis type I after kidney transplantation: A 17-year single-center experience. *Transplantation, 99,* 1172–1177.

Kawasaki, Y., Kanno, S., Ono, A., Suzuki, Y., Ohara, S., Sato, M., . . . Hosoya, M. (2016). Differences in clinical findings, pathology, and outcomes between C3 glomerulonephritis and membranoproliferative glomerulonephritis. *Pediatr Nephrol, 31,* 1091–1099.

Lorenz, E. C., Sethi, S., Leung, N., Dispenzieri, A., Fervenza, F. C., & Cosio, F. G. (2010). Recurrent membranoproliferative glomerulonephritis after kidney transplantation. *Kidney Int, 77*(8), 721–728. doi:10.1038/ki.2010.1.

McEnery, P. T., McAdams, A. J., & West. C. D. (1985). The effect of prednisone in a high-dose, alternate-day regimen on the natural history of idiopathic membranoproliferative glomerulonephritis. *Medicine (Baltimore), 64,* 401–424.

Nasr, S. H., Valeri, A. M., Appel, G. B., Sherwinter J, Stokes, M. B., Said, S. M., . . . D'Agati, V. D. (2009). Dense deposit disease: Clinicopathologic study of 32 pediatric and adult patients. *Clin J Am Soc Nephrol, 4,* 22–32.

Nester, C. M., & Smith, R. J. (2016). Complement inhibition in C3 glomerulopathy. *Semin Immunol, 28*(3), 241–249.

Okuda, Y., Ishikura, K., Hamada, R., Harada, R., Sakai, T., Hamasaki, Y., . . . Honda, M. (2015). Membranoproliferative glomerulonephritis and C3 glomerulonephritis: Frequency, clinical features, and outcome in children. *Nephrology (Carlton), 20*(4), 286–292.

Pickering, M. C., D'Agati, V. D., Nester, C. M., Smith, R. J., Haas, M., Appel, G. B., . . . Cook, H. T. (2013). C3 glomerulopathy: Consensus report. *Kidney Int, 84,* 1079–1089.

Salvadori, M., & Rosso, G. (2016). Reclassification of membranoproliferative glomerulonephritis: Identification of a new GN: C3GN. *World J Nephrol, 5*(4), 308–320.

Sethi, S., & Fervenza, F. C. (2012). Membranoproliferative glomerulonephritis—a new look at an old entity. *N Engl J Med, 366,* 1119–1131.

Sethi, S., Fervenza, F. C., Zhang, Y., Nasr, S. H., Leung, N., Vrana, J., . . . Smith, R. J. (2011). Proliferative glomerulonephritis secondary to dysfunction of the alternative pathway of complement. *Clin J Am Soc Nephrol, 6,* 1009–1017.

Sethi, S., Fervenza, F. C., Zhang, Y., Zand, L., Vrana, J. A., Nasr, S. H., . . . Smith, R. J. (2012). C3 glomerulonephritis: Clinicopathological findings, complement abnormalities, glomerular proteomic profile, treatment, and follow-up. *Kidney Int, 82,* 465–473.

Tarshish, P., Bernstein, J., Tobin, J. N., & Edelmann, C. M., Jr. (1992). Treatment of mesangiocapillary glomerulonephritis with alternate-day prednisone: A report of the International Study of Kidney Diseases in Children. *Pediatr Nephrol, 6,* 123–130.

Wei, C. C., Wang, W., Smoyer, W. E., & Licht, C. (2012). Trends in pediatric primary membranoproliferative glomerulonephritis costs and complications. *Pediatr Nephrol, 27,* 2243–2250.

Yanagihara, T., Hayakawa, M., Yoshida, J., Tsuchiya, M., Morita, T., Murakami, M., & Fukunaga, Y. (2005). Long-term follow-up of diffuse proliferative membranoproliferative glomerulonephritis type 1. *Pediatr Nephrol, 20,* 585–590.

V

SECONDARY GLOMERULAR DISORDERS

DIABETIC KIDNEY DISEASE

Lori Shah and Anna Burgner

1. Define the terms *diabetic nephropathy* (DN) and *diabetic kidney disease* (DKD).
   The terms DN and DKD are used interchangeably to describe a set of characteristic clinical and pathologic findings. The main clinical findings of DKD are the presence of albuminuria, progressive chronic kidney disease (CKD), and less commonly microscopic hematuria. Diabetes is the most common cause of the nephrotic syndrome. Proteinuria is first detected by screening for albumin in the urine. A normal urine albumin level is less than 30 mg/day. Abnormal urine protein is defined in two stages. Moderately increased albuminuria (formerly known as microalbuminuria) is defined as 30 to 300 mg/day. Severely increased albuminuria (formerly known as macroalbuminuria) is defined as greater than 300 mg/day and is also known as overt proteinuria or overt nephropathy. The pathologic features of DKD are outlined in question 4.

2. How is DN from type 1 diabetes mellitus (DM) similar/different from type 2 DM?
   See Table 31.1. Of note, young adults diagnosed with type 2 DM before the age of 20 are at a higher risk for DN, retinopathy, peripheral neuropathy, and hypertension than patients with type 1 DM who are diagnosed at the same age.

3. What is the natural history of the progression of DN to end-stage renal disease (ESRD)?
   This question is most clearly answered in patients with nephropathy from type 1 DM, given the readily identifiable onset of DM. The earliest change of kidney function in DM is kidney hypertrophy and glomerular hyperfiltration occurring in the first 1 to 2 years after diagnosis. The degree of hyperfiltration correlates with the risk of developing nephropathy. The onset of albuminuria is on average 15 years after the diagnosis of DM and increases in severity over time. Patients with type 1 DM who have not developed nephropathy after 25 years have a very low risk of developing nephropathy. End-stage kidney disease (ESKD) occurs 20 to 30 years after the onset of diabetes.

Table 31.1. Comparison of Type 1 Diabetes Mellitus to Type 2 Diabetes Mellitus

	TYPE 1	TYPE 2
Onset of overt nephropathy	Mean onset at 15 years after initial diagnosis of DM	Can be present at time of diagnosis of DM.
Hypertension association	Often occurs after nephropathy develops due to diabetic renal parenchymal disease	Often predates development of diabetic nephropathy as part of the metabolic syndrome
Findings on kidney biopsy	No difference (See Question 4)	No difference (See Question 4)
Cumulative incidence of overt nephropathy	Approximately 25% of patients will develop nephropathy within 25 years of diagnosis of DM	Approximately 30% of patients will develop nephropathy within 20 years of diagnosis of DM
Correlation with retinopathy	More than 95% of patients with nephropathy also have retinopathy	Only approximately 60% of patients with nephropathy also have retinopathy
Risk of cardiovascular disease	Increased risk occurs approximately 2 decades after the diagnosis of type 1 DM and shortly after the development of overt nephropathy	Increased risk is already present at diagnosis of type 2 DM

DM, Diabetes mellitus

Due in part to the unknown time of onset for patients with type 2 DM, moderately increased albuminuria can be seen as early as at the time of diagnosis. In addition, it does not always progress as it does in type 1 DM, because some patients develop diabetes-related loss of kidney function without albuminuria. Patients with DN and type 2 DM are at increased risk of both ESKD and death from cardiovascular disease. Due to increased comorbidities, most patients will die before reaching the need for dialysis.

4. How and when should physicians screen for DKD?

After DM is diagnosed, consideration for screening of DKD must commence. Screening consists of annual measurements of creatinine and urine albumin-to-creatinine ratio (ACR). It should begin 5 years after diagnosis in type 1 DM and at the time of diagnosis in type 2 DM. Moderately increased albuminuria (ACR between 30 mg/g and 300 mg/g) that persists for more than 3 months means the patient is at risk for progression to overt nephropathy.

5. What are the findings seen on kidney biopsy in DN?

Three classic features seen on kidney biopsy:
1. Mesangial expansion leading to wide-appearing glomeruli
2. Thickening of the glomerular basement membrane (GBM) with the notable absence of GBM deposits
3. Nodular glomerulosclerosis. Nodular glomerulosclerosis typically presents as rounded tufts of acellular matrix in the mesangium. These are called Kimmelstiel-Wilson nodules.

Other findings include hyaline deposition within Bowman capsule and the afferent and efferent arterioles. This arteriolar deposition can distinguish DN from hypertensive nephropathy, in which hyalinosis is limited to the afferent arteriole.

Although nodular glomerulosclerosis is typically found in diabetic patients, it can also be seen in monoclonal immunoglobulin deposition disease, amyloidosis, membranoproliferative glomerulonephritis, and in idiopathic nodular sclerosis, a disease of older Caucasian patients with history of hypertension and tobacco use.

6. Is a kidney biopsy indicated in the diagnosis of DN?

The presence of proteinuria in a patient with DM does not necessarily equate with a diagnosis of DN and could in fact represent another glomerular disease. Major clues that suggest another cause of proteinuria include:
- Signs of another systemic disease
- Onset of proteinuria less than 5 years after diagnosis of type 1 DM
- Absence of retinopathy in a patient with type 1 DM
- Rapid deterioration of kidney function or sudden increases in proteinuria
- Presence of hematuria, red or white blood cell urine casts, pyuria, or abnormal protein chains in the urine

A study by Mazzucco et al. found that using restrictive criteria such as these to determine the need for a kidney biopsy may lead to more than 50% of kidney biopsies having another glomerular disease present.

7. What is the role of glycemic control in the treatment of DN?

Type 1 DM and type 2 DM have a different pathogenesis, but both are associated with hyperglycemia. Hyperglycemia activates the intrarenal renin-angiotensin system that plays an important role in the development of DN. However, the role of glycemic control in treatment of established DN is controversial.

The best evidence for preventing DN is in patients with type 1 DM. Tight glycemic control in patients with type 1 DM decreases the risk of development of albuminuria. In individuals with type 1 DM and moderately increased albuminuria, tight glycemic control also reduces the risk of progression to nephropathy. In addition, once severely increased albuminuria is present, small studies have found that return to euglycemia by performing a pancreas transplant led to improvement of biopsy findings 10 years post transplant.

In type 2 DM the data is less certain. Tight glycemic control appears to decrease the risk for development of moderately and severely increased albuminuria but does not decrease the risk for doubling of serum of creatinine or of renal death. In addition, tight blood glucose control to a hemoglobin A1c (HbA1C) less than 6.5% resulted in increased mortality. The current goal HbA1c in patients with DKD is less than 7%, with liberalized goals for elderly patients or those prone to hypoglycemia.

8. What is the current treatment of DN?

In addition to glycemic control as noted previously, inhibition of the renin-angiotensin-aldosterone system, sodium restriction, and blood pressure control are important parts of treating DN.

Renin-Angiotensin System (RAS) Inhibition: Angiotensin-converting enzyme (ACE) inhibitors and angiotensin receptor blockers (ARBs) have been a critical component of treating DN for more than 2 decades. Intrarenal RAS activation plays a major role in the pathogenesis and progression of DN. ACE inhibitors have been studied both early and late in the course of type 1 DN and have been shown to slow the rate of estimated glomerular filtration rate (eGFR) decline and decrease the risk of ESKD. Both ARBs and ACE inhibitors have been shown to do the same in patients with type 2 DN. In addition, since the importance of RAS inhibition in treatment of DN was discovered, there appears to be a slowing of the incidence of ESKD from DN in multiple regions of the world.

Sodium Restriction: High dietary sodium intake can cause hypervolemia and hypertension, leading to adverse cardiovascular outcomes. In addition, sodium restriction has been found to enhance the antiproteinuric effects of RAS inhibition.

Blood Pressure Control: Lowering blood pressure, even without using RAS inhibition, has been shown to decrease the rate of albumin excretion. Current guidelines from the 2017 American College of Cardiology/American Heart Association (ACC/AHA) Task Force suggest a goal blood pressure of less than 130/80 mm Hg for diabetic patients. This recommendation is based on the assumption that the vast majority of adults with DM (and CKD) have a 10-year atherosclerotic cardiovascular disease (ASCVD) risk $\geq$ 10%. This is a departure from the 2014 Joint National Committee on Prevention, Detection, Evaluation, and Treatment of High Blood Pressure (JNC 7) which recommended a goal blood pressure of less than 140/90 mm Hg.

9. **Is there any benefit in using the combination of an ACE inhibitor and an ARB in treatment of DN?**
   Given the significant role of activation of the RAS in the development of DN, many have theorized that combining ACE inhibitors and ARBs would slow the progression of DN more than either alone. Several small early studies supported this theory. However, in large trials such as The Veterans Affairs Nephropathy in Diabetes study (VA NEPHRON-D), combination therapy did not further slow the progression of kidney disease compared with monotherapy and was associated with significant increases in risk, including acute kidney injury, severe hyperkalemia, and hypotension. Thus there is no role for combining ACE inhibitors and ARBs for the treatment of DN.

10. **Do genetics play a role in the development DN?**
    The pathogenesis of DN is multifactorial. Genetic susceptibility certainly seems to play a role in both the development and severity of DN. The likelihood of developing DN, in both type 1 and type 2 DM, is increased in individuals with a first-degree relative with DN. This has perhaps been best described in Pima Indians, for whom an offspring had a 14% chance of developing proteinuria if neither parent had proteinuria. This risk increased to 23% if one parent had proteinuria and to 46% if both parents had proteinuria. There have been numerous genetic variants that have been implicated as potentially increasing the risk of DN, and this remains an area of ongoing study.

11. **Are there any special considerations for kidney transplantation in a patient with DN?**
    Cardiovascular disease is the most common cause of death in patients with diabetes following kidney transplantation. Thus, in addition to typical pretransplant candidacy screening, all patients with diabetes should undergo coronary artery disease screening. They do not necessarily need screening for cerebrovascular disease unless there is history of a transient ischemic attack or cerebrovascular attack. Peripheral vascular disease (PVD) can prevent a successful anastomosis of the allograft, thus screening for PVD should be considered, particularly if there are any signs or symptoms of PVD. Another important consideration is the presence of diabetic foot wounds, which need to be completely healed prior to a transplantation.
    The risk for histopathologic recurrence of DN in the transplanted kidney is high at 80% to 100%, with changes being seen as early as 2 to 3 years post transplant. For this reason, meticulous glycemic control is important before and after transplantation. The use of glucocorticoids should be avoided, when possible, to decrease the risk of uncontrolled DM.
    Patients with ESKD from type 1 DM should be considered for pancreas transplantation. This is often done in the form of simultaneous kidney-pancreas (SPK) transplant, although pancreas after kidney (PAK) transplant is also performed in patients who already have a kidney transplant. Recurrent and de novo DN is prevented with a successful pancreas transplant.

12. **How does treatment of DM change once kidney disease has developed?**
    As significant CKD develops, treatment of DM becomes complicated due to many factors. CKD is associated with increased insulin resistance. At the same time the kidneys are responsible for one-third of exogenous insulin degradation. In addition, the kidneys play a role in the metabolism and excretion

of many of the oral antidiabetic medications. With all of these factors contributing, it is difficult to estimate what a patient will need. Close monitoring is recommended to ensure ongoing good glycemic control. The following treatments have special considerations in the setting of DKD.

Metformin: A first-line therapy for diabetics, metformin was originally contraindicated for patients with kidney disease. However, the U.S. Food and Drug Administration (FDA) has amended this exclusion and now advises to continue giving metformin in patients with an eGFR greater than 30 to 45 mL/min per 1.73 m^2 if already on the therapy. If a patient currently taking metformin has a drop in eGFR less than 45 mL/min per 1.73 m^2, the risks of possible lactic acidosis must be compared with the benefit of glycemic control in that particular patient.

Glucagon-like Peptide-1 (GLP-1) Receptor Agonists and Dipeptidyl Peptidase 4 (DPP-4) Inhibitors: GLP-1 agonists were first isolated from the saliva of the Gila monster. GLP-1 agonists are classified as incretins secondary to their ability to promote insulin and inhibit glucagon secretion. Likewise, DPP-4 inhibitors inhibit glucagon. Due to side effects of nausea and vomiting, as well as increasing sodium excretion in the urine, there are numerous case reports of kidney failure due to volume depletion associated with these drugs. However, early studies suggested a possible nephroprotective effect with these agents. This is supported by findings from the Liraglutide Effect and Action in Diabetes (LEADER) study that examined the GLP-1 agonist liraglutide. This study of almost 10,000 patients demonstrated in prespecified secondary outcomes reduced the composite of new-onset persistent macroalbuminuria, persistent doubling of serum creatinine, ESKD, or death from kidney disease compared with usual care. There is limited evidence in using these agents in individuals with severe kidney disease with an eGFR of less than 30 mL/min per 1.73 m^2.

Sodium-Glucose Cotransporter-2 (SGLT-2) Inhibitors: The use of SGLT-2 inhibitors in patients with diabetes has shown improvements in mortality and cardiovascular events. Early studies suggest that they may slow the progression of DKD by decreasing hyperfiltration and by decreasing the inflammatory and fibrotic response to hyperglycemia. Canagliflozin's kidney outcomes were not considered significant, but it did reduce the composite of a 40% drop in eGFR, need for dialysis, or death from kidney disease (hazard ratio [HR] 0.6, 95% confidence interval [CI] 0.47 to 0.77). Its applicability for use in patients with DKD is still under study, and there are ongoing clinical trials assessing SGLT-2 inhibitors' ability to treat DKD as a primary outcome. Currently these agents are contraindicated with an eGFR less than 30 mL/min per 1.73 m^2 and are not recommended to be initiated at an eGFR of less than 60 mL/min per 1.73 m^2.

13. Name some other agents currently being investigated for treatment of DKD.
    There are multiple other therapies currently being investigated for treatment of DKD. Further studies are needed for all of the following agents before these agents can be recommended for treatment of DKD.

Endothelin A Receptor Antagonists: The endothelin system plays an important role in the pathogenesis of DKD. Endothelin receptor 1 stimulation increases renal vasoconstriction, extracellular matrix accumulation, and interstitial fibrosis. Endothelin A receptor antagonists have shown promise in the treatment of DKD, along with the use of ACE inhibitors in animal studies. Human trials are ongoing; however, one clinical trial studying avosentan was terminated early due to increased cardiovascular events of fluid overload and congestive heart failure. Another endothelin antagonist, atrasentan, was shown to reduce proteinuria in a short study. Longer and larger trials are in progress.

Phosphodiesterase Inhibitors: Phosphodiesterase inhibitors block inflammatory cytokines and leukotrienes associated with DM. They might also play a role in augmenting glomerular hypertrophy occurring in DM. Small studies suggest that phosphodiesterase inhibitors can slow the rate of eGFR decline in DKD. However, large randomized multicenter studies have not been performed.

Mineralocorticoid Antagonists (MRAs): MRAs reduce proteinuria when used alone and have an additive effect when used with an ACE inhibitor or ARB in the treatment of DKD. There are no long-term data evaluating the benefit of adding an MRA to an ACE inhibitor or ARB on hard kidney outcomes such as slowing loss of eGFR and preventing ESRD. Furthermore, worsening hyperkalemia by combining these agents may limit the usefulness of MRAs.

Transforming Growth Factor-β (TGF-β) Inhibitors: The role of TGF-β–induced mesangial matrix expansion and tubular fibrosis in DKD is well established. Early human trials have found a significant increase in eGFR in individuals with DKD treated with TGF-β inhibitors.

Selective Serotonin Receptor Antagonists: Serotonin is a proinflammatory mediator released by activated platelets. Stimulation of the Serotonin receptors is associated with mesangial proliferation, increased type IV collagen deposition, platelet aggregation, and regulation of tissue vasculature. Serotonin receptor subtype 2A (5-HT2A) is found on mesangial cells and is believed to play a role in DKD. Small studies have shown that 5-HT2A antagonists decrease albuminuria in humans with DKD.

14. **Are there any additional markers of DKD?**
Urinary ACR is the traditional biomarker tested when screening for DKD. However, novel biomarkers are being studied to aid in the diagnosis and prognosis of DKD. Inflammatory markers such as tumor necrosis factor (TNF)-α, markers of tubular injury and glomerular damage, markers of endothelial dysfunction, and urinary and plasma microRNAs are all possible future tests of kidney function. Panels of multiple biomarkers are also being investigated to help diagnose early DKD, as well as assess for the risk of progression.

KEY POINTS

1. All adults with newly diagnosed type 2 diabetes mellitus should be screened for nephropathy by serum creatinine and urine albumin testing.
2. Consider kidney biopsy for any patient with diabetes whose kidney disease does not follow the typical progression of diabetic nephropathy.
3. Treat diabetic nephropathy with a combination of blood glucose control, blood pressure control, and renin-angiotensin system inhibition.
4. Patients with diabetes and chronic kidney disease are most likely to die from a cardiovascular cause.

BIBLIOGRAPHY

Adler, A. I., Stevens, R. J., Manley, S. E., Bilous, R. W., Cull, C. A., Holman, R. R., & UKPDS GROUP. (2003). Development and progression of nephropathy in type 2 diabetes: The United Kingdom Prospective Diabetes Study (UKPDS 64). *Kidney International, 63*(1), 225–232.

Coca, S. G., Ismail-Beigi, F., Haq, N., Krumholz, H. M., & Parikh, C. R. (2012). Role of intensive glucose control in development of renal end points in type 2 diabetes mellitus: Systematic review and meta-analysis. *Archives of Internal Medicine, 172*(10), 761–769.

Danovitch, G. M. (2010). *Handbook of kidney transplantation* (5th ed.). Philadelphia: Lippincott Williams & Wilkins.

Dabelea, D., Stafford, J. M., & Meyer-Davis, E. J. (2017). Association of type 1 diabetes vs type 2 diabetes diagnosed during childhood and adolescence with complications during teenage years and young adulthood. *Journal of the American Medical Association, 317*(8), 825–835.

Fogo, A. B., & Kashgarian, M. (2017). *Diagnostic atlas of renal pathology* (3rd ed.). Philadelphia: Elsevier.

James, P. A., Oparil, S., Carter, B. L., Cushman, W. C., Dennison-Himmelfarb, C., Handler, J., . . . Ortiz, E. (2014). 2014 evidence-based guideline for the management of high blood pressure in adults report from the panel members appointed to the Eighth Joint National Committee (JNC 8). *Journal of the American Medical Association, 311*(5), 507–520.

Lee, S.- Y., & Choi, M. (2015). Urinary biomarkers for early diabetic nephropahy: Beyond albuminuria. *Pediatric Nephrology, 30*(7), 1063–1075.

Mann, J. F. E., Ørsted, D. D., Brown-Frandsen, K., Marso, S. P., Poulter, N. R., Rasmussen, S., . . . LEADER Steering Committee and Investigators. (2017). Liraglutide and renal outcomes in type 2 diabetes. *New England Journal of Medicine, 377,* 839–848.

Mazzucco, G., Bertani, T., Fortunato, M., Bernardi, M., Leutner, M., Boldorini, R., & Monga G. (2002). Different patterns of renal damage in type 2 diabetes mellitus: A multicentric study on 393 biopsies. *American Journal of Kidney Diseases, 39*(4), 713–720.

McMahon, E. J., Campbell, K. L., Mudge, D. W., & Bauer, J. D. (2012). Achieving salt restriction in chronic kidney disease. *International Journal of Nephrology,* 720–749.

Molitch, M. E., Adler, A. I., Flyvbjerg, A., Nelson, R. G., So, W. Y., Wanner, C., . . . Mogensen, C. E. (2015). Diabetic kidney disease—a clinical update from Kidney Disease: Improving Global Outcomes (KDIGO). *Kidney International, 87*(1), 20.

Montero, R. M., Covic, A., Gnudi, L., & Goldsmith, D. (2016). Diabetic nephropathy: What does the future hold? *International Urology and Nephrology, 48*(1), 99–113.

Neal, B., Perkovic, V., Mahaffey, K. W., de Zeeuw, D., Fulcher, G., Erondu, N., . . . CANVAS Program Collaborative Group. (2017). Canagliflozin and cardiovascular and renal events in type 2 diabetes. *New England Journal of Medicine, 377,* 644–657.

ONTARGET Investigators. (2008). Telmisartan, ramipril, or both in patients at high risk for vascular events. *New England Journal of Medicine, 358,* 1547–1559.

Pavkov, M. E., Knowler, W. C., Hanson, R. L., & Nelson, R. G. (2008). Diabetic nephropathy in American Indians, with a special emphasis on the Pima Indians. *Current Diabetes Reports, 8*(6), 486–493.

Roscioni, S. S., Lambers Heerspink, H. J., & de Zeeuw, D. (2014). The effect of RAAS blockade on the progression of diabetic nephropathy. *Nature Reviews Nephrology, 10*(2), 77–87.

Skyler, J. S., Bergenstal, R., & Sherwin, R. S. (2009). Intensive glycemic control and the prevention of cardiovascular events: Implications of the ACCORD, ADVANCE, and VA diabetes trials. *Diabetes Care, 32*(1), 187–192.

Whelton, P.K., Carey, R.M., Aronow, W.S., et al. (2017). ACC/AHA Guideline for the Prevention, Detection, Evaluation, and Management of High Blood Pressure in Adults; A Report of the ACC/AHA Task Force on Clinical Practice Guidelines. *Journal of the American College of Cardiology* 24430; DOI: 10.1016/j.jacc.2017.11.006.

CHAPTER 32

LUPUS NEPHRITIS

Pravir V. Baxi and William L. Whittier

1. How common is systemic lupus erythematosus (SLE) and how often is lupus nephritis present in patients with this disease?

   The prevalence of SLE in the United States is around 40/100,000 (0.04%); it has a peak age of onset of 20 to 40 years and is more common in women and certain ethnic groups (especially African Americans). Kidney involvement occurs in 40% of patients with SLE, and the kidney is the most common major organ affected.

2. What is the single most important test to order to determine if a patient with SLE needs further evaluation for lupus nephritis?

   A urinalysis should be performed at every visit in patients with SLE, because lupus nephritis may be asymptomatic or intermittent. The presence of protein or blood on dipstick and/or the presence of red blood cells (RBCs) or RBC casts on microscopic examination requires further workup for lupus nephritis. Glycosuria (with a normal plasma glucose) and sterile pyuria can also represent kidney involvement. Proteinuria, if present on dipstick, should be quantified. The presence of any blood, protein, or casts in the urine warrants further nephrologic evaluation.

3. How does a patient with lupus nephritis present clinically?

   Although kidney involvement may be the first sign of SLE in an individual patient, lupus nephritis typically becomes clinically apparent as a manifestation of the systemic disease. In the Systemic Lupus International Collaborating Clinics classification criteria, patients with biopsy-proven lupus nephritis in the presence of antinuclear antibodies (ANA) or antibodies to double-stranded DNA (anti-dsDNA) satisfy criteria for a diagnosis of SLE. Some patients with lupus nephritis are asymptomatic, but classically patients will have a variety of systemic manifestations including but not limited to the following:
   - Cutaneous abnormalities
   - Fever
   - Malaise
   - Weight loss
   - Synovitis
   - Raynaud phenomenon
   - Serositis
   - Pericarditis
   - Retinopathy
   - Thrombotic microangiopathy (TMA)
   - Neuropsychiatric involvement
   - Hematologic abnormalities
     - Leukopenia
     - Anemia
     - Thrombocytopenia

   Evidence of immunologic activity in the serum is usually present as ANA, anti-dsDNA and Smith (anti-Sm), and hypocomplementemia (see Serologic Evaluation, further on). The pattern of clinical activity varies between patients but characteristically is one of relapsing and remitting disease. Only 10% of patients with discoid lupus will develop SLE; if so, they seldom develop nephritis. Certain medications, such as hydralazine or procainamide, may cause drug-induced systemic lupus, but they are only rarely associated with lupus nephritis.

   In patients with kidney involvement, presentation can range from subtle disease such as asymptomatic microscopic hematuria and proteinuria on urinalysis with normal kidney function to nephritic and/or nephrotic syndrome and rapidly progressive glomerulonephritis with kidney failure and hypertension. Nephrotic syndrome is present in approximately 25% of patients during their disease course. Microscopic hematuria is commonly associated with proteinuria and rarely found in isolation. Kidney failure, defined by an elevated serum creatinine, is present in approximately 40% of patients with lupus nephritis.

4. If my patient with lupus has hematuria or proteinuria, what immunologic serology should I order to determine if lupus nephritis is present or active?
The only definitive way to determine if lupus nephritis is present or active is to perform a kidney biopsy. However, certain types of immunologic serology are useful to establish parameters of activity that can be helpful to diagnose SLE and/or monitor relapses or response to treatment. Serologic evaluation should include
* ANA
* anti-Smith (anti-Sm)
* anti-Sjögren Syndrome A antigen (anti-Ro/SSA)
* anti-Sjögren Syndrome B antigen (anti-La/SSB)
* antiribonucleoprotein
* anti-dsDNA
* Complement components
* Rheumatoid factor
* Antiphospholipid antibodies
    This serology may be positive in a variety of diseases other than SLE, but anti-Sm is quite specific for SLE. Anti-dsDNA antibodies, when present, are strongly associated with lupus nephritis. Hypocomplementemia and anti-dsDNA antibodies will typically correlate with disease activity.

5. When does a kidney biopsy need to be performed in the setting of SLE?
Any patient suspected of having lupus nephritis should be further evaluated with a kidney biopsy. This procedure is considered when abnormalities—such as protein, blood, or casts—are present on urinalysis, often coupled with abnormal serology or reduced kidney function. Severe involvement, such as nephrotic syndrome or nephritic syndrome with or without kidney failure, will require a kidney biopsy for further evaluation. Even when subtle abnormalities are present clinically (i.e., normal kidney function with or without hematuria and less than 1 g of proteinuria/day), severe lupus nephritis may be present on kidney biopsy. Thus a kidney biopsy should be performed to establish a diagnosis, determine prognosis, and guide therapy. Many patients may require more than one biopsy during their disease course. This procedure may be necessary to alter therapy, because the characteristics of lupus nephritis may change over time or to determine if there is late progression of the disease, which may not be amenable to further immunosuppressive treatment.

6. What are the pathologic features of lupus nephritis?
The Renal Pathology Society/International Society of Nephrology (RPS/ISN) classification system divides kidney biopsies into six groups based on pathologic features in the glomeruli (Table 32.1). The number of active and/or chronic (or inactive) lesions guides treatment and is important in determining the patient's long-term kidney prognosis. Common active and chronic lesions in patients with lupus nephritis are listed in Box 32.1. Immunofluorescence is characterized by the presence of glomerular deposits of immune reactants that stain for IgG (dominantly), IgA, IgM, C3, and C1q (known as the "full house" pattern). Electron-dense deposits representing immune complexes are seen on electron microscopy in the mesangium and are found in the subepithelial and/or subendothelial locations. The presence of tubuloreticular inclusions in the glomerular capillary endothelial cell on electron microscopy is relatively specific for lupus nephritis.

Table 32.1.	The International Society of Nephrology/Renal Pathology Society Classification of Lupus Nephritis
I	Minimal mesangial lupus nephritis
II	Mesangial proliferative lupus nephritis
III	Focal lupus nephritis (<50% of glomeruli)
IV	Diffuse lupus nephritis (≥50% of glomeruli)
IV-S	Diffuse segmental lupus nephritis (<50% glomerular surface area)
IV-G	Diffuse global lupus nephritis (≥50% glomerular surface area)
V	Membranous lupus nephritis
VI	Advanced sclerosing lupus nephritis

Box 32.1. Active and Chronic Histologic Lesions in Patients With Systemic Lupus Erythematosus

Active Lesions
Endocapillary hypercellularity or proliferation
Wire loops (subendothelial deposits)
Karyorrhexis
Fibrinoid necrosis
Crescents (cellular or fibrocellular)
Rupture of glomerular basement membranes

Hematoxyphil bodies
Hyaline thrombi (rare)

Chronic Lesions
Glomerular sclerosis
Adhesions
Fibrous crescents

7. Does the lupus nephritis classification provide information on treatment, pathogenesis, and/or prognosis?
The RPS/ISN classification provides valuable information on how to treat patients with lupus nephritis. Treatment of severe lupus requires aggressive immunomodulatory therapy. Severe lupus encompasses classes III, IV, and V (if it has concomitant features of III and IV). Pure mesangial (II) or pure membranous (V) lupus typically require less aggressive immunomodulatory therapy. Class III and class IV disease are further subdivided based on the inflammatory activity or chronicity of the lesions on kidney biopsy. The World Health Organization (WHO) classification was commonly used prior to the RPS/ISN classification. The advantage of the WHO classification is that it categorized information about the pathogenesis of the lesions (i.e., immune complex–mediated or non-immune complex–mediated). The WHO classification also helps delineate prognosis, because patients with severe lupus nephritis have a worse prognosis than those with less severe disease. In addition, those with diffuse proliferative lesions are generally more likely to achieve a remission and less likely to progress to end-stage kidney failure than those with severe segmental lesions, but both have a much higher risk of progression compared with mesangial or pure membranous disease.

8. What nephropathology occurs in patients with SLE that is not part of the classic lupus nephritis?
Although glomerular inflammatory involvement is the prototypical example of lupus nephritis, the tubules, interstitium, and vasculature of the kidney can also be affected.
- Tubulointerstitial disease: proximal tubular dysfunction and hyperkalemic renal tubular acidosis can be seen in patients with lupus. Acute interstitial nephritis including active tubulitis (infiltration and invasion of the tubules) can be seen with or without glomerular disease.
- Podocytopathy: the epithelial cells in the glomerular capillaries may become effaced, termed *podocytopathy*, which typically gives rise to the dramatic onset of the nephrotic syndrome, similar to the clinical presentation of minimal change disease.
- Antiphospholipid syndrome (APS): antiphospholipid antibodies (aPL) can be seen in up to 40% of SLE patients, and about 50% of these patients can develop APS. APS is characterized by a combination of arterial and/or venous thrombosis in the setting of positive aPL. Thus patients are at risk for renal artery stenosis and thrombosis, renal vein thrombosis, and renal infarction. Antiphospholipid nephropathy (APSN) refers to the vascular lesions in glomeruli, small arteries, arterioles, and interlobular arteries seen in patients with persistent aPL (with or without APS). TMA is the distinct histologic finding in acute lesions. Chronic vascular lesions include arterial fibrous intimal hyperplasia, arteriosclerosis, and organized thromboses. Kidney manifestations of APS can occur in the presence or absence of lupus nephritis, and APSN can be associated with all classes of lupus nephritis.
- Acute tubular necrosis and interstitial nephritis can be seen in patients taking nonsteroidal anti-inflammatory agents for arthritis.

9. How is lupus nephritis managed?
Although the clinical presentation (signs, symptoms, serologic and urine tests) is an important part of determining the therapy of lupus nephritis, the information gained from a kidney biopsy is the most useful determinant of a treatment decision for this disease. The biopsy will differentiate severe active lupus nephritis (diffuse or segmental proliferative glomerulonephritis with or without membranous disease) from milder (mesangial glomerulonephritis) or inactive forms.
Treatment of severe active lupus nephritis (Box 32.2) is separated into an induction phase, of which the goal is to induce a remission, and a maintenance phase, of which the goal is to maintain remission and prevent relapse. Because lupus nephritis is a rare and heterogeneous disease,

Box 32.2. Immunomodulatory Treatment Options for Severe Lupus Nephritis

Induction

High-dose steroids (e.g., intravenous methylprednisolone initially or oral prednisone 1 mg/kg not to exceed 80 mg daily, tapering at 4–8 weeks depending on response) plus one of the following:
Oral cyclophosphamide[a] 2 mg/kg daily (not to exceed 150 mg daily) for 6–12 weeks. Dose to be adjusted based on white blood cell count
High-dose IV cyclophosphamide[a] 0.5–1.0 g/m^2 body surface area (BSA) monthly for 6 months. Dose to be adjusted based on white blood cell count
Low-dose IV cyclophosphamide[a] 500 mg every 2 weeks for six doses. Dose to be adjusted based on white blood cell count

Oral mycophenolate mofetil 2–3 g daily in two divided doses for 6 months

Maintenance

Choices of maintenance therapy are as follows:
Oral mycophenolate mofetil 0.5–2 g daily in two divided doses with prednisone taper
Oral azathioprine 1–3 mg/kg daily with prednisone taper
Cyclosporine dosed 2–4 mg/kg daily to keep trough levels 75–200 ng/mL with prednisone taper
Low-dose prednisone is continued with goal to slowly taper off or to attain the minimal dose required to control symptoms

[a]Dose adjustment for kidney dysfunction is recommended.

a standard treatment algorithm does not exist, and treatment is currently individualized. However, based on evidence from clinical trials, the therapeutic options for the induction phase are high-dose prednisone coupled with cyclophosphamide or mycophenolate mofetil (MMF). Cyclosporine is another option for induction, typically when membranous glomerulonephritis is present. To date, there is insufficient data to support the use of rituximab as initial induction therapy for severe lupus nephritis. However, rituximab may be effective in patients with severe lupus nephritis with refractory or relapsing disease. Plasmapheresis has been proven to be ineffective when added to induction with cyclophosphamide and prednisone. The length of induction depends on the method of administration and the response or side effects to the therapy but is typically from 2 to 12 months of therapy. Therapeutic choices for the maintenance phase, which occurs after successful induction and lasts several years (perhaps for life), include MMF, azathioprine, or rarely cyclosporine. Low-dose prednisone is continued with goal of slowly tapering off or attaining the minimal dose required to control symptoms.

Extrarenal manifestations and symptoms should be identified and treated appropriately. Use of an angiotensin-converting enzyme inhibitor (ACEI) or angiotensin II receptor blocker (ARB) to control blood pressure is essential. Managing sequelae of the nephrotic syndrome, such as hyperlipidemia and edema, can be achieved with lipid-lowering agents and diuretics coupled with a low-sodium diet.

10. What tests are useful to monitor response to treatment?
    Urine studies that should be routinely followed include a urinalysis (dipstick and microscopic evaluation) to monitor for hematuria and proteinuria. The urine protein should also be routinely quantified, because lack of improvement may be a sign of unresponsiveness. Serum chemistries, kidney function, albumin, and immune serology (dS-DNA, complement components) should be assessed at every visit.

11. What is the typical response to treatment?
    There are many variables predictive of outcome, but with severe lupus nephritis and normal kidney function, 60% to 85% of patients will achieve a complete or partial remission in 3 to 6 months with induction therapy. This response rate is less likely with abnormal kidney function. Because kidney function correlates directly with response to therapy, early diagnosis of lupus nephritis with a kidney biopsy is imperative. Overall, about 10% of patients with lupus nephritis will progress to end-stage kidney disease. Clinical factors associated with progression of kidney failure are:
    - Failure to achieve an initial remission
    - Nephrotic-range proteinuria
    - Hypertension
    - Anemia
    - Anti-Ro/SSA antibodies
    - African American or Hispanic ethnicity
    - Crescents on the biopsy
    - Severe lupus lesions with or without membranous nephritis
    - Extensive tubulointerstitial disease (Box 32.3)

Box 32.3. Factors Predictive of Progression to Kidney Failure in Lupus Nephritis

Clinical Factors at Baseline:
Elevated serum creatinine
Hypertension
Nephrotic-range proteinuria
Anemia
Race: African American or Hispanic
Anti-Ro/SSA antibodies

Clinical Factors on Follow-up:
Delay in treatment
Frequency and severity of relapse
Failure to achieve complete or partial remission
Increasing serum creatinine

Histopathologic:
Severe lupus nephritis lesions
  Membranous lesions with either focal or diffuse
    proliferative lesions have higher risk than isolated
    membranous lesions
Presence of crescents
Tubulointerstitial disease
High chronicity index
Thrombotic microangiopathy

---

12. **What are common complications of immunomodulatory therapy?**
    - Cyclophosphamide: gonadal failure, hemorrhagic cystitis, infection, bone marrow suppression, and malignancy. Acrolein is an unsaturated aldehyde metabolite of cyclophosphamide that causes urotoxicity. Long-term complications are generally correlated with a higher cumulative dose of cyclophosphamide; thus prior exposure to cyclophosphamide needs to be taken into consideration.
    - If possible, prior to initiation of treatment with cyclophosphamide, patients should be counseled regarding the risks of treatment. The following should be considered as well:
        - Patients interested in having children should be referred to a fertility specialist for cryopreservation and consideration for gonadotropin-releasing hormone agonists (leuprolide).
        - Hepatitis B, hepatitis C, and tuberculosis status should be screened prior to starting therapy (infectious disease consultation may be needed in some patients).
        - No specific cancer screening is currently recommended; however, age-appropriate cancer screening should be completed.
        - *Pneumocystis jiroveci* (PJP) prophylaxis is needed once therapy is started.
        - Patients started on oral cyclophosphamide should be instructed to take the dose in the morning and maintain adequate hydration (adjusted timing of the dose is needed if the patient works exclusively during evening/night shifts). Mesna (2-mercaptoethane sodium sulfonate) has been shown to reduce risk of cystitis in cancer patients receiving high-dose intravenous (IV) cyclophosphamide or ifosfamide; however, this has not been extensively studied in patients with rheumatologic diseases such as SLE. Thus, the use of Mesna remains nephrologist-dependent. Microscopic hematuria, if present at disease onset, can persist during treatment. New-onset microscopic and/or gross hematuria following cyclophosphamide treatment requires further workup, including urologic consultation.
    - MMF: gastrointestinal toxicity, such as early satiety, nausea, and diarrhea. In comparison to cyclophosphamide, MMF treatment does not carry the risk of infertility. However, there remain the risks of bone marrow suppression, infection, and neoplasia. PJP prophylaxis is not routinely given in patients receiving MMF. MMF is associated with birth defects; female patients who may become pregnant must be aware of this and should be on an effective form of birth control.
    - High-dose prednisone: sequelae may include cushingoid features, weight gain, cutaneous changes such as striae and acne, hypertension, osteopenia, and exacerbation of peptic ulcer disease. Long-term complications include avascular necrosis and osteopenia.

13. **Are there gender and/or racial differences in the prognosis and treatment of lupus nephritis?**
    SLE is much more common in female patients. The effect of increased estrogen has been hypothesized to explain these gender differences. Although less common, several studies have demonstrated a relatively higher prevalence of kidney disease in male patients. In a cohort of 315 patients including 45 males, the male patients had lower remission rates, higher relapse rates, and worse long-term kidney outcomes.

    Patient survival is worse in African American patients with SLE as compared with other subgroups. Lupus nephritis is almost twice as frequent in African American patients and carries a poor kidney prognosis. The incidence of ESKD is up to sevenfold higher among African Americans than in any other subgroup. Predictors of ESKD in African American patients include high levels of serum creatinine, the presence of anti-Ro antibodies, and severe segmental lesions on biopsy. Studies have also shown that Hispanic patients have worse outcomes as compared with non-Hispanic Caucasian patients.

In the Aspreva Lupus Management Study, there were differences in the treatment (induction) response across racial and ethnic groups. Specifically, more African American and Hispanic patients responded to MMF than to IV cyclophosphamide. Asian and Caucasian patients showed similar response rates to both MMF and IV cyclophosphamide.

14. **Is there a role for plasmapheresis in SLE?**
In patients with lupus nephritis, the addition of plasmapheresis to treatment with immunosuppressive agents has shown no proven benefit. However, plasmapheresis has been beneficial in patients with lupus cerebritis, SLE-associated thrombotic thrombocytopenic purpura, and diffuse alveolar hemorrhage. The American Society for Apheresis lists severe systemic lupus as a category II recommendation (accepted as second-line therapy, either as a stand-alone treatment or in conjunction with other modes of treatment), whereas lupus nephritis is listed as a category IV recommendation (disorders in which published evidence demonstrates or suggests apheresis to be ineffective or harmful).

15. **Is it advisable for my patient with lupus nephritis to get pregnant? How should pregnant patients be managed differently?**
Both SLE and lupus nephritis commonly occur in women of childbearing age. Women with lupus nephritis have higher rates of maternal complications during pregnancy, including preeclampsia (difficult to distinguish from a lupus flare) and preterm delivery. Fetal complications are also more common, such as low birth weight or even fetal loss. Patients with antiphospholipid antibodies are prone to develop spontaneous abortions and fetal loss. Anti-Ro/SSA and anti-La/SSB antibodies can cross the placenta and cause cutaneous neonatal lupus and/or congenital heart block.

Prepregnancy counseling is recommended. The maternal-fetal risk of complication is lower in patients with normal kidney function, normal blood pressure, a lack of antiphospholipid antibodies, and inactive disease.

If pregnancy is a consideration or if it occurs, a multidisciplinary approach with an obstetrician who specializes in high-risk pregnancies is recommended. Assessment for lupus serology, proteinuria, kidney function, and systemic and pulmonary hypertension is necessary. Medications should be carefully reviewed and, if possible, those that have high teratogenic potential should be discontinued in favor of those that have less. Medications used frequently that exhibit teratogenicity include cyclophosphamide, MMF, ACEIs and ARBs, and hydroxymethylglutaryl-CoA (HMG-CoA) reductase inhibitors. However, the outcome of the pregnancy is directly related to maternal health, and if severe lupus nephritis develops or flares during pregnancy, these medications may be considered so as to prevent the onset of kidney failure.

16. **Can lupus nephritis recur following transplantation?**
Yes. In transplanted patients with ESKD from lupus nephritis undergoing transplant biopsy for kidney failure, hematuria, or proteinuria, recurrent lupus nephritis can be present but rarely leads to graft loss unless there is concomitant chronic allograft nephropathy. In addition, based on the larger series, recurrent lupus nephritis does not have an impact on patient survival.

17. **How often will patients with ESKD from lupus nephritis experience extrarenal flares?**
Extrarenal flares were initially thought to be extremely infrequent once a patient starts dialysis, a process termed "burnout." This may be related to the relative immunodeficiency of uremia and/or dialysis, or it may just characterize the progressive course of lupus. However, in general, patients receiving peritoneal dialysis do not experience fewer extrarenal flares, and modern epidemiologic studies have revealed a persistence of lupus activity, both symptomatically and serologically, in patients undergoing hemodialysis. This may be related to improved dialysis techniques and biocompatibility of dialysis membranes.

KEY POINTS

1. A urinalysis should be performed on every patient with systemic lupus erythematosus (SLE) at each visit. Abnormal urinalysis should lead to an evaluation by a nephrologist. Immunologic serology for SLE and serum chemistries are also useful in determining whether lupus nephritis is present.
2. Early diagnosis of lupus nephritis is imperative because kidney function at the time of biopsy correlates with remission.

3. A kidney biopsy can be performed to determine diagnosis, treatment, and/or prognosis. A biopsy can help differentiate between severe and mild lupus glomerulonephritis, which requires different therapy.
4. Therapy of severe active lupus nephritis is with immunosuppressive medications. Prednisone, cyclophosphamide, mycophenolate mofetil, azathioprine, or cyclosporine are choices that may be used to induce or maintain remission.
5. Because SLE and lupus nephritis frequently occur in women of childbearing age, special considerations and counseling should be given prior to pregnancy if possible. A multidisciplinary approach is recommended.

BIBLIOGRAPHY

Appel, G. B., Contreras, G., Dooley, M. A., Ginzler, E. M., Isenberg, D., Jayne, D., . . . Aspreva Lupus Management Study Group. (2009). Mycophenolate mofetil versus cyclophosphamide for induction treatment of lupus nephritis. *Journal of the American Society of Nephrology, 20,* 1103–1112.

Austin, H. A., III, Illei, G. G., Braun, M. J., & Balow, J. E. (2009). Randomized, controlled trial of prednisone, cyclophosphamide, and cyclosporine in lupus membranous nephropathy. *Journal of the American Society of Nephrology, 20,* 901–911.

Behara, V. Y., Whittier, W. L., Korbet, S. M., Schwartz, M. M., Martens, M., & Lewis, E. J. (2010). Pathogenetic features of severe segmental lupus nephritis. *Nephrology Dialysis Transplantation, 25,* 153–159.

Contreras, G., Pardo, V., Leclercq, B., Lenz, O., Tozman, E., O'Nan, P., & Roth, D. (2004). Sequential therapies for proliferative lupus nephritis. *New England Journal of Medicine, 350,* 971–980.

Ginzler, E. M., Dooley, M. A., Aranow, C., Kim, M. Y., Buyon, J., Merrill, J. T., . . . Appel, G. B. (2005). Mycophenolate mofetil or intravenous cyclophosphamide for lupus nephritis. *New England Journal of Medicine, 353,* 2219–2228.

Houssiau, F. A., Vasconcelos, C., D'Cruz, D., Sebastiani, G. D., de Ramon Garrido, E., Danieli, M. G., . . . Cervera, R. (2010). The 10-year follow-up data of the Euro-Lupus Nephritis Trial comparing low-dose and high-dose intravenous cyclophosphamide. *Annals of the Rheumatic Diseases, 69,* 61–64.

Korbet, S. M., Schwartz, M. M., Evans, J., Lewis, E. J., & Collaborative Study Group. (2007). Severe lupus nephritis: Racial differences in presentation and outcome. *Journal of the American Society of Nephrology, 18,* 244–254.

Korbet, S. M., Whittier, W. L., & Lewis, E. J. (2016). The impact of baseline serum creatinine on complete remission rate and long-term outcome in patients with severe lupus nephritis. *Nephron Extra, 6,* 12–21.

Kraft, S. W., Schwartz, M. M., Korbet, S. M., & Lewis, E. J. (2005). Glomerular podocytopathy in patients with systemic lupus erythematosus. *Journal of the American Society of Nephrology, 16,* 175–179.

Lewis, E. J., Hunsicker, L. G., Lan, S. P., Rohde, R. D., & Lachin, J. M. (1992). A controlled trial of plasmapheresis therapy in severe lupus nephritis. The Lupus Nephritis Collaborative Study Group. *New England Journal of Medicine, 326,* 1373–1379.

Lewis, E. J., Schwartz, M. M., Korbet, S. M., & Chan, T. M. (Eds.), (2010). *Lupus nephritis* (2nd ed.). Oxford: Oxford Clinical Nephrology Series.

Moroni, G., Quaglini, S., Banfi, G., Caloni, M., Finazzi, S., & Ambroso, G. (2002). Pregnancy in lupus nephritis. *American Journal of Kidney Diseases, 40,* 713–720.

Petri, M., Orbai, A. M., Alarcón, G. S., Gordon, C., Merrill, J. T., Fortin, P. R., . . . Magder, L. S. (2012). Derivation and validation of the Systemic Lupus International Collaborating Clinics classification criteria for systemic lupus erythematosus. *Arthritis & Rheumatology, 64,* 2677–2686.

Rovin, B. H., Furie, R., Latinis, K., Looney, R. J., Fervenza, F. C., Sanchez-Guerrero, J., . . . LUNAR Investigator Group. (2012). Efficacy and safety of rituximab in patients with active proliferative lupus nephritis: The Lupus Nephritis Assessment with Rituximab study. *Arthritis & Rheumatology, 64,* 1215–1226.

CHAPTER 33

VASCULITIDES

Vimal K. Derebail and Patrick H. Nachman

1. **Which of the vasculitides are most often associated with glomerular disease?**
   The small-vessel vasculitides are most often associated with glomerular disease (Fig. 33.1). Immuno-globulin (Ig)A vasculitis (Henoch-Schölein-purpura) and cryoglobulinemic vasculitis are associated with immune complex deposition. Pauci-immune glomerulonephritis demonstrates little to no immune deposits and is seen in the antineutrophil cytoplasmic antibody (ANCA)-associated vasculitides, including granulomatosis with polyangiitis (GPA, formerly Wegener granulomatosis), microscopic polyangiitis (MPA), and eosinophilic granulomatosis with polyangiitis (EGPA, formerly Churg-Strauss syndrome), as well as kidney-limited pauci-immune necrotizing and crescentic glomerulonephritis (NCGN).

   Polyarteritis nodosa (PAN), a medium-vessel vasculitis typically affecting medium-sized or small arteries and sparing arterioles, capillaries, and venules, does not cause glomerulonephritis but may cause ischemic kidney injury via inflammation of the larger kidney vessels.

2. **What features distinguish the small-vessel vasculitides?**
   The small-vessel vasculitides have significant overlap in their manifestations and affect small vessels including intraparenchymal arteries, arterioles, capillaries, and venules. Features that distinguish them have been used in proposed classification schemes:
   GPA is associated with granulomatous inflammation that may affect the lower and upper respiratory tracts, often causing sinus symptoms, in addition to glomerulonephritis.

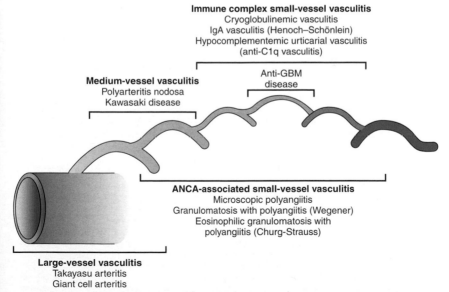

Immune complex small-vessel vasculitis
Cryoglobulinemic vasculitis
IgA vasculitis (Henoch–Schönlein)
Hypocomplementemic urticarial vasculitis
(anti-C1q vasculitis)

Anti-GBM
disease

Medium-vessel vasculitis
Polyarteritis nodosa
Kawasaki disease

ANCA-associated small-vessel vasculitis
Microscopic polyangiitis
Granulomatosis with polyangiitis (Wegener)
Eosinophilic granulomatosis with
polyangiitis (Churg-Strauss)

Large-vessel vasculitis
Takayasu arteritis
Giant cell arteritis

Figure 33.1. Distribution of vessel involvement by large-vessel vasculitis, medium-vessel vasculitis, and small-vessel vasculitis. There may be substantial overlap with respect to arterial involvement, and an important concept is that all three major categories of vasculitis can affect any size of artery. The diagram depicts *(from left to right)* aorta, large artery, medium artery, small artery/arteriole, capillary, venule, and vein. *Anti-GBM*, Anti-glomerular basement membrane; *ANCA*, antineutrophil cytoplasmic antibody; *Anti-GBM*, anti-glomerular basement membrane. (Modified and reproduced with permission from Jennette, J. C., Falk, R. J., Bacon, P. A., et al. (2013). 2012 revised International Chapel Hill Consensus Conference Nomenclature of Vasculitides. *Arthritis & Rheumatology, 65,* 1–11.)

MPA also leads to necrotizing vasculitis of small vessels and often leads to glomerulonephritis as well as pulmonary capillaritis and pulmonary hemorrhage. Notably, granulomatous inflammation is *absent.*

EGPA also demonstrates granulomatous inflammation of small- and medium-sized vessels and involves the respiratory tract. The distinguishing histologic feature is that of eosinophil-rich inflammation with peripheral eosinophilia. Patients also have associated asthma. ANCA are found in about 40% of patients with EGPA compared with about 90% of patients with MPA, GPA, or pauci-immune NCGN.

IgA vasculitis (Henoch-Schölein purpura) demonstrates IgA1 immune deposits with vasculitis affecting small vessels. In addition to glomeruli, skin and gastrointestinal involvement are common. Patients often have arthralgias or arthritis.

Cryoglobulinemic vasculitis leads to skin and glomerular lesions with cryoglobulin immune deposits in affected small vessels. Neurologic involvement may also occur. Cryoglobulins may be present in serum.

3. **What findings in the urinalysis suggest kidney involvement from vasculitis?**
Microscopic hematuria, typically with dysmorphic red blood cells and red blood cell casts, suggests kidney vasculitis. Proteinuria is often present but is usually subnephrotic. Inflammation in the form of white blood cells in the urine may also be an accompanying feature.

4. **What serologic markers may be helpful in the distinguishing the kidney vasculitides?**
Complement levels may be depressed in patients with cryoglobulinemic vasculitis and other vasculitides, including systemic lupus erythematosus (SLE) and postinfectious glomerulonephritis. Complement levels are typically normal in the other small-vessel vasculitides. Although technically difficult to measure, cryoglobulins can be directly measured in serum. Antinuclear antibodies suggest connective-tissue-related disorders, such as SLE, and may be further distinguished by extractable nuclear antigen panel testing. Patients with the small-vessel vasculitides (GPA, MPA, and EGPA) often have positive anti-neutrophil cytoplasmic antibodies (ANCAs) directed to either myeloperoxidase (MPO, MPO-ANCA) or proteinase 3 (PR3, PR3-ANCA). Anti-glomerular basement membrane (anti-GBM) antibodies are detected in patients with anti-GBM disease whether limited to the kidney or associated with diffuse alveolar hemorrhage.

There is a broad overlap in the clinical presentation of the various small-vessel vasculitides. In addition, overlap syndromes can occur. For instance, one-third to one-half of patients with anti-GBM disease will also have circulating ANCA, which is more often directed against MPO. In addition to the clinical presentation and serologic studies, a kidney biopsy is usually indicated to provide a definitive diagnosis and valuable information on the extent of glomerular injury and glomerular and interstitial scarring.

5. **What is the relevance of ANCAs?**
ANCAs are present in 90% of patients with pauci-immune glomerulonephritis, seen in GPA, MPA, and kidney-limited disease. ANCAs are also present in about 40% of patients with EGPA. They are typically absent in patients with PAN. Immunofluorescence is most sensitive to the detection of ANCAs and demonstrates distinct patterns, either a cytoplasmic pattern (C-ANCA) or perinuclear pattern (P-ANCA).

The antigen specificity of C-ANCA is usually directed to a neutrophil and monocyte protease -proteinase-3 (PR3), while P-ANCAs are usually directed to myeloperoxidase (MPO). While both MPO and PR3 may be seen in any of the described manifestations, MPO-ANCA (P-ANCA) is more common in patients with MPA, and PR3-ANCA (C-ANCA) is more common in GPA. Approximately 40% of patients with EGPA will manifest ANCAs, and may be directed to either MPO or PR3. Again, 10% of patients with pauci-immune glomerulonephritis do not demonstrate ANCAs despite kidney biopsy findings consistent with this diagnosis. MPO-ANCA and PR3-ANCA rarely coexist in a patient with idiopathic ANCA vasculitis (<5%). The coexistence of high-titer MPO- and PR3-ANCA has been reported in patients with drug-associated vasculitis, such as that associated with levamisole-adulterated cocaine.

Both *in vitro* and *in vivo* studies support a pathogenic role of ANCAs in vasculitis and glomerulonephritis. Neutrophils and monocytes primed by inflammation express ANCA antigens near or on cell surfaces. Interaction between these antigens and ANCAs activate neutrophils and monocytes, leading to degranulation at the vessel wall and resulting in endothelial cell damage. *In vivo,* the transfer of mouse anti-MPO IgG to MPO-competent mice results in NCGN and pulmonary vasculitis, which is similar to the human disease, thus demonstrating the ability of these antibodies to confer disease. This same mouse model has demonstrated a role for complement activation via the alternative pathway in the pathogenesis of MPO-ANCA glomerulonephritis.

Other antigens besides MPO and PR3 that interact with ANCAs have also been reported. ANCAs directed to elastase have been reported in drug-induced ANCA vasculitis. Antibodies directed to lysosomal membrane protein-2 have also been reported, although their association with small-vessel vasculitis is controversial. In patients with inflammatory bowel diseases, ANCAs have also been described directed to catalase, α-enolase, lactotransferrin, and bactericidal permeability-increasing protein.

6. **Which of the kidney vasculitides are associated with pulmonary-renal syndrome?**
   Pulmonary-renal syndrome describes the presentation of acute glomerulonephritis with alveolar hemorrhage, as demonstrated by radiographic demonstration of pulmonary infiltrates and varying degrees of hypoxia, hemoptysis, and anemia. It is a life-threatening complication of small-vessel vasculitis. The ANCA small-vessel vasculitides are the most common cause of pulmonary-renal syndrome. Anti-GBM disease, or Goodpasture's disease, may also present with pulmonary hemorrhage and concomitant rapidly progressive glomerulonephritis. This syndrome may also be seen in patients with SLE and similar connective tissue diseases, IgA vasculitis (Henoch-Schölein purpura), and in cryoglobulinemic vasculitis.
   Patients with this presentation should also be evaluated for other conditions accompanying kidney failure that may have similar presentations, including pneumonia and pulmonary embolus.

7. **What primary rapidly progressive glomerulonephritis may occur in conjunction with ANCA glomerulonephritis?**
   Anti-GBM disease (Goodpasture's disease) may occur concurrently with ANCA small-vessel vasculitis. About 45% of patients with anti-GBM disease also have positive ANCA testing, more commonly MPO-ANCA. In patients with a history of anti-GBM disease who develop recurrent signs of disease, ANCA testing should be obtained, even if originally negative, as relapsing anti-GBM disease is rare. The kidney survival of patients with both antibodies appears to be worse than those with ANCA disease alone, but it is better than those with anti-GBM disease alone.

8. **What are the histologic findings of a kidney biopsy in patients with ANCA vasculitis?**
   Kidney biopsy usually demonstrates the presence of focal segmental to global fibrinoid necrosis and crescent formation affecting variable proportions of glomeruli. By both immunoflorescence and electron microscopy, glomeruli demonstrate few or no immune depositions, lending to the term pauci-immune glomerulonephritis, and distinguishing ANCA vasculitis from other diseases that may produce similar features by light microscopy, such as anti-GBM disease or immune complex-mediated glomerulonephritis (e.g., lupus nephritis). The glomerular lesions are usually associated with little or no endocapillary proliferation.

9. **What drugs have been implicated in inducing ANCA vasculitis?**
   The development of vasculitis with ANCAs has been associated with many agents. The most commonly implicated drug is the anti-thyroid medication, propothiouracil (PTU), with other thyroid agents, including methimazole and carbimazole, also implicated. Other agents reported to be associated with ANCA vasculitis include hydralazine, minocycline, allopurinol, phenytoin, and penicillamine, among others. Both PTU and hydralazine are typically associated high-titer MPO antibodies, and the latter also with antibodies directed to elastase and lactoferrin. Withdrawal of the offending agent is, at times, sufficient to prompt resolution of the vasculitis, while, in some instances, immunosuppressive therapy is necessary, depending on the severity of the presentation.
   Levamisole, originally utilized as an anti-helminthic, has been used as an adulterant to "cut" cocaine. Reports of vasculitis associated with the use of this agent have emerged over the last decade with a severe presentation of vasculitis that may also present with necrotizing skin lesions, glomerulonephritis, or pulmonary hemorrhage. Patients with levamisole-associated ANCA vasculitis may often be "dual positive" for both MPO- and PR3-ANCA.

10. **What are the medical therapies for the treatment of ANCA vasculitis?**
    Treatment of the ANCA vasculitis centers on the use of immunosuppressive therapies. Initial therapy, or induction, for organ-threatening or life-threatening disease involves the use of corticosteroids in combination with either cyclophosphamide (a cytotoxic agent) or rituximab (a B-cell–depleting agent). Compared to a regimen of daily oral cyclophosphamide, pulse intravenous cyclophosphamide is associated with a similar rate of remission. Although it is associated with a higher rate of relapse, the long-term patient and kidney survival are not significantly different between these two approaches. The pulse intravenous cyclophosphamide regimen results in a significantly lower cumulative dose, which is desired, as the long-term risk of cancer is commensurate with the life-long cumulative exposure to this drug. In a landmark randomized, controlled, clinical trial, induction therapy with

a combination of corticosteroids plus rituximab was not inferior to corticosteroids plus oral cyclophosphamide followed by azathioprine in patients with mild or moderately severe disease. However, data on the use of rituximab in lieu of cyclophosphamide in patients with severe pulmonary hemorrhage or severe kidney failure are relatively scant. In patients with relapsing ANCA vasculitis, the use of rituximab was associated with a greater rate of remission, and avoids repeated exposure to cyclophosphamide.

For patients with non-organ- or non-life-threatening disease and well-preserved kidney function, glucocorticoids in combination with methotrexate or mycophenolate mofetil have been studied for induction therapy. Relapse rates may be higher with these agents, and they should not be used in the setting of kidney dysfunction or pulmonary hemorrhage. The use of these agents is currently supplanted by that of rituximab for induction therapy.

Following induction of remission after 3 to 6 months initial therapy, rituximab or azathioprine can be used as maintenance therapy. In a trial of maintenance therapy, the use of rituximab 500 mg every 6 months was associated with a lower relapse rate than with azathioprine. Mycophenolate mofetil or methotrexate (in patients with good kidney function) can also be considered for use as maintenance therapy in patients who are intolerant to rituximab or azathioprine. No data is currently available to guide the duration of maintenance therapy. Generally, maintenance therapy is suggested for 18 to 24 months after a remission is attained.

Relapses of disease should be treated as new disease presentation, with corticosteroids combined with cyclophosphamide or rituximab in the setting of severe disease. For those patients who initially received cyclophosphamide therapy, the use of rituximab for relapse is favored to minimize lifetime cumulative cyclophosphamide dose. Upon remission after relapse, the prior maintenance therapy should be modified or intensified.

Disease that is refractory to corticosteroids and cyclophosphamide or rituximab may benefit from the addition of the other agent (i.e., adding rituximab to patients who have received cyclophosphamide, and vice versa), plamapheresis, or intravenous immunoglobulin. However, data for the use of these measures in this fashion have been primarily in the form of case reports or case series.

11. What are the indications for the use of plasma exchange therapy in the treatment of ANCA vasculitis?

Plasma exchange or plasmapheresis is thought to rapidly clear ANCAs, coagulation factors, and inflammatory cytokines that may be pathogenic in vasculitis. At present, plasma exchange is recommended in addition to corticosteroids and cyclophosphamide for patients presenting with severe kidney failure in the setting of rapidly progressive glomerulonephritis and/or those presenting with severe pulmonary hemorrhage. The role of plasmapheresis as adjunctive therapy is not established for patients with less severe disease. The use of plasmapheresis in ANCA vasculitis is the focus of a large ongoing clinical trial (Clinicaltrial.gov PEXIVAS). Those patients also presenting with concomitant anti-GBM disease (identified with kidney biopsy demonstrating linear IgM staining of glomerular basement membrane) should receive early initiation of plasma exchange.

12. What is the prognosis of patients with ANCA vasculitides?

Most patients with pauci-immune glomerulonephritis have a good response to present induction therapy, with nearly 85% achieving remission. With corticosteroids and cyclophosphamide, overall survival rates at 1 and 5 years are 85% and 75%, respectively. Mortality is significantly greater in older patients, reaching approximately 23% at 1 year for those over the age of 60 and nearly 44% for those over the age of 70. The presence of diffuse alveolar hemorrhage is associated with an 8-fold risk of death, whereas the serum creatinine level at presentation is the major predictor of kidney outcome. Although pulmonary hemorrhage is a major cause of death in the early weeks after presentation, the major causes of "late" death are infections and cardiovascular disease.

Patients who present with severe kidney failure have a decreased chance of recovering kidney function compared to those with better-preserved GFR. Histopathologic chronicity index score and baseline estimated glomerular filtration rate (greater than or less than 10 mL/min per 1.73 m^2) were associated with treatment response by 4 months. However, there was no identifiable threshold of kidney function at presentation or histopathologic chronicity index score below which treatment could be deemed futile. Among patients who remain dialysis-dependent at 4 months, only 5% subsequently recover kidney function. In the absence of extra-kidney active vasculitis, the risks of continued immunosuppressive therapy beyond 4 months likely outweigh any potential benefit.

Relapsing disease, unfortunately, occurs in almost 50% of patients at 5 years; most respond to therapy but do receive recurrent exposure to immunosuppression and cytotoxic agents. Approximately 20% of patients that survive initial disease presentation eventually will go on to develop end-stage kidney disease (ESKD).

13. Which features are associated with an increased risk of relapse of the ANCA vasculitis?

Patients with PR3-ANCA are more than 1.5 times as likely to relapse when compared to those with MPO-ANCA. Additionally, pulmonary involvement has been associated with higher rates of relapse. Upper airway involvement has also been implicated as a risk factor for relapse, which was linked to the nasal carriage of *Staphylococcus aureus*, which is also suggested as a risk factor for relapsing disease. Although increases in PR3-ANCA or MPO-ANCA levels are generally associated with an increased likelihood of subsequent relapse, such relapses occur in a minority of patients within 12 months. It is currently not recommended to increase or resume immunosuppressive therapy based on an increase in ANCA titer alone, in the absence of clinical signs or symptoms of active ANCA vasculitis.

14. What is the recurrence rate of ANCA disease following kidney transplantation?

Recurrent ANCA vasculitis may occur following kidney transplantation despite anti-rejection therapy. However, the rate of recurrence is low, reported at 0.02 per patient-years, and does not seem to be influenced by the disease phenotype, the ANCA serotype, or the duration of remission for more or less than a year prior to transplantation. Whether a positive ANCA test alone at the time of transplantation (in the absence of clinical signs of active vasculitis) is associated with a greater risk of relapse remains uncertain, and was not associated with decreased graft survival. In such a circumstance, the risk of relapse should be weighed against the morbidity and risk of mortality associated with ESKD.

15. Is venous thromboembolism (VTE; deep venous thrombosis or pulmonary embolus) a concern in patients with ANCA disease?

Venous thrombosis is an increasingly recognized complication of ANCA vasculitis. A higher rate of events has been reported in both PR3- and MPO-ANCA disease, with about 10% of patients developing symptomatic VTE and an incidence of approximately 7 events/100-person years. VTE events appear to occur more frequently at time of active disease. The pathogenesis of VTE in this population remains unclear, but there is speculation that ANCA disease may induce endothelial damage and hypercoagulability.

16. What is associated risk of malignancy for ANCA patients treated with cyclophosphamide?

The increased risk for cancer among ANCA patients treated with cyclophosphamide has been relatively well established. The most current data have demonstrated an increased risk for non-melanomous skin cancers, bladder cancer, and acute myelogenous leukemia (AML). Both bladder cancer and AML appear to occur primarily among those treated with a cumulative cyclophosphamide dose >36 g and have a latency period of 7 years or more.

Additionally, bladder and skin cancers seemed to present more commonly among those treated with azathioprine of mycophenolate mofetil maintenance therapy.

KEY POINTS

1. Microscopic hematuria, typically with dysmorphic red blood cells and red blood cell casts, suggests kidney vasculitis.
2. Anti-neutrophil cytoplasmic autoantibodies, or ANCA, are present in 90% of patients with pauci-immune glomerulonephritis, seen in GPA, MPA, and kidney-limited disease.
3. Anti-GBM disease, or Goodpasture's disease, may occur concurrently with ANCA small-vessel vasculitis.
4. Induction therapy in ANCA vasculitis consists of a combination of corticosteroids and cyclophosphamide or rituximab.
5. In ANCA vasculitis, plasma exchange is currently recommended in addition to corticosteroids, and cyclophosphamide or rituximab for patients presenting with *advanced kidney failure* and/or *pulmonary hemorrhage*.
6. A higher rate of VTE has been reported in ANCA disease, with about 10% of patients developing symptomatic events, particularly at the time of active disease.
7. ANCA patients treated with cyclophosphamide demonstrate an increased risk for non-melanoma skin cancers, bladder cancer, and acute myelogenous leukemia (AML).

BIBLIOGRAPHY

Allenbach, Y., Seror, R., Pagnoux, C., Teixeira, L., Guilpain, P., & Guillevin, L. (2009). High frequency of venous thromboembolic events in Churg-Strauss syndrome, Wegener's granulomatosis and microscopic polyangiitis but not polyarteritis nodosa: A systematic retrospective study on 1130 patients. *Annals of the Rheumatic Diseases, 68,* 564–567.

Faurschou, M., Sorensen, I. J., Mellemkjaer, L., Loft, A. G., Thomsen, B. S., Tvede, N., & Baslund, B. (2008). Malignancies in Wegener's granulomatosis: Incidence and relation to cyclophosphamide therapy in a cohort of 293 patients. *Journal of Rheumatology, 35,* 100–105.

Geetha, D., Eirin, A., True, K., Valentina Irazabal, M., Specks, U., Seo, P., . . . Fervenza, F. C. (2011). Renal transplantation in antineutrophil cytoplasmic antibody-associated vasculitis: A multicenter experience. *Transplantation, 91,* 1370–1375.

Guillevin, L., Pagnoux, C., Karras, A., Khouatra, C., Aumaître, O., Cohen, P., . . . Mouthon, L.; French Vasculitis Study Group. (2014). Rituximab versus azathioprine for maintenance in ANCA-associated vasculitis. *New England Journal of Medicine, 371*(19), 1771–1780.

Huugen, D., van Esch, A., Xiao, H., Peutz-Kootstra, C. J., Buurman, W. A., Tervaert, J. W., . . . Heeringa, P. (2007). Inhibition of complement factor C5 protects against anti myeloperoxidase antibody mediated glomerulonephritis in mice. *Kidney International, 71,* 646–654.

Jayne, D. (2009). The diagnosis of vasculitis. *Best Practice & Research Clinical Rheumatology, 23,* 445–453.

Jayne, D. (2009). Treatment of ANCA-associated systemic small-vessel vasculitis. *APMIS Supplement,* 127, 3–9.

Jennette, J. C., & Falk, R. J. (2014). Pathogenesis of antineutrophil cytoplasmic autoantibody-mediated disease. *Nature Reviews Rheumatology, 10,* 463–473.

Jennette, J. C., Falk, R. J., Bacon, P. A., Basu, N., Cid, M. C., Ferrario, F., . . . Watts, R. A. (2013). 2012 Revised international Chapel Hill consensus conference nomenclature of vasculitides. *Arthritis & Rheumatology, 65,* 1–11.

Kemna, M. J., Damoiseaux, J., Austen, J., Winkens, B., Peters, J., van Paassen, P., & Cohen Tervaert, J. W. (2015). ANCA as a predictor of relapse: Useful in patients with renal involvement but not in patients with nonrenal disease. *Journal of the American Society of Nephrology, 26,* 537–542.

Lee, T., Gasim, A., Derebail, V. K., Chung, Y., McGregor, J. G., Lionaki, S., . . . Nachman, P. H. (2014). Predictors of treatment outcomes in ANCA-associated vasculitis with severe kidney failure. *Clinical Journal of the American Society of Nephrology, 9,* 905–913.

McAdoo, S. P., Tanna, A., Hruskova, Z., Holm, L., Weiner, M., Arulkumaran, N., . . . Pusey, C. D. (2017). Patients double-seropositive for ANCA and anti-GBM antibodies have varied renal survival, frequency of relapse, and outcomes compared to single-seropositive patients. *Kidney International, 92*(3), 693–702. http://clx.cloi.org/10.1016/j.kint.2017.03.014.

Niles, J. L., Bottinger, E. P., Saurina, G. R., Kelly, K. J., Pan, G., Collins, A. B., & McCluskey, R. T. (1996). The syndrome of lung hemorrhage and nephritis is usually an ANCA-associated condition. *Archives of Internal Medicine, 156,* 440–445.

Pagnoux, C., Hogan, S. L., Chin, H., Jennette, J. C., Falk, R. J., Guillevin, L., & Nachman, P. H. (2008). Predictors of treatment resistance and relapse in antineutrophil cytoplasmic antibody-associated small-vessel vasculitis: Comparison of two independent cohorts. *Arthritis & Rheumatology, 58,* 2908–2918.

Pendergraft, W. P., III, & Niles, J. L. (2014). Trojan horses: Drug culprits associated with antineutrophil cytoplasmic autoantibody (ANCA) vasculitis. *Current Opinion in Rheumatology, 26,* 42–49.

Stassen, P. M., Derks, R. P., Kallenberg, C. G., & Stegeman, C. A. (2008). Venous thromboembolism in ANCA-associated vasculitis—incidence and risk factors. *Rheumatology (Oxford), 47,* 530–534.

Stone, J. H., Merkel, P. A., Spiera, R., Seo, P., Langford, C. A., Hoffman, G. S., . . . Specks, U.; RAVE-ITN Research Group. (2010). Rituximab versus cyclophosphamide for ANCA-associated vasculitis. *New England Journal of Medicine, 363*(3), 221–232.

Watts, R., Lane, S., Hanslik, T., Hauser, T., Hellmich, B., Koldingsnes, W., . . . Scott, D. (2007). Development and validation of a consensus methodology for the classification of the ANCA-associated vasculitides and polyarteritis nodosa for epidemiological studies. *Annals of the Rheumatic Diseases, 66,* 222–227.

Xiao, H., Schreiber, A., Heeringa, P., Falk, R. J., & Jennette, J. C. (2007). Alternative complement pathway in the pathogenesis of disease mediated by anti-neutrophil cytoplasmic autoantibodies. *American Journal of Pathology, 170,* 52–64.

Yates, M., Watts, R. A., Bajema, I. M., Cid, M. C., Crestani, B., Hauser, T., . . . Mukhtyar, C. (2016). EULAR/ERA-EDTA recommendations for the management of ANCA-associated vasculitis. *Annals of the Rheumatic Diseases, 75,* 1583–1594.

VI
INFECTION-ASSOCIATED GLOMERULONEPHRITIDES

STREPTOCOCCAL- AND STAPHYLOCOCCAL-RELATED GLOMERULONEPHRITIS

Warren Kupin

CHAPTER 34

1. **Wasn't this category previously called postinfectious glomerulonephritis (PIGN)?**
There has been considerable effort to reclassify glomerular diseases that occur as a result of an infection. PIGN describes a unique clinical and pathogenic sequence of events that lead to an immune complex–mediated glomerulonephritis after resolution of an acute infection. Specifically, the acute glomerulonephritis develops after (post) a latent period of variable duration from the time the infection has completely cleared. Since the infection has completely resolved, antibiotic therapy is ineffective for treating the kidney disease. The only infection known to cause this scenario of events is streptococcal disease. Therefore the category of PIGN is better termed *poststreptococcal glomerulonephritis* (PSGN), as no other microorganism leads to this pathologic phenomenon.
   Compared with PSGN, all other infections (viral, bacterial, and fungal) can be "associated" with the development of glomerulonephritis through a separate pathogenic pathway. For these infections, the onset of glomerulonephritis is almost synchronous with the presence of active infection, and the immune complexes are completely dependent on the availability of ongoing antigenemia generated from the infection. In this circumstance as opposed to PSGN, eradication of the infection through antibiotic therapy will halt the ongoing immune complex deposition in the kidney. Staphylococcal-associated acute glomerulonephritis (SAAG) is now as common as PSGN in adults and represents the classic example of this paradigm of infection-associated glomerulonephritis. It is essential to understand the differences between PSGN and SAAG not only in regard to pathophysiology but more importantly in regard to therapeutic intervention. Key points in differentiating PSGN from SAAG and other glomerular diseases are shown in Table 34.1.

2. **Does the site of infection or strain of streptococcal infection affect whether a patient will develop PSGN?**
Infections at any site in the body have the potential to cause PSGN. Since the original description of this disease appeared after an episode of streptococcal pharyngitis, most physicians primarily associate this site of infection with the development of PSGN; they may not be aware that skin infections, pneumonia, visceral abscesses, urinary tract infections, periodontitis, and endocarditis as a result of streptococcal infection can also lead to the same kidney lesion. The important point to keep in mind is that it is not the location of the streptococcal infection that is important, but rather infection with a specific nephritogenic strain.
   Certain nephritogenic group A beta-hemolytic streptococcal strains cause kidney disease only after an upper respiratory infection, whereas other nephritogenic strains are exclusive to the development of glomerulonephritis after skin infections.

3. **What is the typical time for presentation of PSGN after an infection?**
The course of PIGN has been well documented for both pharyngitis and skin infections. Typically kidney disease begins 7 to 14 days after the onset of streptococcal pharyngitis, whereas it takes about 21 days or longer for the development of glomerulonephritis after a skin infection such as impetigo. The onset of glomerulonephritis after infection in other sites of the body also follows a course of between 2 and 4 weeks postinfection. These time patterns are critical because the infection has healed and been forgotten; only later on does the patient present with kidney disease. A careful history and laboratory workup (described later) may help identify the cause of the kidney disease and the unrecognized existence of a preceding streptococcal infection. During community outbreaks of group A beta hemolytic streptococcal infection, the incidence of PSGN ranges between 5% and 10% for upper respiratory infections to 15% to 25% for skin infections.

231

Table 34.1. Clinical and Pathologic Features of Infection-Related Glomerular Diseases

	PSGN	SAAG	IGA NEPHROPATHY	C3 GLOMERULOPATHY
Location of infection	Pharyngitis Skin	Skin Lung Urinary tract	Pharyngitis	Pharyngitis
Latent period	Pharyngitis: 7–14 days Skin: 14–21 days	None	None	None
Primary histology on kidney biopsy	Diffuse proliferative and exudative glomerulonephritis	Diffuse proliferative and exudative glomerulonephritis	Mesangial proliferative glomerulonephritis	Membranoproliferative glomerulonephritis
Site of immune deposits	Subepithelial Some subendothelial and mesangial	Subepithelial Some subendothelial and mesangial	Mesangial	Subendothelial Mesangial Intr. membranous Subepithelial
Serum complement	Low C3	Primarily low C3 but often with both low C3 and C4	Normal	Low C3
Immunofluorescence	IgG and C3 "Starry sky" or "garland" pattern	IgA dominant C3 and IgG in lower intensity	IgA and C3	C3
Treatment	None—spontaneous resolution	Antibiotics	Variable protocols of immunosuppression	Variable—centered on immunosuppression—complement inhibition

PSGN, Poststreptococcal glomerulonephritis; SAAG, staphylococcal-associated acute glomerulonephritis; URI, upper respiratory illness.

4. **How does PSGN present clinically?**

A wide variety of clinical presentations can occur with PSGN, but most children with transient microhematuria (dysmorphic red cells) remain asymptomatic. However, full-blown nephritic syndrome even with nephrotic-range proteinuria can occur. Kidney function is often significantly impaired, with concomitant hypertension and peripheral/pulmonary edema. Severe, uncontrolled hypertension is a common feature in patients with acute PSGN and requires immediate control and management. Many patients with PSGN present with "dark or tea-colored" urine due to gross hematuria. The color is indicative of the effect of pH on the free hemoglobin molecule, with alkaline urine being more bright red and acidic urine being a darker brownish hue.

5. **What laboratory findings are characteristic of PSGN?**

The development of glomerulonephritis results from immune complex deposition in the basement membrane of the glomerulus, leading to loss of the filtration area and increased permeability to protein. These immune complexes consist of an antigen from the infection and usually an immunoglobulin G (IgG) antibody. The damage to the basement membrane from these complexes is often a result of local complement activation exclusively through the alternative pathway. This pathway leads to C3 cleavage and then the production of the membrane attack complex C5-9. Bypassed in this pathway is the activation of C4, which is used only in activation of the classic complement pathway. Therefore when PSGN is suspected, the measurement of serum complement both C3 and C4 is crucial. In PSGN, the C3 level will be low, but the C4 level will typically be normal. If both C3 and C4 are low, the diagnosis of PSGN is suspect, and another source of immune complexes—such as SAAG, cryoglobulinemia, or systemic lupus erythematosus—may be present that activates the classic complement pathway.

Microbiologic and radiologic tests for infection are frequently negative but should still be done. These studies include a chest x-ray as well as blood, sputum, pharyngeal, and urine cultures in addition to a careful examination of the skin, anogenital region, and oral cavity for signs of inflammation. If a streptococcal infection is suspected, specific serologic assays are available, such as the anti-streptolysin O (ASO) titer. However, this test may be falsely negative and lacks the sensitivity to be used as a stand-alone test for streptococcal infection. A more sensitive screen for a recent streptococcal infection is the streptozyme test, which includes five different antibodies that develop to this infection. These include ASO titer, antihyaluronidase (AHase), antistreptokinase, anti–nicotinamide adenine dinucleotidase, and anti-DNAse B antibodies. This test is important because the source of the streptococcal infection will determine what pattern of antibodies will develop; for skin infections, only the anti-DNAse and AHase are positive, whereas for a pharyngeal infection, all five antibodies are usually present in various concentrations. An ASO test alone would miss the previous presence of a streptococcal skin infection.

6. **What does the kidney biopsy show in PSGN?**

The most common histology seen with all forms of PSGN is diffuse proliferative glomerulonephritis with significant endocapillary proliferation. By light microscopy, this lesion is characterized by involvement of almost all glomeruli, with an influx of neutrophils into the glomerular capillaries and a proliferation of the capillary endothelial cells. The capillary lumens are virtually obliterated, reducing the area for ultrafiltration, which leads to a loss of glomerular filtration rate (GFR). By electron microscopy, the etiology for the inflammation is seen by the presence of immune complexes in the subepithelial space. The subepithelial deposits are often called "humps" because they protrude outward on top of the basement membrane. The presence of these immune complexes results in a "granular" appearance by immunofluorescence using IgG and C3, with additional terminology for this phenomenon being "starry sky" or "garland" patterns.

Additional immune deposits can be noted in the subendothelial space and mesangium. It should be noted that a kidney biopsy is usually not done in straightforward cases of PSGN because the treatment will not differ (as noted later). A kidney biopsy is recommended only for those atypical cases where the clinical and laboratory features are not compatible with PSGN.

7. **Is there any treatment for PSGN?**

The treatment for PSGN is primarily supportive because the infection is no longer present and the immune complex deposition in the kidney resolves spontaneously over time. For supportive therapy, the major focus is on blood pressure and volume control. Importantly, the tubules are relatively unaffected by the glomerular disease, and there is a sodium-avid state that accompanies the glomerular inflammation. The absorption of sodium and water leads to significant volume overload and salt-sensitive hypertension. Therefore in addition to the use of regular antihypertensive medications along with salt and water restriction, the early inclusion of loop diuretics is particularly efficacious in PSGN.

The use of steroids or more aggressive forms of immunosuppression for PSGN has not been shown to alter the natural history of the disease and exposes the patient to the potential short- and long-term risks of immunosuppression. The only exception to this rule is the presence of severe crescentic glomerulonephritis. This subset of PSGN includes the standard features of diffuse proliferative glomerulonephritis coupled with the presence of crescents that arise from the parietal epithelium. Often these patients have been treated with bolus steroids, and there are anecdotal reports of the use of cytotoxic therapy, but there are no well-designed studies supporting the benefit of these therapies.

8. Do patients eventually go into remission or is there evidence for permanent kidney injury after PSGN?

The recovery of the kidney from PSGN follows a different time sequence when looking at the GFR, hematuria, and proteinuria. Of note, the acute kidney injury begins to improve within 1 to 2 weeks of onset and the serum creatinine returns to its baseline level after 3 to 4 weeks. This improvement in GFR usually parallels the clearance of infiltrating neutrophils in the glomerulus and the decrease in the proliferation of endothelial cells.

The proteinuria in PSGN is a result of the *subepithelial* immune complexes and will improve only as these complexes are removed. As a result of their location, these immune complexes are cleared very slowly, and proteinuria may persist for months or years after the initial episode. The hematuria seen in PSGN is a result of the *subendothelial* immune complexes, and these are more rapidly removed from the basement membrane. Consequently, hematuria will resolve within 3 to 6 months. Complement levels of C3 should return to normal within 6 weeks after the onset of kidney disease. It is recommended that failure to resolve the hematuria or proteinuria or normalize the C3 level should warrant a biopsy to determine if a kidney disease other than PSGN is present.

The risk of developing chronic kidney disease and eventually end-stage kidney disease from PSGN is extremely low in children. In adults, however, this can be seen in a minimum of 10% to 15% of cases, especially in third-world countries, where impaired nutrition may lead to immune dysregulation and progressive kidney injury.

9. How does SAAG present compared with PSGN?

In direct contrast to PSGN, SAAG presents almost simultaneously with an active staphylococcal infection. There are no specific nephritogenic strains of staphylococci, but most cases are associated with *Staphylococcus aureus*. Moreover, compared with PSGN, few cases of SAAG develop following an upper respiratory infection; the most common sites of staphylococcal infection are skin, lung, heart, urinary tract, and viscera.

SAAG affects older adults with preexisting morbid conditions such as diabetes or malignancy; it rarely, unlike PSGN, presents in children.

SAAG, like PSGN, presents with the nephritic syndrome, with the nephrotic syndrome being described infrequently. Gross hematuria can also be seen in both syndromes.

10. What does the kidney biopsy show in SAAG?

By light microscopy it may be difficult to distinguish PSGN from SAAG, as both present with a diffuse exudative glomerulonephritis with extensive neutrophilic infiltrate. The key histologic finding in SAAG is seen on immunofluorescence, which demonstrates predominant IgA staining at the site of the deposits. IgG may also be present, but it is often overshadowed by the IgA staining. Other infections causing glomerulonephritis may be associated with a predominant IgA response, but *S. aureus* accounts for the vast majority of these cases. In some instances, only C3 is present on immunofluorescence, which can confuse the differential diagnosis by adding C3 glomerulopathy.

Electron microscopy shows subepithelial deposits similar to PSGN as well as scattered sub-endothelial and mesangial deposits. Both SAAG and PSGN share similar findings on electron microscopy.

11. What serologic tests should be done to diagnose SAAG?

There are no tests similar to the streptozyme analysis for the diagnosis of staphylococcal infections. The key to diagnosis is to document by blood, urine, sputum, or aspiration sample a positive culture for staphylococcal infection in the setting of acute glomerulonephritis. The activation of the complement pathway is present in 82% of cases, with the alternate pathway (low C3) being the most common, but activation of the classic pathway (low C3 and C4) can also be found.

12. What is the treatment and long-term prognosis of SAAG?

Since SAAG is a result of active infection, appropriate selection of antibiotic therapy is the key to stopping the ongoing antigenemia that is fueling the production of immune complexes. The use of immunosuppressive therapy would be absolutely contraindicated, given the fact that these patients are actively infected with *Staphylococcus* and that sepsis could ensue if their immune systems were compromised.

The immune complexes in PSGN are short-lived and often resorb without long-term sequelae. In SAAG, depending on the timing and elimination of the bacteria, significant residual kidney disease is often present in more than 50% of patients. This consists of proteinuria, hematuria, and a persistently lower GFR, with some patients progressing to dependence on dialysis. Advanced age and the presence or absence of diabetes play major roles in determining the outcome of SAAG.

13. When glomerulonephritis follows an upper respiratory illness (URI), are any other differential diagnoses important to consider, other than PSGN or SAAG?

One of the most difficult diagnostic situations occurs when patients develop kidney disease after a URI. In addition to PSGN and rarely SAAG, there are two important differential diagnoses to consider: IgA nephropathy and C3 glomerulopathy. As previously discussed, PSGN occurs approximately 7 to 14 days or more after the infection has started, and there may not be any evidence of the URI at the time kidney disease develops. Alternatively, IgA nephropathy is called "synpharyngitic" because it is exacerbated at the time of the URI, usually within the first few days of onset. It is at this time that the patient will present with gross hematuria, hypertension, and signs of acute kidney injury, such as edema.

Clinically, IgA nephropathy relapses during the episode of URI and then settles back to a background level of low-grade microhematuria and nonnephrotic proteinuria. Many patients have had unsuspected IgA nephropathy prior to the onset of the URI, and it was the gross hematuria from the exacerbation of IgA nephropathy that brought the patient to the physician. The serum complement levels are normal in IgA nephropathy, whereas they are low in PSGN and SAAG, and the biopsy shows a predominant mesangial proliferative histology and not the diffuse proliferative exudative lesion seen with PSGN and SAAG.

C3 glomerulopathy is an immune complex disorder with activation of the alternate pathway of complement (low C3). It can be exacerbated by a URI but is usually present persistently in noninfected patients. The histology of C3 glomerulopathy is a membranoproliferative pattern with more mesangial and subendothelial deposits and basement membrane duplication, which are not the typical patterns seen in PSGN and SAAG. C3 levels remain consistently low compared with SAAG and PSGN, where the levels eventually return to normal with resolution of the kidney lesion.

KEY POINTS

1. Postinfectious glomerulonephritis (PIGN) describes a unique sequence of events consisting of an infection followed by complete resolution with a subsequent latent period of 1 or more weeks before the development of an immune complex–mediated glomerulonephritis. Only streptococcal infections can conclusively cause this pattern; therefore the term *poststreptococcal glomerulonephritis* (PSGN) is preferred over PIGN. However, the two terms can be used interchangeably.
2. The course of PSGN begins 7 to 14 days after the onset of streptococcal pharyngitis, whereas it takes about 21 days for the development of glomerulonephritis after a skin infection.
3. The use of steroids or more aggressive forms of immunosuppression for PSGN has not been shown to alter the natural history of the disease and exposes the patient to the potential short- and long-term risks of immunosuppression.
4. In older adults, staphylococcal-associated acute glomerulonephritis (SAAG) is more common than PSGN, especially after skin and lung infections, with *Staphylococcus aureus* being the primary species cultured.
5. SAAG occurs coincident with the active infection, and there is no latent period.
6. Complement activation of the alternate pathway is found in both PSGN and SAAG.
7. Diffuse proliferative and exudative glomerulonephritis with subepithelial and scattered subendothelial and mesangial deposits is seen with both PSGN and SAAG.
8. IgA-dominant immunofluorescence is seen exclusively with SAAG and not with PSGN.
9. The immunofluorescent pattern in both SAAG and PSGN is described as a "garland" or "starry sky" appearance because of the subepithelial deposits.
10. SAAG has a significantly worse prognosis than PSGN, with more than half the patients developing chronic kidney disease or requiring dialysis.
11. The treatment of SAAG is strictly antibiotic therapy—immunosuppression is contraindicated due to active staphylococcal infection.

Bibliography

Glassock, R. J., Alvarado, A., Prosek, J., Hebert, C., Parikh, S., Satoskar, A., . . . Hebert, L. A. (2015). Staphylococcus-related glomerulonephritis and poststreptococcal glomerulonephritis: Why defining "post" is important in understanding and treating infection-related glomerulonephritis. *American Journal of Kidney Diseases, 65*(6), 826–832.

Kambham, N. (2012). Postinfectious glomerulonephritis. *Advances in Anatomic Pathology, 19*(5), 338–347.

Kanjanabuch, T., Kittikowit, W., & Eiam-Ong, S. (2009). An update on acute postinfectious glomerulonephritis worldwide. *Nature Reviews Nephrology, 5,* 259–269.

Nadasdy, T., & Hebert, L. A. (2011). Infection-related glomerulonephritis: Understanding mechanisms. *Seminars in Nephrology, 31*(4), 369–375.

Naicker, J., Tablan, J., Naidoo, G., Wadee, S., Paget, G., & Goetsch, S, (2007). Infection and glomerulonephritis. *Seminars in Immunopathology, 29,* 397–414.

Nasr, S. H., & D'Agati, V. D. (2011). IgA-dominant postinfectious glomerulonephritis: A new twist on an old disease. *Nephron Clinical Practice, 119*(1), c18–c25. [discussion: c26].

Nasr, S. H., Radhakrishnan, J., & D'Agati, V. D. (2013). Bacterial infection-related glomerulonephritis in adults. *Kidney International, 83*(5), 792–803.

Nast, C. C. (2012). Infection-related glomerulonephritis: Changing demographics and outcomes. *Advances in Chronic Kidney Disease, 19*(2), 68–75.

Stratta, P., Musetti, C., Barreca, A., & Mazzucco, G. (2014). New trends of an old disease: The acute post infectious glomerulonephritis at the beginning of the new millenium. *Journal of Nephrology, 27*(3), 229–239.

Wang, S. Y., Bu, R., Zhang, Q., Liang, S., Wu, J., Liu, X. G., . . . Chen, X. M. (2016). Clinical, pathological, and prognostic characteristics of glomerulonephritis related to staphylococcal infection. *Medicine (Baltimore), 95*(15), e3386. doi:10.1097/MD.0000000000003386.

VIRAL HEPATITIS-ASSOCIATED GLOMERULONEPHRITIS

Warren Kupin

CHAPTER 35

1. **What types of viral hepatitis are associated with glomerulonephritis?**
   Chronic carriers of hepatitis B (HBV; 400 million people worldwide) or hepatitis C (HCV; 170 million people worldwide) are at increased risk of developing a variety of glomerular diseases linked directly to active viral replication. By definition, a carrier state for these viruses would be characterized by a positive quantitative polymerase chain reaction (PCR) assay.

   For HBV, the common serologic markers used for identification of a chronic carrier state includes the presence of circulating hepatitis B surface antigen (HbsAg) and in some cases hepatitis B e antigen (HbeAg) and the absence of hepatitis B surface antibody (HbsAb). For HCV, the most common initial screening test is the enzyme-linked immunosorbent assay (ELISA) for hepatitis C IgG antibodies. In stark contrast to the importance of HbsAb as an indicator of previous exposure and their absence during a chronic carrier state for HBV, the presence of HCV ELISA antibodies usually means the presence of active viremia, since this HCV antibody is non-neutralizing.

   Importantly, here is a small subgroup of patients (5% to 7%) who do not mount an antibody response to HCV, yet are chronic carriers by PCR. This is especially true for patients with end-stage kidney disease; therefore if a kidney lesion is suspicious for HCV related-glomerulonephritis, then a PCR should be done even if the ELISA is negative.

2. **Are the usual measurements of the glomerular filtration rate (GFR) and proteinuria applicable to patients with chronic hepatitis?**
   We know that the serum creatinine concentration results from the metabolism of creatine, which is a nitrogenous organic acid stored in muscles, which functions as an energy-providing catalyst. There are two sources of creatine: endogenous liver production and exogenous oral ingestion. About half the creatine comes from each source, which is extremely important when it comes to evaluating kidney function in patients with chronic hepatitis. Most patients who are chronic carriers of either hepatitis B or C have significant inflammatory injury to the liver and may even have various stages of cirrhosis. Creatine production in the liver will be significantly reduced, and this will lead to a lower serum creatinine. In the presence of cirrhosis, the synthesis of creatine can be reduced by more than 50%, and the oral intake of creatine will also be reduced as a result of malnutrition in these patients. The typical serum creatinine is usually 0.5 to 0.6 mg/dL in patients with cirrhosis, which is well below the normal for the general population (1.2 mg/dL for women and 1.5 mg/dL for men). Patients with liver disease of any cause, not just HCV or HBV, can have significant loss of GFR with a serum creatinine level within "the normal range" for the general population.

   For this reason, all physicians managing patients with chronic hepatitis should be cautious in interpreting kidney function using serum creatinine and should consider monitoring kidney function with either a 24-hour creatinine clearance or an estimated GFR (eGFR). The eGFR is calculated using the Chronic Kidney Disease Epidemiology Collaboration (CKD EPI) formula, and is always included on all automated reports that have a serum creatinine.

   The use of cystatin C to measure the GFR in place of the serum creatinine may be of value, especially in patients with cirrhosis, since it is not affected by muscle mass, bilirubin levels, gender, or age. However, cystatin C is affected by albumin levels and by an inflammatory state, both of which are present in cirrhotic patients. While creatinine-based formulas have overestimated GFR in cirrhotic patients, cystatin-C-based formulas have consistently underestimated the GFRs. Studies have introduced a modified CKD-EPI formula that incorporates both the serum creatinine and cystatin C levels together, and this has shown to be superior in estimating the GFR compared to either creatinine-based or cystatin-C-based formulas alone.

   In addition, all patients who are chronic hepatitis carriers should be screened for proteinuria. A random urine protein/creatinine ratio or a 24-hour urine protein collection is an equally valid way to quantify the degree of proteinuria. In patients with severe jaundice, the colorimetric dipstick may give false readings for protein because of the bilirubin pigment in the urine, so every positive urine dipstick test for protein should be confirmed with a quantitative measurement.

3. **What types of glomerular lesions are seen with a chronic hepatitis B carrier state?**
The most common glomerular pathology seen with HBV carriers is membranous nephropathy (MN; Table 35.1). These patients can also develop an immune complex form of polyarteritis nodosa, membranoproliferative glomerulonephritis (MPGN), IgA nephropathy, and focal segmental glomerulosclerosis (FSGS).

4. **How does HBV cause each of these types of kidney disease?**
The most common lesion seen worldwide with chronic HBV is MN. This lesion is a result of the formation of immune complexes in the sub-epithelial space of the basement membrane of the glomerulus forming "spikes" on electron microscopy similar to idiopathic MN, and demonstrates the classic "granular" immunofluorescence pattern with IgG and C3. The immune complex located in the sub-epithelial space most likely represents a sequential deposition of antigen followed by attachment by antibodies (as opposed to the circulating antigen–antibody complex being deposited in the sub-epithelial space). The only antigen that consistently fits the size limitation to deposit in this area of the basement membrane is HbeAg. Consistent with that observation is the fact that the vast majority of patients with chronic HBV who develop MN are positive for the HbsAg.

For HBV carriers who are HbsAg positive but HbeAg negative, the kidney lesion is usually not MN but MPGN, because the HbsAg is too large to deposit in the sub-epithelial space and is restricted to the sub-endothelial location. The subsequent local inflammation leads to cellular proliferation and histologically appears as Type I MPGN.

IgA nephropathy may result from three separate etiologies in HBV patients:
1. Since the liver is responsible for the metabolism of immunoglobulin A (IgA), in the presence of significant liver injury, the circulating levels of IgA increase and may deposit in the kidney. These complexes first embed in the mesangium, but may also be in the peripheral capillary loops. Clinically significant kidney disease from this "secondary" deposition of IgA in the glomeruli in any patient with liver disease regardless of etiology is extremely rare.
2. IgA antibodies have been shown to co-localize with HBV antigens in the mesangium, indicating HBV can directly cause IgA nephropathy.
3. Because HBV is present worldwide, especially in Asia where IgA is extremely prevalent, it is possible that HBV and IgA can occur independent of each other in certain populations.

Polyarteritis nodosa is a necrotizing vasculitis of medium-sized vessels that is not a direct form of glomerulonephritis. Rather, it affects the inflow circulation of the kidney and, as a result of fibrinoid necrosis and thrombosis of the larger muscular arteries of the kidney, there is severe hypertension, glomerular ischemia, and progressive kidney failure. The etiology for the vasculitis is the presence of HbsAg-antibody-immune complexes in the blood vessel walls, causing local complement activation and necrosis. The presence or absence of HbeAg is not important in the genesis of this lesion.

Finally, reports have shown a higher than expected incidence of FSGS in patients with chronic HBV. Because there are no immune complexes in the kidney with FSGS, it is not clear why this pathologic entity develops. Some studies have shown that HBV may enter and deposit in kidney tissue and through unknown mechanisms lead to FSGS.

5. **Can you determine the specific kidney disease without a kidney biopsy in patients with chronic HBV?**
Ultimately, a kidney biopsy is needed to be certain of the diagnosis. However, among the different possibilities, both MN and FSGS are associated with the nephrotic syndrome while MPGN and IgA

Table 35.1. Kidney Lesions Caused by Hepatitis B

	HBeAg + HBsAg +	HBeAg − HBsAg +	HBeAg − HBsAg +	HBeAg − HBsAg +
Kidney lesion	Membranous nephropathy	Membrano-proliferative glomerulonephritis	Polyarteritis Nodosa	IgA Nephropathy
Location of immune complexes	Sub-epithelial space	Sub-endothelial space	Blood vessel wall Medium size	Mesangium

HBeAg, Hepatitis B e antigen; HBsAg, hepatitis B surface antigen; IgA, immunoglobulin A.

present with a nephritic urinary sediment. Polyarteritis nodosa (PAN) does not cause changes in the urinalysis, since the lesion is a vasculitis in larger blood vessels extrinsic to the glomerulus. When the diagnosis is MN on biopsy, the question arises as to whether this could be idiopathic MN occurring by chance in a patient with HBV. Treatment options are contingent on which one is the cause. Patients with idiopathic MN are predominantly positive for anti-phospholipase A2 receptor antibodies compared to mostly negative results in HBV MN. However, there is enough overlap in published studies to raise a question about the predictive accuracy of this assay.

In spite of HBV-related immune complexes being present in MN, MPGN, and PAN, systemic complement activation is not seen, and C3 and C4 levels remain normal. Low complement levels should raise concern for unsuspected co-infection with HCV.

6. **Is HBV glomerular disease treatable?**
The immune complexes in all HBV kidney lesions require active viral replication, so the primary goal of therapy is to treat the source of the antigens: the active HBV. Lamivudine can suppress the viral load but needs to be continued indefinitely to maintain a sustained viral response. Patients experiencing a complete suppression of viral replication have a remission of MN with normalization of their proteinuria, improved kidney function, and a prolonged kidney survival. Unfortunately, as many as 50% of patients develop resistance to lamivudine and have a relapse of viremia. Current guidelines recommend entecavir as the primary agent for treatment of active hepatitis B antigenemia. For MN, this is the only therapy that is needed along with the typical antiproteinuria therapy, such as angiotensin-converting enzyme inhibitors or angiotensin receptor blockers. No immunosuppression is recommended, although short-term immunosuppression may be used in severe cases of nephrotic syndrome with only a transient increase in systemic viremia.

For patients with MPGN, the data are not as clear; however, theoretically, control of viremia would be essential. Again, the use of steroids or other immunosuppressant agents are not efficacious in the treatment of this lesion. IgA nephropathy, as mentioned, is rarely clinically important, and the IgA deposits are a result of advanced liver disease; unless liver function improves, there will be a continuous presence of IgA in the kidney. If the IgA is directly related to active HBV, then antiviral therapy could lead to a stabilization of kidney function.

PAN is a systemic vasculitis that causes life-threatening widespread organ dysfunction. It results from HBV immune complexes, so once again, control of viremia is essential. However, if there is significant systemic vasculitis, then a temporary use of steroids and even immunosuppressive therapy may be needed. The risks of this option would be a further increase (temporarily) in the hepatitis B viral load at the expense of reducing end-organ damage. This decision must be weighed carefully based on the severity of the vasculitis.

7. **What types of glomerular disease are caused by HCV?**
The most common histologic change in the glomerulus of patients with chronic HCV infection is type I MPGN due to type II cryoglobulinemia. These patients may also develop MN, fibrillary glomerulonephritis, IgA nephropathy, and diabetic nephropathy.

8. **What is type I MPGN as a consequence of type II cryoglobulinemia?**
MPGN is a specific type of glomerular injury in which there is damage to the basement membrane from electron-dense deposits and an increase in the proliferation of endothelial cells and mesangial cells. Therefore, compared to MN, in which there is only thickening of the basement membrane due to immune complexes without cellular proliferation, MPGN is a more aggressive kidney injury. MN typically causes only the nephrotic syndrome, whereas MPGN causes nephrotic syndrome with an "active" urinary sediment showing red cells casts, granular casts, dysmorphic red cells, and kidney tubular epithelial cells.

The MPGN histology is type I MPGN, with immune complexes selectively located in the subendothelial space and mesangium. A reclassification of MPGN has occurred, and this category is now called immune complex mediated MPGN as compared to a separate category called complement mediated MPGN. Hepatitis C results in a unique production of cryoglobulin immune complexes that deposit in the subendothelial space, classifying this as a subset of immune complex MPGN.

The cryoglobulins in hepatitis C are so large that they cannot filter through the basement membrane, so they are trapped in the subendothelial space. Their size forces them to protrude into the lumen of the capillary, and it almost looks like there are thrombi in the glomeruli capillaries. The entire capillary lumen may become filled with the cryoglobulin complex.

Cryoglobulins are immune complexes comprising certain combinations of antibodies and antigens that precipitate on cooling and are classified based on the composition of the antibody involved and its target. When the antibody is composed of a single subtype (monoclonal), such as only an IgG or IgM, and precipitates in the cold, it is called type I cryoglobulinemia. This often results from a hematopoietic malignancy. If there is an antibody that is monoclonal (IgM or IgG) and it targets another antibody that is polyclonal (IgG), this is called type II cryoglobulinemia. This category used to be called essential cryoglobulinemia and is a characteristic of HCV. If there are two different polyclonal antibodies present that interact and form an immune complex, this is called type III cryoglobulinemia.

Once a patient is infected with hepatitis C, the immune system tries to neutralize the virus by producing IgG antibodies against the surface antigens of the viral capsid. Unfortunately, these antibodies do not neutralize the virus, but they do circulate in the blood of patients chronically infected with HCV. This is what is measured with the ELISA: non-neutralizing IgG antibodies against the hepatitis C capsid. What is unusual in HCV is that the patient will make a unique type of monoclonal IgM antibody (IgMk) that directly targets the IgG the person has made against the viral envelope proteins. When one antibody attacks another antibody, this is called an anti-idiotypic antibody. The IgM that is made in patients with HCV is anti-idiotypic because it is directed against the IgG molecule. The cryoglobulin in HCV is composed of a monoclonal IgMk linking together polyclonal IgG and viral capsid envelope proteins. This crosslinking of antibodies to antibodies is why cryoglobulin is so large and obstructs the capillary lumen. It is unique from typical immune complexes in autoimmune syndromes like systemic lupus erythematosus, which are only composed of one antibody and one antigen. It is not known why only the clonal IgM heavy chain and only the kappa light chains are made by the stimulated B cells from hepatitis C.

9. **Why do cryoglobulins form with HCV and not HBV?**
HBV is a hepatotropic virus, meaning it selectively and primarily enters hepatic tissue, possibly infects kidney tissue, but does not invade immunocompetent cells. HCV is not only hepatotropic but also lymphotropic, having an affinity to bind to select receptors on B cells and even enter the cell itself. The viral capsid antigens appear to be able to target B-cell receptors that are responsible for cell proliferation, and disrupt the normal cell cycle. Infected B cells in HCV become clonal and produce the IgMk antibody that has anti-idiotypic capacity. HBV and no other form of viral hepatitis has this propensity to bind to and stimulate B cells, which is why cryoglobulins are common in 50% of HCV patients and extremely rare in HBV.

Over time, patients with HCV who have cryoglobulinemia are at higher risk for the development of B-cell lymphoma. The finding of type II cryoglobulinemia in HCV should be regarded as a premalignant disease. Approximately 6% will develop lymphoma.

10. **Do cryoglobulins cause damage to other organ systems?**
Absolutely! The circulation and deposition of type II cryoglobulins leads to inflammatory damage in the vascular system throughout the body, which is characterized by medium-sized vessel vasculitis. Specifically, these patients develop lower extremity skin lesions (palpable purpura); cerebral/cardiac/pulmonary/peripheral nerve infarction; and a constant inflammatory state characterized by failure to thrive, malaise, and myalgias. HCV-related kidney disease may appear as the only systemic manifestation of type II cryoglobulinemia, but more often appears in the context of systemic disease. Once diagnosed with MPGN, a patient with HCV should undergo a careful screening for systemic complications of vasculitis.

11. **Other than a kidney biopsy, is there any other way to make the diagnosis of MPGN and cryoglobulinemia from hepatitis C?**
Because the kidney disease cannot occur in the absence of active HCV viral replication, the first question to ask is as follows: "What is the status of the patient's HCV?" Many patients are being treated with the new direct acting antivirals (DAA) and have achieved viral remission. If these patients are nephrotic or have impaired kidney function, then there will have to be an alternative explanation, because it is not likely a result of MPGN from HCV, and an alternative investigation is needed.

If the patient has active viral replication, then certain serologic testing may help confirm the diagnosis of HCV-related MPGN/cryoglobulinemia. When immune complexes, such as cryoglobulins, deposit and initiate an inflammatory response, they activate the complement cascade. Cryoglobulins activate the classical complement pathway and lead to reduced serum concentrations of C3 and C4. It is improbable that a patient could have kidney disease because of type II cryoglobulins and not show complement activation. Ordering a C3 and C4 is essential in the work-up of these patients. Usually, both C3 and C4, but sometimes just the C4, is markedly depressed.

A serum cryoglobulins level can be checked, but the turnaround time for this assay is often not quick enough to help with the immediate diagnosis. More commonly, an indirect marker for the presence of cryoglobulins, called the rheumatoid factor, is measured. An IgM antibody directed against another IgG antibody is said to be anti-idiotypic, and if there are no other antigens involved, this is said to possess "rheumatoid factor" activity. In patients with rheumatoid arthritis, these immune complexes likely result in the pathogenesis of the disease. In other diseases that manifest antibodies that are anti-idiotypic, the test for the "rheumatoid factor" will be positive. A positive rheumatoid factor assay coupled with a low C3 and C4 is typical of active cryoglobulinemia.

12. **What is the treatment for MPGN in hepatitis C?**
The development of cryoglobulinemia is contingent on viral interaction with B cells and subsequent B-cell IgM production to form cryoglobulins. Therefore reducing the viral load is the most critical step in controlling this disease process. Initially, the only effective therapy for hepatitis C was the use of interferon with or without adjunctive ribavirin. Interferon was poorly tolerated and rarely led to a sustained viral response.
The development of DAAs has revolutionized the therapy of HCV. These drugs inhibit the assembly of non-structural viral capsid proteins and after a 12-week course of therapy often result in a sustained viral remission of >95% regardless of HCV genotype.
In certain circumstances, additional, more aggressive immunosuppressive therapy may be warranted in HCV-related MPGN. These exceptions include the following: (1) a rapid decline of kidney function with biopsy evidence of crescentic changes; or (2) systemic vasculitis with life-threatening organ dysfunction. In these cases, simply controlling the virus will not modify the damage occurring from the cryoglobulins that are already formed and circulating. The strategy will need to target removing the systemic cryoglobulins so ongoing tissue injury can be attenuated, and then the DAAs can inhibit the new production of IgMk type II cryoglobulins.
Plasmapheresis has become the treatment of choice for severe cases of cryoglobulinemia and will effectively remove these immune complexes from the circulation. Concomitantly, treatment should target the B cells that are producing the abnormal IgMk antibodies. In past years, chemotherapy, such as the use of cyclophosphamide, was used to inhibit B-cell proliferation. This therapy was not specific to B cells and resulted in potentially serious collateral effects on other cell lines. The use of the monoclonal anti-CD20 antibody, rituximab, selectively removes B cells from the circulation and has revolutionized the therapy of B-cell lymphomas and cryoglobulinemia. Rituximab binds to a surface antigen only found on B cells (CD20) and leads to their peripheral destruction and elimination. This assists in stopping cryoglobulin production while plasmapheresis removes the antibodies already present.

13. **Why is diabetic nephropathy listed as a cause of nephrotic syndrome for patients with HCV?**
In addition to the lymphotropic effect of HCV, this virus also binds to bb-islet cells. The interaction of the virus surface antigens with bb-islet cells in the pancreas initiates a sequence of events that leads to islet dysfunction and secondary type II diabetes. In addition, viral structural proteins interfere with the post-receptor response to insulin, leading to a combination of type I and type II diabetes in these patients.
Over years, the end-organ complications of diabetes can accrue, especially the development of diabetic nephropathy. Therefore in a patient with HCV and diabetes who presents with nephrotic syndrome and kidney dysfunction, the differential diagnosis needs to include diabetic nephropathy. Clinically, the presence of low complement levels (C3 and C4) and an active urinary sediment possibly associated with systemic manifestations of vasculitis would all be supportive of HCV-related cryoglobulinemia as opposed to diabetes as the cause of kidney dysfunction.
The treatment of diabetic nephropathy in patients with HCV is similar to that of diabetic nephropathy in the general population and includes inhibition of the renin-angiotensin-aldosterone system (RAAS), blood pressure control, and glycemic control.

14. **Can patients with HBV or HCV glomerulopathies eventually undergo kidney transplantation?**
As discussed earlier, both types of glomerulopathies that occur with HCV and HBV are directly related to active viral replication. In the case of HBV, it results from immune complexes, whereas in the case of HCV, it is associated with the development of cryoglobulinemia. If transplantation is considered in these cases, one of the first questions to ask is: "What is the status of the liver involvement from these viruses?"
The answer to this question is crucial in order to define whether the patient needs a combined liver–kidney transplant or a kidney transplant only. The presence of cirrhosis on biopsy would

automatically mandate that a combined transplant be performed. Without a liver biopsy it is not always possible to estimate whether or not cirrhosis is present. Evaluation of liver function studies, clotting parameters, and the presence or absence of portal hypertension are all useful in the clinical assessment for the presence of cirrhosis.

If the patient has stable liver function and no evidence of cirrhosis, then a kidney transplant alone can be considered. The second question to answer is: "How active is the viral disease?"

It would be counterproductive to perform a transplant on a patient and provide intensive immunosuppression if there is uncontrolled viral proliferation. The risks of exacerbating viral activity can lead to either post-transplant immune complex kidney disease or post-transplant liver disease. One of the most common causes of death in patients with HCV after transplantation is liver disease. There is an increased risk of hepatoma in patients with active HCV or HBV, and routine monitoring of alpha fetoprotein levels is required during follow-up.

In the case of HCV, as long as there is no sign of cirrhosis, a new strategy in the use of DAAs is not to treat the patient while they are on the waiting list, and sign them up to receive an HCV positive donor kidney. Then after the transplant they are started on DAA therapy. The waiting list for an HCV-positive organ donor is significantly shorter than waiting for a routine cadaver donor.

15. What are the really important secrets I need to know about HBV and HCV related glomerulopathies? Table 35.2 summarizes the key aspects of these two lesions.

16. Is there anything else I need to know about hepatitis-induced kidney disease?
Yes. Not every patient with HBV and HCV who develops kidney disease has a viral-induced glomerulopathy. Because these viruses cause kidney disease due to viral replication, it is not surprising that advanced liver disease is usually present when they lead to glomerulonephritis. Consequently, these patients often have portal hypertension and cirrhosis, which adds another differential diagnosis into the picture including hepatorenal syndrome (HRS).

Acute kidney injury in patients with cirrhosis is often related to prerenal azotemia from diuretics used for the mobilization of ascites and lower extremity edema, and at the extreme can result in HRS. It is essential that physicians evaluating a patient with cirrhosis and known HBV or HCV who has developed acute kidney injury take into consideration the possibility of HRS. Differentiating HBV or HCV glomerulonephritis from HRS can be done using routine laboratory and urinalysis tests. The following questions should be asked:

- **Is there proteinuria?** Patients with HRS have less than 500 mg of protein excretion in 24 hours, as compared to patients with either hepatitis B- or C-related glomerulonephritis where the nephrotic syndrome is common.
- **What does the urine sediment show?** In patients with HRS, the urine sediment is bland with no cells or casts. In HCV-related MPGN, the urine will be nephritic with red-cell casts, dysmorphic red blood cells, white blood cells, and kidney tubular epithelial cells. In hepatitis B MN the urine will be nephrotic with fatty casts and oval fat bodies.

Table 35.2. Key Aspects of Hepatitis B and Hepatitis C –Related Glomerulopathies

	HEPATITIS C	HEPATITIS B
Primary glomerular disease	Type I membranoproliferative glomerulonephritis	Membranous nephropathy
Pathophysiology	Type II cryoglobulinemia	Hepatitis B e Ag-antibody immune complexes
Clinical findings	Nephritic syndrome	Nephrotic syndrome
Systemic manifestations	Vasculitis	None
Laboratory features	Low C3, C4 Positive rheumatoid factor	Normal complement levels
Treatment	Direct acting antivirals	Entecavir
Malignancy potential	Hepatoma B-cell lymphoma	Hepatoma

- **Is the FENa (fractional excretion of sodium) helpful?** Unfortunately, the FENa in patients with HRS or any form of glomerulonephritis will be less than 1%, indicating a sodium avid state. The FENa is not useful in differentiating between these diagnoses.
- **What about serum complement levels?** In HCV-related MPGN, the levels of C3 and C4 will be very low, indicating active consumption by the type II cryoglobulins, and the rheumatoid factor will be elevated. For HBV, MN, and HRS, the serum complement levels and rheumatoid factor will all be within normal limits.

KEY POINTS

1. The typical serum creatinine is usually 0.5 to 0.6 mg/dL in patients with cirrhosis, which is well below the normal expected maximum range for the general population: 1.2 mg/dL for women and 1.5 mg/dL for men. Patients with liver disease can have a significant loss of GFR with a serum creatinine level within "the normal range" for the general population.
2. The most common lesion seen worldwide with chronic HBV is MN. This lesion is a result of the formation of immune complexes in the sub-epithelial space of the basement membrane of the glomerulus forming "spikes" on electron microscopy like idiopathic MN, and demonstrates the classic "granular" immunofluorescence pattern with IgG and C3.
3. For those patients who are carriers of hepatitis B but are only HbsAg positive and negative for HbeAg, the kidney lesion is usually not MN but MPGN. This is because the HbsAg-antibody immune complex is too large to filter through the basement membrane, so it lodges in the inner surface of the capillary wall (sub-endothelial space).
4. The most common histologic change in the glomerulus of patients with chronic HCV infection is type I MPGN due to type II cryoglobulinemia. These patients may also develop MN, fibrillary glomerulonephritis, IgA nephropathy, and diabetic nephropathy.
5. Hepatitis C-induced MPGN should be primarily treated with anti-viral therapy. In some cases patients may need additional treatments targeted at reducing antibodies, such as rituximab and plasmapheresis.
6. Not all patients with viral hepatitis and new onset kidney disease have viral-induced glomerulonephritis. HRS is not uncommon in this population.

BIBLIOGRAPHY

Böckle, B. C., & Sepp, N. T. (2010). Hepatitis C virus and autoimmunity. *Autoimmunity Highlights, 1*(1), 23–35.

Dammacco, F., Racanelli, V., Russi, S., & Sansonno, D. (2016). The expanding spectrum of HCV-related cryoglobulinemic vasculitis: A narrative review. *Clinical and Experimental Medicine, 16*(3), 233–242.

Fabrizi, F., Martin, P., Cacoub, P., Messa, P., & Donato, F. M. (2015). Treatment of hepatitis C-related kidney disease. *Expert Opinion on Pharmacotherapy, 16*(12), 1815–1827.

Ferri, S., Muratori, L., Lenzi, M., Granito, A., Bianchi, F. B., & Vergani, D. (2008). HCV and autoimmunity. *Current Pharmaceutical Design, 14*(17), 1678–1685.

Gill, K., Ghazinian, H., Manch, R., & Gish, R. (2016). Hepatitis C virus as a systemic disease: Reaching beyond the liver. *Hepatology International, 10*(3), 415–423.

Ozkok, A., & Yildiz, A. (2014). Hepatitis C virus associated glomerulopathies. *World Journal of Gastroenterology, 20*(24), 7544–7554.

Saadoun, D., Terrier, B., Semoun, O., Sene, D., Maisonobe, T., Musset, L., ... Cacoub, P. (2011). Hepatitis C virus-associated polyarteritis nodosa. *Arthritis Care & Research (Hoboken), 63*(3), 427–435.

Shire, N. J., & Sherman, K. E. (2015). Epidemiology of Hepatitis C virus: A battle on new frontiers. *Gastroenterology Clinics of North America, 44*(4), 699–716.

Sise, M. E., Bloom, A. K., Wisocky, J., Lin, M. V., Gustafson, J. L., Lundquist, A. L., ... Chung, R. T. (2016). Treatment of hepatitis C virus-associated mixed cryoglobulinemia with direct-acting antiviral agents. *Hepatology, 63*(2), 408–417.

Tasleem, S., & Sood, G. K. (2015). Hepatitis C Associated B-cell Non-Hodgkin Lymphoma: Clinical features and the role of antiviral therapy. *Journal of Clinical and Translational Hepatology, 3*(2), 134–139.

Terrier, B., Marie, I., Lacraz, A., Belenotti, P., Bonnet, F., Chiche, L., ... Cacoub, P. (2015). Non HCV-related infectious cryoglobulinemia vasculitis: Results from the French nationwide CryoVas survey and systematic review of the literature. *Journal of Autoimmunity, 65*, 74–81.

Tong, X., & Spradling, P. R. (2015). Increase in nonhepatic diagnoses among persons with hepatitis C hospitalized for any cause, United States, 2004–2011. *Journal of Viral Hepatitis, 22*(11), 906–913.

Yau, A. H., & Yoshida, E. M. (2014). Hepatitis C drugs: The end of the pegylated interferon era and the emergence of all-oral interferon-free antiviral regimens: A concise review. *Canadian Journal of Gastroenterology and Hepatology, 28*(8), 445–451.

Zignego, A. L., Gragnani, L., Piluso, A., Sebastiani, M., Giuggioli, D., Fallahi, P., ... Ferri, C. (2015). Virus-driven autoimmunity and lymphoproliferation: The example of HCV infection. *Expert Review of Clinical Immunology, 11*(1), 15–31.

CHAPTER 36

HUMAN IMMUNODEFICIENCY VIRUS–ASSOCIATED KIDNEY DISORDERS

Warren Kupin

1. **How do you begin the evaluation of kidney disease in the setting of human immunodeficiency virus (HIV) infection?**

   The differential diagnosis of kidney disease in the setting of HIV infection covers a wide spectrum of kidney disorders including acid-base and electrolyte abnormalities, glomerular disease, acute kidney injury (AKI), and chronic kidney disease (CKD). There is no difference in the initial basic approach in the evaluation of a patient with HIV compared to that of a patient who does not have HIV. If patients with HIV develop kidney disease, the specific site of involvement (e.g., glomerular, interstitial, or vascular) should be identified. Treatment options are dependent on proper identification and classification of the various HIV-associated kidney diseases.

2. **How is kidney disease first detected in patients with HIV?**

   Standard recommendations for screening HIV patients have been established and require a measurement of kidney function (creatinine and glomerular filtration rate [GFR] calculation), urine dipstick with microscopy, and a urine protein to creatinine ratio at the time of initial evaluation. This is repeated annually, or more often, depending on whether the patient has risk factors for kidney disease, such as exposure to nephrotoxic drugs or co-morbidities including hypertension, diabetes, or concurrent hepatitis C (HCV) or B (HBV). It is not necessary to measure the GFR by 24-hour urine collections; it can be accurately estimated glomerular filtration rate (eGFR) from the creatinine level using conventional estimating formulas.

   The standard National Kidney Foundation and Kidney Disease: Improving Global Outcomes (KDIGO) definitions for CKD should be applied to patients with HIV as well as the Acute Kidney Injury Network definition of AKI.

3. **How accurate is creatinine for detecting kidney disease in patients with HIV?**

   It is now clear that the serum creatinine has significant limitations in many HIV patients as a result of:
   1. The dependence of creatinine on gender, age, and underlying nutritional status. Patients with active HIV who are not receiving combination anti-retroviral therapy (cART) may have marked reductions in muscle mass as a result of malnutrition, and will have lower baseline serum creatinine levels than in the general population. It would not be unusual for a patient with advanced, untreated HIV to have a seemingly normal serum creatinine level of 0.9 mg/dL and yet have a significant reduction in eGFR.
   2. Interference of HIV therapy with the laboratory measurement of creatinine. Some cART drugs interferes with the tubular secretion of creatinine. Since creatinine is both filtered and secreted, impairment of tubular secretion will increase the serum creatinine even without a change in the GFR. This will cause the eGFR to fall and may lead to an erroneous diagnosis and inappropriate work-up for acute or chronic kidney injury. This process is similar to the spurious elevations of creatinine seen with cimetidine and trimethoprim. Specifically in cART, the integrase strand inhibitors characteristically impede the secretion of creatinine, and it is expected that the creatinine will be higher in these patient by 0.5 mg/dL. Cobicistat, used as a booster for the other cART medications, has also been shown to have the same effect on creatinine secretion. The absence of other markers of kidney injury—that is, abnormal urinary sediment, a normal blood urea nitrogen, and stable clinical course—all support a benign drug-induced elevation of creatinine.

4. **How is proteinuria used as a marker for HIV kidney disease?**

   In addition to an impaired GFR as a sign of kidney disease in patients with HIV, often a patient with HIV will first present with only proteinuria and even microalbuminuria. Proteinuria represents one of the pathognomonic hallmarks of HIV-induced glomerular disease, but also could represent early onset of cART-related kidney tubular injury. All patients with HIV should have a dipstick urinalysis performed for detection of proteinuria. The finding of proteinuria is an accurate and significant predictor of increased morbidity and mortality in patients with HIV. If the dipstick test result is positive, then a spot urine test for protein/creatinine ratio should be done to estimate the degree of proteinuria with a ratio >300 mg/g being a key cut-off level that requires further investigation.

Studies have shown that microalbuminuria may be an important indicator of the presence of kidney disease in patients with HIV, which is similar to the use of microalbuminuria in patients with diabetes. However, current guidelines do require the measurement of microalbuminuria in this population.

5. **What are the common causes of AKI in HIV patients?**
Approximately 5% to 10% of hospitalized patients with HIV will experience AKI, with a mortality risk that is five times higher than the general AKI population without HIV. The most important approach in the assessment of AKI in a patient with HIV requires answers to the following questions:
   - Is the patient receiving cART?
   - What is the viral control of HIV?

The approach to AKI will be different based on the answers to these questions. If a patient is not receiving cART and has uncontrolled HIV viremia, the most common causes of kidney injury are related to systemic infection and volume depletion leading to prerenal azotemia and possible acute tubular necrosis (ATN). Uncontrolled infectious diarrhea with fever and large insensible fluid losses is a common presenting scenario in a patient with HIV who is cART naïve. Patients with HIV frequently develop sepsis from pneumonia and other opportunistic infections complicated by hypotension, which may also lead to ATN. In patients with infection who are cART-naïve, multiple antibiotics are often used to cover bacterial, viral, fungal, and atypical infectious agents. Many of these antibiotics can result in AKI, as noted in Table 36.1.

If the patient is receiving cART therapy with a controlled viral load, then the development of AKI may be secondary to drug-induced tubular dysfunction. Patients on cART have been shown to have a significantly higher risk of AKI, particularly in the setting of volume depletion. It is essential that all physicians treating patients with HIV be familiar with the potential nephrotoxicity of cART.

6. **How does cART cause kidney disease?**
cART involves multiple classes of agents, including protease inhibitors (PI), reverse transcriptase inhibitors, integrase strand inhibitors, and entry blockers. Distinct syndromes are associated with certain classes of cART that must be kept in mind during the evaluation of each patient (Table 36.2). PI can be associated with three main kidney side effects:
   1. They can crystallize in the urinary tract and form either macroscopic stones, resulting in urinary obstruction (hydronephrosis), or they may crystallize inside the tubules, causing microtubular obstruction and ATN (no hydronephrosis).

Table 36.1. Antibiotics Can Result in Acute Kidney Injury

ANTIBIOTIC	KIDNEY SYNDROME(S)
Amphotericin	ATN, type I kidney tubular acidosis
Trimethoprim-sulfamethoxazole	Crystal-induced ATN, allergic interstitial nephritis
Penicillin/cephalosporin agents	Allergic interstitial nephritis
Aminoglycosides	ATN
Foscarnet	ATN
Pentamidine	ATN
Vancomycin	ATN
Ciprofloxacin	Crystal-induced ATN, allergic interstitial nephritis
Acyclovir	Crystal-induced ATN, allergic interstitial nephritis
Azole class antifungals	Potentiate NRTI and calcineurin-induced nephrotoxicity

ATN, Acute tubular necrosis; NRTI, nucleaside reverse transcriptase inhibitors.

Table 36.2. Kidney Syndromes Associated With HAART

cART CLASS	REPRESENTATIVE DRUGS	KIDNEY SYNDROME(S)
Protease inhibitors	Indinavir, atazanavir, nelfinavir, saquinavir, ritonovir, amprenavir	Urolithiasis: obstructive uropathy, ATN Interstitial nephritis CKD
Nucleoside reverse transcriptase inhibitors	Stavudine, zidovudine, didanosine, lamivudine	Mitochondrial cytopathy: hepatic steatosis, lactic acidosis, rhabdomyolysis, acute tubular necrosis
Nucleotide reverse transcriptase inhibitors	Tenofovir, adefovir	Fanconi syndrome, ATN, CKD
Integrase strand inhibitors	Raltegravir, Dolutegravir	—

ATN, Acute tubular necrosis; *CKD*, chronic kidney disease.

2. They may lead to acute interstitial nephritis.
3. They inhibit the cytochrome P450 system, which may lead to nephrotoxicity from other drugs, especially in transplant patients on calcineurin inhibitors (CNI). In the presence of PIs, CNIs may need only once-a-week dosing due to impaired P450 metabolism.
    Nucleaside reverse transcriptase inhibitors (NRTI) cause direct proximal tubular injury with tenofovir as the prototypic agent. Because the tubular injury is localized to the proximal tubule, a Fanconi syndrome may develop with typical Type II renal tubular acidosis and phosphaturia causing hypophosphatemia. Long-term use of tenofovir may also lead to CKD with the development of irreversible interstitial fibrosis, especially in combination with PIs. CKD is now developing in 10% to 15% of long-term cART patients, and this growing global burden of CKD in this population is clinically important. HIV patients with CKD have the same increased mortality from cardiovascular disease as any CKD patient in the general population. The development of a safer delivery form of tenofovir, called tenofovir alafenamide, instead of tenofovir disoproxil fumarate has significantly reduced the risk of nephrotoxicity of this agent, and may replace the previous version as the standard of care.

7. What glomerular diseases are seen in patients with HIV?
    Proteinuria in patients with HIV is often a sign of glomerular disease, even if it is not within the nephrotic range, since it depends on when during an HIV infection the proteinuria is measured. HIV-related glomerular disease goes through an initial phase of microalbuminuria (30 to 300 mg/24 hours) followed by macroalbuminuria (>300 mg/24 hours), culminating in nephrotic syndrome. Any level of proteinuria in a patient with HIV would be considered highly suspicious for one of the glomerular lesions described below:
    - HIV-associated nephropathy (HIVAN): collapsing variant of focal segmental glomerular sclerosis (FSGS)
    - HIV immune complex disease of the kidney (HIVICK): membranous nephropathy (MN), immunoglobulin (Ig)A nephropathy, diffuse proliferative glomerulonephritis
    - HCV-related membranoproliferative glomerulonephritis (MPGN) associated with cryoglobulinemia: Approximately 30% of patients with HIV are co-infected with HCV and may develop glomerular disease from HCV-related immune complex disease
    - HBV-associated MN: Approximately 10% to 20% of HIV are co-infected with HBV and can manifest typical HBV glomerular syndromes
    - Thrombotic microangiopathy; typically seen in advanced untreated HIV patients
    - FSGS: This is the typical perihilar or tip form of FSGS seen in the general population
    - Diabetic nephropathy; diabetes is a frequent complication of cART, and since HIV patients are living 10 to 20 years with controlled HIV disease, contemporary biopsy series now show an increasing burden of diabetic nephropathy
    - Infection-related glomerulonephritis: immune complex proliferative glomerular disease from opportunistic infections such as Streptococci, Staphylococci, Gram-negative bacteria, etc.

When developing a differential diagnosis of glomerular disease in a patient with HIV, the following questions are important to ask:

- Does the patient have active HIV viremia? If yes, consider HIVAN or HIVICK.
- Is the patient co-infected with HCV or HBV? If yes, consider MPGN or MN, respectively.
- Is the patient on cART and well controlled? If yes, consider typical FSGS, especially in black patients.
- Is the patient receiving cART with secondary diabetes? If yes, consider diabetic nephropathy.
- Is the patient septic? If yes, consider an infection-related glomerulonephritis.

8. **What exactly is HIVAN?**
   HIVAN is a unique glomerular disease that is a result of the effects of active HIV viral replication within kidney tissue. This is in direct contrast to HIVICK, which represents an immune complex medicated injury to the kidney. It is characterized by four pathologic changes in the kidney:
   1. Collapsing variant of focal sclerosis: hypertrophy and hyperplasia of the podocytes to the point that it "caves in" the capillary tuft and reduces the filtration area of the glomerulus
   2. Microcystic dilation of the tubules: markedly enlarged dilated tubules in the absence of obstruction
   3. Interstitial nephritis: infiltration of the interstitial space of the kidney with CD8 + T cells
   4. Tubulo-reticular inclusion bodies: the presence of arrays of coagulated proteins in the endoplasmic reticulum in proximal renal tubular cells that result from high levels of cytokines, such as γ-interferon. This is not pathognomonic of HIV and can be seen in systemic lupus erythematosis (SLE).

9. **How does HIVAN present clinically?**
   HIVAN is almost exclusively found in patients of African ancestry (90%) who have active HIV viral replication. It is rarely an early presentation in the course of HIV, and most patients with HIVAN have a CD4 count <200 and a viral load of >400 copies/mL. How HIV was acquired in the first place is not important; however, the degree of HIV activity is the key to developing HIVAN.

10. **Why is HIVAN restricted to patients of black race origin?**
    The single most important risk factor for HIVAN is the presence of active HIV infection (high viral load, low CD4 count) in a susceptible host (African ancestry). The role for a genetic risk in the development of HIVAN has been substantiated by the discovery of the APOL1 (Apolipoprotein L1) gene on chromosome 22. Variants of this gene (called G1 and G2) are protective from Trypanosomiasis Rhodesiense. However, patients homozygous for these variants unfortunately have a significantly increased risk of developing many forms of kidney disease, especially HIVAN (but not HIVICK). It is estimated that 15% of the U.S. black population is homozygous for APOL1 variants, which, in the setting of an HIV infection, markedly increases the risk of HIVAN.

11. **Are there any special clinical features of HIVAN that may help in establishing this diagnosis from others?**
    There are two additional clinical findings (other than race) that are often reported to favor a diagnosis of HIVAN as opposed to the other types of glomerular disease. The first is the absence of hypertension in the setting of kidney disease and proteinuria. Typically, FSGS and the glomerulopathies related to viral hepatitis (HCV or HBV), HIVICK, or diabetes are associated with moderate to marked hypertension, but not HIVAN. Patients with HIVAN have unexpectedly normal blood pressure because of the presence of vasodilatory cytokines that are produced in response to the HIV infection, and a salt-losing state in the kidney, which is also related to active HIV infection. More than 80% of patients with HIVAN have normal blood pressures in the setting of significant kidney injury. Based on these data, the presence of hypertension in a patient with HIV with kidney disease should prompt a reconsideration of the diagnosis of HIVAN to an alternative etiology.
    The second suggestive feature that may point to HIVAN is the presence of large echogenic kidneys on ultrasound. Most patients with nephrotic syndrome and progressive CKD will have loss of kidney size and mild echogenicity due to interstitial fibrosis. In HIVAN, the presence of microcystic dilation may result in larger than expected kidney size at any level of kidney function, and the degree of echogenicity is significantly more than that seen in other kidney lesions. Since HIVAN may increase the size and echogenicity of the kidneys and HIVICK will not, many studies that question the predicative reliability of these findings in HIV patients may be biased, because the patient population may be a mixture of these two diagnoses. Therefore the initial evaluation by ultrasound of a patient with HIV with proteinuria may already lead to a tentative diagnosis of HIVAN if these characteristic findings are reported. The ultrasound radiologist may be the first one to suggest a differential diagnosis of HIVAN based on these characteristic findings.

12. How common is HIVAN?

The natural history of untreated HIV in the United States and Africa has shown that approximately 3% to 12% of black patients will develop HIVAN. Most recent series show that HIVAN and HIVICK are almost equal in their frequency in untreated HIV patients.

13. What is the etiology of HIVAN?

HIVAN is a direct result of active HIV infection in kidney tissue. Current research shows that the HIV virus gains entry into kidney tissue including the podocytes, mesangial cells, and tubular epithelial cells. Once inside the cells, the viral genome is translated and the gene products lead to alterations of cellular function and development. Some of the candidate genes whose products are responsible for HIVAN include negative factor for viral replication (NEF), transactivating factor, and virus protein R. Research studies are still investigating what types of receptors the virus uses to enter kidney tissue. The viral gene proteins lead to an interruption of normal cell maturation, and the infected cells de-differentiate into an immature cell phenotype. The delicate balance between cell growth and apoptosis is offset and, being unable to control their own proliferation, the podocytes—as well as the infected parietal epithelial cells—increase in number and cause collapsing FSGS followed by tubular dilation from proliferating epithelial cells, forming the large microcysts.

14. What is HIVICK?

HIVICK represents a group of histologically different glomerular diseases in HIV patients that share a similar pathogenesis: immune complex injury. The types of glomerular histology within the HIVICK family include membranous, IgA nephropathy, diffuse proliferative glomerulonephritis (SLE-like), and a membranoproliferative pattern. The immune complexes in all these lesions contain HIV antigens, which confirm the dependence of the lesion on active viremia. A second group of immune complex diseases that represent part of HIVICK is glomerulonephritis secondary to the infections that superimpose themselves in advanced HIV. In these cases, the bacterial, viral, or fungal antigens (but not the HIV antigens) form the immune complex. Both of these groups are classified as HIVICK.

In contrast to HIVAN, there is no association of the APOL1 variants and the development of HIVICK.

15. Are HIVICK and HIVAN the most common lesions found in patients with HIV with proteinuria?

Before the development and widespread use of cART therapy, HIVAN was by far the most common cause of nephrotic syndrome in patients with HIV. However, this pattern has changed dramatically in the cART era. HIVAN now accounts for only <40% of all cases of nephrotic syndrome, with HIVICK, classic FSGS, and viral hepatitis-induced glomerulopathies accounting for the remaining proportion. A kidney biopsy is usually recommended for patients with HIV with proteinuria, because a kidney lesion other than HIVAN is usually found.

16. Is there a treatment for HIVAN or HIVICK?

Successful therapy of any kidney disease is dependent on the degree of reversible or irreversible lesions that are present. The most important predictor of response to therapy is the degree of interstitial fibrosis, which can only be ascertained from a kidney biopsy. HIVAN is considered a treatable and potentially reversible disease if diagnosed at an early stage. Because HIVAN is a result of the direct infection of kidney tissue and the gene products of the HIV genome, eradication of active viremia improves kidney function.

cART reverses glomerular and tubular lesions, and patients achieve remission of proteinuria and improved kidney function. This benefit lasts only as long as viremia is controlled, and relapses with the discontinuation of cART and a resurgence of viremia.

Although HIVICK lesions also result from active HIV infection, they do not appear equally responsive to cART therapy. HIVICK-mediated immune complex injury more commonly causes permanent kidney damage, and, unlike HIVAN, complete histologic reversal is not seen.

In addition to cART, short-term steroid therapy may have a role in patients with significant interstitial infiltrates on biopsy. Steroids do not affect the collapsing glomerular lesion of FSGS, but they do reduce the inflammatory cytokine production in the interstitium, and can improve kidney function while cART is initiated. Steroids have not been shown to be effective in HIVICK, most likely because of the lack of a significant component of interstitial nephritis in these patients.

Adjunctive therapy for nephrotic syndrome with inhibitors of the renin-angiotensin system—angiotensin-converting enzyme inhibitors and angiotensin receptor blockers—are effective in reducing proteinuria and delaying the progression of kidney disease in HIVAN. These agents can be used at the time of diagnosis but are not considered to be first-line therapy. The most important initial treatment for HIVAN and HIVICK is cART.

17. **If treatment fails, can a patient with HIV undergo long-term dialysis?**
Currently <1.6% of the U.S. end-stage kidney disease (ESKD) population has HIV as a cause of ESRD, and their survival is similar to those patients without HIV if they are receiving cART. Both types of dialysis modalities, hemodialysis, or peritoneal dialysis, are equally effective options for patients with HIV.

18. **Can a patient with HIV be considered for kidney transplantation?**
The National Institutes of Health have sponsored a multicenter trial to evaluate the efficacy of transplantation in patients with HIV. The prerequisite for transplantation includes the use of cART therapy with a CD4 count >200 and an undetectable viral load. There is experience with the use of both liver and kidney transplants in patients with HIV. The data show acceptable graft and patient survival with a higher risk of rejection, making transplantation a viable option in select patients with HIV. The pharmacologic interaction of cART and immunosuppressive therapy is challenging (as discussed previously) because of the effect of PIs on inhibiting the hepatic P450 enzyme system, thereby reducing the clearance of CNI and the risk of NRTIs, especially tenofovir, on potentiating calcineurin nephrotoxicity. More recent studies have advocated for the use of HIV-positive donors for HIV-positive recipients—a concept that would significantly increase the donor pool for these patients.

KEY POINTS

1. HIVAN results from direct HIV infection of podocytes and tubular cells.
2. HIVICK results from the development of peripheral immune complexes containing HIV antigens that deposit in the glomerulus.
3. Patients with HIV are frequently co-infected with HCV and/or HBV and may develop glomerulonephritis from these infections.
4. Patients with HIVAN are unexpectedly normotensive, often demonstrating large echogenic kidneys on ultrasound.
5. In cART, proteosome inhibitors cause ATN by stone formation and intratubular precipitation and by interstitial nephritis, and directly inhibit the P450 system in the liver.
6. In cART, NRTIs, like tenofovir, cause Fanconi's syndrome and ATN through proximal tubular injury.
7. In cART, integrase strand inhibitors reduce the secretion of creatinine leading to a false diagnosis of AKI.
8. Dialysis and transplantation are viable options for patients with cART controlled HIV.
9. AKI is extremely common in patients with HIV because of cART.
10. Guidelines require all patients with HIV to be regularly screened for kidney disease with a GFR and urinalysis for proteinuria.

BIBLIOGRAPHY

AIDS Working Group (GESIDA) of the Spanish Society of Infectious Diseases and Clinical Microbiology (SEIMC), Spanish Society of Nephrology (S.E.N.), Spanish Society of Clinical Chemistry and Molecular Pathology (SEQC), Górriz, J. L., Gutiérrez, F., Trullas, J. C., Arazo, P., … Miró, J. M. (2014). Consensus document on the management of renal disease in HIV-infected patients. *Nefrologia, 34*(Suppl. 2), 1–81.
Chen, T. K., Estrella, M. M., & Parekh, R. S. (2016). The evolving science of apolipoprotein-L1 and kidney disease. *Current Opinion in Nephrology and Hypertension, 25*(3), 217–225.
Fogo, A. B., Lusco, M. A., Najafian, B., & Alpers, C. E. (2016). AJKD atlas of renal pathology: HIV-associated immune complex kidney disease (HIVICK). *American Journal of Kidney Diseases, 68*(2), e9–e10.
Kumar, N., & Perazella, M. A. (2014). Differentiating HIV-associated nephropathy from antiretroviral drug-induced nephropathy: A clinical challenge. *Current HIV/AIDS Reports, 11*(3), 202–211.
Locke, J. E., Mehta, S., Reed, R. D., MacLennan, P., Massie, A., Nellore, A., … Segev, D. L. (2015). A national study of outcomes among HIV-infected kidney transplant recipients. *Journals of the American Society of Nephrology, 26*(9), 2222–2229.
Milburn, J., Jones, R., & Levy, J. B. (2017). Renal effects of novel antiretroviral drugs. *Nephrology, Dialysis, Transplantation, 32*(2), 434–439.
Muller, E., Barday, Z., Mendelson, M., & Kahn, D. (2015). HIV-positive-to-HIV-positive kidney transplantation—results at 3 to 5 years. *New England Journal of Medicine, 372*(7), 613–620.
Nobakht, E., Cohen, S. D., Rosenberg, A. Z., & Kimmel, P. L. (2016). HIV-associated immune complex kidney disease. *Nature Reviews Nephrology, 12*(5), 291–300.
Wearne, N., & Okpechi, I. G. (2016). HIV-associated renal disease—an overview. *Clinical Nephrology, 86*(13), 41–47.
Yombi, J. C., Pozniak, A., Boffito, M., Jones, R., Khoo, S., Levy, J., & Post, F. A. (2014). Antiretrovirals and the kidney in current clinical practice: Renal pharmacokinetics, alterations of renal function and renal toxicity. *AIDS, 28*(5), 621–632.

VII

ONCONEPHROLOGY

CHAPTER 37

ONCONEPHROLOGY

Rimda Wanchoo and Kenar D. Jhaveri

1. **What is Onconephrology?**
   Onconephrology focuses on all aspects of kidney disease in patients with malignancy, as well as areas where nephrology intersects with hematology. As the name implies, nephrologists and oncologists are well positioned to collaborate on this area of medicine.

2. **What does this field of nephrology include?**
   1. Electrolyte disorders of malignancy
   2. Secondary glomerular diseases of malignancy
   3. Chemotherapy-related kidney complications
   4. Targeted therapies and the kidney
   5. Paraproteinemia (see Chapter 39)
   6. Thrombotic microangiopathy (TMA) and all its causes and treatment strategie (see Chapter 41)
   7. Bone marrow transplant–related kidney diseases
   8. Radiation nephropathy
   9. Tumor lysis syndrome (TLS (see Chapter 38)
   10. Acute kidney injury (AKI) in the hospitalized patient with malignancy
   11. The ethics of dialysis during end of life in malignanc (see Chapter 80)
   12. Dosing of chemotherapy in chronic kidney disease (CKD) and end-stage kidney disease ESKD)
   13. Malignancy-associated obstructive kidney disease
   14. Renal cell carcinoma and related complications post-nephrectom (see Chapter 40)

3. **What are the major causes of AKI in the patients with malignancy?**
   AKI may occur by at least two mechanisms:
   1. A complication of a particular cancer treatment:
      a. TLS
      b. Drug-induced nephropathy
      c. Post-transplant-related kidney diseases
      d. Surgical procedures
   2. Related to the neoplasm itself
      a. Renal cell cancer
      b. Anatomic obstruction due to a metastatic lesion or obstructing mass
      c. Myeloma/amyloid affecting the kidney
      Patients with AKI and malignancy have a worse prognosis than AKI without malignancy.

4. **How common is AKI in the patients with malignancy?**
   The answer depends on the sub-population of patients with a particular malignancy, as well as the clinical setting, for example, intensive care unit (ICU) versus general inpatient service versus outpatient. Four main points may be deduced from major studies:
   1. The incidence of AKI among hospitalized patients with malignancy is higher than that of patients without cancer
   2. Acutely ill patients with cancer admitted to the ICU have an even higher risk of AKI
   3. Some cancers are associated with a higher risk of AKI than others:
      a. Kidney
      b. Gall bladder
      c. Liver
      d. Myeloma
      e. Pancreas
   4. Treatment with a hematopoetic stem cell transplant (HSCT), especially myeloablative allogenic HSCT, further raises the risk of AKI associated with malignancies

5. **What are the common causes of AKI in the cancer patient?**
   Table 37.1 summarizes the pre-renal, intrinsic, and post-renal causes of AKI in the cancer patient.

6. **What is lymphomatous kidney infiltration (LKI)?**
   LKI is common, albeit underdiagnosed, among patients with cancer. In most studies, LKI was found to have a high incidence. While the incidence is high, the association with kidney failure is low. The mechanism of LKI-induced AKI is not completely established. The tubules and glomeruli usually appear morphologically normal on biopsy; it has been proposed that interstitial and intraglomerular pressure elevation due to lymphocytic infiltrations of these compartments is the underlying mechanism of the AKI. Diagnosis can be made via a kidney ultrasound and computed tomography scan imaging in some cases, but a kidney biopsy is required for a definite diagnosis. The management of LKI is focused on the treatment of the underlying malignancy.

7. **What is the most common kidney-related oncologic emergency?**
   TLS is the most common oncologic emergency with an incidence as high as 26% in high-grade B-cell acute lymphoblastic leukemia. TLS results from rapid release of intracellular contents of dying cancer cells into the bloodstream, either spontaneously or in response to cancer therapy. It is biochemically characterized by hyperuricemia, hyperkalemia, hyperphosphatemia, and hypocalcemia. Cardiac arrhythmias, seizures, and superimposed AKI are common clinical presentations. The pathophysiology of TLS-mediated AKI involves intratubular obstruction and inflammation by the precipitation of crystals of uric acid, calcium phosphate, and/or xanthine. Consensus recommendations for TLS prophylaxis include volume expansion for all risk groups, the use of allopurinol in medium- and high-risk groups, and the use of recombinant urate oxidase (rasburicase) in high-risk groups. See Chapter 13.

8. **What are the risk factors for chemotherapy-induced AKI?**
   Patient risk factors for chemotherapy-induced nephrotoxicity include: older age, underlying AKI or CKD, and pharmacogenetics favoring drug toxicity. Volume depletion can enhance innate drug toxicity due to increased drug or metabolite concentration in the kidney and may involve formation of intra-tubular crystals by insoluble drug or metabolites. Kidney hypoperfusion can be due to decreased oral intake, over-diuresis, chemotherapy-induced cardiomyopathy, malignant ascites, or pleural effusion. Tumor-related factors predisposing to chemotherapy-induced nephrotoxicity include the presence of toxic tumor proteins, as with myeloma-related kidney injury, kidney infiltration by lymphoma, and cancer-associated glomerulopathies.

9. **What is the connection between cancer and CKD?**
   CKD and cancer are connected in several ways. Cancer can lead not only to the development of CKD and ESRD—often indirectly, from multiple causes (chemotherapy, HSCT)—but also to the presence of CKD can be associated with cancer. Although the overall incidence and prevalence of CKD among patients with cancer is still uncertain, there is growing evidence to suggest that the risk is high and

Table 37.1. Pre-renal, Intrinsic and Post-renal Causes of Acute Kidney Injury in the Cancer Patient

PRE-RENAL	INTRINSIC	POST-RENAL
Kidney hypo-perfusion due to sepsis, ascites, and effusions	Acute tubular necrosis due to	Obstruction due to
Volume depletion ($\downarrow$ oral intake, diarrhea, over-diuresis)	• Protracted ischemia	• Primary or metastatic abdominal or pelvic malignancy
Impaired cardiac output	• Nephrotoxic agents: for example, IV contrast,	• Retroperitoneal fibrosis
Hepatic sinusoid obstructive syndrome	• Ifosfamide, cisplatin, amino-glycoside	• Crystals (Acyclovir, urate, methotrexate)
Hypercalcemia	Lymphomatous infiltration of the kidney	
Non-chemotherapeutic drugs (NSAIDS, ACEi/ARB, calcineurin inhibitors)	Acute interstitial nephritis	
	Tumor lysis syndrome	
Capillary leak syndrome (e.g., due to IL2, CAR-T therapy)	Cast nephropathy	
	Thrombotic microangiopathy	
	Calcineurin inhibitor toxicity	

ACEi, Angiotensin converting enzyme inhibitor; ARB, angiotensin receptor blocker; CAR-T, chimeric antigen receptor–T-cell therapy; IL, interleukin; IV, intravenous; NSAIDS, non-steroidal anti-inflammatory drugs.

still increasing. The risk for developing CKD varies depending on whether the cancer is solid or hematologic in nature, whether the patient underwent nephrectomy or HSCT, or whether nephrotoxic chemotherapy was administered.

10. **Which cancers are common as the glomerular filtration rate declines?**
Men with CKD are more at risk for lung and urinary tract cancers. In one analysis, the estimated glomerular filtration rate (eGFR) <60 mL/min per 1.73 m^2 appears to be a significant risk factor for death from cancer. The excess cancer mortality in those with reduced kidney function varied with site, with the greatest risk in those with breast and urinary tract cancer. Each decrease in eGFR by 10 mL/min per 1.73 m^2 increased the risk of cancer by 29% in men. Lung and urinary tract cancers comprised most of the excess cancer risk. No increased cancer risk in women with CKD was seen in the same study.

11. **What is the most common paraneoplastic glomerular disease seen with solid tumors and hematologic malignances?**
Membranous nephropathy (MN) remains the most common glomerular pathology reported in patients with solid tumors. The true prevalence of malignancy with MN is unknown. Minimal change disease (MCD) is the most common glomerular disease associated with hematologic malignancies. Table 37.2 summarizes the published list of paraneoplastic glomerular diseases seen with various types of cancer.

12. **How do you differentiate primary MN from cancer-associated secondary MN?**
It has been recently identified that the circulating auto-antibody to podocyte transmembrane glycoprotein M-type phospholipase A_2 receptor (PLA$_2$R) is the cause of adult primary MN in majority of the cases (see Chapter 28). These autoantibodies were not found in cases of secondary MN. Table 37.3 helps summarize the potential ways one can differentiate primary MN from secondary MN associated with cancer.
Thrombospondin type 1 domain containing 7A (THSD7A) is a target antigen in membranous glomerulonephritis associated with cancer. THSD7A was found in 2.6% of 1200 patients with MN. These patients were mostly women. In this cohort, the percentage of patients with THSD7A-associated MN and malignant disease significantly exceeded that of patients with PLA2R-associated MN and malignant disease. In all cohorts, they identified 40 patients with THSD7A-associated MN, 8 of whom developed a malignancy within a median time of 3 months from the diagnosis of MN. In one patient with THSD7A-associated MN and metastases of an endometrial carcinoma, the immunohistochemistry showed THSD7A expression on the metastatic cells and within follicular dendritic cells of the metastasis-infiltrated lymph node. Patients with THSD7A-associated MN should get more intensive screening for the presence of malignancies.

13. **What types of adverse kidney events are associated with traditional chemotherapy agents?**
Chemotherapeutic agents can cause kidney disease that fits the traditional grouping into pre-renal, intrarenal, and post-renal states. However, most of these agents cause intrinsic kidney injury at various parts of the nephron (Table 37.4), with a couple of notable exceptions. For example, interleukin-2 (IL-2) is associated with capillary leak syndrome, which can cause intravascular volume depletion and prerenal azotemia. Post-renal injury is rare with chemotherapy agents, but case reports have linked cyclophosphamide with bladder outlet obstruction from vesicular thrombi in the setting of hemorrhagic cystitis. Intrinsic causes can be tubular, interstitial toxicities, but TMA and glomerular diseases have been reported as well.

14. **What are the commonly reported kidney toxicities associated with targeted therapies?**
In the past decade, advances in cell biology have led to the development of anti-cancer agents that target specific molecular pathways. The National Cancer Institute defines targeted therapies as "drugs or substances that block the growth and spread of cancer by interfering with specific molecules involved in tumor growth and progression." Targeted therapies are now commonly used in cancer treatment, and it is vital that their kidney toxicities be recognized and investigated. Kidney adverse effects of targeted therapies occur through several complex mechanisms. Early reports suggested that targeted therapies were associated with a range of toxicities from hypertension to AKI. Table 37.5 and Fig. 37.1 summarize the kidney effects of targeted therapies.

15. **Where is vascular endothelial growth factor (VEGF) located in the kidney? What are the kidney manifestations of anti-angiogenic therapy?**
VEGF is produced by the glomerular podocytes and tubular epithelial cells in the kidney and bind to the VEGF receptors (a tyrosine kinase receptor) located in the mesangium, glomerular, and peritubular capillaries. VEGF is involved in proliferation, differentiation, and survival of mesangial and endothelial

Table 37.2. Glomerular Diseases Associated With Solid Tumors and Hematologic Malignancies

TYPE OF CANCER	ASSOCIATED PARANEOPLASTIC GLOMERULAR DISEASE
Lung cancer (includes small cell, non-small-cell, squamous cell, and bronchogenic cancers)	MN, MCD, MPGN, IgAN, FSGS, CGN, HSP, TMA
Renal cell cancer	AAA, CGN, IgAN, MCD, FSGS, MPGN, HSP
Colon cancer	MN, MCD, CGN
Gastric cancer	MN, MPGN, CGN, HSP, TMA
Prostate cancer	MN, CGN, HSP
Pancreatic cancer	MN, MCD, IgAN
Breast cancer	MN, FSGS, MPGN, HSP, TMA
Esophageal cancer	MPGN, FSGS
Head and neck cancer	MN, IgAN
Ovarian cancer	MN, MCD
Cervical cancer	MN
Endometrial cancer	MN
Melanoma	MN, MPGN, MN
Hodgkin's lymphoma	MCD, MN, MPGN, IgAN, FSGS, CGN, AAA, Anti-GBM disease, HSP
Non-Hodgkin's lymphoma	MN, MCD, MPGN, IgAN, FSGS, HSP
Chronic lymphocytic leukemia	MPGN, MN, MCD, FSGS, CGN
Acute myelogenous leukemia	MN, FSGS
Chronic myelogenous leukemia	FSGS, MN, MCD, MPGN
MGUS	MPGN, TMA, C3GN
T-cell leukemia	FSGS

AAA, AA amyloidosis; *C3GN*, complete C3 glomerulonephritis; *CGN*, crescentic glomerulonephritis; *FSGS*, focal segmental glomerulosclerosis; *GBM*, glomerular basement membrane; *HSP*, Henoch–Schonlein purpura; *IgAN*, immunoglobulin A nephropathy; *MCD*, minimal change disease; *MGUS*, monoclonal gammopathy of unclear significance; *MN*, membranous nephropathy; *MPGN*, membranoproliferative glomerulonephritis; *TMA*, thrombotic microangiopathy.
Modified from Jhaveri, K. D., Shah, H. H., Calderon, K., Campenot, E. S., & Radhakrishnan, J. (2013). Glomerular diseases seen with cancer and chemotherapy: A narrative review. *Kidney International, 84*(1), 34–44.

cells, and plays a vital role in the maintenance of the structure and function of the glomerular filtration barrier.

Anti-VEGF therapy comprises of drugs such a bevacizumab, which is a recombinant humanized monoclonal antibody to VEGF. Highly vascular tumors with VEGF expression and a high density of VEGF receptors (VEGFR) respond to anti-VEGF therapy (Fig. 37.2). Tyrosine kinase inhibitors of VEGFR, such as sorafenib, sunitinib, and axitinib, have anti-VEGF properties by inhibiting downstream signaling once VEGF binds to its receptors. In women with pregnancies complicated by pre-eclampsia, high levels of soluble VEGFR-1 are seen, which decreases the VEGF level and, in turn, generates the proteinuria and hypertension. Tyrosine kinase inhibitors (sunitinib, sorafenib) used in renal cell cancer, and other solid and liquid tumors, also have anti-VEGF effects and have similar kidney complications.

VEGF antagonism leads to hypertension, proteinuria, TMA, and interstitial nephritis. TMA related to anti-VEGF therapy can present with both kidney limited or systemic findings including thrombocytopenia and presence of microangiopathic hemolytic anemia. The kidney limited TMA findings are more common with anti-VEGF agents compared to other drug induced TMA. For example,

Table 37.3. Clinical Pathologic Features Differentiating Primary from Malignancies Associated Membranous Nephropathy

CLINICOPATHOLOGIC PARAMETERS	PRIMARY MN	SOLID TUMOR ASSOCIATED MN
Historical clues	Younger age, no history of smoking	Age over 65 years, smoking for more than 20 pack years
Serological testing	Presence of circulating anti-PLA2R autoantibodies in serum	Absence of circulating anti-PLA2R autoantibodies in serum
Pathological findings	Predominance of glomerular IgG4 deposition, enhanced glomerular PLA2R staining, presence of less than 8 inflammatory cells per glomeruli	Predominance of IgG1,2 deposition, normal glomerular PLA2R staining, presence of more than 8 inflammatory cells per glomeruli

IgG, Immunoglobulin G; MN, membranous nephropathy; PLA2R, phospholipase A2 receptor.

TMA from gemcitabine or mitomycin is more aggressive, with more severe hematological abnormalities, both glomerular and arteriolar kidney localizations, and worse kidney survival—even after stopping the offending agent.

16. **What is the management of patients who develop kidney complications with anti-angiogenic therapy?**
It is important to monitor blood pressure and proteinuria in these patients. Angiotensin converting enzyme inhibitor (ACEi) or angiotensin receptor blocker is usually the first-line treatment of hypertension in these patients. The non-dihydropyridine calcium channel blockers (verapamil, diltiazem) interact with the cytochrome P450 pathway and can increase tyrosine kinase inhibitor levels. The drugs can continue unless the patient develops nephrotic syndrome, AKI, or TMA.

17. **What is the most common adverse kidney effect seen with immune checkpoint inhibitors?**
Immune checkpoint inhibitors include the anti-cytotoxic T-lymphocyte-associated protein 4 (CTLA-4) antibody as well as anti-programmed death antibodies (programmed cell death [PD]-1). These antibodies serve to enhance the innate anti-tumor T-cell immunity leading to tumor regression and the stabilization of solid tumors. Immune checkpoint inhibitor kidney toxicity is an immune-mediated process. Acute interstitial nephritis (AIN) is the most common biopsy finding reported with PD-1 inhibitors. Ipilimumab, a CTLA4 inhibitor, is also associated with AIN; however, podocytopathies, such as MN, MCD, and TMA, have also been reported. Hyponatremia related to hypophysitis (inflammation of the pituitary gland) is also seen with CTLA4 antagonists. The time of onset usually differs in the two drugs. CTLA4-antagonist-mediated injury usually occurs earlier within the first 2 to 3 months of use, while PD-1-inhibitor-mediated injury is usually seen later, 2 to 10 months into treatment. Treatment usually involves the interruption of therapy and the use of high-dose steroids.

18. **What are the most common electrolyte abnormalities seen in patients with cancer?**
Electrolyte disorders in patients with cancer are common. They could be as a result of the cancer, chemotherapeutic agent, or patient-related factors. Hyponatremia and hypercalcemia are the most common electrolyte abnormalities noted, although others, such as hypernatremia, hypomagnesemia, hypophosphatemia, hyperphosphatemia, hyperkalemia, and hypokalemia, are also seen.

19. **What is the mechanism of hypercalcemia in malignancy?**
Hypercalcemia of malignancy is caused by two mechanisms:
1. Osteolytic release of calcium from bone due to direct invasion of the neoplasm, as seen in skeletal metastasis of solid tumors of breast, lung, kidneys, and multiple myeloma. The release of calcium from the bone is mediated by the receptor activator of nuclear factor kappa B (RANK) and receptor activator of nuclear factor kappa B ligand (RANK-L) interaction. The RANK-L is produced by the bone marrow stromal cells and osteoblasts. The binding of RANK present on osteoclast progenitor cells to its ligand results in osteoclast activation, proliferation, and bone resorption, resulting in the release of calcium. The neoplastic environment with activated T cells, inflammatory cytokines (IL-6, IL-1B0, tumor necrosis factor-alpha) all promote the RANK-L-driven bone resorption and disturb the RANK/RANK-L/osteoprotegerin balance.

Table 37.4. Chemotherapeutic Agents Associated With Acute Kidney Injury and Other Forms of Kidney Injuries.

CHEMOTHERA-PEUTIC AGENT	MECHANISM OF INJURY	CLINICAL PRESENTATION	PROPHYLAXIS
Azacytidine	Proximal and distal tubular injury	Fanconi syndrome, and polyuria	None established. Self-limiting
Bisphosphonate (Pamidronate, Zoledronate)	Acute tubular injury, collapsing FOGG, MOD	AKI	Avoid use of zoledronate in patients with CrCl <35 mL/min. In those patients, reduced doses of pamidronate
Cisplatin	Toxic damage to renal tubule	AKI, magnesium wasting, diabetes insipidus, Fanconi syndrome	Volume expansion, magnesium replacement
Clofarabine	ATN, FSGS	Sudden onset AKI	None established
Cyclophosphamide	Increased ADH activity	Hyponatremia	None established. Self-limiting after discontinuation of drug
Gemcitabine (cell cycle-specific pyramidine antagonist)	TMA	HTN, TMA, proteinuria, and AKI ± Edema	None established
Ifosfamide	Proximal ± distal tubular injury	ATN (often subclinical); Type 2 RTA with Fanconi syndrome; severe electrolyte disarray; nephrogenic diabetes insipidus.	Moderate-severe nephrotoxicity generally occur with cumulative doses >100 g/m² Avoid concurrent use of cisplatin
Interferon (alpha, beta, or gamma)	Podocyte injury resulting in MCD or FSGS	Nephrotic syndrome, AKI	None established
Interleukin-2	Kidney hypoperfusion due to capillary leak, kidney vasoconstriction	AKI, Hypotension, proteinuria, pyuria	None established
Methotrexate	Nonoliguric AKI	Tubular obstruction by precipitation of methotrexate and 7-hydroxymethotrexate	Volume expansion; urinary alkalization; leucovorin rescue; dose reduction for GFR 10–50 mL/min
Mitomycin C	AKI	TTP and HUS (associated with cumulative dose >60 mg)	None established
Nitrosoureas	Glomerular sclerosis and tubulointerstitial nephritis	Insidious, often irreversible kidney injury	Volume expansion

ADH, Antidiuretic hormone; AKI, acute kidney injury; ATN, acute tubular necrosis; CrCl, Creatinine Clearance; FSGS, focal segmental glomerulosclerosis; GFR, glomerular filtration rate; HTN, hypertension; HUS, hemolytic uremic syndrome; MCD, minimal change diseases; RTA, renal tubular acidosis; TMA, thrombotic microangiopathy; TTP, thrombotic thrombocytopenic purpura.

Table 37.5. Kidney Known Side Effects of Various Targeted Therapies

NAME OF AGENT	MECHANISM OF ACTION OF THE TARGETED THERAPY	REPORTED NEPHROTOXICITIES
Bevacizumab	VEGF inhibitor	HTN, proteinuria, nephrotic syndrome, pre-eclampsia like syndrome, kidney limited TMA
Aflibercept	VEGF inhibitor	HTN, proteinuria
Sunitinib	Multi-kinase TKI	HTN, proteinuria, MCD/FSGS, AIN, Chronic interstitial nephritis
Pazopanib	Multi-kinase TKI	HTN, proteinuria
Axitinib	Multi-kinase TKI	HTN, proteinuria
Sorafenib	Multi-kinase TKI	HTN, proteinuria, MCD/FSGS, AIN, chronic interstitial nephritis, hypophosphatemia
Imatinib	Cellular TKI(BCR-ABL)	ATN, HTN, hypocalcemia, hypophosphatemia
Dasatinib	Multi-kinase TKI	Proteinuria
Nilotinib	Multi-kinase TKI	HTN
Ponatinib	Multi-kinase TKI	HTN
Cetuximab	EGFR inhibitor	Hypomagnesaemia, Hypokalemia, AKI, Hyponatremia, glomerulonephritis
Panitumumab	EGFR inhibitor	Hypomagnesaemia, AKI, Hypokalemia
Erlotinib	EGFR inhibitor	AKI, Hypomagnesaemia
Afatinib	EGFR inhibitor	AKI, Hyponatremia
Gefitinib	EGFR inhibitor	AKI, hypokalemia, fluid retention, minimal change disease, proteinuria
Vemurafenib	B-RAF inhibitor	AIN, ATN, hypophosphatemia, Fanconi syndrome
Dabrafenib	B-RAF Inhibitor	AIN, ATN, hypophosphatemia
Crizotinib	ALK Inhibitor	ATN, kidney cysts
Ipilumumab	CTLA-4 inhibitor	AIN, MN, MCD, hyponatremia, TMA
Nivolumab	PD-1 Inhibitor	AIN
Pembrolizumab	PD-1 Inhibitor	AIN
Temsirolimus	mTOR inhibitor	ATN, FSGS
Carfilzomib	Proteasome inhibitor	Prerenal, ATN, TMA
Bortezomib	Proteasome inhibitor	TMA
Lenalidomide	Immunomodulators	Fanconi syndrome, AIN, MCD
Trametinib	MEK inhibitor	AKI

AIN, Acute interstitial nephritis; *AKI*, acute kidney injury; *ALK*, Anaplastic lymphoma kinase; *ATN*, acute tubular necrosis; *BCR-ABL*, breakpoint cluster region-abelson; *BRAF*, B-Raf proto-oncogene serine/threonine-protein kinase; *CTLA-4*, cytotoxic T lymphocyte antigen-4; *EGFR*, epidermal growth factor receptor; *FSGS*, focal segmental glomerulosclerosis; *HTN*, hypertension; *MCD*, minimal change disease; *MEK*, mitogen-activated protein kinase; *MN*, membranous nephropathy; *mTOR*, mechanistic target of rapamycin (also known as the mammalian target of rapamycin); *PD*, programmed cell death; *TKI*, tyrosine kinase inhibitor; *TMA*, thrombotic microangiopathy; *VEGF*, vascular endothelial growth factor.

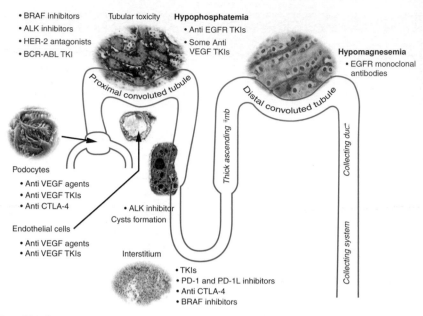

Figure 37.1. Summary of kidney adverse events noted with targeted therapies. *ALK*, Anaplastic lymphoma kinase; *BCR-ABL*, breakpoint cluster region-abelson; *CTLA*, cytotoxic T lymphocyte antigen-4; *EGFR*, epidermal growth factor receptor; *HER-2*, human epidermal growth factor-2; *PD*, programmed cell death; *TKI*, tyrosine kinase inhibitors; *VEGF*, vascular endothelial growth factor. (Modified from Jhaveri, K. D., Wanchoo, R., Sakhiya, V., Ross, D., & Fishbane, S. (2016). Adverse renal effects of novel molecular oncologic targeted therapies: A narrative review. *Kidney International Reports.* doi: http://dx.doi.org/10.1016/j.ekir.2016.09.055, with permission.)

2. Stimulation of osteoclast activity by the release of tumor-derived endocrine factors. In this PTHrP and 1,25-dihydroxyvitamin D play an important role. PTHrP is secreted by squamous cell cancer of the lung, head and neck, renal cell, ovarian, breast, and esophageal cancer. It causes stimulation of the osteoclasts, increases calcium absorption in the loop of Henle and the distal convoluted tubule. Activated vitamin D, in turn, is secreted by lymphomas, or tumor-associated macrophages that possess 1-alpha hydroxylase activity.

20. What is the treatment of hypercalcemia of malignancy?
    The primary goal in the management of hypercalcemia is to enhance the urinary excretion of calcium and to decrease the osteoclast-mediated bone resorption. The first goal is achieved by aggressive volume repletion with a goal urine output of 100 to 150 mL/hour. Furosemide should only be used once the patient is made adequately volume replete. Calcitonin inhibits bone resorption and osteoclast maturation and acts quickly within 4 to 6 hours of administration. Tachyphylaxis prevents its long-term use. In volume overloaded or anuric patients, dialysis with a low dialysate calcium may be needed.
    Bisphosphonates, namely zoledronate and pamidronate, have become the cornerstone of treatment of hypercalcemia of malignancy. Bisphosphonates reduce the osteoclast activity by preventing the osteoclasts from adhering to the bone surface, and preventing the production of their proteins, which are responsible for continued bone resorption. They also result in decreased osteoclast progenitor development and promote their apoptosis. RANKL inhibitors, such as denosumab, play a role in the management of bisphosphonate-resistant hypercalcemia of malignancy even though it does not yet have U.S. Food and Drug Administration approval.

21. What is the most common cause of hyponatremia in cancer patients? What are the other causes?
    The syndrome of inappropriate anti-diuretic hormone (SIADH) is the most common cause of hyponatremia in cancer patients, with higher rates among patients with small-cell lung cancer and head and neck cancers compared to others. The other potential causes of SAIDH are the release of

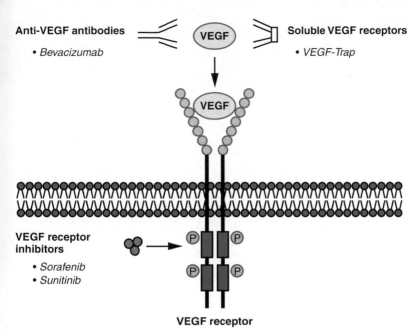

Anti-VEGF antibodies

• *Bevacizumab*

VEGF

Soluble VEGF receptors

• *VEGF-Trap*

VEGF

VEGF receptor inhibitors

• *Sorafenib*
• *Sunitinib*

VEGF receptor

Figure 37.2. Vascular endothelial growth factor (VEGF), the VEGF receptor, and the various mechanisms by which therapies block VEGF effect are demonstrated. Included are an antibody against the VEGF molecule (bevacizumab), soluble receptors that bind VEGF and remove it from the circulation (VEGF-trap), and VEGF receptor inhibitors (sorafenib, sunitinib). (Reproduced with permission from Gurevich, F., & Perazella, M. A. (2009). Kidney effects of anti-angiogenesis therapy: Update for the internist. *American Journal of Medicine, 122*(4), 322–328.)

the anti-diuretic hormone, which is not mediated by an osmotic or volume stimulus, and includes pain, nausea, and medications (cisplatin, cyclophosphamide, vinblastine, and vincristine).

22. Which chemotherapeutic agent/disease state is responsible for salt wasting?
Cisplatin and ifosfamide directly injure the kidney tubular cells and impair the kidney sodium absorption and cause renal salt wasting. Cerebral salt wasting has been described in metastatic central nervous system disease. In hyponatremia from SIADH and salt wasting, urine sodium and urine osmolality are elevated; however, these patients are volume depleted on exam as opposed to SIADH where patients tend to be euvolemic.

KEY POINTS

1. Onconephrology is an evolving subspecialty that focuses on all aspects of kidney disease in cancer patients.
2. AKI in patients with cancer may occur by at least two mechanisms:
   a. It could arise as a complication of a particular cancer treatment:
      i. Tumor lysis syndrome
      ii. Drug-induced nephropathy
      iii. Post-transplant related kidney diseases
      iv. Surgical procedures
   b. Or it could be related to the neoplasm itself:
      i. Renal cell cancer
      ii. Anatomic obstruction due to a metastatic lesion or obstructing mass
      iii. Myeloma/amyloid affecting the kidney
3. TLS is the most common renal oncologic emergency with an incidence as high as 26% in high-grade B-cell acute lymphoblastic leukemia.
4. Novel targeted therapies, such as immune checkpoint inhibitors, can lead to immune-mediated acute interstitial nephritis.

BIBLIOGRAPHY

Flombaum, C. D. (2000). Metabolic emergencies in the cancer patient. *Seminars in Oncology, 27*(3), 322–334.

Gurevich, F., & Perazella, M. A. (2009). Renal effects of anti-angiogenesis therapy: Update for the internist. *American Journal of Medicine, 122*(4), 322–328.

Jhaveri, K. D., Shah, H. H., Calderon, K., Campenot, E. S., & Radhakrishnan, J. (2013). Glomerular diseases seen with cancer and chemotherapy: A narrative review. *Kidney International, 84*(1), 34–44.

Jhaveri, K. D., Wanchoo, R., Sakhiya, V., Ross, D., & Fishbane, S. (2016). Adverse renal effects of novel molecular oncologic targeted therapies: A narrative review. *Kidney International Reports, 2*(1), 108–123. doi:http://dx.doi.org/10.1016/j.ekir.2016.09.055.

Lam, A. Q., & Humphreys, B. D. (2012). Onco-nephrology: AKI in the cancer patient. *Clinical Journal of the American Society of Nephrology, 7*(10), 1692–1700.

Perazella, M. A. (2012). Onco-nephrology: Renal toxicities of chemotherapeutic agents. *Clinical Journal of the American Society of Nephrology, 7*(10), 1713–1721.

Rosner, M. H., & Dalkin, A. C. (2015). Onconephrology. The pathophysiology and treatment of malignancy associated hypercalcemia. *Clinical Journal of the American Society of Nephrology, 7,* 1722–1729.

Salahudeen, A. K., Doshi, S. M., Pawar, T., Nowshad, G., Lahoti, A., & Shah, P. (2013). Incidence rate, clinical correlates, and outcomes of AKI in patients admitted to a comprehensive cancer center. *Clinical Journal of the American Society of Nephrology, 8*(3), 347–354.

Wanchoo, R., Karam, S., Uppal, N. N., Barta, V. S., Deray, G., Devoe, C., ... Cancer and Kidney International Network Workgroup on Immune Checkpoint Inhibitors. (2017). Adverse renal effects of immune check point inhibitors: A narrative review. *American Journal of Nephrology, 45*(2), 160–169.

TUMOR LYSIS SYNDROME

Scott D. Bieber and Jonathan Ashley Jefferson

CHAPTER 38

1. **What is tumor lysis syndrome (TLS)?**
   TLS is a condition in which widespread necrosis of tumor cells releases toxic amounts of intracellular contents into the circulation, resulting in acute hyperuricemia, hyperkalemia, hyperphosphatemia, hypocalcemia, and acute kidney injury (AKI).

2. **What causes TLS?**
   TLS is usually caused by chemotherapeutic agents in patients with cancer resulting in rapid cell necrosis. Common agents implicated include cisplatin, etoposide, fludarabine, cytosine arabinoside, methotrexate, paclitaxel, rituximab, and corticosteroids. Radiation therapy may rarely cause TLS. Occasionally spontaneous TLS may arise in rapidly growing tumors that outgrow their blood supply.

3. **What are the risk factors for the development of TLS?**
   TLS typically occurs following the chemotherapeutic treatment of hematologic malignancies, in particular Burkitt lymphoma and acute B-cell lymphoblastic leukemia. TLS has only rarely been described following the treatment of solid organ tumors. Specific risk factors for the development of TLS include:
   Host-related factors
   • Volume depletion
   • Preexisting kidney disease
   Disease-related factors
   • Large tumor burden, "bulky" disease, or extensive bone marrow involvement
   • High tumor proliferation rate
   • Highly chemo- or radiosensitive tumors
   • Lactate dehydrogenase (LDH) levels greater than 1500 IU (or twice the upper limit of normal)
   • Uric acid level greater than 8.0 mg/dL

4. **What laboratory findings are associated with TLS?**
   Laboratory analysis in TLS typically reveals hyperkalemia, hyperphosphatemia, hypocalcemia, hyperuricemia, and elevated LDH levels. In TLS, the uric acid and LDH levels are often quite elevated. Malignant cells can be very metabolically active, with large amounts of adenosine triphosphate, and can contain up to four times the amount of phosphorus found in normal cells. If AKI develops, decreased kidney clearance of phosphorus and potassium can worsen the hyperphosphatemia and hyperkalemia. Hypocalcemia develops in tumor lysis when calcium complexes with phosphorus.
      Hyperuricemia develops in TLS as purine nucleic acids are released from cells that are often rich in nucleic acid material due to their high turnover rates. Purines are sequentially metabolized into hypoxanthine, then xanthine, and finally uric acid (Fig. 38.1). The intracellular enzyme LDH is often increased in TLS. The pretreatment LDH level is a risk factor for developing TLS because it is a marker of increased tumor burden.

5. **What are the findings on urine microscopy in a patient with TLS?**
   Urine sediment examination in a patient with acute TLS may reveal uric acid or calcium phosphate crystals, although the lack of crystalluria does not rule out TLS. When AKI develops, there will typically be evidence of tubular injury, with kidney tubular epithelial cells and granular or muddy-brown casts.

6. **What is the mechanism of uric acid formation?**
   As illustrated in Fig. 38.1, purines from nucleic acids (DNA, RNA) are metabolized to xanthine and hypoxanthine. Xanthine oxidase catalyzes their conversion to uric acid, which is less water soluble, especially in acidic urine. In other species, urate oxidase catalyzes the conversion of uric acid to the much more soluble allantoin, which is readily excreted by the kidneys. In humans and higher primates, a missense mutation in the gene encoding urate oxidase occurred during early hominid evolution, and the nitrogenous waste is excreted as uric acid.

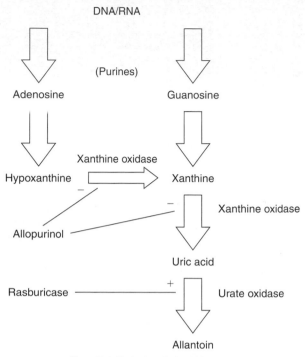

Figure 38.1. Mechanism of uric acid formation.

7. **How does TLS cause AKI?**

The primary mechanism of AKI in TLS is a crystal-induced nephropathy, usually due to uric acid. Glomerular filtration of uric acid followed by fluid reabsorption results in high concentrations within the tubular fluid, leading to the intratubular precipitation of uric acid crystals. Uric acid crystallization is further promoted by volume depletion (nausea and vomiting, diarrhea, poor sodium intake) and low urinary pH (from metabolic acidosis, diuretics, and volume depletion). The intratubular uric acid crystals cause tubular obstruction and may also cause tubular injury by stimulating an inflammatory response. Even if it does not crystalize, soluble uric acid may act as a kidney vasoconstrictor, exacerbating kidney hypoperfusion.

Uric acid is not the only nephrotoxin in TLS. Hyperphosphatemia may lead to the precipitation of calcium phosphate crystals, causing acute phosphate nephropathy. This is especially relevant where alkalinization of the urine is being used to protect against uric acid nephropathy, as alkaline urine promotes the precipitation of calcium phosphate stones.

8. **Can we prevent TLS in patients at high risk?**
   - **Hydration:** The amount of hydration a patient requires is based on a clinical evaluation of volume status and should take into account comorbidities. Vigorous hydration is ideal, but it should be avoided in patients with impaired cardiac function or those with preexisting hypervolemia. In general, patients should receive at least 2 L/m^2 per day beginning 24 hours prior to the administration of chemotherapy, with a goal urine output of greater than 100 mL/h. Increased hydration increases tubular flow, thus enhancing uric acid and phosphate excretion and decreasing intratubular concentrations.
   - **Alkalinization:** Acidic urine promotes the crystallization of uric acid. By contrast, in alkaline environments, uric acid is converted to urate salts, which are more soluble. In theory, the administration of bicarbonate would increase the solubility of uric acid and diminish crystal-induced injury. Maximal uric acid solubility occurs at a urine pH greater than 7.0. However, it should be noted that calcium phosphate crystals precipitate readily in alkaline environments and

that xanthine and hypoxanthine crystals also precipitate at a higher urine pH. Thus the role of alkalinization in TLS is controversial and it is not routinely used.

- **Allopurinol:** Allopurinol and its metabolite oxypurinol are competitive inhibitors of xanthine oxidase. Xanthine oxidase is an enzyme found predominantly in the liver, which converts xanthine and hypoxanthine to uric acid. The blocking of xanthine oxidase decreases the production of uric acid. Allopurinol does not decrease the amount of uric acid already present; it only prevents the generation of additional uric acid and therefore should be started 48 to 72 hours prior to the initiation of chemotherapy.
- **Rasburicase:** This recombinant urate oxidase enzyme converts uric acid to allantoin, replacing the deficient enzyme in humans. Allantoin is 5 to 10 times more soluble than uric acid and is easily excreted by the kidneys. In high-risk patients, the drug should be given at least 4 hours prior to chemotherapy and continued for 3 to 5 days following initiation of chemotherapy. Rasburicase is very expensive; lower-dose and shorter-duration protocols are also used. Rasburicase will lower serum uric acid levels dramatically within 24 hours, and clinical studies have shown it to be effective in the prevention of TLS.

9. **When should a patient get prophylaxis for TLS?**
Clinical judgment should be used to categorize patients as either low or high risk. Risk assessment should take into account the whole patient, keeping in mind the presence or absence of underlying kidney compromise, the type of malignancy, the tumor burden, and the prescribed chemotherapy. In general, patients at high risk have one or more of the risk factors described previously. Patients at low risk should receive intravenous hydration and allopurinol. Patients at high risk for TLS may receive intravenous hydration and rasburicase. Allopurinol and rasburicase are not given together because allopurinol blocks xanthine oxidase, thus decreasing the substrate for rasburicase.

10. **How should the electrolyte abnormalities be managed in TLS?**
Hyperkalemia is a frequent laboratory abnormality in TLS as a consequence of potassium release from lysed tumor cells. If the amount of tumor lysis is massive, hyperkalemia can be life-threatening. Associated oliguria or anuria can worsen the clearance of potassium as urine flow drops off. Hyperkalemia in TLS is managed no differently than hyperkalemia from other causes (see Chapter 77).
   In the absence of symptoms, it is not necessary to treat hypocalcemia in TLS. Worrisome clinical signs of symptomatic hypocalcemia include paresthesias, cramping, tetany, seizures, and a prolonged QT interval on electrocardiography. Symptomatic hypocalcemia is rare in TLS. Electrocardiographic changes such as a prolonged PR interval, widened QRS complex, or peaked T waves in the setting of hyperkalemia would also be an additional indication for calcium therapy. Hyperphosphatemia in TLS may be difficult to manage, as phosphate binders only decrease phosphorus absorption but do not decrease hyperphosphatemia from intracellular release.

11. **Once a patient has developed TLS, is there any therapy available to help protect the kidneys?**
Treatment of the metabolic sequelae of tumor lysis by increasing urinary flow with intravenous hydration and lowering uric acid with rasburicase are the keys to preventing AKI in TLS. Dialysis may be necessary to reverse the metabolic derangements in TLS.

12. **What is the role of renal replacement therapy in the treatment and/or prevention of TLS?**
In general, indications for dialysis in patients with AKI secondary to TLS are similar to indications for dialysis in AKI from other causes. Indications include life-threatening hyperkalemia, volume overload refractory to diuretics, uremic pericarditis, or severe uremic encephalopathy. Dialysis has the added benefit of being able to clear uric acid and phosphorus, which may help prevent further kidney damage. If rasburicase is not available, early hemodialysis for uric acid clearance should be considered and has been shown to increase urine output in oliguric AKI. Clearance rates of uric acid with hemodialysis (70 to 145 mL/min) are much greater than with peritoneal dialysis (6 to 10 mL/min), making it the renal replacement therapy of choice.

KEY POINTS

1. Tumor lysis syndrome typically occurs following chemotherapy in the treatment of acute hematologic malignancies with a large tumor burden.
2. Tumor lysis syndrome can cause profound electrolyte abnormalities (hyperkalemia, hyperphosphatemia, hypocalcemia, and hyperuricemia) as a result of the release of intracellular constituents.
3. Rasburicase, a recombinant uric oxidase, rapidly lowers uric acid levels; although expensive, it is commonly used in the prevention of acute kidney injury associated with tumor lysis syndrome.

BIBLIOGRAPHY

Howard, S. C., Jones, D. P., & Pui, C. H. (2011). The tumor lysis syndrome. *New England Journal of Medicine, 364*(19), 1844–1854.

Howard, S. C., Trifilio, S., Gregory, T. K., Baxter, N., & McBride, A. (2016). Tumor lysis syndrome in the era of novel and targeted agents in patients with hematologic malignancies: A systematic review. *Annals of Hematology, 95*(4), 563–573.

Lopez-Olivo, M. A., Pratt, G., Palla, S. L., & Salahudeen, A. (2013). Rasburicase in tumor lysis syndrome of the adult: A systematic review and meta-analysis. *American Journal of Kidney Diseases, 62*(3), 481–492.

Wilson, F. P., & Berns, J. S. (2012). Onco-nephrology: Tumor lysis syndrome. *Clinical Journal of the American Society of Nephrology, 7*(10), 1730–1739.

CHAPTER 39

DYSPROTEINEMIAS OR LIGHT CHAIN DISEASES

Ashley Bruce Irish and Rajalingam Sinniah

DYSPROTEINEMIAS

1. **What is myeloma?**
   Myeloma is a hematologic malignancy comprising about 1% of all cancers. It consists of an excess of clonally expanded cytogenetically heterogeneous bone marrow-derived plasma cells with two cardinal features: a monoclonal immunoglobulin (the paraprotein or M-protein) and/or associated light chains (LCs; kappa [κ] and lambda [λ]) with bone destruction that usually manifests as osteolytic lesions. All myeloma derives from a preclinical phase known as monoclonal gammopathy of unknown significance (MGUS). Myeloma is diagnosed when there is clonal expansion of bone marrow plasma cells >10% and any one myeloma-defining event using the CRAB criteria:
   - **H**yper**c**alcemia
   - **R**enal insufficiency
   - **A**nemia
   - **B**one lesion

   The most common class of whole immunoglobulin (Ig) is IgG followed by IgA and IgD. In approximately 20% of patients only an associated LC component is detected. It is a disease of the elderly, with the median age of diagnosis being older than 65 years of age. At diagnosis, there is evidence of kidney damage in nearly half of patients and up to 10% will have severe kidney failure requiring urgent dialysis. Kidney failure is most common in patients with IgD and LC myeloma.

2. **How does myeloma cause acute kidney injury (AKI)?**
   - Cast nephropathy
   - Hypercalcemia-induced volume depletion
   - Monoclonal immunoglobulin deposition disease (MIDD)
   - Amyloidosis
   - Proximal tubulopathy/Fanconi syndrome
   - Cryoglobulinemia

   The use of kidney biopsy to distinguish between these potential etiologies and to guide therapy is frequently required.

3. **What is cast nephropathy?**
   The most common histologic finding in myeloma is cast nephropathy (MCN), which is characterized by eosinophilic acellular fractured casts, with brittle cracks commonly in the distal tubules and collecting ducts, and—to a lesser extent—in the proximal tubules with epithelial cell necrosis and thinning and dilatation of the lumina. The casts are surrounded by inflammatory cells including macrophages, multinucleated giant cells, and polymorphonuclear neutrophils. There is interstitial edema and inflammation, and in the later stages interstitial fibrosis (Fig. 39.1). The casts usually stain for a monoclonal LC. In some cases, casts are absent but the interstitial inflammation and fibrosis are present.

4. **What can precipitate AKI in myeloma?**
   Patients with myeloma are particularly vulnerable to factors that cause volume depletion or sudden reductions in glomerular filtration. This is because these changes reduce tubular flow and increase the exposure of the tubule to high LC concentrations. Classically, hypercalcemia related to plasma cell-mediated bone destruction and the release of calcium causes volume depletion and vasoconstriction, and is present in around 15% of patients at diagnosis. Non-steroidal agents prescribed for bone pain and intravenous contrast agents used for diagnostic investigations also abruptly reduce glomerular filtration and are associated with AKI, which is sometimes irreversible. Sepsis resulting from chemotherapy and reduced Ig levels may cause AKI.

267

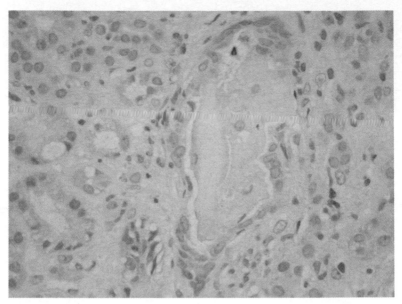

Figure 39.1. Myeloma/light chain cast nephropathy. The tubular cast shows attached giant and inflammatory cells and distension of the lumen. There is interstitial inflammatory cellular infiltration (hematoxylin and eosin ×40).

5. What clinical and laboratory clues suggest myeloma as the cause of AKI?
   The signs/symptoms of AKI due to myeloma are similar to typical AKI with a few additions. They may have malignant bone pain, which is often low back pain resistant to rest or simple analgesics. Myeloma should be suspected when the patient has any severe cytopenia (anemia, thrombocytopenia, or pancytopenia resulting from marrow invasion by plasma cells), relatively preserved albumin-corrected calcium (from bone release of calcium), immunoparesis (when all Ig classes are reduced), or an increased globulin fraction. Urinalysis, although important, may be misleading, because the increased urinary excretion of LCs associated with myeloma is not detected by testing for albumin (e.g., Albustix) but only for total protein (e.g., sulfosalicylic acid test) or by specific urine electrophoresis and immunofixation. The diagnosis of myeloma in AKI is now rapidly and preferentially made by the measurement of the serum free light chain (sFLC) ratio (see Question 12).

6. What specific laboratory diagnostic tests are used for the diagnosis of myeloma?
   Serum protein electrophoresis (SPE) by separation of protein upon an agarose gel can detect the whole Ig in the range of 1 to 5 g/dL, but it only detects increased LC in patients who have very high levels of LC-only myeloma, and it is semi-quantitative. Serum immunofixation electrophoresis (IFE) is around 10 times more sensitive for Igs and LC, but it is not quantitative. Urine IFE requires concentrated urine samples for the detection of FLCs and can detect low levels of LC. The detection of urine LC by the primitive techniques of boiling and precipitation was one of the earliest descriptions of myeloma disease "mollities ossium" and its manifestations published in 1847 by Dr. Henry Bence-Jones. Subsequently Korngold and Lapiri (designated Kappa and Lambda) raised antisera against the two LC domains. Bence-Jones proteins are urinary FLCs detected by urinary protein electrophoresis and immunofixation.

7. Why measure serum FLCs?
   Historically, the biochemical methods to diagnose myeloma, and especially LCs, via protein chemistry have been problematic, slow to perform, and lacked both sensitivity and specificity. In contrast, the measurement of serum FLC by nephelometry is rapid (hours); more sensitive (1 to 3 mg/L); and, along with an SPE (to determine the presence or a whole Ig component), will diagnose the majority of patients with myeloma, amyloidosis, and other MIDD and is now the preferred diagnostic test. An abnormal sFLC ratio (normal κ/λ 0.26 to 1.65) is due to an overproduction of a single κ or λ clone

(with suppression of the other) and this excess is detectable in the serum before urinary tubular catabolism is exceeded and before the SPE or IFE is abnormal. In patients with chronic kidney disease (CKD), significant accumulation of sFLC occurs (approximately fivefold) due to reduced excretion; so the normal range is adjusted to reflect this (κ/λ 0.37–3.17) and reduces the over-diagnosis of monoclonal gammopathy in CKD. In patients with myeloma and severe AKI from MCN the sFLC always exceeds 1000 mg/L and the ratio is always abnormal. The measurement of urine FLC does not improve diagnostic yield, and the measurement of sFLC instead of urine IFE is now incorporated into hematologic guidelines. Serial measurements of FLC also provide real-time and quantitative monitoring of the response to chemotherapy and dialysis because of the short half-life (hours) of the sFLC compared to whole Igs (3 weeks) when measured by SPE.

8. **Why are LCs toxic to the kidney?**
Kidney injury is principally related to the LC component of myeloma because, unlike Igs, LC are freely filtered at the glomerulus and reabsorbed in the proximal tubule. Under normal conditions only small amounts of LC are filtered and reabsorbed, but in myeloma the amount of LC may rise to extreme levels that overwhelm the capacity and function of the proximal tubular cell (and induce proximal tubular injury) and pass to the distal tubule where they interact with uromodulin (Tamm-Horsfall protein) to form insoluble casts that obstruct the tubule, rupture the basement membrane, and induce an inflammatory response.

Recent data suggest that the cysteine residues present at the N and C termini of the FLC-binding domain are linked through an intramolecular disulfide bridge, which places the two histidine residues in close proximity to permit potential ionic interaction with the CDR3 domain of FLC. Capitalizing on this observation, a study analyzed this interaction and showed that the secondary structure and key amino acid residues on the CDR3 of the FLCs were critically important determinants of the molecular interaction with Tamm–Horsfall glycoprotein. These findings permitted the development of a strongly inhibiting cyclized competitor peptide. When used in a rodent model of cast nephropathy, this cyclized peptide construct inhibited cast formation and the associated functional manifestations of AKI in vivo. *However,* not all LC are toxic, and some patients can excrete large quantities without AKI. Specific molecular variants of the LC molecule form specific forms of kidney injury, such as myeloma cast nephropathy or amyloidosis.

9. **What is the value of a bone marrow biopsy in patients with myeloma and AKI?**
Bone marrow biopsy is performed to confirm marrow involvement by clonally expanded plasma cells and for the determination of cytogenetic abnormalities, which provide important prognostic information regarding treatment and outcome. The bone marrow shows displacement of the normal marrow by plasma cells, which ranges from complete replacement by sheets of tumor cells or as nodular aggregates. The mature plasma cells have eccentric nuclei with "clock-face" chromatin and plentiful cytoplasm, and the immature forms are pleomorphic with abnormal nuclear forms. Immunoperoxidase stains show the tumor cells to stain positive with CD138 and a monoclonal LC restriction (Fig. 39.2).

10. **When should I perform a kidney biopsy in patients with myeloma and AKI?**
In patients with biochemically proven myeloma and AKI who do not show a prompt response to hydration and the correction of precipitants, a diagnostic kidney biopsy to determine the cause of kidney injury is suggested because of the variability in kidney etiology and the importance of ensuring a correct histologic diagnosis. In patients with an excess of albuminuria rather than the expected LC proteinuria, a biopsy is necessary to establish the presence of amyloidosis or other glomerular disorders associated with LCs. The type and stage of disease (especially the degree of tubular fibrosis) may influence the choice of chemotherapy and the consideration of adjunctive treatments such as high cut-off (HCO) dialysis. Sometimes, the diagnosis of myeloma is made or suggested by the kidney biopsy as the first investigation and subsequently confirmed with protein chemistry.

11. **How do I treat myeloma cast nephropathy?**
Myeloma cast nephropathy is a medical emergency and requires immediate diagnosis and early institution of therapy to prevent irreversible kidney failure. There are two key treatment strategies.
- The first is to remove any precipitants (e.g., sepsis, non-steroidal antiinflammatory drugs, hypercalcemia) and increase urine flow to reverse or prevent oliguria. The toxicity of LC in the tubules in part relates to their concentration, and increasing tubular flow reduces this. Volume expansion with normal saline (or sodium bicarbonate in the presence of acidosis) and the maintenance of a high urine flow (ideally 3 L a day) with adequate oral fluids are required. The

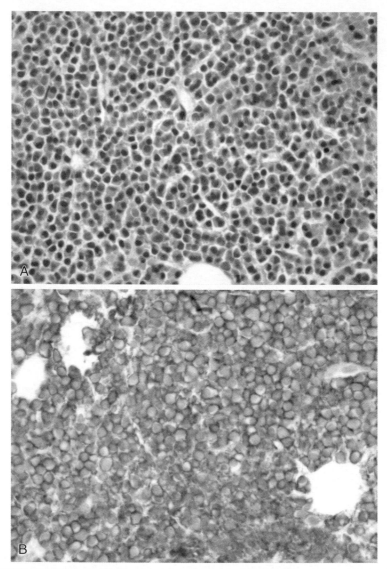

Figure 39.2. (A) Multiple myeloma. The bone marrow is replaced by plasma cells showing nuclear chromatin clumping and eccentric nuclei (hematoxylin and eosin ×40). (B) Multiple myeloma. Immunoperoxidase staining for CD138 and monoclonal antibodies will show membrane and cytoplasm staining (immunoperoxidase stain with monoclonal antibody ×20).

reversal of hypercalcemia with volume expansion and bisphosphonates with reduced dosing and infusion rates (as a result of tubular toxicity in kidney injury) is also indicated. An alternative to bisphosphonates is denosumab, which is not nephrotoxic. The use of furosemide may worsen cast formation and induce volume depletion; it should be used with caution or avoided.
- The second key strategy is the early use of chemotherapy (see Question 12) to reduce the LC load. In all patients, dexamethasone, 20 mg bid, which induces apoptosis of plasma cells, can be immediately commenced to rapidly lower the serum LC load.

12. **What chemotherapy is used in patients with myeloma and AKI?**
Although myeloma and AKI are incurable, chemotherapy and the use of autologous stem cell transplantation (ASCT) have improved patient survival significantly. ASCT is now the procedure of choice for eligible patients and the avoidance of alkylating agents, such as melphalan, that impair stem cell harvest is preferred. Chemotherapy targeting rapid plasma cell killing and LC lowering should include the reversible proteasome inhibitor bortezomib (which does not need dose adjustment in kidney failure) alone or in conjunction with other agents. Lenalidomide, a derivative of thalidomide, has also shown great benefit for rapid lowering of LC, but it requires dose adjustment in kidney failure because of myelosuppression. Determining the optimal chemotherapy requires close collaboration between nephrologists and hematologists to individualize management decisions according to age and comorbidity, suitability for ASCT, eligibility for trials, and consideration of HCO dialysis.

13. **Does plasmapheresis remove free LCs in myeloma?**
Patients with AKI from myeloma cast nephropathy have very high circulating and tissue FLC because of uncontrolled production and impaired excretion. The reduction of this burden by enhanced non-kidney clearance while awaiting clinical benefit from chemotherapy may allow kidney recovery. Conventional dialysis has very low FLC clearance, and plasmapheresis was used to improve plasma clearance. The modeling of clearance suggests that plasmapheresis can reduce the FLC load, but because there is a high extravascular refilling and exchanges are limited to around 3.5 L volumes, it requires daily treatment. Comparison with daily dialysis using HCO membranes (see Question 14) suggests plasmapheresis is inferior, and clinical trials have not shown a benefit of plasmapheresis in MCN. Plasma exchange should be used only in patients with symptoms and signs of hyperviscosity (e.g., in IgA myeloma and Waldenström macroglobulinemia [WM]) when rapid lowering of whole Igs is required to alleviate symptoms.

14. **What form of dialysis is best for patients with myeloma?**
The use of dialysis is required in up to 10% of new patients with myeloma and AKI. Most often this is hemodialysis via central venous catheters. Until recently, only 15% of patients recovered kidney function, and there was a high mortality. However, long-term use of both peritoneal dialysis and hemodialysis has been used, and survival on dialysis, although reduced, depends on myeoma control by chemotherapy. Survival on dialysis is improved with increased response to newer chemotherapy agents. Kidney recovery with freedom from dialysis is associated with an even greater survival benefit. The use of HCO membranes for hemodialysis offers a novel method to remove large amounts of sFLC over extended dialysis (8 hours duration). In conjunction with chemotherapy, especially bortezomib, it is associated with kidney recovery rates of more than 70%. However, the true independent benefit of HCO, and its additional cost, when compared with the introduction of chemotherapy associated with rapid LC lowering alone, remains unproven by randomized clinical trial and therefore cannot be routinely recommended.

15. **What is MGUS?**
MGUS is defined as a paraprotein <3 g/dL, with <10% plasma cells in the bone marrow and no evidence of end-organ damage (no anemia, lytic bone lesions, hypercalcemia, or kidney disease attributable to the paraprotein). Nearly 3% of individuals older than age 70 have MGUS. About 1% of patients with MGUS progress to symptomatic myeloma each year, so annual follow-up is required. Patients with a higher level of paraprotein (>1.5 g/dL), non-IgG paraproteins, and an abnormal sFLC ratio at diagnosis are more likely to progress. Patients with MGUS usually have no or low levels of Bence-Jones proteins.

16. **What is smoldering myeloma?**
Smoldering myeloma is an intermediate clinical stage of disease between MGUS and myeloma that has a much higher risk of progression to myeloma than MGUS (10% year or more). It is defined as a serum monoclonal protein (IgG or IgA) >3g/dL or a urinary monoclonal protein >500 mg/24 h, and/or clonal bone marrow plasma cells between 10% and 60% AND the absence of any CRAB feature. The early initiation of chemotherapy in this patient group may be considered to reduce the risk of organ damage by progression to myeloma.

17. **If I screen a patient with newly found kidney impairment and find a monoclonal protein, how do I know if he or she has myeloma-induced kidney disease?**
Of people older than 70 years, 3% have MGUS; this age group also has a high disease prevalence of diabetes and hypertension. Therefore, screening for alternative causes for kidney dysfunction in this age group will find patients with MGUS. The duration of the clinical history of kidney impairment and

the extent of diabetic complications are helpful in differentiating the cause. In general, patients with MGUS have low levels of monoclonal protein ($<$3 g/dL), a normal FLC ratio, an absence or low level of urine LCs, and no clinical evidence of myeloma (no osteolytic lesions, anemia, or hypercalcemia). In some cases, bone marrow or kidney biopsy may be required.

18. **What is Monoclonal Gammopathy of Renal Significance (MGRS)?**
MGRS is now used to define a group of B cell lymphoproliferative disorders and plasma cell disorders that do not meet criteria for myeloma, WM, or lymphoma/leukemia, yet lead to a histologically defined pattern of kidney injury directly attributable to the paraprotein or LC. In MGRS, the clonal expansion is often low and below any diagnostic threshold for malignancy yet the paraprotein or the LC component is associated with clinical disease of a heterogeneous and significant nature (e.g., amyloidosis, MIDD). Because they have not been previously considered a malignant disorder, this has restricted their access to therapy required for control of the clonal disorder and caused confusion with diagnosis and management. Separating them into a separate group allows better clinical management options and research focus.

19. **What is Waldenstrom Macroglobulinemia (WM) and does it cause AKI?**
WM is an IgM monoclonal-protein-secreting lymphoid and plasma cell malignancy. It usually manifests with anemia and fatigue, but it also may cause constitutional symptoms of fever, weight loss, and sweats; organ involvement with hepatosplenomegaly and lymphadenopathy; peripheral neuropathy; and features of hyperviscosity and cryoglobulinemia (rash). The diagnosis requires a monoclonal IgM protein and a bone marrow with $>$10% lymphoplasmacytic cell infiltration. Usually, the FLC component is kappa only, and urinary kappa LCs can be found in around 70% of cases. Kidney involvement with WM is uncommon and classic myeloma cast nephropathy is rare. Kidney involvement is glomerular and presents with hematuria/proteinuria, impaired kidney function, and rarely nephrotic syndrome. Histologically it takes the form of an immune-mediated glomerulonephritis with IgM deposition and/or features of cryoglobulinemia with intraglomerular thrombi. Treatment is delayed until patients develop significant end-organ damage or symptoms. Plasma exchange, rituximab, alkylating agents (chlorambucil), and the purine nucleoside analogues (fludarabine, cladribine) alone or in combination can be used.

20. **Do plasmacytomas involve the kidneys?**
Plasmacytomas are solitary lesions of clonal plasma cells in bone or soft tissues (especially the upper respiratory tract) without plasma cell involvement of the bone marrow or any other features of myeloma. Approximately 50% have a small monoclonal serum protein. They do not involve the kidneys, although they can progress to myeloma. Elevated sFLC ratio at diagnosis is associated with a higher risk of progression.

21. **What is POEMS syndrome?**
The acronym POEMS refers to
- **P**olyneuropathy
- **O**rganomegaly
- **E**ndocrinopathy
- **M**onoclonal protein
- **S**kin involvement

POEMS is a very rare disease and requires a monoclonal plasma cell disorder with a progressive sensorimotor peripheral neuropathy and at least one other key criterion, particularly the presence of Castleman's disease (angiofollicular lymph node hyperplasia) or osteosclerotic myeloma. In general, kidney involvement is not a usual feature, but when kidney involvement is present, it is unrelated to LC deposition. Definitive therapy is uncertain but may involve radiotherapy and chemotherapy regimens directed toward the myeloma component.

22. **What is amyloidosis?**
Amyloidosis describes diseases characterized by the abnormal deposition of fibrils in extracellular tissues derived from an abnormal protein that is bound to serum amyloid P protein. When this abnormal protein is a LC (usually λ), it is known as primary or AL amyloidosis. Other causes include the hereditary/genetic (AH; e.g., transthyretin) or secondary amyloidosis when chronic inflammation (e.g., familial Mediterranean fever) is associated with increased serum amyloid A protein (AA amyloid). These fibrils form tissue deposits within the body, especially the kidney, heart, liver, nerves, and gut. Although associated with myeloma in around 10% of patients, the majority present with organ dysfunction as a result of tissue infiltration rather than bone destruction.

23. **What are the histologic features of amyloidosis?**
Macroscopically the kidneys are enlarged, firm, and pale, and may be waxy. On light microscopy AA and AL amyloid have the same morphologic features and involve mainly the glomerulus and blood vessels, with less involvement from the tubulointerstitium. The glomerular deposits are seen predominantly in the mesangium as amorphous acidophilic deposits, weakly periodic acid–Schiff positive and negative or weakly positive with Silver stain (Fig. 39.3A). There is usually extension of the deposits along the peripheral capillary wall and the deposits form delicate spikes on the outer surfaces. The classical diagnostic test is the Congo red stain, which shows an orange-red color and apple-green birefringence when examined by polarized microscopy. Potassium permanganate bleaches AA amyloid. Specific immunohistochemistry tests identify Ig LCs or amyloid A protein, with the majority of AL amyloidosis caused by lambda LC deposits. Electron microscopy shows the distinctive amyloid fibrils, which are non-branching, are randomly arranged, measure 9 to 12 nm, and have electrolucent cores but cannot distinguish between AA, AL, and AH amyloidosis (see Fig. 39.3B).

24. **How does amyloidosis present?**
Patients with amyloidosis usually present with edema and nephrotic syndrome. However, restrictive cardiomyopathy, hepatomegaly (from infiltration), and peripheral neuropathy (carpal tunnel syndrome) are also common presentations. Severe edema, often with anasarca and pleural effusions, is common, and other clinical signs include easy bruising and macroglossia. Involvement of the adrenal glands can cause primary hypoadrenalism. In some cases, amyloid is confined to a single organ including bowel, bladder, and upper airways; these localized disorders are not usually associated with kidney disease. AA amyloid is usually associated with a chronic illness such as rheumatoid arthritis, bronchiectasis, or familial Mediterranean fever.

25. **What is the diagnostic test for amyloidosis?**
Although the diagnosis is suggested by the finding of heavy albuminuria and bland urine sediment, a tissue biopsy is required to diagnose amyloidosis and distinguish between the various types (AL, AA, and AH). Amyloid deposits can also be found in virtually all other organs including the rectum, abdominal fat pad, and the bone marrow, and these are sometimes biopsied in preference to the kidney. The combination of SPE and serum FLC will be abnormal in 98% of patients with primary amyloidosis as a result of an LC disorder because of the increase in the abnormal (usually λ) sFLC.

26. **How can we treat amyloidosis?**
Primary amyloidosis frequently occurs in elderly patients, and therapy requires chemotherapy and/or ASCT to effect survival by reducing or eliminating the plasma cell clone responsible. Survival is based on the patient's age and the extent of tissue involvement, with cardiac involvement suggesting a particularly poor prognosis. Prednisolone and melphalan have modest benefits on survival, and newer LC-focused strategies, including ASCT derived from studies in myeloma, are now recommended. The management of AA amyloidosis requires treatment of the underlying secondary disorder; AH treatment depends on the specific genetic mutation, and liver transplantation may be curative in some cases.

27. **What are the MIDD?**
The MIDD (which are now considered within the MGRS classification of disease) describe another histologic and clinical variant of abnormal tissue deposition resulting from a monoclonal-free LC (or, rarely, the heavy chain [HC] component of Ig alone or in combination with LC), which has some characteristics similar to amyloidosis in that abnormal extracellular protein deposition occurs, yet the microstructure differs because these proteins do not form fibrils and the deposits do not stain with Congo red. Typically, light chain deposition disease (LCDD) (also known as Randall's disease) is associated with specific variants of the κ-LC variable region domain (types I and IV), which bind strongly and accumulate along the tubular and glomerular basement membrane, but also deposit in the mesangium where they induce the production of extracellular matrix and typical nodular glomerular lesions. The clinical presentation of both LCDD and heavy chain deposition disease (HCDD) is similar, and is usually with a glomerulonephritis or nephritic picture: hypertension, hematuria, and proteinuria with kidney impairment. Cardiac and hepatic involvement may also occur. Therapy is directed toward treatment of the LC with steroids and myeloma chemotherapy including ASCT, and clinical response is variable. Kidney transplantation has a high risk of recurrent disease.

28. **What are the features of LCDD on kidney biopsy?**
LCDD, HCDD, and light and heavy chain deposition disease show the same morphologic features. The glomerular changes are heterogeneous and range from mild mesangiopathic changes to a mesangiocapillary (membranoproliferative) pattern with features similar to diabetic nodular

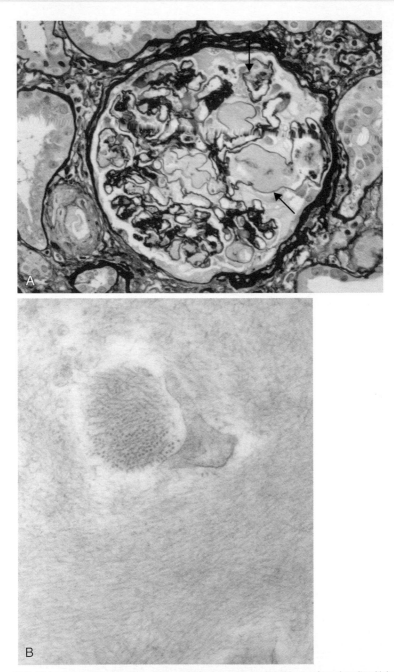

Figure 39.3. (A) Amyloidosis. The glomerulus shows marked mesangial expansion with amorphous deposits with loss of mesangial argyrophilia *(arrows)*. Similar deposits are present in the arteriole (methenamine silver with periodic acid–Schiff counter stain ×40). (B) Amyloidosis. Electron microscopy shows randomly arranged parallel bundles of straight fibrils (magnification ×12,500).

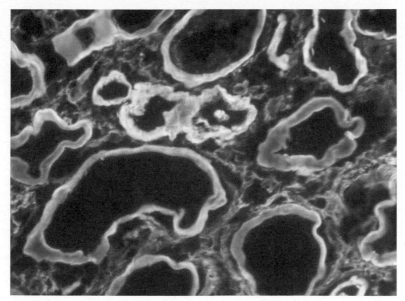

Figure 39.4. Light chain deposition disease. There is a heavy concentration of single light chain deposits along the outer aspect of the tubular basement membrane (immunofluorescence microscopy with antibody to single light chain ×25).

glomerulosclerosis (Kimmelstiel-Wilson type) but do not stain strongly positive with Silver stains. They are Congo red negative, and immunofluorescence microscopy shows monoclonal LC deposits in the glomerular basement membrane, the Bowman capsule, and the cortical and medullary tubular basement membranes (Fig. 39.4). Electron microscopy shows a band of dense granules usually in the inner position of the lamina densa of the glomerular basement membrane and the outer aspect of the tubular basement membrane.

29. What are fibrillary and immunotactoid glomerulonephritis?

Fibrillary and immunotactoid glomerulonephritis are very uncommon non-amyloid (Congo red negative) forms of Ig-associated kidney disease with abnormal tissue deposits from fibrils. Similar to LCDD, they usually present with a glomerulonephritis picture (hematuria and proteinuria, hypertension, and kidney impairment). They can only be distinguished from LCDD by kidney biopsy and especially electron microscopy, where the size and characteristics of the deposits differ (Table 39.1). Fibrillary glomerulonephritis does not usually associate with a paraprotein and has polyclonal IgG deposits, whereas immunotactoid disease may be associated with hematologic disorders (lymphoma, leukemia) and have monoclonal IgGλ or IgG κ deposits and in some cases a circulating paraprotein. The treatment of fibrillary disease is often attempted with steroids and cytotoxics, but the response is poor. Immunotactoid disease may respond to treatment of the underlying hematologic disorder. Progression to end-stage kidney disease is frequent and can occur within a few years.

30. Can patients with CKD and dysproteinemias receive a kidney transplant?

Despite significant advances in diagnosis and chemotherapy, most patients with myeloma, amyloidosis, or LCDD are older and have significant comorbidity. Since the disease remains incurable with a high chance of recurrence, kidney transplant is rarely considered appropriate. A smaller group of younger patients with myeloma, after successful induction therapy and ASCT, may be considered suitable if prolonged disease remission (approximately 3 years) by standard criteria and if normalization of the sFLC ratio are achieved. In the absence of active LC myeloma, the risk of recurrent cast nephropathy is low. Surveillance after kidney transplant for disease recurrence is indefinite and would involve regular estimation of sFLC ratio because this is the most sensitive and specific marker of disease recurrence and provides an estimate of the risk of allograft injury. The results for LCDD suggest a very high risk of early and aggressive disease recurrence after kidney transplant in the absence of prolonged disease remission and ASCT. Rare cases of kidney transplantation in primary amyloidosis after chemotherapy and ASCT are also reported.

Table 39.1. The Clinical and Histologic Characteristics of the Dysproteinemias

	MYELOMA	AMYLOIDOSIS (AL/AA/AH)	LCDD	FIBRILLARY GLOMERULONEPHRITIS	IMMUNOTACTOID GLOMERULONEPHRITIS	WALDENSTRÖM MACROGLOBULINEMIA
Clinical presentation	Acute kidney injury	Nephrotic syndrome	Nephrotic syndrome	Nephritic syndrome	Nephritic syndrome	Nephritic or nephrotic hyperviscosity
Urinalysis	Bland or proteinuria (no or minimal albumin)	Bland predominant albuminuria	Hematuria Proteinuria casts	Hematuria Proteinuria casts	Hematuria Proteinuria casts	Hematuria Proteinuria casts
Serum paraprotein class	IgD/IgA/IgG	None	None	Uncommon	IgG	IgM
Serum free light chains	κ and λ	λ > κ (primary) None (secondary/hereditary)	κ > λ (LCDD)	Unknown	Unknown	λ
Histology						
Light microscopy	Interstitial fibrosis, edema, inflammation, and giant cells with distal casts	All show similar features with acidophilic deposits in the mesangium, peripheral capillaries, and blood vessels	Heterogeneous most severe pattern is membranoproliferative (mesangiocapillary) with nodularity	Heterogeneous mesangial to membrano-proliferative pattern	Heterogeneous proliferative to membrano-proliferative pattern	Subendothelial deposits and thrombi
Congo red stain	Negative	All positive	Negative	Negative	Negative	Negative
Immunofluorescence	κ or λ only	λ > κ	κ > λ	Polyclonal IgG κ and λ	Monoclonal IgGκ or IgGλ ± IgM	IgM ± IgG
Complement C3	Negative	All negative	Negative	Positive	Positive	Positive
Electron microscopy	Tubular crystals	All show similar random fibrils 8–12 nm	Amorphous dense deposits	Random fibrils 15–30 nm	Parallel microtubules 10–90 nm	Dense deposits ± cryoglobulin microtubules

Nephrotic syndrome = edema, hypoalbuminemia, and heavy albuminuria.
Nephritic syndrome = hematuria and proteinuria, hypertension, kidney impairment.
LCDD, Light chain deposition disease.

KEY POINTS: MYELOMA

1. Patients with myeloma are particularly vulnerable to factors that cause volume depletion or sudden reductions in glomerular filtration. This is because these changes reduce tubular flow and increase the exposure of the tubule to high single-nephron light chain (LC) concentrations.
2. Patients with myeloma most frequently present with the signs and symptoms of kidney failure, anemia, or malignant bone pain, typically low back pain unrelieved by rest or simple analgesics.
3. Urinalysis by dipstix preferentially detect albumin and may be negative in the presence of significant quantities of LCs (Bence-Jones proteinuria).
4. Myeloma cast nephropathy is a medical emergency and requires immediate diagnosis and early institution of therapy in order to prevent irreversible kidney failure.
5. Dcxamethasone 20 mg bid, which induces apoptosis of plasma cells, can be immediately commenced to rapidly lower the serum LC load.
6. Bortezomib-based chemotherapy regimens are recommended as the optimal management of acute kidney injury and myeloma

KEY POINTS: LIGHT CHAINS

1. Kidney injury is principally related to the light chain (LC) component of myeloma because, unlike immunoglobulins, LCs are freely filtered at the glomerulus and reabsorbed in the proximal tubule.
2. The measurement of serum free light chain by nephelometry is both rapid and sensitive, and will diagnose all patients with myeloma and acute kidney injury due to LC excess.

KEY POINTS: MONOCLONAL GAMMOPATHY OF UNKNOWN SIGNIFICANCE, MONOCLONAL GAMMOPATHY OF RENAL SIGNIFICANCE AND WALDENSTRÖM MACROGLOBULINEMIA

1. Patients with monoclonal gammopathy of unknown significance (MGUS) have low levels of monoclonal protein (<3 g/dL), a normal free light chain (LC) ratio, an absence or low level of urine LCs, and no clinical evidence of myeloma (no osteolytic lesions, anemia, or hypercalcemia).
2. Monoclonal gammopathy of renal significance defines patients with biochemical features of MGUS *and* an associated kidney disease directly attributable to the associated paraprotein on kidney histology.
3. Kidney involvement with Waldenström macroglobulinemia is uncommon, and classic myeloma cast nephropathy rare.

KEY POINTS: AMYLOIDOSIS

1. Amyloidosis is due to deposition of fibrils within the body, especially the kidney, heart, liver, nerves, and gut.
2. Primary amyloidosis is associated with myeloma in <10% of patients and the majority present with edema and nephrotic syndrome.
3. The combination of serum protein electrophoresis and serum free light chain (sFLC) will be abnormal in 98% of patients with primary amyloidosis because of the increase in the abnormal (usually λ) sFLC.

BIBLIOGRAPHY

Bradwell, A. R. (2008). *Serum free light chain analysis* (5th ed.). Birmingham, UK: The Binding Site Ltd.
Dimopoulos, M. A., Sonneveld, P., Leung, N., Merlini, G., Ludwig, H., Kastritis, E., ... Terpos, E. (2016). International Myeloma Working Group Recommendations for the diagnosis and management of myeloma-related kidney impairment. *J Clin Oncol, 34,* 1544–1557.
Heher, E. C., Spitzer, T. R., & Goes, N. B. (2009). Light chains: Heavy burden in kidney transplantation. *Transplantation, 87*(7), 947–952.

Hutchison, C. A., Basnayake, K., & Cockwell, P. (2009). Serum free light chain assessment in monoclonal gammopathy and kidney disease. *Nat Rev Nephrol, 5*, 621–627.

Jennette, J. C., Olson, J. L., Schwartz, M. M., & Silva, F. G. (Eds.). (2007). *Heptinstall's pathology of the kidney*. Philadelphia: Lippincott Williams & Wilkins.

Ludwig, H., Drach, J., Graf, H., Lang, A., & Meran, J. G. (2007). Reversal of acute renal failure by bortezomib-based chemotherapy in patients with multiple myeloma. *Haematologica, 92*(10), 1411–1414.

Motwani, S. S., Herlitz, L., Monga, D., Jhaveri, K. D., Lam, A. Q., & American Society of Nephrology Onco-Nephrology Forum. (2016). Paraprotein-related kidney disease: glomerular diseases associated with paraproteinemias. *Clin J Am Soc Nephrol, 11*(12), 2260–2272.

Rajkumar, S. V., Dimopoulos, M. A., Palumbo, A., Blade, J., Merlini, G., Mateos, M. V., … Miguel, J. F. (2014). International Myeloma Working Group updated criteria for the diagnosis of multiple myeloma. *Lancet Oncol, 15*, e538–e548.

Rajkumar, S. V., & Kumar, S. (2016). Multiple myeloma: Diagnosis and treatment. *Mayo Clin Proc, 91*(1), 101–119.

Rosner, M. H., Edeani, A., Yanagita, M., Glezerman, I. G., Leung, N., & American Society of Nephrology Onco-Nephrology Forum. (2016). Paraprotein-related kidney disease: Diagnosing and treating monoclonal gammopathy of renal signficance. *Clin J Am Soc Nephrol, 11*(12), 2280–2287. doi:10.2215/CJN.02920316.

Sanders, P. W., & Booker, B. B. (1992). Pathobiology of cast nephropathy from human Bence-Jones proteins. *J Clin Invest, 89*, 630–639.

Yadav, P., Hutchison, C. A., Basnayake, Stringer, S., Jesky, M., Fifer, L., … Cockwell, P. (2016). Patients with multiple myeloma have excellent long-term outcomes after recovery from dialysis-dependent acute kidney injury. *Eur J Haematol, 96*(6), 610–617.

CHAPTER 40

KIDNEY NEOPLASIAS

Carol Nadai, Alexander Novakovic, Sumanta Kumar Pal and Robert A. Figlin

1. Describe the demographics of renal cell carcinoma (RCC). How many cases of RCC are diagnosed annually, and how many deaths are attributable to this disease? Is RCC more common in males or females? What is the median age at diagnosis of RCC?

   In 2016, an estimated 62,700 cases of RCC were diagnosed, and 14,240 deaths were attributable to the disease. Approximately 63% and 65% of diagnoses and deaths, respectively, occurred in males. The median age at diagnosis is 65.

2. What are the three most common histologic subtypes of RCC, and what proportion of RCC cases do they account for?

   Clear cell RCC accounts for approximately 80% of cases, while papillary and chromophobe histologies represent 10% and 5% of cases, respectively.

3. What are the clinical features of collecting duct (Bellini duct) carcinoma? What clinical disorder is associated with the medullary variant of collecting duct carcinoma?

   Collecting duct carcinoma comprises less than 1% of RCC cases, and has a particularly aggressive phenotype. Medullary RCC represents a variant of collecting duct carcinoma, and was first noted to occur among patients with sickle-cell trait.

4. What are common presenting signs of RCC?

   Often, RCC presents as an incidental finding on radiographic imaging of the abdomen. With respect to symptoms, common complaints include hematuria and flank pain. In the setting of metastatic disease, patients may note bone pain, palpable adenopathy, or pulmonary complaints (i.e., shortness of breath secondary to bulky lung disease or pleural effusions).

5. What paraneoplastic syndromes are associated with RCC? What is Stauffer's syndrome?

   Nearly 40% of patients with RCC develop paraneoplastic syndromes. RCC produces a range of ectopic hormones, including parathyroid-like hormone, erythropoietin, insulin, gonadotropins, renin, and placental lactogen. Clinically, this may manifest in a range of symptoms and laboratory abnormalities including, but not limited to, hypertension (24%), hypercalcemia (10% to 15%), and erythrocytosis (4%). Stauffer's syndrome, which occurs in roughly 6% of patients, implies liver function test abnormalities but absent hepatic metastases. This reversible liver dysfunction is pathognomonic for RCC.

6. What gene is disrupted in the majority of sporadic cases of RCC?

   The *VHL* gene is disrupted in up to 70% of sporadic cases of RCC. In approximately 50% of cases, somatic mutations occur, and in 10% to 20% of cases, the gene is hypermethylated. A consequence of *VHL* mutation is upregulation of hypoxia-induced genes, leading to increased production of moieties such as vascular endothelial growth factor (VEGF). This, in turn, causes increased tumor angiogenesis.

7. Describe the features of (1) hereditary papillary renal cell carcinoma, (2) Birt-Hogg-Dubé syndrome, and (3) hereditary leiomyomatosis/renal cell carcinoma (HLRCC).

   Hereditary papillary renal cell carcinoma is characterized by mutations in the *MET* proto-oncogene, located at 7q31. The mutations are highly penetrant and autosomal dominant. The resulting tumors are classified as papillary type 1 and are often multifocal and bilateral. Birt-Hogg-Dubé syndrome is characterized by the triad of hair follicle hamartomas, lung cysts, and renal neoplasia. The disorder is caused by mutations in the *BHD* gene, located at 17p11.2. While the disorder is highly penetrant with respect to lung and skin findings (>85%), renal neoplasia only occurs in 25% to 35% of patients. Finally, HLRCC is characterized by mutations in the gene-encoding fumarate hydratase (*FH*, located at 1q24-43). The resulting phenotype includes type 2 papillary RCC, along with cutaneous and uterine leiomyomas.

8. What is the staging workup for RCC?

   Guidelines from the National Comprehensive Cancer Network (NCCN) suggest that the initial workup for RCC should include a complete history and physical, comprehensive laboratories (including a low-density lipoprotein [LDH] and urinalysis), and abdominal/pelvic computed tomography (CT) or magnetic resonance imaging (MRI). If clinically indicated, an MRI of the brain and bone scan should be ordered. If urothelial carcinoma is suspected, urine cytology or ureteroscopy should be considered.

9. **For patients with localized RCC (stage I to III), what treatment is recommended after surgical resection of the tumor? What follow-up exams are recommended after surgical resection?**
At present, no adjuvant therapy is recommended for patients with resected RCC. Follow-up (per NCCN guidelines) is guided by risk stratification according to tumor, node, and metastasis (TNM) staging. For example, patients with T1a disease are recommended to receive history and physical and labs every 6 months for 2 years, and annually up to 5 years. Abdominal CT or MRI is recommended within 6 months, and then at least annually. Imaging of the chest is recommended annually for surveillance of metastases. In much higher-risk disease (e.g., stage II or III disease), history and physical is recommended every 3 to 6 months for 3 years, then annually up to 5 years. Baseline CT or MRI of the abdomen is recommended within 3 to 6 months, then every 3 to 6 months for 3 years, and annually up to 5 years. Baseline CT of the chest is recommended on essentially the same frequency. Bone scan is recommended as clinically indicated.

10. **In which patients is nephron-sparing surgery appropriate?**
Nephron-sparing surgery is appropriate in selected patients who have multiple primaries, a uninephric state, or kidney disease. Nephron-sparing techniques may also be used in selected patients with small unilateral tumors.

11. **What are common sites of metastasis of RCC?**
RCC classically spreads to the lung, bone, brain, liver, and adrenal gland. With improvements in systemic therapy, the rates of brain metastasis are steadily increasing. This is because the brain remains a "sanctuary site," where penetration of systemic therapy is highly variable.

12. **What are the two classes of agents used to treat metastatic RCC?**
The two broad classes of agents used to treat metastatic RCC include (1) immunotherapy and (2) targeted therapy. Immunotherapy may be divided into the more classical cytokine-based treatments such as interferon-α (IFN-α) and high-dose interleukin-2 (IL-2), and novel checkpoint inhibitors such as nivolumab. Nivolumab inhibits programmed death-1 (PD-1), which sits at the T-cell and antigen presenting cell interface and induces T-cell anergy. Targeted therapies include inhibitors of VEGF, including the monoclonal antibody bevacizumab and the small-molecule tyrosine kinase inhibitors such as sunitinib, pazopanib, sorafenib, and axitinib. Also U.S. Food and Drug Administration (FDA) approved are two inhibitors of the mammalian target of rapamycin (mTOR), namely everolimus and temsirolimus. Two multikinase inhibitors with affinity for a number of oncogenic drivers are lenvatinib and cabozantinib. Beyond VEGF receptor, lenvatinib inhibits signaling through the fibroblast growth factor receptor (FGFR), while cabozantinib inhibits signaling through MET and AXL.

13. **What proportion of patients responds to front-line VEGF-directed therapy? What is the typical delay in cancer growth with these treatments?**
VEGF-directed therapy still represents the mainstay of therapy for most patients with newly diagnosed metastatic RCC. FDA-approved agents with category 1 recommendations include sunitinib, pazopanib, and bevacizumab/IFN-α. Response rates range from 30% to 40% in the pivotal phase III studies assessing these agents in the front-line setting, with a delay in cancer growth (or progression-free survival, PFS) ranging from 9 to 12 months. Importantly, these therapies are not curative—however, with the advent of new treatments for metastatic RCC, median survival has improved to roughly 3 years.

14. **What proportion of patients respond to therapy with high-dose IL-2? What are some of the side effects of therapy?**
In a series of 259 patients treated at the NIH between 1986 and 2006, an overall RR of 20% was noted with IL-2 therapy. All patients who experienced a partial response (12%) were noted to relapse, with a median duration of response of 15.5 months. In contrast, 19 of 23 patients who experienced a complete response remained disease free with a median follow-up ranging between 24 and 221 months. This experience is representative of others, suggesting that while the complete response rate associated with high-dose IL-2 is relatively low, those patients who do develop a complete response may experience a durable remission. The side effects of high-dose IL-2 weigh heavily in the risk-benefit discussion with the patient. High-dose IL-2 causes vasodilatation, diarrhea, and a capillary leak syndrome, all of which can contribute to hypotension and oliguria. Hematologic and hepatic laboratory abnormalities are also frequently seen with IL-2 therapy.

15. **What are common side effects associated with VEGF-directed therapies?**
The most commonly reported moderate-to-severe side effects in the pivotal trial of sunitinib were hypertension, fatigue, diarrhea, and hand-foot syndrome. Similarly, diarrhea, rash, fatigue, and hand-foot skin reactions were the most frequently reported adverse events in the pivotal trial of sorafenib. Early results from the phase III randomized trial comparing pazopanib and placebo suggested the most frequent adverse events with pazopanib were diarrhea, hypertension, hair color change, nausea, and anorexia. Liver enzymes were also abnormally elevated in a large proportion of patients.

16. **How are mTOR inhibitors applied in metastatic RCC?**
Two mTOR inhibitors, everolimus and temsirolimus, have been approved for use in metastatic RCC. Everolimus was compared to placebo in a phase III study including patients who were refractory to sunitinib and/or sorafenib. In this study, everolimus therapy was associated with an improvement in PFS. As such, everolimus has been approved for use after failure of VEGF tyrosine kinase inhibitor therapy. In a randomized, phase II experience, the combination of lenvatinib and everolimus showed superiority over everolimus alone. For this reason, this combination may supplant everolimus monotherapy in the previously treated setting. In contrast, temsirolimus was approved based on a study comparing temsirolimus, IFN-γ, and the combination of agents in patients with poor risk metastatic RCC. In the context of this study, poor risk was defined as having $\geq$3 of the following predictors of short survival:
* LDH > 1.5 × the upper limit of normal
* Hemoglobin < lower limit of normal
* Corrected serum calcium >10 mg/dL
* Interval of <1 year from original diagnosis to the start of systemic therapy
* Karnofsky performance score <70, and (6) $\geq$2 sites of organ metastases.
Among the three treatment arms, temsirolimus was associated with improved overall survival. Considering this data, temsirolimus has been approved for the first-line treatment of poor-risk metastatic RCC.

17. **What side effects are associated with everolimus and temsirolimus?**
Class effects of the mTOR inhibitors include stomatitis, rash, fatigue, hyperglycemia, and hypertriglyceridemia. Pneumonitis (potentially severe) has also been noted with use of these agents.

18. **What side effects are associated with nivolumab (a PD-1 inhibitor) in RCC?**
The practitioner should be aware of potential autoimmune sequelae with novel checkpoint inhibitors. These include, for instance, autoimmune colitis, hepatitis, hypophysitis, thyroiditis, arthritis, and hepatitis. It is recommended that, in addition to surveillance for clinical manifestations of these symptoms, patients have frequent monitoring of hepatic and thyroid function. Prompt institution of steroids is recommended if these symptoms are recognized and other pertinent causes are excluded. Consultation with specialists is recommended. Salient to the theme of this text is autoimmune nephritis, which occurs sporadically but can be marked by rapid decline in kidney function. Biopsy can be used to diagnose autoimmune nephritis, with heavy immune infiltration of nephrons seen on pathology. Again, steroids may be used to treat this phenomenon.

KEY POINTS

1. The incidence of renal cell carcinoma has been steadily increasing with increased use of computerized tomography and other radiographic studies for diagnosing abdominal conditions.
2. Management of localized renal cell carcinoma largely entails surgical resection of the primary site and possibly adjacent lymph nodes.
3. Systemic therapy for metastatic renal cell carcinoma can be broadly divided into two categories: targeted therapy and immunotherapy. Targeted therapy entails agents that block the vascular endothelial growth factor signaling pathway, while novel immunotherapies target programmed death inhibitor-1, thereby decreasing T-cell anergy.
4. Vascular endothelial growth factor pathway inhibitors can cause hypertension and proteinuria.
5. Novel immunotherapeutic agents, such as programmed death-1 inhibitors, can cause a wide range of immune-related side effects, including autoimmune nephritis. Prompt initiation of steroids should occur if this is suspected.

BIBLIOGRAPHY

Escudier, B., Bellmunt, J., Negrier, S., Bajetta, E., Melichar, B., Bracarda, S., . . . Sneller V. (2010). Phase III trial of bevacizumab plus interferon Alfa-2a in Patients With Metastatic Renal Cell Carcinoma (AVOREN): Final analysis of overall survival. *Journal of Clinical Oncology, 28,* 2144–2150.

Escudier, B., Eisen, T., Stadler., W.M., Szczylik, C., Oudard, S., Siebels, M., . . . TARGET Study Group. (2007). Sorafenib in advanced clear-cell renal-cell carcinoma. *The New England Journal of Medicine, 356,* 125–134.

Hudes, G., Carducci, M., Tomczak, P., Dutcher, J., Figlin, R., Kapoor, A., . . . Global ARCC Trial. (2007). Temsirolimus, interferon alfa, or both for advanced renal-cell carcinoma. *The New England Journal of Medicine, 356,* 2271–2281.

Karumanchi, S. A., Merchan, J., & Sukhatme, V. P. (2002). Renal cancer: Molecular mechanisms and newer therapeutic options. *Current Opinion in Nephrology and Hypertension, 11,* 37–42.

Kim, W. Y., & Kaelin, W. G. (2004). Role of VHL gene mutation in human cancer. *Journal of Clinical Oncology, 22,* 4991–5004.

Klapper, J. A., Downey, S. G., Smith, F. O., Yang, J. C., Hughes, M. S., Kammula, U. S., . . . Rosenberg, S. (2008). High-dose interleukin-2 for the treatment of metastatic renal cell carcinoma. *Cancer, 113,* 293–301.

Motzer, R. J., Escudier, B., McDermott, D. F., George, S., Hammers, H. J., Srinivas, S., . . . Sharma, P. (2015). Nivolumab versus everolimus in advanced renal-cell carcinoma. *New England Journal of Medicine, 373,* 1803–1813.

Motzer, R. J., Escudier, B., Oudard, S., Hutson, T. E., Porta, C., Bracarda, S., . . . RECORD-1 Study Group. (2008). Efficacy of everolimus in advanced renal cell carcinoma: A double-blind, randomised, placebo-controlled phase III trial. *Lancet, 372,* 449–456.

Motzer, R. J., Hutson, T. E., Glen H., Michaelson, M. D., Molina, A., Eisen, T., . . . Larkin, J. (2015). Lenvatinib, everolimus, and the combination in patients with metastatic renal cell carcinoma: A randomised, phase 2, open-label, multicentre trial. *Lancet Oncology, 16,* 1473–1482.

Motzer, R. J., Hutson, T. E., Tomczak, P., Michaelson, M. D., Bukowski, R. M., Rixe, O., . . . Figlin, R. A. (2007). Sunitinib versus interferon alfa in metastatic renal-cell carcinoma. *The New England Journal of Medicine, 356,* 115–124.

National Comprehensive Cancer Network Clinical Practice Guidelines. *Renal Cell Carcinoma.* Available at http://www.nccn.org; last accessed March 29, 2016.

Ooi, A., Dykema, K., Ansari, A., Petillo, D., Snider, J., Kahnoski, R., . . . Furge, K. A. (2013). CUL3 and NRF2 mutations confer an NRF2 activation phenotype in a sporadic form of papillary renal cell carcinoma. *Cancer Research, 73,* 2044–2051.

Rini, B. I., Escudier, B., Tomczak, P., Kaprin, A., Szczylik, C., Hutson, T. E., . . . Motzer, R. J. (2011). Comparative effectiveness of axitinib versus sorafenib in advanced renal cell carcinoma (AXIS): A randomised phase 3 trial. *Lancet, 378,* 1931–1939.

Schmidt, L. E., & Linehan, W. M. (2009). When should genetic syndromes be considered? In *2009 Genitourinary Cancers Symposium Abstract Book* (p. 62). Alexandria, VA: American Society of Clinical Oncology.

Siegel, R. L., Miller, K. D., & Jemal, A. (2016). Cancer statistics, 2016. *CA: A Cancer Journal for Clinicians, 66,* 7–30.

Sternberg, C. N., Davis, I. D., Mardiak, J., Szczylik, C., Lee, E., Wagstaff, J., . . . Hawkins, R. E. (2010). Pazopanib in locally advanced or metastatic renal cell carcinoma: Results of a randomized phase III trial. *Journal of Clinical Oncology, 28,* 1061–1068.

Yap, T. A., Olmos, D., Brunetto, A. T., Tunariu, N., Barriuso, J., Riisnaes, R., . . . de Bono, J. S. (2011). Phase I trial of a selective c-MET inhibitor ARQ 197 incorporating proof of mechanism pharmacodynamic studies. *Journal of Clinical Oncology, 29,* 1271–1279.

CHAPTER 41

THROMBOTIC MICROANGIOPATHIES

Harpreet Singh, Matthew A. Sparks, and Hermann Haller

1. **Define thrombotic microangiopathy.**
   Thrombotic microangiopathy (TMA) is a pathologic description characterized by arteriole and capillary endothelial vessel wall damage that results in platelet activation, thrombosis, and damaged erythrocytes (schistocytes) leading to ischemia and organ failure. Several different clinical syndromes can present with the characteristic features of TMA.

2. **What are the clinical features associated with thrombotic microangiopathy?**
   The main clinical features of all TMA syndromes include microangiopathic hemolytic anemia (anemia with the presence of schistocytes), thrombocytopenia, and altering degrees of renal and neurologic dysfunction. Due to the hemolysis, patients will have an elevated lactate dehydrogenase (LDH) and a low haptoglobin. The direct antiglobulin test (Coombs test) is negative because the anemia is nonimmune in nature.

3. **What are the most common clinical syndromes associated with thrombotic microangiopathy?**
   - Shiga toxin–associated hemolytic uremia syndrome (ST-HUS)
   - Thrombotic thrombocytopenic purpura (TTP)
   - Atypical hemolytic uremic syndrome (aHUS)

4. **Are there clinical features that may help distinguish between these clinical syndromes?**
   Yes and no. HUS often presents with kidney injury, whereas TTP is associated with more neurologic dysfunction and less often kidney injury. Although these associations are "classic," patients with TTP can have kidney injury and patients with HUS can have neurologic manifestations. The platelet count in aHUS as compared with TTP is rarely less than 80,000. The classic clinical pentad of TTP includes:
   - microangiopathic hemolytic anemia
   - thrombocytopenia
   - acute kidney injury
   - neurologic symptoms
   - fever

5. **What are the underlying pathophysiologic mechanisms of the major TMA syndromes?**
   - ST-HUS: This is caused by Shiga toxin secreted from strains of *Escherichia coli* (most common is *E. coli* O157:H7) or *Shigella dysenteriae*. Shiga toxin binds to vascular endothelial cells, renal mesangial cells, and renal epithelial cells, leading to cell damage.
   - TTP: This is caused by a deficiency in von Willebrand factor–cleaving metalloprotease (A Disintegrin And Metalloproteinase with ThromboSpondin Motifs 13 [ADAMTS13]) that cleaves von Willebrand factor. The deficiency leads to large multimers of von Willebrand factor that increase the risk of platelet thrombi in small vessels.
   - aHUS: This is caused by uncontrolled activation of the alternative complement pathway, leading to increased formation of the membrane attack complex injuring normal cells.

6. **What is the incidence of the varying clinical syndromes of TMA?**
   - ST-HUS: 60 cases for 1,000,000/year in children <5 years of age; 10 to 20 cases for 1,000,000/year in overall population including adults >18 years of age.
   - TTP: 0.1 case for 1,000,000/year in children; 3 cases for 1,000,000/year in adults.
   - aHUS: 1 case for 1,000,000/year in the overall population

7. **Does Shiga toxin–associated HUS occur more often in children or adults?**
   ST-HUS occurs more frequently in children. When ST-HUS occurs in adults, the clinical manifestations are often more severe.

8. Describe the presentation and clinical course of patients with ST-HUS.
Patients often develop prodromal hemorrhagic diarrhea with associated abdominal pain after eating Shiga toxin–contaminated food. The kidney failure and other clinical manifestations (including thrombocytopenia and neurologic manifestations) develop after the diarrhea has begun to resolve. Among patients who develop Shiga toxin enteritis, 5% to 15% develop HUS. If neurologic abnormalities and hypertension occurred, they can persist even after the acute phase is over. End-stage kidney disease (ESKD) is rare.

9. What are the treatment options for patients with ST-HUS?
The mainstay of treatment for patients with ST-HUS is supportive care. This entails aggressive supportive care including hydration with intravenous fluids, supporting the anemia, and managing the renal failure with renal replacement therapy, if needed. There are no randomized clinical trial data to support plasmapheresis or eculizumab, but they have been used in severe ST-HUS with reported success, especially in Germany after the *E. coli* 0157:H7 outbreak from contaminated bean sprouts in 2011 (Fig. 41.1).

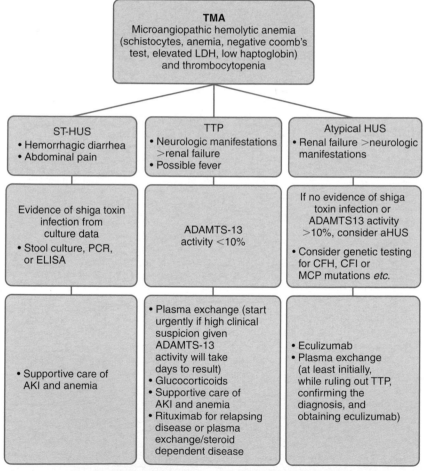

Figure 41.1. Thrombotic microangiopathy *(TMA)*, approach to differential diagnosis, clinical characteristics, diagnostics, and management. *CFH,* Complement factor H; *CFI,* complement factor I; *HUS,* hemolytic uremia syndrome; *ST-HUS,* Shiga toxin–associated hemolytic uremia syndrome; *TTP,* thrombotic thrombocytopenic purpura.

10. Should patients with Shiga toxin infection be treated with antibiotics?

No. This has remained a controversial subject for many years. A recent meta-analysis revealed that the use of antibiotics in Shiga toxin infections was not associated with increased risk of developing HUS. When the authors excluded papers that were at a high risk of bias and did not have an acceptable definition of HUS, there was a significant association between antibiotic use for Shiga toxin infections and the development of HUS.

11. What is the pathway that is dysregulated in atypical HUS (aHUS)?

The alternative pathway of the complement system is dysregulated in aHUS. In a steady state the alternative pathway is always active. There is continuous production of C3b from C3 (called "C3 tickover"). C3b deposition in tissues leads to formation of the C5b-9 terminal complement complex, which in turn leads to injury of normal cells. In atypical HUS the alternative pathway is dysregulated, leading to increased C3b production. This allows for increased terminal complement complex and thereby cell injury.

12. What are the genetic mutations/other causes of aHUS?

Hereditary aHUS is caused by loss of function mutations in regulatory genes, such as complement factor H (CFH), complement factor I (CFI), thrombomodulin (THBD), membrane cofactor protein (MCP), as well as gain-of-function mutations in effector genes complement factor B (CFB) and C3. CFH mutations are the most prevalent. Currently, more than 30 mutations have been described.

Autoantibodies to CFH can result in a functional deficiency of CFH. These autoantibodies reduce CFH binding to C3b, leading to a decrease in C3b activation. CFH antibodies account for approximately 10% of atypical HUS. Autoantibodies are mostly seen in children with aHUS.

13. Do all mutations in the genes regulating the complement pathway cause phenotypic disease of atypical HUS (i.e., penetrance)?

No. The majority of complement mutations associated with aHUS are heterozygous with many family members remaining asymptomatic. Penetrance of hereditary aHUS is estimated to be 50% in carriers. This suggests that both genetic and environmental insults are required for disease expression of atypical HUS.

14. Does the underlying genetic defect impact clinical outcomes in aHUS?

Yes. CFH mutations carry the worst prognosis, with approximately 70%–80% of patients developing ESKD or dying from complications of aHUS. Mutations in CFI, CFB, C3, and THBD have a rate of ESKD or death in the 60%–70% range. In contrast, patients with MCP mutations rarely develop ESKD or death (<20%). Complement genetic studies are now commercially available and may be helpful to confirm the diagnosis, as well as provide prognostic information.

15. What are known triggers and associations of aHUS?

Patients with aHUS have a genetic defect that renders them susceptible to end-organ damage. Hence several triggers and associations have been identified. Infections with human immunodeficiency virus, as well as bacterial infections with *Streptococcus pneumoniae* and *Mycoplasma pneumoniae,* are known triggers of aHUS. Pregnancy and malignancy are also known triggers. Medications such as calcineurin inhibitors (tacrolimus and cyclosporine), chemotherapeutic agents (i.e., mitomycin C, cisplatin, and gemcitabine), and antiplatelet agents (clopidogrel, ticlopidine) have all been associated with atypical HUS.

16. What are the treatments available for atypical HUS?

Anticomplement therapy is now the standard of care for the treatment of aHUS. Eculizumab is a humanized monoclonal antibody directed against C5 of the complement cascade and thereby inhibits the formation of C5a and C5b-9 membrane attack complex. Its use may be limited in patients with C5 mutations. In patients with autoantibodies to CFH, eculizumab can be used in addition to the consideration of immunosuppression with corticosteroids. The ongoing considerations with regards to eculizumab use are the high cost of the medication and no clear criteria of when to stop the medication. Plasmapheresis remains a part of initial therapy because there may be a delay in diagnosis and/or obtaining the drug.

17. How do ST-HUS and aHUS vary with regard to kidney transplant outcome?

The outcomes for kidney transplant secondary to ST-HUS are good, whereas the outcomes for aHUS are worse. In patients with prior history of aHUS, the disease recurs in approximately 50% of patients who are transplanted. Graft failure occurs in 80% to 90% of patients with recurrent aHUS. Living related renal transplantation is contraindicated in aHUS even if genetic screening is negative, because of the risk of unidentified genetic susceptibility factors. Prophylactic treatment with eculizimab has been discussed as a therapeutic option.

18. **Does the type of underlying genetic defect in aHUS impact transplant outcome?**
Yes. Patients with an MCP mutation have the best outcome, with low rates of aHUS recurrence (<20%) and long-term graft survival similar to patients who underwent transplantation for other etiologies. Patients with CFH and CFI mutations have the worse outcome with transplantation; 70% to 90% have a recurrence.

19. **What are the two major causes of ADAMTS13 deficiency in TTP?**
The first cause is in an inherited form of TTP secondary to homozygous or compound heterozygous mutations in ADAMTS13 gene, hereditary TTP. The second, more common cause is autoantibody to ADAMTS13, acquired TTP.

20. **What tests can be used to help diagnose TTP?**
In hereditary TTP, a genetic mutation of ADAMTS13 in the absence of an autoantibody is required for a diagnosis. In TTP, an assay to detect ADAMTS13 activity can be obtained. A level indicating less than 10% normal enzyme activity helps support the clinical diagnosis of TTP. The level is not sufficiently sensitive or specific and therefore needs to be used in addition to the patient's clinic presentation (see Fig. 41.1).

21. **What is the mainstay of treatment for patients with TTP?**
Prompt initiation of plasmapheresis with fresh frozen plasma is the most important treatment for TTP. In acquired TTP, plasmapheresis has the benefit of removing the autoantibodies in the patient's blood. In hereditary TTP, plasma infusion as opposed to plasmapheresis is indicated. Glucocorticoids may be of benefit in patients with acquired TTP (decrease the production of autoantibodies to ADAMTS13).

22. **Is rituximab indicated in patients with acquired TTP?**
Yes. Rituximab is an anti-CD20 monoclonal antibody. Its use in TTP is mainly indicated in adult TTP patients who are refractory to plasmapheresis and corticosteroids and in patients who have a relapsing course.

KEY POINTS ✓

1. HUS and TTP are clinical syndromes of TMA that present with microangiopathic hemolytic anemia, thrombocytopenia, and organ failure, typically of the kidney or the brain.
2. aHUS is caused by dysregulation of the alternative pathway of the complement system, resulting in increased activation of the complement pathway and cell damage. The overactivation of the pathway occurs either via a genetic mutation or autoantibodies to a regulatory protein.
3. The renal outcome, clinical course, and success of transplantation in aHUS is influenced by the type of underlying genetic mutation. *CFH* mutations are associated with the worse prognosis and *MCP* mutations with the best prognosis.
4. Typical or ST-HUS occurs most commonly in children who consume food contaminated with Shiga toxin–producing *E. coli*. ST-HUS rarely progresses to ESKD.
5. TTP is caused by a genetic mutation in *ADAMTS13* or an autoantibody to ADAMTS13. ADAMTS13 is an enzyme that cleaves vWF. The result of a genetic or functional deficiency in this enzyme leads to large multimers of vWF leading to platelet aggregation and thrombi formation.

BIBLIOGRAPHY

Barbour, T., Johnson, S., Cohney, S., & Hughes, P. (2012). Thrombotic microangiopathy and associated renal disorders. *Nephrology Dialysis Transplant, 27*, 2673–2685.

Freedman, S., Xie, J., Neufeld, M. S., Hamilton, W. L., Hartling, L., & Tarr, P. I. (2016). Shiga toxin-producing Escherichia coli infection, antibiotics, and risk of developing hemolytic uremic syndrome: A meta-analysis. *Clinical Infectious Diseases, 62*, 1251–1258.

George, J. (2010). How I treat patients with thrombotic thrombocytopenic purpura: 2010. *Blood, 116*, 4060–4069.

George, J., & Nester, C. (2014). Syndromes of thrombotic microangiopathy. *New England Journal of Medicine, 371*, 654–666.

Laurence, J., Haller, H., Mannucci, P. M., Nangaku, M., Praga, M., & Rodriguez de Cordoba, S. (2016). Atypical hemolytic uremic syndrome (aHUS): Essential aspects of an accurate diagnosis. *Clinical Advances in Hematology & Oncology, 14*(Suppl. 11), 2–15.

Noris, M., Mescia, F., & Remuzzi, G. (2012). STEC-HUS, atypical HUS and TTP are all disease of complement activation. *Nature Review Nephrology, 8*, 622–633.

Noris, M., & Remuzzi, G. (2009). Atypical hemolytic-uremic syndrome. *New England Journal of Medicine, 361*, 1676–1687.

Trachtman, H. (2013). HUS and TTP in children. *Pediatric Clinics of North America, 60*, 1513–1526.

VIII
OTHER RENAL PARENCHYMAL DISEASES

FABRY DISEASE

Robert J. Desnick

CHAPTER 42

1. What is Fabry disease?

Fabry disease is a systemic, X-linked, lysosomal storage disorder that results from the deficient activity of the enzyme α-galactosidase A (α-Gal A) and the lysosomal accumulation of its primary glycolipid substrate, globotriaosylceramide (GL-3). The progressive GL-3 accumulation, particularly in vascular endothelial lysosomes, leads to ischemia and occlusion of small vessels throughout the body. Clinical onset in affected males with the Type 1 Classic phenotype occurs in childhood or adolescence and is characterized by painful acroparesthesias, gastrointestinal dysfunction, corneal dystrophy, absent or decreased sweat (anhidrosis or hypohidrosis), and cutaneous lesions (angiokeratomas). With advancing age, the progressive glycolipid accumulation, especially in podocytes and cardiomyocytes, leads to kidney failure, cardiac disease, ischemic strokes, and early demise. Patients typically develop end-stage kidney disease (ESKD) in the third to fifth decades of life. Female heterozygotes from Type 1 Classically affected families can be as severely affected as Type 1 Classically affected males, or may be asymptomatic throughout life, primarily as a result of random X-chromosomal inactivation. Patients with the Type 2 Later-Onset phenotype lack the childhood manifestations of the Type 1 Classic early-onset phenotype and often are unrecognized. Previously undiagnosed males with both Types 1 and 2 Fabry disease have been identified in hemodialysis, cardiac, and stroke clinics by screening patients for markedly deficient plasma α-Gal A activity. Such studies have identified that ~0.2% of males on hemodialysis have unrecognized Fabry disease. Since the disease is X-linked, at-risk family members should be screened, and affected patients should receive genetic counseling, medical evaluations, and early therapeutic intervention, especially in males with the Type 1 Classic phenotype.

2. What are the two major subtypes of Fabry disease?

The two major subtypes of Fabry disease are the Type 1 Classic and Type 2 Later-Onset phenotypes. The **phenotypic subtypes** are determined by the specific α-Gal A mutation; thus, all affected family members will have the same phenotypic subtype. Affected males with the Type 1 Classic phenotype have little, if any, α-Gal A enzyme activity (<1% of mean normal), whereas males with the Type 2 Later-Onset phenotype have residual enzymatic activity, typically >1% of mean normal activity. Heterozygous females from Type 1 Classic Fabry families have a wide range of clinical manifestations from asymptomatic to severely affected, whereas heterozygous females from Type 2 Later-Onset families may have symptoms later in life, including cardiac and kidney manifestations. Heterozygotes from Type 2 Later-Onset families are likely to be less involved clinically, but can have as severe manifestations as their affected male relatives. Newborn screening studies have revealed that the Type 2 Later-Onset patients are more commonplace than patients with the Type 1 Classic phenotype.

3. What is the genetic basis of Fabry disease?

All cases of Fabry disease are caused by mutations in the gene *GLA* encoding the lysosomal hydrolase α-Gal A. The *GLA* gene is located on the X-chromosome, and the disease is inherited as an X-linked disorder. To date, more than 950 *GLA* gene mutations have been described. Type 1 Classically affected males have mutations that result in essentially no enzymatic activity, whereas patients with the Type 2 Later-Onset phenotype have mutations that retain low levels of residual enzyme activity. There are no common *GLA* mutations, and most *GLA* gene mutations are private, occurring in only one or a few families. For both phenotypes, the sons of affected males will not have the disease, whereas all daughters will be heterozygotes. For heterozygous females, there is a 50% risk of passing the *GLA* gene mutation onto their children with each pregnancy:

- 50% of sons will be affected and 50% will not inherit the disease
- 50% of daughters will be heterozygotes and 50% will not inherit the disease gene

4. What is the metabolic abnormality in Fabry disease?

The deficient or absent α-Gal A activity results in the accumulation of glycolipids with terminal α-linked galactose molecules. As noted above, the major accumulated glycolipid is GL-3. In addition, galabiosylceramide, the blood group B glycolipid, and lyso-GL-3 accumulate in the lysosomes of various cell types. The major pathology leading to kidney failure results from the glycosphingolipid accumulation in the kidney microvascular endothelial cells, interstitial, mesangial, tubular cells, and particularly in the podocytes. In the Type 2 Later-Onset patients the kidney pathology results primarily from glycolipid accumulation in the podocytes.

5. What are the clinical findings in males with Type 1 Classic and Type 2 Later-Onset Fabry disease?
Clinical manifestations in Type 1 Classically affected males begin in childhood or adolescence. Most often, the first symptoms are painful acroparesthesias (especially during febrile illnesses); hypohidrosis; and gastrointestinal symptoms, including postprandial abdominal cramping, bloating, and diarrhea. Small petechial-like angiokeratomas, the classic cutaneous vascular lesions, typically are present in the umbilical and swimsuit regions in childhood. Type 1 Classically affected males also have a distinctive corneal dystrophy observed by slit-lamp microscopy, which does not affect vision. Microvascular involvement of the kidney begins in childhood; progresses to isothenuria, proteinuria, and tubular dysfunction; then, with advancing age, results in progressive kidney disease and ESKD typically by age 35 to 45 years. Dialysis and kidney transplantation are effective in correcting the kidney disease, and kidney transplants are not affected by the disease. All potential family donors should be evaluated to ensure that they are not affected or heterozygotes.

Other manifestations include lower extremity edema in the absence of significant kidney disease, hypoproteinemia, or varices; the lymphedema results from the accumulation of GL-3 in the lymphatic vessels and nodes. Cardiac manifestations include arrhythmias (initially sinus bradycardia), valvular abnormalities, and left ventricular hypertrophy, which may lead to hypertrophic cardiomyopathy. Cerebrovascular disease manifests as transient ischemic attacks and stroke; the strokes often result from the cardiac arrhythmias. Progressive high-frequency hearing loss occurs in Type 1 Classically affected males in the third to fifth decades of life.

In contrast, males with the Type 2 Later-Onset phenotype lack the microvascular endothelial glycolipid deposition that leads to the early manifestations in Type 1 Classic males. Type 2 males develop renal disease and/or heart disease in their third decade of life, or later. The renal disease is characterized by increasing proteinuria due to progressive podocyte glycolipid accumulation, and can progress to renal failure. The heart disease is characterized by progressive cardiomyocyte glycolipid accumulation and typically results in the development of left ventricular hypertrophy (LVH) leading to hypertrophic cardiomyopathy (HCM). Type 2 males also may develop transient ischemic attacks (TIA) and strokes primarily due to cardiac arrhythmias.

6. What are the clinical findings in female heterozygotes with Fabry disease?
The clinical manifestations in heterozygous females from Type 1 Classically affected families range from as severely affected as males to asymptomatic throughout life. The variation in manifestations is primarily a result of random X-chromosomal inactivation. Kidney manifestations in heterozygotes can include isosthenuria, proteinuria, and the presence of leukocytes, erythrocytes, and hyaline and granular casts in the urinary sediment. Approximately 15% of heterozygotes will progress to ESKD, according to US and European registry data. Cardiac involvement, transient ischemic attacks, and strokes may occur in older heterozygotes. Heterozygotes from Type 2 Later-Onset families typically are asymptomatic for decades, but can develop kidney, cardiac, or cerebrovascular disease later in life.

7. What is the "kidney variant" of Fabry disease?
The screening of patients undergoing hemodialysis by determining their plasma α-Gal A activity revealed that about 0.04% to 1.7% of males had unrecognized Fabry disease. Most of these males lacked the acroparesthesias, angiokeratomas, hypohidrosis, and corneal opacities that typically brought Type 1 Classically affected males to medical attention. In contrast, 41% of the hemodialysis patients had the Type 2 Later-Onset phenotype with *GLA* missense or alternative splicing mutations both encoding residual α-Gal A activity. These Type 2 Later-Onset males presented with kidney manifestations as early as the third or fourth decades of life. They were originally called "Kidney Variants," but they also may have cardiac involvement, typically left ventricular hypertrophy. These patients are now more correctly designated as having the Type 2 Later-Onset phenotype.

8. What other abnormalities may be associated with Fabry disease?
Pulmonary involvement can manifest as dyspnea and wheezing, and pulmonary function tests may reveal an obstructive pattern. Most Type 1 Classically affected males and older heterozygotes may have tinnitus, bilateral hearing loss, and/or vertigo. Depression, anxiety, and fatigue are also seen in affected individuals.

9. **What are the characteristic kidney biopsy findings in Fabry disease?**
   In patients with the Type 1 Classic Phenotype, chronic kidney disease is due to GL-3 accumulation primarily in the microvascular endothelium and podocytes. The typical concentric lamellar lysosomal inclusions, which appear like "onion skin" or "zebra bodies," are best seen by electron microscopy. They also can be seen histologically as foamy periodic acid–Schiff positive inclusions on frozen sections. The podocytopathy causes proteinuria. To a lesser extent, and in later stages of disease, the proximal tubules, histiocytes, mesangial, and interstitial cells all develop glycolipid accumulation. Lipid-laden distal tubular epithelial cells and podocytes desquamate and can be detected by urine microscopy. Nonspecific pathologic changes such as arteriolar sclerosis, glomerular atrophy and fibrosis, tubular atrophy, and diffuse fibrosis can be seen in the later stages of disease. Biopsies early in the disease course will show histologically the foamy inclusions in most cell types, and early podocyte effacement is an important sign of kidney disease requiring treatment. The histology of the ESKD is not diagnostic, and electron microscopy is needed to visualize the characteristic lamellar cytoplasmic inclusions in the kidney lysosomes.
   Of note, kidney glycosphingolipid accumulation in Type 2 Later-Onset males occurs primarily in the podocytes with little involvement of the glomerular vascular endothelial, interstitial, or mesangial cells.

10. **What treatment is available for Fabry disease?**
    Enzyme replacement therapy (ERT) has been shown to be safe and effective treatment for Fabry disease. Two preparations are available: agalsidase-alfa (Replagal; Shire Pharmaceuticals, Lexington, MA) and agalsidase-beta (Fabrazyme; Genzyme Corp., Cambridge, MA). Only agalsidase-beta is US Food and Drug Administration approved and commercially available in the United States. Agalsidase-beta delivered intravenously at 1 mg/kg every 2 weeks has been shown in randomized, double-blind, placebo-controlled, clinical trials to clear the accumulated glycolipids from interstitial capillary endothelial cells of the kidney and to stabilize the estimated glomerular filtration rate. ERT with agalsidase-beta also cleared the GL-3 from the vascular endothelial cells in the heart and skin. A phase IV randomized, double-blind, placebo-controlled study in advanced patients with Fabry disease with mild to moderate kidney insufficiency demonstrated that agalsidase-beta slowed the progression of kidney dysfunction. Subsequent studies have shown that the addition of angiotensin-converting enzyme inhibitors or angiotensin II receptor blockade augments the kidney protective effects of enzyme replacement. Studies have compared the effect of dose in patients with Type 1 Classic disease.

11. **When should ERT be started, and what are the risks?**
    Published guidelines suggest that ERT be initiated at the time of diagnosis in males older than 16 years and at the onset of significant symptoms in males younger than 16 years, and should be considered in asymptomatic males between the ages of 10 and 13 years. ERT is considered safe for use in children based on a pediatric trial. ERT should be started in heterozygous females with clinical symptoms or when there is evidence of organ involvement (i.e., proteinuria, cardiac dysfunction). ERT has been associated with infusion-related reactions for which pre-medication with an antipyretic and antihistamine is recommended. Type 1 Classically affected males typically develop IgG antibodies to ERT, and the titers tend to decrease with continued treatment. These antibodies may be neutralizing but have not affected efficacy based on kidney biopsies after 5 years of treatment.

KEY POINTS

1. Patients undergoing hemodialysis may have unrecognized Fabry disease, a treatable X-linked kidney disease. The plasma α-galactosidase A (α-Gal A) assay reliably diagnoses affected males but not heterozygous females, who require mutation analysis for accurate diagnosis.
2. Enzyme replacement therapy in Fabry disease can clear the kidney glycolipid accumulation and stabilize kidney function; early treatment and adequate dose (1 mg/kg every other week) are important.
3. Females in families with X-linked Fabry disease can develop proteinuria and kidney failure.
4. The differential diagnosis of postpartum proteinuria should include Fabry disease.
5. Males undergoing hemodialysis can be screened for Fabry disease by identifying those with deficient plasma α-Gal A activity, and then confirming the diagnosis by mutation analyses. At-risk family members can then be diagnosed for genetic counseling, medical evaluations, and early therapeutic intervention.

BIBLIOGRAPHY

Banikazemi, M., Bultas, J., Waldek, S., Wilcox, W. R., Whitley, C. B., McDonald, M., ... Fabry Disease Clinical Trial Study Group. (2007). Agalsidase-beta therapy for advanced Fabry disease: A randomized trial. *Annals of Internal Medicine, 146*, 77–86.

Desnick, R. J., Ioannou, Y. A., & Eng, C. M. (2014). Galactosidase A deficiency: Fabry disease. In D. Valle, A. L. Beaudet, B. Vogelstein, K. W. Kinzler, S. E. Antonarakis, A. Ballabio, ... G, Mitchell (Eds.), *The online metabolic and molecular bases of inherited disease.* New York: McGraw-Hill. http://ommbid.mhmedical. com/content.aspx?bookid=971&Sectionid=62644837.

Eng, C. M. Germain, D. P., Banikazemi, M., Warnock, D. G., Wanner, C., Hopkin, R. J., ... Wilcox, W. R. (2006). Fabry disease: Guidelines for the evaluation and management of multi-organ system involvement. *Genetics in Medicine, 8*, 539–548.

Eng, C. M., Guffon, N., Wilcox, W. R., Germain, D. P., Lee, P., Waldek, S., ... International Collaborative Fabry Disease Study Group. (2001). Safety and efficacy of recombinant human alpha-Galactosidase A replacement therapy in Fabry's disease. *New England Journal of Medicine, 345*, 9–16.

Germain, D. P., Charrow, J., Desnick, R. J., Guffon, N., Kempf, J., Lachmann, R. H., ... Wilcox, W. R. (2015). Ten-year outcome of enzyme replacement therapy with agalsidase beta in patients with Fabry disease. *Journal of Medical Genetics, 52*, 353–358.

Germain, D. P., Waldek, S., Banikazemi, M., Bushinsky, D. A., Charrow, J., Desnick, R. J., ... Guffon, N. (2007). Sustained, long-term renal stabilization after 54 months of agalsidase beta therapy in patients with Fabry disease. *Journal of the American Society of Nephrology, 18*, 1547–1557.

Hwu, W. L., Chien, Y. H., Lee, N. C., Chiang, S. C., Dobrovolny, R., Huang, A. C., ... Hsu, L. W. (2009). Newborn screening for Fabry disease in Taiwan reveals a high incidence of the Later-Onset GLA mutation c.936 + 919G > A (IVS4 + 919G > A). *Human Mutation, 30*, 1397–1405.

Linthorst, G. E., Bouwman, M. G., Wijburg, F. A., Aerts, J. M., Poorthuis, B. J., & Hollak, C. E. (2010). Screening for Fabry disease in high risk populations: A systematic review. *Journal of Medical Genetics, 47*, 217–222.

Nakao, S., Kodama, C., Takenaka, T., Tanaka, A., Yasumoto, Y., Yoshida, A., ... Desnick, R. J. (2003). Fabry disease: Detection of undiagnosed hemodialysis patients and identification of a "renal variant" phenotype. *Kidney International, 64*, 801–807.

Spada, M., Pagliardini, S., Yasuda, M., Tukel, T., Thiagarajan, G., Sakuraba, H., ... Desnick, R. J. (2006). High incidence of Later-Onset Fabry disease revealed by newborn screening. *American Journal of Human Genetics, 79*, 31–40.

Tøndel, C., Bostad, L., Larsen, K. K., Hirth, A., Vikse, B. E., Houge, G., & Svarstad, E. (2013). Agalsidase benefits renal histology in young patients with Fabry disease. *Journal of the American Society of Nephrology, 24*, 137–148.

Tøndel, C., Kanai, T., Larsen, K. K., Ito, S., Politei, J. M., Warnock, D. G., & Svarstad, E. (2015). Foot process effacement is an early marker of nephropathy in young classic Fabry patients without albuminuria. *Nephron, 129*, 16–21.

Wraith, J. E., Tylki-Szymanska, A., Guffon, N., Lien, Y. H., Tsimaratos, M., Vellodi, A., & Germain, D. P. (2008). Safety and efficacy of enzyme replacement therapy with agalsidase beta: An international open-label study in pediatric patients with Fabry disease. *Journal of Pediatrics, 152*, 563–570.

CYSTIC DISEASES OF THE KIDNEYS

Maria V. Irazabal and Vicente E. Torres

CHAPTER 43

1. **What are cystic diseases of the kidneys?**
   Cystic diseases of the kidney are a heterogeneous group of disorders that can be inherited, developmental, or acquired (Box 43.1).
   Kidney cysts are fluid-filled cavities lined by epithelial cells that derive primarily from the tubules or collecting duct, losing its connection with their origin tubule once developed. Various imaging techniques can identify kidney cysts, which, depending on their characteristics and distribution and together with clinical and genetic information on the patient, can aid in the differential diagnosis (Fig. 43.1). In some the kidney cysts are the prominent abnormality, whereas in others the cysts are part of a more complex phenotype.

2. **Which kidney cystic diseases are the most common ones?**
   Acquired simple kidney cysts are the most common abnormality and can be single or multiple. They are rare in children and individuals less than 30 years old, but the frequency increases with age.
   Among the inherited cystic diseases, autosomal dominant polycystic kidney disease (ADPKD) is the most frequent one followed by autosomal recessive polycystic kidney disease (ARPKD).

3. **What are the genetic features of ADPKD?**
   ADPKD is a genetically heterogeneous disease, for which two different genes have been identified. *PKD1*, located on the short arm of chromosome 16, is responsible for approximately 85% of the cases in which a mutation has been identified, whereas *PKD2*, located on chromosome 4, accounts for nearly 15% of remaining cases with an identified mutation. *PKD1* and *PKD2* encode for polycystin-1 and polycystin-2, respectively. These membrane-bound glycoproteins are located in the plasma membrane of the primary cilia and regulate calcium homeostasis. PKD1 is associated with more

---

Box 43.1. Classification of Cystic Kidney Diseases

Autosomal dominant polycystic kidney disease (ADPKD)
Autosomal recessive polycystic kidney disease
Autosomal dominant or X-linked diseases in the
differential diagnosis of ADPKD
• Tuberous sclerosis complex
• von Hippel-Lindau syndrome
• Hepatocyte nuclear factor-1 associated nephropathy
• Familial renal hamartomas associated with
hyperparathyroidism–jaw tumor syndrome
• Orofaciodigital syndrome
Autosomal dominant medullary cystic kidney disease
(autosomal dominant tubulointerstitial kidney disease)
Hereditary recessive ciliopathies with interstitial
nephritis and/or cysts
• Nephronophthisis
• Joubert syndrome
• Meckel-Gruber syndrome
• Bardet-Biedl syndrome
• Alström syndrome

• Nephronophthisis variants associated with skeletal
defects
Renal cystic dysplasias
• Multicystic kidney dysplasia
Other cystic kidney disorders
• Simple cysts
• Localized or unilateral renal cystic disease
• Medullary sponge kidney
• Acquired cystic kidney disease
Renal cystic neoplasms
• Cystic renal cell carcinoma
• Multilocular cystic nephroma
• Cystic partially differentiated nephroblastoma
• Mixed epithelial and stromal tumor
Cysts not of tubular origin
• Cystic disease of the renal sinus
• Perirenal lymphangiomas
• Subcapsular and perirenal urinomas
Pyelocalyceal cysts

Modified from Torres, V. E., & Harris, P. C. (2016). Cystic diseases of the kidney. In B. M. Brenner (Ed.), *The kidney* (10th ed.). Philadelphia: W. B. Saunders.

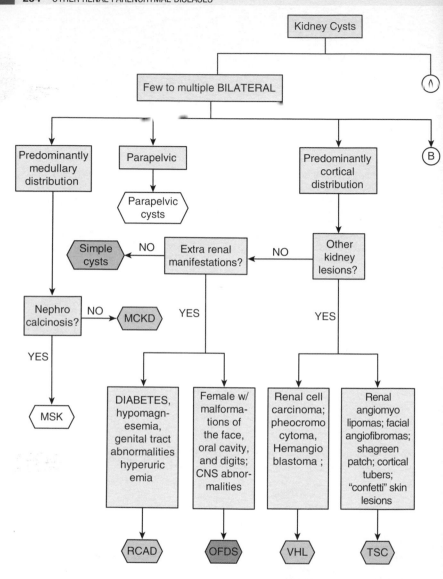

Figure 43.1. Algorithm diagnosis of cystic diseases of the kidney based on imaging characteristics, clinical presentation, and pattern of inheritance. *(Reproduced from Kim, B., King, B. F., Jr., Vrtiska, T. J., Irazabal, M. V., Torres, V. E., & Harris, P. C. (2016). Inherited renal cystic diseases. Abdom Radiol (NY), 41, 1035–1051, with permission of Springer.)*

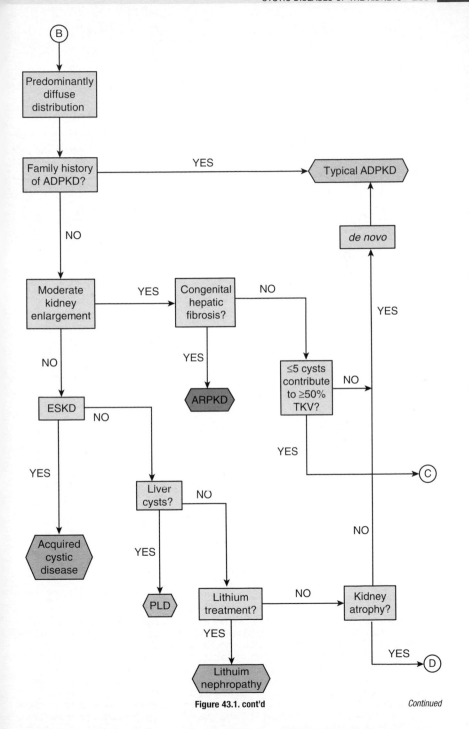

Figure 43.1. cont'd

Continued

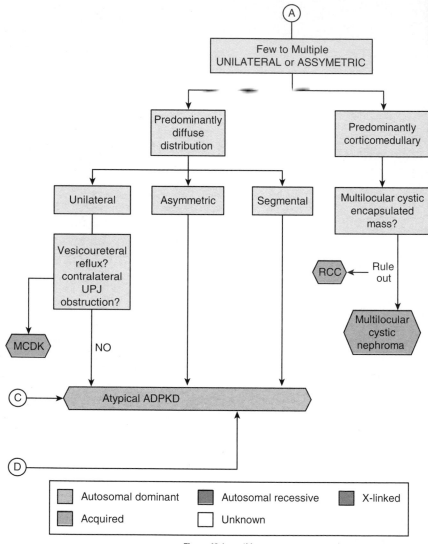

Figure 43.1. cont'd

severe disease compared with PDK2. This is due to the fact that patients with PKD1 develop more cysts at an early age rather than faster cyst growth. There have been hundreds of different pathogenic mutations identified in *PKD1* and *PKD2*. It is thought that kidney cysts may develop from loss of functional polycystin with somatic inactivation of the normal allele consistent with a "two-hit" mechanism, but other genetic mechanisms may play a role. Between 7% and 10% of ADPKD cases remain genetically unresolved after genetic screening. Data suggest that mutations in *GANAB*, a coding gene that encodes for a glucosidase-II alpha subunit, may account for approximately 3% of the genetically unresolved ADPKD cases. However, due to the mild phenotype presentation of patients with mutations in *GANAB*, it is possible that this account for a larger proportion of the missing genetic causes of ADPKD and may be underdiagnosed.

4. How is ADPKD diagnosed?

In patients older than 18 years with a family history of ADPKD, the diagnosis is primarily established by imaging studies. Patient counseling should always be done before performing imaging studies. Ultrasound is commonly used because it is noninvasive and inexpensive. Diagnostic criteria for ADPKD by ultrasound are summarized in Table 43.1. There are no preestablished diagnostic criteria for computed tomography (CT) or magnetic resonance imaging (MRI), but ultrasound criteria could reasonably be applied to CT or MRI if restricted to cysts measuring ≥1 cm in diameter. Contrast-enhanced CT and MRI provide better anatomic definition than ultrasonography and are more helpful to ascertain the severity and prognosis of the disease. In addition, both techniques are used to better characterize cystic lesions and complications. MRI is the preferred imaging modality for following disease progression in these patients. It provides great cystic-parenchyma definition without requiring intravenous (IV) contrast. CT with contrast is also highly sensitive (detects cysts as small as 3 mm), and both techniques may provide useful information regarding extrarenal manifestations of the disease (liver, pancreas, spleen, and other organs). CT with contrast should be avoided if there is evidence of significant risk of contrast nephropathy (see Chapter 13). CT (with and without contrast) is also helpful in assessing and identifying complications, such as nephrolithiasis, complex cysts, or cyst wall calcifications from old cyst hemorrhage. Kidneys, ureter, and bladder scan and tomograms may be helpful to differentiate uric acid stones from calcium stones, whereas dual energy computed tomography may help discriminate uric acid stones from other kidney stones. Indium 111 (^{111}In) scans may be useful to identify infected kidney or liver cysts. Likewise, positron emission tomography (PET) scans may identify infected liver cysts.

Genetic testing (linkage analysis and direct DNA sequencing) is available as a clinical test and can detect *PKD1* and *PKD2* mutations in approximately 90% of confirmed cases. The ADPKD Mutation Database (http://pkdb.mayo.edu) lists known mutations of the *PKD1* and *PKD2* genes. Counseling should be done before genetic testing. Evaluation of family history may also provide important clues about the genetic variant, which has prognostic implications. For example, the presence of at least one affected family member who reached end-stage kidney disease (ESKD) at or before 55 years old is highly suggestive of a *PKD1* mutation. Contrarily, the presence of at least one affected family member with either preserved kidney function or ESKD developed after 70 years old is highly indicative of a *PKD2* mutation. Lastly, in patients with multiple bilateral cysts (10 or more per kidney) but negative family history, a presumptive diagnosis of ADPKD may be considered.

Table 43.1. Ultrasound Criteria for the Diagnosis of Autosomal Dominant Polycystic Kidney Disease

	CRITERIA	PKD1	PKD2	UNKNOWN ADPKD GENE TYPE
Revised Unified Diagnostic Criteria for ADPKD				
15–29	≥3 cysts, unilateral or bilateral	SEN = 94.3%	SEN = 69.5%	SEN = 81.7%
30–39	≥3 cysts, unilateral or bilateral	SEN = 96.6%	SEN = 94.9%	SEN = 95.5%
40–59	≥2 cysts in each kidney	SEN = 92.6%	SEN = 88.8%	SEN = 90%
>60	≥4 cysts, in each kidney	SEN = 100%	SEN = 100%	SEN = 100%
Revised Ultrasound Criteria for Exclusion of ADPKD				
15–29	≥1 cyst	SPEC = 97.6%	SPEC = 96.6%	SPEC = 97.1%
30–39	≥1 cyst	SPEC = 96.0%	SPEC = 93.8%	SPEC = 94.8%
40–59	≥2 cyst	SPEC = 98.4%	SPEC = 97.8%	SPEC = 98.2%

Note: These criteria if applied to magnetic resonance imaging or computed tomography will result in false-positive diagnoses.
ADPKD, Autosomal dominant polycystic kidney disease; PKD, polycystic kidney disease; SEN, sensitivity; SPEC, specificity.

5. Can we rule out ADPKD in individuals with normal kidney ultrasounds?
   No, because the utility of ultrasound to exclude ADPKD is limited in individuals under 30 years old with a family history of the disease, particularly those with *PKD2* mutations. In these individuals, MRI, CT, or genetic testing should be considered. Nevertheless, most ADPKD cases can be confirmed or ruled out on imaging testing. Furthermore, a study has shown that fewer than five kidney cysts on MRI are sufficient for excluding ADPKD in at-risk subjects between 16 and 40 years of age.

6. Which are the most common extrarenal manifestations of ADPKD?
   Besides kidney cysts, patients with ADPKD frequently present extrarenal disease, including hepatic cysts, cysts in other organs, cardiovascular manifestations, diverticular disease, and abdominal hernias.

   Polycystic liver disease (PLD) is the most common extrarenal manifestation of ADPKD and is characterized by multiple cysts distributed throughout the liver parenchyma. Hepatic cysts are commonly seen in patients with ADPKD, and their prevalence is as high as 90% on screening MRI. In a minority of patients, it can result in severe PLD requiring surgical intervention. The disease is usually found in association with ADPKD but can occur in isolation, with only a small number of kidney cysts (or even the total absence of cysts). Mutations in protein kinase C substrate 80K-H (PRKCSH) gene on chromosome 19p13 and SEC63 homologue, protein translocation regulator on chromosome 6q, account for more than 30% of isolated cases. Although most patients remain asymptomatic with preserved liver function, abdominal pain, distension, and liver decompensation may occur due to compressive effects of enlarged cysts.

   Pancreatic cysts have been found in approximately 10% of patients with ADPKD. These are more prevalent with increasing age. Pancreatic cysts are nearly always asymptomatic, but in very rare occasions, cyst compression of the main pancreatic duct may cause recurrent pancreatitis. In addition, a few cases of combined ADPKD and pancreatic carcinoma have been reported, suggesting genetic interactions between ADPKD and pancreatic carcinogenesis. Asymptomatic arachnoid membrane cysts and spinal meningeal cysts have been reported in a small proportion of patients with ADPKD (8% and 2%, respectively). Arachnoid membrane cysts can increase the risk of subdural hematomas, and spinal meningeal cysts can leak and present with orthostatic headache due to intracranial hypotension.

   Ovarian cysts are not associated with ADPKD, whereas cysts of the seminal vesicles occur in 40% to 60% of men with ADPKD but rarely result in infertility.

   Vascular manifestations are the most important noncystic complications and include intracranial aneurysms (IAs), dolichoectasias, thoracic aortic and cervicocephalic artery dissections, and coronary artery aneurysms. They are caused by alterations in the vasculature directly linked to mutations in *PKD1* or *PKD2*. Polycystin-1 and polycystin-2 are known to be expressed in vascular smooth muscle cells. IAs represent the most feared vascular manifestation of ADPKD because their rupture carries a 35% to 55% risk of combined severe morbidity and mortality. The rate of IA in ADPKD patients ranges from 6% (negative family history of IA) to 16% (positive family history of IA), approximately five times more common than in the general population (1% to 2%). They are often asymptomatic (Irazabal et al., 2015). However, focal findings such as cranial nerve palsy or seizure may result from compression of local structures.

   Cardiac valvular abnormalities are common in patients with ADPKD. Mitral valve prolapse is the most frequent valvular abnormality found in up to 25% of patients on echocardiography, whereas aortic regurgitation and tricuspid prolapse may occur in a small proportion. Nevertheless, they rarely require valve replacement, and screening echocardiography is not indicated unless a cardiac murmur is detected on clinical examination.

   The prevalence of colonic diverticulosis and diverticulitis in patients with ESKD with ADPKD is significantly higher than in individuals with other kidney diseases (83% vs. 32%). However, whether ADPKD patients with preserved kidney function show propensity for diverticular disease remains unknown. The mechanisms implicated in the development of colonic diverticula may include alterations in polycystin function, which can exacerbate aging-induced smooth muscle dysfunction.

   Abdominal hernias (inguinal, incisional, and paraumbilical) are frequent in the ADPKD population. Importantly, hernias are associated with complications (intestinal incarceration or strangulation) and may cause problems in patients undergoing peritoneal dialysis.

7. What are the most frequent complications of ADPKD?
   - *Hypertension:* The majority of patients with ADPKD present with abnormal blood pressure levels. Studies have shown that hypertension is diagnosed 15 years earlier in ADPKD patients compared

with those with essential hypertension. Indeed, the prevalence of hypertension reaches 50% in patients aged 20 to 30 years, representing the initial presentation for 30% of ADPKD patients, but increases to 100% of those with ESKD.

- The pathogenesis of hypertension in ADPKD is complex, and the most plausible hypotheses include activation of the renin-angiotensin-aldosterone system, cyst expansion, intrarenal ischemia, and decreased expression levels of polycystin-1 and 2, and nitric oxide (NO) availability. Importantly, uncontrolled blood pressure is associated with increased mortality rates from valvular heart disease and aneurysms, increases the risk of proteinuria and hematuria, and increases speed of decline of kidney function. Therefore earlier detection and treatment of hypertension and more rigorous blood pressure control are important on these patients.
- *Pain:* Approximately 60% of patients with ADPKD suffer from pain, the most common symptom reported by adults with ADPKD. Pain is most commonly located in the flank, back, and abdomen and is primarily attributed to cystic compression of the kidney capsule and parenchyma, but it can also be caused by hemorrhage into a cyst, cyst rupture, or infection. Importantly, kidney stones or tumor should be always ruled out. Acute causes of kidney pain include renal hemorrhage, passage of stones, and urinary tract infections (UTIs). Cyst hemorrhages often resolve within a week, but if it is prolonged or if the initial episode occurs after the age of 50 years, screening to exclude neoplasm should be done. Although most patients with hepatic cysts are asymptomatic, cystic enlargement of the liver may also cause mechanical back pain.
- *Nephrolithiasis:* Kidney stones occur in 20% to 36% of patients with ADPKD. The most common types of stones are composed of uric acid or calcium oxalate. Metabolic factors such as low urine citrate and urine pH, and decreased ammonia excretion may predispose to stone formation, yet urinary stasis due to distorted kidney anatomy may also prompt stone formation. Abdominal CT before and following contrast enhancement is important to detect renal calculi. Stones may be missed if only a contrast-enhanced CT is performed.
- *Urinary infections:* In ADPKD, UTIs are more frequent in women than in men, as in the general population. UTIs are usually caused by gram-negative enteric bacteria *(Enterobacteriaceae).* Although CT and MRI can detect cyst complications and provide anatomic definition, none of these findings are specific for infection. Alternatively, nuclear imaging with [67]Ga- or ^{111}In-labeled leukocyte scans may be used, but false negative and false positive may occur. An 18-F-fluorodeoxyglucose PET scan is a promising agent for detection of infected cysts. However, its efficacy for diagnosing UTI is limited. When a kidney cyst infection is suspected, delayed images should be obtained. Finally, in the event that the clinical setting and imaging are suggestive of infection, but blood and urine cultures are negative, cyst aspiration should be considered.
- *ESKD:* ADPKD is the leading inheritable cause of ESKD, with 45% of patients with ADPKD developing ESKD by 60 years of age. Men tend to progress faster than women, which may be partly attributed to a greater prevalence and severity of hypertension. There is a strong relationship between kidney volume growth and glomerular filtration rate (GFR) decline.

8. Is there a way to identify disease severity and predict disease progression in patients with ADPKD?

Several factors contribute to kidney function decline. Cyst development is a continuous process that starts in utero and continues through the patient lifetime. The Consortium of Radiologic Imaging Studies of PKD has shown that higher kidney volumes are associated with faster declines in kidney function qualifying as a prognostic biomarker. As a result, total kidney volume (TKV) has been widely used as a primary or secondary end point in clinical trials. However, TKV has limitations as a surrogate marker for disease progression and does not always predict changes in kidney function. TKV is particularly inaccurate in patients with few large cysts or in patients with kidney atrophy secondary to ischemia or urinary tract obstruction. Furthermore, a higher TKV at an earlier age probably indicates a faster kidney growth rate. An imaging classification of ADPKD has been developed to identify patients with various degrees of disease severity and risks for progression to guide in the selection of patients for clinical trials or patients likely to benefit from effective therapies directed to slowing kidney growth. This classification uses CT and MR images and prespecified findings (Table 43.2) to assign patients as:

- Class 1: typical, bilateral diffuse presentation
  - Class 1 is further divided into A to E based on height-adjusted TKV and age.
  - Risk for declining GFR and ESKD increased progressively from class A to class E (Fig. 43.2).
- Class 2: atypical, asymmetric cyst distribution

Table 43.2. Classification of Autosomal Dominant Polycystic Kidney Disease Patients by Prespecified Imaging Findings

CLASS	SUBCLASS	TERM	DESCRIPTION
1 Typical ADPKD			Bilateral and diffuse distribution, with mild, moderate, or severe replacement of kidney tissue by cysts, where all cysts contribute similarly to TKV.
2 Atypical ADPKD	A	Unilateral	Diffuse cystic involvement of one kidney causing marked kidney enlargement with a normal contralateral kidney defined by a normal kidney volume (<275 mL in men; <244 mL in women) and having no or only 1–2 cysts.
		Segmental	Cystic disease involving only one pole of one or both kidneys and sparing the remaining kidney tissue.
		Asymmetric	Diffuse cystic involvement of one kidney causing marked kidney enlargement with mild segmental or minimal diffuse involvement of the contralateral kidney defined by a small number of cysts (i > 2 but <10) and volume accounting for <30% of total kidney volume.
		Lopsided	Bilateral distribution of kidney cysts with mild replacement of kidney tissue with atypical cysts where five cysts or less account for at least 50% TKV.
	B	Bilateral presentation with acquired unilateral atrophy	Diffuse cystic involvement of one kidney causing mod-severe kidney enlargement with contralateral acquired atrophy. (The largest cyst diameter is used to estimate individual cyst volume).
		Bilateral presentation with bilateral kidney atrophy	Impaired kidney function (SCr ≥ 1.5 mg/dL) without significant enlargement of the kidneys, defined by an average length <14.5 cm, and replacement of kidney tissue by cysts with atrophy of the parenchyma.

ADPKD, Autosomal dominant polycystic kidney disease; TKV, total kidney volume.
Reproduced from Irazabal, M. V., Rangel, L. J., Bergstralh, E. J., Osborn, S. L., Harmon, A. J., Sundsbak, J. L., . . . CRISP Investigators. (2015). Imaging classification of autosomal dominant polycystic kidney disease: A simple model for selecting patients for clinical trials. *Journal of the American Society of Nephrology, 26*(1), 160–172 with permission of the Journal of the American Society of Nephrology.

Class 2 includes patients who present with unilateral, segmental, asymmetric, or bilateral atypical presentation (class 2A) but also patients who present with bilateral distribution with acquired unilateral atrophy or bilateral kidney atrophy (class 2B). Patients qualifying as class 2A presented low risk for estimated glomerular filtration rate (eGFR) decline, and patients classified as 2B may not benefit from therapies directed to slowing kidney growth. For prognostic enrichment design in randomized clinical trials, it was proposed to exclude class 1A and 2 and to follow class 1B patients to more precisely define their risk for progression. An online tool to estimate height-adjusted total kidney volume and classify patients with typical ADPKD is available (http://www.mayo.edu/research/documents/pkd-center-adpkd-classification/doc-20094754).

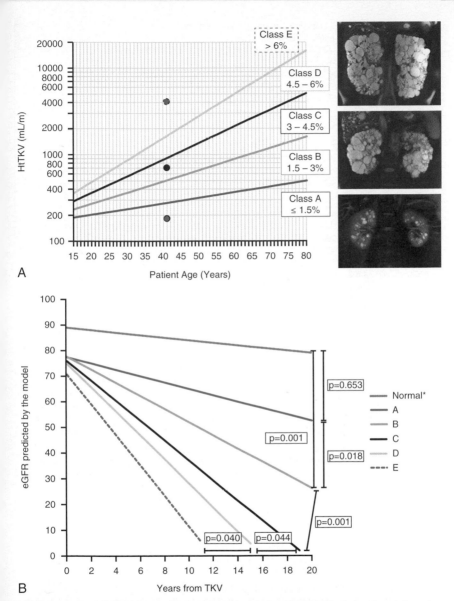

Figure 43.2. Imaging classification identifies groups of disease severity and predicts change in estimated glomerular filtration rate over time in patients with typical autosomal dominant polycystic kidney disease. **(A)** Classification of typical autosomal dominant polycystic kidney disease patients based on height-adjusted total kidney volume (HtTKV) limits for their age, assuming estimated kidney growth rates of 1.5%, 3.0%, 4.5%, and 6.0%, and three patient examples at the same age and their corresponding HtTKV. **(B)** Estimated glomerular filtration rate (eGFR) slopes derived from a longitudinal mixed effect prediction model were significantly different among all class 1 (typical) patients and were all significantly different from a control population of healthy kidney donors, except 1A. *(Reproduced from Irazabal, M. V., Rangel, L. J., Bergstralh, E. J., Osborn, S. L., Harmon, A. J., Sundsbak, J. L., . . . CRISP Investigators. (2015). Imaging classification of autosomal dominant polycystic kidney disease: A simple model for selecting patients for clinical trials. Journal of the American Society of Nephrology, 26(1), 160–172. With permission of the Journal of the American Society of Nephrology.)*

9. **What other prognostic tools besides imaging are available?**
   - The mutated gene *(PKD1 is worse than PKD2)*
   - Type of mutation in PKD1 (truncating mutations are worse than nontruncating)
   - Male sex
   - Diagnosis before the age of 30 years
   - First episode of hematuria before age 30 years
   - Onset of hypertension before age 35 years
   - Hyperlipidemia
   - Low high-density lipoprotein
   - Sickle cell trait

   Prognostic Model to Predict Survival to ESRD in ADPKD scoring system (PRO-PKD score) (ranging from 0 to 9) has been developed on the basis of PKD mutation and clinical parameters. A score of ≤3 has been shown to exclude progression to ESKD before the age of 60 years, and a score >6 predicts ESKD onset before the age of 60 years. The prognosis is uncertain in patients with an intermediate score (4 to 6 points).

10. **What are the most important treatment strategies for ADPKD?**
    Patients with ADPKD should be advised to adopt a healthy lifestyle. Early detection of hypertension, strict blood pressure control (130/80 mm Hg or lower) and low sodium intake (<2 g/day) are recommended because cardiovascular complications remain the most common cause of morbidity and mortality in ADPKD. Antihypertensive therapy with angiotensin-converting enzyme inhibitors or angiotensin II receptor blockers is recommended. Dual blockade (lisinopril-telmisartan), although safe, did not show a benefit, as compared with lisinopril alone, with regard to the change in TKV or eGFR in The Polycystic Kidney Disease Treatment Network (HALT PKD) study. Protein intake should be restricted to 0.8 g/kg of ideal body weight per day. Likewise, a low cholesterol (<200 mg/day) diet is recommended in patients with hypercholesterolemia. Caffeine consumption should also be limited because it may increase cyclic adenosine monophosphate levels.

    Advancements in understanding the pathophysiologic mechanisms responsible for the disease have provided a foundation for the development and testing of potential new therapies. Among them, vasopressin 2 receptor antagonist (tolvaptan) has been the most successful pharmacologic intervention at reducing the rate of TKV increase and kidney function decline in patients with ADPKD. The somatostatin analogues octreotide and lanreotide have shown a reduction in the average rate of TKV growth in the initial 6 or 12 months of treatment. Larger studies with somatostatin analogues are underway. mTOR inhibitors have been effective in slowing or arresting the progression of ADPKD in preclinical models, yet clinical trials in patients with ADPKD have been largely disappointing.

11. **Which antibiotics are indicated for ADPKD patients with UTI?**
    UTIs in ADPKD patients should be treated promptly because they may be complicated with septic shock or perirenal abscess and accelerate its progression to ESKD. Most UTI in patients with ADPKD are caused by *Enterobacteriaceae*. Intravenous antibiotics are needed initially for presentations with sepsis, acute pyelonephritis, or cyst infection, and the choice of antibiotics is dictated by antimicrobial susceptibilities whenever possible. Switching to oral antibiotics with good penetration into the cysts, such as quinolones and trimethoprim-sulfamethoxazole, can be considered after an initial favorable response with resolution of fever and pain. Prolonged antibiotic treatment for several weeks may be needed to eradicate the infection. Complications (e.g., obstruction, cyst infection, or infected stone) need to be excluded if there are relapses after completing antibiotic therapy. Percutaneous or surgical drainage may be required in some cases.

12. **Should patients with ADPKD be screened for IAs?**
    Despite the relatively higher prevalence of IA in patients with ADPKD, widespread screening for IA in asymptomatic patients without personal or family history of IA or subarachnoid hemorrhage (SAH) is not recommended. Presymptomatic screening for IA is specially indicated in patients with family history of IA or SAH or high-risk occupations (e.g., pilots), as well as in those undergoing major surgical procedures (i.e., kidney transplant, liver resection) with risk of hemodynamic instability.

    Magnetic resonance angiography is the gold standard for the screening of IA in patients with ADPKD. However, a thin-cut noncontrast CT is more sensitive than MRI for detecting SAH. Therefore CT should be performed in patients with known ADPKD who present with new-onset or severe headache or other troubling central nervous system symptoms. Other treatable causes of headache (e.g., cervicocephalic artery dissection, subdural hematoma, leaking spinal meningeal diverticulum, or uncontrolled hypertension) should be considered.

13. **Is nephrectomy indicated in ADPKD?**

    Indications for nephrectomy in patients with ADPKD include recurrent and/or severe infection, severe renal hemorrhage, intractable pain, and renal carcinoma. Pretransplant nephrectomy is not usually performed, to avoid the anephric state. Pretransplant nephrectomy should be considered only if an ADPKD kidney is sufficiently enlarged to interfere with the site of implantation of the donor kidney; in the event of frequent, recurrent infection or hemorrhage in the native kidneys; or when solid tumor cannot be ruled out. Hand-assisted laparoscopic nephrectomy is a feasible and safe procedure compared with open nephrectomy, which is associated with significant morbidity and mortality.

14. **Is renal cell carcinoma (RCC) more frequent in patients with ADPKD than in the general population?**

    No, the incidence of RCC is similar in ADPKD compared with the general population. However, patients with ADPKD may develop RCC at an earlier age and have an increased risk for developing sarcomatoid, bilateral, multicentric, and metastatic tumors. MRI and contrast-enhanced CT can be useful in the diagnosis. RCC appears on MRI as solid masses and may present restricted diffusion. On CT, speckled calcifications and contrast enhancement are highly suspicious for RCC. Thrombosis and lymphade-nopathy can be seen in rare cases of RCC. Because of the multiple cysts, some necrotic or cystic RCC can be difficult to detect.

15. **What are the clinical features of ARPKD?**

    ARPKD, an inherited disorder that affects 1 in 20,000 live births, is an important cause of chronic kidney disease in children. The disease commonly presents in neonates; in some individuals it is diagnosed later in life but is rarely diagnosed in adults. Typically, the severity of the kidney and hepatic manifestations is inversely correlated and depends on the age at diagnosis. ARPKD is caused by mutations in the polycystic kidney and hepatic disease 1 *(PKHD1)* gene and is characterized by massively enlarged cystic kidneys, hepatic fibrosis, and pulmonary hypoplasia secondary to oligohydramnios, which may lead to respiratory insufficiency and death in one-third of affected newborns. Although siblings may suffer from ARPKD, the disease does not occur in their parents. More than half of the patients are detected during late pregnancy, and those who are undetected on prenatal evaluation usually survive the perinatal period.

    The liver disease consists of enlargement and fibrosis of portal areas, bile duct proliferation, and hypoplasia of portal vein branches leading to portal hypertension; some patients have non-obstructive intrahepatic bile duct dilatation (Caroli disease). A minority of affected individuals can present for the first time as older children or adolescents, usually with manifestations of portal hypertension as a result of congenital hepatic fibrosis (CHF) (gastrointestinal bleeding from varices, hepatosplenomegaly, or hypersplenism) or episodes of cholangitis resulting from Caroli disease. ARPKD is rarely diagnosed in adults. Genetic testing for ARPKD is available, with a mutation detection rate of approximately 95%. All reported associated gene mutations are archived in the ARPKD mutation public database.

16. **Can we clinically distinguish ADPKD from ARPKD?**

    Besides their different inheritance pattern, ADPKD and ARPKD exhibit important clinical differences. Despite cyst development starting in utero, ADPKD is typically an adult-onset disease. The disease is characterized by progressive bilateral cystic development and enlargement of the kidneys. GFR is preserved for many decades until it starts declining rapidly (4.4 to 5.9 mL/min/m^2 per year). The mean age of onset of ESKD is 59 years, but approximately 15% of patients present with normal kidney function by the age of 80 years. In a small number of patients, ADPKD may present as very-early-onset disease with kidney enlargement in children younger than 18 months of age. In this setting, ADPKD may be confused with ARPKD. Unlike ADPKD, ARPKD typically presents in the neonatal period with enlarged echogenic kidneys with loss of corticomedullary differentiation on ultrasound. Clinically, ARPKD presents with nephromegaly, hypertension, and CKD. The kidney enlargement is characterized by fusiform dilatation of the collecting ducts and may be associated with renal calcifications. More than 50% of them progress to ESKD within the first 10 years of life. Liver involvement is characterized by hepatomegaly and CHF.

17. **What is medullary cystic kidney disease (MCKD)?**

    Autosomal dominant tubulointerstitial kidney disease, also known as MCKD, is a new term that has been proposed for a group of diseases with an autosomal dominant pattern of inheritance, character-ized by small to normal size kidneys, cysts primarily located at the corticomedullary junction, associ-ated with irregular thickening of the tubular basement membrane, tubular atrophy, and interstitial fibrosis. The disease is caused by mutations in at least four genes: *MUC1* (chromosome 1q22) encoding mucin-1, *UMOD* (chromosome 16p12.3) encoding uromodulin, *HNF1β* (chromosome 17q12) encoding hepatocyte nuclear factor-1b, *REN* (chromosome 1q32.1) encoding renin.

Clinical presenting symptoms include polydipsia and polyuria, low-grade proteinuria, benign urine sediment, and subsequent development of CKD. These patients are commonly diagnosed and develop ESKD at a later age compared with those with nephronophthisis (NPHP). In addition, MCKD patients do not have extrarenal involvement, with the exception of gout. A history of gout at an early age or a strong family history of gout is suggestive of mutations in *UMOD*, whereas a history of anemia in childhood and mildly elevated serum potassium concentrations is suggestive of mutations in *REN*. If none of the preceding clinical characteristics is present, *MUC1* molecular genetic testing should be considered.

Kidney transplantation is the preferred treatment for MCKD-induced ESKD. Exhaustive diagnostic evaluation should be performed in living related donors.

18. **What are the main characteristics of the tuberous sclerosis complex (TSC)?**
TSC is an inherited disorder that affects 1:6000 newborns and is characterized by the potential for hamartoma formation in several organs, including the brain, heart, skin, eyes, kidney, lungs, liver, and gastrointestinal tract. Its inheritance is autosomal dominant with almost complete penetrance and is caused by mutations in the *TSC1* (chromosome 9q34) or *TSC2* (chromosome 16p13.3) genes, which encode the tumor suppressor proteins hamartin and tuberin, respectively. *TSC2* and *PKD1* genes are in close relationship and lie adjacent to each other on chromosome 16 at 16p13.3. Deletions inactivating *TSC2* and *PKD1* are associated with polycystic kidneys diagnosed during the first year of life or early childhood, also known as *TSC2/PKD1* contiguous gene syndrome. Therefore TSC should be considered in children with kidney cysts and no family history of PKD.

A definite diagnosis of TSC includes at least two major features (renal angiomyolipoma [AML], facial angiofibromas or forehead plaques, nontraumatic ungual or periungual fibroma, three or more hypomelanotic macules, shagreen patch, multiple retinal nodular hamartomas, cortical tuber, subependymal nodule, subependymal giant cell astrocytoma, cardiac rhabdomyoma, lymphangioleiomyomatosis) or one major feature plus two minor features (multiple kidney cysts, nonrenal hamartoma, hamartomatous rectal polyps, retinal achromic patch, cerebral white matter radial migration tracts, bone cysts, gingival fibromas, "confetti" skin lesions, multiple enamel pits).

Kidney manifestations, present in 50% to 80% of patients, include multiple AMLs, kidney cysts, and rarely (2% to 3%) RCCs. AMLs are the most common benign tumors of the kidney and are composed of abnormal vessels, immature smooth muscle cells, and fat cells. These tumors are the second most common cause of retroperitoneal hemorrhage, and they may also cause clinical problems secondary to compression and replacement of kidney tissue, leading to ESKD. Patients suffering from contiguous gene syndrome commonly develop ESKD at an earlier age compared with those with ADPKD alone. Genetic testing for *TSC1* and *TSC2* is clinically available.

19. **What are the clinical features of von Hippel-Lindau (VHL) disease?**
VHL disease is a rare autosomal dominant syndrome that affects 1:30,000 to 1:50,000 live births and is associated with germline mutations in the VHL tumor suppressor gene, located on the short arm of chromosome 3 (3p25-26). Clinical features include hemangioblastomas in the retina, brain, and spine, tumors of the endolymphatic sac, pheochromocytomas, and pancreatic cysts. In the kidney, VHL presents with multiple, bilateral, clear cell–lined cysts in 70% to 80% and multifocal and bilateral renal clear cell carcinoma in 40% to 60% of patients. Genetic testing for VHL is available as a clinical test.

20. **What is a medullary sponge kidney (MSK)?**
MSK is a disorder characterized by dilated collecting ducts (precalyceal ducts) that may or may not contain calculi and/or nephrocalcinosis, and classic "papillary blush" or "paint brush" linear striations on intravenous urography (IVU) or CT urography. This characteristic appearance is the result of pooling contrast material within dilated collecting ducts in the tips of the renal papilla.

Although the prevalence in the general population is unknown, it is well represented among kidney stone patients (12% to 20% of calcium stone formers). MSK is incidentally diagnosed when IVU is performed for flank pain or indications other than renal colic. It can be seen in 1 in every 200 IVUfs and is more frequent in women than men. Because conventional CT has almost completely replaced IVU, the diagnosis of MSK may now be made less often since the finding of medullary nephrocalcinosis on CT are suggestive, but is not diagnostic, of MSK. A multidetector-row CT using high-resolution three-dimensional volume rendering late urographic images is required for a diagnosis of MSK by CT.

The disease may affect one, both, or only portions of the kidneys and is characterized by dilation (3 to 8 mm) of medullary collecting ducts, which in 50% of patients contain calcium deposits or stones and is the most common presentation of this disease. However, usually patients with MSK are asymptomatic and therefore remain undiagnosed for life. Other associated symptoms include macro-hematuria and microhematuria and UTI.

21. **What is acquired renal cystic disease (ARCD)?**
ARCD is a noninherited condition characterized by multiple small cysts (three or more per kidney) filled with serous fluid distributed throughout the renal parenchyma of patients with ESKD. Therefore family and clinical history are often helpful for distinguishing ARCD from ADPKD. The prevalence of ARCD varies as a function of serum creatinine levels, being 7% to 22% in patients with CKD and serum creatinine greater than 3 mg/dL, 35% in patients with less than 2 years of dialysis, 58% with 2 to 4 years, 75% with 4 to 8 years, and 92% in those undergoing dialysis for 8 or more years.

ARCD usually affects both kidneys equally, and the affected kidneys are typically small (<100 g), although a few exceptional cases may growth resembling ADPKD. Most patients with ARCD are asymptomatic, but hemorrhage may occur. Cysts often regress after kidney transplantation but may occasionally develop in chronically rejected kidneys. Importantly, patients with ESKD and ARCD have 50-times higher risk of developing RCC during dialysis or after kidney transplantation compared with the general population. Risk factors for coexisting ARCD and RCC in ESKD patients include uremic toxins (p-cresol), ischemia, viral infections, tubular obstruction, and increased secretion of parathyroid hormone and growth factors. Carcinomas in patients undergoing dialysis are three times more common in the presence than in the absence of ARCD, and it is six times more common in large cystic kidneys than in small cystic kidneys. Therefore ultrasonography or MRI screening has been recommended after 3 years of dialysis, followed by screening for neoplasm at 1- or 2-year intervals thereafter.

KEY POINTS

1. Cystic diseases of the kidney are a heterogeneous group of disorders with different origins. The presence of multiple bilateral kidney cysts should raise suspicion of inherited kidney cystic disease.
2. Most of the time the differential diagnosis of cystic diseases can be made based on clinical presentation, family history, and imaging studies; genetic testing can be helpful in equivocal cases.
3. ADPKD, the most common inherited cystic disease of the kidney, is a multisystem disease characterized by the progressive development of bilateral kidney cysts but can additionally present with a wide variety of extrarenal manifestations that need to be recognized.
4. Patients with ADPKD present with large phenotypic variability due to heterogeneity at the gene (*PKD1* and *PKD2*) and mutation level but also genetic and environmental modifying factors.
5. The vasopressin 2 receptor antagonist tolvaptan has been the most successful pharmacologic intervention thus far at reducing the rate of TKV increase and kidney function decline in patients with ADPKD.

BIBLIOGRAPHY

Chapman, A. B., Bost, J. E., Torres, V. E., Guay-Woodford, L., Bae, K. T., Landsittel, D., . . . Grantham, J. J. (2012). Kidney volume and functional outcomes in autosomal dominant polycystic kidney disease. *Clinical Journal of the American Society of Nephrology, 7*(3), 479–486.
Cornec-Le Gall, E., Audrezet, M. P., Rousseau, A., Hourmant, M., Renaudineau, E., Charasse, C., . . . Le Meur Y. (2016). The PROPKD score: A new algorithm to predict renal survival in autosomal dominant polycystic kidney disease. *Journal of the American Society of Nephrology, 27*(3), 942–951.
Irazabal, M. V., Huston, J., 3rd, Kubly, V., Rossetti, S., Sundsbak, J. L., Hogan, M. C., . . . Torres V. E. (2011). Extended follow-up of unruptured intracranial aneurysms detected by presymptomatic screening in patients with autosomal dominant polycystic kidney disease. *Clinical Journal of the American Society of Nephrology, 6*(6), 1274–1285.
Irazabal, M. V., & Torres, V. E. (2013). Experimental therapies and ongoing clinical trials to slow down progression of ADPKD. *Current Hypertension Reviews, 9*(1), 44–59.

Irazabal, M. V., Rangel, L. J., Bergstralh, E. J., Osborn, S. L., Harmon, A. J., Sundsbak, J. L., . . . CRISP Investigators. (2015). Imaging classification of autosomal dominant polycystic kidney disease: A simple model for selecting patients for clinical trials. *Journal of the American Society of Nephrology, 26*(1), 160–172.

Pei, Y., Hwang, Y. H., Conklin, J., Sundsbak, J. L., Heyer, C. M., Chan, W., . . . Haider, M. A. (2015). Imaging-based diagnosis of autosomal dominant polycystic kidney disease. *Journal of the American Society of Nephrology, 26*(3), 746–753.

Pei, Y., Obaji, J., Dupuis, A., Paterson, A. D., Magistroni, R., Dicks, E., . . . Ravine, D. (2009). Unified criteria for ultrasonographic diagnosis of ADPKD. *Journal of the American Society of Nephrology, 20*(1), 205–212.

Porath, B., Gainullin, V. G., Cornec-Le Gall, E., Dillinger, E. K., Heyer, C. M., Hopp, K., . . . Harris, P. C. (2016). Mutations in GANAB, encoding the glucosidase IIalpha subunit, cause autosomal dominant polycystic kidney and liver disease. *American Journal of Human Genetics, 98*(6), 1193–1207.

Schrier, R. W., Abebe, K. Z., Perrone, R. D., Torres, V. E., Braun, W. E., Steinman, T. I., . . . HALT-PKD Trial Investigators. (2014). Blood pressure in early autosomal dominant polycystic kidney disease. *New England Journal of Medicine, 371*(24), 2255–2266.

Torres, V. E., Chapman, A. B., Devuyst, O., Gansevoort, R. T., Grantham, J. J., Higashihara, E., . . . TEMPO 3:4 Trial Investigators. (2012). Tolvaptan in patients with autosomal dominant polycystic kidney disease. *New England Journal of Medicine, 367*(25), 2407–2418.

OTHER HEREDITARY KIDNEY DISORDERS

Beth A. Vogt

CHAPTER 44

1. **What is familial or inherited hematuria?**
   Familial (inherited) hematuria is defined as a group of genetic kidney disorders that are clinically characterized by the onset of persistent microscopic hematuria during childhood. The unifying feature of these conditions is an abnormality in the network of type IV collagen in the glomerular basement membrane (GBM). The major forms of familial hematuria are Alport syndrome and thin basement membrane nephropathy (TBMN).

2. **How common is Alport syndrome?**
   Alport syndrome is a rare condition, occurring in 1 in 50,000 individuals.

3. **What are the major clinical features in males with Alport syndrome?**
   Males with Alport syndrome have persistent microscopic hematuria beginning in infancy. Episodes of macroscopic hematuria may occur, but they become less frequent after adolescence. Proteinuria and progressive chronic kidney disease develop as early as the second decade of life but may not be present until well into adulthood. End-stage kidney disease (ESKD) develops in virtually all affected males, but the rate of progression of kidney disease is variable between families. Overall, about 50% of males reach ESKD by age 25, 90% by age 40, and 100% by 60 years.

4. **What are the major clinical findings in females with Alport syndrome?**
   Females with Alport syndrome have a much milder course than do males, but should be characterized as "affected individuals" rather than "carriers" who have an "at risk" state. Microscopic hematuria is present in 95% of females, but significant proteinuria and progressive kidney dysfunction occur in 15% of females by the age of 60 years.

5. **What other abnormalities may be associated with Alport syndrome?**
   High-frequency, sensorineural hearing loss typically begins in late childhood and ultimately develops in 70% of males with Alport syndrome by the age 40 years. Deafness ultimately develops in 80% of affected males. A minority of females with Alport syndrome develop hearing loss. About 40% of males with Alport syndrome exhibit characteristic ocular abnormalities. Twenty percent of patients have white or yellow perimacular flecks, which increase in number with age. Twenty percent of patients have anterior lenticonus, a protrusion of the central area of the lens into the anterior chamber, which can result in recurrent corneal erosion. Leiomyomatosis and platelet abnormalities are occasionally seen.

6. **What are the characteristic kidney biopsy findings in Alport syndrome?**
   The pathognomonic kidney biopsy finding in Alport syndrome is diffuse thickening of the GBM with splitting of the lamina densa, giving a basket-weave appearance on electron microscopy. In young patients, both thickening and thinning of the GBM may be present, causing difficulty in distinguishing the early stages of Alport syndrome from TBMN. Light microscopy shows segmental or global glomerulosclerosis, interstitial fibrosis, and tubular atrophy.

7. **How is Alport syndrome inherited?**
   The most common form of Alport syndrome is X-linked Alport syndrome (XLAS), which comprises 80% of cases. Autosomal-recessive Alport syndrome (ARAS) comprises 15% of cases, and autosomal-dominant Alport syndrome (ADAS) is rare, comprising only 5% of cases. Of children with XLAS, 10% to 15% have no family history of hematuria or kidney disease and are felt to represent de novo mutations.

8. **What are the genetic abnormalities in Alport syndrome?**
   XLAS results from one of a variety of mutations in the gene for the alpha-5 chain of type IV collagen (*COL4A5*) on the X chromosome. The result is an alteration in the structure of the alpha-5 collagen chain, preventing normal incorporation of alpha-3 and alpha-4 collagen chains into basement

membranes. ARAS results from homozygous or compound heterozygous mutations in both copies of either the *COL4A3* or *COL4A4* gene on chromosome 2. ADAS is caused by heterozygous mutations in either the *COL4A3* or *COL4A4* gene.

9. What treatment is available for Alport syndrome?
Currently, there is no definitive therapy for Alport syndrome. Treatment remains supportive in nature and should focus on the control of hypertension and the reduction of proteinuria to slow the progressive loss of kidney function over time. Angiotensin-converting enzyme inhibitors (ACEi) and/or angiotensin receptor blockers are useful agents and are recommended in patients with Alport syndrome with proteinuria greater than 200 mg/day, although there is some thought that the earlier initiation of ACEi before proteinuria develops may prove helpful. The metabolic consequences of chronic kidney disease should be carefully managed, and all affected family members should be identified by urine screening or genetic testing, if indicated.

10. Are there any special complications in patients with Alport syndrome following kidney transplantation?
Patients with XLAS who undergo transplant have survival rates similar to or better than those with other inherited kidney diseases. However, 3% to 5% of transplanted males with Alport syndrome develop post-transplant anti-GBM nephritis, leading to rapid decline in allograft function despite aggressive therapy. This condition results from an immunologic response by the recipient to the alpha-5 chain of type IV collagen, a previously unrecognized antigen in the transplant recipient. The subset of patients with Alport syndrome at highest risk for this complication includes males with significant deafness and the onset of ESKD before the age of 30 years.

11. What is TBMN?
TBMN is a form of inherited hematuria estimated to occur in 1% of the population. TBMN is characterized by persistent microscopic hematuria and occasionally episodic macroscopic hematuria. Proteinuria, hypertension, progressive loss of kidney function, and extrarenal abnormalities are not part of the clinical picture. The family history reveals individuals with persistent hematuria but none with associated ESKD or hearing loss.

12. What is the inheritance pattern of TBMN?
TBMN follows an autosomal-dominant pattern of inheritance. Heterozygous mutations in the type IV collagen gene (*COL4A3* and *COL4A4*) are causative, although the penetrance rate is only 70%.

13. What are the kidney biopsy findings in TBMN?
The pathognomonic kidney biopsy finding in TBMN is uniform thinning of the GBM ($<$250 nm) on electron microscopy, with attenuation of the lamina densa. Light and immunofluorescence microscopic analyses are usually normal.

14. What is the natural history of TBMN?
In the majority of patients, TBMN is a benign condition in which progressive kidney failure does not occur. Rarely, patients may develop more significant kidney disease. For this reason, it is recommended that patients with persistent microscopic hematuria due to suspected TBMN have yearly follow-up with plans for diagnostic kidney biopsy if they develop proteinuria greater than 1 g/day and/or impairment in kidney function. The biopsy is to confirm the diagnosis of TBMN and rule out other conditions, such as Alport syndrome and immunoglobulin-A nephropathy.

15. What is nephronophthisis?
Nephronophthisis (NPHP) is an autosomal recessive cystic kidney disease that is now known to be included in a growing class of disorders called ciliopathies. NPHP is characterized by chronic tubulointerstitial nephritis with eventual progression to ESKD. NPHP is believed to account for 5% of pediatric ESKD in the United States and 10% to 25% of pediatric ESKD in Europe, and is therefore the most frequent genetic cause of ESKD in the first three decades of life. The three forms of NPHP include infantile (NPHP2), juvenile (NPHP1), and adolescent (NPHP3), with variable ages of onset. Juvenile NPHP accounts for the majority of affected individuals.

16. What are the clinical features of NPHP?
Children with NPHP1 may have a subtle presentation, with progressive polyuria, polydipsia, secondary enuresis, impaired growth, fatigue, and pallor. Anemia is a prominent finding even before significant reduction in kidney function occurs. Progression to ESKD occurs on average at 13 years of age in children with juvenile NPHP, at age 1 year in infantile NPHP, and at age 19 years in adolescent NPHP. Hematuria, proteinuria, urinary tract infection, and hypertension are uncommon.

17. What is the genetic basis of NPHP?

NPHP is inherited in an autosomal recessive fashion. To date, 20 genes for NPHP have been identified, each coding for a nephrocystin expressed in the primary cilia of kidney epithelial cells and other cell types. Ciliary dyfunction leads to abnormalities in their flow, osmolal, or chemosensor functions. *NPHP1,* the most common gene for juvenile NPHP, is found in 20% to 40% of cases.

18. What extrarenal findings have been associated with NPHP?

Of patients with NPHP, 10% to 15% have extrarenal symptoms, including retinitis pigmentosa (Senior-Loken syndrome), cerebellar ataxia (Joubert syndrome), developmental delay, skeletal anomalies (Jeune syndrome), and hepatic fibrosis. These findings are felt to be related to the presence of abnormal cilia in photoreceptors, chondrocytes, cholangiocytes, and other cells.

19. What are the ultrasound findings in NPHP?

The kidney ultrasound of patients with NPHP may initially be normal; however, with time, it shows small, hyperechoic kidneys with small, 1 to 2 mm corticomedullary cysts. The absence of medullary cysts does not rule out the diagnosis of NPHP.

20. What are the kidney biopsy findings in NPHP?

Kidney biopsy in NPHP shows tubular basement membrane disruption, tubulointerstitial nephropathy, interstitial fibrosis, and corticomedullary cysts.

21. What is the treatment for NPHP?

There is currently no definitive treatment for NPHP. Treatment is focused on supportive therapy for progressive kidney dysfunction, control of hypertension, and early identification of affected family members. Kidney transplantation is successful, and recurrent disease in the kidney allograft has not been reported.

22. What is autosomal dominant tubulointerstitial kidney disease (ADTKD)?

ADTKD is a new terminology for a collection of rare inherited kidney diseases characterized by autosomal dominant inheritance, bland urinalysis, tubulointerstitial fibrosis, and slowly progressive kidney dysfunction. These disorders often present in young adulthood, between the ages of 20 and 50 years. The diagnosis of ADTKD must be considered in any adult with chronic kidney disease unrelated to hypertension and diabetes, a bland urinalysis, and a positive family history of ESKD.

23. What is the genetic basis of ADTKD?

Four forms of ADTKD have been identified, based on specific abnormalities in genes expressed in the tubular cells of the distal nephron. ADTKD-UMOD, the most common disorder, is associated with a mutation in the *UMOD* gene, which expresses uromodulin (Tamm-Horsfall protein). A cardinal feature of ADTKD-UMOD is hyperuricemia and early-onset gout. ADTKD-MUC1 is related to a mutation in the mucin-1 gene *(MUC1),* which codes for a transmembrane protein expressed in the distal nephron. ADTKD-REN, a rare disorder associated with a mutation in the gene for preprorenin *(REN),* is characterized by reduced renin production and mild hypotension. ADTKD-HNF1B is a disorder that involves a mutation in hepatocyte nuclear factor 1B *(HNF-1B),* a transcription factor that regulates multiple genes expressed in the kidney, pancreas, and liver. This disorder is associated with maturity-onset diabetes of the young (MODY-5), uterine malformations, gout, hypomagnesemia, liver abnormalities, and other systemic findings. There is a 30% to 50% de novo mutation rate in ADTKD-HNF1B.

24. What is the treatment for ADTKD?

Treatment of patients with ADTKD remains supportive in nature and should include blood pressure control, hydration, avoidance of nephrotoxins, and management of the complications of chronic kidney disease. In patients with ADTKD-UMOD, allopurinol may be used to control hyperuricemia, although its effectiveness at slowing the progression of kidney disease is uncertain.

KEY POINTS

1. The major forms of familial (inherited) hematuria are Alport syndrome and TBMN.
2. XLAS results from mutations in the gene for the alpha-5 chain of type IV collagen (*COL4A5*) on the X chromosome.
3. NPHP is an autosomal recessive cystic kidney disease characterized by chronic tubulointerstitial nephritis and progression to ESKD.
4. ADTKD are a group of rare monogenic kidney diseases characterized by interstitial fibrosis and slowly progressive kidney dysfunction.

BIBLIOGRAPHY

Eckardt, K. U., Alper, S. L., Antignac, C., Bleyer, A. J., Chauveau, D., Dahan, K., ... Devuyst O. (2015). Autosomal dominant tubulointerstitial kidney disease: Diagnosis, classification, and management—A KDIGO consensus report. *Kidney International, 88*(4), 676–683.

Savige, J., Gregory, M., Gross, O., Kashtan, C., Ding, J., & Flinter, F. (2013). Expert guidelines for the management of Alport syndrome and thin basement membrane nephropathy. *Journal of the American Society of Nephrology, 24*, 364–375.

Wolf, M. T. F. (2015). Nephronophthisis and related syndromes. *Current Opinion in Pediatrics, 27*, 201–211.

CHAPTER 45

TUBULOINTERSTITIAL DISEASES
Rupali S. Avasare

ACUTE TUBULOINTERSTITIAL NEPHRITIS

1. **What is acute tubulointerstitial nephritis?**
   Acute tubulointerstitial nephritis (ATIN) is characterized by inflammation and edema in the kidney tubulointerstitium and can cause acute kidney injury (AKI). Definitive diagnosis is established by kidney biopsy, though this may not be necessary if the index of suspicion for ATIN is high. A retrospective study done by Goicoechea showed that the incidence of ATIN, particularly ATIN in the elderly, has increased over the past decade due to a higher biopsy rate and/or an increased use of causative drugs, such as nonsteroidal antiinflammatory drugs (NSAIDs) and antibiotics.

2. **What are the most common causes of ATIN?**
   The most common causes of ATIN are classified as below:
   - Drugs
   - Infection
   - Autoimmune systemic diseases
   - Idiopathic
   Drugs account for most ATIN cases. Drug-induced ATIN is not dose dependent, but rather is an idiosyncratic reaction. Repeat exposure to the same drug or a closely related agent can lead to recurrence of the disease process (Table 45.1).

3. **Describe the pathogenesis of ATIN.**
   ATIN is caused by an immune reaction in the kidney. Drug-induced ATIN is caused by a cell-mediated, delayed-hypersensitivity type of immune response characterized by infiltration of CD4+ T cells. In addition, an antibody-mediated response may play a role given high serum immunoglobulin (Ig)E levels and, rarely, anti–tubular basement membrane (anti-TBM) staining on kidney biopsy.

4. **What are the characteristic histopathologic findings in ATIN?**
   - Presence of an inflammatory cell infiltrate in the interstitium
   - Interstitial edema
   - Tubulitis
   - Other findings may include:
     - Granulomas in the interstitium. As seen in sarcoidosis, Sjögrens, and tubulointerstitial nephritis and uveitis (TINU)
     - Anti-TBM antibodies
     - Diffuse foot process effacement. As seen in NSAID-induced minimal change disease.
   - Normal glomeruli and vessels. This, in particular, distinguishes tubulointerstitial nephritis from inflammatory glomerular diseases (e.g., glomerulonephritides)

5. **What are the clinical manifestations of ATIN?**
   ATIN may be asymptomatic, but in some patients it presents with fatigue, fever, nausea, vomiting, rash, or arthralgias. The classic triad of fever, maculopapular rash, and peripheral eosinophilia that was originally described with methicillin-induced ATIN is seen in less than 10% of ATIN cases.

6. **What are the laboratory manifestations of ATIN?**
   - Azotemia (elevated blood urea nitrogen and serum creatinine)
   - Peripheral eosinophilia
   - Eosinophiluria
   - Sterile pyuria (occasionally, white blood cell [WBC] casts)
   - Microscopic hematuria (very rarely, red blood cell [RBC] casts)
   - Proteinuria (usually <3.5 g/day, with the exception of NSAID-induced ATIN)
   - Renal tubular acidosis (RTA; varies depending on which segment of the renal tubule is affected)

311

Table 45.1. Drugs Causing Acute Tubulointerstitial Nephritis

Antimicrobial Agents
Acyclovir
Ampicillin[a]
Amoxicillin
Aztreonam
Carbenicillin
Cefaclor
Cefamandole
Cefazolin
Cephalexin
Cephaloridine
Cephalothin
Cephapirin
Cephradine
Cefoxitin
Cefotetan
Cefotaxime

Ciprofloxacin
Cloxacillin
Colistin
Cotrimoxazole[a]
Erythromycin
Ethambutol
Foscarnet
Gentamicin
Indinavir
Interferon
Isoniazid
Lincomycin

Methicillin[a]
Mezlocillin
Minocycline
Nafcillin
Nitrofurantoin[a]
Norfloxacin
Oxacillin[a]

Penicillin G[a]
Piperacillin
Piromidic acid
Polymyxin acid[a]
Quinine
RIFAMPICIN[a]
Spiramycin[a]

Sulfonamides
Teicoplanin
Tetracycline
Vancomycin

NSAIDs, Including Salicylates
Alclofenac
Azapropazone
Aspirin
Benoxaprofen
Diclofenac
Diflunisal[a]
Fenclofenac
Fenoprofen
Flurbiprofen
Ibuprofen
Indomethacin
Ketoprofen
Mefenamic acid
Meloxicam
Mesalazine (5-ASA)
Naproxen
Niflumic acid
Phenazone
Phenylbutazone
Piroxicam
Pirprofen
Sulfasalazine
Sulindac
Suprofen
Tolemetin
Zomepirac
Analgesics
Aminopyrine
Antipyrine
Antrafenin
Clometacin[a]
Floctafenin[a]
Glafenin[a]
Metamizol
Noramidopyrine
Anticonvulsants
Carbamazepine
Phenobarbital
Phenytoin[a]
Valproate sodium

Diuretics
Chlorthalidone
Ethacrynic acid
Furosemide[a]
Hydrochlorothiazide[a]
Indanamide
Tienilic acid[a]
Triamterene[a]
Others
Allopurinol[a]
Alpha-methyldopa
Azathioprine
Bismuth salts
Captopril[a]
Carbimazole
Chlorpropamide[a]
Cyclosporine
Cimetidine
Clofibrate
Clozapine
D-penicillamine
Fenofibrate[a]
Gold salts
Griseofulvin
Interferon
Interleukin-2
Omeprazole
Phenindione[a]
Phenothiazine
Phenylpropanolamine
Probenecid
Propranolol
Propylthiouracil
Ranitidine
Streptokinase
Sulphinpyrazone
Warfarin

[a]Drugs that can induce granulomatous acute interstitial nephritis.
Drugs most commonly involved are shown in capital letters.

Wu et al. investigated the use of urine biomarkers in the evaluation of drug-induced ATIN and found that urinary monocyte chemotactic peptide-1 (MCP-1) levels showed the closest correlations with interstitial inflammation when compared to other urine biomarkers, such as neutrophil gelatinase-associated lipocalin (NGAL), a1-microglobulin (a1-MG), and N-acetyl-B-D-glucosaminidase (NAG).

7. **What is the importance of eosinophiluria in ATIN?**

Eosinophiluria is a nonspecific finding that can be seen in a variety of conditions (e.g., acute pyelonephritis, acute glomerulonephritis, acute cystitis, and prostatitis). Muriithi et al. found that even at a 5% cut-off, urine eosinophils are poorly discriminated between ATIN and other forms of kidney disease.

8. **What drugs cause ATIN?**

The three most common drug classes that cause ATIN are: NSAIDs, proton-pump inhibitors, and antibiotics. Different drug classes are associated with different manifestations of ATIN. For example, while beta-lactam antibiotics may be associated with a systemic allergic response (fever, rash, and/or peripheral eosinophilia), NSAID-induced ATIN is not typically associated with extrarenal symptoms. ATIN secondary to NSAIDs may manifest 6 to 18 months after initiation of the medication. A large percentage of patients with NSAID-induced ATIN have nephrotic syndrome. Withdrawal of NSAIDs leads to recovery in most cases, though recovery may take up to 12 months.

9. **Which autoimmune diseases are associated with ATIN?**

Lupus nephritis, sarcoidosis, Sjögren disease, ANCA-associated vasculitis, and Crohn disease. See more on this in the section "Chronic tubulointerstitial disease" below.

10. **What is the role of gallium scanning in the diagnosis of ATIN?**

The presence of an active interstitial inflammatory infiltrate in ATIN leads to a diffuse, intense kidney uptake of the gallium67 radioisotope. This finding is nonspecific and can be seen in many causes of AKI. Note that acute tubular necrosis (ATN) is characterized by decreased uptake of gallium67, thus the gallium scan may be useful in distinguishing ATIN from ATN.

11. **What is the most definitive means to diagnose ATIN?**

Definitive diagnosis is made by kidney biopsy. Because it is common practice to withdraw the suspected etiologic agent and carefully observe the kidney function in the ensuing days, kidney biopsies are not always performed in suspected cases of ATIN.

The most common indications for doing a kidney biopsy in suspected ATIN are as follows:
- Unexplained AKI
- Absence of improvement after withdrawal of suspected offending agent
- Consideration of immunosuppression for treatment of suspected ATIN

12. **What are the treatment options for ATIN?**
- Withdrawal of offending agent
- Corticosteroid therapy
- Steroid-sparing immunosuppressive therapy

To date, the optimal treatment for ATIN is unclear. There have been no randomized, controlled trials investigating the use of immunosuppressive therapy for treatment of ATIN.

Corticosteroids may be considered in patients with biopsy-proven ATIN in whom there is prolonged and/or progressive kidney dysfunction despite withdrawal of the offending agent. There is no standardized treatment regimen for ATIN. Typically oral prednisone is started at 1 mg/kg per day and tapered off over 8 to 12 weeks.

Preddie et al. reported the use of mycophenolate mofetil (MMF) for 13 to 34 months in a group of patients who were steroid dependent for up to 6 months.

For now, one may consider the use of MMF for those who have biopsy-proven ATIN, who are either intolerant of, dependent on, or resistant to corticosteroids.

13. **What is the typical course of ATIN?**

The majority of suspected cases of ATIN, whether treated by withdrawal of the suspected offending agent alone or with immunosuppression, result in the recovery of kidney function in a few days to weeks. Prolonged kidney dysfunction (>3 weeks) and the presence of interstitial fibrosis and tubular atrophy on histopathology are considered poor prognostic features.

CHRONIC TUBULOINTERSTITIAL NEPHRITIS

14. What is chronic tubulointerstitial nephritis?

Chronic tubulointerstitial nephritis is characterized by the presence of chronic interstitial inflammation, interstitial fibrosis, and tubular atrophy, which leads to chronic kidney disease (CKD). Causes of chronic tubulointerstitial nephritis are listed in Box 45.1. Different diseases affect different segments of the tubule. The functional abnormalities depend on the tubular site of involvement. For example, Sjögrens leads to distal tubular injury and is associated with metabolic acidosis (type 1 RTA) and hypokalemia. Injury involving the kidney medulla is characterized by impaired ability to concentrate urine, as seen in sickle cell nephropathy (Box 45.2).

Box 45.1. Causes of Chronic Tubulointerstitial Nephritis

Primary or Idiopathic
Epstein-Barr virus

Secondary
Infections
Polyomavirus
Pyelonephritis (acute and chronic)

Drugs
Analgesic abuse nephropathy
Lithium-induced kidney disease
Acyclic nucleoside inhibitors
Calcineurin inhibitors
Aristolochic acid/Chinese herb nephropathy
Chemotherapeutic agents: cisplatin, ifosfamide, carmustine

Heavy Metals
Lead nephropathy
Cadmium

Hematologic Diseases
Multiple myeloma
Lymphoproliferative disorders
Light chain disease
Sickle cell nephropathy

Obstructive Uropathy
Reflux nephropathy

Immune-Mediated Diseases
Sarcoidosis
Lupus
IgG4-related disease
Primary Sjögren's syndrome
Tubulointerstitial nephritis with uveitis
Idiopathic hypocomplementemic interstitial nephritis

Metabolic Disorders
Hyperoxaluria
Hypercalcemia/hypercalciuria
Hypokalemic nephropathy

Genetic Disorders
Cystinosis
Dent disease

Miscellaneous
Endemic (Balkan) nephropathy
Radiation nephritis

Box 45.2. Clinical Features of Chronic Tubulointerstitial Nephritis

Electrolyte and Acid-Base Disorders
Proximal RTA or Fanconi Syndrome
Myeloma
Dent disease
Cystinosis

Distal RTA
Bacterial pyelonephritis
Reflux nephropathy
Lithium
Lead
Myeloma
Light chain disease

Lupus nephritis
Hypercalcemia
Sjögrens disease

Hyperkalemia (Type 4) RTA
Reflux nephropathy
Lead
Lupus nephritis
Sickle cell nephropathy
Sodium wasting

Clinical Syndromes
Kidney Stones
Hypercalcemia
Hyperoxaluria
Uric acid nephropathy

Box 45.2. Clinical Features of Chronic Tubulointerstitial Nephritis—cont'd

Dent disease
Sarcoidosis

Nephrogenic Diabetes Insipidus
Lithium
Cisplatin
Hypokalemia
Hypercalcemia
Dent disease

Acute Kidney Injury
Pyelonephritis
Analgesic nephropathy
Lithium

Calcineurin inhibitors
Cisplatin
Myeloma
Lymphoma
Lupus nephritis
Hypercalcemia
Uric acid nephropathy
Radiation nephritis

Papillary Necrosis
Acute pyelonephritis
Analgesic nephropathy
Sickle cell nephropathy

RTA, Renal tubular acidosis.

15. What common infections cause chronic tubulointerstitial nephritis?
- Chronic pyelonephritis
  - Chronic bacterial infections of the urinary tract are among the most common causes of chronic tubulointerstitial nephritis. The majority of these cases are associated with vesicoureteral reflux (VUR)—hence the term "reflux nephropathy." For those not associated with VUR, however, the disease is termed "chronic pyelonephritis."
  - Clinically, patients with chronic pyelonephritis present with symptoms consisting of fever and chills, dysuria, vague flank or back pain, and hypertension. Some patients may present with tubular abnormalities, such as impaired urinary concentrating ability, hyperkalemia, and salt wasting, all of which reflect distal tubular dysfunction. Chronic or repeated urinary tract infections are predisposing risk factors.
  - Examination of the urine often reveals an active urinary sediment consisting of WBCs and WBC casts.
  - Grossly, the kidneys may appear contracted.
  - Histopathologically, findings are similar to other forms of chronic tubulointerstitial nephritis, with tubular atrophy and interstitial fibrosis. Lymphocytes and mononuclear cells predominate the chronic inflammatory infiltrative population.
- Xanthogranulomatous pyelonephritis
  - Persistent chronic pyelonephritis can progress to a localized infection called "xanthogranulo-matous pyelonephritis." Typically, this is associated with urinary tract obstruction. There is ischemia and destruction of kidney parenchymal tissue, granuloma formation, and subsequent accumulation of lipid deposits. These lipid deposits are actually lipid-laden macrophages called foam cells.
  - Symptoms are similar to those of chronic pyelonephritis. Characteristically, a distinct mass may be palpable over the affected "nonfunctioning" kidney.
  - Urine cultures are usually positive for *E. coli,* other gram-negative bacilli or *Staphylococcus aureus.*
  - Computed tomography, the imaging modality of choice, may show the source of obstruction (stone), an enlarged kidney, and dilated calyces. Neoplasm must be excluded.
  - On intravenous pyelography, the involved kidney may contain a localized abscess-like area, which may look like a complex cyst or tumor.
  - Current treatment recommendations consist of antibiotic therapy combined with total or partial nephrectomy.

16. What medications are commonly associated with chronic tubulointerstitial nephritis?
Analgesics, lithium, calcineurin inhibitors, Chinese herbs, chemotherapeutic agents, and heavy metals are associated with chronic tubulointerstitial nephritis.

17. What is analgesic abuse nephropathy?
Prolonged use of analgesic mixtures containing phenacetin, paracetamol, aspirin, and/or NSAIDs may cause analgesic nephropathy.

The main site of kidney injury in analgesic nephropathy is the vascular endothelial cells in the kidney medulla, primarily because of low oxygen tension and toxin accumulation.

Occasionally, patients may present with flank pain or gross hematuria due to papillary necrosis. Papillary calcification and characteristic "bumpy" kidney contours may be seen on imaging. In some instances, the kidneys may appear bilaterally atrophic or asymmetric in size. Urinalysis may show sterile pyuria, microscopic or macroscopic hematuria, and mild proteinuria.

Patients with analgesic nephropathy are at increased risk for transitional cell carcinoma of the uroepithelium.

Management is primarily supportive and includes discontinuation of the culprit analgesic agent. Close monitoring, especially for development of new symptoms, such as gross hematuria, is recommended because of the increased risk of uroepithelial tumors.

18. How is lithium associated with chronic tubulointerstitial nephritis?

Long-term lithium ingestion may cause chronic tubulointerstitial nephritis, nephrogenic diabetes insipidus (NDI), RTA, and hypercalcemia. Lithium enters the collecting tubule cells via the luminal epithelial sodium channels and accumulates intracellularly where it interferes with antidiuretic hormone (ADH)-mediated water reabsorption. An incomplete distal (type 1) RTA, secondary to lithium-induced decreased $H+ATPase$ pump activity in the distal tubule, has been described. Lithium has also been associated with hypercalcemia caused by morphologic changes in the parathyroid glands.

Lithium-induced nephropathy is characterized by the formation of microcysts in the distal convoluted tubules and collecting ducts.

Typically, kidney dysfunction secondary to chronic lithium use is mild to moderate. Amiloride, a potassium-sparing diuretic, has been shown to reduce polyuria and to block lithium uptake in the sodium channels of the collecting duct. Those with serum creatinine levels greater than 2.5 mg/dL at the time of presentation may progress to end-stage kidney disease (ESKD) even after the cessation of lithium. The average latent period between the initiation of lithium therapy and the onset of ESKD is 20 years.

For those patients receiving chronic maintenance therapy with lithium, regular follow-up of serum creatinine is recommended. Elevations in creatinine should lead to either dose reduction or complete withdrawal of the drug.

19. How are calcineurin inhibitors associated with chronic tubulointerstitial nephritis?

Calcineurin inhbitors (CNIs), namely cyclosporine and tacrolimus, are used as antirejection therapy after organ transplantation and as immunosuppressive therapy for various autoimmune diseases. CNIs can cause acute and chronic nephrotoxicity.

Acutely, CNIs may cause vasoconstriction of the afferent and efferent arterioles and decreased kidney blood flow. Chronically, there is vascular damage leading to glomerular and tubular injury. On histology, there is vacuolization of the tubules and focal areas of tubular atrophy and interstitial fibrosis leading to a "striped fibrosis" pattern.

Laboratory evaluation is notable for hyperkalemia, nonanion gap metabolic acidosis, hypomagnesemia, hypophosphatemia, and hyperuricemia.

Treatment of CNI toxicity consists of lowering the dose or discontinuing the CNI when possible. Calcium channel blockers may protect against CNI-induced vasoconstriction.

20. How are Chinese herbs associated with chronic tubulointerstitial nephritis?

Chinese herbs nephropathy was described in a group of Belgian women using Chinese herbs for weight loss. The weight loss tea was contaminated with aristolochic acid, which is also a known carcinogen.

Histopathologically, a hypocellular interstitial fibrosis with marked tubular atrophy is seen.

If untreated, patients may rapidly progress to ESKD. A short course of oral steroids has been shown to slow the progression of kidney failure.

21. Describe the association between chemotherapeutic agents and tubulointerstitial nephritis.

Cisplatin can cause selective injury to proximal tubular cells, where it is taken up by organic cation transporters and accumulates intracellularly. Clinically, this can manifest as decreased glomerular filtration rate (GFR), Fanconi-like syndrome, salt-wasting, and hypomagnesemia.

Ifosfamide can cause tubular toxicity also resulting in a Fanconi-like syndrome and polyuria due to solute (mainly sodium) diuresis.

High-dose methotrexate can cause ATN secondary to methotrexate crystal precipitation.

22. Describe the association between heavy metals and chronic tubulointerstitial nephritis.

Prolonged environmental or occupational exposure to cadmium may lead to chronic tubulointerstitial nephritis and eventual progression to kidney failure. Proximal tubular dysfunction, presenting as Fanconi syndrome, characterized by glycosuria, aminoaciduria, and tubular proteinuria, is common.

Increased urinary cadmium excretion is characteristic. Currently, the treatment for cadmium nephrotoxicity is primarily supportive.

Similar to cadmium, the proximal tubule cells tend to be the site of accumulation for lead, thereby leading to a Fanconi-type picture. Chronic tubulointerstitial nephritis secondary to lead exposure for several years is characterized histopathologically by progressive tubular atrophy and widespread fibrosis.

Lead nephropathy also reduces urinary excretion of uric acid, thereby leading to hyperuricemia and gout. This syndrome, called "saturnine gout," gained prominence with increased ingestion of moonshine.

The diagnosis of lead nephropathy is established by increased urinary excretion of chelated lead (i.e., after the administration of ethylenediamine tetraacetic acid [EDTA]). Cumulative body stores of lead are estimated by doing an EDTA mobilization test or by performing an x-ray fluorescence, which determines bone lead content. In the EDTA mobilization test, 2 g of EDTA are administered either by the intravenous or intramuscular route, and then patients collect a 24-hour urine for lead. Urinary lead greater than 0.6 g/day is considered abnormal. One major limitation of the EDTA mobilization test is that it cannot mobilize lead deposits in bone.

Lead decreases the enzymatic activity of erythrocyte delta-aminolevulinic acid dehydratase (ALAD). Thus, peripheral blood ALAD is a good biomarker for lead toxicity. Since uremia can also decrease ALAD activity, reduced levels of ALAD compared with levels of ALAD "restored" by the addition of dithiothreitol may be even more efficient in detecting increased body lead burden in patients with chronic kidney failure.

It is important to note that serum levels of lead, although elevated during acute exposure, are not very helpful in the chronically exposed. The explanation for this is that, during acute exposure, lead is concentrated in the RBCs, which later die and the lead then moves to the bones and other tissues. A kidney biopsy shows nonspecific findings seen in chronic tubulointerstitial nephritis.

The treatment of lead nephropathy is EDTA chelation therapy or oral succimer, which has been shown to slow the progression of CKD.

23. What are immune-mediated causes of chronic tubulointerstitial nephritis?
- Sarcoidosis
  - Kidney involvement in sarcoidosis can occur in a variety of ways. Most commonly, patients have hypercalcemia secondary to increased production of 1, 25-dihydroxyvitamin D_3 by activated macrophages residing in granulomatous tissues. Hypercalcemia can lead to NDI, hypercalciuria-related nephrolithiasis, and, in some cases, kidney failure.
  - Sarcoidosis can also present as a form of interstitial nephritis with associated noncaseating granulomas.
  - Typical tubular manifestations include mild proteinuria, sterile pyuria, and impaired ability to concentrate urine.
  - Treatment is with high-dose corticosteroids (prednisone up to 1 mg/kg per day).
- **Sjögren syndrome:** Sjögren syndrome–associated chronic interstitial nephritis characteristically presents as type 1 RTA with hypokalemia and a normal anion gap metabolic acidosis. Although the mechanism for this is incompletely understood, it is believed to be related to autoantibodies against carbonic anhydrase II. Treatment with immunosuppression may be helpful.
- **Lupus nephritis:** Isolated tubulointerstitial disease secondary to lupus is exceedingly rare. More commonly, tubulointerstitial disease is accompanied by glomerular involvement.
- **IgG4 related disease:** Kidney involvement is reported in up to one-third of patients with IgG4-related disease. The disease is characterized by a lymphoplasmacytic infiltrate, with increased numbers of IgG4-positive plasma cells, in the affected organ. A majority of patients also have elevated serum IgG or IgG4 levels. Patients with kidney involvement also may have hypocomplementemia. Most patients also have radiographic abnormalities consisting of small low-attenuation lesions. Raissian et al. have proposed diagnostic criteria for IgG4-related tubulointerstitial nephritis that includes histologic (>10 IgG4 staining plasma cells/hpf), imaging, serologic, and other organ involvement parameters.

- **Tubulointerstitial nephritis and uveitis syndrome:** Tubulointerstitial nephritis and uveitis (TINU) was first described by Dobrin et al. in 1975. It usually affects young females.
  - The exact pathogenesis remains unclear, but the predominance of T lymphocytes in affected tissues and possible association with chlamydia and Epstein-Barr virus suggest that delayed-type hypersensitivity and cell-mediated immunity may play major roles.
  - Clinically, patients present with nonspecific signs and symptoms (i.e., fever, generalized malaise, anemia, asthenia). Uveitis of the anterior chamber is seen bilaterally, presenting as redness and pain over the eyes. Uveitis may occur 2 months prior to, simultaneously, or up to 14 months after the onset of interstitial nephritis.
  - Kidney manifestations include both proximal and distal tubular dysfunction. Increased urine β2 microglobulin (a marker of tubulointerstitial disease) has been noted. Ultrasonography may reveal enlarged, swollen kidneys.
  - Definitive diagnosis is established by demonstrating typical findings of interstitial nephritis (i.e., tubulointerstitial edema with infiltration of lymphocytes, plasma cells, and histiocytes). Infiltration of CD4 and CD8 T lymphocytes, monocytes, and macrophages has been described. Eosinophils and noncaseating granulomas also may be seen.
  - Other oculorenal syndromes include sarcoidosis and Sjögren's (see above).
  - Kidney disease frequently resolves spontaneously over the course of 12 months without steroid therapy. However, for those with moderately advanced CKD, prednisone 1 mg/kg per day may be given for 3 to 6 months. Although the kidney manifestations may resolve spontaneously and respond well to a course of systemic steroids, the uveitis often has a chronic or relapsing course that may require more aggressive therapy.
- **Idiopathic hypocomplementemic interstitial nephritis:** This disease entity is in older men with hypocomplementemia in the absence of lupus or Sjögren's syndrome. Histopathology reveals extensive tubulointerstitial involvement and a predominantly lymphocytic infiltrate.

24. What are the metabolic causes of chronic tubulointerstitial nephritis?
  - Oxalate nephropathy
    - Dietary: Star fruit, rhubarb, peanuts, and black tea contain high levels of oxalate and are known to cause oxalate nephropathy when consumed in large quantities. Vitamin C is metabolized to oxalate, and thus high doses of vitamin C may also cause oxalate deposition in the kidney.
    - Enteric hyperoxaluria: This occurs when there is fat or bile acid malabsorption. The free fatty acids bind to calcium and thereby decrease the availability of calcium to bind to oxalate. Free soluble oxalate is then absorbed in the gut and excreted by the kidney. The most common causes of enteric hyperoxaluria are inflammatory bowel disease, Roux-en-Y gastric bypass surgery, and pancreatic insufficiency.
    - Ethylene glycol toxicity results in the formation of calcium oxalate crystals that precipitate in the kidney tubules.
    - Genetic: Primary hyperoxaluria types 1, 2, and 3 are each caused by a different enzyme deficiency that leads to the overproduction of oxalate. This leads to nephrocalcinosis, kidney stones, and/or tubulointerstitial disease. When the glomerular filtration rate (GFR) decreases to less than 30 to 45 mL/min per 1.73 m^2, plasma levels of oxalate exceed saturation and oxalate deposits in other tissues.
  - **Hypercalcemia/hypercalciuria:** Hypercalcemia (resulting from hyperparathyroidism, sarcoidosis, multiple myeloma, etc.) affects the kidney in a variety of ways.
    - NDI: This may occur secondary to tubulointerstitial injury and disruption of the interstitial osmotic gradient. Furthermore, activation of the calcium-sensing receptor may also affect the osmotic gradient by decreasing sodium chloride absorption in the loop of Henle.
    - Vasoconstriction.
    - Distal (type 1) RTA.
    - Nephrolithiasis.
  - **Hypokalemia:** Chronic hypokalemia is associated with proximal tubular cell vacuolization, dilated intercellular spaces, and medullary cysts; this clinically correlates with impaired ability to concentrate urine (NDI) and conserve salt, and with the development of hypertension. However, it remains unclear how often chronic tubulointerstitial nephritis occurs secondary to chronic hypokalemia.

25. What is Balkan (endemic) nephropathy?
  As the name implies, this disease is particularly endemic in the so-called Balkan states or the former Yugoslavia, plus Bulgaria and Romania. No specific etiologic cause has yet been identified, but as a result of its specific geographic distribution, environmental factors have long been suspect. Genetic and immune-related factors have also been identified.

Balkan nephropathy is a slow yet progressive form of chronic tubulointerstitial nephritis that eventually leads to ESKD.

There is a strong link between dietary consumption of aristolochic acid (see previous discussion above on Chinese herb nephropathy) with this disease and its attendant risk of uroepithelial cancer. Interestingly, aristolactam-DNA adducts were identified in kidney and urothelial tissues of affected patients.

Clinically, a characteristic early feature is that of normochromic normocytic anemia, which is disproportionate to the stage of CKD. Urinalysis usually shows mild proteinuria with few RBCs and WBCs. Patients tend to be normotensive in the earlier stages of the disease, with eventual progression to hypertension toward more advanced stages.

26. **What is radiation nephritis?**
Radiation nephritis is classified into two categories based on the onset of symptom presentation: (1) acute radiation nephritis and (2) chronic radiation nephritis.

Acute radiation nephritis usually presents within 6 to 12 months of exposure to radiation. Patients may present with edema, hypertension (may be malignant), proteinuria, and anemia. Often, this progresses to secondary chronic radiation nephritis. Angiotensin-converting enzyme inhibitors (ACE-I) are the antihypertensive agents of choice for treatment of hypertension associated with radiation nephritis.

Primary chronic radiation nephritis presents after more than 18 months of radiation exposure and is characterized by proteinuria, hypertension, and progression of CKD.

Although the exact pathogenesis remains elusive, it is believed that exposure of the kidneys to greater than 1500 to 2500 rad leads to endothelial cell injury. Radiation can also cause direct injury to the tubular epithelial cells. Furthermore, patients receiving radiation therapy for some underlying malignancy also receive concomitant chemotherapy, which may potentiate radiation's toxic effects on the kidneys.

Histopathologically, there is characteristic thickening of the capillary walls, which may also demonstrate "splitting." Interposition of deposits between the split layers of the glomerular basement membrane is noticeably similar to that seen in hemolytic uremic syndrome and thrombotic thrombocytopenic purpura.

Proper shielding of the kidneys, especially in those with preexisting CKD, should be pursued when possible. Fractionizing the total irradiation dose into several small doses over several days may also be protective.

27. **What is acute phosphate nephropathy?**
Acute phosphate nephropathy is seen in patients after exposure to oral sodium phosphate solutions (OSPS), which was used as a bowel cleanser in preparation for a colonoscopy. Histopathologically, there is evidence of acute and chronic tubular injury with interstitial edema, accompanied by tubular atrophy and interstitial fibrosis. The distinctive feature of this entity is the presence of abundant calcium phosphate deposits in the distal tubules and collecting ducts. The following factors predispose patients to acute kidney failure: volume depletion, advanced age, hypertension, concurrent treatment with ACE-I or angiotensin receptor blockers, diuretics and NSAIDs, baseline creatinine elevation, or inappropriate use of OSPS in those with underlying CKD. In 2008, the US Food and Drug Administration released a boxed warning regarding the use of oral sodium phosphate products for bowel cleansing and the risk of AKI.

KEY POINTS

1. ATIN accounts for up to one-third of AKI cases.
2. The classical triad of fever, maculopapular rash, and peripheral eosinophilia is seen in only a minority of cases (<10%) of ATIN.
3. The absence of eosinophiluria does not necessarily exclude the diagnosis of ATIN.
4. Drug-induced ATIN is not dose dependent. A repeat exposure to the same drug can potentially lead to a recurrence of the disease process. The most common offending drugs are NSAIDs, proton pump inhibitors, and antibiotics.
5. The majority of suspected cases of ATIN result in the recovery of kidney function in a few days to weeks.
6. Patients who do not recover kidney function within a few weeks of withdrawal of the offending agents may benefit from corticosteroids.
7. In chronic tubulointerstitial nephritis, depending on the culprit agent, the disease may have a particular predilection for either the proximal tubules or the distal tubules or both; the consequent functional abnormalities depend on the tubular site of involvement. The involvement of the proximal tubule often leads to hypophosphatemia, glycosuria, aminoaciduria, and hypomagnesemia.
8. Lithium-induced nephropathy is characterized by the formation of microcysts (cortical and medullary tubular cysts) in the distal convoluted tubules and collecting ducts.

BIBLIOGRAPHY

Appel, G. B. (2008). The treatment of acute interstitial nephritis: More data at last. *Kidney Int, 73*, 905.

Appel, G. B., & Bhat, P. (2007). Tubulointerstitial diseases. In D. C. Dale (Ed.), *ACP medicine*. Philadelphia: American College of Physicians.

Bossini, N., Savoldi, S., Franceschini, F., et al. (2000). Clinical and morphological features of kidney involvement in primary Sjögren's syndrome. *Nephrol Dial Transplant, 16*, 2328.

Boton, R., Gaviria, M., & Batlle, D. C. (1987). Prevalence, pathogenesis, and treatment of renal dysfunction associated with chronic lithium therapy. *Am J Kidney Dis, 10*, 329.

Braden, G. L., O'Shea, M. H., & Mulhern, J. G. (2005). Core curriculum in nephrology: Tubulointerstitial diseases. *Am J Kidney Dis, 46*, 560–572.

Clarkson, M. R., Giblin, L., O'Connell, F. P., et al. (2004). Acute interstitial nephritis: Clinical features and response to corticosteroid therapy. *Nephrol Dial Transplant, 19*, 2778.

Dobrin, R. S., Vernier, R. L., & Fish, A. L. (1975). Acute eosinophilic interstitial nephritis and renal failure with bone marrow-lymph node granulomas and anterior uveitis: A new syndrome. *Am J Med, 59*(3), 325–333.

Fontanellas, A., Navarro, S., Moran-Jimenez, M. J., et al. (2002). Erythrocyte aminolevulinate dehydrase activity as a lead marker in patients with chronic renal failure. *Am J Kidney Dis, 40*, 43–50.

Goicoechea, M., Rivera, F., & López-Gómez, J. M. (2013). Increased prevalence of acute tubulointerstitial nephritis. *Nephrol Dial Transplant, 28*(1), 112–115.

Gonzalez, E., Gutierrez, E., Galeano, C., et al. (2008). Early steroid treatment improves the recovery of renal function in patients with drug-induced acute interstitial nephritis. *Kidney Int, 73*, 940.

Grollman, A. P., Shibutani, S., Moriya, M., et al. (2007). Aristolochic acid and the etiology of Balkan (endemic) nephropathy. *Proc Natl Acad Sci USA, 104*(29), 12129–12134.

Kambham, N., Markowitz, G. S., Tanji, N., et al. (2001). Idiopathic hypocomplementemic interstitial nephritis with extensive tubulointerstitial deposits. *Am J Kidney Dis, 37*, 388–399.

Markowitz, G. S., Radhakrishnan, J., Kambham, N., et al. (2000). Lithium nephrotoxicity: A progressive combined glomerular and tubulointerstitial nephropathy. *J Am Soc Nephrol, 11*, 1439.

Markowitz, G. S., Stokes, M. B., Radhakrishnan, J., et al. (2005). Acute phosphate nephropathy following oral sodium phosphate bowel purgative: An underrecognized cause of chronic renal failure. *J Am Soc Nephrol, 16*, 3389–3396.

Martinez, M. C. M., Nortier, J., Vereerstraeten, P., et al. (2002). Progression rate of Chinese herb nephropathy: Impact of Aristolochia fungchi ingested dose. *Nephrol Dial Transplant, 17*, 408–412.

Michel, D. M., & Kelly, C. J. (1998). Acute interstitial nephritis. *J Am Soc Nephrol, 9*, 506.

Muntner, P., He, J., Vupputuri, S., et al. (2003). Blood lead and chronic kidney disease in the general US population: Results from NHANES III. *Kidney Int, 63*, 1044.

Muriithi, A. K., Nasr, S. H., & Leung, N. (2013). Utility of urine eosinophils in the diagnosis of acute interstitial nephritis. *Clin J Am Soc Nephrol, 8*(11), 1857–1862.

Perazella, M., & Markowtiz, G. (2010). Nature reviews. *Nephrology, 6*, 461–470.

Pirani, C., Valeri, A., D'Agati, V., & Appel, G. (1987). Renal toxicity of nonsteroidal anti-inflammatory drugs. *Contr. Nephrol, 55*, 159–175.

Preddie, D. C., Markowitz, G. S., Radhakrishnan, J., et al. (2006). Mycophenolate mofetil for the treatment of interstitial nephritis. *Clin J Am Soc Nephrol, 1*, 718.

Presne, C., Fakhouri, F., Nöel. L. H., et al. (2003). Lithium-induced nephropathy: Rate of progression and prognostic factors. *Kidney Int, 64*, 585–592.

Raissian, Y., Nasr, S., Cornell, L., et al. (2011). Diagnosis of IgG4-related tubulointerstitial nephritis. *J Am Soc Nephrol, 22*(7), 1343–1352.

Ramesh, G., & Reeves, W. B. (2004). Salicylate reduces cisplatin nephrotoxicity by inhibition of tumor necrosis factor-alpha. *Kidney Int, 65*(2), 490–499.

Wu, Y., Yang, L., Li, X. M., et al. (2010). Pathological significance of a panel of urinary biomarkers in patients with drug-induced tubulointerstitial nephritis. *Clin J Am Soc Nephrol, 5*(11), 1954–1959.

CHAPTER 46

URINARY TRACT INFECTION

Lindsay E. Nicolle

1. **What is a urinary tract infection (UTI)?**
   UTI is the presence of microorganisms in the urine or tissues of the normally sterile genitourinary tract. Infection may be localized to the bladder alone or involve the kidneys and, in men, the prostate. Acute uncomplicated UTI occurs in women with a normal genitourinary tract and usually manifests as acute cystitis (bladder infection or lower tract infection). These same women experience, less frequently, kidney (upper tract or kidney parenchymal) infection, referred to as acute uncomplicated or acute non-obstructive pyelonephritis. Complicated UTI occurs in individuals with structural or functional abnormalities of the genitourinary tract, including those with indwelling devices, such as urethral catheters. Recurrent urinary infection may be reinfection, with a new organism, or relapse, when the same organism is isolated posttherapy.

2. **What is asymptomatic bacteriuria?**
   Asymptomatic bacteriuria is isolation of bacteria from the urine culture in quantitative counts consistent with infection but with no genitourinary signs or symptoms attributable to infection.

3. **Who gets UTIs?**
   UTI occurs primarily in two groups of individuals.
   - The first group is healthy girls and women with normal genitourinary tracts. About 10% of all women experience at least one episode of infection in a given year, and 20% to 45% of young women will have a recurrence within 1 year following a first infection.
   - The second group at risk for UTI are individuals with underlying functional or structural abnormalities of the genitourinary tract, such as obstruction, diverticula, vesicoureteral reflux, or indwelling devices. This group includes infants and most men who experience UTIs, as well as women.

4. **What is the pathogenesis of UTI?**
   Urinary infection usually occurs following colonization of the periurethral area by organisms from the normal gut flora and subsequent ascension of these bacteria into the bladder. This is facilitated by sexual intercourse in women, by urologic procedures including catheter insertion, or by turbulent urine flow in men with prostate hypertrophy. Vesicoureteral reflux, if present, facilitates the ascension of organisms from the bladder to the kidneys. Rarely, UTI follows hematogenous spread from another source, and may present as kidney abscesses. Indwelling urethral catheters and other urologic devices uniformly acquire a surface biofilm composed of microorganisms growing within an extracellular mucopolysaccharide material that they produce. This biofilm incorporates urine components, such as magnesium and calcium ions, and Tamm Horsfall protein. Organisms persist and multiply within the protected environment provided by this biofilm, where there is restricted diffusion of antibiotics and impaired access of host defenses, such as neutrophils.

5. **What risk factors are associated with increased frequency of UTI?**
   Healthy women and girls have both genetic and behavioral risks for UTI. Genetic variables include polymorphisms of genes for the innate immune response and or being a nonsecretor of the blood group substances so bacteria may adhere more avidly to mucosal surfaces. For premenopausal women, 75% to 90% of episodes of infection are attributable to sexual intercourse. Other risk factors include use of spermicides, which disrupt the normal vaginal flora and promote colonization by potential uropathogens, or a new sexual partner within 1 year, which is associated with colonization with new organisms.
   A wide variety of functional and structural genitourinary abnormalities contribute to complicated urinary infection, through promoting increased access of bacteria to the bladder or by interfering with normal voiding to allow organisms to persist in the urine (Table 46.1). For patients with indwelling devices, the major risk factor for infection is the duration the device remains in situ.

6. **Which are the common infecting organisms in UTI?**
   Escherichia coli is isolated in 80% to 85% of episodes of acute cystitis and 85% to 90% of episodes of acute uncomplicated pyelonephritis. Uropathogenic *E. coli* are characterized by the expression of

TABLE 46.1. Abnormalities of the Genitourinary Tract Which May Promote Complicated Urinary Tract Infection

Congenital	
Obstruction	Congenital urethral valves
	Ureteric stricture
	Urethral stricture
	Prostate hypertrophy
	Pelvi calyceal junction
	Extrinsic compression
Other urologic abnormalities	Urolithiasis
	Bladder diverticulae
	Cystoceles
	Tumor
	Neurogenic bladder
	Vesicouretral reflux
	Ileal conduit
	Augmented bladder
Comorbidities	Diabetes
	Nephrocalcinosis
	Medullary sponge kidney
	Polycystic kidney
	Kidney transplant
Indwelling devices	Indwelling catheter
	Ureteric stent
	Nephrostomy tube

diverse virulence factors including adhesins, iron sequestration systems, and toxins. Pyelonephritis is consistently associated with expression of the P pilus, a Gal-$\propto$(1-4), Gal-β disaccharide galabiose adhesin. *Staphylococcus saprophyticus,* a coagulase negative staphylococcus, is isolated from 5% to 10% of cystitis episodes. It is virtually only identified as a pathogen in acute cystitis.

A greater variety of organisms are isolated from complicated urinary infection. *E. coli* remains an important pathogen, but *Klebsiella pneumoniae, Citrobacter* spp., *Proteus mirabilis, Pseudomonas aeruginosa, Enterococcus* spp., and other bacteria or yeast are also isolated. These bacteria are more likely to be resistant to antimicrobials. This is attributed to prior antimicrobial exposure or the acquisition of health care–associated organisms following urologic interventions. Urease-producing organisms, such as *P. mirabilis, Morganella morganii,* and *Providencia stuartii,* are common in the biofilm on indwelling devices.

7. **What are the usual symptoms of UTI?**
   Bladder infection presents with one or more symptoms of acute dysuria, frequency, urgency, stranguria, hematuria, and suprapubic discomfort. Women with recurrent cystitis can reliably self-diagnose a UTI in more than 90% of cases. Kidney infection presents with costovertebral angle pain or tenderness with or without fever, which is frequently also accompanied by lower tract symptoms. Patients with complicated UTI may present with symptoms of either bladder or kidney infection. Urinary infection in infants is more common in boys and presents as fever and failure to thrive. Patients with an indwelling urethral catheter also usually present with fever without localizing genitourinary findings, although hematuria, catheter obstruction, or costovertebral angle pain and tenderness may be present. Acute prostatitis is a severe systemic illness characterized by high fever, bacteremia, and, often, acute urinary obstruction. Chronic bacterial prostatitis may present as relapsing acute cystitis in older men.

8. **How is a laboratory diagnosis of UTI made?**
   A urine culture confirms the diagnosis and identifies the specific infecting organism and susceptibilities. A urine specimen for culture should be obtained prior to initiating antimicrobial therapy for all presentations of symptomatic urinary infection, with the exception of women with

acute uncomplicated cystitis in whom the characteristic clinical presentation is reliable for diagnosis. However, these women should have a urine culture obtained if presenting symptoms are not characteristic, or when there is failure to respond to antibiotics or the recurrence of infection within 1 month of antimicrobial therapy. A voided urine specimen, collected using a method to minimize contamination, is usually appropriate. If a voided specimen cannot be obtained, an in-and-out catheter specimen is recommended.

Patients with a short-term indwelling urinary catheter should have the urine specimen obtained by puncture through the catheter port. When a long-term indwelling catheter is present, the catheter should be replaced and a specimen collected through the replacement catheter to obtain a sample of bladder urine not contaminated by microorganisms present in the biofilm.

9. **How is a quantitative urine culture interpreted?**
   Isolation of $\geq 10^5$ colony-forming unit (CFU)/mL of an organism generally distinguishes bacteria causing infection from contaminants. However, 25% to 30% of young women with acute cystitis have organisms isolated in quantitative counts $< 10^5$ CFU/mL; any gram-negative organism isolated in counts $\geq 10^2$ CFU/mL is considered relevant for this presentation. Lower quantitative counts are also occasionally isolated from patients with other clinical presentations of urinary infection. When this occurs, the diagnosis should be critically reassessed, considering the specimen collection method (i.e., the likelihood of contamination) and the number and species of organisms grown. Isolation of multiple organisms or gram-positive organisms from voided specimens is more likely to be contaminants. Any quantitative count $\geq 10^2$ CFU/mL is considered diagnostic of infection for specimens obtained by in-and-out catheter, including intermittent catheterization, as these collection methods are less subject to contamination.

10. **Is pyuria a useful diagnostic test?**
    The presence of pyuria is not, by itself, diagnostic of urinary infection. Pyuria has low specificity for identification of asymptomatic or symptomatic infection in older individuals, or in patients with underlying genitourinary abnormalities or indwelling devices. However, the absence of pyuria in a symptomatic patient is reliable for excluding urinary infection.

11. **How do you diagnose urinary infection in an elderly resident of a nursing home?**
    For some elderly individuals, ascertainment of clinical signs and symptoms may be difficult because of dementia, impaired communication, or coexisting chronic genitourinary symptoms. In the absence of an indwelling catheter, a clinical diagnosis of urinary infection in an elderly person should be made only if localizing genitourinary symptoms—such as frequency, urgency, hematuria, or costovertebral angle pain or tenderness—are present. Nonlocalizing or nonspecific signs or symptoms in elderly individuals, such as increased confusion or falls, should not be attributed to urinary infection. For the 30% to 50% of male or female nursing home residents with bacteriuria at any time, 90% will also have pyuria. The presence of pyuria, "foul-smelling urine," or other urinalysis findings, such as bacteriuria or hematuria, are not indications for antimicrobial therapy in the absence of other localizing signs or symptoms.

12. **How do you diagnose urinary infection in residents with chronic indwelling catheters?**
    Residents with chronic catheters uniformly have bacteriuria and pyuria. Urinalysis abnormalities, such as pyuria and smelly or cloudy urine, are not sufficient for diagnosis of symptomatic urinary infection in a resident with an indwelling catheter. For the elderly resident with an indwelling urethral catheter, fever, by itself, may be a presentation of symptomatic urinary infection if there are no apparent alternate sources. Localizing symptoms, such as obstruction, hematuria, or suprapubic or costovertebral pain or tenderness, are present in only a minority of patients. If symptomatic urinary infection is suspected, the indwelling catheter should be replaced and a urine specimen for culture should be obtained through the new catheter before initiating antimicrobial therapy.

13. **How should acute uncomplicated urinary infection be treated?**
    Acute cystitis is a mucosal infection effectively treated with relatively short courses of antimicrobial agents that achieve high urinary concentrations. Recommended first-line empiric regimens are antimicrobials to which the infecting organism is susceptible and which will have limited impact on the gut flora. These include nitrofurantoin macrocrystals/monohydrate, fosfomycin or, where available, pivmecillinam (Table 46.2). Trimethoprim/sulfamethoxazole (TMP/SMX) 160/800 mg bid for 3 days or TMP 100 mg bid for 3 days is effective but not recommended if local resistance prevalence of TMP/SMX for community-acquired organisms exceeds 20%. The fluoroquinolones—norfloxacin, ciprofloxacin, and levofloxacin—are effective given as a 3-day course, but are not recommended for first-line therapy

TABLE 46.2. Antimicrobial Regimens for Empiric Treatment and for Prevention of Acute Uncomplicated Urinary Tract Infection

Treatment	
First line	Nitrofurantoin 50–100 mg or nitrofurantoin macrocrystals 100 mg bid × 5 days Fosfomycin 3 g single dose Pivmecillinam 400 mg bid × 5 days
Second line	TMP/SMX 160/800 mg bid × 3 days Trimethoprim 100 mg bid × 3 days Ciprofloxacin 250 or 500 mg bid × 3 days Levofloxacin 250 or 500 mg bid × 3 days Norfloxacin 400 mg bid × 3 days Cephalexin 250–500 mg qid × 7 days Amoxicillin/clavulanic acid 500 mg tid or 875 mg bid × 7 days Cefixime 400 mg qod × 7 days Doxycycline 100 mg bid × 7 days
Prophylaxis	
Postintercourse (single dose)	Nitrofurantoin 50 mg or nitrofurantoin macrocrystals 100 mg TMP/SMX 40/200 mg Trimethoprim 100 mg Ciprofloxacin 125 mg Norfloxacin 200 mg Cephalexin 250 mg
Long-term low dose: (at bedtime)	Nitrofurantoin 50 mg qod or nitrofurantoin macrocrystals 100 mg qod TMP/SMX 40/200 mg qod Trimethoprim 100 mg od Norfloxacin 200 mg qod Ciprofloxacin 125 mg Cephalexin 500 mg qod

TMP/SMX, Trimethoprim/sulfamethoxazole.

because of concerns of safety and resistance emergence. They are contraindicated in children because of adverse effects on cartilage development. The beta-lactam antimicrobials, such as amoxicillin, amoxicillin/clavulanic acid, and cephalosporins, are all 10% to 20% less effective for susceptible organisms than first-line agents and require a longer course of therapy, usually 7 days.

14. How do you prevent acute uncomplicated UTI?
   Prophylactic antimicrobial therapy given as a long-term, low-dose regimen or as a single dose postintercourse prevents up to 95% of episodes of recurrent cystitis (see Table 46.2). This approach is recommended for women who experience frequent reinfections, usually defined as two infections within 6 months or three infections within 1 year. Patient self-treatment with a 3-day course of TMP/SMX, norfloxacin, or ciprofloxacin is also effective. This is a useful approach for the management of women who are concerned about developing infection while traveling, or who experience severe but less frequent episodes.
   Women with recurrent urinary infection should be advised not to use spermicides. Other behavioral interventions, such as changing their type of underwear, showering rather than bathing, postintercourse voiding, and postvoiding hygiene, are not helpful. The use of probiotics, including yogurt, to reestablish normal vaginal flora is not effective. Daily cranberry tablets or juice have limited, if any, efficacy in decreasing the frequency of recurrent symptomatic infection. The role of topical vaginal estrogen to prevent recurrent infection in postmenopausal women requires further evaluation; vaginal estrogen is not currently recommended solely for the prevention of recurrent urinary infection.

15. How is uncomplicated pyelonephritis treated?
   Acute nonobstructive pyelonephritis is a serious infection requiring prompt investigation and treatment. If the patient is clinically stable and can tolerate oral therapy, ciprofloxacin 500 mg twice a day for

7 days or levofloxacin 750 mg once a day for 5 days is a recommended empiric regimen. An initial single parenteral dose of ceftriaxone or an aminoglycoside may be considered. Two regular-strength tablets of TMP/SMX twice a day for 14 days is also effective for susceptible organisms, but is not recommended for empiric therapy because of the high prevalence of TMP/SMX resistance in many regions. Effective parenteral antimicrobial regimens include ceftriaxone 1 to 2 g daily or gentamicin or tobramycin 3 to 5 mg/kg daily. Where resistant strains are likely, alternate regimens, such as a carbapenem, should be initiated. The clinical status and urine culture results should be reviewed at 48 to 72 hours following the initiation of antimicrobial therapy. Patients receiving parenteral therapy who have an adequate clinical response are then switched to appropriate oral therapy to complete a therapeutic course. If the infecting organism is resistant to the empiric antimicrobial therapy initiated, the regimen should be changed to an effective agent, irrespective of clinical response.

16. What is the antimicrobial treatment of complicated UTI?

The treatment of complicated UTI requires consideration of the underlying abnormality and recognition of the wide spectrum of potential infecting organisms and the increased likelihood of antimicrobial resistance. When symptoms are mild, antimicrobial therapy should be delayed pending urine culture results so specific therapy can be prescribed. Empiric antimicrobial therapy, when indicated, is selected considering recent antimicrobial therapy, any previous urine culture results, patient tolerance, and kidney function. The antimicrobial should have good urinary excretion and provide coverage for the presumed infecting organism and susceptibility. A fluoroquinolone is often prescribed for empiric therapy. When parenteral therapy is indicated, aminoglycosides (gentamicin, tobramycin) are effective for patients without kidney failure because most gram-negative organisms remain susceptible to these agents. If aminoglycosides cannot be used, an extended spectrum cephalosporin (cefotaxime, ceftriaxone, ceftazidime), penicillin (piperacillin/tazobactam), or carbapenem (meropenem, ertapenem) are other options.

17. How is complicated UTI, including catheter-acquired UTI, prevented?

The most important intervention to prevent complicated UTI is to characterize and correct the underlying genitourinary abnormality. If the underlying abnormality persists, such as in a patient with spinal cord injury, the goal of management is to optimize voiding and to limit the use of indwelling devices wherever possible. Prophylactic antimicrobial therapy is not effective to prevent recurrence, as there is usually rapid reinfection with resistant organisms. Cranberry products are also not effective in preventing reinfection.

The most important intervention to prevent catheter-acquired urinary infection is to avoid catheter use. These devices should be used only when essential, and catheters must be removed promptly once no longer needed. Optimal practices for catheter care and maintenance should be followed. Replacement of a chronic indwelling catheter immediately prior to initiating antimicrobial therapy decreases the frequency of early posttherapy symptomatic relapse and leads to more rapid defervescence.

18. When should imaging studies be obtained?

Patients who present with severe systemic manifestations, including sepsis, should have urgent imaging to exclude obstruction, abscess, or other abnormalities that may require surgical intervention for immediate source control. For patients with less severe presentations, imaging to identify underlying abnormalities that may require urologic intervention should be considered if the initial clinical response after 48 to 72 hours is not satisfactory, or if there is an early relapse posttherapy and the infecting organism is susceptible to the antimicrobial given. The optimal imaging modality is a contrast-enhanced computed tomography scan.

19. Why are pregnant women at risk for pyelonephritis?

Women with asymptomatic bacteriuria identified in early pregnancy who are not treated have a 20% to 30% risk of developing pyelonephritis in later pregnancy. The high risk of pyelonephritis is attributed to urine stasis from hormone-induced dilation of the smooth muscle of the urinary tract and, later in pregnancy, ureteric obstruction by pressure of the fetal head at the pelvic brim. Pyelonephritis, as with any febrile illness in later pregnancy, may lead to premature labor and delivery with adverse fetal outcomes.

20. How is pyelonephritis prevented and treated in pregnant women?

Pregnant women are screened for bacteriuria by urine culture in early pregnancy. Asymptomatic women with a positive urine culture ($\geq 10^5$ CFU/mL of a single gram-negative organism on two or more consecutive urine cultures) or women with symptomatic infection at any time are treated and then screened for recurrent bacteriuria, usually monthly, for the duration of the pregnancy. If a second episode of urinary infection occurs, prophylactic antimicrobial therapy is given until the end of the pregnancy. The preferred regimen is a beta-lactam antibiotic, which is safe for the fetus. Nitrofurantoin is also safe and effective. TMP/SMX is avoided because of a small but well-documented association with fetal abnormalities when given in the first trimester, and fluoroquinolone antimicrobials are contraindicated because of potential detrimental effects on fetal cartilage. For prophylactic therapy, either cephalexin 500 mg or nitrofurantoin 50 or 100 mg daily are recommended.

A pregnant woman who presents with pyelonephritis should be hospitalized for initial management. The recommended empiric regimen is ceftriaxone 1 to 2 g once daily. A carbapenem or aminoglycoside, usually gentamicin, may be used if there is antimicrobial resistance or patient intolerance to ceftriaxone.

21. **When should asymptomatic urinary infection be treated?**
Asymptomatic bacteriuria may be transient or persistent and is common in women, the elderly, and individuals with complicated UTI. The prevalence reaches 25% to 50% of long-term care facility residents and 50% of patients with spinal cord injury managed with intermittent catheters. Screening for and treatment of asymptomatic bacteriuria is indicated for pregnant women. The only other indication for treatment is to prevent bacteremia and sepsis following invasive genitourinary procedures associated with mucosal trauma and bleeding. For these procedures, treatment of antimicrobial therapy is, conceptually, surgical prophylaxis. Usually a single dose initiated immediately prior to the intervention is adequate. Screening for and treatment of asymptomatic bacteriuria is not recommended for other populations, including kidney transplant patients, because this strategy will not decrease subsequent episodes of symptomatic infection or other morbidity, but is associated with increased adverse drug reactions and reinfection with more resistant bacteria.

22. **How do you diagnose and treat bacterial prostatitis?**
Acute bacterial prostatitis is a urologic emergency. Patients are severely ill with high fever and prominent voiding symptoms. Broad-spectrum parenteral antimicrobial treatment is initiated following collection of urine and blood cultures. Obstruction to voiding is usually present and is managed with a short-term indwelling catheter. Initial broad-spectrum parenteral treatment is stepped down to oral therapy, preferably a fluoroquinolone, once clinically indicated and when culture results are available. The total recommended duration of the antimicrobial course is 30 days.

Chronic bacterial prostatitis is diagnosed when the voided urine culture is negative but bacterial growth and pyuria are documented in expressed prostate secretions. Only 10% of men presenting with chronic pelvic pain syndrome/chronic prostatitis symptoms have chronic bacterial prostatitis confirmed as the cause of these symptoms, so microbiologic documentation of infection is necessary. A clinical presentation in older men is recurrent cystitis when bacteria that persist in the prostate reenter the urine. Treatment for documented chronic bacterial prostatitis is 4 weeks of ciprofloxacin or levofloxacin for susceptible organisms. This regimen is 70% to 80% effective for long-term cure.

23. **What is emphysematous pyelonephritis, and how this is managed?**
Emphysematous pyelonephritis is an unusual presentation of acute necrotizing renal infection. It is characterized by gas formation in kidney tissue and the perinephric space, which is usually associated with Enterobacteriaceae infection. Patients with this presentation usually have diabetes, and obstruction is often present. Management requires effective antimicrobial therapy together with glucose control, correction of the obstruction, and drainage of any abscesses. Percutaneous drainage is the recommended initial approach, if possible. Delayed elective nephrectomy may subsequently be required for some patients.

24. **How do you diagnose and treat fungal UTI?**
Risk factors for fungal UTI include exposure to broad-spectrum antimicrobial therapy, the presence of diabetes, and the use of chronic indwelling catheters. *Candida albicans* is the most common organism; other *Candida* spp. may also be isolated. Most of these patients are asymptomatic, and asymptomatic funguria should not be treated. Fluconazole has good urinary excretion and is the treatment of choice for symptomatic infection. For species, such as *C. glabrata,* which are resistant to fluconazole, the recommended alternate treatment is amphotericin B deoxycholate. 5-flucytosine may also be effective but has substantial side effects and requires monitoring of drug levels when used. Other azoles and echinocandins do not achieve therapeutic concentrations in the urine and are not recommended for treatment of urinary infection. Patients with an inadequate therapeutic response to appropriate antifungal therapy should have imaging studies to exclude a fungus ball which, if present, requires surgical intervention.

25. **What is suppressive antimicrobial therapy, and when should this be used?**

Suppressive antimicrobial therapy is long-term antimicrobial therapy given to prevent symptomatic relapsing infection in selected patients with recurrent complicated UTI in whom infection cannot be eradicated. Some examples include its use in men with frequent recurrent cystitis from a persistent prostate source; in kidney transplant patients with recurrent symptomatic infection from an infected native kidney; or or an individual with an inoperable infection stone to prevent further stone enlargement and preserve kidney function. Antimicrobial therapy is selected based on the organism isolated from urine culture and considering patient tolerance. Initial treatment is for 2 to 4 weeks at the full therapeutic dose. If this is effective and well tolerated, therapy is usually continued indefinitely at the lowest effective dose, which is usually one-half or less of the standard dose, or until the underlying abnormality is corrected.

KEY POINTS

1. Acute uncomplicated urinary tract infection (UTI) is common in women of any age. These women have a normal genitourinary tract and can usually be effectively treated with short courses of antimicrobial therapy.
2. Complicated UTI occurs in individuals with structural or functional abnormalities of the genitourinary tract, including those with indwelling devices, such as urethral catheters. A principal goal of therapy in these patients is the characterization and correction of abnormalities that promote infection.
3. *Escherichia coli* is the most common cause of UTI. *E. coli* isolated from women with acute uncomplicated urinary infection express diverse virulence factors. *E. coli* strains isolated from individuals with complicated UTI or asymptomatic bacteriuria less frequently express virulence factors.
4. Pyuria is not, by itself, diagnostic of UTI or an indication for antimicrobial therapy. However, the absence of pyuria may exclude UTI.
5. Asymptomatic bacteriuria should be screened for and treated only in pregnant women or individuals who are to undergo an invasive genitourinary procedure likely to be associated with mucosal bleeding.

BIBLIOGRAPHY

Chenoweth, C. E., Gould, C. V., & Saint, S. (2014). Diagnosis, management, and prevention of catheter-associated urinary tract infections. *Infectious Disease Clinics of North America, 28*, 105–119.

Geerlings, S. E., Beerepoot, M. A., & Prins, J. M. (2014). Prevention of recurrent urinary tract infections in women: Antimicrobial and nonantimicrobial strategies. *Infectious Disease Clinics of North America, 28*, 135–147.

Grigoryan, L., Trautner, B. W., & Gupta, K. (2014). Diagnosis and management of urinary tract infections in the outpatient setting: A review. *Journal of the American Medical Association, 312*, 1677–1684.

Gupta, K., Hooton, T. M., Naber, K. G., Wullt, B., Colgan, R., Miller, L. G., ... European Society for Microbiology and Infectious Diseases. (2010). International clinical practice guidelines for the treatment of acute uncomplicated cystitis and pyelonephritis in women: A 2010 update by the Infectious Diseases Society of America and the European Society for Microbiology and Infectious Diseases. *Clinical Infectious Diseases, 52*, e103–e120.

Lipsky, B. A., Bryen, I., & Hoey, C. T. (2010). Treatment of bacterial prostatitis. *Clinical Infectious Diseases, 50*, 1641–1652.

Mody, L., & Juthani-Mehta, M. (2014). Urinary tract infections in older women: A clinical review. *Journal of the American Medical Association, 311*, 844–854.

Nicolle, L. E., Bradley, S., Colgan, R., Rice, J. C., Schaeffer, A., Hooton, T. M., ... American Geriatric Society. (2005). IDSA guideline for the diagnosis and treatment of asymptomatic bacteriuria in adults. *Clinical Infectious Diseases, 40*, 643–654.

Schaeffer, A. J., & Nicolle, L. E. (2016). Clinical practice: Urinary tract infections in older men. *New England Journal of Medicine, 374*, 562–571.

Schwenger, E. M., Tejani, A. M., & Loewen, P. S. (2015). Probiotics for preventing urinary tract infections in adults and children. *Cochrane Database of Systematic Reviews*, (12), CD008772. doi:10.1002/14651858.CD008772.pub2.

Stein, R., Dogan, H. S., Hoebeke, P., Kočvara, R., Nijman, R. J., Radmayr, C., ... European Society for Pediatric Urology. (2015). Urinary tract infections in children: EAU/ESPU guidelines. *European Urology, 67*, 546–558.

IX
KIDNEY DISEASES IN SPECIAL POPULATIONS

KIDNEY DISEASE AND HYPERTENSION IN PREGNANCY

Susan Hou

CHAPTER 47

1. **What changes take place in the kidney during pregnancy?**
   The kidney undergoes anatomic and physiologic changes during normal pregnancy. The length of the kidney increases by 1 to 1.5 cm and there is hormonally mediated dilatation of the collecting system to a volume of about 300 cc. The resulting physiologic hydronephrosis makes it difficult to diagnose obstruction by ultrasound. The glomerular filtration rate increases by 50% during the first trimester so that the serum creatinine is expected to be 0.5 to 0.7 mg/dL. Pregnancy is also characterized by a reset osmotstat where the serum sodium is normally in the range of 134 mEq/L, but a water load can be excreted normally. Additionally, pregnancy is characterized by respiratory alkalosis with a compensatory drop in bicarbonate, making the normal bicarbonate in pregnancy 18 to 20 mEq/L.

2. **How often do urinary tract infections occur during pregnancy?**
   Urinary stasis from the dilated collecting system predisposes to urinary tract infections. Asymptomatic bacteriuria occurs in 5% of pregnancies. Untreated, 30% of asymptomatic bacteriuria leads to pyelonephritis, which in pregnant women is frequently complicated by decreased kidney function/acute kidney injury, sepsis, and even acute respiratory distress syndrome (ARDS). Only 2% of healthy women with a negative urine culture on the first screening will develop a urinary tract infection (UTI) later in pregnancy, but women with preexisting kidney disease should be screened monthly.

3. **What is the importance of preeclampsia?**
   Preeclampsia is the most common and important of the hypertensive disorders of pregnancy, affecting between 5% and 7% of pregnancies. Preeclampsia is a multisystem disease. The American College of Obstetrics and Gynecology does not require proteinuria if other end-organ disease is present. Severe preeclampsia is denoted by its most common symptoms, microangiopathic Hemolytic anemia, Elevated Liver enzymes and Low Platelets (HELLP syndrome). It can be accompanied by severe manifestations including acute kidney injury, stroke, blindness from vasoconstriction in the occipital lobe or retinal detachment, disseminated intravascular coagulation, hepatic rupture, or pulmonary edema. Preeclampsia may progress to seizures, a progression that changes the designation to eclampsia. The hypertension in preeclampsia is identified relative to prepregnancy blood pressure. A rise in systolic blood pressure of 30 mm Hg or a rise in diastolic blood pressure of 15 mm Hg raises the possibility of preeclampsia. The definitive treatment of preeclampsia is delivery of the baby and placenta, but depending on the severity of the preeclampsia, efforts may be made to postpone delivery if it occurs in the second trimester or early in the third trimester. Anticonvulsants, most commonly magnesium in the U.S., and antihypertensive drugs are usually required while getting the mother ready for delivery.

   Over the last decade, long-term follow-up of large populations of women with preeclampsia has shown a subsequent increased risk of cardiovascular disease, kidney biopsy, and end-stage kidney disease (ESKD).

4. **What is the pathophysiology of preeclampsia?**
   The initiating factor in preeclampsia is incomplete remodeling of uterine spiral arteries, which results in placental ischemia. The ischemic placenta produces high levels of the antiangiogenic factors, soluble Fms-like tyrosine kinase (sFlt1) and soluble endoglin which are released into the circulation. Levels of placental growth factor (PIGF) and vascular endothelial growth factor (VEGF) are low. sFlt1 antagonizes the angiogenic activity of VEGF and PIGF, causing diffuse vasoconstriction and glomerular endothelial damage. Therapies targeting antiangiogenic factors to treat preeclampsia are an ongoing area of investigation. A different pathogenesis has been proposed for late-onset preeclampsia (more than 34 weeks gestation). In late preeclampsia, the problem may be maternal endothelial dysfunction in response to oxidative stress in the placenta.

331

5. **What are the other hypertensive disorders of pregnancy?**

   The three other hypertensive disorders of pregnancy are chronic hypertension, chronic hypertension with superimposed preeclampsia, and gestational hypertension. Women with preexisting hypertension may become pregnant so that essential hypertension is seen during pregnancy. The diagnosis of essential hypertension is made by a blood pressure ≤140/90 before 20 weeks gestation with no other explanation or a diagnosis of essential hypertension before pregnancy. These women are at increased risk for preeclampsia, giving rise to essential hypertension with superimposed preeclampsia in 25%. Gestational hypertension is hypertension that occurs late in pregnancy and is not accompanied by proteinuria or other end organ disease or preeclampsia. It resolves postpartum but is a predictor of future essential hypertension.

6. **What antihypertensive drugs can be used to treat hypertension in pregnancy?**

   Use of angiotensin converting enzyme inhibitor (ACEi) in the second and third trimester is associated with renal dysplasia, oligohydramnios, and neonatal death from hypoplastic lungs. Using ACEis in the first trimester may cause cardiac anomalies in the neonate. There are less data on angiotensin receptor blockers (ARBs), but they are avoided because of concern that their effects will be similar to those of ACEis. Direct renin inhibitors, such as aliskiren, should also be avoided.

   Alpha methyldopa has been used for more than 50 years to treat hypertension in pregnant women and careful follow-up on children support its safety. Labetalol, hydralazine, and calcium channel blockers are safe. Calcium channel blockers may cause severe hypotension when used with magnesium. Hydralazine is ineffective as a single oral agent, but may be effective when used with a sympatholytic drug. Beta blockers, particularly atenolol, have been reported to have adverse effects on fetal growth and labetalol can usually be used as an alternative. They are not considered contraindicated. Diuretics have been associated with less than normal expansion of plasma volume but may be necessary in women with underlying kidney disease. Intravenous hydralazine and labetalol are the drugs most commonly used for hypertensive emergencies.

7. **What are the causes of acute kidney injury in pregnancy?**

   In underdeveloped countries, sepsis from illegal abortion and preeclampsia are the most common causes of acute kidney injury. With improved health care systems, pregnancy-associated acute kidney injury is rare, on the order of 1 in 10,000 to 20,000 pregnancies. Preeclampsia is occasionally associated with acute kidney injury, especially in the setting of the HELLP syndrome. Pregnancy can be complicated by hemolytic uremic syndrome, which presents in a manner similar to hemolytic uremic syndrome (HUS) in other settings. It can be distinguished from preeclampsia by the elevated transaminases and abnormal clotting parameters seen in preeclampsia. Acute kidney injury can complicate acute fatty liver of pregnancy. Despite the rarity of acute kidney injury in pregnancy, pregnancy makes the kidney more susceptible to cortical necrosis. When acute kidney injury occurs in the setting of an obstetric catastrophe such as abruptio placentae, amniotic fluid embolus, or hemorrhage from other causes, there may be residual kidney dysfunction after recovery.

8. **What is the effect of chronic kidney disease (CKD) on fertility and pregnancy?**

   Fertility is decreased in women with preexisting kidney disease. Since the denominator (number of women with kidney disease trying to become pregnant) is not known, it is impossible to know how much fertility is decreased, but it is unusual to see a pregnancy in a woman with a serum creatinine >2.5 mg/dL. In women with kidney disease and preserved glomerular filtration rate (GFR), pregnancy carries an increased risk of hypertension and premature delivery. If proteinuria is present, it is likely to increase during pregnancy. It can be difficult to distinguish between hypertension associated with kidney disease and preeclampsia, since increased proteinuria, increased uric acid, and increased creatinine may be seen in both. One complication of pregnancy in a woman with kidney disease is worsening kidney function. The likelihood of worsening kidney function depends on the level of kidney function before conception. Most studies rely on serum creatinine to assess kidney function. The risk of worsening kidney function increases when the serum creatinine is >1.4 mg/dL. If the serum creatinine is >2 mg/dL, the risk of worsening kidney function is 30% to 50%. Imbasciati et al. used eGFR and proteinuria in assessing kidney disease. Worsening kidney function was seen only in women with both a GFR of <40 cc/min and at least 1 g of proteinuria in 24 hours. The formulas used to calculate GFR have not been validated in pregnancy.

9. **Is successful pregnancy possible in patients on renal replacement therapy?**

   Fertility is markedly decreased in dialysis patients with frequency of conception ranging from 0.3% to 1.5% per dialysis patient per year. One exception is a 15% conception rate among women treated with nocturnal dialysis. There are no data on whether or not women were trying to become pregnant. Outcomes are better with increased dialysis hours. In women with less than 20 hours of dialysis per week, infant survival is about 50%. Infant survival increases to 75% with 20 or more hours of dialysis. The most encouraging outcomes originate from women receiving nocturnal dialysis (48 h/week) where 84.6% of infants survived. Prematurity is decreased in the pregnancies of nocturnal dialysis patients with a mean gestational age of 36 weeks. Life-threatening hypertension can occur up to 6 weeks postpartum in dialysis patients. There are no data on the ideal time to start dialysis in pregnant women, but fetal loss appears to increase when the serum creatinine is between 3 and 4 mg/dL.

For pregnancies in women with kidney insufficiency severe enough to require starting dialysis during pregnancy, infants survival is around 75%. With lesser degrees of kidney insufficiency, infant survival is above 80%. There are two studies in women with serum creatinine over 2 mg/dL where fetal survival was 100%.

10. **Can erythropeietin (ESAs) be used during pregnancy?**
Erythropoiesis stimulating agents are continued in dialysis patients during pregnancy and the dose has to be increased to achieve the same hemoglobin level. They can be started in non-dialysis patients if the hemoglobin drops to 8 g/dL.

11. **Should a woman with a kidney transplant become pregnant?**
Fertility is usually restored by kidney transplant. Three broad areas of concern are:
• The effect of pregnancy on the kidney allograft.
• The effect of immunosuppressive medication on the fetus.
• The risk of opportunistic infection.
Women are advised to wait a year after transplant, and to only become pregnant if they have stable kidney function with a serum creatinine of less than 2 mg/dL. As in other kidney diseases, the most important risk factor for worsening kidney function is poor kidney function prior to pregnancy. Statins and angiotensin-converting enzyme (ACE) inhibitors must be stopped before conception. Mycophenolate mofetil is associated with increased congenital anomalies and should also be stopped prior to conception. About 50% of pregnancies in women taking mycophenolate end in spontaneous abortion and 30% of live born infants have congenital anomalies. Cyclosporine and tacrolimus are associated with small-for-gestational-age babies. Prednisone and azathioprine are widely used without major problems. There is no information on sirolimus, everolimus, and belatacept.
Infectious diseases such as cytomegalovirus (CMV), toxoplasmosis, herpes simplex, and listeria, which are seen in transplant recipients, pose a risk for the fetus. Transplant recipients are at increased risk for CMV during pregnancy. CMV is a leading cause of developmental delay and sensorineural hearing loss. Of women who are seronegative at conception, 1% to 4% will develop a primary infection during pregnancy. There are case reports of successful use of valganciclovir in women with CMV during pregnancy. The data are scant and more data are needed regarding both efficacy and safety. CMV hyperimmune globulin has also been used, but again, data are limited. Treatment with ganciclovir should be used if maternal disease requires treatment.

12. **What is the effect of lupus nephritis on pregnancy and vice versa?**
Lupus occurs most frequently in women of child-bearing age and may be diagnosed during pregnancy. When the onset of lupus nephritis occurs during pregnancy, the kidney histology is often World Health Organization (WHO) class IV, which requires prompt treatment. New-onset lupus is one of the indications for a kidney biopsy in a pregnant woman, since the drugs most commonly used for severe lupus nephritis such as cyclophosphamide should not be used in early pregnancy. In a woman with diffuse proliferative lupus nephritis, high-dose steroids can be used initially. Oral cyclophosphamide has been used in women beyond 20 weeks gestation, but long-term follow-up is limited. Lupus nephritis, including membranous lupus nephritis, carries the risk of relapse during pregnancy. The risk of relapse is lowest if the woman has been in remission 6 months before pregnancy but even then, one-third of women have a flare during pregnancy and during the first 6 weeks postpartum. The greatest risks may come from extrarenal lupus. Many antibodies associated with lupus are immunoglobulin G (IgG) and cross the placenta. They may cause rash and thrombocytopenia in the infant during the first 6 months of life. Anti-Sjögren's-syndrome-related antigen A (anti-Ro) (anti-SSA) antibody is associated with congenital heart block.

13. **What are the indications for and risks of kidney biopsy during pregnancy?**
Indications for kidney biopsy during pregnancy include newly diagnosed lupus, unexplained acute kidney injury, and nephrotic syndrome severe enough to require treatment. In most cases, biopsy can be postponed until the postpartum period. Because of the increased kidney blood flow associated with pregnancy, the risk of bleeding is higher than in nonpregnant patients. Packham and Fairly reported biopsies of 111 pregnant women with few complications during the first and second trimesters.

Table 47.1. Causes of AKI in Pregnancy

	HUS	HELLP	LUPUS NEPHRITIS	AFLP	CORTICAL NECROSIS
Creatinine	↑	↑ or nl	↑ or nl	↑ or nl	↑
Platelets	↓	↓	↓ or nl	↓ or nl	nl
Transaminases	nl	↑↑	nl	↑	nl
LDH	↑	↑	nl	↑	nl
PT/PTT	nl	↑ or nl	nl	↑	nl
Schistocytes	†	†	No	No	No
BP	↑	↑	↑ or nl	↓ or nl	↓↑ or nl
Progression	Frequent	Rare	Variable	No	Frequent

AFLP, Acute fatty liver of pregnancy; *AKI,* acute kidney injury; *BP,* blood pressure; *HELLP,* hemolytic anemia, elevated liver enzymes and low platelets; *HUS,* hemolytic uremic syndrome; *LDH,* lactate dehydrogenase; *PT,* prothrombin time; *PTT,* partial thromboplastin time.

However, the complication rate is higher in smaller series. Biopsy should be postponed until after delivery unless management will be determined by biopsy results.

14. **What is diabetes insipidus of pregnancy?**
    Diabetes insipidus of pregnancy is a rare disorder that occurs in the third trimester and resolves within a few weeks postpartum. It is characterized by polyuria, polydipsia, and, if inadequate free water is provided, hypernatremia. It is resistant to exogenous vasopressin and vasopressin levels may be normal or high. A second problem with urinary concentration may occur in women with partial central diabetes insipidus. The placenta makes vasopressinase, which breaks down endogenous native ADH but not 1-desamino-8d-arginine vasopressin (DDAVP), so that the DDAVP dose may need to be increased to offset accelerated breakdown of residual native antidiuretic hormone (ADH).

15. **How does pregnancy affect nephrolithiasis?**
    Nephrolithiasis is the most common nonobstetric cause of abdominal pain during pregnancy. Pregnancy is characterized by factors that promote (increased urinary calcium and uric acid, decreased peristalsis of the ureter, and dilatation of the collecting system) and prevent (increased urinary magnesium, citrate, and acid glycoproteins) stone formation. Stones may be difficult to diagnose because hydronephrosis is normal in pregnancy, and use of computed tomography (CT) scans is generally contraindicated in pregnancy. Additionally, on kidneys, ureters, bladder (KUB) x-rays, radiopaque stones may be obscured by the fetal skeleton, especially in the third trimester when stones are most common. Indications for intervention include intractable pain, infection, complete obstruction, or obstruction of a solitary kidney. Treatments include extraction of the stone by a skilled urologist or placement of percutaneous nephrostomy tubes. Pregnancy is considered a contraindication to lithotripsy.

16. **How do we distinguish among different causes of acute kidney injury (AKI) in pregnancy?**
    See Table 47.1.

KEY POINTS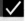

1. Normal pregnancy is associated with decreased serum creatinine and respiratory alkalosis, causing a decrease in serum bicarbonate.
2. The pathogenesis of preeclampsia is thought to be the consequence of the abnormal development of uterine spiral arteries and placental ischemia leading to increased levels of antiangiogenic factors and low levels of angiogenic growth factors.
3. There is a high rate of fetal loss among pregnant dialysis patients, but this has improved with prolonged dialysis. The outcome of pregnancy in transplant recipients with stable, well-preserved kidney function is good despite immunosuppressive medication.
4. Pregnancy is possible after kidney transplant. A stable immune status and good kidney function is essential. Modification of the immunosuppression will likely be needed.

BIBLIOGRAPHY

Armenti, V. T., Radomski, J. S., Moritz, M. J., Gaughn, W. J., Phillips, L., McGrory, C. H., & Coscia, L. A. (2001). Report from the National Transplantation Pregnancy registry: Outcomes of pregnancy after transplantation. In J. M. Cecka & P. I. Terasaki (Eds.), *Clinical transplants* (pp. 97–105). Los Angeles: UCLA Immunogenetics Center.

Barron, W. M., Cohen, L. H., Ulland, L. A., Lassiter, W. E., Fulghum, E. M., Emmanouel, D., . . . Lindheimer, M. D. (1984). Transient vasopressin resistant diabetes insipidus of pregnancy. *New England Journal of Medicine, 310,* 442–444.

Barua, M., Hladunewick, M., Keunen, J., Pierratos, A., McFarlane, P., Sood, M., & Chan, C. T. (2008). Successful pregnancies on nocturnal home hemodialysis. *Clinical Journal of the American Society of Nephrology, 3,* 392–396.

Hladunewich, M. A., Hou, A., Cornelis, T., Pierratos, A., Goldstein, M., Tennakore, K., . . . Chan, C. T. (2014). Intensive hemodialysis associates with improved pregnancy outcomes: A Canadian and United States cohort comparison. *Journal of the American Society of Nephrology, 25,* 1103–1109.

Hou, S. (1999). Lupus in pregnancy. In E. J. Lewis, M. M. Schwartz, & S. M. Korbet (Eds.), *Lupus nephritis.* Oxford: Oxford University Press.

Jones, D. C., & Hayslett, J. P. (1996). Outcome of pregnancy in women with moderate or severe renal insufficiency. *New England Journal of Medicine, 335,* 226–232.

Matnard, S. E., Min, J. Y., Merchan, J., Lim, K. H., Li, J. Y., Mondal, S., . . . Sukhatme, V. P. (2003). Excess placental fms-like tyrosine kinase 1(sFlt1) may contribute to endothelial dysfunction, hypertension and proteinuria in preeclampsia. *Journal of Clinical Investigation, 111,* 649–658.

McKay, D. B., Josephson, M. A., Armenti, V. T., August, P., Coscia, L. A., Davis, C. L., . . . Women's Health Committee of the American Society of Transplantation. (2005). Reproduction and transplantation: Report of the AST consensus conference on reproductive issues and transplantation. *American Journal of Transplantation, 5,* 1592–1599.

Okundaye, I. B., Abrinko, P., & Hou, S. H. (1998). A registry for pregnancy in dialysis patients. *American Journal of Kidney Diseases, 31,* 766–773.

Phipps, E., Prasanna, D., Brima, W., & Jim, B. (2016). Preeclampsia: Updates in pathogenesis, definitions and guideline. *Clinical Journal of the American Society of Nephrology, 11,* 1102–1113.

Podymow, T., & August, P. (2011). Antihypertensive drugs in pregnancy. *Seminars in Nephrology, 31,* 70–85.

Sibai, B. M., Ramadan, M. K., Chari, R. S., & Friedman, S. A. (1995). Pregnancies complicated by HELLP syndrome (hemolysis, elevated liver enzymes and low platelets): Subsequent pregnancy outcome and long term prognosis. *American Journal of Obstetrics and Gynecology, 172,* 125–129.

CHAPTER 48

SICKLE CELL NEPHROPATHY

Phuong-Chi T. Pham and Phuong-Thu T. Pham

1. **What is the pathophysiology of sickle cell disease (SCD)?**
   Hemolysis, vasoocclusion, and ischemia reperfusion are the clinical hallmarks of SCD. The substitution of glutamate for valine at position 6 of the hemoglobin β-chain is the mutation defining hemoglobin S (HbS). HbS polymerizes when the concentration of its deoxygenated form exceeds a critical threshold. Conditions that promote HbS polymerization and red blood cell sickling include low local oxygen tension, acidemia (reduces HbS affinity for oxygen), and hyperosmolality (dehydrates red blood cells and increases HbS concentration).

   Extensive HbS polymerization, red blood cell sickling, cell membrane injury, and associated cell membrane adhesive interactions with the endothelium contribute to vasoocclusion leading to multiorgan damage.

2. **What is the pathophysiology of sickle cell nephropathy (SCN)?**
   Increased blood viscosity and red blood cell sickling promoted by the renal medullary milieu of low oxygen tension, low pH, and high osmolality lead to vasoocclusion and hypoperfusion in the medullary microcirculatory beds, and result in local ischemia and infarction. Severe medullary hypoperfusion can lead to papillary necrosis, sloughing, and obstructive uropathy.

   In contrast to medullary hypoperfusion, glomerular ischemia appears to promote compensatory increase in kidney blood flow and the glomerular filtration rate (GFR). Glomerular hyperfiltration is mediated by glomerular hypertrophy and increased activity of vasodilatory factors including prostaglandins, kallikrein, carbon monoxide, and possibly nitric oxide (NO).

   Proximal tubular secretory and absorptive hyperfunctioning are characteristic of SCD. Tubular hyperfunctioning is thought to reflect glomerulotubular balance in the face of glomerular hyperfiltration, and is evidenced by increased proximal tubular secretion of uric acid and creatinine and increased tubular reabsorption of low-molecular-weight protein (β2-microglobulins) and phosphate. Hypersecretion of creatinine causes an overestimation of the true GFR when using serum creatinine-based estimated GFR equations.

   Chronic hemolysis and hemoglobinuria involving HbS can induce oxidant-mediated tubular injury, proliferation of mesangial cells, and upregulation of proinflammatory and profibrogenic responses to promote glomerulosclerosis and tubulointerstitial fibrosis.

   Progressive kidney failure occurs due to:
   - Increased glomerular growth
   - Heme-induced injury to mesangial cells with chronic hemolysis
   - Repetitive vascular congestion and vasoocclusion-induced endothelial injury
   - Capillary rarefaction (reduced capillary density)
   - Ischemia-reperfusion-induced proinflammatory and profibrogenic responses
     Contributing factors to kidney vascular congestion and dysfunction include:
   - Endothelin-1: increases kidney vascular congestion, inflammation, and vasoconstriction induced by hypoxia
   - Thrombospondin: induces shedding of microparticles from red blood cells that can lead to oxidant-mediated endothelial injury, red blood cell adhesion to the endothelium, and worsening of kidney vasoocclusive disease
   - Adenosine: promotes red blood cell sickling by increasing levels of 2,3-diphosphoglycerate in red blood cells.

3. **In addition to proximal tubular hyperfunctioning, what other tubular abnormalities may be seen in patients with SCD?**
   - Diminished concentrating ability: Red blood cell sickling and congestion in the vasa recta leads to ischemia and associated impairment of solute reabsorption by the ascending limb of Henle loop and the vasa recta function as countercurrent exchangers. The suboptimal maintenance of the high interstitial osmolality in the inner medulla reduces effective water reabsorption across the

collecting ducts, hence the reduced kidney concentrating ability. A diminished concentrating ability leads to hypo- or isosthenuria where urine osmolality typically does not exceed 450 mosm/Kg. Affected adults present with polyuria, nocturia, and volume depletion and children with enuresis. Blood transfusions of HbA-containing red blood cells can improve concentrating ability in children younger than age 15, but not thereafter due to permanent injury.

- Renal tubular acidosis: Patients may develop incomplete distal renal tubular acidosis via reduced H+-ATPase activity due to hypoxemia, selective aldosterone deficiency, distal nephron resistance to aldosterone, reduced ammonium availability, or, in rare cases, hyporenin hypoaldosteronism.

4. What are the common abnormal urinary findings in SCD?
   - Hematuria: Both microscopic and macroscopic hematuria may be observed. The left kidney is affected four times greater than the right due to the increased venous pressure within the longer left vein that is compressed between the aorta and the superior mesenteric artery. This is known as the "nutcracker phenomenon." The increased venous pressure leads to increased relative hypoxia in the renal medulla, hence sickling. In 10% of cases, hematuria occurs bilaterally. Hematuria may also indicate the presence of papillary necrosis and, in rare cases, renal medullary carcinoma. The latter is predominantly observed in sickle cell trait rather than SCD.
   - Proteinuria: The prevalence of albuminuria and proteinuria is 30% within the first three decades of life and increases up to 70% in older patients. Proteinuria may be associated with defects in glomerular permselectivity, tubular injury, and/or specific single nucleotide polymorphisms in the *APOL1* genes.
   - Bacteriuria: Patients with SCD may be at increased risk for urinary tract infections from encapsulated organisms due to autosplenectomy, abnormally dilute and alkaline urine (more favorable for bacterial growth compared with hypertonic and acidic urine), and papillary necrosis. However, significant bacteriuria generally occurs in less than 10% of sickle cell patients, half of whom are asymptomatic.

5. What are the common causes of acute kidney injury (AKI) in patients with SCD?
   - AKI may occur more frequently among patients with acute chest syndrome than those with a painful crisis. Predisposing factors leading to AKI include volume depletion due to concentrating defects, sickling process, and hemolysis. Patients may present with acute tubular necrosis from volume depletion or sepsis, tubular injury from ischemia-induced rhabdomyolysis, hemosiderin accumulation, or chronic use of nonsteroidal antiinflamatory drugs, kidney vein thrombosis, or, in rare cases, hepatorenal syndrome due to liver failure associated with the sickling process per se or transfusion-associated complications.
   - Kidney infarction and papillary necrosis: Severe ischemia can lead to kidney infarction and papillary necrosis. Papillary necrosis typically presents as painless gross hematuria, but may be complicated by obstructive uropathy and urinary tract infections. Current data suggest that hematuria and papillary necrosis do not portend greater risk for kidney failure. Acute segmental or total kidney infarction may present with flank or abdominal pain, nausea, vomiting, fevers, and presumably renin-mediated hypertension.

6. How does SCD affect blood pressure?
   Patients with SCD generally have lower blood pressure compared with their healthy unaffected counterparts due to presumed reduced vascular reactivity, compensatory systemic vasodilatation associated with microvascular disturbances from the sickling of red blood cells and thrombotic complications, elevated levels of prostaglandins and nitric oxide, and possibly kidney sodium and water wasting associated with suboptimal medullary concentrating activity. Blood pressures in the "normal" range defined for the general population may thus represent hypertension in patients with SCD. Whether the lower blood pressure reduces long-term cardiovascular disease risks is not known as the median survival for patients with SCD is only 40 years.

7. How do SCD and sickle cell trait (SCT) differ with respect to common kidney manifestations?
   Kidney manifestations are generally more common and severe in SCD compared with those seen in sickle cell trait. However, one notable exception is the increased frequency of aggressive renal medullary carcinoma seen among patients with sickle cell trait. Renal medullary carcinoma occurs almost exclusively in patients with sickle cell trait (not SCD). Renal medullary carcinoma typically presents in young patients (20 to 30 years old) as an aggressive metastatic disease at the time of diagnosis. Median survival is 3 months following diagnosis. Affected individuals may present with hematuria, flank pain, and/or abdominal mass.

8. **What are the underlying pathogenesis of chronic kidney disease (CKD) and risk factors associated with CKD progression in patients with SCN?**
   - Pathogenesis of CKD: Although glomerular filtration is increased in younger patients with SCD, it progressively declines after the age of 30. The development of CKD is thought to be due to early glomerular hypertrophy and hyperfiltration; tubular hyperfunctioning; endothelial injury with repeated sickling and vasoocclusive episodes; hemolysis and iron-induced proinflammatory and profibrotic changes in endothelial cells; and glomerular mesangium and tubulointerstitium.
   - Risk factors for CKD progression: underlying hypertension, nephrotic range proteinuria, severe anemia, vasoocclusive crisis, acute chest syndrome, stroke, β^S-gene haplotype, genetic variants of *MYH9* and *APOL1*, pulmonary hypertension, and infection with parvovirus B19. Of note, although studies have provided statistical evidence implicating *APOL1* variation in nondiabetic nephropathies, *MYH9* risk variants are still associated with CKD in non–African American populations and in SCD nephropathy. It has been hypothesized that *MYH9* and *APOL1* may be coregulated and interact under anemic stress to induce nephropathy risk.
   - Protective factors: coinheritance with α-thalassemia, higher fetal hemoglobin.

9. **What tests are needed to diagnose SCN?**
   The diagnosis of SCN is based on clinical manifestations and is primarily a diagnosis of exclusion. Routine evaluation for common causes of proteinuria (particularly when severe) and active urinary sediments, obstructive uropathy, and kidney biopsy should be performed as clinically indicated.
   - Routine proteinuria evaluation for both infectious (e.g. HIV, hepatitis B and C) and noninfectious serologies associated with glomerular diseases based on age, gender, and risks.
   - Imaging studies including kidney ultrasound to rule out obstructive uropathy, bladder scanning for postvoid retention or bladder neck obstruction, and possibly a computed tomography scan with or without contrast agent as clinically indicated.
   - Review of recent or current use of nephrotoxic medications.
   - Kidney biopsy as clinically indicated by active urinary sediment, significant proteinuria (e.g., urine protein to creatinine ratio >1 g/g) with predominant albuminuria, or unexplained rapid kidney function deterioration.

10. **What are typical radiographic findings in SCN?**
    - Increased echodensity and "garland" pattern of calcification in the medullary pyramids.
    - Calyceal clubbing on contrast computed tomogram urography seen with papillary necrosis (often described with "egg in a cup" or "golf ball and a club").

11. **Why do patients with SCN develop hyperphosphatemia?**
    - Release of intracellular phosphate from acute hemolysis or rhabdomyolysis.
    - Proximal tubular hyperfunctioning with increased reabsorption of phosphate via sodium phosphate cotransporters in early disease.
    - Reduced filtration of phosphate in advanced kidney disease.

12. **What glomerular disorders are commonly seen in patients with SCN?**
    - Secondary focal segmental glomerulosclerosis (FSGS) and its variants are major glomerular lesions observed in SCD. Both collapsing and noncollapsing patterns of FSGS have been described. The development of FSGS is likely adaptive to the initial glomerular hyperfiltration followed by repeated episodes of ischemia and reperfusion injuries. Glomerular hypertrophy was found to be greater in HbS patients than in idiopathic FSGS. Medullary fibrosis is prominent, suggesting that SCD-associated FSGS mainly affects the juxtamedullary nephrons supplied by the vasa recta.
    - Membranoproliferative glomerulonephropathy and thrombotic microangiopathy may also occur, but at a lower frequency than FSGS. Membranoproliferative glomerulonephritis (MPGN) with mesangial expansion and basement membrane duplication may be seen either as an isolated finding or in association with FSGS. It has been suggested that this rare form of MPGN is caused by fragmented red blood cells lodged in isolated capillary loops and phagocytosed by mesangial cells, stimulating the expansion of the mesangium and new basement membrane deposition. Although MPGN was initially attributed to immune complex injury, subsequent studies demonstrated that MPGN commonly occurred without immune complex deposits. In essence, the absence of immune complexes and electron-dense deposits differentiates SCD-associated MPGN from other forms of MPGN that are associated with lymphoproliferative or autoimmune disorders, chronic infections, or dysregulation of the complement system.
    - Although rare with modern screening for blood borne pathogens, HIV nephropathy and hepatitis-associated glomerulonephropathies may be possible.

13. How is sickle cell anemia managed?
  - Goal hemoglobin for patients with sickle cell anemia and the correction rate of the anemia are recommended to be no more than 10 to 10.5 g/dL and less than 1% to 2% per week, respectively. Higher hemoglobin levels and more rapid correction of anemia may precipitate a vasoocclusive crisis.
  - Anemia correction may be achieved with blood transfusion or the use of erythropoietin stimulating agents (ESA). Blood transfusions provide a higher proportion of HbA compared with stimulating endogenous red blood cells with an ESA. Additionally, the use of ESA may be associated with increased vasoocclusive risk. ESA dosing may need to be higher in individuals receiving hydroxyurea due to the inherent bone marrow suppressive effect of the latter. However, it has also been suggested that the addition of ESA may allow administration of higher doses of hydroxyurea and improved fetal hemoglobin levels. Hydroxyurea is used in the treatment of SCD to increase the synthesis of fetal hemoglobin, which, unlike HbS, does not sickle.

14. How is hematuria managed?
  - Conservative measures, including bedrest and oral hydration, remain the cornerstone in the management gross hematuria.
  - In more severe cases, hydration with alkaline fluids may be used to correct volume depletion, acidemia, or both, to reduce sickling and minimize HbS precipitation. Other considerations include the use of loop diuretic to prevent microtubular obstruction, and blood transfusions to reduce HbS and sickling.
  - Alternative therapeutic options may be considered in refractory cases and include high-dose urea, vasopressin, or epsilon-aminocaproic acid (EACA). High doses of oral or intravenous urea (up to 160 g/day) to achieve blood urea nitrogen greater than 100 mg/dL has been shown to inhibit the polymerization of deoxygenated sickle hemoglobin and are reported to be effective in some refractory cases. Vasopressin is thought to improve clotting via the increase in plasma factor VIII and von Willebrand factor. Vasopressin may be given intravenously over 30 minutes at 0.3 mcg of DDAVP/kg body weight. EACA inhibits fibrinolysis by inhibiting plasmin activity. However, blood clot formation within the collecting system from the use of EACA may lead to tubular obstruction, leading to kidney injury. Note that these alternative therapeutic options lack data and are not without adverse effects. Their use should only be considered for refractory cases. Optimal EACA dosing is not known, but has been suggested to be 2 to 3 g daily (5 to 50 mg/kg every 8 to 12 hours) over several days, not to exceed 12 g daily due to risk of thrombosis.
  - Angiographic embolization of the involved kidney vessel or balloon tamponade for bleeding from papillary necrosis may be considered in cases of failed conservative medical therapies.
  - Unilateral nephrectomy is not recommended, because bleeding can recur in the contralateral kidney.

15. How are patients with CKD managed?
  - Progression of CKD:
    - Although angiotensin-converting enzyme inhibitors (ACEi) and angiotensin receptor blockers (ARB) are commonly used to reduce proteinuria in addition to slowing CKD progression and lowering blood pressures in non–sickle cell nephropathies, significant antiproteinuric benefits have not been proven in patients with SCD. Nonetheless, the most updated Cochrane database review (in 2015) revealed a potential for reduction in microalbuminuria and proteinuria with the use of captopril among patients with SCD compared with those without the disease. Confirmatory studies using other ACEi and ARB are lacking.
    - Hydroxyurea may have a role in reducing proteinuria and hyperfiltration. It has been suggested that the increase in fetal Hb with the use of hydroxyurea reduces sickling, which would lead to improved tissue oxygenation, decreased cardiac output, and reduced kidney blood flow, and therefore decreased hyperfiltration, glomerular injury, and proteinuria.
  - End-stage kidney disease (ESKD): All forms of kidney replacement may be beneficial to patients with ESKD from sickle cell anemia.
  - Dialysis: Both hemo and peritoneal dialytic therapies may be offered to patients reaching ESKD if there is no modality-specific contraindication. Both modalities confer their own theoretical advantages.
    - Hemodialysis: Readily available vascular access may be used for the urgent or emergent need for standard and exchange blood transfusions.
    - Peritoneal dialysis: The slow rate of ultrafiltration minimizes any acute rise in hematocrit, and therefore leads to a lower risk of vasoocclusive crisis.
  - Kidney transplantation:
    - Kidney transplantation may be hindered by high levels of panel reactive antibody due to numerous previous blood transfusions. There is also a higher infection risk due to autosplenectomy. Sickle

cell transplant patients have higher risks of avascular necrosis with chronic steroid use and precipitating sickle cell crises due to anemia correction following a successful transplant.
- Kidney transplant may be also complicated by allograft venous thrombosis, deep vein thrombosis, and vasoocclusive crises.

16. What is the prognosis of patients with SCN
    - In general, patients with SCD have life expectancy reduced by 25 to 30 years.
    - Patients with SCD and kidney failure: Median survival among patients with and without kidney failure is 29 and 51 years, respectively. Survival is substantially worse among patients with SCD and ESKD compared with their counterpart without the disease.
    - Kidney transplant recipients: Although survival of transplant recipients with SCD is inferior to that of matched African American recipients without the disease, survival of SCD patients is comparable with that of matched diabetic patients. One-year graft survival exceeds 60% to 80%.

KEY POINTS

1. The clinical hallmarks of sickle cell disease are:
   - Hemolysis
   - Vasoocclusion
   - Ischemia reperfusion

   The underlying mechanisms of kidney injury or sickle cell nephropathy (SCN) primarily relate to hypoxia and ischemia.
2. SCN encompasses a wide range of kidney abnormalities indicating that all segments of the nephron can be affected. The clinical presentation of SCN includes:
   - Hyposthenuria
   - Isothenuria
   - Hematuria
   - Proteinuria
   - Hyperkalemia
   - Papillary necrosis
   - Rental tubular acidosis
   - Nephrogenic diabetes insipidus
   - Glomerulonephritis
   - Acute kidney injury
   - Progressive decline in glomerular filtration rate and eventual development of end-stage kidney disease (ESKD)
3. Goal hemoglobin and correction rate of anemia should be no more than 10 to 10.5 g/dL and less than 1% to 2% per week, respectively. Higher hemoglobin levels and more rapid correction of anemia may precipitate a vasoocclusive crisis.
4. All forms of renal replacement may be beneficial to patients with ESKD from sickle cell anemia. These include hemodialysis, peritoneal dialysis, and kidney transplantation.

BIBLIOGRAPHY

Alhwiesh, A. (2014). An update on sickle cell nephropathy. *Saudi Journal of Kidney Diseases and Transplantation, 25*(2), 249.

Anderson, B. R., Howell, D. N., Soldano, K., Garrett, M. E., Katsanis, N., Telen, M. J., ... Ashley-Koch, A. E. (2015). In vivo modeling implicates APOL1 in nephropathy: Evidence for dominant negative effects and epistasis under anemic stress. *PLoS Genetics, 11*(7), e1005349.

Ashley-Koch, A. E., Okocha, E. C., Garrett, M. E., Soldano, K., De Castro, L. M., Jonassaint, J. C., ... Telen, M. J. (2011). MYH9 and APOL1 are both associated with sickle cell disease nephropathy. *British Journal of Haematology, 155*(3), 386.

Aygun, B., Mortier, N. A., Smeltzer, M. P., Shulkin, B. L., Hankins, J. S., & Ware, R. E. (2013). Hydroxyurea treatment decreases glomerular hyperfiltration in children with sickle cell anemia. *American Journal of Hematology, 88*(2), 116–119.

Bergmann, S., Zheng, D., Barredo, J., Abboud, M. R., & Jaffa, A. A. (2006). Renal kallikrein: A risk marker of nephropathy in children with sickle cell disease. *Journal of Pediatric Hematology/Oncology, 28*(3), 147.

Boyle, S. M., Jacobs, B., Sayani, F. A., & Hoffman, B. (2016). Management of the dialysis patient with sickle cell disease. *Seminars in Dialysis, 29*(1), 62.

De Gracia-Nieto, A. E., Samper, A. O., Rojas-Cruz C, Gascón, L. G., Sanjuan, J. B., & Mavrich, H. V. (2011). Genitourinary manifestations of sickle cell disease. *Archivos Españoles de Urología, 64*(7), 597.

Gargiulo, R., Pandya, M., Seba, A., Haddad, R. Y., & Lerma, E. V. (2014). Sickle cell nephropathy. *Disease-a-month,* 60, 494.

Gladwin, M. T. (2016). Cardiovascular complications and risk of death in sickle-cell disease. *Lancet, 387,* 2565–2574.

Guasch, A., Navarrete, J., Nass, K., & Zayas, C. F. (2006). Glomerular involvement in adults with sickle hemoglobinopathies: Prevalence and clinical correlates of progressive renal failure. *Journal of the American Society of Nephrology, 17,* 2228.

Haymann, J. P., Stankovic, K., Levy, P., Avellino, V., Tharaux, P. L., Letavernier, E., ... Lionnet, F. (2010). Glomerular hyperfiltration in adult sickle cell anemia: A frequent hemolysis associated feature. *Clinical Journal of the American Society of Nephrology, 5,* 756.

Huang, E., Parke, C., Mehrnia, A., Kamgar, M., Pham, P. T., Danovitch, G., & Bunnapradist, S. (2013). Improved survival among sickle cell kidney transplant recipients in the recent era. *Nephrology Dialysis Transplantation,* 28(4), 1039.

Kiryluk, K., Jadoon, A., Gupta, M., & Radhakrishnan, J. (2007). Sickle cell trait and gross hematuria. *Kidney International, 71,* 706–710.

Nath, K. A., & Hebbel, R. P. (2015). Sickle cell disease: Renal manifestations and mechanisms. *Nature Reviews Nephrology, 11*(3), 161.

Nath, K. A., & Katusic, Z. S. (2012). Vasculature and kidney complications in sickle cell disease. *Journal of the American Society of Nephrology, 23*(5), 781.

Pham, P. T., Pham, P. C., Wilkinson, A. H., & Lew, S. Q. (2000). Renal abnormalities in sickle cell disease. *Kidney International, 57,* 1.

Scheinman, J. I. (2009). Sickle cell disease and the kidney. *Nature Clinical Practice Nephrology,* 5(2), 78.

Wang, W. C. (2016). Minireview: Prognostic factors and the response to hydroxurea treatment in sickle cell disease. *Experimental Biology and Medicine (Maywood), 241*(7), 730.

CHAPTER 49

KIDNEY DISEASES IN THE ELDERLY

Devasmita Choudhury and Moshe Levi

1. **What is the prevalence of chronic kidney disease in the elderly?**
   Approximately 11% of patients older than age 65 years are noted to have chronic kidney disease (CKD) as estimated by using the Modification of Diet in Renal Disease (MDRD) study equation in those participating in National Health and Nutrition Examination Survey III. As the proportion of elderly increases in the population as a whole, the number of elderly patients with CKD is also expected to increase.

2. **What structural changes occur in the kidney with age?**
   A progressive decrease in kidney weight and size occurs with increasing age as the glomeruli and the interstitium undergo fibrosis and sclerosis, tubules atrophy with drop in number and size, and vasculature scleroses and simplifies (Fig. 49.1). Individual rates of kidney senescence may vary as various factors that are known to mediate fibrosis such as angiotensin II, transforming growth factor, nitric oxide, advanced glycosylated end products, oxidative stress, and factors associated with reducing sclerosis such as Klotho (antiaging transmembrane protein) and autophagy are altered as the kidney ages.

3. **How does age affect kidney function?**
   Functional changes in the kidney occur in parallel to changes in structure.
   - **Decreased effective renal plasma flow (ERPF):** ERPF decreases approximately 10% per decade with age in relation to progressive vascular sclerosis and loss of nephron number. Both changes in the number of functioning glomeruli and altered intrarenal signal and response to vasodilatory and vasoconstrictive mediators may affect renal plasma flow in the elderly.
   - **Decrease in glomerular filtration rate (GFR):** An estimated drop of 0.8 to 1.0 mL/min per 1.73 m^2/year in GFR is noted with progressive age depending on methodology used to measure clearance. Decreases in GFR with age may also be affected by race, gender, genetic variation, and underlying comorbidities including hypertension, diabetes, and cardiovascular disease.

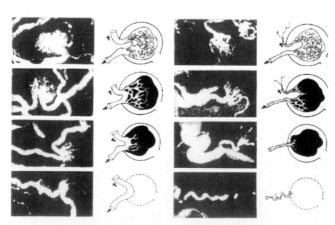

Figure 49.1. Stages of progressive vascular simplification and glomerular degeneration of cortical and juxtamedullary glomeruli and arterioles with associated microangiograms. *(From Takazakura, E., Sawabu, N., Handa, A., et al. (1972). Intravascular changes with age and disease.* Kidney international, 2, *224. Reprinted by permission from Macmillan Publishers Ltd.)*

342

- **Decreased ability to conserve filtered sodium:** An increase in solute load per nephron in the face of decreased nephron number and increased medullary flow, and lower levels of plasma renin and aldosterone with age, likely contribute to individuals 60 years and older taking nearly twice the number of hours (31 vs. 18 hours) compared to those 30 years and younger to reach appropriate distal tubular sodium reabsorption when sodium restriction is imposed.

- **Decreased natriuretic ability:** Individuals older than 40 years also handle a salt load less efficiently, as seen by taking a longer time to excrete 2 L of saline than those younger than 40 years. Although levels of the natriuretic hormone atrial natriuretic peptide appropriately increase, an incremental increase in urine sodium excretion is not evident in older compared to younger subjects, suggesting a possible decreased tubular sensitivity to natriuretic stimuli.

- **Abnormal tubular concentrating and diluting capacity:** The older individual may not be able to reach maximal urinary concentration despite 12 hours of overnight water deprivation. Studies in aged animals indicate a decrease in tubular transporters, Na-K-2Cl, and ENaC beta and gamma subunits, urea transporters UT-A1, UT-B1, and intrarenal resistance to arginine vasopressin may be reasons for decreased urinary concentration. Similarly, maximally dilute urine is also not found with increasing age given that appropriate solute extraction, suppression of arginine vasopressin, and distal delivery of the filtered load is necessary.

- **Decreased net acid excretion:** A diminished capacity for net acid excretion is found in older adults as both renal mass and GFR decrease are particularly noted when there is increased acid generation or acid load.

- **Changes in potassium handling:** Although total body potassium is lower given a decrease in muscle mass in older individuals, lower plasma renin and aldosterone levels and decreased aldosterone response to potassium load in the elderly predispose to decreased tubular excretion of potassium. In the face of a sudden potassium load, older individuals may have a decreased ability to shift potassium into cells because Na-K-ATPase activity is decreased with increasing age.

- **Decreased kidney phosphate reabsorption:** With phosphate restriction, older kidneys display evidence for decreased tubular phosphate absorption.

- **Tubular calcium excretion:** Remains unchanged in the kidney with increasing age.

4. Why are the elderly subjects more susceptible to osmolar disorders such as hyponatremia and hypernatremia?

With inability to maximally dilute urine, the elderly subjects face a greater likelihood for hyponatremia when situations lead to increased arginine vasopressin (AVP) secretion or response. Medications such as morphine (high dose), nicotine, vincristine, and cyclophosphamide can enhance, whereas chlorpropamide, tolbutamide, nonsteroidal agents, and lamotrigine may promote AVP action. Age-associated decreased prostaglandin synthesis inhibits water diuresis and also predisposes the older individual to hyponatremia.

Hyponatremia with thiazide-type diuretics, commonly used to treat hypertension, is more common in the elderly. Similarly, the presence of a decreased thirst response in addition to a urinary-concentrating defect can predispose older individuals to dehydration and hypernatremia. Medications associated with decreased AVP secretion such as morphine (low dose), fluphenazine, promethazine, carbamazepine, and Haldol, or decreased AVP response including propoxyphene, demeclocycline, glyburide, and lithium, may increase likelihood of developing hypernatremia in older patients.

5. What makes older kidneys susceptible to kidney injury?

Acute kidney injury occurs with 3.5 times greater incidence in those older than 70 years. Approximately one-third of those $\geq$65 years of age are unable to regain kidney function defined as independence from dialysis therapy, or return of kidney function at or near baseline kidney function after an episode of acute injury. Loss of nephron number and function and decreased vascular response to vasodilation in aging contributes to decreased kidney reserve. Thus any process that further compromises kidney perfusion or loss of nephron function, including pre-renal, intrinsic, or post-renal causes, increases susceptibility to kidney injury. Volume loss, marked vasoconstriction, or decreased cardiac output are frequent pre-renal processes in the elderly with numerous comorbidities such as hypertension, diabetes, heart failure, malignancy, or atherosclerosis. Medications, including angiotensin-converting enzyme inhibitors or angiotensin receptor blockers, and nonsteroidal agents or contrast infusion, can exacerbate the prerenal process, thereby requiring careful volume assessment before use. Intrinsic kidney processes such as toxin-associated tubular dysfunction (i.e., aminoglycosides), interstitial inflammation (i.e., antibiotic or other drug-mediated), or manipulation of the arterial tree leading to cholesterol embolization are often evident in the older individuals undergoing diagnoses and treatment of comorbid illnesses. Urinary tract obstruction can present with acute decline in kidney function in the elderly given laxity or overgrowth of pelvic structures with age and enlarged or prolapsed uterus in females and prostatic hypertrophy in male patients.

6. **What are the best ways to estimate kidney clearance in the elderly?**
Given loss of muscle mass with age, serum creatinine may not be the most useful marker for estimating kidney clearance. When appropriately collected, 24-hour urine creatinine clearances can be useful to measure steady-state clearances in the elderly. Formulas derived from 24-hour urine collections of populations of elderly with and without kidney disease are frequently used to estimate GFR at the bedside, minimizing frequent cumbersome 24 hour urine clearances in the elderly. Radioisotopes including iothalamate or iohexol X-ray fluorescence can be accurate; however, expense, radioactivity exposure, and availability limit these procedures for routine GFR measurements (see Chapter 3).

7. **How does age affect blood pressure?**
Data from the National Health and Nutrition Examination Survey (NHANES) report 67% of adults ≥60 years have hypertension. Changes in vascular elasticity with altered extracellular matrix cross-linking, fibrosis, and calcium deposition with age lead to stiffness and decreased capacity in the larger elastic vasculature. Older adults are thus noted to have high systolic blood pressure (SBP) and low diastolic blood pressure (DBP) with subsequent widened pulse pressure. Isolated systolic hypertension (ISH), defined as SBP >160 mm Hg and DBP <90 mm Hg, can be found in 75% of elderly patients with hypertension.

8. **What is the importance of isolated systolic hypertension in the elderly?**
ISH is associated with a twofold to fourfold increase in the risk of myocardial infarction, left ventricular hypertrophy, kidney dysfunction, stroke, and cardiovascular mortality. Even in patients who also have diastolic hypertension, the cardiovascular risk correlates more closely with the systolic than the diastolic BP. Among elderly patients, coronary heart disease risk varies directly with the systolic and pulse pressures and inversely with the diastolic pressure.

9. **Should target blood pressure in the elderly be the same as in younger patients?**
Treatment of elevated blood pressure in the elderly including those older than 80 years of age is clearly beneficial. Current studies indicate that intensive blood pressure lowering (systolic <120 mm Hg) can decrease both cardiovascular outcomes and mortality in nondiabetics including those 75 years or older. Intensive BP lowering in patients ≥50 years of age does not significantly impact chronic kidney disease progression; however, intensive BP lowering may increase risk for acute kidney injury events and incidence of hypotension in the elderly. While recommended BP goal is SBP <140 mm Hg for the general population and more intensive control of SBP <120 mm Hg considered for nondiabetics with increased cardiovascular risk, no clear data provide guidance related to the minimum diastolic BP that can be tolerated when treating elderly patients with isolated systolic hypertension (ISH). An analysis from the Systolic Hypertension in the Elderly Program (SHEP) trial found significant increases in cardiovascular events in the active treatment group when the diastolic BP was ≤60 mm Hg. Among patients being treated for ISH, the post-treatment diastolic blood pressure should be >60 mm Hg overall or, in patients with known coronary artery disease, >65 mm Hg unless symptoms attributable to hypo-perfusion occur at higher pressures. SBP goals should not be reached at the expense of excessive DBP reduction.

10. **What are important considerations in treating hypertension in the elderly?**
BP reduction should always be gradual in elderly patients. All patients should receive nonpharmacological therapy, particularly dietary salt restriction and weight loss in patients who are obese. Drug therapy should be started if lifestyle changes are not sufficient. A potential limiting factor to the use of antihypertensive drugs is orthostatic (postural) and/or postprandial hypotension, common symptoms among elderly patients with hypertension. A long-acting dihydropyridine or a thiazide diuretic is generally preferred in elderly patients because of increased efficacy in blood pressure lowering.

11. **Does revascularization in atherosclerotic renovascular disease improve outcomes in comparison to medical therapy alone?**
With age, vascular changes, and as part of generalized atherosclerosis, atherosclerotic renovascular disease (ARVD) prevalence is estimated at 6.8% in community-dwelling patients older than age 65. Heightened suspicion for ARVD in older patients should occur when sudden increase in blood pressure or worsening of kidney function is noted. Screening methodologies including duplex ultrasonography, computed tomographic angiography, or magnetic resonance angiography, in conjunction with functional significance for underlying stenotic lesions, should be utilized based on patient tolerance and test availability. Medical therapy with antihypertensive medications, particularly agents blocking the renin-angiotensin system, is useful, although careful follow-up is necessary in the face of high-grade

bilateral stenotic lesions given an associated drop in GFR. Although concern for loss of kidney mass or poorly controlled hypertension with risk for increased cardiovascular events endorses need for a revascularization procedure either percutaneous or surgical, multiple randomized trials show no evidence for increased clinical benefit in the initial years after revascularization in patients with atherosclerotic renal-artery stenosis when compared to medical therapy. No significant improvements in blood pressure or reductions in kidney or cardiovascular events or mortality were seen.

12. **What glomerular diseases are common in the elderly?**
    Elderly patients presenting with nephritic sediment and acute or rapidly progressive kidney failure often have pauci-immune glomerulonephritis, although anti-glomerular basement membrane and post-infectious glomerulonephritis should also be considered.

    A nephrotic presentation, particularly not diabetes related, is commonly associated with membranous glomerulopathy. Although minimal change disease is most common in children, it can be seen in 1 out of 10 older adults with nephrosis. Amyloidosis should also be suspected in older adults with marked proteinuria. Secondary etiologies such as malignancy for these presentations should also be investigated in the older adults given increased association of solid tumors with membranous kidney lesions, Hodgkin and non-Hodgkin lymphoma with minimal change disease, and the presence of paraproteinemia with amyloidosis.

13. **What is the most common cause for mortality in the elderly with chronic kidney disease?**
    The presence of CKD adds further burden to underlying cardiovascular risks and disease noted with age. As prevalence of hypertension increases with age, lipid abnormalities are also seen with aging and CKD. Dyslipidemia in the elderly is characterized by increased triglyceride levels, small high-dense low-density lipoprotein (LDL), and a low concentration of high-density lipoprotein (HDL), characteristics similar to CKD. Therefore it is not unusual that mortality in elderly with CKD results more from cardiovascular causes than in the progression of kidney disease and kidney failure. Cardiovascular risk management in elderly with CKD becomes particularly important.

14. **Does modality of kidney replacement affect outcome in the elderly?**
    A clear survival advantage in the elderly is not associated with either modality choice of hemodialysis or peritoneal dialysis. Some epidemiologic studies, however, suggest a higher mortality for elderly patients, particularly with diabetes, undergoing peritoneal dialysis. At this time, modality choice in the elderly should be individualized based on the ability to reach adequate clearance and tolerability of the procedure, considering both medical and psychosocial factors for each person.

15. **What is the best hemodialysis access in elderly patients with end-stage kidney disease (ESKD)?**
    While arteriovenous fistula is considered the optimal access for long-term hemodialysis, benefits and risk assessment including comorbidity, frailty, nutritional status, performance status, life expectancy, vascular disease, ability to undergo surgical access, risk for infection, and quality of life are important factors to assess for older individuals in determining the optimal access for each person. With numerous factors contributing to overall success in arteriovenous access, those with low comorbidities, expected longer survival, and good functional status may benefit from arteriovenous fistula placement, whereas those older individuals with lower functional status and increased comorbidities may benefit from arteriovenous graft survival. However, older individuals with high comorbidity status, poor functional status, and overall decreased long-term expected survival may benefit from tunneled central venous catheter placement.

16. **What are considered major contraindications to dialysis in the elderly?**
    The major contraindications to dialysis are advanced malignancy, irreversible dementia, or advanced liver disease. Observational studies of elderly with poor functional status as determined by inability to achieve some independence in performing activities of daily living as well as increased numbers of comorbid conditions, including high cardiovascular disease burden, particularly those dependent on nursing home care, appear to have little survival advantage or improved quality of life with dialysis over conservative management of no dialysis. Therefore, while not a contraindication, weighed benefits of survival and quality of life with dialysis to risks of infection, access surgery, hemodynamic shifts, as well as resource efforts should be individually and carefully considered and conveyed to elderly patients and or family and surrogates making decisions for dialysis initiation in the elderly.

17. **Does transplant have advantages over dialysis in the elderly?**
    Comparison of patients ≥ 70 years who remained on wait list for kidney transplantation to those patients transplanted indicated transplanted patients had 41% decreased risk of death. Mortality benefit was also seen in those elderly with diabetes and those that received extended criteria donors. These findings confirm similar comparisons in those aged 60 to 74 years with noted 61% lower mortality for

transplanted elderly compared to wait-listed elderly with a calculated 4-year increase in life expectancy. Prediction models on nearly 129,000 adults ≥65 years with Medicare-primary incident ESKD from United States Renal Data System and nearly 7000 Medicare-primary first-kidney transplant recipients of the United Network Organ Sharing evaluating post-transplant outcomes suggest that 9.1% of the patients are excellent candidates with 3-year post-kidney transplant survival of 87.6% or higher. While living donation is ideal, older donors may face difficulty in receiving a standard-criteria donor transplant, given current allocation based on Kidney Donor Profile Index. Patients ≥60 years who receive older donor kidneys and extended-criteria donor continue to have lifetime benefits of allograft function and should be encouraged. While frailty as a state of decreased physiologic reserve with unintentional weight loss, loss of grip strength weakness, slow walking speed, low physical activity, and self-noted exhaustion affects mortality in the elderly, lower frailty scores are beneficial for survival in elderly whether initiating dialysis or after transplantation. These data suggest continued advantage of kidney transplant over dialysis maintenance in the elderly, and older individuals should be considered for kidney transplant referral if medically eligible.

18. **What is the major cause of kidney transplant graft loss in the elderly?**
Kidney transplant graft loss in the elderly is related primarily to patient death. Main causes of morbidity and mortality in the elderly following kidney transplantation are cardiovascular disease, infection, and malignancy.

19. **What are the important considerations for immunosuppression in the elderly?**
Immunosuppressive therapy must be modified in the elderly transplant recipient because immune-competence lessens, thereby resulting in a decreased likelihood of immunologic rejection, but increasing the risk of infection. The other important consideration is altered pharmacokinetics and effects of drugs in the elderly. Some studies suggest that lower levels of immunosuppression may be sufficient in elderly patients to achieve adequate patient and graft survival.

20. **What is the patient and graft survival in the elderly kidney transplant recipient?**
Recipient survival is affected by allograft type. Recipient survival at 1, 3, and 5 years from 2007 registry data are reported to be 99%, 96%, and 79%, respectively, for living donor recipients ≥65 years; 97%, 92%, and 67%, respectively, for deceased nonextended-criteria donor; and 95%, 88%, and 58%, respectively, for deceased extended-criteria donor grafts.
Registry data of 2007 also note excellent allograft survival for recipients ≥65 years after 1, 3, and 5 years with living donor allografts having better outcome with 97%, 94%, and 73%, respectively; followed by deceased nonextended criteria donor graft survival of 94%, 86%, and 60%, respectively; and 91%, 81%, and 49% for deceased extended criteria donors, respectively.

21. **What is the prevalence of simple cysts in older people?**
The prevalence of simple cysts increases with age. Presence of at least one or more simple cysts is found in approximately 11.5% of those aged 50 to 70 years. The prevalence appears to double to 22.1% in those older than age 70 years and has been reported as high as 36.1% in those older than age 80 years, with a 2:1 frequency in men compared to women.

KEY POINTS

1. Both effective kidney plasma flow and glomerular filtration rate decrease in parallel to progressive sclerotic changes seen in glomeruli, interstitium, and vasculature of the aging kidney.
2. A decrease in both concentrating and diluting ability can predispose elderly patients to osmolar disorders of hyponatremia and hypernatremia.
3. Decreased kidney reserve with aging increases susceptibility for acute kidney injury.
4. Isolated systolic hypertension is most common in the elderly.
5. Blood pressure reduction should always be gradual in older patients.
6. Membranous nephropathy is common in older patients presenting with nephrotic syndrome, and pauci-immune glomerulonephritis can be a common presentation of rapidly progressive glomerulonephritis in older patients.
7. Revascularization for atherosclerotic renal artery lesions may not add benefit to treatment with medical therapy alone.
8. Elderly patients with chronic kidney disease die primarily from cardiovascular disease.
9. Kidney transplant graft loss in the elderly is primarily from patient death.
10. Prevalence of simple cysts increases with age.

Bibliography

Alfaadhel, T. A., Soroka, S. D., Kiberd, B. A., Landry, D., Moorhouse, P., & Tennankore, K. K. (2015). Frailty and mortality in dialysis: Evaluation of a clinical frailty scale. *Clinical Journal of the American Society of Nephrology, 10*(5), 832–840.

Choudhury, D., & Levi, M. (2011). Kidney aging—inevitable or preventable? *Nature Reviews Nephrology, 7*(12), 706–717.

Concepcion, B. P., Forbes, R. C., & Schaefer, H. M. (2016). Older candidates for kidney transplantation: Who to refer and what to expect? *World Journal of Transplantation, 6*(4), 650–657.

Crowe, M. J., Forsling, M. L., Rolls, B. J., Phillips, P. A., Ledingham, J. G., & Smith, R. F. (1987). Altered water excretion in healthy elderly men. *Age Ageing, 16*(5), 285–293.

Davison, A. M., & Johnston, P. A. (1996). Glomerulonephritis in the elderly. *Nephrology, Dialysis, Transplantation, 11*(Suppl. 9), 34–37.

Epstein, M., & Hollenberg, N. K. (1976). Age as a determinant of renal sodium conservation in normal man. *Journal of Laboratory and Clinical Medicine, 87*(3), 411–417.

Frassetto, L. A., Morris, Jr., R. C., & Sebastian, A. (1996). Effect of age on blood acid-base composition in adult humans: Role of age-related renal functional decline. *American Journal of Physiology, 271*(6 Pt 2), F1114–F1122.

Kurella Tamura, M., Covinsky, K. E., Chertow, G. M., Yaffe, K., Landefeld, C. S., & McCulloch, C. E. (2009). Functional status of elderly adults before and after initiation of dialysis. *The New England Journal of Medicine, 361*, 1539–1547.

Martins, P. N., Pratschke, J., Pascher, A., Fritsche, L., Frei, U., Neuhaus, P., & Tullius, S. G. (2005). Age and immune response in organ transplantation. *Transplantation, 79*(2), 127–132.

McAdams-DeMarco, M. A., Isaacs, K., Darko, L., Salter, M. L., Gupta, N., King, E. A., . . . Segev, D. L. (2015). Changes in frailty after kidney transplantation. *Journal of the American Geriatrics Society, 63*(10), 2152–2157.

Ostchega, Y., Dillon, C. F., Hughes, J. P., Carroll, M., & Yoon, S. (2007). Trends in hypertension prevalence, awareness, treatment, and control in older U.S. adults: Data from the National Health and Nutrition Examination Survey 1988 to 2004. *Journal of American Geriatric Society, 55*(7), 1056–1065.

Schmitt, R., Coca, S., Kanbay, M., Tinetti, M. E., Cantley, L. G., & Parikh, C. R. (2008). Recovery of kidney function after acute kidney injury in the elderly: A systematic review and meta-analysis. *American Journal of Kidney Diseases, 52*(2), 262–271.

Staessen, J. A., Gasowski, J., Wang, J. G., Thijs, L., Den Hond, E., Boissel, J. P., . . . Fagard, R. H. (2000). Risks of untreated and treated isolated systolic hypertension in the elderly: Meta-analysis of outcome trials. *Lancet, 355*(9207), 865–872.

Takazakura, E., Sawabu, N., Handa, A., Takada, A., Shinoda, A., & Takeuchi, J. (1972). Intravascular changes with age and disease. *Kidney International, 2*, 224–230.

Wheatley, K., Ives, N., Gray, R., Kalra, P. A., Moss, J. G., Baigent, C., . . . ASTRAL Investigators. (2009). Revascularization versus medical therapy for renal-artery stenosis. *New England Journal of Medicine, 361*(20), 1953–1962.

Wright J. T., Jr., Williamson, J. D., Whelton, P. K., Snyder, J. K., Sink, K. M., Rocco, M. V., . . . SPRINT Research Group. (2015). A randomized trial of intensive versus standard blood-pressure control. *The New England Journal of Medicine, 373*(22), 2103–2116.

CHAPTER 50

KIDNEY DISEASES IN AFRICAN AMERICANS

Keith C. Norris

1. **What is the incidence of end-stage kidney disease (ESKD) in African Americans?**
   African Americans represent about 13% of the United States population but account for more than one-third of the ESKD population. African American adults are almost four times as likely as non-Hispanic Caucasians to develop ESKD. Among men aged 20 to 39, African Americans are approximately 15 times more likely to develop ESKD secondary to hypertension than age-matched Caucasian men.

2. **What are the risk factors for ESKD among African Americans?**
   Many biologic and socioeconomic variables might influence the onset and progression of kidney disease among African Americans. Hypertension, diabetes, and obesity are associated with increased risk for ESKD and are more highly prevalent in African Americans. High blood pressure (BP) accounts for nearly one-third, and diabetes accounts for nearly half, of new cases of ESKD among this population group. The social position of African Americans in the United States and the lingering effects of legalized residential segregation place most African Americans in neighborhoods with poor health assets. They are more likely to suffer from low socioeconomic status, being uninsured or under-insured, and have low health literacy. These factors and others, such as a lack of awareness of chronic kidney disease (CKD) risk factors, contribute to the increased risk of ESKD among this group. These factors may adversely affect BP and blood glucose control in patients with hypertension and diabetes, respectively, accelerating the onset and progression of kidney disease.

   Biological factors that originated as a result of shared evolutionary ancestry, such as variant *APOL1* gene polymorphisms, which emerged in West Africa to protect against trypanosomiasis, and the presence of two risk alleles (present in approximately 12% of African Americans) is associated with an increased risk of developing ESKD. Other biologic markers, such as certain polymorphisms of the *GSTM1* gene, an oxidative stress regulator, are associated with a reduced risk of CKD and are more prevalent among African Americans. Thus, the role of social determinants of health juxtaposed with an array of risk and resilience genes may conspire differently in varying settings to influence CKD and ESKD in African Americans.

3. **What is the role of diabetes in kidney disease among African American patients?**
   High BP and diabetes account for nearly three-quarters of the new cases of ESKD. Diabetes alone accounts for nearly half of new ESKD cases. Increased rates of poor diabetes control among African Americans accelerate diabetes-related kidney injury. Increased rates of hypertension and poor BP control further contribute to the high prevalence of kidney disease among this patient group with diabetes.

4. **What are some of the key lifestyle changes to optimize BP and blood sugar control and preserve kidney function in African American patients?**
   Healthy diet
   • Low fat, low sodium, high potassium, and adequate calcium intake.
   Regular physical activity
   • Increase physical activity as part of the daily routine by undertaking an enjoyable physical activity for 30 to 45 minutes per day for 3 to 5 days per week.
   Weight maintenance
   • Monitor body weight and maintain a healthy body mass index.
   • Maintain weight by making permanent changes in the daily diet.
   Stress reduction
   • Develop coping skills for specific stressors in work and/or home environment with meditation, relaxation, yoga, biofeedback, etc.
   Smoking cessation
   • Ensure a smoke-free environment.

5. What are some of the key approaches to achieve healthy dietary changes in African American patients?
   - Recommend nutritional substitutions with foods that an individual will likely eat
   - Eat more broiled (grilled) and steamed foods
   - Eat more grains, fresh fruits, and vegetables
   - Eat fewer fats and use healthier fats, such as olive oil
   - Eat fewer processed foods, fast foods, and fried foods
   - Read labels and pay attention to the sodium, potassium, and fat content of foods
   - Do not season foods with smoked meats, such as bacon and ham hocks
   - If lactose intolerant, try lactose-free milk or yogurt, or drink calcium-fortified juices or soy milk
   - Limit alcohol consumption to <2 beers, 1 glass of wine, or 1 shot of hard liquor per day
   - Limit the intake of sugar-sweetened beverages and juices

6. When should antihypertensive drug therapy be initiated in African American patients with kidney disease?
   Pharmacotherapy should be initiated promptly for persistent elevation in BP in spite of the therapeutic lifestyle changes. Many guidelines recommend both pharmacotherapy and therapeutic lifestyle intervention if BP is greater than 140/100 mm Hg. If below that level, a 3-month trial of therapeutic lifestyle intervention to achieve a BP less than 140/90 mm Hg—and if that is not achieved then pharmacotherapy—should be initiated. In the presence of proteinuria and/or comorbidities, a more aggressive approach with targeting a BP below 130/80 mm Hg is recommended by some guidelines. This approach would be supported as safe and likely effective by the findings of the Systolic Blood Pressure Intervention Trial (SPRINT) that demonstrated improved outcomes in nondiabetic patients with hypertension with an even lower systolic BP target of less than 120 mm Hg, including the subset with reduced estimated glomerular filtration rate (eGFR).

7. What is the relationship between BP level and kidney disease among African American patients?
   African Americans suffer from one of highest prevalence rates of high BP in the world. High BP predisposes to kidney disease and kidney disease predisposes to high BP. This vicious cycle among African Americans, in part, accounts for the substantially higher incidence of hypertension-related ESKD compared to non-Hispanic Whites. Aggressive and appropriate screening for elevated BP and kidney disease among African Americans will minimize the role of this vicious cycle in the rapid progression of kidney disease.

8. What are some of the effective antihypertensive drugs for controlling BP in African American patients with kidney disease?
   Among a subset of participants in the Antihypertensive and Lipid-Lowering Treatment to Prevent Heart Attack Trial (ALLHAT) with reduced eGFR, it was reported that diuretics, renin–angiotensin system inhibitors, and calcium channel blockers were similar in efficacy. By contrast, the African American Study of Kidney Disease and Hypertension Study (AASK) found participants who received renin–angiotensin system inhibitors had the best outcomes, followed by beta blockers, then calcium channel blockers. Almost all patients in AASK had concomitant diuretic use. In addition, both ALLHAT and AASK had an alpha blocker arm that was stopped early, making it the drug class of last resort for African Americans with hypertension and kidney disease. A sequential approach to using different classes of antihypertensive therapies based on AASK is provided below.
   1. Diuretics (loop diuretics if GFR < 30 mL/min)
   2. Renin–angiotensin system inhibitors
   3. Beta blockers
   4. Calcium channel blockers
   5. Centrally acting sympatholytic agents
   6. Direct vasodilators

9. What should the goal be of BP treatment among African American patients with kidney disease?
   At a population level, the risk of cardiovascular (CV) mortality doubles for every 20 mm Hg increase in systolic blood pressure from 120 to 180 mm Hg. There is no distinct cutoff for the ideal BP in the general population, and, similarly, there is no ideal BP level for African Americans. In general, treatment is recommended when BP exceeds 140/90 mm Hg. The recommended BP treatment goal in patients with hypertension and kidney disease has changed over time from <130/80 mm Hg to <140/90 mm Hg. The AASK trial found no difference in outcomes between participants randomized to the <140/90 arm and the <125/75 arm, but a secondary analysis of participants with albuminuria (>300 mg/day) found improved outcomes with the lower BP target. Thus, several clinical guidelines recommend a

target BP of <130/80mm Hg in patients with CKD and proteinuria. Many patients will require three to four medications to achieve this treatment goal. Achieving the lower target BP of <130/80 mm Hg in African Americans with kidney disease and proteinuria should provide the best clinical outcomes.

10. **What is the role of the low renin status in kidney disease among African Americans?**
Low serum renin levels are more prevalent among African Americans and the elderly, and are associated with salt sensitivity. A suboptimal BP response to weight loss has also been associated with low renin status. Animal studies suggest low systemic renin status may be due to an increase in intrarenal renin–angiotensin activity leading to downregulation of systemic renin. The increased intrarenal renin–angiotensin activation may place people with low systemic renin levels at an increased risk of kidney damage.

11. **Do African American patients with ESKD have a higher mortality rate?**
Although African Americans in the general population have higher rates of overall premature morbidity and mortality, including cardiovascular diseases, those with ESKD who are on dialysis actually have a lower mortality rate than their age-adjusted non-Hispanic Caucasian counterparts. The reasons for this are not clear, but may be linked to a survival bias of
   i. Who reaches dialysis (the smaller group of surviving African Americans may be more resilient)
   ii. Better adaptation to a high-stress environment based on higher rates of prior exposure to stressors
   iii. Reverse epidemiology of cardiovascular disease where major cardiovascular disease (CVD) risk factors, such as obesity, poorly controlled BP, and diabetes (which are more prevalent in African Americans) now appear to be protective
   iv. Potential biologic polymorphisms of cell stress regulation
   All of these may be protective in this setting.

12. **Does the use of recombinant human erythropoietin predispose African American patients with ESKD to cardiovascular disease?**
What is not commonly appreciated is that African Americans have approximately 0.5 g/dL lower adjusted mean hemoglobin (Hb) levels than Caucasians in the general and CKD populations. This may be due, in part, to variant hemoglobin phenotypes and/or higher rates of inflammation. Therefore African Americans have lower Hb levels at the initiation of dialysis. Despite these population differences, the hemoglobin goals in ESKD are the same for African Americans and Caucasians, which results in the greater use of erythropoiesis-stimulating agents (ESAs) to achieve target Hb levels. The need for higher doses of recombinant human erythropoietin in the management of anemia in African American patients with ESKD may worsen high BP and increase vascular thrombosis. This could lead to accelerated cardiovascular disease and premature death. However, African American patients with ESKD do not have an increased risk for cardiovascular death. It is possible that the better survival rates of African Americans on dialysis might be even greater if there was less use of ESAs. An analysis found no difference in cardiovascular outcomes among Caucasians fee-for-service Medicare patients on dialysis before and after the reduced use of ESA driven by the Centers for Medicare & Medicaid Services reimbursement policy implemented 2011, while there was an 18% reduction in cardiovascular events observed in their African American peers, which supports the possibility of better survival rates of African Americans on dialysis with less ESA use.

13. **What is a practical approach for treating high BP in African American patients with kidney disease?**
A practical target BP for African American patients with proteinuric kidney disease, based on existing evidence, is less than 130/80 mm Hg and is expected to use at least two agents to achieve this goal. Therapy should include an angiotensin-converting enzyme inhibitor or an angiotensin receptor blocker along with a diuretic. If hypertension is refractory to therapy, adverse events should be monitored, sociocultural factors (e.g., insurance status and medication plan should be evaluated, secondary causes of hypertension should be considered, and adherence to medication and sodium restriction (perhaps by use of 24 hours urine sodium collection) should be assessed. The diuretic should be thiazide-type if eGFR > 30 mL/min and a loop diuretic (usually administered two to three times/day) if eGFR is <30 mL/min.

CONTROVERSY

14. **Is blood pressure response to antihypertensive therapy different in African Americans?**
African Americans have been shown to exhibit lesser BP reductions on monotherapy with renin–angiotensin system inhibition compared to Caucasians; however, there are no differences in the cardiorenal benefits of renin–angiotensin system inhibition across racial/ethnic categories. Controlling

BP to target levels with a regimen that includes renin–angiotensin system inhibition in both African Americans and Caucasians with CKD is associated with comparable improvements in cardiorenal outcomes, including a similar decrease in kidney protein excretion.

15. **Is there evidence of ethnic differences in clinical outcomes based on hypertensive treatment regimens in people with kidney disease?**

No clinically relevant ethnic differences in outcomes have been noted in patients with hypertension and CKD following most randomized controlled evidence-based pharmacologic interventions for BP control. Among participants in the ALLHAT with reduced eGFR, there were no differences in clinical outcomes by race/ethnicity. However, the paucity of data with adequate numbers of African American study participants reinforces the need to achieve greater ethnic diversity in clinical trials. In addition to considering the clinical evidence when treating hypertensive kidney disease, clinicians should pay detailed attention to potential cultural and socioeconomic influences that disproportionately affect adherence and/or access to care among ethnic minority patients.

KEY POINTS

1. The incidence and prevalence of kidney disease are highest among African Americans.
2. Kidney disease among African Americans is characterized by an earlier onset and a more rapid progression to ESKD.
3. High BP and diabetes account for more than two-thirds of the new cases of ESKD.
4. Clinical outcomes among African Americans with kidney disease can be improved by appropriate BP and blood sugar control.

BIBLIOGRAPHY

Cushman, W. C., Whelton, P. K., Fine, L. J., Wright, J. T., Jr, Reboussin, D. M., Johnson, K. C., Oparil, S.; SPRINT Study Research Group. (2016). SPRINT Trial Results: Latest news in hypertension management. *Hypertension, 67*(2), 263–265.

Genovese, G., Friedman, D. J., Ross, M. D., Lecordier, L., Uzureau, P., Freedman, B. I., . . . Pollak, M. R. (2010). Association of trypanolytic ApoL1 variants with kidney disease in African Americans. *Science (New York, NY), 329*(5993), 841–845.

Improving Global Outcomes (KDIGO) Blood Pressure Work Group. (2012). KDIGO Clinical Practice Guideline for the Management of Blood Pressure in Chronic Kidney Disease. *Kidney International Supplements, 2,* 337–414.

Ku, E., Gassman, J., Appel, L. J., Smogorzewski, M., Sarnak, M. J., Glidden, D. V., . . . Hsu, C. Y. (2017). BP control and long-term risk of ESKD and mortality. *Journal of the American Society of Nephrology, 28*(2), 671–677.

Martins, D., Agodoa, L., & Norris, K. C. (2012). Hypertensive chronic kidney disease in African Americans: Strategies for improving care. *Cleveland Clinic Journal of Medicine, 79*(10), 726–734.

Nicholas, S. B., Kalantar-Zadeh, K., & Norris, K. C. (2015). Socioeconomic disparities in chronic kidney disease. *Advances in Chronic Kidney Disease, 22*(1), 6–15.

Nicholas, S. B., Vaziri, N. D., & Norris, K. C. (2013). What should be the blood pressure target for patients with chronic kidney disease? *Current Opinion in Cardiology, 28*(4), 439–445.

Rhee, C. M., Kalantar-Zadeh, K., & Norris, K. C. (2016). Why minorities live longer on dialysis: An in-depth examination of the Danish nephrology registry. *Nephrology Dialysis Transplantation, 31*(7), 1027–1030.

SPRINT Research Group, Wright, J. T., Jr., Williamson, J. D., Whelton, P. K., Snyder, J. K., Sink, K. M., . . . Ambrosius, W. T. (2015). A randomized trial of intensive versus standard blood-pressure control. *N Engl Med, 373*(22), 2103–2116.

USRDS. United States Renal Data System. (2015). *2015 USRDS annual data report: Epidemiology of kidney disease in the United States.* Bethesda, MD: National Institutes of Health, National Institute of Diabetes and Digestive and Kidney Diseases.

X
TREATMENT OPTIONS

CHAPTER 51

HEMODIALYSIS

Michael V. Rocco

TECHNICAL ASPECTS OF HEMODIALYSIS

1. **What are the components used during a hemodialysis procedure?**
   The components needed to conduct dialysis include a dialysis machine, a method to access the patient's arterial and/or venous system, a supply of treated water in order to make dialysate, and the dialyzer. The dialysis machine consists of two major components: (1) a blood pump and associated safety equipment for the blood pump to monitor pressures in the system and to ensure that air does not enter the blood circuit; and (2) a dialysate pump, with associated safety devices to ensure that the dialysate is at the correct temperature, has the correct concentration of electrolytes, and has not been exposed to blood from a leak in the dialyzer membrane. The dialysis machine uses the blood pump to move blood through the dialysis circuit, from the patient, through the dialyzer, and back to the patient. The patient needs to have some type of access to allow for the rapid movement of blood through the dialysis circuit. Treated water is needed to make the dialysate used during the dialysis procedure.

2. **What is a dialysis access?**
   A dialysis access allows blood to be removed from the patient, sent to the dialyzer, and then returned to the patient. The minimum blood flow rate that should be delivered is 300 mL/min; thus, peripheral intravenous (IV) lines, Hickman catheters, and peripherally inserted central catheter lines cannot be used for this purpose because none of these devices can deliver a high blood flow rate. There are three different types of vascular access that can be used for hemodialysis: an arteriovenous (AV) fistula, a synthetic graft, or a catheter. The preferred type of vascular access is an AV fistula.

3. **What is an AV fistula?**
   The AV fistula is created by making a surgical anastomosis between an artery in the forearm or upper arm with an adjacent vein. Over a period of 4 to 8 weeks, the increased pressure that the vein is exposed to from the arterial bed causes the vein to dilate and develop a thicker vessel wall. Once the fistula has matured—defined as a blood flow rate of at least 600 mL/min and a diameter of at least 6 mm—the fistula can be cannulated with dialysis needles to allow for the removal and return of blood. Typically, 15-gauge needles are used as dialysis needles, although smaller needles may be used at first if the fistula is not fully mature.

4. **What is a synthetic graft and why is it not the optimal type of dialysis access?**
   A synthetic graft (e.g., GORETEX graft) is created by the surgical interposition of a synthetic blood vessel between an artery and a vein. Both the AV fistula and the synthetic graft are below the skin. An AV fistula is preferred over a synthetic graft because the AV fistula has fewer complications and a longer primary patency rate (intervention free access survival) and secondary patency rate (access survival until abandonment). Specifically, there is a much higher rate of intimal hyperplasia at the vein anastomosis in grafts versus fistulas, resulting in stenosis and ultimately obstruction with thrombosis. Grafts also have higher infection rates due to the presence of a foreign body. Nonetheless, about 30% to 50% of fistulas that are placed are abandoned prior to use due to thrombosis, inadequate blood flow, or complications from access placement.

5. **When is a catheter used for dialysis access?**
   A catheter is used for hemodialysis access when a patient requires dialysis and does not have a mature AV fistula or graft. This circumstance can occur if either the patient needs dialysis acutely and does not have a functional AV fistula or graft in place, or if the patient has no suitable site to place an AV fistula or graft and thus uses the catheter for permanent hemodialysis access. In observational studies, catheters are the least desirable, because patients with this access have a higher rate of morbidity and mortality than do patients with either AV grafts or AV fistulas. Permanent catheters are usually placed into the superior vena cava through the internal jugular vein using a subcutaneous tunnel to decrease the risk of infection. Temporary catheters can be placed without a subcutaneous tunnel into an internal jugular vein or into a femoral vein.

6. **What is a dialyzer?**

A dialyzer consists of a container that contains a semipermeable membrane that separates the dialysate from the blood that has been removed from the patient. A hollow fiber dialyzer, the type most commonly used today, consists of a cylinder that contains more than 10,000 hollow fibers that are made of a semipermeable material. To maximize the diffusion that takes place between the blood and dialysate, blood travels through the hollow fibers, and dialysate flows around the outside of these hollow fibers in a countercurrent direction from the blood. The size of the dialyzer is measured by the surface area of the semipermeable membrane and is expressed in square meters. Most adult hemodialysis membranes have a surface area between 1.5 and 2.5 m^2; pediatric dialyzers are often less than 1 m^2. A number of different materials are used for the semipermeable membranes. These materials vary in the degree to which small and middle molecules can pass through the membrane, which, in turn, is determined by the number and size of the pores in the dialyzer membrane. In the United States, most membranes are composed of either semisynthetic or synthetic materials that allow for the removal of larger molecules to some degree. Typical dialyzer membranes consist of polysulfone, polyethersulfone, cellulose acetate, biacetate or triacetate, or polyamides.

7. **What is dialysate?**

Dialysate is a physiologic solution that consists of both inorganic ions found in the body and glucose. The dialysate concentration of sodium and chloride is usually physiologic, whereas the concentration of magnesium and phosphorus is usually less than physiologic to allow for the removal of these substances on dialysis. The bicarbonate concentration is usually higher than the physiologic concentration to allow for the treatment of metabolic acidosis, which is common in patients undergoing dialysis. Typically, several different potassium and calcium concentrations are available so that the rate of removal of these ions can be varied as clinical circumstances dictate. The dialysate flows through the dialyzer in a countercurrent direction, preferably at a rate that is 1.5 times the blood flow rate to maximize diffusion. The temperature of the dialysate is usually set at just below the patient's body temperature, as this setting will allow for vasoconstriction and thus minimize the risk of hypotension with volume removal on dialysis. The dialysate temperature can be adjusted by 1°C to 2°C to assist with volume removal.

8. **What occurs during the dialysis procedure?**

The two processes that occur during a hemodialysis session are diffusion and ultrafiltration. Diffusion refers to a process by which small and middle molecules move, based on concentration gradients, between the blood and dialysate compartments of a dialyzer via a semipermeable membrane. Molecules can move through the semipermeable membrane by both diffusion and ultrafiltration. Small molecules move across the semipermeable membrane from an area of higher concentration (usually the blood) to an area of lower concentration (usually the dialysate). The overall effect is to remove small molecules that are likely to be toxins in high concentrations (such as potassium, phosphorus, and urea) while repleting those small molecules that are likely to be deficient (such as calcium or bicarbonate). Larger molecules do not move as readily across the membrane, and molecules that are bound to protein are unlikely to be removed by dialysis. In addition, fluid can be removed during the dialysis procedure via the process of ultrafiltration (see Question 10).

9. **What determines the rate of toxin removal?**

The rate of toxin removal is traditionally measured by the removal of urea. The removal of urea during the hemodialysis session is increased by any of these factors:

- **Higher blood flow rate and dialysis flow rate:** The higher the blood flow rate, the more urea diffusion that will occur per unit time. The limiting factor is the dialysis access, with a fistula usually being able to deliver the highest flow rates (up to about 550 mL/min) and a catheter usually being able to deliver the lowest flow rates (300 to 350 mL/min).
- **Higher efficiency of the dialyzer:** A higher-efficiency dialyzer typically has a large surface area, a thin membrane, and increased porosity. This efficiency is expressed as the dialyzer mass transfer area coefficient or KoA of the dialyzer.
- **Longer time on dialysis:** The longer the time for a single dialysis treatment, the more urea diffusion will occur. However, the urea removal per hour diminishes with each additional hour of dialysis provided.
- **Frequency of dialysis:** The standard form of in-center hemodialysis is three sessions per week, but increasing frequency increases the amount of urea and other uremic toxins that can be removed.

10. **How does fluid removal occur during the dialysis procedure?**
The removal of water during the dialysis treatment is referred to as ultrafiltration. During a hemodialysis treatment, a transmembrane hydrostatic pressure gradient develops between the blood and dialysate compartments. The total pressure difference between these two compartments determines the rate of ultrafiltration. The removal of fluid during the hemodialysis session is increased by any of these factors:

- **Higher transmembrane hydrostatic pressure:** In most modern dialysis machines, the amount of fluid to be removed during the dialysis session is set on the dialysis machine, and the machine will automatically adjust the pressures to allow for the appropriate amount of fluid to be removed. A higher transmembrane pressure results in more fluid being removed per unit time.
- **Higher ultrafiltration coefficient (K_{uf}) of the dialysis membrane:** The value of this coefficient is dependent on the dialyzer surface area, composition, thickness, and porosity.
- **Longer duration of a dialysis session.** Ultrafiltration will vary based on K_{uf} and transmembrane pressure. This will result in a set amount of ultrafiltration per minute; by extending the number of minutes, one can get more ultrafiltration.

11. **How does one determine the amount of fluid to remove during a hemodialysis session?**
Typically, a patient will gain between 1% and 5% of their body weight from fluid accumulation between dialysis sessions. Patients receiving chronic hemodialysis are assigned a dry weight by their nephrologist. A common definition of dry weight is the weight below which patients become hypotensive on dialysis. A more precise physiologic definition of dry weight is the body weight at a physiologic extracellular volume state. Practically speaking, the dry weight is the weight at which the patient is euvolemic on a minimal number of blood pressure medications. The dry weight is set based on clinical findings and by patient response to removing additional fluid. The patient's dry weight will vary over time as a result of changes in appetite, the presence of diarrhea, and the like; thus, the patient's dry weight should be reassessed on a regular basis.

12. **How does one prevent clotting of blood in the blood circuit system during hemodialysis?**
Heparin is routinely given during the hemodialysis treatment to prevent thrombosis in the extracorporeal circuit. Heparin is usually given as a bolus at the initiation of dialysis, followed by a constant infusion. The initial dose of heparin required is weight based; however, over time, it is individualized for each patient receiving dialysis to prevent complications. The appropriate dose of heparin is generally the amount that prevents clotting in the extracorporeal circuit but, at the same time, does not lead to bleeding from the needle puncture sites for more than 10 minutes after the needles are removed at the end of the hemodialysis treatment. In patients who are at high risk for bleeding, such as in postoperative patients or those with gastrointestinal bleeding, no heparin is given with monitoring of the dialyzer to ensure that it does not clot.

13. **What are the difference types of hemodialysis that can be performed?**
The most common type of hemodialysis performed in the United States is in-center hemodialysis. Other types of hemodialysis include in-center nocturnal hemodialysis and home hemodialysis. In-center hemodialysis is typically performed three times per week, with a session duration of 3 to 4.5 hours. A fourth treatment per week is sometimes added if additional fluid needs to be removed due to excess weight gain between dialysis treatments.

14. **What are the different types of home hemodialysis?**
Home hemodialysis is performed by about 1% of patients receiving chronic hemodialysis in the United States. Patients performing home hemodialysis need a partner to assist with the dialysis procedure (or at a minimum to assist with emergencies) and will need about 4 to 8 weeks of training to learn the home hemodialysis procedure. Patients can perform dialysis with a catheter or by self-cannulation using a fistula. Several different hemodialysis modalities can be performed at home, including conventional three times per week dialysis, short (2 to 3 hours per session) daily (six times per week) hemodialysis, and overnight or nocturnal (6 to 8 hours per session) hemodialysis performed three to six times per week. For the latter method, several different types of alarms are used to assess for blood or dialysate leakage as patients typically sleep during this form of hemodialysis.

15. **How is in-center nocturnal hemodialysis performed?**
Nocturnal in-center hemodialysis is performed in an outpatient hemodialysis center overnight for 6 to 8 hours per treatment, and is typically performed three times per week. Patients typically perform dialysis in bed and sleep during the dialysis session.

ASSESSING THE DOSE OF DIALYSIS

16. How is the dose of dialysis determined?

    The dose of dialysis is determined by measuring the urea concentration in the blood at the start and end of the dialysis procedure to determine the amount of urea that is removed during the dialysis session and concurrently determining the amount of fluid removed during a single hemodialysis session. Once these values are available, a variety of techniques can be used to determine the dose of dialysis provided to the patient.

17. What are the methods for measuring the dose of dialysis?

    The dose of dialysis can be expressed as the urea reduction ratio (URR), the single pool Kt/V, the double pool or equilibrated Kt/V, or the weekly or standard Kt/V. The first expressions can be used only for patients who receive hemodialysis three times per week, whereas the standard or weekly Kt/V can be used to estimate the dose of dialysis regardless of the number of times per week that the patient receives hemodialysis.

    1. The **URR** is expressed as follows:

    $$URR = 100\% \times [1 - (C_t/C_0)]$$

    where C_t and C_0 represent postdialysis and predialysis serum urea levels. Because the URR equation does not account for volume removal during a dialysis treatment, it is considered less accurate than any of the Kt/V formulas.

    2. **Single pool Kt/Vurea** (spKt/Vurea) is a unitless parameter that can be used to estimate the dose of dialysis provided to the patient, where K is the dialyzer blood water urea clearance (L/hour), t is the dialysis session length (hours), and V is the volume of distribution of urea (L). Because both K and V are difficult to measure accurately in vivo, several regression equations have been developed to estimate spKt/V. The most commonly used equation is the Daugirdas II equation:

    $$spKt/V = -\ln\ [(R - 0.008 \times t] + [(4 - 3.5\ R] \times 0.55\ (UF/V)]$$

    where R is the postdialysis over predialysis serum urea level (C_t/C_0), t is the time of dialysis (in hours), UF is ultrafiltration volume in liters (amount of fluid removed by dialysis), and V is the body water volume in liters. The first part of the equation represents the effects of urea generation during dialysis, whereas the second part of the equation represents the additional urea removed with volume removal during dialysis. A modification of the Daugirdas formula can be used to estimate spKt/V for dialysis frequencies other than three times per week (see link under #4 below).

    3. **Equilibrated Kt/Vurea** (eKt/Vurea) values accounts for urea release from sequestered tissue sites into the blood that occurs in the first 30 to 60 minutes after dialysis. The eKt/V is usually about 0.2 units less than the spKt/V. The formula for eKt/V depends on whether the patient is using a catheter for hemodialysis access:

    $$\text{Arterial access}: eKt/V = spKt/V - 0.6 \times (spKt/V)/t + 0.03$$
    $$\text{Venous access}: eKt/V = spKt/V - 0.47 \times (spKt/V)/t + 0.02$$

    4. **Standard or weekly Kt/V** can be used to estimate the dose of dialysis regardless of the number of days per week that the patient receives dialysis. The formula for the weekly Kt/V is complex; calculators are available that can provide the value for the weekly Kt/V (including HYPERLINK "http://www.hdcn.com/ukm/" http://www.hdcn.com/ukm/).

18. How often should the dose of dialysis be measured?

    The National Kidney Foundation's (NKF) Kidney Outcomes Quality Improvement Initiative (KDOQI) guidelines for hemodialysis adequacy recommend that the dose of dialysis be measured on a monthly basis in patients receiving chronic hemodialysis. Note that if residual kidney function is being included in calculating the dose of dialysis (see Question 21), then this residual kidney function should be measured every 3 months and any time that an event has occurred that could reduce the patient's residual kidney function (e.g., contrast load, prolonged hypotension).

19. What technical factors should be considered when measuring the dose of dialysis?

    The method by which the predialysis and postdialysis blood samples are obtained is important in ensuring accurate results. Blood urea nitrogen (BUN) levels are subject to rebound of three different types: access recirculation, cardiopulmonary recirculation, and remote compartment rebound. By following a specific technique for blood drawing, the effect of access recirculation on the postdialysis BUN sample is minimized. Both the predialysis and postdialysis samples should be drawn during the same dialysis session. The postdialysis BUN samples should be obtained using either the slow flow or stop flow technique. With the slow flow technique, the dialysate flow is turned off and the blood pump is slowed to about 100 mL/min for about 15 seconds prior to obtaining the sample from the sampling port. Alternatively, with the stop flow technique, after the aforementioned procedures are performed, the blood pump is stopped and the arterial and venous blood lines are clamped prior to obtaining the sample.

20. **What factors can cause the differences between the prescribed and delivered Kt/V?**
The factors that can cause a discrepancy between the prescribed and delivered dose of dialysis can be categorized into factors resulting from compromised urea clearance (Table 51.1) and factors resulting from a decrease in the effective dialysis session length (Table 51.2).

Table 51.1. Reasons for Compromised Urea Clearance

PATIENT-RELATED REASONS	STAFF-RELATED REASONS	MECHANICAL PROBLEMS

Decreased effective time on dialysis
• Decreased BFR
• Access clotting
  • Use of intravenous catheters (instead of arteriovenous graft or fistula)
  • Inadequate flow through vascular access
Recirculation
• Use of catheters
  • Inadequate access for prescribed BFR
  • Stenosis, clotting of access
	Decreased effective time
	Decreased BFR
	• Less than prescribed
	• Difficult cannulation
	Decreased dialysate flow rate
	• Less than prescribed
	• Inappropriately set
	Dialyzer
	• Inadequate quality control of "reuse"
		Dialyzer clotting during reuse
		• Blood pump calibration error
		Dialysate pump calibration error
		Inaccurate estimation of dialyzer performance by the manufacturer
		Variability in blood tubing

BFR, Blood flow rate.
Modified from Parker, T. F. (1992). Trends and concepts in the prescription and delivery of dialysis in the United States. *Seminars in Nephrology, 12,* 267–275.

Table 51.2. Reasons for Decreased Effective Time on Dialysis

PATIENT-RELATED REASONS	STAFF-RELATED REASONS	MECHANICAL REASONS
Late start (patient tardy) • Early sign off • With consent (i.e., symptoms) • Against advice (i.e., social) Medical complications (e.g., hypotension) No show	Late start (staff tardy) Wrong patient taken off Time calculated incorrectly Time on/off read incorrectly Clinical deficiencies (i.e., no time registered) Premature discontinuation for unit convenience • Scheduling conflicts • Emergencies Incorrect assumptions of continuous treatment time (e.g., failure to account for interruptions of treatment such as repositioning needles or accidental removal) Inaccurate assessment of effective time by using variable timepieces	Clotting of dialyzer Dialyzer leaks Machine malfunction

Modified from Parker, T. F. (1992). Trends and concepts in the prescription and delivery of dialysis in the United States. *Seminars in Nephrology, 12,* 267–275.

21. What dose of dialysis is considered adequate for in-center hemodialysis?

For patients receiving hemodialysis three times per week, the 2016 NKF-KDOQI Hemodialysis Adequacy guidelines recommend "a target single pool Kt/V (spKt/V) of 1.4 per hemodialysis session for patients treated thrice weekly, with a minimum delivered spKt/V of 1.2 (Grade 1B) and a minimum treatment time of 3 hours if residual kidney function is less than 2 mL/min (Grade 1D)." These guidelines also note that "for hemodialysis schedules other than thrice weekly, we suggest a target standard Kt/V of 2.3 per week with a minimum delivered dose of 2.1 using a method of calculation that includes the contributions of ultrafiltration and residual kidney function (Not Graded)." A higher dose of dialysis, achieved by either additional hemodialysis sessions or longer hemodialysis treatment times, should be considered for patients with large weight gains, high ultrafiltration rates, poorly controlled blood pressure, difficulty achieving dry weight, or poor metabolic control (such as hyperphosphatemia, metabolic acidosis, and/or hyperkalemia (Not Graded).

22. How does one achieve an adequate dose of dialysis in an individual patient?

The actual delivered dose of dialysis is usually less than the predicted dose of dialysis. A variety of calculators can be used to estimate the dose of dialysis once the patient's size and dialyzer type are inputted into the program. Factors that influence the dose of dialysis that can be adjusted include the size of the dialyzer, the blood and dialysate flow rates, and the time per dialysis session. Increasing any of these parameters should increase the delivered dose of dialysis.

23. Are there other uremic toxins that are present in patients with end-stage kidney disease?

There are hundreds of toxins that accumulate in kidney failure. Some of these toxins are middle or large molecules, some are charged particles, and others are protein bound. Many of these compounds are not well removed by conventional hemodialysis. Urea is a surrogate marker for uremic toxins, although the removal of urea is a poor model for most other uremic toxins. Additional research is needed in this area to determine the extent and effects of these other uremic toxins on morbidity and mortality of patients with ESRD. A database of uremic toxins may be found on this website: http://www.uremic-toxins.org/DataBase.html.

COMPLICATIONS OF HEMODIALYSIS

24. What are some of the common complications that are seen during a hemodialysis session?

Hypotension is the most common complication of the dialysis procedure. The reported prevalence of hypotension varies widely, depending on the definition used and the patient population studied, with prevalence ranging from 10% to 40%. Other common complications include cramping (5% to 30%), nausea and vomiting (5% to 10%), headache (5% to 10%), pruritus (1% to 5%), chest pain (1% to 5%), back pain (1% to 5%), and fever and chills (<1%).

25. What are the symptoms associated with intradialytic hypotension?

Intradialytic hypotension is often accompanied by lightheadedness, dizziness, cramping, and nausea. At times, there may be no symptoms until the patient's blood pressure has dropped to very low, and potentially dangerous, levels. To help monitor for hypotension, blood pressure is monitored during the dialysis treatment on a regular basis, usually every 30 to 60 minutes.

26. What is the etiology of hypotension during hemodialysis?

The causes of intradialytic hypotension can be divided into four broad categories, including volume-related issues, inadequate vasoconstriction, cardiac factors, and other causes. Volume-related issues center around a high ultrafiltration rate, an incorrectly low dry weight, or a low sodium level in the dialysate. Vasoconstrictive factors include the use of antihypertensive medications just prior to dialysis, autonomic neuropathy, a dialysate temperature higher than the patient's body temperature, and eating during dialysis. Cardiac factors include cardiac ischemia, heart failure, and arrhythmias. Other, less common causes include a number of complications of dialysis that are described in more detail later, including dialyzer reactions, hemolysis, air embolism, septicemia, myocardial infarction, pericardial tamponade, and severe anemia.

27. What are some of the treatments used to help minimize intradialytic hypotension?

The incidence of hypotension can be minimized by assessing dry weight on a regular basis and counseling the patient on avoiding large fluid gains between dialysis treatments, using a combination of a fluid-restricted and low-salt diet. Additional measures that may be beneficial include increasing the dialysis treatment time to decrease the hourly ultrafiltration rate, decreasing the dialysate temperature by 0.5°C to 2.0°C, avoiding intradialytic food ingestion, and using midodrine (an alpha-adrenergic agonist) in patients who do not have active cardiac ischemia. Midodrine is ineffective if the patient is prescribed alpha-adrenergic blockers.

28. **What is the dialysis dysequilibrium syndrome and how can it be prevented?**
    The dialysis dysequilibrium syndrome can occur when patients who are acutely uremic and have a high (>150 mg/dL) BUN level are subjected to a prolonged hemodialysis session. It is thought that the syndrome develops from an acute increase in brain water content from an abrupt decrease in plasma tonicity leading to the movement of water from the plasma to brain tissue. Mild manifestations of the dialysis dysequilibrium syndrome are nonspecific and include restlessness, headache, nausea, and vomiting; severe cases result in seizures, obtundation, or coma. For severe dysequilibrium, the dialysis session should be stopped, consideration should be given to prescribing IV mannitol, and the airway should be controlled if needed. The risk of dysequilibrium syndrome can be minimized by performing short (2- to 2.5-hour) hemodialysis sessions initially and by prescribing mannitol during these initial sessions.

29. **What are some of the life-threatening complications that can occur during a hemodialysis session?**
    See Table 51.3.

30. **How do anaphylactic dialyzer reactions present and how are they treated?**
    There are type A or anaphylactic reactions and type B or nonspecific dialyzer reactions. Anaphylactic reactions are medical emergencies and are commonly manifested by dyspnea, a feeling of warmth, and a sense of impending catastrophe, and can be followed by cardiac arrest and death. Milder symptoms include watery eyes, sneezing, cough, abdominal cramping, diarrhea, itching, and urticaria. Symptoms usually develop during the first several minutes of dialysis, although the symptoms can be delayed for more than 30 minutes. There is a diverse etiology of anaphylactic reactions including an allergy to ethylene oxide (used to sterile dialyzers), AN-69 dialysis membranes, contaminated dialysis solutions, and heparin or dialyzer reuse. Management is to stop dialysis immediately, clamp the blood lines, disconnect the patient from the dialysis circuit, and discharge the blood lines and dialyzer without returning the blood to the patient. The patient may need emergency treatment for anaphylaxis if the reaction is severe. Avoidance of the offending agent is needed to prevent recurrent reactions.

31. **What other dialyzer reactions can occur?**
    Type B reactions are usually much less severe than type A reactions and are usually manifested by chest or back pain, with an onset 20 to 60 minutes after the start of dialysis. Management of type B reactions is supportive; consideration should be given to using a different dialyzer to prevent in the future.

32. **How does hemolysis occur during a hemodialysis session?**
    Acute hemolysis is a medical emergency and can result from either problems with the blood tubing or needles or problems with the dialysate. Any obstruction or narrowing of the blood line, as a result of kinks, manufacturing defects, or the use of small-gauge needles in the presence of high blood flow rates, can cause hemolysis. Likewise, dialysate that has an incorrect electrolyte concentration, is too hot, or is contaminated with chemicals also can cause hemolysis. Contaminants include chloramine

Table 51.3. Life-Threatening Reactions

REACTION	RISK FACTORS
Dialyzer reaction	See Question 30
Arrhythmias	Preexisting cardiovascular disease, hypotension, electrolyte imbalances, acidosis
Myocardial infarction	Preexisting cardiovascular disease, hypotension
Pericardial effusion	Recurrent or unexpected hypotension
Seizures	Severe hypertension, markedly elevated blood urea nitrogen levels
Intracranial bleeding	Preexisting vascular disease, hypertension
Hemolysis	Blood line obstruction/narrowing, problem with dialysate
Air embolism	Inadvertent air entry into the blood circuit

added to the city water supply; formaldehyde or bleach used to reuse dialyzers; or inadequate water treatment resulting in the presence of fluoride, nitrate, zinc, or copper.

33. What are the manifestations of hemolysis and how is it treated?
Hemolysis may be suspected if the blood in the venous line is port wine in color or if plasma is pink in centrifuged samples, or with a marked drop in hemoglobin without an obvious source of bleeding. If hemolysis is suspected, the dialysis session should be stopped immediately and the blood in the dialyzer and blood tubing should be discarded because it may have a markedly elevated potassium level as a result of potassium release from hemolyzed erythrocytes. Patients will need to be hospitalized to monitor the extent of hemolysis and to treat hyperkalemia.

34. How is an air embolism detected and treated?
Air embolism is a medical emergency that can lead to death if it is not recognized and promptly treated. The manifestations of air embolism depend on the positioning of the patient, and, thus, where the air embolism travels to. In seated patients, air enters the cerebral circulation, leading to central nervous system events, including loss of consciousness and death. In recumbent patients, air enters the cardiopulmonary system, leading to dyspnea, cough, arrhythmias, chest tightness, and acute cardiac and neurologic events. This emergency should be managed by immediately clamping the blood line, stopping the blood pump, placing the patient in a recumbent position on the left side with the head and chest tilted downward, and administering 100% oxygen by mask or endotracheal tube.

KEY POINTS

1. The rate of uremic toxin removal is determined by the time on dialysis, the blood and dialysate flow rates, and the efficiency of the dialyzer.
2. The dose of dialysis can be expressed as the URR, the single pool Kt/V, the double pool or equilibrated Kt/V, or the weekly or standard Kt/V.
3. For patients receiving hemodialysis three times per week, it is recommended that the minimum delivered single pool Kt/V dose of dialysis is 1.2 and that the minimum treatment time is 3 hours if residual kidney function is less than 2 mL/min.
4. Hypotension is the most common complication of the dialysis procedure, seen in 10% to 50% of treatments.
5. Dialysis dysequilibrium syndrome occurs when patients who are acutely uremic and have a high (>150 mg/dL) BUN level are subjected to a prolonged hemodialysis session.

BIBLIOGRAPHY

Chertow, G. M., Levin, N. W., Beck, G. J., Daugirdas, J. T., Eggers, P. W., Kliger, A. S., . . . the Frequent Hemodialysis Network (FHN) Trials Group. (2016). Long-term effects of frequent in-center hemodialysis. *Journal of the American Society of Nephrology, 27*(6), 1830–1836.
Davenport, A. (2015). Complications of hemodialysis treatments due to dialysate contamination and composition errors. *Hemodialysis International, 19*(Suppl. 3), S30–S33.
Drew, D. A., & Lok, C. E. (2014). Strategies for planning the optimal dialysis access for an individual patient. *Current Opinion in Nephrology and Hypertension, 23*(3), 314–320.
Ebo, D. G., Bosmans, J. L., Couttenye, M. M., & Stevens, W. J. (2006). Haemodialysis-associated anaphylactic and anaphylactoid reactions. *Allergy, 61*(2), 211–220.
Eknoyan, G., Beck, G. J., Cheung, A. K., Daugirdas, J. T., Greene, T., Kusek, J. W., . . . Toto, R. (2002). Effect of dialysis dose and membrane flux in maintenance hemodialysis. *New England Journal of Medicine, 347*(25), 2010–2019.
National Kidney Foundation. (2015). KDOQI Clinical Practice Guideline for Hemodialysis Adequacy: 2015 update. *American Journal of Kidney Diseases, 66*(5), 884–930.
Rocco, M. V., Daugirdas, J. T., Greene, T., Lockridge, R. S., Chan, C., Pierratos, A., . . . Kliger, A. S. (2015). Long-term effects of frequent nocturnal hemodialysis on mortality: The Frequent Hemodialysis Network (FHN) Nocturnal Trial. *American Journal of Kidney Diseases, 66*(3), 459–468.

CHAPTER 52

HOME DIALYSIS

John V. Duronville and Ruediger W. Lehrich

1. **What is home hemodialysis (HHD)?**
   HHD is a kidney replacement modality for patients with end-stage kidney disease (FSKD) that can be performed safely in the patient's home environment. Assistance of a trained caregiver or qualified hemodialysis nurse is a requirement. The frequency of treatment for HHD can vary per individual patient. HHD can be performed as conventional HHD, with treatments 3 days a week for 3 to 4 hours or longer each time. It can also be performed as short daily HHD, occurring 5 to 7 times a week for shorter duration. Lastly, it can be performed overnight as nocturnal NHHD where treatments normally last 6 to 8 hours.

2. **How many people today use HHD?**
   The 2010 United States Renal Data System (USRDS) report showed that 0.51% of incident dialysis patients were undergoing HHD. Based on the 2015 USRDS report, the use of HHD by incident ESKD patients increased by 222% from 2007 to 2013. Even with the large relative rise in HHD, its overall utilization as a home dialysis modality is significantly lower than that of peritoneal dialysis (PD). Home dialysis, either HHD or PD, was utilized by 9.1% of all patients undergoing dialysis as of 2013.

3. **What machines are used for HHD?**
   In the United States HHD is performed with a "low-flow systems" (L-FS) machine. The most frequently used L-FS machine in the United States is the NxStage System. The NxStage machine is portable; it weighs 32 kg (71 lbs) and is 15 × 15 inches. Dialysate for the machine is provided in two ways. Delivery of 5-L dialysate bags can be made to a patient's home, with four to six bags needed for short daily dialysis. These bags are convenient when patients are traveling. Alternatively, there is a fluid generator (PureFlow) that can prepare up to 60 L of dialysate (enough for two to three treatments) using a filtering system within the machine and connection to a tap water source.

4. **How is HHD technically performed when compared with conventional hemodialysis?**
   The common conventional in-center dialysis machine is a "single-pass system" (SPS) machine. A SPS machine produces dialysate within the machine by proportionally mixing acid and base concentrates with a purified water source. The dialysate then moves as a single-pass, high-flow fluid to the dialyzer for transmembrane contact with the patient's blood. A SPS machine typically uses a dialysate flow to blood flow (Qd:Qb) ratio of 2:1. With an L-FS machine (like the NxStage), the flow rates are reversed so that Qd:Qb is between 1:2 and 1:3. This permits a more complete equilibrium between dialysate and patient's blood, ultimately allowing for the use of less dialysate.

5. **What type of access is used for HHD?**
   Patients are able to use a tunneled central venous catheters (CVCs) or arteriovenous fistulae (AVF) to connect themselves to an HHD machine. As in conventional in-center hemodialysis, an AVF is preferred over a CVC, given the increased risk of blood stream infections associated with CVCs.

6. **Describe the "buttonhole" method and why it is used.**
   The conventional method of repeated cannulation of an AVF involves using sharp-tip needles and rotating needle puncture sites ("rope-ladder technique") with each successive dialysis treatments. A "buttonhole" is a constant fibrous tract established by repeated puncture followed by small eschar formation of the same site. Recannulation of the same two sites eventually allows access with a blunt-tip needle.

7. **What are the advantages and disadvantages of buttonholes?**
   Some observational studies suggest that the buttonhole method helps minimize patient discomfort and adverse effects of repeated cannulation attempts and provides a predictable location for repeated puncture. Buttonholes can allow for greater ease of cannulation by the patient or caregiver. It has also been reported to reduce the pain associated with sharp-needle puncture, although this claim has been disputed with a more recent randomized controlled trial. The primary limitation of buttonhole use

is its increased risk of infections. Studies have shown that buttonhole cannulation results in higher rates of both local and systemic infections. In particular, it increases the risk of *Staphylococcus aureus* bacteremia. The use of the buttonhole technique thus may be more appropriate in some cases, such as for patients with short AVF segments.

8. **What are clinical benefits of HHD?**
   There are randomized and nonrandomized trials that have shown several benefits to more frequent hemodialysis. Daily hemodialysis has been shown to improve cardiovascular parameters such as a reduction in left ventricular (LV) mass, a decrease in systolic blood pressure, and mean arterial pressure. Other surrogate markers of clinical improvement attributed to daily hemodialysis include a reduction in antihypertensive medication use, improved adequacy of dialysis, improved serum phosphate control, and improved quality of life. Some key limitations to these studies deal with the selection bias of home dialysis patients. Patients performing their own dialysis treatments at home tend to have greater social support, financial resources, greater health literacy, motivation, and might be overall healthier than their in-center dialysis counterparts.

9. **Describe the clinical outcomes of HHD versus in-center hemodialysis.**
   One retrospective cohort study showed that patients receiving "intensive" dialysis (five to seven sessions per week) compared with patients receiving in-center hemodialysis (three treatments per week) showed a strong association with improved survival. During the 4-year follow-up period 13% of the intensive HHD group died, compared with 21% of the conventional in-center dialysis group.

10. **What was the Frequent Hemodialysis Network (FHN) Trials?**
    The FHN trials are the largest to-date prospective randomized controlled trials to study the safety, feasibility, and efficacy of frequent in-center (Daily Trial) and frequent home-based nocturnal (Nocturnal Trial) hemodialysis. The first arm (FHN-Daily Trial) randomized 245 patients from 10 regional centers to receive six (frequent) or three (conventional) in-center hemodialysis sessions per week for 12 months. The second arm (FHN-Nocturnal Trial) randomized 87 patients from 9 regional centers to 12 months of 6 times per week (frequent) home nocturnal hemodialysis versus 3 times a week (conventional) HHD. All patients were receiving conventional thrice-weekly in-center dialysis prior to the time of randomization.

11. **What did we learn from the FHN trials?**
    The coprimary composite outcomes examined in both daily and nocturnal trials were (1) death or change in LV mass death or (2) change in physical health composite (PHC) score. Secondary outcomes analyzed were cognitive performance, self-reported depression, laboratory markers of nutrition, mineral metabolism and anemia, blood pressure and rates of hospitalization, and vascular access interventions. The FHN-Daily Trial showed a statistically significant benefit of more frequent hemodialysis (HD) for both coprimary composite outcomes (death/LV mass or death/PHC). The FHN-Nocturnal Trial (HHD patients) did not show a definitive benefit of more frequent nocturnal HD for either coprimary outcome. Both arms showed improvement in phosphorus and systolic blood pressure control. Neither trial showed significant benefit among the other main secondary outcomes. Long-term survival (median 3.6 years follow-up) was significantly better in the group of patients who were initially randomized to the frequent dialysis arm of the FHN-Daily trial. In contrast, long-term survival (median 3.7 years follow-up) was worse for the frequent dialysis HHD patients in the FHN-nocturnal trial.

12. **Are there studies that compare overall mortality between HHD to PD?**
    There are few comparative effectiveness studies to help better answer this question. One of the first studies to examine this was an observational cohort analysis using the Australia and New Zealand Dialysis and Transplant Registry (ANZDATA). The primary outcome of mortality between conventional in-center dialysis, PD, and HHD was examined with all patients starting dialysis over a 1-year period. HHD had a 49% lower mortality rate when compared with patients receiving conventional in-center HD. In contrast, patients receiving PD had similar mortality as the conventional in-center HD cohort. However, patients in the HHD group were younger, with fewer comorbid conditions, and hence "healthier" than their PD and in-center HD counterparts.

13. **Are there differences between the rates of hospitalization or technique failure with HHD versus PD?**
    An observational study compared the relative mortality, hospitalization rate, and technique failure of HHD versus PD. Technique failure in this setting was defined as switching to a different dialysis modality. An incident cohort of HHD patients (NxStage System One Registry) was matched to a cohort of incident PD patients from USRDS database between 2007 and 2010. Overall, HHD was associated with decreased mortality, fewer hospitalizations, and less technique failure.

Table 52.1. A Comparison of Peritoneal Dialysis and Home Hemodialysis

PERITONEAL DIALYSIS	HOME HEMODIALYSIS
Mobile dialysis machine	Mobile dialysis machine
Highly efficient use of dialysate	Highly efficient use of dialysate
Physiologic perfusion of peritoneal membrane	High blood flow
115–140 L lactate buffered dialysate per week.	100–180 L lactate buffered dialysate per week.
6–7[a] doses per week	5–6[a] doses per week

[a]Typical frequency prescribed to achieve optimal clearance.

14. How are PD and HHD similar?
    See Table 52.1.

15. What are the primary reasons for hospitalization in HHD patients?
    Studies have shown that HHD patients have significantly lower rates of hospitalization due to cardiovascular disease (specifically heart failure and hypertension related causes) when matched to conventional in-center HD patients. When compared with PD, HHD patients have a significantly lower composite (combined causes being infection, cardiac, access related, or bleeding) hospitalization rates. HHD patients when compared with in-center HD patients have significantly higher rates of infection-associated hospitalizations, specifically sepsis and metastatic infections of the bone and heart.

16. Are there psychosocial benefits to choosing HHD?
    Patients along with their care partner who choose home dialysis modalities have greater autonomy over their treatments. Patients do not have to travel 3 times a week and adhere to a strict in-center dialysis schedule. Patients on home dialysis have greater flexibility with work and lifestyle schedule. Depression has been found to be significantly less prevalent in patients undergoing HHD (8%) versus in-center hemodialysis patients (42.3%). In comparison, patients receiving short-daily in-center HD in the FHN trial did not experience an improvement in depression.

17. What are some barriers to HHD?
    Barriers to selecting HHD include patients' fear of isolation and having to manage their care independent of a facility with similar patients and medical staff. Furthermore, patients may have anxiety about self-cannulation or risk of a catastrophic event during dialysis without the assistance of trained medical personnel. HHD requires a care partner to assist with dialysis. Patients may not have a suitable home environment (insufficient space, hygiene, plumbing, or electricity). Some patients are intimidated by the perceived complexity of the process. For some patients, operating the machine may seem overwhelming. Though overall costs for HHD may be less than in-center HD, some of the costs may be shifted from the dialysis unit to the individual patient. Providers who are unfamiliar or dialysis centers that do not have the appropriate resources can also become barriers to patients choosing HHD.

18. What challenges do caregivers of HHD face?
    All patients who undergo HHD are required to have a care partner present in the home when dialysis occurs. Some patients dialyze at home independently, not needing help, while caregivers/partners aid others. Caregivers tend to be a patient's spouse, parent, child, other relative, or friend. The caregiver's burden presents another major challenge to patients undergoing HHD. Caregivers are typically trained with the patient and need to be present during the entirety of a patient's treatment. One systemic review of qualitative studies showed that caregivers experienced great strain with the demands and responsibilities of assisting with HHD. Caregivers with partners with more comorbidities may feel a greater strain both physically and financially. The emotional and physical strain from daily dialysis can create "burnout" in the patient or caregiver.

19. What is the training for HHD?
    There is no standardized method for training patients to undergo HHD. Nonetheless, there are key elements of the training process that are integral in producing a successful HHD patient:
    1. Selecting the right patient. Though most patients can undergo HHD, some contraindications to HHD include unstable medical conditions (i.e., seizure disorder), unstable behavioral problems

(i.e., intravenous (IV) drug use, uncontrolled psychosis), and conditions that may cause abrupt loss of consciousness.
2. The patient's home must be suitable for HHD. There must be a proper water supply, electrical source, and appropriate hygiene.
3. Nurses/trainers must be motivated, knowledgeable, and understand the principles of adult learning.
4. Training usually takes 4 to 6 weeks, with the involvement of a care partner.
5. There should be an adequate assessment of the patient's ability to safely perform HHD at home independently or with a care partner.
6. Patients should also be able to understand and manage other aspects related to their ESKD, such as diet, nutrition, medications, and obtaining appropriate lab work.

20. **Is HHD safe?**
There is a paucity of literature available on the rate of adverse events and technical complications associated with HHD. Adverse events associated with conventional hemodialysis are also present with HHD. Life-threatening emergencies like exsanguination and air embolism are rare. Other complications like access-related infections, hemolysis, hemodynamic instability associated with aggressive ultrafiltration, or dialysate leak and acute electrolyte derangements associated with treatments are more common. Nonetheless, HHD is safe. One retrospective multicenter study out of Canada found that among 190 HHD patients, life-threatening adverse events occurred at a rate of 0.060 per 1000 treatments. Another study out of New Zealand and Australia found after comparing HHD pts to conventional in-center dialysis the relative risk of death from angioaccess bleeding or infection was 0.27 (0.20 to 0.37). Effective training/retraining, routine evaluation of access stability, wet sensors, and machine alarms, along with other safety measures, are utilized to reduce adverse events associated with HHD.

KEY POINTS

1. HHD is usually prescribed as more frequent and shorter dialysis seasons compared to conventional in-center dialysis. As such, HHD has been shown to improve several important surrogate outcomes like phosphorus and BP control. It likely is associated with improved patient survival as well.
2. HHD is convenient, allows for greater patient autonomy, and provides a portable platform to perform kidney replacement therapy.
3. HHD is a safe dialysis modality that has multiple safety mechanisms incorporated into the machine and patient training. This leads to life-threatening adverse events being very rare occurrences.
4. Key barriers to HHD include patients' fears, anxiety toward managing their dialysis outside of a medicalized facility, and the dialysis provider's lack of familiarity with the modality.

BIBLIOGRAPHY
Agar, J. W., Perkins, A., & Heaf, J. G. (2015). Home hemodialysis: Infrastructure, water, and machines in the home. *Hemodialysis International, 19*(Suppl. 1), S93–S111.
Annual Data Report. (2015). *United States Renal Data System.* Available at: https://www.usrds.org/2015/view/Default.aspx.
Bennett, P. N., Schatell, D., & Shah, K. D. (2015). Psychosocial aspects in home hemodialysis: A review. *Hemodialysis International, 19*(Suppl. 1), S128–S134.
Chertow, G. M., Levin, N. W., Beck, G. J., Daugirdas, J. T., Eggers, P. W., Kliger, A. S., . . . Greene, T. (2016). Long-term effects of frequent in-center hemodialysis. *Journal of the American Society of Nephrology, 27*(6), 1830–1836.
Daugirdas, J. T., Blake, P. G., & Ing, T. S. (Eds.). (2015). *Handbook of dialysis* (5th ed.). Riverwoods, IL: Wolters Kluwer Health.
Home Hemodialysis. National Kidney Foundation. (2015). A to Z health guide: home hemodialysis. Available at: https://www.kidney.org/atoz/content/homehemo. Accessed August 2017.
Marshall, M. R., Hawley, C. M., Kerr, P. G., Polkinghorne, K. R., Marshall, R. J., Agar, J. W., & McDonald, S. P. (2011). Home hemodialysis and mortality risk in Australian and New Zealand populations. *American Journal of Kidney Diseases, 58*(5), 782–793.
Masterson, R. (2008). The advantages and disadvantages of home hemodialysis. *Hemodialysis International, 12*(Suppl. 1), S16–S20.
Nadeau-Fredette, A. C., & Johnson, D. W. (2016). Con: Buttonhole cannulation of arteriovenous fistulae. *Nephrology Dialysis Transplantation, 31*(4), 525–528.

Nesrallah, G. E. (2016). Pro: Buttonhole cannulation of arteriovenous fistulae. *Nephrology Dialysis Transplantation, 31*(4), 520–523.

Nesrallah, G. E., Lindsay, R. M., Cuerden, M. S., Garg, A. X., Port, F., Austin, P. C., . . . Suri, R. S. (2012). Intensive hemodialysis associates with improved survival compared with conventional hemodialysis. *Journal of the American Society of Nephrology, 23*(4), 696–705.

Pauly, R. P., Eastwood, D. O., & Marshall, M. R. (2015). Patient safety in home hemodialysis: Quality assurance and serious adverse events in the home setting. *Hemodialysis International, 19*(Suppl. 1), S59–S70.

Rioux, J. P., Marshall, M. R., Faratro, R., Hakim, R., Simmonds, R., & Chan, C. T. (2015). Patient selection and training for home hemodialysis. *Hemodialysis International, 19*(Suppl. 1), S71–S79.

Rocco, M. V., Lockridge, R. S., Jr, Beck, G. J., Eggers, P. W., Gassman, J. J., Greene, T., . . . Kwok, S. (2011). The effects of frequent nocturnal home hemodialysis: The Frequent Hemodialysis Network Nocturnal Trial. *Kidney International, 80*(10), 1080–1091.

Walker, R. C., Hanson, C. S., Palmer, S. C., Howard, K., Morton, R. L., Marshall, M. R., & Tong, A. (2015). Patient and caregiver perspectives on home hemodialysis: A systematic review. *American Journal of Kidney Diseases, 65*(3), 451–463.

Weinhandl, E. D., Gilbertson, D. T., & Collins, A. J. (2016). Mortality, hospitalization, and technique failure in daily home hemodialysis and matched peritoneal dialysis patients: A matched cohort study. *American Journal of Kidney Diseases, 67*(1), 98–110.

Wienhandl, E. D., Nieman, K. M., Gilbertson, D. T., & Collins, A. J. (2015). Hospitalization in daily home hemodialysis matched thrice-weekly in-center hemodialysis patients. *American Journal of Kidney Diseases, 65*(1), 98–108.

Wong, B., Zimmerman, D., Reintjes, F., Courtney, M., Klarenbach, S., Dowling, G., & Pauly, R. P. (2014). Procedure-related serious adverse events among home hemodialysis patients: A quality assurance perspective. *American Journal of Kidney Diseases, 63*(2), 251–258.

CHAPTER 53

PERITONEAL DIALYSIS

James A. Sloand

TECHNICAL ASPECTS OF PERITONEAL DIALYSIS

1. **What is peritoneal dialysis (PD), and how does it work?**

   PD is a means of removing waste (such as urea, creatinine, and phosphate), other solutes (i.e., sodium and chloride), and excess fluid from the body when the kidneys have failed. A sterile solution (PD fluid) containing a balanced concentration of electrolytes and an osmotically active agent is introduced into the patient's peritoneal cavity by a PD catheter or tube. The latter is placed surgically (laparoscopic or open) or by interventional (bedside or radiologic) technique. The introduced PD fluid bathes the expansive network of capillaries covering the surface area of the peritoneum. As the PD fluid is devoid of any waste, solutes move down concentration gradients across peritoneal capillaries into the PD fluid over time until near-equilibrium of uremic solute concentrations is reached between the blood and the PD fluid. Once this occurs, the PD fluid ("dialysate effluent") is drained, again through the PD catheter. The process is then repeated with fresh PD fluid. The osmotically active agent present in the PD fluid draws fluid, called ultrafiltrate, across the peritoneal capillaries into the PD fluid. Wastes and excess fluid are removed when "spent" PD fluid effluent is drained. The cycle of infusion of PD fluid, followed by its dwell in the peritoneum, and subsequent drainage from the patient is referred to as an "exchange."

2. **What are the indications for and clinical benefits of PD?**

   PD can be performed in any patient who has end-stage kidney disease (ESKD) and has intact peritoneal anatomy and function. Specific contraindications are discussed later (see Question 9).

   The main clinical benefit of PD is that it allows patients the flexibility and lifestyle choices inherent in a home-suitable kidney replacement therapy. It also has an advantage in providing continuous removal of waste and fluid, similar to the continuous function provided by the kidneys. The resulting physiologically gentle means of dialysis is thought to contribute to better preservation of existing residual kidney function (RKF). Maintenance of RKF has been shown to provide survival advantage for patients with ESKD. The continuous nature of PD also affords greater hemodynamic stability and avoids rapid transcellular shifts of fluids and electrolytes. These features help maintain circulatory integrity and tissue perfusion, factors potentially compromised by intermittent renal replacement therapies.

   Initiating renal replacement therapy (RRT) with PD also helps preserve vasculature for future vascular access as part of an "integrated therapy" strategy for patients anticipated to require multiple RRTs (PD, transplant, home hemodialysis [HD], in-center HD) over their lifetime. As such, a RRT strategy of "PD first" is one advocated by an increasing number of clinicians when a preemptive kidney transplant is not available. This approach could also reduce the need for central venous catheters (CVCs) in patients needing an unplanned dialysis start.

   Better preservation of RRF, avoidance of compromised cardiac, brain, and gut perfusion, as well as avoidance of CVCs may help explain the apparent survival advantage reported in retrospective observational analyses of propensity matched-PD and HD-treated incident ESKD cohorts.

3. **What is peritoneal membrane transport, and why is it important?**

   Bidirectional transport of solutes and water occurs across the capillary walls of peritoneal membrane. Solute concentration gradients between the peritoneal capillary blood and the PD fluid are the primary drivers of net transport. However, the intrinsic transport characteristics of the peritoneal membrane capillary network are variable between patients and have a significant impact on patient outcome. Understanding an individual patient's peritoneal membrane transport type is therefore critical to appropriate tailoring of their PD prescription.

   Membrane transport is classified as slow, slow average, fast average, or fast, according to the peritoneal equilibration test (PET), as described in the following sections. In general, patients with fast to fast average membrane transport characteristics should be prescribed shorter dialysis dwell times to enhance fluid and small solute removal. Patients with slow and slow average membrane transport should generally be prescribed longer dwell times.

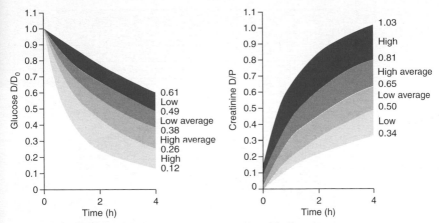

Figure 53.1. Interpretation of the peritoneal equilibration test. Changes in solute concentration during a peritoneal equilibration test allow classification into different transport types. Creatinine is corrected for glucose interference in this assay. *(Modified from Twardowski, Z. J., Nolph, K. D., Khanna, R., Prowant, B. F., Ryan, L. P., Moore, H. L., & Nielsen, M. P. (1987). Peritoneal equilibration test.* Peritoneal Dialysis Bulletin, 7, *138–147.)*

4. **What is the PET?**
   The PET is a standardized procedure for assessing the permeability and efficiency of a patient's membrane to exchange small solutes and fluid. The PET uses a series of dialysate (D) and plasma (P) samples obtained over a 4-hour period to measure solute equilibration (D/P creatinine), rate of glucose absorption, and net fluid removal or "ultrafiltration" (UF; Fig. 53.1). After determining these values, the patient's peritoneal membrane is categorized into one of the four membrane transport classifications. Each membrane classification (slow, slow average, fast average, fast) has specific characteristics that guide the clinician in tailoring the patient's dialysis prescription. An example of results from a typical standard PET is included (Fig. 53.2). In general, patients found to have fast to fast average membrane transport characteristics should be prescribed shorter dialysis dwell times to enhance fluid and small solute removal. Rapid equilibration of waste between dialysate and plasma, along with absorption of the osmotic agent (dextrose) by abundant peritoneal capillaries, are the reason for this.
   The standard PET is usually done with a 2.5% (2.27% anhydrous) dextrose PD solution, but a 4.25% (3.86% anhydrous) dextrose solution can be used as an alternative. The benefit of using the latter is that it produces near-identical diffusive results to a 2.5% solution and provides additional information about maximal UF capacity of the peritoneal membrane being tested. Reproducible and accurate results have been demonstrated with either solution.

5. **What is the "Three-Pore Model," and what is its relevance to peritoneal membrane transport?**
   Fluid and solute are transported between the blood and the peritoneal cavity across the peritoneal membrane. The capillary endothelial membrane provides the primary hindrance to this exchange. Mathematical modeling to describe, understand, and simulate this transport was captured by Bengt Rippe in his 1991 description of the "Three-Pore Model." The accuracy of the model has been validated in clinical studies and is used extensively to predict solute and fluid removal using different PD prescriptions for given peritoneal transport characteristics. As implied, transport across the peritoneal capillary is characterized to occur across three distinct endothelial "pores":
   1. Intracellular aquaporins or water channels. Aquaporins are affected by osmotic pressure and are exclusively permeable to water.
   2. Inter-endothelial cell or "small" pores. Small pores respond to both crystalloid and colloid osmotic forces and are permeable to both water and solutes smaller than albumin.
   3. Large inter-endothelial cellular pores. Large pores account for less than 0.01% of all capillary pores. While these are capable of passing larger molecules and proteins, they are effectively unresponsive to osmotic forces given their large size (precluding a transcellular gradient). Transport across these is unidirectional from plasma to peritoneal cavity and occurs by hydrostatic pressure. Large pores are responsible for leakage of protein into the peritoneal cavity.

Hours	Plasma creatinine (mg/dL)	Dialysate creatinine	D/P $_{creat}$	Dialysate glucose (mg/dL)	Dt/DO $_{Glucose}$
0	–	0.9	0.1	2071.5	1.0
2	9.70	5.2	0.56	1050.0	0.51
4	–	6.6	0.71	698.00	0.34

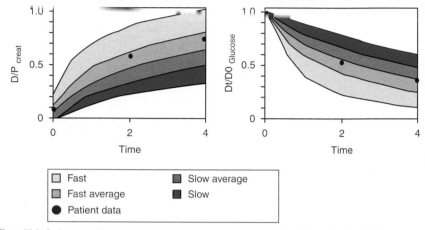

Figure 53.2. Peritoneal equilibration test example. Membrane transport of creatinine is determined by the rate of creatinine removal from the blood. This determination utilizes the ratio between dialysate creatinine concentration (D) after a 2- or 4-hour dwell and plasma creatinine concentration (P), represented as D/Pcreatinine. The greater the value of D/Pcreatinine (maximum of 1), the more creatinine has been transported into the dialysate. Similarly, membrane transport of glucose is determined by the rate of glucose absorption from the dialysate. The determination utilizes the ratio between the dialysate glucose concentration after 2- or 4-hour dwell times (Dt) and the dialysate glucose concentration at 0 hour (D0), represented as Dt/D0glucose. The lower the value of Dt/D0 glucose, the more rapidly glucose has been absorbed into the circulation. The sample values are indicated by black indicators (•). As apparent, values would classify this patient has having fast average peritoneal membrane characteristics. While D/Pcreatinine and Dt/D0glucose values are usually in agreement, the latter is more subject to error given the influence of blood glucose variability.

The Three-Pore Model is a fairly accurate mathematical tool used to predict solute and water transport for specific peritoneal membrane transport characteristics in response to different PD solutions with varying osmotic contents.

6. **What are the different methods of PD catheter placement?**
   There are currently three techniques for catheter placement:
   1. The dissective technique involves surgical placement of the catheter by mini-laparotomy. This is typically done under general anesthesia.
   2. The modified Seldinger technique involves "blind" insertion of a needle into the abdomen, placement of a guidewire, dilation of a tract, and insertion of the catheter through a sheath, all without visualization of the peritoneal cavity.
   3. Laparoscopic insertion using a small optical peritoneoscope for direct inspection of the peritoneal cavity. The latter can be performed as an outpatient procedure under local anesthesia with gas insufflation.
   The advantage of the Seldinger approach is that it can be placed acutely at the bedside or in the interventional radiology/nephrology suite without the need for general anesthesia. Conversely, superior results have been demonstrated using the advanced laparoscopic technique. Though some of the success may be operator dependent, the technique benefits from:
   - Rectus sheath tunneling, during which the transmural segment of the catheter is obliquely placed through a long musculofascial tunnel in the abdominal wall. This effectively maintains pelvic orientation of the catheter tip and reduces the risk of both exit site leak and hernia.

- Direct visualization of the PD catheter into the pelvic cavity
- Ability to address other abdominal peritoneal issues such as occult hernias, adhesions, redundant omentum, and epiploic appendices that may influence short- and long-term catheter success

The insertion technique used is determined by availability of expertise and economics. Success of the catheter after implantation is driven by the following of best demonstrated practices (BDPs), operator expertise, and patient comorbidities. To ensure the best patient outcomes, there needs to be cooperation among surgeons, radiologists, and nephrologists, irrespective of who places the PD catheter. These operators need to work collaboratively to develop common pathways and techniques to provide timely peritoneal access and resolve complications.

7. **Can elderly, obese, diabetic, and pediatric patients receive PD?**
PD can be used successfully in the majority of patients with kidney disease requiring dialysis. PD has been shown to be effective for patients with large body size or obesity, polycystic kidney disease, advanced age, diabetes, or other comorbidities (e.g., liver failure, ascites), and in patients without clinically significant kidney function (called *anuria*; see Question 8).

PD is also the preferred form of dialysis for most pediatric patients with ESKD, including neonates and infants. Benefits include no need for vascular access or venous puncture, association with good blood pressure control, fewer hospital visits for dialysis and associated care, facilitation of full-time school attendance, and better psychosocial adjustment for both patients and caregivers.

Assisted PD describes support of individuals unable to perform their own PD with assistance for all or part of their dialysis procedure. Assistance is provided by a health care technician, community nurse, family member, or a trained partner. Assisted PD is an option for elderly or disabled patients, allowing them to initiate or continue to use PD despite mental or physical limitations.

8. **Can patients continue receiving PD after they are anuric?**
Although maintenance of even a minimal amount of kidney function has been demonstrated to have a survival benefit in patients treated with either PD or HD, patients with anuria do fine on PD. Adequate nutritional intake and UF appear to be key elements to good outcome in patients who are anuric and receiving PD.

9. **What are the absolute contraindications to PD?**
The definition of absolute contraindication is the presence of a clinical condition that makes a treatment either unsafe or unlikely to be effective. There are few absolute contraindications for PD. PD is contraindicated in patients with:
- Diaphragmatic defects (e.g., pleuroperitoneal abnormalities)
- Abdominal defects (e.g., unfixable hernia) or processes (e.g., acute diverticulitis) that prevent effective PD or increase the risk of infection
- Situations where the patient and/or caregiver are unable or unwilling to learn the therapy. As noted previously, assisted PD has provided a solution for the later problem.

10. **Why would a patient want to do PD?**
- PD is generally provided in the patient's home, precluding the need to commute to and from dialysis on a fixed schedule.
- PD provides patients an active role in their own care
- Greater independence
- More flexibility in dialysis prescription to accommodate school, work, travel, and recreation
- Unlike conventional HD, PD is a needleless form of RRT.

11. **Are there requirements that would limit certain patients from being able to do PD?**
PD is typically performed in the home, a setting in which either the patient or home caregiver is responsible for setup, connections, and execution of the treatment. While this may limit the ability of certain patients with visual, tactile, or motor restrictions from performing PD on their own, for most patients, "where there is a will, there is a way." Patients are enabled by the flexibility to do either continuous ambulatory peritoneal dialysis (CAPD) or automated peritoneal dialysis (APD; see definitions that follow), family and/or caregivers (i.e., see the section on "Assisted Peritoneal Dialysis" that follows), and PD nursing teams knowledgeable about innovative care accessories that help overcome most limitations. Notably, many nursing homes offer PD, offloading any burden from the patient. Similarly, while space limitations or the presence of pets (i.e., cats) may at first seem to be a barrier to PD use, smaller, more frequent home supply deliveries and the use of CAPD, respectively, help circumvent these issues. PD should ideally be performed in a dedicated area of the living quarters that is kept clean (not sterile), and is free from blowing dust or dander.

12. **Which is better: PD or HD?**

PD, HD, and kidney transplant offer alternative and complementary means to treat ESKD. Most comparative analyses of observational registry studies have demonstrated similar outcomes for PD and HD in patients. A number of studies have shown better early survival (6 to 24 months) for patients treated with PD compared with those treated with HD (lower relative risk of death or higher survival probability favoring PD). While patient involvement in the decision-making process is key, clinician guidance in development of an integrated "ESKD Life Plan" can optimize clinical and lifestyle outcomes when the full spectrum of renal replacement therapies is appropriately sequenced. When possible, initial treatment with PD has the potential to improve early survival, improve transplant results, preserve vasculature for future access, and maintain more downstream renal replacement options. A "PD First" or preferred policy exists in many countries based on clinical as well as economic benefits.

13. **What do CAPD, APD, CCPD, NIPD, and "high-dose" mean?**

CAPD is the abbreviation for continuous ambulatory peritoneal dialysis. Typically patients manually infuse and drain 2 to 3 L of PD fluid three to four times a day. The PD fluid is allowed to dwell in the peritoneal cavity for a period of 4 to 6 hours per each of three daytime exchanges and 8 to 10 hours during the overnight exchange. Patients will usually carry PD fluid in the peritoneum *continuously,* 24 hours a day. Depending on the individual circumstance, a dry period may be allowed for reasons of patient comfort or convenience.

APD is the abbreviated term for automated peritoneal dialysis. This refers to use of a cycler (see Question 14) to assist in administration and drainage of PD fluid. Typically this is utilized to administer several dialysis exchanges at night while the patient is sleeping, with a final filling of the abdomen in the morning before the patient disconnects from the device. When APD is programmed to provide dialysis cycles both at night and for a "last fill" of fresh PD fluid that will remain in the peritoneal cavity during the day, it is called continuous cyclic PD, or CCPD. When a "last fill" is not programmed and the cycler only provides nocturnal dialysis exchanges, the APD is termed nocturnal intermittent PD, or NIPD. NIPD, where patients have a "dry day," should only be considered for patients who have residual kidney function (RKF). RKF is associated with improved survival in PD patients thought perhaps to be related to removal of larger molecular weight substances (i.e., B2 Microglobulin). When kidney function is lost, removal of these larger molecular weight solutes by PD is time-dependent and therefore is enhanced with a long dwell. As such, anuric patients should be prescribed either CCPD or CAPD where there is no "dry" period (neither a "dry day" or a "dry night," respectively).

Use of APD does not preclude additional manual exchanges from being done during the daytime hours, if needed. When a "last fill" is drained in the late morning or in the afternoon followed by infusion of an additional "midday" exchange with the intent of augmenting fluid and solute removal, the term "high-dose" is used.

14. **What is acute PD?**

Many patients need urgent or emergent dialysis. This occurs in patients who are not previously known to have chronic kidney disease (CKD) or when dialysis is started in situations of progressively deteriorating, but known, CKD without a permanent access (i.e., a fistula or a PD catheter). Urgent or emergent dialysis also occurs in situations of acute kidney injury (AKI). In the United States, Canada, and Europe, these patients are usually started on HD after placement of a CVC. However, there is movement to increase use of PD in these situations, with the goal of avoiding CVCs (tunneled and untunneled) and the morbidity and mortality associated with them.

PD can be used in many patients who have an unplanned start for dialysis. In a retrospective analysis comparing the outcomes of a group of patients started acutely on PD and a nonmatched group of patients with a planned start on chronic PD, there was no difference in infectious complications or technique survival rate, although mechanical complications were significantly more common in the acute group. In another small study in France, patients were nonrandomly selected for unplanned start with either PD or HD. Median time from PD catheter insertion to PD start was 4 days. The 1-year survival adjusted for comorbidity (79% survival on HD compared with 83% on PD) and the rehospitalization rate were similar. In a more recent observational cohort study from Germany, groups started on either unplanned acute PD or HD had equivalent mortality rates. HD patients had a significantly higher risk of bacteremia, presumably due to CVC use. PD was initiated within 12 hours after PD catheter implantation in this study, delivered nocturnally thrice weekly. Urgent start PD has also been proven effective in the elderly population. It should be noted that these are all single-center studies where the norm is HD. One would anticipate that increasing experience using PD for unplanned starts would improve outcomes.

Published experience with PD for AKI is limited. Ponce et al. demonstrated that high-volume PD (weekly Kt/V ~ 3.5) could achieve adequate metabolic and fluid control in AKI patients without severe fluid overload or hypercatabolism. A prospective randomized experience of 120 patients comparing high-volume PD to six times per week HD showed both similar survival (58% and 53%) and recovery of kidney function (28% and 26%). Although results here are encouraging, experience with acute placement of PD catheters and PD therapy itself is a critical factor for success. Acute abdominal processes would be a contraindication to using acute PD.

15. **What is a cycler, and who can or should use it?**
A cycler is a mechanized device made to assist in the administration and drainage of PD fluid. Use of the cycler to administer part or all of the PD prescription is termed APD. Although the cycler is primarily used by patients to administer their PD prescription at home, it can also be used in settings outside the home such as acute care, chronic care, or rehabilitation facilities to provide dialysis. The automation provided by APD allows a wider range of PD prescription options (both dwell volume and exchange frequency), allowing the ability to tailor prescriptions to accommodate individual patient needs. Accordingly, patients with "fast" peritoneal membrane transport characteristics have improved survival using APD compared with CAPD. Use of the cycler also reduces the number of manual connections the patient or care provider needs to perform. This lowers the risk for touch contamination. Patients treated with APD have similar or lower rates of peritonitis and similar or better technique survival compared with patients not using the cycler (e.g., CAPD).

16. **What are the contents of PD solutions?**
All PD solutions are sterile fluids containing physiologically balanced amounts of electrolytes and an osmotically active agent. The latter is needed to draw fluid across the peritoneal capillaries into the PD fluid (UF). There is a variety of commercial PD solutions available, with the main differences related to one of two things: the base buffer (and accompanying solution pH) and the osmotically active agent (Table 53.1).
    The electrolyte composition of PD solutions is roughly
- Sodium 132 mEq/L
- Chloride 95 to 105 mEq/L
- Calcium 2.5 to 3.5 mEq/L
- Magnesium 0.5 mEq/L

    Potassium is not in any PD fluid, but it can be manually added using sterile technique if necessary. Standard PD solutions contain lactate rather than bicarbonate as the base buffer to prevent precipitation of calcium and magnesium in the PD fluid. The usual concentration of lactate is approximately 40 mEq/L, and the resulting pH is 5.2 to 5.5. The pH rises rapidly to a physiologic level above 7.0 within about 15 minutes of infusion into the peritoneal cavity. Lactate absorbed from the PD fluid is converted to bicarbonate by a healthy liver. PD solutions containing exclusively lactate as the base buffer are contraindicated in patients with preexisting severe lactic acidosis.
    Alternatively, bicarbonate can be used as the primary base buffer, enabling a final solution pH of 7.4. This can be done by separating bicarbonate from calcium and magnesium using a dual-chambered PD container, with the separation maintained until just before infusion into the peritoneum. This reduces or even eliminates the pain during infusion of PD fluid that is experienced by some patients. It also has other theoretical advantages based on the more physiologic or "biocompatible" nature of the solution (discussed later).
    Both standard PD solutions and dual-chambered bicarbonate buffered PD solutions utilize dextrose (D-glucose) as an osmotic agent. Dextrose-containing solutions are usually available in three concentrations: 1.5 g/dL, 2.5 g/dL, and 4.25 g/dL (concentrations based on dextrose in its monohydrous, rather than anhydrous, form*). Manufacturers of some brands of dual-chambered solutions contain 10% more dextrose, however. Increasing the glucose content of PD solutions increases their osmolality, thus augmenting their ability to remove fluid (UF). The osmolalities associated with the previous standard dextrose concentrations are 346, 396, and 478 mOsm/kg, respectively. The osmotic gradient generated by dextrose-containing PD solutions dissipates over time as the dextrose is absorbed by the peritoneal capillaries. This gradient will dissipate more rapidly when lower concentrations of dextrose are used (e.g., 1.5 g/dL or 1.36 g/dL dextrose-containing solution, monohydrous or anhydrous, respectively) and in patients who have a larger peritoneal capillary network (e.g., fast membrane transport). Long exchange dwell times (e.g., >6 hours) can result in poor fluid removal, or even net negative fluid balance, because lymphatic absorption of PD fluid occurs at a constant rate (typically 1 to 2 mL/min), and can exceed transcapillary UF, particularly toward the end of a long exchange.
    Both icodextrin (Extraneal) and amino acids (Nutrineal) have been used as alternative osmotic agents to dextrose. Icodextrin is a polyglucose molecule having a very large molecular weight, a property that increases colloidal osmosis (oncotic pressure) of the containing PD solution (as opposed

---

* The same dextrose content of solutions is used in Europe, but dextrose is referred to in its anhydrous form. Respective dextrose concentrations are therefore 1.36%, 2.27%, and 3.86%.

Table 53.1. Contents of Peritoneal Dialysis Solutions

	DIANEAL PD1	DIANEAL PD2	DIANEAL PD4	PHYSIONEAL 35	PHYSIONEAL 40	EXTRANEAL	NUTRINEAL	PLASMA (ADULT)
Electrolytes (mmol/L)								
Sodium	132	132	132	132	132	133	132	136–145
Calcium	1.75	1.75	1.25	1.75	1.25	1.75	1.25	1.12–1.32
Magnesium	0.75	0.25	0.25	0.25	0.25	0.25	0.25	0.65–1.05
Chloride	102	96	95	101	95	96	105	98–107
Buffer (mmol/L)								
Lactate	35	40	40	10	15	40	40	0.6–1.7
Bicarbonate	—	—	—	25	25	—	—	21–30
pH	5.5	5.5	5.5	7.4	7.4	5.5	6.7	7.4
Osmotic Agent, Osmolarity (mOsm/L)								
1.36% glucose	347	345	344	345	344	—	—	—
2.27% glucose	398	396	395	396	395	—	—	—
3.86% glucose	486	484	483	484	483	—	—	—
7.5% icodextrin	—	—	a	—	—	284	—	—
1.1% amino acids	—	—	—	—	—	—	365	—

PD, Peritoneal dialysis.

to crystalloid osmotic pressure generated by dextrose-containing solutions). Extraneal does not contain any dextrose, has an osmolality of 282 mOsm/kg, and has a pH of 5.2. The fluid-removing capacity of this novel solution is not attenuated over time, making it ideal for long daytime (APD) or nighttime (CAPD) exchanges. Nutrineal also has the benefit of being glucose-free, utilizing 1.1 g/dL of amino acids as an osmotic agent. It has a pH of 6.4 and an osmolality of 365 mOsm/L.

17. **What are "biocompatible" PD solutions, and what is their clinical impact?**
PD solutions whose composition more closely mirrors physiologic conditions in terms of pH, osmolality, osmotic agent, manufacturing-induced breakdown products of osmotic agents, and buffer are generally considered "biocompatible" PD solutions. The intent of "biocompatibility" is "to leave the anatomical and physiological characteristics of the peritoneum unchanged in time." Conventional PD solutions are considered "bioincompatible" because they are glucose-containing, hyperosmolar, lactate-buffered, and generally below physiologic pH. They also contain glucose degradation products (GDPs) that develop as consequence of heat sterilization of the glucose contained in the PD solutions. Fibrotic and microvascular changes are observed to occur in the peritoneal membrane over the time of chronic exposure to these solutions. The association has led to the conclusion of their presumed culpability for these histologic changes, which are linked to increased small solute permeability, reduced UF, and attenuated technique success. Relevant to this discussion is the fact that UF failure accounts for less than 10% of PD technique failure at 2 to 3 years.
Production of more "biocompatible" PD solutions employing alternative osmotic agents (e.g., icodextrin, amino acids), buffers (e.g., lactate/bicarbonate or pure bicarbonate), and dual-chambered containers to reduce GDP content has therefore ensued. The composition of the latter includes a low pH, calcium/ magnesium, and glucose-containing compartment. GDP production is minimized during heat sterilization of glucose at low pH. The adjacent buffer-containing compartment contains either bicarbonate/lactate or bicarbonate alone. Precipitation of calcium or magnesium with these buffers is prevented by their separation until just prior to peritoneal infusion, at which time the seal between the two adjacent chambers is broken.
The clinical impact of neutral-pH, low-GDP PD solutions in comparison to conventional PD solutions was assessed in a recent systematic Cochrane review. No significant effects were seen on peritonitis, technique survival, and patient survival, nor were harms identified with their use. In addition, while extended time to anuria and greater urine output was noted in several studies, this effect may have been influenced by diminished UF capacity of some of the neutral-pH, low-GDP solutions. Reduced UF could result in expanded effective arterial volume, augmenting urine output. Studies examining the potential benefit of "biocompatible" solutions on preservation of peritoneal membrane solute transport and UF capacity are ongoing.

18. **Can icodextrin interfere with results of "Point of Care" glucometer results?**
"Point of Care" (POC) glucometers and test strips that do not use glucose-specific methodologies cannot discern the difference between glucose and other sugars in the blood (e.g., maltose). While icodextrin is not absorbed across the peritoneal membrane, some is absorbed via peritoneal lymphatics and eventually reaches the systemic circulation. There it undergoes metabolism by amylase, with the main metabolite being maltose. Given limited kidney excretion in patients with ESKD, plasma levels of icodextrin and maltose metabolites with once daily use reach stable levels that do not return to baseline values for at least 2 weeks following complete cessation of icodextrin use. As such, nonglucose-specific POC glucometers may result in falsely elevated blood glucose readings in patients on icodextrin. This could either result in the masking of true hypoglycemia or provide falsely elevated blood glucose reading, situations that could lead to erroneous clinician action and potentially life-threatening events. Patients on icodextrin should therefore have blood glucose measurements done exclusively with glucose-specific POC monitors or, if hospitalized, have their blood glucose values ascertained by the clinical chemistry laboratory.

19. **What are the elements of a PD prescription, and how is it determined?**
Elements of a PD prescription include:
- Total number of exchanges per day
- Dwell duration, dwell volume, and PD fluid content (dextrose, icodextrin, amino acid) of each exchange
- The method of PD (CAPD or by cycler [APD], and whether the peritoneum is dry for any part of the day, is also included in the prescription.
The PD prescription is individualized for each patient based on his or her physiologic needs and desired lifestyle. The former is determined by the size of the patient (either volume of distribution of urea or body surface area), their peritoneal membrane transport characteristics, and their RKF. Further adjustment can be made based on dietary and fluid intake of the patient. The prescription can then be

modified to accommodate their work, school, or social schedule using either CAPD or APD. In general, patients with fast peritoneal membrane transport require shorter dwell times (as equilibration happens quickly), whereas those with slower membrane transport require longer dwell times. Although minor differences are apparent, icodextrin is handled similarly, irrespective of membrane transport type.

20. **What is tidal APD?**

Tidal APD is a technique whereby a constant *residual volume* of PD fluid (e.g., 200 mL) is left in the peritoneal cavity following the first APD cycle and dwell. Partial fill volumes delivered for subsequent cycles (e.g., 1800 mL) are reduced proportionate to this prescribed residual volume, so that the total peritoneal volume does not exceed the prescribed dwell volume (e.g., 2000 mL). Accommodation in cycler prescription must be made for the anticipated UF. Failure to do so will result in progressive increases in peritoneal volume and intraperitoneal pressure, an effect that could result in adverse abdominal wall or cardiopulmonary events. Intermediate full drains are possible and programmable in the cycler. Tidal PD is usually prescribed for reasons of drain pain, to provide a "cushion" of PD fluid between the PD catheter and pelvic organs. A constant residual volume provided through tidal PD can also help manage slow PD catheter drainage occurring toward the end of drain attributable to pelvic structures impeding flow at low peritoneal fluid volumes.

21. **How long can patients stay on PD?**

There is no defined time limit to a patient being able to stay on PD. Technique survival of patients treated with PD (defined as the proportion of patients who remain on PD and have not transferred to HD) is highly variable (45% to 84% after 3 years of therapy and 25% to 75% after 5 years of therapy), given large local and regional differences in PD catheter placement expertise, peritonitis rates, preservation of peritoneal transport function, transplantation rates, and supportive home assistance. To some extent, lack of evidence-based international care standards, or of adherence to them, has contributed to this variation. Introduction of the Peritoneal Dialysis Outcomes Practice Patterns Study (PDOPPS) in 2013 should hopefully provide some solution at least to identification of best practice. Adequate nutritional intake, maintenance of a normal volume status, avoidance of infection, and reducing patient care burden are key elements to successful longevity (technique survival) on PD.

22. **Does PD affect kidney transplantation?**

Patients receiving PD as their means of RRT are much more likely to receive a kidney transplant. Although this may be explained by demographics of the PD population, there may be other contributing factors. Infectious and cardiovascular challenges inherent to intermittent HD could potentially result in the removal of prospective transplant patients from an "active" transplant list, delaying transplantation.

Patients receiving PD as their pretransplant means of RRT have a similar or better overall posttransplant patient survival, and a similar or lower incidence of delayed graft dysfunction compared with those treated with CHD. Conversely, the risk of graft failure was similar or higher in the population treated with PD before transplant; some studies also demonstrated a higher risk of graft thrombosis.

23. **What dietary restrictions are required for PD?**

In general, there are fewer dietary restrictions for patients on PD than there are for those on thrice-weekly HD because of the continuous nature of PD as a RRT. Patients on PD can be allowed a reasonably liberal intake of potassium. Conversely, unrestricted sodium and water intake should be discouraged unless the patient has an excellent urine output and little need for high-concentration dextrose PD solutions. Chronic exposure to consistently high dextrose–containing PD solutions may contribute to the development of hypokalemia, adverse changes to the peritoneal membrane, and weight gain by the patient.

KDOQI recommends that all patients with ESKD on RRT be encouraged to ingest a diet high in protein, particularly protein with high biologic value. This helps offset the catabolic effects of dialysis related to HD and amino acids and/or protein lost in the spent hemodialysate or peritoneal dialysate. Approximately 5 to 15 g of protein can be lost in PD effluent over a 24-hour period, highlighting the importance of a recommended intake of 1.2 to 1.3 g/kg per day of dietary protein.

KEY POINTS: TECHNICAL ASPECTS OF PERITONEAL DIALYSIS

1. The main clinical benefit of peritoneal dialysis (PD) is that it allows for greater flexibility and lifestyle choices inherent in home-suitable kidney replacement therapy.
2. Initiating incident patients on PD (i.e., "PD First") offers survival and other clinical benefits, particularly in situations where renal replacement is unplanned or a central venous catheter would otherwise be used.

3. The continuous nature of PD affords greater hemodynamic stability by avoiding rapid shifts in intravascular volume and rapid transcellular shifts of electrolytes. These features help maintain circulatory integrity and tissue perfusion, factors potentially compromised by intermittent renal replacement therapies.
4. Residual kidney function is associated with survival benefits and is better preserved with PD than intermittent hemodialysis.
5. Initiating incident patients on PD preserves the vasculature for future access, maintaining more downstream kidney replacement options.

ASSESSING THE DOSE OF DIALYSIS

24. What is dialysis adequacy, how is it measured in PD, and what are the current minimum targets in PD?

Accumulation of uremic wastes not removed by the failing kidneys contributes to poor outcome in patients with ESKD, although this may be a simplistic view, given a number of other neurohormonal changes that accompany loss of kidney function. Ideally the removal of a threshold or *adequate* amount of waste with dialysis would result in improved outcome, with any incremental amount removed above this amount having little impact on improving clinical outcome. Previous and more recent studies have primarily focused on the relationship between clearance of only small solutes, in particular urea and creatinine, and outcome. It is important to recognize the limitations of this conventional and "convenient" assumption, however. Many important uremic toxins with much larger molecular weight and water solubility behave quite differently than urea and creatinine do and are therefore not removed effectively by standard dialysis, either HD or PD. Despite this, the use of urea and creatinine removal by dialysis has remained the primary metric of dialysis adequacy, with expectation that increased removal of these using augmented dialysis treatment intensity will result in improved clinical outcomes. To date, results of randomized controlled interventional trials comparing distinct tiers of urea removal have failed to demonstrate this. Conversely these studies have shown that poor outcomes can occur if minimum amounts of urea are *not* removed. Based on these results, both the National Kidney Foundation Kidney Disease Outcomes Quality Initiative and the International Society of Peritoneal Dialysis guidelines for PD recommend that *adequacy* be assessed by total (peritoneal and kidney) clearance of urea (termed "Kt"), normalized to its volume of distribution (V_{urea}). Assessment of this requires collection and measurement of urea present in 24-hour collections of both drained PD effluent and urine. Although the current *weekly* standardized Kt/V_{urea} target recommended by both the Kidney Disease Outcome Quality Initiative (KDOQI) and the International Society for Peritoneal Dialysis (ISPD) is 1.7, both guidelines recognize the importance of clinical assessment of the individual patient in determining need for more dialysis. In recent years, there has been doubt cast on the validity of Kt/V_{urea} as a valuable metric of clinical outcome, much less a payment-required "reportable" one. Other factors possibly important in patient outcome include volume status, sodium, phosphate, and middle molecule (e.g., beta-2-microglobulin) removal, as well as inflammation. The means to address these are currently being considered.

25. Why is there so much difference in the minimum Kt/V_{urea} targets for PD (i.e., *weekly* $Kt/V \geq 1.7$) and conventional thrice-weekly HD (i.e., *per treatment* or *equilibrated* $Kt/V_{urea} \geq 1.2$)?

PD provides continuous removal of uremic solute, therefore resulting in a relatively constant concentration of urea and other uremic wastes. Conversely, because of its intermittent nature, thrice-weekly HD results in uremic solute levels that are highly variable, with peak levels occurring just prior to treatment, nadirs during and immediately upon cessation of treatment, followed by progressively increasing levels over the next 48 to 72 hours until the next therapy. To account for these differences, *time-averaged* blood urea nitrogen levels are used to formulate a weekly *standardized* Kt/V_{urea}. Based on these calculations, an *equilibrated* Kt/V_{urea} of 1.2 obtained at *thrice weekly* with intermittent HD is equivalent to a *weekly standardized* Kt/V_{urea} of 1.7 to 2.0, values comparable to that achieved with PD.

26. Is peritoneal clearance equivalent to that provided by the kidneys?

Peritoneal clearance is not equivalent to that afforded by the kidneys. While PD clearance of small solutes is reasonable, that of larger molecular weight solutes and protein-bound toxins pales in comparison to what renal clearance provides. Thus the value of Kt provided by dialysis is inferior to a similar numerical value of Kt provided by the kidneys.

27. **Why is residual kidney function (RKF) important in patients with PD?**

RKF is strongly associated with a survival advantage for patients receiving both peritoneal and HD. Postulated reasons for this association include better

- Removal of phosphate
- Removal of middle molecular and protein-bound wastes
- Salt and water balance
- Removal of inflammatory mediators

Therefore it is important to protect RKF in patients receiving dialysis. PD is superior to HD in preserving RKF. This is probably related to the hemodynamic factors associated with its continuous nature. It is important to protect RKF, irrespective of their chosen modality of kidney replacement therapy. This includes the use of agents to block the renin-angiotensin-aldosterone system, avoidance of nonsteroidal inflammatory drugs and radiocontrast agents, volume depletion, and sodium phosphate bowel preparations. Prolonged use of aminoglycosides and other nephrotoxins should also be avoided. Short-term use of aminoglycosides in patients with ESKD is safe and can be used, pending identification and sensitivity of organisms causing peritonitis with subsequent change to an alternative nonaminoglycoside agent later.

28. **How important is volume control in patients treated with PD, and how is it best managed?**

Attainment of euvolemia has been demonstrated to be important to clinical outcome in patients with ESKD, whether treated with PD or HD. Although determination of dry weight is challenging for any patient, observational analyses have demonstrated that enhanced UF in patients treated with PD is associated with improved survival.

Conservative management is the cornerstone of volume management and includes kidney protective measures, sodium restriction, and optimal use of diuretics. Peritoneal UF using icodextrin (Extraneal) is superior to dextrose-based solutions for the long dwell exchange (8 to 16 hours). Icodextrin also removes greater amounts of sodium per volume of ultrafiltrate than dextrose-based solutions (i.e., 130 mEq/L vs. 100 mEq/L of UF, respectively) related to its mechanism of action. Specifically, Icodextrin is an iso-osmolar solution that acts exclusively on the small pores of the peritoneal capillaries, drawing near isotonic ultrafiltrate (by colloid osmosis) into the peritoneal cavity from the blood. Conversely, nearly half of ultrafiltrate obtained by dextrose-based solutions (crystalloid osmosis) is sodium-free water derived from the osmolality-sensitive aquaporins. The use of icodextrin also simplifies the PD prescription, as UF and sodium removal with icodextrin is relatively independent of patient transport type (Fig. 53.3). It also helps reduce peritoneal glucose exposure and systemic glucose absorption, particularly for fast and fast average transport patients.

29. **Does the peritoneal membrane transport status impact the prescribed dose of PD?**

"Fast transporters" typically have no problem achieving adequate clearance of small solutes, given rapid equilibration of these substances across the peritoneal capillary membranes. Conversely, rapid absorption of glucose from the PD fluid and dissipation of the glucose-associated osmotic gradient occurs simultaneously, impacting adequate removal of both fluid and sodium. The latter is presumed to account for an increased risk of death and technique failure in "fast transport" patients treated with CAPD and longer dwell times. Modeling studies have suggested, and clinical studies have confirmed, that UF and sodium removal can be achieved in faster membrane transport through the prescription of shorter dwells (most conveniently done with APD) and icodextrin for the long dwell. Notably these prescriptive changes are also associated with significantly improved outcomes. An appropriate PD prescription, tailored to the patient's peritoneal membrane transport, is imperative for optimal clinical outcome.

KEY POINTS: ASSESSING THE DOSE OF DIALYSIS

1. An appropriate peritoneal dialysis (PD) prescription, tailored to the patient's peritoneal membrane transport, is imperative for optimal clinical outcome.
2. Although determination of dry weight is challenging for any patient, observational analyses have demonstrated that enhanced ultrafiltration (UF) in patients treated with PD is associated with improved survival. Peritoneal UF and sodium removal using icodextrin (Extraneal) has been shown to be superior compared to dextrose-based solutions.
3. Residual kidney function is strongly associated with survival advantage for patients receiving both peritoneal and hemodialysis. As such, strong attention should be paid to protecting kidney function for all patients on dialysis.
4. Icodextrin used as a cornerstone to the initial PD prescription simplifies the PD prescription for both patients and prescribers and minimizes the impact of patient membrane transport type on UF and sodium removal.

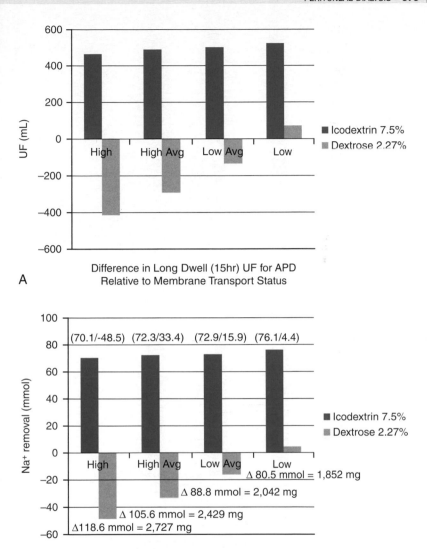

A, Difference in Long Dwell (15hr) UF for APD Relative to Membrane Transport Status

B, Difference Long Dwell (15hr) Sodium Removal for APD Relative to Membrane Transport Status

Figure 53.3. Estimation of ultrafiltration volumes and sodium removal difference using either icodextrin or 2.5% (monohydrous) glucose-containing dialysate during simulated automated peritoneal dialysis and continuous ambulatory peritoneal dialysis therapies for the long dwell (15 hours and 9 hours, respectively). **A,** Difference in long dwell UF for APD relative to membrane transport status. **B,** Difference in long dwell sodium removal for APD relative to membrane transport status.

Continued

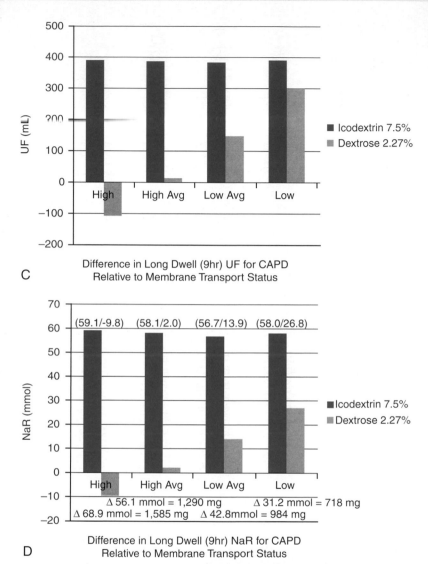

Figure 53.3. cont'd C, Difference in long dwell UF for CAPD relative to membrane transport status. **D,** Difference in long dwell sodium removal for CAPD relative to membrane transport status. *(Modified from Akonur, A., Sloand, J., Davis, I., & Leypoldt, J. (2016). Icodextrin simplifies PD therapy by equalizing UF and sodium removal among patient transport types during long dwells: A modeling study. Peritoneal Dialysis International, 36, 79–84.)*

COMPLICATIONS OF PERITONEAL DIALYSIS

30. What are the risks of infection with PD compared with HD?

The overall incidence of infection among patients with PD is no greater than among patients with HD. According to data collected by USRDS, patients on PD are significantly less likely to have dialysis-associated bacteremia or sepsis, a complication almost completely associated with HD. Conversely, the most serious infection and one almost exclusively occurring in patients on PD is peritonitis. Technical advances in the past decade around "patient-to-dialysate connectology" and infection control strategies have reduced the peritonitis infection rates markedly. While infection-related hospitalizations rates are higher for patients on PD than for those on HD, this is likely related to the ability to treat infections for the HD population in the dialysis outpatient setting using a permanent vascular access. Notwithstanding, in recent years, infection-related hospitalizations have declined more among patients on PD than among those on HD.

31. **What are an exit site infection and a tunnel infection?**
The presence of purulent drainage, with or without erythema on the skin around the catheter exit site, indicates the existence of an exit site infection. Redness around the catheter may be an early heralding sign of infection or simply local irritation. The latter is more likely if it occurs shortly after catheter placement, trauma, or traction about the catheter exit site. A positive culture in the absence of abnormal exit site appearance is suggestive of colonization, not infection.
    A tunnel infection is defined by involvement of the catheter tunnel beyond the superficial cuff. The presence of catheter tunnel infection can occur in the setting of an exit site infection. This is suggested by erythema, edema, and tenderness over the subcutaneous course of the PD catheter. A fluid collection demonstrated by ultrasound can facilitate diagnosis (and adequate duration of treatment) of a tunnel infection.

32. **How is an exit site infection prevented?**
Prevention of exit site infections (and peritonitis, described later) starts with proper placement of the PD catheter. The exit site of the catheter should be in a location that can be clearly seen by the patient, downward or laterally facing to preclude funneling of dirt or cellular debris into the catheter exit site, and not buried in a panniculus or abdominal skinfold. Prophylactic antibiotics given prior to PD catheter placement have value in preventing subsequent peritonitis. Avoidance of anchoring sutures at the PD exit site and allowing the PD catheter to remain covered, clean, dry, and undisturbed until well healed are additional key factors in preventing an infectious nidus from being seeded about the catheter exit site or tunnel. Consistent, steadfast training of the patient and staff regarding sterile technique, observation of meticulous handwashing, and daily exit site care is then required. Application of either mupirocin or gentamycin cream to the exit site prevents infections.

33. **What is the appropriate initial empiric antibiotic therapy for PD catheter exit site infection?**
Staphylococcus aureus, coagulase-negative *staphylococcus*, and other gram-positive organisms are the most frequent causes of exit site infection, followed in frequency by *Pseudomonas aeruginosa* and other gram-negative organisms. As with peritonitis, however, knowledge of both the epidemiology of exit site/tunnel infections and the local antibiotic sensitivities in each PD unit is imperative to guide therapy in that unit. After identification of an exit site or tunnel infection, empiric antibiotic therapy may be initiated, or therapy can be deferred until the results of the culture of the exit site drainage can guide the choice of agent. Empiric therapy should always cover *S. aureus* and consider *P. aeruginosa*, because these are common causes of infection and are associated with peritonitis. An oral *Penicillinase*-resistant penicillin (i.e., dicloxacillin 500 mg four times a day) or a first-generation cephalosporin (i.e., cephalexin 500 mg twice a day) provide good gram-positive coverage, and oral quinolones can provide gram-negative (including antipseudomonal) and some gram-positive coverage. Documented *P. aeruginosa* may require two antipseudomonal drugs, given its relative resistance to therapy. Antimicrobial agents should be continued for 2 weeks or until the exit site appears normal, whichever is longer. Ultrasound may be helpful in determining the presence, response, and duration of therapy in the case of a tunnel infection. Failure to adequately eradicate the infection should prompt replacement of the PD catheter. Dosing recommendations of other commonly used antibiotics and details useful in the treatment of exit site and tunnel infection can be found at www.ISPD.org.

34. **What is peritonitis?**
Peritonitis is inflammation of the peritoneal membrane. Although this most often results from infection, peritonitis can also result from noninfectious cause. Entry of infectious organisms into the peritoneum can occur from
    • Touch contamination by the patient because of improper technique
    • Extension of infection from around the PD catheter
    • Transluminal migration of bacteria across the bowel wall
    • Hematogenous seeding in the case of bacteremia or sepsis from another source
        Patients usually present with symptoms of abdominal pain and cloudy PD effluent.

35. **What is the appropriate diagnostic workup of peritonitis in a patient undergoing PD?**
Upon presentation by any patient on PD with symptoms of either abdominal pain or cloudy effluent, a diagnosis of peritonitis should be entertained and ruled out. However, the clinician should also be

mindful of other non-PD-related causes of these symptoms, such as a ruptured viscus, diverticulitis, cholecystitis, ischemic bowel, or pancreatitis. Prompt diagnosis and treatment are imperative for best outcomes in PD-related peritonitis and any of the other conditions.

A sample of PD effluent that has ideally been dwelling in the peritoneum for at least 1 to 2 hours should be obtained by the patient or health care provider. The effluent fluid is sent to the laboratory for cell count, gram stain, and microbial culture. The diagnosis of peritonitis requires at least two of the following three features:

1. Peritoneal fluid leukocytosis ($>100/mm^3$ and at least 50% polymorphonuclear cells)
2. Abdominal pain
3. Positive culture of the dialysis effluent

36. Why should a gram stain and microscopy of the peritoneal effluent be performed with suspected peritonitis?

The primary reason for microscopy is to identify the presence of budding yeast or hyphae, indicative of fungal peritonitis. These findings should prompt immediate removal of the PD catheter, an action that may have a significant impact on patient survival.

37. How should peritonitis be prevented and treated?

A team-based, multifaceted approach to continuous quality improvement with regular audit of infection rates and outcomes is essential to improving peritonitis rates. Training and retraining of both patients and nurse patient-educators is a cornerstone of this effort.

A number of peritonitis episodes are the result of direct extension of an infection associated with the exit site, in particular when the infecting organism at the exit site is either *S. aureus* or *P. aeruginosa*. All BDPs in reducing exit site infections will decrease peritonitis episodes. Another measure to reduce peritonitis is "flush before fill" connectology, a technology that washes any bacteria introduced at the tubing–catheter interface during an exchange into the drainage bag rather than into the patient's peritoneum. Avoidance of constipation reduces the risk of peritonitis by attenuating transmigration of enteric bacteria across the bowel wall.

Observational studies have suggested benefits in draining the peritoneum dry and providing appropriate prophylactic antibiotics prior to dental, gastrointestinal, and genitourinary procedures. Adequate 25-hydroxyvitamin D levels have also been associated with lower peritonitis rates.

Once a presumptive diagnosis of peritonitis is made, prompt treatment with antibiotics capable of covering both gram-negative and gram-positive organisms is implemented. Although antibiotics can be given orally or intravenously, intraperitoneal (IP) administration has the benefit of providing immediate delivery of bacteriocidal concentrations of antibiotics. PD fluid culture results should then help narrow the spectrum and guide the duration of antimicrobial therapy. Attention to achieving a consistent mean inhibitory concentration (MIC) of antibiotics in the PD fluid, particularly if the patient is receiving APD or if intermittent antibiotic therapy is being used, is critical to successful treatment. Continuous rather than intermittent antibiotic therapy should ensure that a therapeutic MIC is achieved. While intermittent vancomycin dosing appears to be acceptable, it is prudent to obtain serum levels to ensure adequate MIC levels, particularly in the presence of significant RKF. Serum vancomycin levels should be kept >15 mmg/mL.

The signs and symptoms of peritonitis usually resolve within 48 hours after appropriate antimicrobial therapy. Persistent pain, cloudy fluid, and elevation of peritoneal fluid white blood cell (WBC) count should prompt reevaluation of the infectious cause and whether antibiotic therapy is suitable. Peritonitis refractory to treatment, defined as failure of the effluent to clear within 5 days of appropriate antibiotic therapy, should result in removal of the catheter. The ISPD has published guidelines for the prevention, diagnosis, and treatment of peritonitis.

38. What is the appropriate initial empiric antibiotic therapy for suspected PD-related peritonitis?

Initial empiric therapy should reflect knowledge of both the epidemiology of peritonitis and the antibiotic sensitivities in the local PD unit. In general, ISPD recommends initial coverage of both gram-positive and gram-negative microorganisms. Use of a third-generation cephalosporin or an aminoglycoside for gram-negative coverage *and* vancomycin or a first-generation cephalosporin for gram-positive coverage would accomplish these goals. This should provide coverage against the majority of organisms that cause peritonitis, including *Pseudomonas* and *S. aureus*. Initial and subsequent doses of antibiotics for IP administration can be found at www.ISPD.org.

39. Are there concerns with intermittent IP antibiotic dosing for peritonitis?

The goal of treating peritonitis is to ensure that a consistent MIC of antibiotics is maintained in the PD fluid. This prevents inadequate treatment, relapsing and repeat peritonitis, and development of microbial resistance. The principle behind intermittent IP antibiotic therapy is that antibiotics allowed to dwell in the peritoneal cavity for a period of at least 6 hours are absorbed into the bloodstream, where their volume of distribution serves as an "antibiotic depot." Antibiotics from this systemic depot then move down their concentration gradient from the blood into the peritoneum during subsequent PD exchanges, which are devoid of added antibiotics. Achieving an MIC in those exchanges depends on the blood antibiotic concentration, the length of the exchange, and the rapidity of clearance of the systemic antibiotic depot. The latter may be augmented with more frequent exchanges, fast membrane transport status, and greater levels of RKF. Given these issues, there is a risk of suboptimal dosing and treatment when intermittent antibiotic therapy is used, particularly in APD. As such, antimicrobial therapy should be carefully thought out and individualized.

40. **How do you approach fungal peritonitis?**
Fungal peritonitis is a serious disease that can lead to death in up to 25% of patients affected. Diagnosis either by microscopy or culture requires removal of the PD catheter, along with initiation of dual therapy with intravenous amphotericin B (dose adjusted to weight) and oral flucytosine 1000 mg/day. Given poor peritoneal penetration with intravenous use and chemical peritonitis with IP use, amphotericin should be replaced with another antifungal agent after fungal susceptibilities are determined. Most peritoneal fungal infections are a result of either *Candida albicans* or *Candida parapsilosis*, but can result from an assortment of fungi.

Recent antibiotic treatment has been shown to be a predisposing factor associated with subsequent development of fungal peritonitis. As such, antifungal prophylaxis is recommended for PD patients treated with a course of antibiotics, as per ISPD guidelines.

While fungal peritonitis is associated with a high frequency of technique failure, a third of patients were able to return to PD in a recent observational analysis.

41. **What are the indications for removal of a PD catheter?**
Removal of the PD catheter should be strongly considered in cases of the following:
- Refractory peritonitis, defined as failure of the peritoneal effluent to clear after 5 days of appropriate antibiotics
- Relapsing peritonitis, defined as redevelopment of peritonitis with the same organism or after an episode of sterile peritonitis occurring within 4 weeks of completion of therapy of the previous episode
- Repeat peritonitis, defined as redevelopment of peritonitis with the same organism more than 4 weeks after completion of therapy for the previous episode; this may also be an indication for removal given presumed similarities in cause to relapsing peritonitis.
- An exit site and/or tunnel infection failing to respond to recommended treatment with appropriate antibiotics
- Fungal peritonitis
- Peritonitis associated with the growth of multiple enteric organisms, particularly anaerobic organisms; the risk of intraabdominal pathology is raised in this setting

42. **What is difference between relapsing and repeat peritonitis?**
Relapsing peritonitis describes redevelopment of peritonitis with the same organism *within* 4 weeks of completion of therapy for a previous episode; repeat peritonitis describes redevelopment of peritonitis with the same organism, but occurring *more than* 4 weeks after completion of therapy for the previous episode. Both suggest inadequate treatment (i.e., low MIC with the first episode of peritonitis) or a continued nidus of infection (i.e., catheter biofilm, need for catheter removal).

43. **What is pericatheter leakage?**
Pericatheter leakage describes a complication of PD where administered dialysis fluid and ultrafiltrate is not confined to the peritoneal cavity, but rather escapes or leaks around the entrance site or across the abdominal wall tissue planes crossed by the PD catheter. Leakage around the PD catheter exit site commonly presents as moisture or drainage of clear fluid. Alternatively, leakage can occur around the rectus muscle sheath or Scarpa's fascia, resulting in pericatheter edema. The technique of PD catheter placement (median as opposed to paramedian location), factors related to initiation of PD (excessive volume of PD fluid relative to timing of the PD catheter placement), or intrinsic abdominal wall weakness (children, excessive physical straining, obesity, or long-term therapy with steroids) are the causative factors associated with peri-catheter leak.

PD fluid can also leak into fluid spaces outside of the peritoneum related to intrinsic peritoneal, abdominal wall, or diaphragmatic defects. A patent processus vaginalis; inguinal or periumbilical hernias can result in edema in genital and other respective areas. Conversely, tendinous defects in the diaphragm can result in collection of fluid within the thoracic cavity. Positive abdominal and negative intrathoracic pressure contributes to the collection of fluid in the chest cavity in the setting of a diaphragmatic defect. Leak or extravasation of fluid outside the peritoneum can present with decreased UF, increased weight, localized swelling, or shortness of breath. The latter is particularly true in the case of transthoracic infiltration of fluid, which, if sizeable, can result in a unilateral decrease in breath sounds, dullness to percussion on the involved side, and a pleural effusion on chest imaging. An increased glucose content of fluid leaking from the area around the PD catheter or obtained by thoracentesis (in the case of a presumed diaphragmatic defect) relative to the blood glucose level provides a helpful diagnostic clue. Suspicion of internal leakage of PD fluid into tissue planes can be confirmed with imaging studies. If magnetic resonance imaging (MRI) is used, it should be done without gadolinium. The PD fluid itself can serve as the "contrast" for MRI diagnosis of internal leaks.

PD should usually be interrupted, if possible, for 1 to 2 weeks when early external or subcutaneous leaks develop to allow more time for healing around the catheter. An alternative is to reduce the dwell volume coupled with use of supine dialysis, leaving the abdomen dry when the patient is sitting, upright, or ambulatory. Antibiotics should be strongly considered in the presence of an external leak to reduce the risk of a tunnel infection or peritonitis. Recurrence of a leak after a several week period of peritoneal rest or modified, supine PD should prompt strong consideration of surgical intervention. Temporary transfer to HD to allow for primary healing or after correction of an abdominal wall defect may be necessary depending on the presence and the amount of RKF in addition to the clinical scenario. Late leaks, defined as those occurring more than 30 days after catheter insertion, are more likely to require surgical correction of the defect to achieve resolution. It is notable that successful continuation of PD using a regimen of supine-attenuated PD has been described.

Discontinuation of PD is appropriate in the case of PD-related hydrothorax. Successful surgical correction of the diaphragmatic defect after surgical repair or pleurodesis may allow the patient to return to PD after a judicious interval to allow for complete healing.

44. **What is inflow/outflow pain?**
Occasionally, patients complain of pain upon infusion or drainage of PD fluid. Infusion pain can result from infusion of an inappropriately cool or warm PD solution, peritoneal sensitivity to the lower than physiologic pH of PD solution (i.e., 5.2 to 6.4), visceral sensitivity to a directed jet stream of PD fluid from the PD catheter, or a malpositioning of the PD catheter against the viscera. Discomfort during drainage ("drain pain") of PD effluent usually relates to a siphoning effect on the viscera or peritoneum and may therefore also relate to catheter positioning. The effect of constipation on expansion of intestinal diameter and resultant crowding of the viscera around the catheter should not be minimized as a cause of either fill or drain pain.

Timing and duration of the pain usually provide the diagnostic clues as to which of the aforementioned issues are causative and therefore crucial to discerning appropriate treatment. Transient pain related to inappropriate temperature can be adequately managed with proper patient instruction. Pain related to the lower pH of the PD solution is also transient in nature, given the rapid increase in the PD fluid pH to physiologic levels. The use of neutral pH PD solutions can address this issue if available. Although addition of bicarbonate to the PD solution prior to peritoneal infusion can also help reduce pain, introduction of any exogenous substance to the PD fluid theoretically may increase infection risks. Alternatively, patients can leave a small residual volume of PD fluid in the abdomen at the end of the drain phase of the exchange. This residual volume serves as a buffer to the inflowing dialysate and reduces the tugging sensation associated with the last phase of the drain. Use of "tidal" therapy with APD accomplishes the same effect. Tidal PD can also reduce nightly alarms during cycler treatment related to sluggish PD catheter outflow. However, caution should be taken to avoid too large of a residual volume so as to avoid a total IP volume that may cause clinical problems. Effective treatment of constipation should always be undertaken as a simpler means to relieve either fill or drain pain prior to considering leaving a residual volume after each exchange.

45. **What is poor or slow inflow/outflow?**
Poor or slow inflow or outflow of PD fluid is a problem that more frequently occurs during the initial break-in period of a PD catheter, but can occur at any time in the course of treatment. The most common cause is constipation, and the first step is to effectively clear the bowel of excessive stool. If this is not effective at resolving the problem, then other causes need to be investigated.

Discernment as to whether the flow problem is bidirectional or unidirectional (only poor outflow) helps determine the cause of the problem. Bidirectional flow problems usually indicate obstruction of the catheter lumen by clot, fibrin, or a kink or bend in the catheter. Conversely, unidirectional poor outflow suggests either of the following:

- Malposition of the PD catheter in a place where the PD fluid cannot be drained (i.e., migration of the catheter out of the true pelvis).
- Encumbrance of catheter drainage pores by tissue or viscera. Although the force of PD fluid inflow can more easily push bowels engorged with stool, epiploic appendices, omental wraps, or adhesions aside, the negative pressure of outflow results in collapse of these organs and tissues on the draining catheter.

Plain-film roentgenographic imaging of the abdomen provides diagnostic assistance in determining the presence of constipation or malposition or kinking of the PD catheter. Catheters can be repositioned by trocar or laparoscopy. By exclusion, outflow occlusion not related to constipation is most likely related to adhesions, omental wrapping, or epiploic appendices, and would require surgical or laparoscopic intervention and correction. Injection of catheters with sterile contrast by radiology can facilitate diagnosis. Inability to resolve these issues with the existing or new PD catheter would be an indication for transfer to HD.

The presence of fibrin or blood occluding a PD catheter at times can be signaled by the appearance of these substances in the PD catheter or effluent. Heparin should be added in a concentration of 500 to 2000 U/L to each dialysate exchange and continued for at least 24 to 48 hours after the effluent is clear.

A catheter obstructed with blood or fibrin can be treated with push–pull infusion of dialysate or sterile saline under moderate pressure with a 50-mL syringe. The procedure should be discontinued if the patient has any pain or cramping. Alternatively there are several anecdotal reports of success utilizing different regimens of tissue plasminogen activator (tPA) infused with sterile saline or sterile water into the PD catheter. No controlled studies demonstrate the safety or efficacy of this methodology, however.

46. **Why is hypokalemia common in patients with PD?**
In contrast to patients treated with intermittent HD, patients on PD generally do not have problems with hyperkalemia. This gives patients on PD therapy greater dietary choice and clinicians treating these patients greater flexibility in prescribing of medications that influence potassium balance (i.e., angiotensin-converting enzyme inhibitors, angiotensin receptor antagonists, or aldosterone antagonists) compared with treatment with HD. Conversely, when dietary intake is suboptimal, hypokalemia can develop. More than 25% of patients on PD have potassium levels <4.0 mEq/L, which may impact infectious and cardiovascular risk. Hypokalemia may be related to poor nutritional intake, transcellular shifts induced by insulin release from absorption of peritoneal glucose, or the continuous nature of the therapy (maintenance of a diffusion gradient between dialysate and plasma).

Hypokalemia should be treated with a more liberal diet for potassium or oral potassium supplements. If necessary, IP potassium can be administered under sterile conditions at a concentration up to 4 mEq/L of PD fluid. Careful monitoring of serum potassium levels is important in these situations.

47. **Why is hypoalbuminemia common in patients with PD, what are the causes, and how should it be addressed?**
Hypoalbuminemia is a frequent finding in patients treated with either peritoneal and HD and is associated with increased overall morbidity and mortality. Serum albumin levels in patients with PD are a function of synthesis, catabolism, volume of distribution, and loss, usually in urine or the peritoneal effluent. Albumin is also a negative acute phase reactant, so inflammation will decrease levels. As such, all these factors should be considered in evaluation and targeted for correction in patients with hypoalbuminemia.

PD patients typically lose about 6 to 8 g/day of albumin in the effluent, more during peritonitis episodes. This process probably contributes to generally lower serum albumin levels in PD compared to HD patients. However, for every specific level of serum albumin, the risk of all-cause and cardiovascular mortality is lower in PD patients than in patients treated with HD. This suggests that the decrease in serum albumin level related to peritoneal protein losses does not result in a higher risk of adverse events. It is also important to note that treatment with HD increases loss of amino acids compared to that seen with PD.

As changes in serum albumin over time impact mortality, therapeutic interventions to improve nutritional status should be undertaken. When nutritional intake is deemed inadequate, attempts should be made to increase intake of protein. Depression and medications should always be considered in the differential of poor dietary intake and should be addressed.

An expanded intravascular volume due to failure to achieve dry weight can cause decreased albumin levels. Therefore, in evaluating hypoalbuminemia, the clinician should look for and treat volume overload.

As albumin is a negative acute-phase reactant, patients should be evaluated for any source of inflammation and treatment should be initiated for this as appropriate.

KEY POINTS

1. Patients on peritoneal dialysis (PD) are significantly less likely to have dialysis-associated bacteremia or sepsis, a complication almost completely associated with hemodialysis. Conversely, the most serious infection and one almost exclusively occurring in patients on PD is peritonitis. Technical advances in "connectology" and infection control strategies have dramatically reduced the peritonitis infection rates.
2. The primary reason for performing gram stain and microscopy when a patient presents with signs and symptoms of peritonitis is to identify the presence of budding yeast or hyphae, indicative of fungal peritonitis. These findings should prompt immediate removal of the PD catheter.
3. When treating peritonitis, it is critical to ensure that mean inhibitory concentrations of antibiotics are achieved in the PD fluid throughout the 24-hour period to attain successful bacterial killing. This may best be achieved with continuous, rather than intermittent, antibiotic therapy, despite logistic challenges for patients receiving automated peritoneal dialysis.

BIBLIOGRAPHY

Akonur, A., Sloand, J., Davis, I., & Leypoldt, J. (2016). Icodextrin simplifies PD therapy by equalizing UF and sodium removal among patient transport types during long dwells: A modeling study. *Peritoneal Dialysis International, 36,* 79–84.

Brown, E. A., Davies, S. J., Rutherford, P., Meeus, F., Borras, M., Riegel, W., . . . EAPOS Group. (2003). Survival of functionally anuric patients on automated peritoneal dialysis: The European APD Outcome Study. *Journal of the American Society of Nephrology, 14,* 2948–2957.

Cho, Y., Johnson, D. W., Craig, J. C., Strippoli, G. F., Badve, S. V., & Wiggins, K. J. (2014). Biocompatible dialysis fluids for peritoneal dialysis. *Cochrane Database of Systematic Reviews,* (3), CD007554. doi:10.1002/14651858.CD007554.pub2.

Finkelstein, F., Healy, H., Abu-Alfa, A., Ahmad, S., Brown, F., Gehr, T., . . . Mujais, S. (2005). Superiority of icodextrin compared with 4.25% dextrose for peritoneal ultrafiltration. *Journal of the American Society of Nephrology, 16,* 546–554.

Johnson, D. W., Hawley, C. M., McDonald, S. P., Brown, F. G., Rosman, J. B., Wiggins, K. J., . . . Badve, S. V. (2010). Superior survival of high transporters treated with automated versus continuous ambulatory peritoneal dialysis. *Nephrology, Dialysis, Transplantation, 25,* 1973–1979.

Keshaviah, P. R., Nolph, K. D., & Van Stone, J. C. (1989). The peak concentration hypothesis: A urea kinetic approach to comparing the adequacy of continuous ambulatory peritoneal dialysis (CAPD) and hemodialysis. *Peritoneal Dialysis International, 9,* 257–260.

Kolesnyk, I., Dekker, F. W., Boeschoten, E. W., & Krediet, R. T. (2010). Time-dependent reasons for peritoneal dialysis technique failure and mortality. *Peritoneal Dialysis International, 30,* 170–177.

Kumar, V. A., Sidell, M. A., Jones, J. P., & Vonesh, E. F. (2014). Survival of propensity matched incident peritoneal and hemodialysis patients in a United States health care system. *Kidney International, 86,* 1016–1022.

Li, P. K., Szeto, C. C., Piraino, B., de Arteaga, J., Fan, S., Figueiredo, A. E., . . . Johnson, D. W. (2016). ISPD Peritonitis Recommendations: 2016 Update on Prevention and Treatment. *Peritoneal Dialysis International, 36*(5), 481–508.

Mehrotra, R., Duong, U., Jiwakanon, S., Kovesdy, C. P., Moran, J., Kopple, J. D., & Kalantar-Zadeh, K. (2011). Serum albumin as a predictor of mortality in peritoneal dialysis: Comparisons with hemodialysis. *American Journal of Kidney Diseases, 58,* 418–428.

Mendelssohn, D. C., Mujais, S. K., Soroka, S. D., Brouillette, J., Takano, T., Barre, P. E., . . . Finkelstein, F. O. (2009). A prospective evaluation of renal replacement therapy modality eligibility. *Nephrology, Dialysis, Transplantation, 24,* 555–561.

Neu, A. M., Richardson, T., Lawlor, J., Stuart, J., Newland, J., McAfee, N., Warady, B. A., & SCOPE Collaborative Participants. (2016). Implementation of standardized follow-up care significantly reduces peritonitis in children on chronic peritoneal dialysis. *Kidney International, 89,* 1346–1354.

Paniagua, R., Amato, D., Vonesh, E., Correa-Rotter, R., Ramos, A., Moran, J., Mujais, S.; & Mexican Nephrology Collaborative Study Group. (2002). Effects of increasing peritoneal clearances on mortality rates in peritoneal dialysis: ADEMEX, a prospective, randomized, controlled trial. *Journal of the American Society of Nephrology, 13,* 1307–1320.

Perl, J., & Bargman, J. M. (2009). The importance of residual kidney function for patients on dialysis: A critical review. *American Journal of Kidney Diseases, 53,* 1068–1081.

Piraino, B., Bernardini, J., Brown, E., Figueiredo, A., Johnson, D. W., Lye, W. C., & Szeto, C. C. (2011). ISPD position statement on reducing the risks of peritoneal dialysis-related infections. *Peritoneal Dialysis International, 31*(6), 614–630.

Torlén, K., Kalantar-Zadeh, K., Molnar, M. Z., Vashistha, T., & Mehrotra, R. (2012). Serum potassium and cause-specific mortality in a large peritoneal dialysis cohort. *Clinical Journal of the American Society of Nephrology, 7,* 1272–1284.

Twardowski, Z. J., Nolph, K. O., Khanna, R., Prowant, B. F., Ryan, L. P., Moore, H. L., & Nielsen, M. P. (1987). Peritoneal equilibration test. *Peritoneal Dialysis Bulletin, 7,* 138–147.

THERAPEUTIC PLASMA EXCHANGE (PLASMAPHERESIS)

Ernesto Sabath and Bradley M. Denker

CHAPTER 54

1. **What is the definition of plasmapheresis, and when is it indicated?**
   The term "apheresis" is Greek for "taking away" and refers to a procedure where the therapeutic removal of macromolecules from the plasma is done for therapeutic reasons. It is indicated for conditions where substances that are not removable with conventional dialysis must be removed from the blood.

2. **Describe the techniques for plasma separation during the plasmapheresis procedure.**
   The two major modalities to separate the plasma from the blood during a plasmapheresis procedure are by centrifugation and membrane filtration. The centrifugation method uses centrifugal force to separate whole blood into plasma and cellular fractions according to their density. The membrane filtration technique is based on a synthetic membrane filter composed of different pore sizes. This filter is similar to a hemodialysis filter and is composed of many hollow fiber tubes with relatively large pore sizes (0.2 to 0.6 μm in diameter) and arranged in parallel.

3. **What are the different modalities of the plasmapheresis procedure?**
   Plasma exchange involves the withdrawal of blood from the circulation and its separation into cellular and plasma fractions by centrifugal separation or perfusion of a synthetic filter. In both methods, the cellular components are returned to the patient and the plasma is removed.

   Double filtration plasmapheresis uses two filters with different pore sizes to separate toxic substances from plasma; the second filtration step is to separate useful substances that are returned to the circulation from higher-molecular-weight pathogenic substances that are removed.

   Plasma adsorption procedure involves plasma exchange followed by delivery to an adsorption column to which pathogenic substances bind and are then removed from circulation.

4. **Define the possible mechanisms of action for plasmapheresis leading to clinical improvement.**
   There are two general mechanisms that may lead to improvement: (1) removal of pathologic substances or (2) replacement of a missing or abnormal plasma component (such as A Disintegrin And Metalloproteinase with a ThromboSpondin type 1 motif (ADAMTS-13) in thrombotic thrombocytopenic purpura [TTP]). The pathologic factors that can be removed by plasmapheresis are:
   - Auto-antibodies
   - Immune complexes
   - Cryoglobulins
   - Complement products
   - Lipoproteins
   - Protein-bound toxins
     The success of plasmapheresis depends on the rate of production of the abnormal protein or antibody and the efficiency of removal with plasmapheresis. Plasmapheresis is most often utilized with other immunosuppressive strategies to decrease production and reduce inflammation. Other additional benefits may include reversal of impaired splenic function to remove immune complexes and improvement of macrophage and monocyte function.

5. **What type of venous access can be used for plasmapheresis?**
   The clinical scenario, especially the possibility for long-term venous access, and the type of plasmapheresis being used are important factors to consider when deciding on peripheral or central venous access. A peripheral vein allows a maximum flow of up to about 50 to 90 mL/min, so a single venous access is adequate for intermittent centrifugation. Continuous centrifugation techniques require two venous access sites or a central venous catheter. If long-term (>1 to 2 weeks) plasmapheresis is planned, a central venous catheter is required.

6. **Which anticoagulants can be used during the plasmapheresis procedure?**
   The most common anticoagulants used are sodium citrate, unfractionated heparin, and hirudin; nafamostat mesylate, a synthetic serine protease inhibitor, has been commonly used in Japan as an anticoagulant in hemodialysis and plasmapheresis procedures.
   There are some reports of plasmapheresis without anticoagulation as a safe and effective procedure in patients at high risk of bleeding.

7. **How much plasma should I remove, and how is the volume calculated?**
   Each plasmapheresis session should remove 1 to 1.5 times the plasma volume, and this can be calculated from the following formula:

   Estimated plasma volume (in liters) $= 0.07$ weight (in kg) $(1 -$ hematocrit [Hct])

8. **What replacement fluid should be used during the plasmapheresis procedure?**
   The choice of replacement fluids includes 5% albumin, fresh-frozen plasma (FFP), and crystalloid (e.g., 0.9% saline, Ringer's lactate) solutions. Albumin is generally combined 1:1 with 0.9% saline, and does not contain calcium, potassium, coagulation factors, or immunoglobulins. FFP contains complement and coagulation factors and is the replacement fluid of choice in patients with TTP, because the infusion of normal plasma may contribute to the replacement of the deficient plasma factor, ADAMTS-13. Plasma may also be preferable in patients at risk of bleeding, or those requiring intensive therapy, because frequent replacements with albumin solution will eventually result in postplasmapheresis coagulopathy and a net loss of immunoglobulins.

9. **What are the main complications of plasmapheresis, and how often do they occur?**
   Plasmapheresis is a relatively (but not entirely) safe procedure. Some registries reported a 4.2% incidence of adverse events, and just 1% of all apheresis procedures had to be interrupted due to an adverse event.
   The most common adverse effects reported are paresthesias (0.52%), hypotension (0.5%), urticaria (0.34%), shivering, nausea, and electrolyte disturbances such as hypocalcemia, hypo- or hypernatremia, metabolic alkalosis, hypokalemia, and rarely hypophosphatemia.
   Death is rare, occurring in less than 0.1% of all the procedures.

10. **Why does citrate cause paresthesias?**
    Paresthesias are often related to hypocalcemia caused by the citrate infusion as anticoagulant for the extracorporeal system or in the FFP administered as a replacement fluid. Citrate binds to free calcium to form soluble calcium citrate, thereby lowering the free but not the total serum calcium concentration.

11. **What are the main clinical indications of plasmapheresis for kidney diseases?**
    Table 54.1 summarizes the most important clinical indications for kidney diseases by category.

Table 54.1. Clinical Indications for Kidney Diseases by Category

DISEASE	CATEGORY
Anti-GBM disease	I
TTP	I
Rapidly progressive glomerulonephritis	II
Cryoglobulinemia	II
Desensitization for kidney transplantation	II
Hemolytic uremic syndrome	III
Recurrent FSGS	III
Systemic lupus erythematosus	III
Kidney transplant rejection	IV

FSGS, Focal and segmentary glomerulosclerosis; *TTP*, thrombotic thrombocytopenia purpura. *Category I*, Standard Primary Therapy; *Category II*, Supportive Therapy; *Category III*, When the evidence of benefit is unclear; *Category IV*, When there is no current evidence of benefit or for research protocols.

12. What is the role of plasmapheresis in anti-glomerular basement membrane (GBM) disease?
   In anti-GBM disease, the role of plasmapheresis is the rapid removal of the pathogenic antibodies. Plasmapheresis in combination with cyclophosphamide (blocks additional antibody production) and corticosteroids (reduces inflammation) may prevent kidney failure. All patients with anti-GBM antibody disease and severe kidney failure who do not require immediate dialysis should be treated with aggressive immunosuppression and intensive plasmapheresis. Plasmapheresis should be initiated in patients with pulmonary hemorrhage regardless of the severity of the kidney failure. However, patients presenting with dialysis dependence only had 8% kidney survival, and if the kidney biopsy showed crescentic lesions in all glomeruli, kidney survival was 0%. Plasmapheresis is usually done for 14 days or until the anti-GBM antibody is no longer detectable.

13. What is the evidence for the use of plasmapheresis in antineutrophil cytoplasmic autoantibody (ANCA)–associated vasculitis?
   There is a beneficial role for plasmapheresis in patients with severe kidney involvement (creatinine >500 μmol/L or 5.7 mg/dL) and ANCA-associated vasculitis. In contrast to anti-GBM disease, the addition of plasmapheresis to treatments including cyclophosphamide, azathioprine, and steroids was associated with better kidney survival. In patients with both ANCA and anti-GBM associated disease, as well as in any patient with diffuse pulmonary alveolar hemorrhage, plasmapheresis is beneficial for recovery and reducing the risk of progression to dialysis. The use of plasmapheresis for less severe kidney disease remains unresolved, but the PEXIVAS (Plasma Exchange and Glucocorticoid Dosing in the Treatment of ANCA Vasculitis) study is currently under way, with the aim to detect the efficacy of plasma exchange (PE) in this population.

14. Is there any evidence for a role of plasmapheresis in lupus nephritis?
   The current literature does not support a benefit for the addition of plasmapheresis to immunosuppressive therapy for lupus nephritis. However, there are refractory individual patients for whom there is anecdotal evidence that it may provide some benefit.
   One retrospective study suggested that plasmapheresis might be effective in improving the recovery and kidney outcomes in patients with lupus nephritis plus thrombotic microangiopathy.

15. Is plasmapheresis indicated as treatment in patients with multiple myeloma and cast nephropathy?
   The role of plasmapheresis in myeloma cast nephropathy is debated. Although early studies demonstrated improvement in kidney function and patient survival, the largest study to date of 104 patients with multiple myeloma and acute kidney failure randomly assigned to conventional therapy plus plasma exchanges or conventional therapy alone did not show differences in the composite outcome of death, dialysis dependence, or severely reduced kidney function. The findings of this study do not support the routine use of plasmapheresis in myeloma patients, but it can be considered in patients with unusually high paraprotein burdens or Waldenstrom macroglobulinemia and hyperviscosity syndromes.

16. What is the efficacy of plasma exchange in the treatment of TTP?
   Plasmapheresis may replenish the levels of ADAMTS-13 protease that is deficient in some cases of TTP. Duration of daily therapeutic plasma exchange (TPE) to achieve a durable remission (e.g., platelet count >150,000 for 3 days and lactate dehydrogenase (LDH) near normal and no neurologic deficit, if initially present) is variable. There is no evidence for a beneficial role of plasmapheresis in patients with TTP secondary to cancer, chemotherapy, or bone marrow transplantation.

17. Can plasmapheresis be used to remove toxic substances?
   Plasmapheresis can be considered for the removal of protein-bound toxins that are not readily removed with dialysis or hemoperfusion. Plasmapheresis is effective in removing highly protein-bound toxins from the blood but not from other fluid compartments. Reports of the successful use of plasmapheresis in the treatment of various drug overdoses and poisonings are generally anecdotal. Amanita poisoning (mushrooms) is the most frequent clinical diagnosis where plasmapheresis has been utilized with success, perhaps showing decreased mortality, especially in children.

18. Is there any indication for plasmapheresis in the treatment of dyslipidemia?
   Low density lipoprotein (LDL) apheresis should be the treatment of choice for patients that are homozygotic for familial hypercholesterolemia (FH). Therapy is initiated from age 7 unless their serum cholesterol can be reduced by more than 50% (or decreased to <9 mmol/L, 350 mg/dL) by drug therapy. It is also indicated in individual patients with either heterozygous FH or a family history of premature cardiac death, progressive coronary disease, and where LDL cholesterol remains higher than 5.0 mmol/L (193 mg/dL) or is decreased by less than 40% with maximal drug therapy.

19. **Is there a role for plasmapheresis in recurrent focal and segmentary glomerulosclerosis (FSGS)?**
    Yes, the mechanisms of recurrent FSGS and early detection of proteinuria after kidney transplantation are unclear, but the early reappearance of proteinuria suggests that a nondialyzable circulating factor that alters glomerular permeability may be present. Removal of a circulating factor by immunoadsorption or plasma exchange may account for the remission of the disease in some patients.

20. **Describe the role of plasmapheresis in kidney transplantation.**
    In addition to reducing the risk of recurrent FSGS in some patients, plasmapheresis is now utilized for ABO blood group incompatible transplants, positive T cell cross-match, and acute humoral rejection.

21. **What are some indications for plasmapheresis in nonkidney diseases that are supported by clinical trials (category I)?**
    - Guillain-Barré syndrome
    - Myasthenia gravis
    - Chronic inflammatory demyelinating polyneuropathy
    - Hyperviscosity in monoclonal gammopathies (Waldeström macroglobulinemia)
    - Cutaneous T cell lymphoma (photopheresis)

22. **Is there any indication for plasmapheresis in pregnancy?**
    Plasmapheresis can be safely performed during pregnancy, and introduction of plasmapheresis for specific indications has improved maternal and fetal survival rates. Plasmapheresis has been safely carried out in myasthenic crisis, Guillain-Barré syndrome, anti-GBM disease, acute fatty liver of pregnancy, and TTP. There is no indication in cardiac neonatal lupus, despite its theoretical benefits.

    Some complications of plasmapheresis are premature delivery due to the removal of essential hormones maintaining pregnancy, hypovolemic reaction, allergy, transitory cardiac arrhythmias, and nausea. During the exchanges, blood pressure must be carefully monitored to avoid hypotension, and after the second trimester, it is preferable to place the patient on her left side to avoid compression of the inferior vena cava by the gravid uterus.

KEY POINTS

1. Plasmapheresis can be effective in removing large toxins and pathogenic antibodies when combined with immunosuppression.
2. Plasmapheresis is the treatment of choice in patients with TTP, anti-GBM disease (without advanced kidney failure), and hemoptysis from ANCA or anti-GBM disease.
3. Plasmapheresis may be beneficial in ANCA disease *with* advanced kidney failure.
4. There is no current indication for plasmapheresis in patients with lupus nephritis.
5. Indications for plasmapheresis in kidney transplant are ABO-incompatible kidney transplantation, recurrent FSGS, and acute humoral rejection.

BIBLIOGRAPHY
Clark, W. F., Huang, S. S., Walsh, M. W., Farah, M., Hildebrand, A. M., & Sontrop, J. M. (2016). Plasmapheresis for the treatment of kidney diseases. *Kidney International, 90*(5), 974–984.

Clark, W. F., Stewart, A. K., Rock, G. A., Sternbach, M., Sutton, D. M., Barrett, B. J., . . . Churchill, D. N. (2005). Plasma exchange when myeloma presents as acute renal failure: A randomized, controlled trial. *Annals of Internal Medicine, 143*, 777–784.

Jayne, D. R., Gaskin, G., Rasmussen, N., Abramowicz, D., Ferrario, F., Guillevin, L., . . . Pusey, C. D. (2007). Randomized trial of plasma exchange or high dosage methylprednisolone as adjunctive therapy for severe renal vasculitis. *Journal of the American Society of Nephrology, 18*, 2180–2188.

Kashgary, A., Sontrop, J. M., Li, L., Al-Jaishi, A. A., Habibullah, Z. N., Alsolaimani, R., & Clark, W. F. (2016). The role of plasma exchange in treating post-transplant focal segmental glomerulosclerosis: A systematic review and meta-analysis of 77 case-reports and case-series. *BMC Nephrology, 17*, 104.

Levy, J. B., Turner, A. N., Rees, A. J., & Pusey, C. D. (2001). Long-term outcome of anti-glomerular basement membrane antibody disease treated with plasma exchange and immunosuppression. *Annals of Internal Medicine, 134*, 1033–1042.

Madore, F. (2002). Plasmapheresis: Technical aspects and indications. *Critical Care Clinics, 18*, 375–392.

Montgomery, R. A., Locke, J. E., King, K. E., Segev, D. L., Warren, D. S., Kraus, E. S., . . . Haas, M. (2009). ABO Incompatible renal transplantation: A paradigm ready for broad implementation. *Transplantation, 87*, 1246–1255.

Reeves, H. M., & Winters, J. L. (2014). The mechanisms of action of plasma exchange. *British Journal of Haematology, 164*, 342–351.

Sarode, R., Bandarenko, N., Brecher, M. E., Kiss, J. E., Marques, M. B., Szczepiorkowski, Z. M., & Winters, J. L. (2014). Thrombotic thrombocytopenic purpura: 2012 American Society for Apheresis (ASFA) consensus conference on classification, diagnosis, management, and future research. *Journal of Clinical Apheresis, 29*, 148–167.

Schwartz, J., et al. (2016). Guidelines on the use of therapeutic apheresis in clinical practice—evidence-based approach from the Writing Committee of the American Society for Apheresis: The seventh special issue. *J Clin Apher. 31*, 149–162.

Walsh, M., Casian, A., Flossmann, O., Westman, K., Höglund, P., Pusey, C., Jayne, D. R., for the European Vasculitis Study Group. (2013). Long-term follow-up of patients with severe ANCA associated vasculitis comparing plasma exchange to intravenous methylprednisolone treatment is unclear. *Kidney International, 84*, 397–402.

XI
TRANSPLANTATION

EPIDEMIOLOGY AND OUTCOMES

Beje Thomas and Matthew R. Weir

CHAPTER 55

1. **What is United Network of Organ Sharing (UNOS)?**
   UNOS is the nonprofit, scientific and educational organization that administrates over the United States national organ registry known as the Organ Procurement and Transplantation Network (OPTN). UNOS originated as an initiative of The South-Eastern Organ Procurement Foundation (SEOPF) in 1977. SEOPF was the first organization to develop a computerized system that used medical information to match potential organ donors and recipients. SEOPF started the Kidney Center in 1982, which evolved into UNOS. The National Organ Transplant Act was passed in 1984 by the US Congress and established the OPTN. UNOS was appointed administrator for OPTN and continues in this role today. UNOS is involved in multiple aspects of organ transplantation and donation, including managing the wait list, matching donors and recipients, maintaining the US national organ transplant database, policy development, ensuring adherence to organ allocation policies, and providing organ transplantation education for the general public and medical professionals. The Scientific Registry of Transplant Recipients (SRTR) does an annual data collection for kidney transplants across the United States, which is available online at www.ustransplant.org.

2. **What is involved in kidney allocation?**
   The process of allocating a kidney to a recipient is an intricate process. The procuring organization accesses the national transplant computer database, UNet^{sm}, through the Internet or contacts UNOS directly. In either situation, information about the kidney donor is entered into UNet^{sm} and a donor/recipient match is determined for each donated kidney.
   All transplant candidates incompatible with the donor for medical factors such as blood type are eliminated from the match list. The match list of potential recipients is then ranked according to objective medical criteria (body habitus, blood type, tissue type, size of the organ, medical urgency of the recipient, time accrued on the waiting list, and distance between donor and recipient). Survival benefit was added as an additional factor in 2015 (see Question 3).
   Using the match of potential recipients, the local organ procurement coordinator or an organ placement specialist contacts the transplant center of the highest-ranked patient and offers the organ to that center. If the kidney is rejected, the next potential recipient's transplant center is contacted. Calls are made to multiple recipients' transplant centers in succession to expedite the organ placement process until the kidney is placed. Once the kidney is accepted for a patient, transportation arrangements are made and the transplant surgery team is notified.

3. **What important factors are weighed in the new kidney allocation score?**
   There were significant changes made to the allocation system in December of 2014.
   - **Estimated Post Transplant Survival Score (EPTS):** This is an estimate of patient longevity. The score is 0% to 100%, with higher scores associated with poorer survival. It is calculated using the patient's age, dialysis time, diagnosis of diabetes, and history of prior transplant. It is not used in pediatric patients. The EPTS score is divided into large two groups, 0% to 20% and those over 20%. Previous organ transplant or long dialysis vintage increase EPTS scores. An individual with an EPTS score of 0% to 20% will be prioritized over candidates with higher scores, but only for the highest-longevity kidneys, which are those kidneys with a Kidney Donor Profile Index (KDPI) of less than or equal to 20%. Patients with an EPTS of 0% to 20% will receive priority for zero mismatches, local offers, as well as regional and national offers. The EPTS score is recalculated regularly.
   - **KDPI:** The KDPI quantifies the health of a donated kidney. It is calculated based on:
     - Age
     - Height
     - Weight
     - Ethnicity
     - History of hypertension or diabetes
     - Cause of death

- Terminal creatinine
- Hepatitis C status
- Whether the donated organ was after circulatory death
- KDPI replaced the terms Standard Criteria Donor (SCD) kidney and Expanded Criteria Donor (ECD) kidney to better estimate kidney longevity. Therefore a kidney with a KDPI <20% based on the calculated factors should survive longer than 80% of the previous years' harvested kidneys. On average, a kidney with a KDPI of <20% for the last 11.5 years, a kidney with a KDPI of 20% to 85% over the last 9 years, and a kidney with a KDPI >85% is expected to function for over 5.5 years. A patient who previously would only accept an SCD kidney would default to accepting a kidney with a KDPI of <85%. If the patient is consented to an ECD kidney, the KDPI of the kidney can be over 85%. Only individuals with an EPTS score <20% have access to a kidney with a KDPI <20%. This is for longevity matching so patients with longer expected survival time receive kidneys with the longest expected survival time.
- **Time on the Wait List:** Patient with longer wait time has priority. Another change to the allocation system made in 2014 was to credit time on dialysis prior to listing. So a patient who has been on dialysis for 2 years prior to getting on the transplant list will start with 2 years of wait time.
- **Age:** In the new allocation policy, pediatric patients will receive priority over adult patients for donors with a KDPI score <35%, regardless of donor age. This is a change from the previous policy where the organ priority for pediatric patients was based on age of the donor (<35 years of age) as opposed to the KDPI score. Age is a factor in calculating KDPI and EPTS.
- **Medical urgency:** Only considered in local kidney allocation
- **Human leukocyte antigen mismatch:** Priority to zero antigen mismatch
- **Degree of panel reactivity antibody (PRA):** In the old system, patients with a calculated PRA (cPRA) >80% received 4 points and those below this cutoff received 0 points. The more of these points a patient accumulates, the more priority they receive for transplant. This puts the patient who has some degree of sensitization at a disadvantage. In other words, though it is more difficult to find an organ for a patient with a cPRA of 70% versus one with a cPRA of 20%, in the old system they were treated the same. In the new allocation system, to help rectify this, the points are assigned when the cPRA is ≥20% according to a sliding scale. The greater the cPRA, the more points awarded, so those with the highest cPRA >98% receive the most points. However, patients with a smaller degree of sensitization do also receive some benefit as compared to before.
- **Blood type:** Patients with blood type B have longer wait times generally than the other blood types. Blood type B is more common in blacks. In the old allocation system, a patient with blood type B could only receive a kidney from a donor that was blood type O or B. In the new allocation system, they can receive an organ from a donor with blood types O, B, A2, or A2B. The patient must have a low anti-A IgG titer prior to transplant if they are to be a candidate for an A2 or A2B kidney (also see Question 8, Chapter 56).

4. What are the most recent trends in kidney transplant survival?
   - The 2015 OPTN/SRTR report showed that though living donor transplants had better survival than deceased donor transplants, both have continued improvement in their 1, 3, 5, and 10 years death-censored graft survival regardless of donation type.
   - The three groups among deceased donor kidney transplants with the lowest 5-year graft survival were those with primary kidney failure from diabetes (70.4%) or hypertension (71.8%), and in patients who received an organ with a KDPI >85% (57.6%, KDPI >85%; 73.3%, KDPI 35% to 85%).
   - There was no significant difference in the 5-year graft survival between kidneys donated after brain death or cardiac death.
   - Living donor transplant recipients >65 years of age at the time of transplant had the lowest 5-year graft survival compared to other age groups.

5. What donor type confers the best outcomes in regard to kidney recipient survival?
   Living donor kidney transplants have the best recipient survival. Among deceased donor kidneys, those with a lower KDPI have better outcomes.

6. What donor type confers the best outcomes in regard to kidney graft survival?
   Living donor kidney transplants have the best allograft survival, followed by deceased donor kidney transplants. Among deceased donor kidney transplants, those organs from a donor with a lower KDPI have greater longevity. To reiterate, it is estimated that a kidney with a KDPI of <20% will last 11.5 years, a kidney with a KDPI of 20% to 85% will last 9 years, and a kidney with a KDPI >85% will last 5.5 years.

7. What is the most recent number of transplants separated by type of transplant?
   In total, 17,611 kidney transplants were done in 2015; this includes adult, pediatric, and combined organ transplantation. Of those, 12,280 transplants were from a deceased donor and 5331 transplants were from a living donor.

8. What are the recent trends affecting the wait list?
   For the first time in 10 years, the overall wait list decreased from 99,120 at the beginning of 2015 to 97,680 at the end of the year. This is due to:
   1. Less inactive patients on the list
   2. Increased transplant rate with the new allocation system
   3. Removal of those medically ineligible
   4. A decrease in number of new listings
       There is no advantage in the new system for listing inactive patients. The number of active patients increased from 47,000 patients in 2005 to 61,000 patients in 2015. In 2015, 31,672 patients were removed from the kidney wait list. Out of those removed from the wait list, 17,611 patients underwent kidney transplantation and about 5000 patients died. In the last 5 years, there has been almost a 3-fold increase in the number of patients removed from the wait list for medical reasons, from 1533 patients in 2010 to 4154 patients in 2015.

9. Has the age of patients on the waiting list changed over the last few years?
   Yes. Patients older than 65 years of age grew from 14.5% of the list in 2005 to 22% in 2015. If this pace continues, patients over 65 years of age will outnumber patients 25 to 49 years of age in about 2020. Patients over 65 now are less willing to accept a kidney with a KDPI score >85%. However, the number of patients being transplanted in this age group has decreased from previous years. This was a concern of the new allocation system; it is also likely secondary to a decreased willingness to accept a kidney with a higher KDPI score.

10. What is the distribution of race among individuals in transplantation?
    The majority of patients that are transplanted from the wait list are Caucasian. This number has been relatively stable since 2008 at 8500 to 8800 transplants per year. The number of blacks being transplanted has grown in the same time period from about 4000 transplants in 2008 to 5136 transplants in 2016. The other group that has seen a significant growth is Hispanic patients—in 2008 there were 2449 transplants versus 3496 patients in 2016. The majority of living donors are Caucasian. The number of black donors has declined by 4% over the last 10 years.

11. What is the most common cause of kidney disease in patients on the wait list?
    Diabetes and hypertension are the most common causes of chronic kidney disease in the general population, so it is not surprising that the both are the main causes of kidney disease of those on the wait list. Glomerular disease as the cause of kidney disease in patients on the wait list has declined over the last decade.

12. What is the definition of an inactive patient on the wait list?
    An inactive patient is defined as a transplant candidate who is considered temporarily unsuitable for kidney transplantation. These patients usually have a medical condition that temporarily makes them unable to receive a kidney transplant. Patients still accrue waiting time. Once the condition is resolved, the patient is reinstated to the active wait list and is eligible for kidney transplant allocation.
       The most common reason for being inactive at time of listing is incomplete medical workup. The changes to the allocation system in 2014 allow for dialysis patients to complete their workup and still receive credit for their time on dialysis (see Question 2, Time on Wait List). This does not help the predialysis patient, so their workup should be completed as quickly as possible.

13. Does a candidate's blood type affect their time on the waiting list?
    Yes.
    • AB: wait time 2 years
    • A: wait time 3 years
    • O: wait time 5 years
    • B: wait time 6 years

14. What is the median time to transplantation for individuals on the waitlist?
    As of 2015, the median wait time for a kidney transplant was 3.6 years.

15. Is the access to kidney transplantation equitable among all persons?

Equal access to kidney transplantation for all who could benefit is a major problem. Disparities exist in patient education, geography, race, and level of pretransplantation nephrology care. UNOS is attempting to make the process of organ accessibility and allocation equitable among all different patient populations.

16. What are the two major causes of long-term kidney allograft failure?

The major causes of long-term kidney allograft failure are chronic rejection and death with a functioning kidney.

17. What are the most common causes of death after kidney transplantation?

The most common cause of death in kidney transplantation is cardiovascular disease, followed by infectious disease and malignancy.

KEY POINTS

1. The UNOS administrates the national transplant registry, the OPTN. They are responsible for equitability in accessibility and adherence to national guidelines for transplantation. Improvements in allograft survival over the past decade have been attributed to a reduction in acute/chronic rejection episodes, shortened cold-ischemia times, and lower plasma reactive antibody levels among recipients.
2. Kidney Donor Exchange is a growing venue to add the availability of organs to potential transplant candidates.

BIBLIOGRAPHY

Hart, A., Smith, J. M., Skeans, M. A., Gustafson, S. K., Stewart, D. E., Cherikh, W. S., . . . Israni, A. K. (2017). OPTN/SRTR 2015 Annual Data Report: Kidney. *American Journal of Transplantation, 17*(Suppl. 1), 21–116. doi:10.1111/ajt.14124.

Organ Procurement and Transplant Network. http://optn.transplant.hrsa.gov.

Sood, A., Abdullah, N. M., Abdollah, F., Abouljoud, M. S., Trinh, Q. D., Menon, M., & Sammon, J. D. (2015). Rates of kidney transplantation from living and deceased donors for blacks and whites in the United States, 1998 to 2011. *JAMA Internal Medicine, 175*(10), 1716–1718. doi:10.1001/jamainternmed.2015.4530.

United Network of Organ Sharing. https://www.unos.org/.

United States Renal Data System. (2016). *2016 USRDS annual data report: Epidemiology of kidney disease in the United States.* Bethesda, MD: National Institutes of Health, National Institute of Diabetes and Digestive and Kidney Diseases.

CHAPTER 56

DONOR AND RECIPIENT EVALUATION

Beje Thomas and Matthew R. Weir

1. **What are the various categories of living-donor transplants?**
   - **Related donors:** Donor and recipient are biologically related.
   - **Unrelated donors:** Donor is not biologically related, but an emotional relationship exists between the donor and recipient (e.g., coworker, classmate, friend).
   - **Directed anonymous donors:** Donor has no relationship to the recipient; the donor learned of the recipient's situation and decided to donate altruistically.
   - **Undirected anonymous donors:** Donor decides to donate his or her kidney to the waiting list.
   - **Paired exchange donors:** A pair of donor–recipient candidates (from the related or unrelated categories) enters into a scheme in which the donor is exchanged with another donor–recipient candidate pair so as to achieve donor–recipient biologic compatibility of the ABO blood group system and/or negative cross-match reactivity.
   - **Multiple paired exchange donors:** A paired exchange donation that involves more than two donor–recipient candidate pairs.

2. **What is the present system that classifies donors into different categories?**
   The Kidney Donor Profile Index is now used to divide up the donor pool. This replaced the old terms Standard and Extended Criteria Donor kidneys.

3. **What percentage of living donor kidneys survive for 10 years?**
   About 60%.

4. **Discuss Transplant Tourism and the Declaration of Istanbul.**
   Transplant Tourism involves organ trafficking and/or transplant commercialism if the resources used for patients from outside a particular country harms the ability of that country to provide transplant services to the native population. Organ trafficking involves living and deceased donors that are coerced, pressured, or in some fashion influenced to donate. The Declaration of Istanbul published in 2008 emphasized that transplant tourism should be prohibited due to ethical considerations and to protect potential donors. There are exceptions; for example, if a donor and recipient are genetically related, they should be allowed to undergo the transplant in a country of their choice. Transplant tourism is legal in China and in Iran. China has a history of procuring organs from executed prisoners, which has been seen as a violation of the Declaration of Istanbul. In Iran, kidney sales are regulated.

5. **What are some contraindications for living kidney donation?**
   The contraindications listed with an asterisk can have further work up, including a kidney biopsy, to determine the candidacy of a potential donor. Other possible contraindications are acceptable depending on the transplant center. For instance, certain centers will accept a Caucasian donor with hypertension if they are over 60 years of age with well-controlled blood pressure on one medication.
   - Chronic kidney disease (glomerular filtration rate <80 mL/min per 1.73 m^2)
   - Proteinuria*
   - Hematuria*
   - Active infection
   - Chronic, active viral infections (e.g., HIV, hepatitis B/C)
   - Active malignancy
   - Family history of renal cell carcinoma
   - Hypertension*
   - Diabetes
   - Urologic abnormalities, including nephrolithiasis*
   - Active substance abuse
   - Obesity (body mass index >35 kg/m^2)*
   - Age younger than 18 years

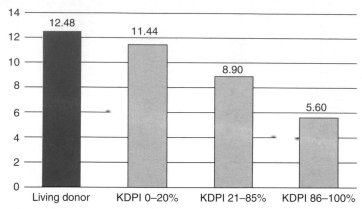

Deceased donor kidney with a Kidney Donor Profile Index (KDPI) of 0% to 20% is expected to function about 11.5 years, compared to over 12 years for a living donor kidney. Deceased donor kidneys with a KDPI from 21% to 85% are expected to function about 9 years and those kidneys with a KDPI exceeding 85% are expected to function for at least 5.5 years.

6. How is a living kidney donor evaluated to be compatible for a specific recipient? If not compatible, what options are available?

The evaluation of a potential living kidney generally begins with an assessment of the donor and recipient blood groups and a cross-match.

- The donor and recipient generally must be ABO compatible. This can occur under one of the following circumstances: the donor and recipient are ABO identical, the donor has blood type O (universal donor), or the recipient is blood type AB (universal recipient). Given the distribution of blood group antigens in the United States, the waiting time on the deceased donor list is prolonged for patients with blood group O and B. A recipient with blood type B and a low anti-A Ag IgG titer can potentially receive a transplant from a donor with blood type A2B or A2 (see Question 8).
- When a potential donor is identified, a cross-match is performed prior to transplantation to evaluate for any evidence of preformed antibodies against the specific donor (human leukocyte antigens [HLA]) that could result in hyperacute and/or acute humoral rejection. A final cross-match using fresh serum is performed in all cases immediately preceding transplantation to ensure compatibility between the donor and recipient. The methods available for cross-match testing include: enzyme-linked immunosorbent assay, flow cytometry, complement-dependent cytotoxicity, and single antigen bead assay. Transplantation has been done with low-level pre-existing donor specific antibody (DSA); however, graft function tends to worsen quicker than in those without pre-existing DSA.
- If the donor is incompatible with the recipient, then Kidney Paired Donor Exchange is the most common solution today; we will discuss this further in the next question. ABO-incompatible or cross-match positive transplantations following desensitization strategies have been performed successfully at some institutions.

7. What is Kidney Paired Donor Exchange?

Barriers against living kidney donation include ABO blood group incompatibility and existence of preexisting HLA antibodies between potential donor-recipient pairs. In a Kidney Paired Donor Exchange (KPDE) program, a medically approved incompatible pair is able to receive and exchange with other incompatible pair(s). This results in compatible organs for all recipients. The first KPDE was established in the United States in 2000. There were a total of 552 kidneys transplanted in 2014 with the KPDE program, amounting to about 10% of all living donor transplants that year.

The five different types of exchange include:

1. Two-way is between two incompatible pairs with the procurement operations occurring simultaneously so that neither donor could back out.
2. k-Way (k is the number of pairs) is exchanges between more than two pairs using the same concept of the two-way exchange. Reciprocally matching donors are not required. For example, Pairs A, B, and C, Pair A donor is compatible with Pair B recipient, but Pair B donor is not a match for the Pair A recipient. However, Pair C donor is a match for Pair A recipient and Pair C recipient is

a match for Pair B donor. Now all three recipients receive a transplant from a compatible donor. Due to logistical reasons of the donors required to be in the operating room at the same time, the number in this exchange is usually limited to 3 to 4 pairs.

3. Unspecified donor chain starts with an unspecified donor (altruistic donor), who, instead of, as previously, donating to the deceased donor list, would now donate to an incompatible pair. The donor in this incompatible pair would donate to another incompatible pair and this pattern would continue, forming a chain. The last donor in the chain would donate to the deceased donor list, ending the chain. This modality of donor exchange is called the domino-paired donation (DPD). Since it is possible to arrange these chains so that no donor-recipient pair had to donate a kidney before receiving a kidney, the requirement for all donors to be in the operating room simultaneously was relaxed. This allowed for the development of the non-simultaneous extended altruistic donor chains. The last donor in a DPD would become a "bridge" donor, which meant instead of donating to the deceased donor list, the donor would donate to another incompatible pair at a later time, thus extending the chain.

4. List exchange is when a donor in an incompatible pair donates to the deceased donor list and their recipient is now given priority for a deceased donor organ transplant.

5. Altruistically unbalanced exchange is between a compatible pair and another incompatible pair. It allows an incompatible pair to find a donor and affords the opportunity for the compatible pair to receive a kidney of higher quality.

8. Explain why organs from an individual with blood type A2 or A2B can be transplanted into a blood type B recipient?

A2 kidneys and A2B kidneys express little A antigen on their surface. If the potential candidate has a low anti-A Ag IgG titer (<4), they are able to receive an A2 or A2B kidney transplant. If the titer is high, then the candidate can only be eligible for a kidney from a donor with a B blood type. This allows for greater access to deceased donor kidneys for those with blood type B. This strategy is not limited to deceased donor kidney transplantation, but can also be used in living donor kidney transplantation.

9. Why are kidney imaging tests performed in living kidney donors prior to transplantation?
   - To ensure the presence of two kidneys
   - To exclude malignancy involving the urinary tract
   - To exclude anatomic abnormalities of the urinary tract
   - To assess the vascular supply to the donor kidney

10. What are some common imaging tests performed to evaluate the donor kidney?
    - Helical computed tomography (CT)
    - CT angiogram
    - Magnetic resonance angiogram

11. What are the short- and long-term outcomes for living kidney donors, including surgical risk?
    A major concern for living donors is the long-term impact of having a solitary kidney, with risk for developing hypertension, proteinuria, and chronic kidney disease. Most of the available data suggests that the risks of living donor donation is low enough to justify such donation. However, this data is limited by several factors including short observation times, lack of racial diversity, insufficient power, and donors lost to follow-up. The operative risk is very low, with studies showing a 90-day mortality rate of 0.03%. Blood transfusions, vascular complications, and returning to the operating room occurred in $<0.5\%$ of cases. The most common complication seen in the immediate postoperative time period is gastrointestinal—specifically, increased reflux, bowel injury, and abdominal hernias.

    The most important risk factor for long-term poor donor outcomes, including the development of diabetes, hypertension, and worsening kidney function, is the development of obesity post-donation. Long-term risks include cardiovascular and kidney complications. Most studies have shown that kidney donation does not portend a greater cardiovascular risk. The average loss of kidney function after donation is about 30%. The risk of hypertension is elevated in donors compared to non-donors by as much as 5% to 20%. Donors who are black, obese, or have high blood pressure are most at risk for progressive CKD after donating a kidney.

    End-stage kidney disease (ESKD) risk in living kidney donors is less than the general population. Donors should be informed that, while there is an increased relative risk of ESKD after kidney donation, the absolute lifetime risk for ESKD in a donor is 0.9% as compared to the 3.2% lifetime risk for the general population.

12. Does living donation increase risk of gestational hypertension and pre-eclampsia?
Yes. Garg et al. compared 131 donor pregnancies with 788 non-donor pregnancies and showed that though the absolute risk of gestational hypertension and pre-eclampsia remains small overall, it is about two times greater than in non-donor pregnancies. In non-donors, 2% developed gestational hypertension versus 5% of donors; 3% of non-donors developed pre-eclampsia versus 6% in the donor group.

13. Are there tools to predict ESKD risk for a living donor candidate?
Yes. Grams et al. used a meta-analysis of seven general non-donor populations and calibrated the population level incidence of ESKD and mortality. This was compared to 15-year projections with the observed risk among 52,998 living donors.
In a 40-year-old non-donor with health characteristics that were similar to those of age-matched kidney donors, the 15-year projections of the risk of ESKD varied according to race and sex; the risk was 0.24% among black men, 0.15% among black women, 0.06% among white men, and 0.04% among white women. Important risk factors influencing the development of ESKD over time included a lower estimated glomerular filtration rate at time of donation, higher albuminuria, hypertension, current or former smoking, diabetes, and obesity. In the model-based lifetime projections, the risk of ESKD was highest among persons in the youngest age group, particularly among young blacks. The 15-year observed risks of ESKD after donation among kidney donors in the United States were 3.5 to 5.3 times as high as the projected risks in the absence of donation.
The ESKD Risk Tool for Kidney Donor Candidates Calculator can be found at *http://www.transplantmodels.com/*

14. What is the potential use of Apolipoprotein L1 (APOL 1) gene variant testing in African American (AA) donors?
APOL1 is located on chromosome 22 and is associated with non-diabetic CKD in AAs. There are two kidney risk variants of APOL1 associated with CKD: 40% of AAs have one variant and 13% have two variants. Those with one variant have a 1.3-fold higher risk and those with two variants have a 7.3-fold higher risk of CKD. The role of APOL1 in evaluating kidney donors is not settled, but given the emerging data, it may be prudent to advise potential donors with APOL1 risk variants to avoid living donation.

15. At what level of kidney dysfunction is it appropriate to refer a patient for kidney transplant evaluation?
If a medically acceptable living donor has been identified, elective kidney transplantation ideally is performed just before dialysis is required ("preemptive"). If a living donor is not available, patients can be evaluated for transplantation at any time, but cannot officially be listed for transplantation until their glomerular filtration rate falls below 20 mL/min.

16. What are some general contraindications for kidney transplantation from a recipient perspective?
- Presence of vascular disease that precludes the arterial and venous anastomoses requisite for a technically successful transplant
- Recent or current malignancy (Box 56.1)
- Chronic illness with short life expectancy
- Active substance abuse
- Active infectious process
- Poor cardiac and pulmonary status
- Psychosocial factors that may hinder future medicine adherence

Box 56.1. Guidelines for Transplantation in Patients With Previous Malignancies

Generally: Advised waiting time is 2 years
No waiting time necessary:
  Incidental renal carcinoma
  In situ carcinoma
  Focal neoplasm (defined as a localized tumor without metastases)
  Low-grade bladder cancer
  Basal cell skin cancer

Waiting time of more than 2 years necessary:
  Melanoma
  Breast carcinoma
  Colorectal carcinoma
  Uterine carcinoma

Data from Penn, I. (1993). The effect of immunosuppression on pre-existing cancers. *Transplantation, 55,* 742–747.

17. What is the recurrence of primary glomerulonephritis and the graft survival if a recurrence occurs at 5 years?
    - Focal segmental glomerulosclerosis recurrence rate of 35% with a 5-year graft survival of 73%
    - Membranous nephropathy recurrence rate of 55% with a 5-year graft survival of 80%
    - Membrano-proliferative glomerulonephritis recurrence rate of 40% with a 5-year graft survival of 54%
    - IgA nephropathy recurrence rate of 51% with a 5-year graft survival of 81%

18. What is a "sensitized" potential recipient?
    A "sensitized" potential recipient is an individual who has detectable preformed HLA antibodies that pose considerable future risk to the allograft survival. Patient sensitization is classically reported as the percent panel reactivity antibody (PRA). PRA is defined as the percentage of donors expected to react with a patient's serum based on known antibody. Highly "sensitized" patients often cross-match positive to multiple potential donors and require a zero antigen mismatch allograft to increase success. Consequently, these "sensitized" patients are less likely to be transplanted or will spend an extended time on the waitlist pending the availability of a suitable donor. The new allocation system, however, does give "points" for these individuals to increase their transplant rate.

19. What are some ways that potential recipients become sensitized?
    - Pregnancy
    - Exposure to antigens from previous transplants
    - Exposure to antigens from blood product exposure (e.g., transfusions)
        Of note, it has not been shown that removal of leukocytes via leukodepletion ("washing" packed red blood cell units) reduces the risk of sensitization or development of HLA antibodies. The erythrocytes actually carry HLA Class I molecules and are in large enough quantity in a unit of packed red blood cells that they can stimulate a HLA Class I sensitization. Despite this evidence, leukodepletion occurs in almost 100% of centers in Europe and 75% of centers in the United States.

20. What are some methods to desensitize potential recipients who possess preformed HLA antibodies?
    - Intravenous immunoglobulin
    - Plasmapheresis
    - Rituximab
    - Splenectomy

KEY POINTS

1. Living kidney donation requires proper counseling and informed consent, as there is an increased risk of hypertension, pre-eclampsia, and ESKD. A major risk factor for the donor developing renal issues is obesity.
2. It is important to understand that certain kidney diseases may recur in the transplant, resulting in graft loss. This should be part of the pre-transplant counseling for the potential recipient.
3. Kidney Donor Exchange is a growing venue to increase availability of organs to potential transplant candidates.

BIBLIOGRAPHY

Annual Data Report of the US Organ Procurement and Transplantation Network (OPTN) and the Scientific Registry of Transplant Recipients (SRTR). (2013). Preface. *American Journal of Transplantation, 13*(Suppl. 1), 1–7. doi:10.1111/ajt.12028.

Axelrod, D. A., McCullough, K. P., Brewer, E. D., Becker, B. N., Segev, D. L., & Rao, P. S. (2010). Kidney and pancreas transplantation in the United States, 1999–2008: The changing face of living donation. *American Journal of Transplantation, 10*(4 Pt 2), 987–1002. doi:10.1111/j.1600-6143.2010.03022.x.

Bryan, C. F., Cherikh, W. S., & Sesok-Pizzini, D. A. (2016). A2/A2 B to B renal transplantation: Past, present, and future directions. *American Journal of Transplantation, 16*(1), 11–20. doi:10.1111/ajt.13499.

Cosio, F. G., & Cattran, D. C. (2017). Recent advances in our understanding of recurrent primary glomerulonephritis after kidney transplantation. *Kidney International, 91*(2), 304–314. doi:S0085-2538(16)30484-7.

Garg, A. X., McArthur, E., & Lentine, K. L., & Donor Nephrectomy Outcomes Research (DONOR) Network. (2015). Gestational hypertension and preeclampsia in living kidney donors. *New England Journal of Medicine, 372*(15), 1469–1470. doi:10.1056/NEJM.

Glorie, K., Haase-Kromwijk, B., van de Klundert, J., Wagelmans, A., & Weimar, W. (2014). Allocation and matching in kidney exchange programs. *Transplant International, 27*(4), 333–343.

Grams, M. E., Garg, A. X., & Lentine, K. L. (2016). Kidney-failure risk projection for the living kidney-donor candidate. *New England Journal of Medicine, 374*(21), 2094–2095. doi:10.1056/NEJMc1603007.

http://optn.transplant.hrsa.gov.

Keith, D. S., & Vranic, G. M. (2016). Approach to the highly sensitized kidney transplant candidate. *Clinical Journal of the American Society of Nephrology, 11*(4), 684–693. doi:10.2215/CJN.05930615.

Kher, A., & Mandelbrot, D. A. (2012). The living kidney donor evaluation: Focus on renal issues. *Clinical Journal of the American Society of Nephrology, 7*(2), 366–371. doi:10.2215/CJN.10561011.

Lefaucheur, C., Loupy, A., Hill, G. S., Andrado, J., Nochy, D., Antoine, C., ... Suberbielle-Boissel, C. (2010). Preexisting donor-specific HLA antibodies predict outcome in kidney transplantation. *Journal of the American Society of Nephrology, 21*(8), 1398–1406. doi:10.1681/ASN.2009101065.

Lentine, K. L., & Segev, D. L. (2017). Understanding and communicating medical risks for living kidney donors: A matter of perspective. *Journal of the American Society of Nephrology, 28*(1), 12–24. doi:10.1681/ASN.2016050571.

Locke, J. E., Reed, R. D., Massie, A., MacLennan, P. A., Sawinski, D., Kumar, V., ... Segev, D. L. (2017). Obesity increases the risk of end-stage renal disease among living kidney donors. *Kidney International, 91*(3), 699–703. doi:S0085-2538(16)30613-5.

Locke, J. E., Sawinski, D., Reed, R. D., Shelton, B., MacLennan, P. A., Kumar, V., ... Lewis, C. E. (2017). Apolipoprotein L1 and chronic kidney disease risk in young potential living kidney donors. *Annals of Surgery.* doi:10.1097/SLA.0000000000002174.

Mahdi, B. M. (2013). A glow of HLA typing in organ transplantation. *Clinical and Translational Medicine, 2*(1), 6. doi:10.1186/2001-1326-2-6.

Obrador, G. T., & Macdougall, I. C. (2013). Effect of red cell transfusions on future kidney transplantation. *Clinical Journal of the American Society of Nephrology, 8*(5), 852–860. doi:10.2215/CJN.00020112.

Pham, P. T., Pham, P. A., Pham, P. C., Parikh, S., & Danovitch, G. (2010). Evaluation of adult kidney transplant candidates. *Seminars in Dialysis, 23*(6), 595–605. doi:10.1111/j.1525-139X.2010.00809.x.

Segev, D. L. (2012). Innovative strategies in living donor kidney transplantation. *Nature Reviews Nephrology, 8*(6), 332–338. doi:10.1038/nrneph.2012.82.

CHAPTER 57

IMMUNOSUPPRESSION

Beje Thomas and Matthew R. Weir

1. **What is the goal of immunosuppression?**
   The central goal of immunosuppression is to prevent rejection of the renal allograft. The intensity of immunosuppression must be weighed against the undesired consequences of immunodeficiency, such as infection or cancer. Close monitoring, knowledge, and expertise are required to balance the efficacy and toxicity of kidney transplantation immunosuppression.

2. **What are the classes of immunosuppressive therapies used in kidney transplantation?**
   See Table 57.1.

3. **What are the different phases of immunosuppression?**
   Induction involves the use of powerful immunosuppressive agents to provide a high degree of immunosuppression immediately post-transplant. This prevents acute rejection and allows time for maintenance immunosuppression to be titrated to appropriate levels.

   Maintenance immunosuppression's objectives are to prevent rejection and safely preserve the function of the kidney allograft. These agents are used for the life of the transplant.

4. **What are desensitization protocols?**
   Desensitization for the highly sensitized patients involves decreasing preformed antibody levels. This occurs prior to induction. There are several different methods that include various medications, including rituximab, bortezomib, intravenous immunoglobulin, plasmapheresis, and early initiation of maintenance immunosuppression weeks before transplantation. The outcomes have been equivocal. In addition, there is a significant financial cost as well as increased malignancy and infectious risk for the patient.

5. **What are the methods of induction therapy?**
   Induction strategies can be classified according to the mechanism of the agent used. The two mechanisms that define these agents are lymphocyte-depleting and non-lymphocyte-depleting agents. The lymphocyte-depleting agents used today are rabbit or equine anti-thymocyte globulin (thymoglobulin) and alemtuzumab (humanized anti-CD52 monoclonal antibody, Campath-1H, approved to treat chronic lymphocytic leukemia). Neither agent is approved for induction by the US Food and Drug Administration, despite their widespread use. The non-lymphocyte-depleting agent used is basiliximab (interleukin-2 receptor antibody, anti-CD25). Large pulse doses of steroids are also commonly used at the time of induction in addition to the lymphocyte- or non-lymphocyte-depleting agent. Overall, 85% of transplant programs use induction therapy, most commonly thymoglobulin followed by campath-1H and then basiliximab. Basiliximab is used in those individuals at lower immunologic risk (e.g., Caucasian race, first transplant, older patient, low panel reactive antibody. The benefit is a better safety profile than lymphocyte-depleting agents—in other words, less risk of infection and cancer. Those patients who are at higher risk for rejection should receive induction with a lymphocyte-depleting agent. The most common lymphocyte-depleting agent used today is thymoglobulin. Campath-H1 was the formulation of alemtuzumab sold up until 2012. It is no longer produced, and the remaining supply is used by certain transplant centers until there is no more available. The new formulation of alemtuzumab now in production is called Lemtrada.

6. **What is the three-signal model of T cell-mediated rejection?**
   - Signal 1: Antigen triggers T-cell receptors and synapse formation occurs.
   - Signal 2: Signal 1 allows co-stimulation of antigen-presenting cells to occur.
   - Signal 3: Signal 1 and signal 2 stimulate a cascade of intracellular events culminating in the initiation of the T-cell cycle; stimulation of the T-cell cycle allows T cells to infiltrate the graft.
   - Summary effect is to inhibit T-cell receptor activation, cytokine production, and subsequent lymphocyte proliferation to prevent rejection.

7. **What are the main drugs used for maintenance therapy?**
   1. Calcineurin inhibitors (CNI): tacrolimus, cyclosporine
   2. Anti-metabolites: azathioprine, mycophenolate mofetil (MMF), and mycophenolic acid (MPA)

Table 57.1. Common Drug I\Interactions

INCREASE METABOLISM DECREASE CNI LEVELS	DECREASE METABOLISM INCREASE CNI LEVELS
Carbamazepine	Ketoconazole
Phenytoin	Erythromycin
Phenobarbital	Clarithromycin
INH	Verapamil
Rifampin	Diltiazem
	Nicardipine

CNI, Calcineurin inhibitor.

3. mTOR (mammalian target of rapamycin) inhibitors: rapamycin and everolimus
4. Corticosteroids
5. Selective co-stimulation blockade: belatacept
   The most frequently used combination today is tacrolimus, anti-metabolite (MMF or MPA), and prednisone.

8. What are CNIs?
   CNIs remain a cornerstone of immunosuppressive regiments in kidney transplantation. This class of drugs works by blocking calcineurin, an intricate protein in the signal transduction pathway that activates signal 3. The two prototypes of the class are tacrolimus and cyclosporine, with tacrolimus being the primary drug of choice today.
   The side effects of the CNIs include:
   • Nephrotoxicity (discussed in next question)
   • Thrombotic microangiopathy (TMA)
   • New onset diabetes after transplant
   • Hypertension
   • Tremor
   • Hypercalciuria, hyperkalemia, and hypomagnesemia
   • Alopecia (Tacrolimus,)
   • Hirsutism, gingival hyperplasia, hyperuricemia, metabolic acidosis, hypophosphatemia (Cyclosporine)

9. Discuss CNI Nephrotoxicity.
   CNI nephrotoxicity can be divided into acute and chronic forms.
   • Acute nephrotoxicity usually involves afferent vascular constriction and lower kidney blood flow, leading to kidney ischemia and damage. This resolves with either removal of the drug or lower drug levels. TMA secondary to CNIs can present acutely as well. TMA can also be seen in antibody-mediated rejection.
   • Chronic CNI nephrotoxicity is seen histologically by global and focal glomerulosclerosis, arteriolar hyaline thickening, isometric tubular vacuolization, and focal areas of tubular atrophy and interstitial fibrosis. The fibrosis is classically seen in bands on biopsy and is called stripped fibrosis.

10. How are CNI levels monitored?
    CNIs require trough monitoring to ensure an adequate degree of immunosuppression. The trough should be 12 hours after the last dose, so it is imperative the patient take the medication regularly at 12-hour intervals and plan for the lab about 30 minutes prior to the next dose. There is also an extended 24-hour release formulation of tacrolimus. In this case, levels are checked 24 hours after the last dose. Desired drug level varies from center to center, depending on the particular immunosuppression strategy, but the goal in the first year is usually 8 to 12 with lower levels desired targeted further out from transplant
    If a drug level is uncharacteristically elevated, when calling the patient, always ask if they had taken the CNI prior to the blood draw to check the level. Another common cause of elevated CNI levels due to increased absorption is diarrhea. If drug levels are either higher or lower than usual, ask if the patient is on any new medications.

11. **How can Tacrolimus be administered?**
Tacrolimus can be given by mouth (PO), intravenously (IV), or sublingual. Oral dosing, when initially given in combination with MMF or MPA, is 0.1 mg/kg per day. It is important to know if the tacrolimus is immediate release (twice daily dosing) or extended release (once daily dosing); the ratio is 1:1. If IV tacrolimus is used the dose is 0.03 to 0.05 mg/kg per day by continuous infusion. The conversion ratio from oral dosing to IV dosing is roughly about 4:1. The maximum IV dose is 4 mg daily. However, the levels are difficult to follow and can be labile with IV dosing. Sublingual dosing is about 50% of oral dosing. If a patient is nothing by mouth (NPO), sublingual is preferable to IV dosing. In a situation where the patient cannot be appropriately dosed, the immunosuppression plan should be discussed with a transplant specialist.

12. **What are the anti-metabolites used for immunosuppression?**
Inosine monophosphate dehydrogenase inhibitors (IMPDH inhibitors) inhibit purine synthesis. Two important drugs in this class are MPA and MMF. MPA directly inhibits IMPDH (a key enzyme in purine synthesis), whereas MMF is a prodrug that releases MPA. The principal side effects of these medications are gastrointestinal (nausea, vomiting, diarrhea) and hematologic (anemia, leukopenia). Azathioprine inhibits interferes with DNA, RNA, and protein synthesis. It is an option for those patients who cannot tolerate the IMPDH inhibitors for reasons such as GI distress.

13. **What are mTOR inhibitors?**
mTOR inhibitors block the mTOR and thus prevent cytokine signals from activating the T-cell cycle (signal 3). Two examples of these medications are sirolimus and everolimus. The principal adverse drug reactions include hyperlipidemia, impaired wound healing, and thrombocytopenia. Additionally, mTOR inhibitors have been linked to mouth ulcers and pneumonitis. The half-life for mTOR inhibitors is about 60 hours, so when changing the dose, the level is usually checked about a week later. Desired drug levels depend on the overall immunosuppression regiment: if an mTOR inhibitor is used by itself, the target level is similar to tacrolimus. On the other hand, if used with a CNI, the target level of both the CNI and mTORinhibitor is lower.

14. **What is Belatacept?**
A biological agent that blocks the co-stimulation necessary for activation of the T-cell (signal 2), Belatacept is associated with less metabolic side effects and nephrotoxicity compared to CNIs and mTOR inhibitors. Drug levels do not need to be checked, allowing for less lab draws. Another advantage is that once loaded, it is typically a once-monthly intravenous infusion, potentially improving patient compliance. Studies comparing Belatacept to CNI (cyclosporine) showed that, though there was improved glomerular filtration rates in the Belatacept arm, this came at the cost of an increased rejection rate. Also, Belatacept was associated with post-transplant lymphoproliferative disease when given in patients who were Epstein-Barr negative. The primary barriers for Belatacept to be a more mainstream agent are the need for the infusion, cost, and the possible higher rate of rejection in high-risk transplant groups.

15. **What are the common drug interactions of concern with immunosuppressants?**
The major drug interactions involve the CNIs (cyclosporine, tacrolimus) and drugs that are metabolized through the cytochrome p450-3A4 system (Box 57.1).

Box 57.1. Classes of Immunosuppressive Drugs Used in Kidney Transplantation

A. Glucocorticoids
B. Small molecule drugs
  1. Immunophilin-binding drugs[a]
    a. Calcineurin inhibitors (cyclosporine, tacrolimus)
    b. Mammalian target of rapamycin inhibitors (sirolimus, everolimus)
  2. Inhibitors of nucleotide synthesis
    a. Purine synthesis (inosine monophosphate dehydrogenase) inhibitors (mycophenolate mofetil, mycophenolic acid
    b. Pyrimidine synthesis inhibitors (Leflunomide)
  3. Anti-metabolites (Azathioprine)

C. Protein drugs
  1. Antibody-depleting agents against T cells, B cells, or both
    a. Polyclonal antibody (thymoglobulin)
    b. Monoclonal antibody (muromonab)
  2. Non-depleting antibodies (basiliximab)
  3. Fusion drugs (Belatacept)
  4. Intravenous immune globulin

[a]Immunophilin is an intracellular protein that, when bound to calcineurin inhibitors, will engage calcineurin.

16. **When should steroids be withdrawn following kidney transplantation?**
The long-term use of steroids is associated with numerous adverse effects, including osteoporosis, new-onset diabetes after transplant, poor wound healing, hypertension, obesity, and dyslipidemia. Patients at lower immunologic risk do well with early steroid withdrawal 3 to 21 days post-transplantation. However, the benefits of early steroid withdrawal may be outweighed in patients at higher immunologic risk, particularly in the black population. Early steroid withdrawal in this group has shown a higher incidence of acute rejection and chronic antibody mediated rejection. There is possibly a subgroup of blacks that could benefit from steroid withdrawal, but this likely is a group with more potent induction therapy and maintenance immunosuppression. This subgroup would also include fewer human leukocyte antigen (HLA) mismatches, living donor, and no delayed graft function. The late withdrawal of steroids has demonstrated conflicting results.
   Steroid-free protocols are increasingly used, despite some controversy over their efficacy and safety. Data from the FREEDOM study group showed a higher rate of acute rejection in the steroid-free group, despite no differences in creatinine, glomerular filtration rate, or graft survival compared to the steroid maintenance arm. The steroid-free group had less statin use, weight gain, and anti-hyperglycemic medicine use. The issue of steroid use post-transplantation remains controversial and requires further investigation to identify the optimal strategy. For now, the use of steroids post-transplantation should be individualized, considering a recipient's comorbidities and overall risk of allograft rejection.

17. **What is the purpose of CNI minimization or avoidance strategies?**
These strategies are meant to avoid the long-term toxicities associated with CNI use—in particular, nephrotoxicity. This must be individualized to the patient and their immune risk for rejection. Various strategies include switching to a lower drug level target for tacrolimus in combination with an mTOR inhibitor with or without steroids. CNIs can be completely switched out for an mTOR inhibitor or Belatacept with an antimetabolite and steroids as well. There is some increased risk of rejection, particularly in high-risk populations when CNIs are minimized. The other concern that has come to light more recently is that CNI nephrotoxicity might not be the main culprit limiting long-term graft survival, but rather chronic alloimmune damage. If this is the case, it might be better to keep a patient on a CNI and not aggressively try to reduce the CNI exposure. Additional studies are needed.

18. **Are there generic versions of transplant medications?**
There are generic versions of Tacrolimus, Cyclosporine, and MMF that are commonly used today. If the patient is switched from a brand name to a generic version, the transplant center should be notified so they can follow closely along. Cyclosporine has different brand names, including Sandimmune and Gengraf. When possible, a patient should be kept on what they have been taking in the past. MMF is interchangeable with MPA (250 mg of MMF is equivalent to 180 mg of MPA).

KEY POINTS

1. The intensity of immunosuppression must be weighed against the undesired consequences of immunodeficiency (infection or cancer).
2. Immunosuppression is divided into the induction phase and maintenance phase. Induction involves lymphocyte and non-lymphocyte depleting agents commonly with pulse dose steroids. Maintenance therapy involves CNIs, anti-metabolites, mTOR inhibitors, steroids, and co-stimulation blockade with Belatacept.
3. CNIs remain a cornerstone of immunosuppressive regiments in kidney transplantation. This class of drugs works by blocking calcineurin, an intricate protein in the signal transduction pathway.
4. Deciding on immunosuppression strategy from induction to maintenance should be individualized as per the patient's individual risk for rejection and metabolic complications.
5. The issue of steroid use post-transplantation remains controversial and requires further investigation to identify the optimal strategy. For now, the use of steroids post-transplantation should be individualized, considering a recipient's comorbidities and overall risk of allograft rejection.

BIBLIOGRAPHY

Brennan, D. C., Daller, J. A., Lake, K. D., Cibrik, D., Del Castillo, D., & Thymoglobulin Induction Study Group. (2006). Rabbit antithymocyte globulin versus basiliximab in renal transplantation. *New England Journal of Medicine, 355*(19), 1967–1977. doi:355/19/1967.

Del Bello, A., Marion, O., Milongo, D., Rostaing, L., & Kamar, N. (2016). Belatacept prophylaxis against organ rejection in adult kidney-transplant recipients. *Expert Review of Clinical Pharmacology, 9*(2), 215–227. doi:10.1586/17512433.2016.1112736.

Haller, M. C., Royuela, A., Nagler, E. V., Pascual, J., & Webster, A. C. (2016). Steroid avoidance or withdrawal for kidney transplant recipients. *Cochrane Database of Systematic Reviews,* (8), CD005632. doi:10.1002/14651858.CD005632.pub3.

Halloran, P. F. (2004). Immunosuppressive drugs for kidney transplantation. *New England Journal of Medicine, 351*(26), 2715–2729. doi:351/26/2715.

Keith, D. S., & Vranic, G. M. (2016). Approach to the highly sensitized kidney transplant candidate. *Clinical Journal of the American Society of Nephrology, 11*(4), 684–693. doi:10.2215/CJN.05930615.

Kidney Disease: Improving Global Outcomes (KDIGO) Transplant Work Group. (2009). KDIGO clinical practice guideline for the care of kidney transplant recipients. *American Journal of Transplantation, 9*(Suppl. 3), S1– S155. doi:10.1111/j.1600-6143.2009.02834.x.

Lim, M. A., Kohli, J., & Bloom, R. D. (2017). Immunosuppression for kidney transplantation: Where are we now and where are we going? *Transplantation Reviews (Orlando), 31*(1), 10–17. doi:S0955-470X(16)30054-4.

Naesens, M., Kuypers, D. R., & Sarwal, M. (2009). Calcineurin inhibitor nephrotoxicity. *Clinical Journal of the American Society of Nephrology, 4*(2), 481–508.

Prashar, R., & Venkat, K. K. (2016). Immunosuppression minimization and avoidance protocols: When less is not more. *Advances in Chronic Kidney Disease, 23*(5), 295–300. doi:S1548-5595(16)30077-5.

Taber, D. J., Hunt, K. J., Gebregziabher, M., Srinivas, T., Chavin, K. D., Baliga, P. K., & Egede, L. E. (2017). A comparative effectiveness analysis of early steroid withdrawal in black kidney transplant recipients. *Clinical Journal of the American Society of Nephrology, 12*(1), 131–139.

Thomas, B., & Weir, M. R. (2015). The evaluation and therapeutic management of hypertension in the transplant patient. *Current Cardiology Reports, 17*(11), 95.

Vincenti, F., Schena, F. P., Paraskevas, S., Hauser, I. A., Walker, R. G., Grinyo, J., & FREEDOM Study Group. (2008). A randomized, multicenter study of steroid avoidance, early steroid withdrawal or standard steroid therapy in kidney transplant recipients. *American Journal of Transplantation, 8*(2), 307–316. doi:10.1111/j.1600-6143.2007.02057.x.

Vlachopanos, G., Bridson, J. M., Sharma, A., & Halawa, A. (2016). Corticosteroid minimization in renal transplantation: Careful patient selection enables feasibility. *World Journal of Transplantation, 6*(4), 759–766.

CHAPTER 58

REJECTION OF THE KIDNEY TRANSPLANT

Beje Thomas and Matthew R. Weir

1. **How to evaluate acute kidney injury (AKI) in the kidney transplant patient?**
   See Fig. 58.1. When deciding the baseline kidney function and using the serum creatinine (Scr), the clinician must be careful. The ideal baseline Scr is based on the most recent trend when the patient was in a steady state. Time after transplantation is also critical in sorting through the differential diagnosis of AKI. The differential changes when the patient is a recent transplant and could have surgical complications, such as a urine leak in the first few months as opposed to a patient several years after transplant in whom that is less likely.

2. **What are the various types of rejection as defined by time?**
   There are three general types of organ rejection:
   1. Hyperacute
   2. Acute
   3. Chronic
      Hyperacute rejection is a complement-mediated response by the recipient with preexisting donor specific antibodies (DSA). Hyperacute rejection occurs almost immediately following organ implantation and necessitates immediate explant of the organ. Hyperacute rejection is uncommon with pre-transplantation cross-matches and screening.
      Acute rejection is associated with a sudden deterioration in allograft function that can occur as early as 1 week post-transplantation. Acute rejection may also be subclinical, associated with a more insidious rise in creatinine. Acute rejection has a major adverse effect on long-term graft survival.
      Chronic rejection, better defined as chronic antibody-mediated rejection (AMR), is the main cause of late allograft loss and is histologically defined as transplant glomerulopathy (TG).

3. **What are the two different types of acute rejection?**
   For diagnosis, both require a kidney transplant biopsy. A patient can have a mixed rejection with features of both cell-mediated acute cellular rejection and AMR (Table 58.1).

4. **What is the Banff criteria for acute cell-mediated rejection?**
   The Banff classification of kidney allograft rejection grades acute tubulointerstitial rejection by severity of tubulitis and acute vascular rejection by severity of arteritis. Types of T-cell-mediated rejection are as follows:
   - **Type IA:** Cases with significant interstitial infiltration by lymphocytes (>25% of parenchyma affected) and foci of *moderate* tubulitis
   - **Type IB:** Cases with significant interstitial infiltration of lymphocytes (>25% of parenchyma affected) and foci of *severe* tubulitis
   - **Type IIA:** Cases with *mild-to-moderate* intimal arteritis
   - **Type IIB:** Cases with *severe* intimal arteritis
   - **Type III:** Cases with transmural arteritis and/or arterial fibrinoid change and necrosis of medial smooth muscle cells with accompanying lymphocytic inflammation

5. **What should be considered when acute rejection is diagnosed?**
   The possibility of inadequate immunosuppression should be considered whenever acute rejection is confirmed. This inadequacy may result from noncompliance, under-dosing of maintenance immunosuppressants, drug interactions, and/or rapid withdrawal of immunosuppressants post-transplantation. A systematic approach to identify the contributing factors for acute rejection should be instituted to mitigate further graft damage and eventual graft failure.

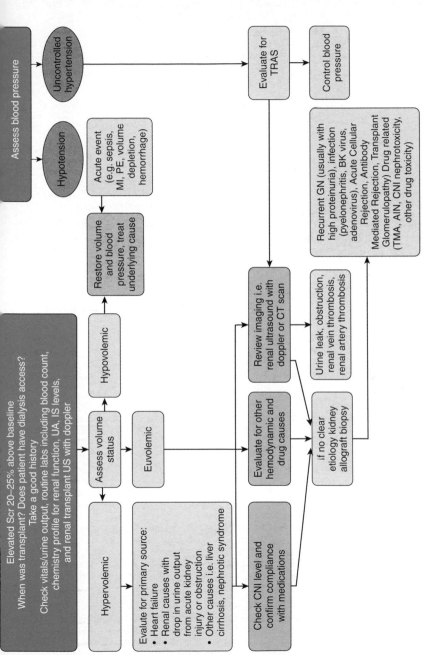

Figure 58.1. Evaluation of Renal Transplant Dysfunction. *AIN,* Acute interstitial nephritis; *CNI,* calcium inhibitor; *CT,* computerized tomography; *GN,* glomerulonephritis; *IS,* immunosuppression; *MI,* myocardial infarction; *PE,* pulmonary embolism; *Scr,* creatine; *TMA,* thrombotic microangiopathy; *TRAS,* transplant renal artery stenosis; *UA,* urinalysis; *US,* ultrasound. (From Colvin, R. B. (2007). Antibody-mediated renal allograft rejection: Diagnosis and pathogenesis. *Journal of the American Society of Nephrology, 18,* 1046–1056)

Table 58.1. Acute Rejection Types

CELL-MEDIATED REJECTION	ANTIBODY-MEDIATED REJECTION
Cell-mediated Adaptive immune system	B-cell mediated Innate immune system Can be activated by a T-cell response
Can occur within the first few weeks of transplant	Can occur within hours to days after transplant
Scr might be stable and can have subclinical rejection, though usually is elevated	When acute, more likely to cause rapid kidney allograft dysfunction Proteinuria
Lymphocyte infiltration, tubulits, arteritis Negative DSA Negative C4d in peritubular capillaries	Intimal arteritis, peritubular capillaritis and glomerulitis, microthrombi Positive DSA Positive C4d in peritubular capillaries (can be negative in AMR; however, have positive DSA and other histological changes consistent with acute AMR
Treatment involves shutting down T-cell response using steroids and lymphocyte-depleting agents Optimize maintenance immunosuppression	Treatment involves removing and shutting down antibody production using steroids, plasmapheresis, intravenous immunoglobulin, lymphocyte-depleting agents, and B-cell (rituxan, boertezomab) or compliment- specific therapies (eculizimab) Optimize maintenance immunosuppression

AMR, Antibody-mediated rejection; *DSA*, donor specific antibodies; *Scr*, serum creatinine.

6. What are the treatment options for cell-mediated rejection?
   - Pulse corticosteroids
   - Anti-T-cell antibody therapies (e.g., thymoglobulin)
   - Cyclophosphamide—(rarely used)

7. What are some general principles when treating acute cell-mediated rejection?
   - Pulse dose corticosteroids, typically methylprednisolone 500 mg daily intravenously for 3 days are considered the first-line therapy for Banff class IA. In higher grades of rejection beyond Banff IA pulse corticosteroids are routinely used as well but in concert with other more potent drugs such as lymphocyte depleting agents.
   - Optimizing maintenance immunosuppression. The calcineurin inhibitor dose should be adjusted if levels preceding the acute rejection episode were sub-therapeutic. If tolerable, the dose of mycophenolate mofetil/mycophenolic acid should be increased. Typically, a steroid taper is given as well.
   - Lymphocyte-depleting agents are used regularly for Grade 1B rejection or a higher grade of rejection. They are used in Grade1A if the rejection is resistant to steroids. Thymoglobulin is the common lymphocyte-depleting agent used.
     If there is no response, the possibility of AMR should be considered. Patients should be assessed for DSA and the biopsy stained for C4d staining. A repeat kidney transplant biopsy should also be considered. If there are no contraindications, an alternate lymphocyte-depleting agent (CampathH-1), plasmapheresis, and/or intravenous immune globulin may be considered. The decision to discontinue therapy should be based on many factors, but mainly the recipient's clinical status and degree of damage on repeat allograft biopsy.

8. What are the Banff criteria for AMR/humoral rejection?
   - Acute AMR: Defined by detection of DSA, C4d staining on the biopsy, and allograft pathology consistent with this diagnosis of AMR. The 2013 Banff Conference changed the definition of AMR. It acknowledges that C4d staining may be negative in AMR, termed C4d negative AMR. In this setting, there are other pathological changes, including intimal arteritis, peritubular capillaritis, and glomerulitis in the setting of positive DSA.
   - Chronic AMR/TG: Defined by the Banff histological term chronic glomerulopathy (CG). CG is the double contouring of the glomerular basement membrane seen on light or electron microscopy.

This is a result of repetitive episodes of endothelial activation, injury, and repair leading to pathological changes of the glomerular basement membrane. TG risk factors include preexisting or de novo anti-HLA antibodies, Hepatitis C infection, and thrombotic microangiopathy. TG prevalence is 5% to 20% in most series, reaching 55% in some high-risk cohorts, and is associated with worse allograft outcomes. Kidney transplant biopsy is the gold standard for diagnosis of TG. One has to be vigilant, as the Scr may not rise until considerable damage is done. A rising level of proteinuria several years after transplant is an indication for kidney transplant biopsy, as this can be sign of developing TG.

9. What are the postulated stages of humoral rejection/transplant glomerulopathy with the development of de novo DSA?
   1. De novo DSA
   2. Peritubular capillaritis
   3. ±C4d positivity
   4. Glomerulitis
   5. Interstitial fibrosis and tubular atrophy
   6. Rise of creatinine and proteinuria

10. What are panel reactive antibody (PRA), DSA, and C4d?
    - Patient sensitization is classically reported as the percent PRA and is an estimate of the likelihood of a positive cross-match to a pool of potential donors and their respective human leukocyte antigens (HLA). In simpler terms, it is a method for determining a patient's risk of organ rejection prior to transplantation. PRA greater than 80% is considered highly sensitized.
    - DSA are immunoglobulin G antibodies targeted against HLAs. DSA may be anti-class I or anti-class II. Anti-donor HLA antibodies against either class I or class II antigens are associated with higher frequency of acute and chronic AMR.
    - C4d is a degradation product of the classic complement pathway. C4d has a high affinity for endothelial and collagen basement membranes and serves as a method of detecting antibody activation within the glomerulus and tubules. C4d is evidence of AMR.

11. What is the treatment algorithm for AMR?
    Pulse dose corticosteroids of 500 mg intravenously daily for a total of three doses with 9 to 10 sessions of plasmapheresis for removal of antibodies and inflammatory mediators. This is followed by the patient receiving intravenous immunoglobulin to decrease activation of the complement system and cell-mediated immunity. The intravenous immunoglobulin can be given after a session of plasmapheresis. In order to avoid an infusion reaction no more than 500 mg is given at one time, the total dose given by the end of treatment is 2 g/kg. The combination of pulse dose steroids, plasmapheresis, and intravenous immunoglobulin is the most common treatment method for AMR. It is also necessary to optimize the patient's maintenance immunosuppression, such as increasing their tacrolimus goal, the dose of the anti-metabolite, or adding prednisone if not on it.

    Other therapies that are available with limited data include B-cell/plasma cell therapy with Rituxan and Bortezomab to prevent antibody formation. Eculizimab is another alternative agent with limited data in AMR. It inhibits formation of C5b-9 attack complex that causes cell lysis in the kidney transplant in AMR.

KEY POINTS

1. Use a systematic, algorithmic approach to AKI in the kidney transplant patient. Remember, not all AKI is rejection.
2. The possibility of inadequate immunosuppression should be considered whenever acute rejection is confirmed.
3. Acute AMR includes documentation of circulating DSA, C4d staining in the peritubular capillaries, and allograft pathology consistent with this diagnosis. However, C4d negative AMR is a recognized form of AMR.
4. Transplant glomerulopathy is a main cause of long-term graft loss. Proteinuria and serum creatinine may be stable and rise only after significant pathological damage has been done.
5. Multiple factors, both alloantigen-dependent and alloantigen-independent, appear to contribute to the pathogenesis of chronic graft dysfunction.

BIBLIOGRAPHY

Bock, H. A. (2001). Steroid-resistant kidney transplant rejection: Diagnosis and treatment. *Journal of the American Society of Nephrology, 12*(Suppl. 17), S48–S52.

Djamali, A., Kaufman, D. B., Ellis, T. M., Zhong, W., Matas, A., & Samaniego, M. (2014). Diagnosis and management of antibody-mediated rejection: Current status and novel approaches. *American Journal of Transplantation, 14*(2), 255–271. doi:10.1111/ajt.12589.

Haas, M. (2014). An updated Banff schema for diagnosis of antibody-mediated rejection in renal allografts. *Current Opinion in Organ Transplantation, 19*(3), 315–322. doi:10.1097/MOT.0000000000000072.

Kumbala, D., & Zhang, R. (2013). Essential concept of transplant immunology for clinical practice. *World Journal of Transplantation, 3*(4), 113–118. doi:10.5500/wjt.v3.i4.113.

Nankivell, B. J., & Alexander, S. I. (2010). Rejection of the kidney allograft. *New England Journal of Medicine, 363*(15), 1451–1462. doi:10.1056/NEJMra0902927.

Remport, A., Ivanyi, B., Mathe, Z., Tinckam, K., Mucsi, I., & Molnar, M. Z. (2015). Better understanding of transplant glomerulopathy secondary to chronic antibody-mediated rejection. *Nephrology Dialysis Transplantation, 30*(11), 1825–1833. doi:10.1093/ndt/gfu371.

Solez, K., Colvin, R. B., Racusen, L. C., Haas, M., Sis, B., Mengel, M., . . . Valente, M. (2008). Banff 07 classification of renal allograft pathology: Updates and future directions. *American Journal of Transplantation, 8*(4), 753–760. doi:10.1111/j.1600-6143.2008.02159.x.

POSTTRANSPLANT MALIGNANCIES

Beje Thomas and Matthew R. Weir

1. **Are transplant recipients at greater risk for the development of malignancies?**
   Yes. The chronic exposure to immunosuppressive agents increases the long-term risk of malignancy by two to threefold compared with the general population of the same age and sex. Kidney transplant recipients have the cancer risk of a nontransplanted individual 20 to 30 years older than them. If a recipient had a cancer prior to transplant, the risk post transplant is increased by 40%. See Fig. 59.1.

2. **What are posttransplant lymphoproliferative diseases (PTLD) and the risk factors?**
   PTLD is a well-recognized complication of the immunosuppression in the kidney transplant patient. Epstein-Barr virus (EBV) is found in two-thirds of PTLD cases. PTLD in kidney transplant patients is mainly a B cell–derived, large cell lymphoma.
   Risk factors for PTLD include:
   - Degree of immunosuppression such as the use of lymphocyte-depleting agents
   - Transplantation between EBV-positive donor and EBV-negative recipient
   - <25-year-old recipient
   - Pretransplant malignancy
   - PTLD occurs in 0.6% to 1.5% of patients after kidney transplantation, with the majority in the first year

3. **How common are lymphoproliferative disorders following transplantation?**
   Excluding nonmelanoma skin cancer and in situ cervical cancer, lymphoproliferative disorders are the most common malignancies complicating organ transplantation. Lymphoproliferative disorders account for 21% of all malignancies in patients who have received transplants, compared with 5% of malignancies in the general population. Lymphoproliferative disorders occur in 5% of patients who have received a kidney transplant.

4. **Does PTLD have the same characteristics as lymphoproliferative disease in the general population?**
   No, the proportion of patients with non-Hodgkin lymphoma (NHL) is much higher in transplant patients (95%), whereas NHL accounts for only 65% of lymphomas in the general population.

5. **What is the clinical presentation of PTLD?**
   PTLD can be divided into "early" and "late." Early PTLD is seen in younger patients who have a de nova EBV infection. The kidney allograft is involved in 57% of cases. This is responsive to immunosuppression reduction. Late PTLD occurs after the first year and is usually more disseminated and does not respond as well to immunosuppression reduction. Most patients present with nonspecific complaints, including fatigue, weight loss, and fever. Some patients present with symptoms resembling infectious mononucleosis. Up to 10% to 15% of PTLD present with central nervous system involvement. A patient may present with lymphadenopathy or palpable masses. Extranodal involvement is common. Given the nonspecific nature of clinical presentation, the diagnosis of PTLD requires a high index of suspicion.

6. **What are the different types of PTLD?**
   - Benign polyclonal lymphoproliferation
   - Polyclonal lymphoproliferation with malignant transformation
   - Monoclonal lymphoproliferation with malignant transformation (Hanson et al., 1996)

7. **What are the treatment options for various PTLDs?**
   The treatment and management of PTLD is varied. Treatment is often dictated by the cell type and stage of the lymphoproliferative process. Treatment strategies are individualized and can include:
   - Reduction of immunosuppression
   - Antiviral therapy

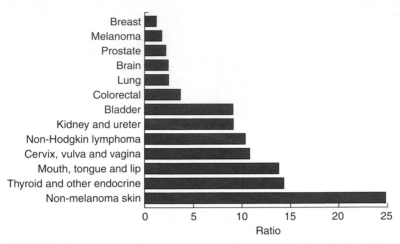

FIGURE 59.1. Risk of developing malignancies in transplant recipients compared with the general population.

- Chemotherapy
- Intravenous immunoglobulin (IVIG)
- Surgical resection
- Radiation
- Interferon therapy
- Anti-CD20 monoclonal antibody therapies

8. Discuss the relationship between EBV and PTLD?
   EBV is present in 95% of the adult US population. Kidney recipients that are EBV negative receiving an organ from an EBV-positive donor are at increased risk of PTLD. After infection, the virus persists in B-cell lymphocytes and can lead to cell transformation. This transformation leads to a persistently activated B cell that is constantly replicating. Normally in the immunocompetent patient, the body's cellular component of the immune system (helper and cytotoxic T cells, natural killer cells) eliminate these "transformed" B cells. However, with immunosuppression, this regulatory process does not respond appropriately, and PTLD can develop. This is why PTLD is more common in the first year post transplant after induction therapy and higher levels of maintenance immunosuppression.

9. Is treatment of EBV with antiviral therapies beneficial for PTLD?
   Despite their widespread use, there is currently no evidence that any antiviral therapy is efficacious for the treatment of PTLD. Given the lack of evidence-based support for antiviral therapies, they are not recommended as a sole treatment. The use of antivirals to reduce the incidence of PTLD following transplantation has not been validated.

10. What is the most common form of skin cancer in transplant recipients?
    Squamous cell carcinoma is the most common, occurring 65 to 250 times more frequently in the transplant population than in the general population. In the general population, basal cell carcinoma is more common than squamous cell skin cancer.

11. How can we reduce the risk of skin cancer in patients who have received kidney transplant?
    All kidney transplant recipients, especially those who have fair skin, live in sun-exposed climates, had significant sun exposure as a child, or have a history of skin cancer, should be educated on their high risk of skin cancer. Minimization of sun exposure (avoiding the sun from 10 a.m. to 4 p.m.), the use of sunscreen, and meticulous skin self-examinations should be instituted to reduce the risk of skin cancers in this high-risk population. An annual skin examination by a dermatologist is recommended in most kidney transplant recipients. In regard to immunosuppression, those on calcineurin inhibitor (CNI) converted to mechanistic target of rapamycin (mTOR) inhibitors have decreased rates of skin malignancies compared with those who remain on CNI. However, there is increased risk of rejection, and not all patients are able to tolerate the mTOR inhibitors.

12. **What is the association of immunosuppression and malignancy?**
It is important to note that a higher degree of immunosuppression confers a higher risk of malignancy. If the patient has an episode of acute rejection after transplant the treatment may include a second round of induction (lymphocyte-depleting) agents which increases the risk of future malignancies as well. CNIs are known to promote carcinogenesis. Azathioprine is associated with higher incidence of lymphoma and skin malignancies. Mycophenolate mofetil (MMF) and mycophenolate acid (MPA) were developed as anticancer drugs; however, there has been no difference in malignancy rates in patients on these drugs or not. However, if they are on the MMF or MPA, there is reduced rejection. mTOR inhibitors have a lower rate of malignancy. Reducing the risk of malignancy is one of the drivers pushing research into lighter immunosuppression protocols. However, this must be balanced against the risk of rejection.

13. **How should the transplant recipient be screened for malignancies?**
- History and physical examination to exclude disseminated or localized organ involvement by PTLD. High-risk kidney transplant patients (EBV-positive donor with EBV-negative recipient) should be screened the first week post transplant, monthly for 3 to 6 months, then every 3 months until the end of the first year, and then annually.
- Skin examinations by dermatologist (every 6 months in patients at high risk, otherwise yearly)
- Ultrasound or computed tomography scan of the native kidneys annually
- Gynecologic examinations, including Pap test and ultrasound of genitourinary organs annually
- Prostate-specific antigen and digital rectal examination annually in men older than 50 years old or younger in high-risk groups
- Fecal occult blood test annually in men older than 50 years old or younger in high-risk groups
- Abdominal ultrasound and serum alpha fetoprotein levels in carriers of hepatitis B or C virus
- Colonoscopy in individuals, as per general population guidelines
- Mammogram in females, as per general population guidelines
- Cystoscopy in individuals with hematuria, particularly with a history of cyclophosphamide therapy
- Hepatic ultrasound and alpha fetoprotein yearly in patients with cirrhosis

KEY POINTS

1. The chronic exposure to immunosuppressive agents increases the long-term risk of many malignancies, particularly when compared with the general population.
2. Lymphoproliferative disorders are the most common malignancies complicating organ transplantation, excluding nonmelanoma skin cancer and in situ cervical cancer.
3. The clinical presentation of posttransplant lymphoproliferative disorder is protean. Most patients present with nonspecific complaints, including fatigue, weight loss, and fever.
4. Squamous cell carcinoma occurs 65 to 250 times more frequently in the transplant population than in the general population.

BIBLIOGRAPHY

Al-Mansour, Z., Nelson, B. P., & Evens, A. M. (2013). Post-transplant lymphoproliferative disease (PTLD): Risk factors, diagnosis, and current treatment strategies. *Current Hematologic Malignancy Reports, 8*(3), 173–183. doi:10.1007/s11899-013-0162-5.
Chapman, J. R., Webster, A. C., & Wong, G. (2013). Cancer in the transplant recipient. *Cold Spring Harbor Perspectives in Medicinie, 3*(7), pii: a015677. doi:10.1101/cshperspect.a015677.
Hanson, M. N., Morrison, V. A., Peterson, B. A., Stieglbauer, K. T., Kubic, V. L., McCormick, S. R., . . . Litz, C. E. (1996). Posttransplant T-cell lymphoproliferative disorders—an aggressive, late complication of solid-organ transplantation. *Blood, 88*(9), 3626–3633.
Kasiske, B. L., Vazquez, M. A., Harmon, W. E., Brown, R. S., Danovitch, G. M., Gaston, R. S., . . . Singer, G. G. (2000). Recommendations for the outpatient surveillance of renal transplant recipients. American Society of Transplantation. *Journal of the American Society of Nephrology, 11*(Suppl. 15), S1–S86.
Kidney Disease: Improving Global Outcomes (KDIGO) Transplant Work Group. (2009). KDIGO clinical practice guideline for the care of kidney transplant recipients. *American Journal of Transplantation, 9*(Suppl. 3), S1–S155. doi:10.1111/j.1600-6143.2009.02834.x.
Le, J., Durand, C. M., Agha, I., & Brennan, D. C. (2017). Epstein-Barr virus and renal transplantation. *Transplantation Reviews (Orlando), 31*(1), 55–60. doi:S0955-470X(16)30073-8. [pii].
Penn, I. (1990). Cancers complicating organ transplantation. *New England Journal of Medicine, 323*(25), 1767–1769. doi:10.1056/NEJM199012203232510.
Webster, A. C., Wong, G., Craig, J. C., & Chapman, J. R. (2008). Managing cancer risk and decision making after kidney transplantation. *American Journal of Transplantation, 8*(11), 2185–2191. doi:10.1111/j.1600-6143.2008.02385.x.

CHAPTER 60

POSTTRANSPLANT INFECTIONS

Beje Thomas and Matthew R. Weir

1. **What type of infections do kidney transplant recipients develop?**
   - Donor-derived infections
   - Recipient-derived infections
   - Nosocomial-acquired infections
   - Community-acquired infections

2. **Is there any pattern to infections that occur post transplantation?**
   Yes. Karuthu et al. reviewed this recently, including the timing of infections post transplant. Infections occur in a generally predictable pattern after kidney transplantation. See Fig. 60.1
   - First month post transplant:
     - Nosocomial and surgery-related infections are the predominant infections
     - Aspiration pneumonia
     - Catheter infections
     - Wound infections
     - Anastomotic leaks
     - Clostridium difficile colitis
     - Resistant organisms such as methicillin-resistant *Staphylococcus aureus*
   - Months post transplantation 1 through 6:
     - Activation of latent infections is most common
     - *Pneumocystis jiroveci* (previously *Pneumocystis carinii*) pneumonia
     - Fungal infections
     - Herpes-related disease
     - BK virus
     - *Clostridium difficile* colitis
     - Hepatitis C virus
     - Adenovirus
     - Influenza
     - *Cryptococcus*
     - *Mycobacterium tuberculosis*.
   - Posttransplant month 6 and beyond:
     - Community-acquired infections are predominant (urinary tract infections [UTIs], pneumonia)
     - Fungal infections, including Nocardia, Aspergillus, and Mucor
     - Late viral infections (cytomegalovirus [CMV], hepatitis B and C, herpes simplex virus, John Cunningham (JC) virus)

3. **What is the most common bacterial infection that leads to hospitalizations in kidney transplant patients?**
   UTIs. The most common bacterial cause is *Escherichia coli*.

4. **What infectious prophylaxis do patients receive post transplant?**
   - Valganciclovir to prevent CMV for 3 to 6 months
   - Trimethoprim-sulfamethoxazole to prevent *Pneumocystis jirovici* and UTIs for 6 months
   - Nystatin or clotrimazole to prevent esophageal candidiasis for 3 months

5. **What is BK virus?**
   BK virus is a ubiquitous, double-stranded DNA polyomavirus with a 5300–base pair genome that replicates in the host nucleus. The polyoma family includes JC virus (infectious cause of progressive multifocal leukoencephalopathy [PML]), SV40, and monkey polyomavirus. Although the human polyomaviruses are highly seroprevalent in humans, they appear to cause clinical disease only in immunocompromised hosts.

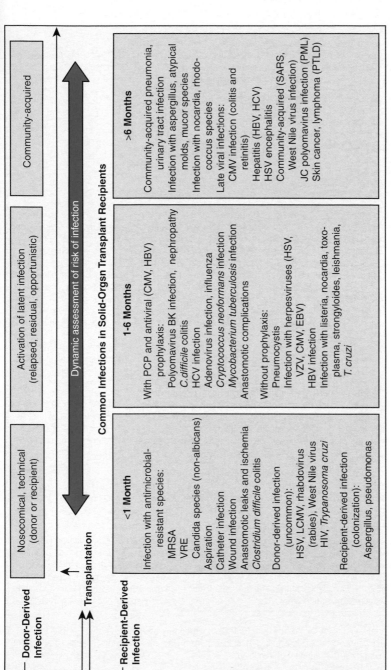

Figure 60.1. Timeline of common infections in transplant recipients. *CMV,* Cytomegalovirus; *EBV,* Epstein-Barr virus; *HBV,* hepatitis B virus; *HCV,* hepatitis C virus; *HSV,* herpes simplex virus; *LCMV,* lymphocytic choriomeningitis; *MRSA,* methicillin-resistant *Staphylococcus aureus; PCP, Pneumocystis jiroveci* pneumonia; *PML,* progressive multifocal leukoencephalopathy; *PTLD,* posttransplant lymphoproliferative disorder; *SARS,* severe acute respiratory syndrome; *VRE,* vancomycin-resistant enterococci; *VZV,* varicella-zoster virus. (From *New England Journal of Medicine,* Fishman, J. A., *Infection in solid-organ transplant recipients,* Volume 357, page 2606, Copyright 2007 Massachusetts Medical Society. Reprinted with permission from Massachusetts Medical Society.)

The figure contains the following text:

Common Infections in Solid-Organ Transplant Recipients

Donor-Derived Infection

Recipient-Derived Infection

| Nosocomical, technical (donor or recipient) | Activation of latent infection (relapsed, residual, opportunistic) | Community-acquired |

Transplantation

Dynamic assessment of risk of infection

<1 Month

Infection with antimicrobial-resistant species:
MRSA
VRE
Candida species (non-albicans)
Aspiration
Catheter infection
Wound infection
Anastomotic leaks and ischemia
Clostridium difficile colitis

Donor-derived infection (uncommon):
HSV, LCMV, rhabdovirus (rabies), West Nile virus
HIV, *Trypanosoma cruzi*

Recipient-derived infection (colonization):
Aspergillus, pseudomonas

1-6 Months

With PCP and antiviral (CMV, HBV) prophylaxis:
Polyomavirus BK infection, nephropathy
C.difficile colitis
HCV infection
Adenovirus infection, influenza
Cryptococcus neoformans infection
Mycobacterium tuberculosis infection
Anastomotic complications

Without prophylaxis:
Pneumocystis
Infection with herpesviruses (HSV, VZV, CMV, EBV)
HBV infection
Infection with listeria, nocardia, toxoplasma, strongyloides, leishmania, *T. cruzi*

>6 Months

Community-acquired pneumonia, urinary tract infection
Infection with aspergillus, atypical molds, mucor species
Infection with nocardia, rhodococcus species
Late viral infections:
CMV infection (colitis and retinitis)
Hepatitis (HBV, HCV)
HSV encephalitis
Community-acquired (SARS, West Nile virus infection)
JC polyomavirus infection (PML)
Skin cancer, lymphoma (PTLD)

6. What is BK-associated nephropathy?
   BK virus damages the transplant kidney. The prevalence of BK nephropathy ranges from 1% to 10%. BK nephropathy is characterized by a tubulointerstitial disease pattern that closely resembles acute rejection.

7. Besides nephropathy, can BK virus cause any other kidney problems?
   Yes. BK virus is associated with ureteral stenosis/strictures, which may lead to obstructive uropathy. Obstructions associated with BK virus usually occurs 2 to 4 months post transplant, whereas ischemia-induced stenosis usually occurs 1 to 2 weeks postoperatively.

8. What are the risk factors for the development of BK-associated nephropathy?
   - Human leukocyte antigen mismatch
   - Previous acute rejection
   - Use of lymphocyte depleting therapy
   - Use of steroid pulses
   - Age >55
   - Male gender
   - White race
   - Diabetes

9. Discuss BK screening.
   BK virus is detectable both in the blood and the urine. The virus first appears in the urine (viruria) and then is detectable in the blood (viremia) several weeks later. The preferred screening test at most transplant centers is the blood BK quantitative viral DNA polymerase chain reaction (PCR). The sensitivity between the serum and urine BK viral testing is the same at 100%, but the specificity of serum testing is 90% versus 80% for urine testing. BK viremia is also a better predictor of BK nephropathy. There is an alternative strategy that does use BK viruria for screening because it appears earlier that BK viremia. Once BK viruria is present, the clinician considers lowering immunosuppression and now switching to BK viremia for screening.
   Recommended screening times are monthly for the first 6 months and then every 3 months up to 24 months post transplant.
   A BK viral load greater than 10,000 copies is strongly associated with BK nephropathy. BK viruria greater than 1,000,000 copies is associated with BK nephropathy. The next step is a kidney transplant biopsy, which is the gold standard to confirm the diagnosis and see the degree of nephropathy.

10. What does the kidney biopsy show in BK-associated nephropathy?
    Biopsy remains the gold standard for the diagnosis of BK-associated nephropathy. BK virus can induce a number of characteristic changes on kidney biopsy, including intranuclear viral inclusions, tubular injury/tubulitis, and tubulointerstitial inflammation. Because none of these kidney biopsy findings are pathognomonic for BK-associated nephropathy, the diagnosis must be confirmed by demonstrating antibodies against BK with immunohistochemistry.

11. What does urine cytology show in BK-associated nephropathy?
    Cytologic examination of the urine can detect BK-infected cells ("decoy cells"). These characteristic cells have enlarged nuclei with a single, basophilic, intranuclear inclusion. Identification of decoy cells is sensitive, but not specific, for the diagnosis of BK-associated nephropathy.

12. What is the treatment for BK-associated nephropathy?
    The goal in treating BK-associated nephropathy is to eradicate the virus while maintaining kidney function and preventing acute or chronic rejection. Most treatments of BK-associated nephropathy involve reducing immunosuppression to permit native, immune-mediated handling of the BK virus. Possible strategies include discontinuation of a single immunosuppressive agent, reduction of dosages, and steroid avoidance. Antiviral therapy with leflunomide or cidofovir has been used in conjunction with decreasing immunosuppressants in some instances. IVIG also has been used, particularly in patients with concomitant acute rejection.

13. Can patients with graft failure resulting from BK nephropathy be retransplanted?
    Yes. Transplant nephrectomy is usually not indicated. Ideally the BK viral load should be undetectable in the serum by PCR at the time of transplant.

14. Discuss CMV, including risk factors for the development of CMV infections post transplantation.
    CMV is a member of the genus *Herpesvirus* and belongs to the family *Herpesviridae*. It is composed of a double-stranded DNA genome. Exposure to the virus, as indicated by immunoglobulin G anti-CMV

antibodies, is present in more than two-thirds of donors and recipients prior to transplantation. CMV can be transmitted from the donor either by blood transfusions or by the transplanted kidney. Symptomatic CMV infection occurs in 20% to 60% of all transplant recipients and is a significant cause of morbidity and mortality.

Risk factors associated with the development of CMV infections post transplantation include lymphocyte-depleting induction therapy, high-dose MMF, and the absence of adequate antiviral prophylaxis.

15. **What groups are at highest risk from CMV infections?**
Historically, groups who are CMV donor positive and CMV recipient negative (CMV D+/R-) are at greatest risk for severe "primary" infection during the first 3 months post transplantation.

16. **Besides infection, what other ways does CMV infection affect the transplant recipient?**
CMV has been associated with atherosclerosis and chronic allograft rejection. CMV is associated with several other vascular injuries, including transplant glomerulopathy, hemolytic uremic syndrome, thrombotic microangiopathy, and transplant renal artery stenosis.

17. **How do you diagnose CMV disease in a kidney transplant recipient?**
CMV infection implies the detection of CMV via culture or PCR. By comparison, CMV disease requires clinical signs and symptoms, in addition to viral detection. The clinical signs and symptoms of CMV disease include fever, leukopenia, or organ involvement (hepatitis, pneumonitis, colitis, chorioretinitis, etc.). The quantitative assessment of viral load via PCR can help determine the clinical phenotype. CMV DNA levels >500 copies/mmg of total DNA in peripheral blood correlates with clinically evident disease.

18. **What are the prophylactic strategies for CMV infection?**
There are two strategies for CMV prevention; antiviral prophylaxis and preemptive monitoring/therapy. Antiviral prophylaxis means giving valganciclovir without any evidence of CMV infection or viremia. Preemptive monitoring/therapy means reserving antiviral therapy for patients who develop CMV viremia. Preemptive monitoring is associated with lower drug costs and adverse toxicities. However, there are increased laboratory surveillance and logistical labor. Antiviral prophylaxis, on the other hand, is more expensive and puts patients at risk for drug toxicity but is associated with decreased reactivation of other herpesvirus, lower rates of opportunistic infections, and allograft loss. The drug of choice for prophylaxis is valganciclovir. The duration of CMV prophylaxis depends on the CMV serology of the donor and recipient. D+/R- prophylaxis lasts 6 months, and all others last 3 months.

19. **What is the treatment for CMV?**
Ganciclovir and valganciclovir are the most commonly used agents for the treatment of CMV infection. Both drugys must be dosed based on renal function. Valganciclovir is indicated in patients with mild to moderate disease. The treatment dose with normal kidney function is 900 mg twice daily. The dose needs to be reduced in kidney failure. Ganciclovir is indicated in more severe disease, those with high viral load, or those with questionable gastrointestinal absorption. Treatment is usually continued until the viral load is undetectable for 2 weeks, then the patient is switched to 1 to 3 months of prophylactic therapy. If the viral load does not change with appropriately dosed ganciclovir after 2 to 3 weeks, then ganciclovir resistance should be assessed by viral genotype testing. If resistance is discovered, the usual strategy is to increase the ganciclovir dose or use foscarnet or cidofovir. However, these are nephrotoxic. The other aspect of treatment is the careful reduction of immunosuppression.

20. **What is Epstein-Barr virus (EBV) and what posttransplantation condition is it associated with?**
EBV is a member of the herpesvirus family and one of the most common human viruses. Most people become infected with EBV sometime during their lives. It can flourish in the setting of immunosuppression and is associated with PTLD.

21. **Discuss vaccinations in reference to kidney transplantation.**
Live vaccines are contraindicated after transplantation and should be administered prior. If a live vaccine is given prior to transplantation, the patient cannot be on immunosuppression and therefore transplanted for a minimum of 4 weeks. Inactivated vaccines can be given post transplant. The time frame to be able to receive a vaccination post transplant is 3 to 6 months. Close contacts should also be appropriately vaccinated. Table 60.1 shows a table of commonly questioned vaccinations.

The inhaled influenza vaccine is a live attenuated vaccine and is contraindicated. Patients traveling abroad should consider visiting a travel clinic for appropriate vaccinations and prophylaxis as needed.

Table 60.1. Vaccine Timing and Transplant

VACCINE	INACTIVATED/LIVE ATTENUATED	GIVE PRIOR OR AFTER TRANSPLANTATION
Influenza (injected)	Inactivated	Both
Hepatitis B	Inactivated	Both but preferably completed prior to transplant
Tetanus	Inactivated	Both
Pertussis (Tdap)	Inactivated	Both
Streptococcus pneumoniae	Inactivated	Both
Neisseria meningitidis	Inactivated	Both
Rabies	Inactivated	Both
Measles-Mumps-Rubella (MMR)	Live Attenuated	Only Prior
Varicella	Live Attenuated	Only Prior
Human Papilloma Virus	Inactivated	Both

22. Is hepatitis C treatable post kidney transplant?
    Yes. Interferon alpha and ribavirin are contraindicated post transplant. Direct-acting antiviral agents (DAAs) can be used in the kidney transplant population with an estimated glomerular filtration rate >30 mL/min. This has also increased the use of hepatitis C–positive kidneys in transplantation, increasing the transplant rate. A patient with hepatitis C, if not overtly cirrhotic, can be listed for a hepatitis C kidney, which has a substantially shorter wait time. They are treated post transplant with DAAs. Studies are being developed to look at transplanting organs from Hepatitis C positive donors to hepatitis C negative recipients. The recipients would be treated for Hepatitis C posttransplant.

23. What are the requirements for a human immunodeficiency virus (HIV)-infected individual to qualify for a transplant?
    Well-controlled HIV with CD4 counts >200 cells/mmL, undetectable viral load, and the absence of untreatable infection or malignancy. There must be great care taken in these patients because their antiretroviral medications have significant interactions with transplant medications.

24. What central nervous system infections are of particular concern in patients who have undergone solid organ transplant?
    • Listeria meningitis
    • Herpes simplex virus encephalitis
    • JC virus–induced PML
    • *Cryptococcus neoformans* meningitis

KEY POINTS

1. Nosocomial and surgery-related infections are the predominant infections that occur within the first month post transplantation.
2. Although the human polyomaviruses are highly seroprevalent in humans, they appear to cause clinical disease only in immunocompromised hosts.
3. The goal in treating BK-associated nephropathy is to eradicate the virus while maintaining kidney function and preventing acute or chronic rejection.
4. CMV-positive donor to CMV-negative recipient (CMV D+/R-) transplants are at greatest risk for severe "primary" infection during the first 3 months post transplantation. However, CMV D+/R+ group and not the D+/R- group has the worst graft and patient survival at 3 years. This could be secondary to increased vigilance in monitoring the CMV D+/- group.
5. Epstein-Barr virus can flourish in the setting of immunosuppression and is associated with the majority of posttransplant lymphoproliferative disorder.
6. Live vaccines are contraindicated post transplant.

Bibliography

Fishman, J. A. (2007). Infection in solid-organ transplant recipients. *New England Journal of Medicine, 357*(25), 2601–2614. doi:357/25/2601. [pii].

Jamboti, J. S. (2016). BK virus nephropathy in renal transplant recipients. *Nephrology (Carlton), 21*(8), 647–654. doi:10.1111/nep.12728.

Karuthu, S., & Blumberg, E. A. (2012). Common infections in kidney transplant recipients. *Clinical Journal of the American Society of Nephrology, 7*(12), 2058–2070. doi:10.2215/CJN.04410512.

Ramanan, P., & Razonable, R. R. (2013). Cytomegalovirus infections in solid organ transplantation: A review. *Infection & Chemotherapy, 45*(3), 260–271. doi:10.3947/ic.2013.45.3.260.

Sawinski, D., & Goral, S. (2015). BK virus infection: An update on diagnosis and treatment. *Nephrology Dialysis Transplantation, 30*(2), 209–217. doi:10.1093/ndt/gfu023.

Sawinski, D., Kaur, N., Ajeti, A., Trofe-Clark, J., Lim, M., Bleicher, M., . . . Bloom, R. D. (2016). Successful treatment of hepatitis C in renal transplant recipients with direct-acting antiviral agents. *American Journal of Transplantation, 16*(5), 1588–1595. doi:10.1111/ajt.13620.

CHAPTER 61

PRIMARY CARE OF THE KIDNEY TRANSPLANT RECIPIENT

Beje Thomas and Matthew R. Weir

1. What are the risk factors for cardiovascular disease (CVD) in patients receiving a kidney transplant? See Table 61.1.

2. Are statins beneficial in patients receiving kidney transplant?
   Statins are the treatment of choice, and studies show there is a benefit to using them in the kidney transplant population. The incidence of dyslipidemia is high in kidney transplant patients secondary to immunosuppressive medications, proteinuria, transplant dysfunction, and the higher incidence of metabolic syndrome and new-onset diabetes after transplant. Various trials have shown improved cardiovascular outcomes with the use of lipid therapy in patient with chronic kidney disease. The Assessment of Lescol in Renal Transplantation (ALERT) study aimed to see if statin therapy reduced the primary outcome of a major cardiovascular event, including cardiac death or a cardiac intervention. The trial did not reach this primary end point due to insufficient power but did show a reduction in nonfatal myocardial infarctions. In the extended follow-up of ALERT participants, the incidence of major adverse cardiac events was reduced in patients treated with statin; however, there was no difference in patient mortality or allograft function. A Cochrane Database review stated that statins may reduce cardiovascular events in kidney transplant patients. However, statin treatment had no clear benefit in affecting overall mortality, stroke rate, kidney function, and toxicity outcomes in kidney transplant patients.
   Statin use is associated with decreased proteinuria, decreased C-reactive protein, and decreased interstitial fibrosis incidence in transplant protocol biopsies, all which may confer additional benefit.

3. Which patients should be started on a statin post transplant?
   If a patient is younger than 30 years without established atherosclerotic cardiovascular disease (ACVD) or diabetes, then based on the benefit-to-risk ratio, the patient can start a statin. Ideally all kidney transplant patients older than 30 years should be considered for a statin.

4. How do we monitor lipid levels?
   Patients should have an initial lipid profile checked. The American College of Cardiology recommends follow-up in 4 to 12 weeks for compliance and then at least yearly lipid profile checks. Kidney Disease Improving

Table 61.1. Risk Factors for Cardiovascular Disease

TRADITIONAL	TRANSPLANT RELATED	CONDITIONAL
Age	Immunosuppression	Homocysteine
Male sex	CKD	CRP
Family history	Proteinuria	AGEs
Obesity	Anemia	
Diabetes		
Hypertension		
Hyperlipidemia		
Tobacco abuse		

AGEs, Advanced glycosylated end products; *CKD,* chronic kidney disease; *CRP,* C-reactive protein.

Global Outcomes (KDIGO) guidelines differ in that they do not require to repeat lipid profiles, because the indication for treatment is the higher cardiovascular risk, not the low-density lipoprotein (LDL) level.

5. What are the goals of lipid lowering therapy?

In the general population, target goals for the lipid profile have been replaced by the aim of therapy being to reduce ACVD risk. As mentioned earlier, KDIGO guidelines follow with this. However, although the KDIGO guidelines do not require repeat lipid profiles, it might be prudent to recheck a lipid profile after statin therapy to confirm compliance, response to therapy, and reevaluation ACVD risk.

6. Are there any risks of statin use in transplant recipients?

Yes. Most statins are metabolized by the same cytochrome P450 system (CP3A4) as calcineurin inhibitors (CNIs). As a consequence, CNIs (particularly cyclosporine) may accumulate in plasma and may be associated with a greater frequency of rhabdomyolysis. Data on tacrolimus are sparse, although pharmacokinetic studies on concomitant atorvastatin and tacrolimus therapy did not demonstrate significant interactions. Fluvastatin and pravastatin may be safer because they are metabolized through non-CP3A4 mechanisms. Fluvastatin, pravastatin, rosuvastatin, simvastatin, and atorvastatin have all been used in kidney transplant patients. These patients should be closely monitored for side effects from statin therapy. It is important to note that cyclosporine inhibits the metabolism of statins, and so the statin dose is usually kept low and not aggressively titrated up.

7. What are the causes of hypertension (HTN) in patients who have undergone kidney transplant?
   - Primary HTN
   - Secondary HTN related to native kidneys
   - Recipient factors, including male gender, genetic profile, metabolic syndrome, and diabetes
   - Donor factors, inducing HTN history, age, allograft quality, and donor-recipient size discrepancy
   - Immunosuppression in particular CNIs
   - Kidney allograft dysfunction
   - Allograft vascular compromise
   - Obstructive sleep apnea
   - Kidney artery stenosis

8. What is the optimal blood pressure medication for kidney transplant recipients?

Because there is no evidence that a particular class of antihypertensive agents is more effective than other classes, the choice of medications should be individualized and based on various comorbidities. Calcium channel blockers (CCBs) are an attractive first-line agent, mainly because they counteract the vasoconstrictive effects of CNIs. CCB use may cause untoward effects, particularly nondependent edema and worsening proteinuria. In addition, CNI doses may need reduction with the use of nondihydropyridine CCBs.

The use of angiotensin-converting enzyme (ACE) inhibitors/angiotensin receptor blockers (ARBs) in kidney transplant recipients is safe. However, the effectiveness has been questioned. Hiremath et al. performed a meta-analysis of eight trials involving a total of 1502 patients, with only two trials going beyond 5 years. The study did not show an improvement in kidney outcomes. Other studies have shown the use of ACE inhibitors/ARBs has been associated with prolonged allograft and patient survival. In summary, ACE inhibitors/ARBs should be used thoughtfully, weighing the pros and cons in the transplant patient.

Because the combination of afferent arteriolar vasoconstriction from CNI and efferent arteriolar vasodilation as a result of renin-angiotensin system (RAS) blockade can predispose to acute kidney injury, we routinely advise our patients to discontinue their ACE inhibitors/ARBs if they are acutely ill and at risk for volume depletion. In addition, we advise postponing the addition of RAS blockers until 3 months post transplantation to avoid superfluous kidney biopsies.

Beta blockers should be considered in all kidney transplant patients with CVD. Diuretics can be used to control volume-mediated HTN and to enhance the antihypertensive effects of ACE inhibitors/ARBs. These drugs help with volume control and augment urine output. Thiazide-type diuretics are particularly effective at countering CNI-induced hyperkalemia. Alpha-1 blockers and centrally acting agents may be necessary to achieve blood pressure goals.

9. What is the blood pressure goal for kidney transplant recipients?

Kidney Disease Outcomes Quality Initiative (K/DOQI) guidelines suggest a blood pressure goal of less than 130/80 mm Hg for all kidney transplant recipients.

10. **What is NODAT?**
    NODAT is an acronym for new-onset diabetes after transplantation. The prevalence of NODAT is anywhere from 15% to 30%, with the majority of cases occurring shortly after transplant. The major risk factors are divided into nonmodifiable (age, male sex, genetics, polycystic kidney, race, previous glucose intolerance) and modifiable (obesity, sedentary lifestyle, metabolic syndrome, immunosuppression with steroids, CNIs, and sirolimus). Oral agents are typically used to manage NODAT. The patient should also be advised on a healthier lifestyle. Goal of therapy is a hemoglobin (HbA1c) less than 7%

11. **Should all patients who have received kidney transplant be screened and counseled on tobacco use?**
    Yes. The same strategies to prevent and treat tobacco use in the general population should be applied to all transplant recipients. Smoking at the time of transplantation is associated with graft failure and death. In addition, smoking has been associated with posttransplantation malignancies. Kidney transplant recipients who stopped smoking more than 5 years before transplantation had a 34% risk reduction in cardiovascular events. There are no interactions between immunosuppressive medications and tobacco cessation medications that would obviate their administration.

12. **Should kidney transplant recipients be screened and counseled on obesity?**
    Yes. Obesity is independently associated with cardiovascular events and mortality in kidney transplant recipients. In addition, obesity can predispose to insulin resistance, diabetes, and reduced graft survival. Diet and other behavior modifications are safe and may help reduce weight, eventually improving long-term graft survival. Weight loss guidance and support is necessary in all transplant recipients who are overweight.

13. **What is the role of acetylsalicylic acid (ASA) prophylaxis in transplant recipients?**
    In the general population, daily ASA (aspirin) use decreases cardiovascular events in patients at high risk of CVD. In patients receiving kidney transplant, low-dose aspirin therapy is associated with improved allograft function and prolonged allograft survival. The current guidelines recommend the use of aspirin dosed from 65 to 325 mg/daily for primary and secondary prevention of CVD in the kidney transplant recipient with CVD, diabetes, or other risk factors. The institution of daily ASA therapy for all patients receiving kidney transplant should be weighed against the higher risk of gastrointestinal bleeding in this population.

14. **What is the significance of proteinuria in kidney transplant recipients?**
    In patients who have received kidney transplant, proteinuria occurs in up to 45% of cases. It is associated with CVD events and mortality. A baseline level of urine protein should be obtained in the first month post transplantation, every 3 months in the first year post transplantation, and then annually. It is important to note the patient's urine output prior to transplant, as diseased native kidneys can be a cause of posttransplant proteinuria. Persistent proteinuria not from the native kidneys is a sign of allograft pathology, including transplant glomerulopathy, interstitial fibrosis and tubular atrophy, de novo or recurrence of a primary nephrotic disease, and rejection. Mammalian target of rapamycin (mTOR) inhibitors may cause proteinuria. The gold standard for diagnosing the cause of the proteinuria is kidney transplant biopsy. In regards to treatment, RAAS blockade should be considered to reduce proteinuria.

15. **Is mineral bone disease common in the kidney transplant population?**
    Yes. Chronic kidney disease–mineral bone disease (CKD-MBD) is common in kidney transplant recipients. Use of corticosteroids as part of the immunosuppressive regiment may further affect CKD-MBD management. Studies have demonstrated a rapid decrease in bone mineral density in the first 6 to 12 months after transplantation. In addition, fractures are common in kidney transplant recipients and are associated with substantial morbidity. Monitoring bone mineral density should be routine for all patients taking chronic corticosteroids. Monitoring parathyroid hormone is also important, particularly in the setting of high calcium. It takes 3 to 6 months for PTH to start to decrease. Bisphosphonate administration is often necessary to maintain and restore bone mineral density, particularly in the setting of chronic steroid and immunosuppressant use. Bisphosphonate use has not shown decreased fracture incidence.

16. **Is nutritional vitamin D deficiency prevalent in the kidney transplant population?**
    It is extremely prevalent. It is estimated that 56% of early kidney transplant patients are vitamin D deficient (12 to 39 nmol/L) and 12% are severely vitamin D deficient (<12 nmol/L). Vitamin D stores should be repleted as per general population guidelines.

17. **When is the best time to vaccinate a transplant recipient?**
Ideally, patients who have received a transplant should receive all vaccinations prior to transplantation to provide the strongest native immunoprotection. If this is not possible, vaccinations should be administered when the immunosuppressant dosages are reduced (usually 6 to 12 months post transplantation). Influenza vaccinations should be given to all patients who have undergone transplant and their close contacts. It is recommended that the influenza vaccine be given prior to the onset of the annual influenza season, provided the recipient is at least 1 month post transplant. If available, H1N1 vaccinations should be administered to all eligible kidney transplant recipients.

18. **What vaccinations should not be given to patients who have undergone kidney transplant?**
In general, all live vaccines are contradicted in patients on Immunosuppression. These include vaccines for varicella zoster; bacille Calmette-Guérin; smallpox; intranasal influenza; measles, mumps, and rubella; oral polio; and yellow fever.

19. **What cancer screening does a kidney transplant patient require?**
Screening recommendations for breast, prostate, and colon cancers in transplant recipients mirror guidelines from the US Preventive Services Task Force. It is imperative, particularly with the higher risk of skin cancer in the kidney transplant patient, that they be seen by a dermatologist once a year.

20. **What is the preferred creatinine-based glomerular filtration rate (GFR) estimation equation for monitoring kidney transplant patients?**
Chronic Kidney Disease Epidemiology Collaboration (CKD-EPI) equation is preferred over the modification of diet in renal disease (MDRD) equation.

KEY POINTS

1. Fluvastatin, pravastatin, and atorvastatin seem to have a more favorable safety profile in kidney transplant recipients.
2. Because there is no evidence that a particular class of antihypertensive agents is more effective than other classes, the choice of medications should be individualized and based on various comorbidities.
3. Kidney Disease Outcomes Quality Initiative (K/DOQI) guidelines suggest goal blood pressure less than 130/80 mm Hg for all kidney transplant recipients.
4. NODAT should be carefully monitored for and develops in up to 54% of kidney transplant patients, particularly in the first 6 months.
5. Studies have demonstrated a rapid decrease in bone mineral density in the first 6 to 12 months after transplantation.

BIBLIOGRAPHY

Baigent, C., Landray, M. J., Reith, C., Emberson, J., Wheeler, D. C., Tomson, C., . . . SHARP Investigators. (2011). The effects of lowering LDL cholesterol with simvastatin plus ezetimibe in patients with chronic kidney disease (Study of Heart and Renal Protection): A randomised placebo-controlled trial. *Lancet, 377*(9784), 2181–2192.

Cimino, F. M., & Snyder, K. A. (2016). Primary care of the solid organ transplant recipient. *American Family Physician, 93*(3), 203–210.

Danziger-Isakov, L., Kumar, D., & AST Infectious Diseases Community of Practice. (2013). Vaccination in solid organ transplantation. *American Journal of Transplantation, 13*(Suppl. 4), 311–317. doi:10.1111/ajt.12122.

Hiremath, S., Fergusson, D. A., Fergusson, N., Bennett, A., & Knoll, G. A. (2017). Renin-angiotensin system blockade and long-term clinical outcomes in kidney transplant recipients: A meta-analysis of randomized controlled trials. *American Journal of Kidney Disease, 69*(1), 78–86. doi:S0272-6386(16)30420-6.

Holdaas, H., Fellström, B., Cole, E, Nyberg, G., Olsson, A. G., Pedersen, T. R., . . . Assessment of LEscol in Renal Transplantation (ALERT) Study Investigators. (2005). Long-term cardiac outcomes in renal transplant recipients receiving fluvastatin: The ALERT extension study. *American Journal of Transplantation, 5*(12), 2929–2936. doi:AJT1105.

Kasiske, B. L., Vazquez, M. A., Harmon, W. E., Brown, R. S., Danovitch, G. M., Gaston, R. S., . . . Singer, G. G. (2000). Recommendations for the outpatient surveillance of renal transplant recipients. American Society of Transplantation. *Journal of the American Society of Nephrology, 11*(Suppl. 15), S1–S86.

Kidney Disease: Improving Global Outcomes (KDIGO) Transplant Work Group. (2009). KDIGO clinical practice guideline for the care of kidney transplant recipients. *American Journal of Transplantation, 9*(Suppl. 3), S1–S155. doi:10.1111/j.1600-6143.2009.02834.x.

Palepu, S., & Prasad, G. V. (2015). New-onset diabetes mellitus after kidney transplantation: Current status and future directions. *World Journal of Diabetes, 6*(3), 445–455. doi:10.4239/wjd.v6.i3.445.

Palmer, S. C., Navaneethan, S. D, Craig, J. C, Perkovic, V., Johnson, D. W., Nigwekar, S. U., . . . Strippoli, G. F. (2014). HMG CoA reductase inhibitors (statins) for kidney transplant recipients. *Cochrane Database of Systematic Review, 1,* CD005019. doi:10.1002/14651858.CD005019.pub4.

Sarnak, M. J., Bloom, R., Muntner, P., Rahman, M., Saland, J. M., Wilson, P. W., & Fried, L. (2015). KDOQI US commentary on the 2013 KDIGO clinical practice guideline for lipid management in CKD. *American Journal of Kidney Diseases, 65*(3), 354–366. doi:10.1053/j.ajkd.2014.10.005.

Shaffi, K., Uhlig, K., Perrone, R. D , Ruthazer R,, Rule, A., Lieske, J. C., . . . Levey, A. S. (2014). Performance of creatinine-based GFR estimating equations in solid-organ transplant recipients. *American Journal of Kidney Diseases, 63*(6), 1007–1018. doi:10.1053/j.ajkd.2014.01.436.

Shamseddin, M. K., & Knoll, G. A. (2011). Posttransplantation proteinuria: An approach to diagnosis and management. *Clinical Journal of the American Society of Nephrology, 6*(7), 1786–1793. doi:10.2215/CJN.01310211.

Stavroulopoulos, A., Cassidy, M. J., Porter, C. J., Hosking, D. J., & Roe, S. D. (2007). Vitamin D status in renal transplant recipients. *American Journal of Transplantation, 7*(11), 2546–2552.

Taler, S. J., Agarwal, R., Bakris, G. L., Flynn, J. T., Nilsson, P. M., Rahman, M., . . . Townsend, R. R. (2013). KDOQI US commentary on the 2012 KDIGO clinical practice guideline for management of blood pressure in CKD. *American Journal of Kidney Diseases, 62*(2), 201–213. doi:10.1053/j.ajkd.2013.03.018.

Thomas, B., & Weir, M. R. (2015). The evaluation and therapeutic management of hypertension in the transplant patient. *Current Cardiology Reports, 17*(11), 95. doi:10.1007/s11886-015-0647-z.

Toth-Manikowski, S. M., Francis, J. M., Gautam, A., & Gordon, C. E. (2016). Outcomes of bisphosphonate therapy in kidney transplant recipients: A systematic review and meta-analysis. *Clinical Transplantation, 30*(9), 1090–1096. doi:10.1111/ctr.12792.

XII
HYPERTENSION

CHAPTER 62

PRIMARY HYPERTENSION

Hillel Sternlicht and George L. Bakris

1. **How is hypertension defined and classified?**

   The Eighth Report of the Joint National Committee on Prevention, Detection, Evaluation, and Treatment of High Blood Pressure (Joint National Committee 8), published in 2014, continues to classify hypertension by the degree of blood pressure (BP) elevation (Table 62.1A and B). The measurement must be based on the average of at least two seated measurements on each of two or more office visits. For children, hypertension is defined as systolic or diastolic BP greater than the 95th percentile of BP for a given age, height, and gender, on repeat measurement.

   While national and international guidelines have largely promoted uniform BP targets for all populations (<140/90 for those younger than 80, <150/90 for those older than 80), there is increasing recognition that "goal" BP is patient and comorbid specific. For those with prior strokes, the range of 125 to 135/70 to 80 is desired, whereas 130 to 135/80 is adequate for those with non-proteinuric kidney disease. Finally, among those at low-to-moderate risk for cardiovascular disease without diabetes, 120 to 125/70 to 80 appears to provide maximal benefit. The 2017 ACC/AHA guidelines define the systolic BP target of <130/80 mm Hg for everyone except those with a <10% 10-year risk for cardiovascular (CV) events where it is still <140/90.

2. **What is the appropriate means of measuring BP?**

   Measuring BP in the office should be performed with individuals seated for at least 5 minutes in a chair with their feet on the ground and an arm supported at the level of the heart. An appropriate-sized cuff with the cuff bladder encircling at least 80% but no more than 100% of the upper arm should be used; attention should be paid to ensure the bladder covers the brachial artery. While the "gold standard" remains a mercury sphygmomanometer, electronic (oscillometric) monitors have grown in popularity, and are being utilized in both clinical trials and office-based practice. Ausculatory oscillometric blood pressure (AOBP) devices were used in trials such as SPRINT and ACCORD, but they provide readings that are 5 to 10 mm Hg systolic lower than conventional office measurements. Electronic units are simpler to use and can be set on a timer, which allows the provider to leave the room (thereby reducing the white coat effect). Moreover, they do not have the environmental concerns of mercury-based devices. However, many offices do not have a separate quiet room nor the time to measure BP in this way.

3. **Is home blood pressure monitoring useful?**

   Home BP monitoring, or ambulatory BP monitoring, is better at predicting cardiovascular events compared to office-based readings. Home BP is documented to improved BP control and patient adherence with medications. It has also been validated against daytime 24-hour ABPM. Therefore home BP should occupy a prominent role in the management of hypertension.

   ABPM is used to rule out both white-coat and masked hypertension; BP readings during periods of dizziness or orthostasis can also aid in assessing the contribution of BP to such symptoms.

   Wrist-based cuff devices are unreliable, and therefore upper arm (brachial) cuff units are preferred. While many units are available, validation and accuracy are not prerequisites for production; therefore only rigorously tested machines should be purchased. The appropriate technique is like that for ausculatory measurements. Machines should be rechecked annually by measuring pressures against a validated unit.

4. **What is the prevalence of hypertension in the United States? How well is hypertension controlled among those with a diagnosis of hypertension?**

   The prevalence of hypertension rises with age so those at age 80 have a 90% chance of being hypertensive. According to the most recent (2014) National Health and Nutrition Examination Survey (NHANES) data, nearly one-third of Americans over the age of 18 suffer from hypertension, with the disease affecting two-thirds of those above age 60. The rates among men and women are similar. Hypertension is more common among African Americans (42%) than among Caucasians, Hispanics, and those of Asian ancestry (25% to 28%).

Table 62.1A. Classification for Adults 18 Years or Older with Elevated Blood Pressure

BP CATEGORY	SBP		DBP
Normal	<120 mm Hg	and	<80 mm Hg
Elevated	120–129 mm Hg	and	<80 mm Hg
Hypertension			
Stage 1	130–139 mm Hg	or	80–89 mm Hg
Stage 2	140–159 mm Hg	or	90–99 mm Hg
Stage 3	≥160 mm Hg	or	≥100 mm Hg

BP, Blood pressure; DBP, diastolic blood pressure; SBP, systolic blood pressure.

Table 62.1B. Classification for Adults 18 Years or Older with Elevated Blood Pressure

HYPERTENSION STAGE	SBP	DBP
Prehypertension	120–139 mm Hg	Or 80–89 mm Hg
Stage I	140–159 mm Hg	Or 90–99 mm Hg
Stage II	≥160 mm Hg	Or ≥100 mm Hg

DBP, Diastolic blood pressure; SBP, systolic blood pressure.

Awareness, treatment, and control of hypertension continue to rise but remain suboptimal. As at 2012, awareness rates were at 80%, treatment at 75%, and control rates at 53%.

5. What is the appropriate initial evaluation for individuals with hypertension?
   In the absence of end organ damage, care should be taken to ensure the patient has sustained elevations in BP. This is particularly important in geriatric patients who are prone to white-coat hypertension and high BP variability due to high sodium intake. Young people, including pregnant women, should be closely evaluated given the lifelong implications of treatment and potential adverse fetal effects of antihypertensive therapy. Home BP readings are an excellent source of collateral information, but 24-hour ambulatory BP monitoring also can be performed.
   Once sustained hypertension is documented, easily correctable causes of hypertension should be sought. The key to this is to evaluate for secondary causes of hypertension, the most common of which is primary hyperaldosteronism. Thus, one should ask about a history of hypokalemia that did not easily correct with supplements. Lifestyle factors, such as a high-salt diet, are a common cause of hypertension and can produce hypokalemia, although this is easily correctable with potassium supplements and low-sodium diet. Excessive alcohol intake, physical inactivity, and sleep/obstructive sleep apnea are important lifestyle issues to note as well, and they contribute to resistant hypertension. Common medications with hypertensive effects include nonsteroidal antiinflamatory drugs, oral contraceptives, stimulants, and perhaps decongestants and herbal supplements. Obesity, while a modifiable risk factor, is usually difficult for the patient to correct.
   Traditional "secondary" causes, such as Cushing disease, primary hyperaldosteronism (most common cause), pheochromocytoma, thyroid disease, and renal artery stenosis, should be evaluated based on clinical suspicion. Finally, it should be standard practice to check the patient's electrolyte levels, kidney function, and urine for albumin; assays for cholesterol and impaired glucose tolerance serve to further stratify the patient's overall CV risk.

6. What is the appropriate initial therapy for individuals with diagnosed hypertension?
   Initial therapy is predicated on age, ethnicity, body habitus, and kidney function. Comorbid conditions may also mandate specific agents as particular classes offer additional salutary effects more than those attributable to BP lowering alone.
   As outlined above, easily correctable causes of hypertension, such as diet, sleeping habits, and medications, should be addressed. Thereafter, among otherwise healthy individuals with persistent stage I hypertension, monotherapy with either a calcium channel blocker, thiazide-like diuretic

(chlorthalidone, indapamide), or a blocker of the renin-angiotensin system are considered first-line therapies. Those with diabetic nephropathy or heart failure should receive ACEi iARB therapy. β-blockers are not indicated for BP-lowering therapy, but they are the preferred agents for those with heart failure, arrhythmia, or recent myocardial infarction.

7. What are the most common side effects of antihypertensive that patients should be alerted to prior to starting therapy?
   While patients should be alerted to and continuously surveyed for the adverse medication effects (listed below), it is important to stress that such effects are uncommon and not to be expected.
   * **Diuretics:** photosensitivity, rash, hypokalemia, hyperuricemia/gout, impaired glucose tolerance, erectile dysfunction, orthostatic hypotension
   * **ACEi:** cough, hyperkalemia, angioedema, small elevations in creatinine due to hemodynamic changes
   * **ARBs:** hyperkalemia, cough (rarely), and angioedema (controversial), elevations in creatinine
   * **Dihydropyridine calcium channel blockers (amlodipine and others):** lower-extremity edema, flushing, headache, gingival hyperplasia
   * **Non-dihydropyridine calcium channel blockers (diltiazem, verapamil):** headache, edema, fatigue, constipation, gingival hyperplasia
   * **β-blockers:** bronchospasm, hypoglycemic unawareness (among those with diabetes), weight gain, unmasking of peripheral vascular disease; it is unclear if β-blockers cause depression or erectile dysfunction
   * **α-blockers:** urinary incontinence, orthostatic hypotension.

8. What is the pathophysiology of primary hypertension?
   The genesis of primary hypertension is not completely understood. Primary hypertension demonstrates a polygenic pattern of inheritance, and it is clear that multiple environmental and genetic factors coalesce. While BP is the product of systemic vascular resistance and cardiac output, the final common pathway is an elevation in systemic vascular resistance. Multiple lines of investigation have linked derangements in the kidney, vasculature, central and systemic nervous system, immune system, and cardiovascular system to the generation and maintenance of systemic hypertension. Heightened sympathetic tone, increases in total body sodium, and excess activation of the renin-angiotensin-aldosterone axis, among others, remain the commonly cited drivers of increased vascular tone. More recently, imbalances between endogenous vasoconstrictors, such as endothelin, and vasodilators such as nitric oxide have been implicated.

9. Why are thiazide-type diuretics one of the first-line agents for stage I primary hypertension?
   Among the current classes of antihypertensive agents, thiazide and thiazide-type diuretics are both the oldest and most evidence-based, showing consistent decreases in morbidity and mortality in large, randomized, controlled trials. While low-dose (12.5 to 25 mg) hydrochlorothiazide (HCTZ) is the most frequently prescribed thiazide at present, landmark and more recent trials demonstrate the superiority of chlorthalidone (25 mg), indapamide (2.5 mg), or higher dose HCTZ (50 to 100 mg) on cardiovascular outcomes. Moreover, given the contributions of sodium to volume-mediated hypertension, particularly in the "salt-sensitive" elderly and African American populations, agents that promote natriuresis are particularly effective.

10. Why are blockers of the renin-angiotensin system preferred in individuals with diabetic nephropathy?
    ACE inhibitors and ARBs are the preferred antihypertensive therapy in those with greater than 300 mg of albuminuria a day from diabetes. Such agents slow the progression of chronic kidney disease (CKD) more than other medication classes despite similar reductions in BP. Clinical trials in patients with Stage 3 and 4 CKD evaluating these agents in both type 1 and type 2 diabetes demonstrated greater slowing than conventional BP-lowering therapy. While there is slightly more evidence for ARB than ACE inhibitor therapies, their efficacy is felt to be related to a similar mechanism of action, so that agents from each class are considered therapeutic equivalents.

11. What is salt-sensitive hypertension? What is the effect of dietary salt restriction on BP?
    Salt resistance/sensitivity refers specifically to the effect of dietary sodium chloride (salt) intake on BP. Increased dietary salt intake promotes an early and uniform expansion of extracellular fluid volume and increased cardiac output. To compensate for these hemodynamic changes and to maintain constant BP with high sodium intake, peripheral vascular resistance falls and is associated with an increase in production of nitric oxide. Among those who are salt sensitive, the decline in peripheral

vascular resistance and the increase in nitric oxide are impaired or absent in salt sensitivity, promoting an increase in BP in these individuals.

Salt-sensitive hypertension has variable definitions, but is conventionally defined as an increase in systolic BP of $\geq$10 mm Hg in response to 6 g of dietary salt loading. Salt-sensitive hypertension is most prevalent in African Americans, the obese, the elderly, those with high pulse pressure (i.e., $\geq$70), and those with CKD. Among those with a salt-rich diet, changing to a sodium-restricted diet has consistently lowered BP. This salt-restricted diet is particularly useful in people with resistant hypertension. It also onhances of the antihypertensive effects of diuretics, ACE inhibitors, and ARBs. Current guidelines recommend diets containing no more than 100 mEq of sodium (2.3 g) per day, a target below the 3.4 g consumed by most Americans.

12. When should a secondary cause of hypertension be suspected and evaluated?

Evaluation for secondary causes of hypertension should be initiated based on history, physical exam, laboratory results, or clinical suspicion.

Anyone with difficult-to-correct or persistent hypokalemia should be suspected of secondary hypertension. Primary hyperaldosteronism is the most common cause of secondary hypertension. It is usually a bilateral adrenal hyperplasia. Not all patients have hypokalemia, and this may present with low normal potassium levels. Hypercortisolism (Cushing's syndrome or disease) is a relatively rare form of secondary hypertension and shows a strong female predominance. It presents with a picture of central obesity and thin extremities, which is different from obesity, and, biochemically, will be associated with hypokalemia and metabolic alkalosis. It can easily be mistaken for primary aldosteronism until the hormone levels for aldosterone and cortisol are obtained. Pheochromocytomas are also an uncommon form of secondary hypertension. Incidental adrenal masses are frequently found by computed tomography scan, but very few have biochemical evidence for a pheochromocytoma. Clinical signs of a pheochromocytomas include labile BP and orthostatic hypotension, findings that are also associated with poor sleep quality, and this should always be sought in the patient's history. Additional symptoms include waking in the night with very high pressures and sweats; in fact, it is the most common secondary cause of hypertension associated with orthostatic hypotension. Apart from fibromuscular dysplasia, renal artery stenosis is a manifestation of atherosclerotic disease found in patients with extensive atherosclerosis either from hypercholesterolemia or from smoking.

13. How does obesity contribute to hypertension?

The association between obesity and hypertension has been known since the days of the Framingham Heart Study. However, a causative role was unclear considering the long-standing view that adipose tissue was a hormonally and metabolically inert substance. More recent evidence suggests a direct role of visceral obesity in the development and maintenance of hypertension—a process driven by elevations in leptin and aldosterone. Leptin is synthesized and secreted by adipocytes and upregulates sympathetic activity. Visceral fat also produces angiotensin, which serves as a substrate in the renin angiotensin aldosterone system, and ultimately leads to higher circulating aldosterone levels. Elevations in aldosterone levels and enhanced sympathetic activity ultimately promote urinary sodium retention, and, thus, hypertension. Finally, obesity suppresses adiponectin, a natriuretic hormone.

In addition to obesity, there are a number of lifestyle issues discussed in this chapter that can directly reduce BP if done consistently (Table 62.2).

Table 62.2. Lifestyle Issues that Can Directly Reduce Blood Pressure

			Approximate Impact on SBP	
	NON-PHARMACOLOGIC INTERVENTION	DOSE	HYPERTENSION	NORMOTENSION
Physical activity	Aerobic	• 90–150 min/ week • 65%–75% heart rate reserve	-5/8 mm Hg	-2/4 mm Hg

Table 62.2. Lifestyle Issues that Can Directly Reduce Blood Pressure—cont'd

NON-PHARMACOLOGIC INTERVENTION		DOSE	*Approximate Impact on SBP*	
			HYPERTENSION	NORMOTENSION
	Dynamic Resistance	• 90–150 min/week • 50%–80% 1 rep maximum • 6 exercises, 3 sets/exercise, 10 repetitions/set	-4 mm Hg	-2 mm Hg
	Isometric Resistance	• 4 × 2 minutes (hand grip), 1 minute rest between exercises, 30%–40% maximum voluntary contraction, 3 sessions/week • 8–10 weeks	-5 mm Hg	-4 mm Hg
Healthy diet	DASH dietary pattern	Diet rich in fruits, vegetables, whole grains, and low-fat dairy products with reduced content of saturated and total fat	-11 mm Hg	-3 mm Hg
Weight loss	Weight/body fat	Ideal body weight is the best goal, but at least 1 kg reduction in body weight for most adults who are overweight	-5 mm Hg	-2/3 mm Hg
Reduced intake of dietary sodium	Dietary sodium	<1500 mg/day is the optimal goal but at least 1000 mg/day reduction in most adults	-5/6 mm Hg	-2/3 mm Hg
Enhanced intake of dietary potassium	Dietary potassium	3500–5000 mg/day, preferably by consumption of a diet rich in potassium	-4/5 mm Hg	-2 mm Hg
Moderation in alcohol intake	Alcohol consumption	In individuals who drink alcohol, reduce alcohol to: • Men: ≤2 drinks daily • Women: <1 drink daily	-4 mm Hg	-3 mm Hg

DASH, Dietary Approaches to Stop Hypertension; *SBP*, systolic blood pressure.

KEY POINTS

1. Traditionally, BP is measured in the office setting by mercury or aneroid BP devices; however, electronic (oscillometric) devices are being used in influential studies and are gaining acceptance as an alternative.
2. Home BP monitoring is better than office BP monitoring and is equivalent to ambulatory daytime BP monitoring for predicting cardiovascular events as well as a useful adjunct to guide management and improve patient adherence.
3. Ambulatory BP monitoring serves an important purpose to:
   a. exclude white coat hypertension
   b. define masked hypertension (BP elevated outside the office under high-stress conditions)
   c. help define the presence of dipping during sleep; and
   d. help define salt-sensitive-related elevations in BP
4. Prior to evaluating for secondary causes of hypertension, a thorough evaluation for more common contributing causes—high-salt diet, sleep apnea—should be conducted.
5. BPs below 140/90 mm Hg consistently reduce cardiovascular risk. More recent evidence suggests further mortality reductions with pressures as low as 120/80 in select populations.

   Patients with advanced proteinuric kidney disease benefit from pressures below 130/80 mm Hg for cardiovascular risk reduction and, to a lesser degree, for additional CKD slowing. Among those with nondiabetic CKD, the high-quality Modification of Diet in Renal Disease and the African American Study of Kidney Disease and Hypertension (AASK) studies showed no benefit of lowering BP below 130/80 mm Hg with respect to the progression of CKD. However, in post hoc analysis of the AASK trial, among those with heavy proteinuria, BPs <130/80 offered additional benefit on slowing CKD progression.

   There are no randomized trials evaluating the effects of different BP goals on the progression of diabetic nephropathy. Post hoc analysis suggests pressures of 130 to 140/80 to 90 are adequate, but prospective trials have yet to test this recommendation.
6. Patients who have a history of hypokalemia while off diuretics and blockers of the renin angiotensin system should have a 24-hour urine for sodium and total creatinine if, after counseling regarding a low-sodium diet, they have recurring hypokalemia. Primary hyperaldosterism should be considered if the patient has <2300 mg/day sodium intake.
7. While agent selection is tailored to the needs of the individual patient, thiazide-like diuretics have the longest track record and are particularly useful in those with salt-sensitive hypertension, such as the elderly, African Americans, the obese, and those with CKD.

BIBLIOGRAPHY

ALLHAT Officers and Coordinators for the ALLHAT Collaborative Research Group. (2002). Major outcomes in high-risk hypertensive patients randomized to angiotensin converting enzyme-inhibitor or calcium channel blocker vs. diuretic: The Antihypertensive and Lipid-lowering Treatment to Prevent Heart Attack Trial. *JAMA, 288*, 2981–2997.

Bakris, G. L. (2016). The implications of blood pressure measurement methods on treatment targets for blood pressure. *Circulation, 134*(13), 904–905.

Bakris, G. L., & Weir, M. R. (2000). Angiotensin-converting enzyme inhibitor-associated elevations in serum creatinine: Is this a cause for concern? *Archives of Internal Medicine, 160*(5), 685–693.

Bakris, G. L., Weir, M. R., Shanifar, S., Zhang, Z., Douglas, J., van Dijk, D. J., Brenner, B. M.; for the RENAAL Study Group. (2003). Effects of blood pressure level on progression of diabetic nephropathy: Results from the RENAAL trial. *Archives of Internal Medicine, 163*, 1555–1565.

Feng, W., Dell'Italia, L., & Sanders, P. (2017). Novel paradigms of salt and hypertension. *Journal of the American Society of Nephrology, 28*, 1362–1369.

James, P. A., Oparil, S., Carter, B. L., Cushman, W. C., Dennison-Himmelfarb, C., Handler, J., . . . Ortiz, E. (2014). 2014 Evidence-Based Guideline for the Management of High Blood Pressure in Adults. *JAMA, 311*(5), 507–520.

Klahr, S., Levey, A. S., Beck, G. J., Caggiula, A. W., Hunsicker, L., Kusek, J. W., Striker, G. (1994). Modification of Diet in Renal Disease Study Group. The effects of dietary protein restriction and blood-pressure control on the progression of chronic renal disease. *New England Journal of Medicine, 330*, 877–884.

Lonn, E. M., Bosch, J., López-Jaramillo, P., Zhu, J., Liu, L., Pais, P., . . . Yusuf, S. (2016). Blood-pressure lowering in intermediate-risk persons without cardiovascular disease. *New England Journal of Medicine, 374*, 2009–2020.

Mallick, S., Kanthety, R., & Rahman, M. (2009). Home blood pressure monitoring in clinical practice: A review. *American Journal of Medicine, 122*, 803–810.

Matthew, B., Patel, S. B., Reams, G. P., Freeman, R. H., Spear, R. M., & Villarreal, D. (2007). Obesity-hypertension: Emerging concepts in pathophysiology and treatment. *American Journal of Medicine Science, 334*, 23–30.

Ozturk, S., Sar, F., Bengi-Bozkurt, O., & Kazancioglu, R. (2009). Study of ACEI versus ARB in managing hypertensive overt diabetic nephropathy: Long-term analysis. *Kidney and Blood Pressure Research, 32,* 268–275.

Sacks, F. M., Svetkey, L. P., Vollmer, W. M., Appel, L. J., Bray, G. A., Harsha, D., . . . for the DASH-Sodium Collaborative Research Group. (2001). Effects on blood pressure of reduced dietary sodium and the Dietary Approaches to Stop Hypertension (DASH) diet. *New England Journal of Medicine, 344,* 3–10.

Sarafidis, P. A., & Bakris, G. L. (2008). Resistant hypertension: An overview of evaluation and treatment. *Journal of the American College of Cardiology, 52,* 1749–1757.

Sowers, J. R., Whaley-Connell, A., & Epstein, M. (2009). Narrative review: The emerging clinical implications of the role of aldosterone in the metabolic syndrome and resistant hypertension. *Annals of Internal Medicine,* 150, 776–783.

Staessen, J. A., Thijs, L., & Fagard, R. (1999). Predicting cardiovascular risk using conventional vs ambulatory blood pressure in older patients with systolic hypertension. *JAMA, 282*(6), 539–546.

Stergiou, G., & Kollias, A. (2017). Home monitoring of blood pressure. In G. L. Bakris & M. Sorrentino (Eds.), *Hypertension: A companion to Braunwald's Heart Disease* (pp. 89–95). Philadelphia: Elsevier.

Sternlicht, H., & Bakris, G. L. (2017). The kidney in hypertension. *Medical Clinics of North America, 101*(1), 207–217.

Sung, S. Y., Fryar, C. D., & Carroll, M. D. (2015, November). *Hypertension Prevalence and Control Among Adults: United States, 2011–2014.* Center for Disease Control. National Center for Data Statistics, No. 220. Retrieved from http://www.cdc.gov/nchs/products/databriefs/db220.htm.

Wright, J. T., Bakris, G., Greene, T., Agodoa, L. Y., Appel, L. J., Charleston, J., . . . Rostand, S. G. (2002). Effect of blood pressure lowering and anti-hypertensive drug class on progression of hypertensive kidney disease: Results from the AASK trial. *JAMA,* 288, 2421–2431.

Wright, J. T., Williamson, J. D., Whelton, P. K., Snyder, J. K., Sink, K. M., Rocco, M. V., . . . Ambrosius W. T. (2015). A randomized trial of intensive versus standard blood-pressure control. *New England Journal of Medicine,* 373, 2103–2116.

CHAPTER 63

KIDNEY PARENCHYMAL HYPERTENSION

Martin J. Andersen and Rajiv Agarwal

1. **What is the epidemiology of hypertension?**

   Hypertension remains a common disease among Americans. Data from the National Health and Nutrition Examination Survey reveal that 29% of Americans are hypertensive; this prevalence rate has remained stable for the past 15 years. African Americans bear the highest burden, as over 41% are hypertensive. Other racial groups (i.e. Whites, Asians, and Hispanics) demonstrate hypertension prevalence of 25% to 28%. During this time period, blood pressure (BP) control has improved, largely through the increased use of angiotensin converting enzyme (ACE) inhibitors, angiotensin receptor blockers (ARB), and thiazide-type diuretics in single-pill or multiple-pill combinations. In 2001 to 2002, only 45% of treated hypertensive patients achieved control, defined as BPs $<140/90$ mm Hg (or $<130/80$ mm Hg for diabetic patients or chronic kidney disease [CKD] patients [patients with estimated glomerular filtration rates (GFR) <60 mL/min per 1.73 m^2 or urinary albumin concentrations >200 mg/g creatinine]). By 2009 to 2010, 60% of treated hypertensive patients had achieved control. However, BP control remains difficult for African Americans, Hispanics, patients with diabetes, and CKD patients. Compared to Caucasians, African Americans and Hispanics are 1.4- and 1.3-fold less likely to achieve control. Again, the greater use of thiazide-type diuretics improves BP control for African Americans. Nearly 70% of treated hypertensive patients without significant comorbidities achieved control by 2009 to 2010, though only approximately 45% of patients with either diabetes mellitus or CKD achieved control.

   Obesity complicates hypertension treatment. A cross-sectional study of German hypertensive patients showed that obese patients (i.e., patients with body mass indices ≥30 kg/m^2) are 1.4- to 2-fold less likely to achieve BP control, compared to normal weight hypertensive patients. While
   - 12% of Americans are currently diabetic
     - by 2050, diabetic prevalence may increase to more than 25%
   - 36.5% of Americans are currently obese
     - by 2030, 41% may be obese, and 11% may be severely obese
   - 15% of Americans suffer from CKD
     - by 2030, the prevalence of CKD in adults over the age of 30 may be close to 50%

   Recent epidemiologic studies confirm the association of albuminuria and poor BP control in patients with CKD. In a study of 232 US veterans with CKD, proteinuria, not estimated GFR, was found to be an independent predictor of systolic BP. Among the independent predictors of hypertension (age, race, and number of antihypertensive medications), proteinuria most strongly correlated with hypertension. Compared to estimated GFR, albuminuria (or proteinuria) is a stronger determinant of hypertension; albuminuria is also a stronger determinant of poor BP control.

2. **What is the cardiovascular disease risk?**

   The World Health Organization estimates that hypertension is directly responsible for 13% of all deaths worldwide, and its effect is largely independent of a country's underlying wealth. The Center for Disease Control and Prevention determined that hypertension-related deaths for Americans 45 years of age and older (i.e., hypertension was listed as a cause of death on death certificates) increased 62% between 2000 and 2013, though, as a primary cause of death, hypertension remained stable during this time period (17.5% of all deaths). The Prospective Studies Collaboration, a meta-analysis of 1 million patients, showed that cardiovascular mortality risk began with BPs as low as 115/75 mm Hg, and, for patients 40 to 69 years old, each 20/10 mm Hg increase in BP increased cardiovascular mortality 2-fold.

   Whether a J-curve—the point at which low BPs treated within the physiologic range increase cardiovascular risk—exists, is controversial. This is of interest, as the coronary arteries receive significant perfusion during diastole; low diastolic BPs may predispose patients to adverse outcomes. The Prospective Studies Collaboration did not note a J-curve, though older studies have, especially in hypertensive patients with underlying cardiovascular disease who achieve diastolic BPs <85 to 90 mmHg.

CKD imparts increased cardiovascular risk as well. A large meta-analysis of nearly 267,000 patients with diabetes mellitus, hypertension, or cardiovascular disease showed that both low estimated GFRs and albuminuria independently increased all-cause and cardiovascular mortality. Compared to patients with an estimated GFR of 95, cardiovascular mortality risk increased 73% in patients with an estimated GFR of 45, and increased 208% in patients with an estimated GFR of 15. Patients with albumin-to-creatinine ratios of 10, 30, and 300 mg/g experienced a 13%, 55%, and 159% increase in cardiovascular mortality risk, compared to patients with an albumin-to-creatinine ratio of 5 mg/g.

3. Should diastolic, systolic, or pulse pressure be used as a treatment target?
   Studies for more than 25 years old have consistently shown that systolic BPs correlate more closely to cardiovascular outcomes and mortality than diastolic BPs, at least for older patients. However, diastolic BPs do provide important prognostic information for younger patients (i.e., those younger than 50 years). As patients age, arterial stiffening occurs, which impairs the buffering of the systolic impulse and causes an increase in the reflected wave. With increased arterial stiffening, systolic pressure rises and diastolic pressure falls.
   - For patients <50 years of age, every 10 mm Hg increase in diastolic BP increases relative cardiovascular risk by 34%.
   - Patients ≥ 60 years of age, every 10 mm Hg increase in pulse pressure increases cardiovascular risk 24%.
   - Diastolic and systolic BPs provide equal cardiovascular risk information for patients 50 to 59 years of age.
     Patients with CKD, despite being younger, often have increased arterial stiffness and systolic hypertension. Arterial stiffness worsens with higher stages of kidney disease. Therefore among patients with CKD, systolic hypertension should be the major target for treatment.

4. What BP measurement technique should be used?
   Hypertension trials use standardized clinic blood measurements to assess the efficacy of treatment regimens and BP targets. Data from these trials have been used to set BP treatment guidelines. Unfortunately, in the day-to-day world of clinical practice, standardized clinic BPs are rarely obtained, as they are technically demanding and time consuming. Improper techniques of measuring BPs correlates poorly with ambulatory BPs, which is currently considered the gold standard for BP measurement. A patient undergoing ambulatory BP monitoring wears a BP cuff for 24 hours. The BP data provided by 24-hour monitoring correlate more closely than clinic BPs, both routine and standardized, to target organ damage and cardiovascular outcomes. Both the United States and the United Kingdom advocate for the use of ambulatory BP monitoring when diagnosing patients with hypertension. Unfortunately, ambulatory BP monitoring, while considered cost effective in hypertension management, still remains largely relegated to clinical trials. An acceptable surrogate for ambulatory BP monitoring is home BP monitoring. Patients performing home BP monitoring obtain BPs in their usual settings. These data provide more information about kidney and cardiovascular risk than clinic BPs. Patients should be advised to use validated monitors. Clinicians may find a list of validated monitors at the Dabl Educational website (http://www.dableducational.org/index.html). A minimum of 12 BP recordings, obtained over 1 week, should be used for clinical decision making.
   A recent development in BP measurement technique is automated office BP monitoring. Automated office BP measurements are obtained using either a BPTru or an Omron HEM-907. BPTru does not require a period of seated rest whereas the Omron device can be programmed to measure BP only after 5 minutes of seated rest is completed. With both devices, however, medical personnel are not in the room during the measurement. Both are validated machines that are capable of measuring clinic BP while a patient is sitting quietly alone in an examination room. Because medical personnel are absent, the white coat effect (i.e., the artificially elevated BP caused by a patient's alerting reaction in the clinical setting) is avoided.
   Automated office BPs are lower than routine and standardized clinic BPs, though each measurement technique correlates poorly to ambulatory BP measurements. However, as a predictor of target organ damage, automated office BP measurements are superior, as recently demonstrated in a trial of 275 veterans with CKD. Routine clinic BPs were measured after study participants had undergone echocardiography, and automated office BPs were measured using the Omron HEM-907 after participants had rested quietly alone for 5 minutes. Three measurements, 30 seconds apart, were obtained and averaged. Both routine clinic and automated office BP measurements did not predict daytime ambulatory BPs particularly well. Routine clinic systolic BPs were, on average, 4.8 mm Hg higher than daytime ambulatory systolic BPs, though they could underestimate daytime ambulatory systolic BPs by nearly 27 mm Hg or overestimate by 36.5 mm Hg. The automated office systolic BP data were not much better. They were, on average, 7.9 mm Hg lower than daytime ambulatory systolic BPs; they could underestimate daytime

ambulatory systolic BPs by 33.2 mm Hg or overestimate 17.4 mm Hg. However, as a predictor of left ventricular hypertrophy, automated office systolic BPs performed significantly better than routine clinic systolic BPs, and they were almost superior to the predictive ability of daytime ambulatory systolic BPs.

5. What are the blood pressure treatment goals?

The optimal blood pressure level for a patient is controversial. The panel that convened for the Eighth Report of the Joint National Committee on Prevention, Detection, Evaluation, and Treatment of High Blood Pressure (JNC 8) published recommendations in early 2014. The members limited themselves to review only randomized, controlled trials. JNC 8 published a number of controversial recommendations:

- Patients with diabetes and chronic kidney disease, the goal clinic blood pressure changed from <130/80 mm Hg to <140/90 mm Hg, as results from trials such as the ACCORD, REIN-2, AASK, and MDRD did not reveal that lower clinic blood pressures improved outcomes in these groups.
- Based upon trials such as the HYVET, Syst-Eur, and SHEP, patients ≥60 years without diabetes mellitus or chronic kidney disease achieve a goal clinic blood pressure <150/90 mm Hg, while those <60 years achieve a blood pressure <140/90 mm Hg.

Many experts found this last recommendation troubling, as they felt it predisposed high-risk patients (e.g., older African Americans with hypertension) to lax blood pressure control and increased cardiovascular risk over time. Most international guidelines recommend changing the 60-year-old cut-off to 80 years of age or older.

In November of 2017, the American College of Cardiology (ACC) and the American Heart Association (AHA) published joint guidelines for the diagnosis and management of hypertension. The following terms were defined based on clinic blood pressures obtained in a standardized manner:

- Normal blood pressure: systolic pressure <120 mm Hg, diastolic pressure is <80 mm Hg
- Elevated blood pressure: systolic pressure 120 to 129 mm Hg, **and** diastolic pressure is <80 mm Hg
- Stage 1 hypertension: systolic blood pressure of 130 to 139 mm Hg, **or** a diastolic blood pressure of 80 to 89 mm Hg
- Stage 2 hypertension: systolic blood pressure ≥140 mm Hg, **or** a diastolic blood pressure of ≥90 mm Hg

All patients should receive nonpharmacological therapy if they have elevated clinic blood pressures, stage 1 hypertension, or stage 2 hypertension. Those patients with ≥10 % risk of developing atherosclerotic cardiovascular disease over 10 years (http://tools.acc.org/ASCVD-Risk-Estimator-Plus/#!/calculate/estimate/) or with known cardiovascular disease should be treated pharmacologically if they have stage 1 hypertension. All patients, regardless of cardiovascular disease status, should receive pharmacological therapy if they have stage 2 hypertension.

The SPRINT trial called attention to the way blood pressure is measured. Automated office blood pressure monitoring was employed in the SPRINT trial by using the Omron HEM-907 device. The study protocol mandated that patients sit quietly for five minutes prior to the machine taking three measurements at one-minute intervals. The blood pressure measurements were then averaged. The trial randomized three groups of hypertensive patients ≥50 years at high risk for cardiovascular events:

1. Chronic kidney disease patients
2. Patients with known cardiovascular disease with an estimated 10-year Framingham risk score >15%
3. Patients with ≥75 years

The two blood pressure targets were either a systolic blood pressure <120 mm Hg or <140 mm Hg. The intensively treated group achieved a systolic blood pressure of 121.5 mm Hg, whereas the control group achieved a systolic blood pressure of 134.6 mm Hg. After a little more than three years of follow-up, the trial was stopped prematurely because of a 25% relative risk reduction among the intensive group in the primary endpoint. The primary endpoint was a combination of cardiovascular outcomes including cardiovascular mortality. Furthermore, a 27% relative risk reduction in all-cause mortality was seen. When interpreting the SPRINT results, one must be cautious not to directly compare these data to other hypertension trials that obtained clinic blood pressures using oscillometric or mercury cuffs operated by medical personnel without the mandated period of five minutes of seated rest. Thus applying either the JNC 8 or the ACC/AHA recommendations in a post-SPRINT world becomes problematic. Automated office blood pressures generally run 5 to 10 mm Hg lower than traditionally obtained clinic blood pressures. The Canadian Hypertension Education Program now recommends that the cutoff for diagnosing hypertension by automated office blood pressure monitoring be <135/85 mm Hg, instead of <140/90 mm Hg. However, it is unlikely that an algebraic manipulation alone will be useful for individual level decision-making.

Out-of-office blood pressures are also generally lower than traditional clinic blood pressures. Recent ambulatory blood pressure thresholds have been published:

For awake ambulatory blood pressures:
- For men without high-risk disease, the goal blood pressure is <135/85 mm Hg
- For women without high-risk disease, the goal blood pressure is <125/80 mm Hg

- For hypertensive patients with diabetes or chronic kidney disease, the goal blood pressure is <120/75 mm Hg
  For home blood pressures the American Heart Association recommends
- Hypertensive patients without high-risk disease a blood pressure goal of <135/85 mm Hg
- Diabetic and chronic kidney disease patients with hypertension a blood pressure goal of <130/80 mm Hg

6. **What is the relationship between end-stage kidney disease (ESKD) risk and hypertension?**
   Of the American population, 15% have kidney disease, and more than 80% of patients with an estimated GFR <60 mL/min per 1.73 m^2 have hypertension. Uncontrolled hypertension predisposes to ESKD. The Multiple Risk Factor Intervention Trial (MRFIT) was a randomized, multicenter trial to prevent coronary artery disease in males by treating hypertension, hyperlipidemia, and tobacco abuse. Investigators followed these patients for several decades. Compared with optimal BPs, those patients with baseline systolic pressures ≥160 mm Hg had at least a 6-fold higher risk of progressing to ESKD. Poor African American men were at particularly high risk for developing ESKD. A more recent trial showed that, compared to optimal BPs, patients with prehypertension had 62% to 98% increased relative risk for developing ESKD. Those patients with stage I and II hypertension had a 2.5-fold and nearly 4-fold risk, respectively. Using predialysis BP recordings, patients who undergo long-term hemodialysis are nearly all hypertensive (86%), and only 30% of these patients have controlled BPs. However, only one-third of hemodialysis patients are hypertensive when ambulatory BP recordings are used.

7. **How does kidney disease cause hypertension?**
   - **Nephron number:** A recent pathologic study noted that middle-aged Caucasians with essential hypertension or left ventricular hypertrophy had significantly fewer nephrons than age-matched controls. The fewer nephrons that develop during fetal life mean less kidney mass for sodium and volume homeostasis, and may predispose these patients to hypertension.
   - **Salt and volume:** African Americans, patients who are obese, and elderly patients nearly all have salt-sensitive hypertension. Conversely, primitive societies that ingest little salt have no hypertension. Usually, when salt is consumed, a pressure natriuresis occurs that excretes the excess salt and volume. Patients who are salt sensitive need higher BPs to excrete a sodium load. One reason for sodium sensitivity could result from kidney tubulointerstitial inflammation and ischemia.
   - **The sympathetic nervous system:** The sympathetic nervous system increases renin secretion, decreases urinary sodium excretion, and decreases kidney blood flow. Increased sympathetic activity may be one of the mechanisms that leads to kidney damage and salt-sensitive hypertension. The sympathetic nervous system is overactive in patients with CKD, and kidney denervation, nephrectomy, or angiotensin-converting enzyme inhibition are possible treatment modalities to decrease sympathetic activation. The recently discovered enzyme renalase, which is mostly produced in the kidney, inactivates circulating catecholamines and may be important for BP regulation.
   - **The renin-angiotensin-aldosterone system:** Renin, secreted by the juxtaglomerular cells of afferent arteriole, cleaves angiotensinogen to angiotensin I (ATI). ATI is converted to angiotensin II (ATII) by ACE. ATII increases kidney sodium reabsorption, kidney arteriolar vasoconstriction, and aldosterone secretion. With kidney damage, increased ACE expression may occur and lead to elevated ATII levels. Pathologic levels of ATII can cause kidney damage and salt-sensitive hypertension.
   - **Oxidative stress:** Reactive oxygen species (ROS) are produced in the kidney in the course of oxidative metabolism. An elegant system of enzymes exists in the kidney to neutralize excess ROS. In patients with CKD, this neutralizing system is impaired. Excess ROS can have deleterious consequences. For example, increased ROS can inactivate nitric oxide (NO), a molecule that causes endothelium-dependent vasodilation. Inactivation of NO occurs in oxidative stress (nitrosative stress), and this can lead to hypertension through increased vasoconstriction. Salt-sensitive hypertensives and patients with CKD also have elevated levels of asymmetric dimethylarginine—an inhibitor of NO synthase—which also leads to the reduced production of NO.

8. **What is the proper antihypertensive regimen?**
   With the epidemics of obesity, diabetes mellitus, and CKD, nearly all patients with hypertension will need multiple medications, and many will require three or more medications. The JNC 8 recommends that non-African American hypertensive patients with or without diabetes mellitus begin therapy with either an ACE inhibitor, ARB, calcium channel blocker, or thiazide-type diuretic, while African American hypertensive patients with or without diabetes mellitus begin therapy with either a thiazide-type diuretic or a calcium channel blocker. All hypertensive CKD patients, regardless of diabetic status or race, should begin therapy with either an ACE inhibitor or ARB. The first goal for physicians is to bring their patients' BPs under good control as quickly as possible, as prompt BP control reduces cardiovascular

risk. Data from the Valsartan Antihypertensive Long-term Use Evaluation (VALUE) trial suggest that BP control should be achieved no later than 6 months after treatment begins. Many patients will already be on complex medication regimens, and fixed-dose combination pills may be more effective in achieving control than using a multiple-pill approach. Nonpharmacologic management, such as sodium restriction, exercise, smoking cessation, and weight loss, should be emphasized. The aforementioned program should be coupled with regular home BP monitoring.

ACE inhibitors and ARBs merit special attention. They are not appropriate for pregnant women or women planning to become pregnant and those with hyperkalemia, liver cirrhosis, or volume depletion. Serum creatinine and potassium should be checked within a week or two of starting either medication or increasing the dose. Labs should be followed periodically thereafter. Patients prone to hyperkalemia (e.g., diabetics) should be given dietary education. Nonsteroidal medications should be discontinued. Creatinine increases within 30% of baseline levels have traditionally been considered acceptable if unaccompanied by volume depletion and symptomatic hypotension. A recent cohort study of over 120,000 British patients calls into question this arbitrary cutoff, which was determined from clinical trials from the 1990s. Patients in this study who were prescribed either ACE inhibitors or ARBs and whose creatinine levels increased at least 30% from baseline within 2 months of treatment were at significantly higher relative risk for ESKD (243%), myocardial infarctions (46%), heart failure (37%), and death (84%) compared to those patients whose creatinine levels increased <30%. However, many patients whose creatinine levels increased <30% from baseline were also at significant risk: patients whose creatinine levels increased only 10% to 19% experienced higher relative risks for ESKD (73%), myocardial infarctions (12%), heart failure (14%), and death (15%) compared to patients whose creatinine levels increased <10%. Physicians must closely follow their patients' kidney function while on these medications and consider the risks and benefits of continuing them in the context of even small creatinine elevations. Certainly, the combination of ACE inhibitors and ARBs is no longer recommended. Spironolactone in combination with either an ACE inhibitor or ARB can reduce proteinuria, though this combination can cause significant hyperkalemia, and a beneficial effect on hard endpoints has not been demonstrated.

KEY POINTS

1. Despite significant improvements in BP control over the past decade, mortality from hypertension remains high.
2. Ambulatory BP monitoring should be considered when diagnosing patients with hypertension.
3. The current blood pressure goal depends on individual patients risk of cardiovascular (CV) events. Patients with a history of CV disease or a 10% risk of atherosclerotic events in the next decade should target a blood pressure below 130/80, all others should target a blood pressure below 140/90.
4. The 2017 ACC/AHA guidelines are largely based on the SPRINT trial which used automated office blood pressure monitoring. There is some concern that using those targets with conventional blood pressure measurements may result in over treatment of blood pressure. If current guidance on BP targets are followed it is important that the BP measurement technique be the same as used in SPRINT.
5. Automated office BP monitoring, a novel way to measure clinic BPs, eliminates the white coat effect.
6. Treatment of hypertension with both an ACE inhibitor and angiotensin receptor blocker (ARB) should be avoided, and a combination of an ACE inhibitor or ARB with spironolactone should only be used with caution.

BIBLIOGRAPHY

Abbas, S., Ihle, P., Harder, S., & Schubert, I. (2015). Risk of hyperkalemia and combined use of spironolactone and longterm ACE inhibitor/angiotensin receptor blocker therapy in heart failure using real-life data: A population- and insurance-based cohort. *Pharmacoepidemiol Drug Saf, 24*(4), 406–413.

Agarwal, R. (2017). Implications of blood pressure measurement technique for implementation of Systolic Blood Pressure Intervention Trial (SPRINT). *J Am Heart Assoc, 6*, e004536.

SPRINT Research Group, Wright, J. T., Jr., Williamson, J. D., Whelton, P. K., Snyder, J. K., Sink, K. M., . . . Ambrosius, W. T. (2015). A randomized trial of intensive versus standard blood-pressure control. *New Engl J Med, 373*(22), 2103–2116.

Boyle, J. P., Thompson, T. J., Gregg, E. W., Barker, L. E., & Williamson, D. F. (2010). Projection of the year 2050 burden of diabetes in the US adult population: Dynamic modeling of incidence, mortality, and prediabetes prevalence. *Popul Health Metr, 8*, 29.

Chronic Kidney Disease Surveillance Project. https://nccd.cdc.gov/ckd/detail.aspx?QNum=Q8.

Daskalopoulou, S. S., Rabi, D. M., Zarnke, K. B., Dasgupta, K., Nerenberg, K., Cloutier, L., . . . Padwal, R. S. (2015). The 2015 Canadian Hypertension Education Program recommendations for blood pressure measurement, diagnosis, assessment of risk, prevention, and treatment of hypertension. *Can J Cardiol, 31,* 549–568.

van der Velde, M., Matsushita, K., Coresh, J., Astor, B. C., Woodward, M., Levey, A., . . . Manley, T. (2011). Lower estimated glomerular filtration rate and higher albuminuria are associated with all-cause and cardiovascular mortality. A collaborative meta-analysis of high-risk population cohorts. *Kidney Int, 79,* 1341–1352.

Finkelstein, E. A., Khavjou, O. A., Thompson, H., Trogdon, J. G., Pan, L., Sherry, B., & Dietz, W. (2012). Obesity and severe obesity forecasts through 2030. *Am J Prev Med, 42*(6), 563–570.

Global Health Risks (The World Health Organization). http://www.who.int/healthinfo/global_burden_disease/GlobalHealthRisks_report_full.pdf.

Gu, Q., Burt, V. L., Dillon, C. F., & Yoon, S. (2012). Trends in antihypertensive medication use and blood pressure control among United States adults with hypertension. *Circulation, 126,* 2105–2114.

Hermida, R. C., Smolensky, M. H., Ayala, D. E., & Portaluppi, F. (2013). 2013 Ambulatory blood pressure monitoring recommendations for the diagnosis of adult hypertension, assessment of cardiovascular and other hypertension-associated risk, and attainment of therapeutic goals. *Chronobiol Int, 30*(3), 355–410.

High Blood Pressure in Adults (US Preventive Services Task Force). http://www.uspreventiveservicestaskforce.org/Page/Document/RecommendationStatementFinal/high-blood-pressure-in-adults-screening.

Hoerger T. J., Simpson, S. A., Yarnoff, B. O., Pavkov, M. E., Ríos, Burrows, N., Saydah, S. H., . . . Zhuo, X. (2015). The future burden of CKD in the United States: A simulation model for the CDC CKD Initiative. *Am J Kidney Dis, 65*(3), 403–411.

Horowitz, B., Miskulin, D., & Zager, P. (2015). Epidemiology of hypertension in CKD. *Adv Chronic Kidney Dis, 22*(2), 88–95.

Hypertension Prevalence and Control among Adults. *United States, 2011–2014* (NCHS Data Brief No. 220). http://www.cdc.gov/nchs/data/databriefs/db220.pdf.

Hypertension-related Mortality in the United States, 2000–2013 (NCHS Data Brief No. 193). http://www.cdc.gov/nchs/data/databriefs/db193.pdf.

James, P. A., Oparil, S., Carter, B. L., Cushman, W. C., Dennison-Himmelfarb, C., Handler, J., . . . Ortiz, E. (2014). 2014 evidence-based guideline for the management of high blood pressure in adults. *JAMA, 311*(5), 507–520.

Menke A., Casagrande, S., Geiss, L., & Cowie, C. C. (2015). Prevalence of and trends in diabetes among adults in the United States, 1988–2012. *JAMA, 314*(10), 1021–1029.

Myers, M. G., Godwin, M., Dawes, M., Kiss, A., Tobe, S. W., Grant, F. C., & Kaczorowski, J. (2011). Conventional versus automated measurement of blood pressure in primary care patients with systolic hypertension: Randomised parallel design controlled trial. *BMJ, 342,* d286.

Prevalence of Obesity among Adults and Youth. *United States, 2011–2014* (NCHS Data Brief No. 219). http://www.cdc.gov/nchs/data/databriefs/db219.pdf.

Schmidt, M., Mansfield, K. E., Bhaskaran, K., Nitsch, D., Sørensen, H. T., Smeeth, L., & Tomlinson, L. A. (2017). Serum creatinine elevation after renin-angiotensin system blockade and long term cardiorenal risk: Cohort study. *BMJ, 356,* j791.

The Clinical Management of Hypertension in Adults (National Institute for Clinical Excellence). https://www.nice.org.uk/guidance/cg127/evidence/full-guideline-248588317.

Wang, W., Li, L., Zhou, Z., Gao, J., & Sun, Y. (2013). Effect of spironolactone combined with angiotensinconverting enzyme inhibitors and/or angiotensin II receptor blockers on chronic glomerular disease. *Exp Ther Med, 6,* 1527–1531.

Wright, J. T., Jr., Fine, L. J., Lackland, D. T., Ogedegbe, G., & Dennison, Himmelfarb, C. R. (2014). Evidence supporting a systolic blood pressure goal of less than 150 mmHg in patients aged 60 Years or older: The minority view. *Ann Intern Med, 160,* 499–503.

CHAPTER 64

RENOVASCULAR DISEASE

Edward J. Horwitz and Mahboob Rahman

1. **What clinical syndromes are associated with renal artery stenosis?**
   Renovascular hypertension, progressive loss of kidney function from ischemic nephropathy, and recurrent episodes of flash pulmonary edema (meaning acute/abrupt onset pulmonary edema) are the clinical syndromes typically associated with renal artery stenosis. However, renal artery stenosis can also be completely asymptomatic. In the case of renovascular hypertension, hemodynamically significant unilateral or bilateral renal artery stenosis leads to decreased perfusion pressure in one or both kidneys. This stimulates activation of the renin-angiotensin-aldosterone system, which increases systemic pressure to restore kidney perfusion distal to the stenotic lesion(s).
   The pathophysiology of ischemic nephropathy is complex and likely relates to activation of multiple pathways triggered by reduced kidney perfusion that promote kidney injury and fibrosis. Flash pulmonary edema in the context of renal artery stenosis tends to occur only with bilateral stenosis (or renal artery stenosis affecting a solitary kidney). In this situation, patients are likely predisposed to episodes of pulmonary edema from enhanced tubular sodium reabsorption and volume expansion from increased renin-angiotensin-aldosterone activity in the absence of a pressure natriuresis phenomenon that would occur within an unaffected kidney.

2. **What are the two main causes of renal artery stenosis?**
   The two important causes of renal artery stenosis are atherosclerosis and fibromuscular dysplasia. Atherosclerotic renal artery stenosis is the more common cause and is often seen in older patients. It occurs in the setting of atherosclerotic disease affecting other vascular beds, such as the coronary, cerebral, and peripheral arterial circulation. These patients often have other risk factors for atherosclerosis, such as diabetes, hypertension, and smoking. In contrast, fibromuscular dysplasia is typically seen in younger female patients.

3. **How common is renal artery stenosis?**
   It depends on the population examined. Some degree of renal artery stenosis will be found incidentally in 19% to 42% of patients with atherosclerotic vascular disease such as coronary artery disease or peripheral vascular disease. Fibromuscular dysplasia causing renal artery stenosis is seen in 3% to 5% of healthy patients being evaluated as potential living kidney donors. In studies examining patients with mild to moderate hypertension, renal artery stenosis has been found in 0.6% to 3% of this population. In patients with refractory hypertension, renal artery stenosis may be found in between 10% and 45% of patients.

4. **How often does renal artery stenosis lead to end-stage kidney disease?**
   In some series of patients receiving dialysis, atherosclerotic renal artery stenosis may lead to end-stage kidney disease in up to 15% of patients. However, in the most recent United States Renal Data Service report, which is a registry that tracks various data on virtually all patients receiving dialysis in the United States, the incidence of renal artery stenosis as the cause for end-stage kidney disease was only 0.6%.

5. **Who is at risk of developing renal artery stenosis?**
   Patients with risk factors for atherosclerotic vascular disease, such as hypertension, dyslipidemia, diabetes, tobacco use, and older age, are at increased risk for atherosclerosis affecting the renal arteries causing stenosis.

6. **Who should be screened for renal artery stenosis?**
   Features suggestive of renal artery stenosis include:
   - Abrupt onset of hypertension at a relatively young age (30 years old) or older age (>50 years old)
   - Worsening control of previously well treated hypertension
   - Recurrent episodes of "flash pulmonary edema"
   - Kidney failure precipitated by initiation of antihypertensive therapy—especially angiotensin-converting enzyme (ACE) inhibitors or angiotensin receptor blockers (ARBs)
   - Unexplained kidney failure
   - Unilateral atrophic kidney

- Abdominal bruit
- Unexplained hypokalemia
- The presence of atherosclerotic disease in other vascular beds.

7. **What diagnostic tests can you use to identify renal artery stenosis? How do you decide which test to use?**

Screening for suspected renal artery stenosis can be done with duplex ultrasonography of the renal arteries, computed tomographic angiography (CTA), or magnetic resonance angiography (MRA). Duplex ultrasonography has the advantage of being noninvasive and does not expose patients to potential toxicities of the contrast agents needed for CTA or MRA. However, accuracy of duplex ultrasound is operator dependent and may be limited in patients who are morbidly obese. CTA is noninvasive and can characterize renal artery stenosis with a high degree of sensitivity (as high as 98%) and specificity (as high as 94%). The main disadvantages of this modality are radiation exposure and the need for iodinated contrast, which is potentially nephrotoxic, particularly in patients with impaired kidney function and diabetes. MRA gives exceptional resolution of lesions, causing renal artery stenosis with a very high sensitivity (up to 100%) and specificity (up to 97%), and it has the benefit of not exposing patients to radiation or the risk of contrast nephropathy because gadolinium is used instead of iodinated contrast. Although gadolinium is generally not considered to be a nephrotoxic agent, its use is not without risk. In patients with advanced chronic kidney disease, especially those with end-stage kidney disease, gadolinium has been associated with nephrogenic systemic fibrosis. In addition, MRA is generally a more expensive noninvasive test to evaluate for renal artery stenosis compared with ultrasound and CTA. The gold standard study to diagnose renal artery stenosis is conventional digital subtraction angiography. However, this is an invasive procedure that exposes patients to radiation and iodinated dye in addition to the risk of cholesterol atheroembolic disease (discussed in detail later).

8. **What is the resistance index, and how may it be useful in managing renal artery stenosis?**

The resistance index is a measure of relative blood flow velocity during systole and diastole within the renal arterial supply using Doppler ultrasonography. It is calculated with the following formula:

$$\text{Resistance index} = [1 - \text{end-diastolic velocity}/\text{maximal systolic velocity}] \times 100$$

It has been shown to correlate with changes in blood pressure following revascularization. Specifically, a high resistance index of >80 suggests extensive atherosclerotic disease of the smaller vessels in the arterial network and is associated with a lack of improvement in blood pressure following revascularization.

9. **What is the natural history of renal artery stenosis?**

Atherosclerotic renal artery stenosis often progresses anatomically (the degree of stenosis increases over time) and is associated with a high mortality. Numerous studies have documented anatomic progression of atherosclerotic lesions over the course of a few years using various imaging methods. For example, in one study angiographic progression was observed in 11% of patients followed an average of approximately 2.5 years, whereas in another study anatomic progression was seen in 44% of a population followed for slightly longer than an average of 4 years. Patients with fibromuscular dysplasia also may have angiographic progression of their renal artery lesions; 33% of patients with fibromuscular dysplasia in one cohort displayed anatomic progression over an average of about 4 years.

10. **What are the long-term outcomes of patients with renal artery stenosis?**

Most of the patients with atherosclerotic renal artery stenosis die of cardiovascular disease before ever developing end stage kidney disease (ESKD). Potential reasons for this increased burden of cardiovascular disease in patients with atherosclerotic renal artery stenosis include the presence of atherosclerosis in other vascular beds, excessive activation of the renin-angiotensin-aldosterone and sympathetic nervous systems, and the coexistence of chronic kidney disease. Mortality rates and incidence of ESKD in atherosclerotic renal artery stenosis depend on the populations examined. For example, in some older cohorts, mortality was reported to be as high 32% at 2 years and 45% at 5 years. However, in more recent randomized controlled trials published within the past 10 years Angioplasty and Stenting for Renal Artery Lesions (ASTRAL) trial, Cardiovascular Outcomes in Renal Atherosclerotic Lesions (CORAL) trial, STent placement and blood pressure and lipid-lowering for the prevention of progression of renal dysfunction caused by Atherosclerotic ostial stenosis of the Renal artery (STAR) trial) comparing medical therapy alone to stenting with medical therapy in patients with atherosclerotic renal artery stenosis, mortality was reported to be approximately 8% at 2 years and then ranged between 14% and 26% over approximately 5 years of follow-up. In contrast, the percentage of patients with atherosclerotic renal artery stenosis requiring dialysis in observational studies ranged from approximately 3% at 2 years to 12% at 5 years. In the more recent randomized controlled trials involving atherosclerotic renal artery stenosis, approximately 2% to 10% of patients with atherosclerotic renal artery stenosis started chronic dialysis over approximately a 5-year period. Kidney failure as a result of fibromuscular dysplasia is felt to be very rare.

11. **What treatment options exist for renal artery stenosis caused by atherosclerosis?**
Atherosclerotic renal artery stenosis may be treated by medical management, angioplasty/stent placement, or surgery.
    Medical management is based on blood pressure control with appropriate antihypertensive medications along with lifestyle modifications and other medical interventions aimed at reducing the high cardiovascular risk associated with atherosclerotic renal artery stenosis. This includes aspirin, statins, smoking cessation, and good glycemic control in patients with diabetes. In addition to this approach, revascularization, now mainly done with percutaneous interventions (angioplasty and stenting) rather than surgery, can be used to treat renovascular hypertension and ischemic nephropathy. However, multiple randomized trials suggest that revascularization does **not** significantly improve blood pressure control, kidney outcomes, cardiovascular outcomes, or mortality compared with medical management alone. The two largest and most recently published studies that randomized participants to either medical management with revascularization or medical management alone:
    1. Angioplasty and STenting for Renal Artery Lesions (ASTRAL) trial in 2009 included more than 800 patients
    2. Cardiovascular Outcomes in Renal Atherosclerotic Lesions (CORAL) study in 2014 included approximately 950 subjects
       Both trials failed to demonstrate a benefit for revascularization toward kidney outcomes, cardiovascular outcomes, and mortality compared with medical management alone. Moreover, in the ASTRAL study, no difference in blood pressure control was observed between the revascularization group and the medical management group. The CORAL trial did find a statistically significant difference in blood pressure between participants who underwent revascularization compared with those receiving only medical management. However, this difference was only 2.3 mm Hg and did not lead to any improvement in clinical outcomes. Of note, periprocedural complications occurred in approximately 9% of patients who underwent revascularization in ASTRAL and in approximately 5% of vessels treated in CORAL.

12. **How should renal artery stenosis caused by fibromuscular dysplasia be managed?**
In contrast to atherosclerotic renal artery stenosis, revascularization of fibromuscular dysplasia generally leads to favorable clinical outcomes and should be considered in many cases. Although there are no randomized trials exclusively involving patients with fibromuscular dysplasia, several case series and a large meta-analysis with these patients have shown that hypertension was improved or even cured in a significant proportion of patients who underwent percutaneous revascularization.

13. **What are the potential benefits and risks associated with percutaneous revascularization of renal artery stenosis?**
Percutaneous revascularization (angioplasty with or without stenting) can potentially correct stenotic lesions in a relatively noninvasive procedure, but it is certainly not without risk. Patients are at risk for bleeding complications, contrast nephropathy, and renal artery dissection, occlusion, or perforation. Acute kidney injury associated with any of these events may require dialysis and is not necessarily reversible. One other potential complication of conventional angiography and percutaneous revascularization procedures that deserves special mention is cholesterol atheroembolic disease. This disorder occurs when cholesterol fragments from atheromatous plaques embolize to distal arterial blood vessels, causing ischemic injury. This embolic event most often occurs in the context of anticoagulation/thrombolytic therapy or some procedure, such as vascular surgery or conventional angiography, where mechanical trauma to the atherosclerotic vessels with vulnerable plaques may be unavoidable. The clinical manifestations vary depending on where the cholesterol-laden fragments embolize and may include stroke, mesenteric ischemia, acute kidney injury, and ischemic digits. Atheroembolic disease affecting the kidneys should be suspected in patients who have a decline in kidney function following an arterial intervention or angiography who also demonstrate any of the following:
- Livedo reticularis
- Ischemic digits
- Peripheral eosinophilia
- Hypocomplementemia
    Patients with cholesterol atheroembolic disease may lose kidney function over the course of weeks to months in a stepwise fashion, and this may not be reversible. Although treatment is mainly supportive,

it is important to avoid anticoagulation if possible because it is believed this may predispose the patient to further embolic events. Cholesterol-lowering agents may be of some benefit.

14. **Should patients with uncontrolled hypertension caused by atherosclerotic renal artery stenosis undergo revascularization?**
   No. Data from randomized trials have not clearly and consistently demonstrated a significant benefit to revascularization compared with medical management alone in regard to renovascular hypertension. The risks and benefits of each option should be discussed with each individual patient, in consultation with a vascular surgeon or interventional radiologist.

15. **Do patients who have chronic kidney disease with significant atherosclerotic renal artery stenosis benefit from revascularization over medical management alone?**
   No. The randomized trials completed to date do not clearly show patients with chronic kidney disease who underwent revascularization compared with those with medical management alone had improved kidney outcomes, cardiovascular outcomes, or overall mortality.

16. **Does it matter which antihypertensive agents are used to control blood pressure in patients with renal artery stenosis?**
   As long as inhibitors of the renin-angiotensin system (RAS) do not precipitate kidney failure, patients with atherosclerotic renal artery stenosis treated with ACE inhibitors seem to have more favorable long-term outcomes compared with those not taking ACE inhibitors. Consequently, this class of medications is preferred in the treatment of hypertension associated with atherosclerotic renal artery stenosis. Moreover, as long as severe bilateral disease is not present, antagonists of the RAS would not necessarily be expected to precipitate acute kidney failure. A rise in serum creatinine of up to 30% from baseline after initiation of an ACE inhibitor or ARB is often observed, particularly in patients with some underlying chronic kidney disease, and should not prompt discontinuation of the medication. In contrast, a more substantial decline in kidney function (creatinine increase of >30%) or significant hyperkalemia (potassium >6) after initiation of a RAS inhibitor should raise some suspicion for concurrent states of decreased effective arterial blood volume such as volume depletion or decompensated heart failure, nonsteroidal antiinflammatory drug use, bilateral renal artery stenosis, or renal artery stenosis of a solitary kidney. In this situation the RAS inhibitor should be at least temporarily held and these possibilities explored.

17. **In what situations may it be appropriate to consider revascularization for atherosclerotic renal artery stenosis?**
   Despite the results of trials that do not suggest patients with ischemic nephropathy or renovascular hypertension benefit from revascularization in general, there still may exist some situations in which revascularization is appropriate to attempt. For example, it may be reasonable to try revascularization in patients with recurrent flash pulmonary edema. Moreover, if a patient is intolerant of many antihypertensive medications or their hypertension cannot be adequately controlled with medications, revascularization would be reasonable to consider. Finally, if a patient were rapidly losing kidney function, believed to be from atherosclerotic renal artery stenosis, it could be argued that because they will likely require dialysis or a transplant very soon if nothing else is done. In this situation the potential benefits of an attempted intervention may outweigh the risks.

KEY POINTS

1. Renal artery stenosis is associated with three main clinical syndromes: ischemic nephropathy, renovascular hypertension, and recurrent flash pulmonary edema. However, it may be completely asymptomatic.
2. Renal artery stenosis should be suspected in patients with resistant hypertension, abrupt onset of hypertension at a relatively young or old age, worsening blood pressure control in someone with previously well-controlled hypertension, recurrent episodes of flash pulmonary edema, unexplained kidney dysfunction, unexplained hypokalemia, an atrophic unilateral kidney, kidney failure precipitated by initiation of blockers of the renin-angiotensin system, an abdominal bruit, and the presence of atherosclerotic disease in other vascular beds.
3. Screening for suspected renal artery stenosis can be done with duplex ultrasonography, magnetic resonance angiography, or computed tomographic angiography. The gold standard diagnostic study is digital subtraction angiography, but this involves an invasive procedure.
4. Atherosclerotic renal artery stenosis commonly progresses anatomically and is associated with high mortality largely from cardiovascular causes.

BIBLIOGRAPHY

Baboolal, K., Evans, C., & Moore, R. H. (1998). Incidence of ESRD-stage renal disease in medically treated patients with severe bilateral atherosclerotic renovascular disease. *American Journal of Kidney Diseases, 31*(6), 971–977.

Bakris, G. L., & Weir, M. R. (2000). Angiotensin-converting enzyme inhibitor-associated elevations in serum creatinine: Is this a cause for concern? *Archives of Internal Medicine, 160*, 685–693.

Bax, L., Woittiez, A. J., Kouwenberg, H. J., Mali, W. P., Buskens, E., Beek, F. J., . . . Beutler, J. J. (2009). Stent placement in patients with atherosclerotic renal artery stenosis and impaired renal function: A randomized trial. *Annals of Internal Medicine, 150*, 840–848.

Cooper, C. J., Murphy, T. P., Cutlip, D. E., Jamerson, K. Henrich, W., Reid, D. M., . . . CORAL Investigators. (2014). Stenting and medical therapy for atherosclerotic renal-artery stenosis. *New England Journal of Medicine, 370*, 13–22. DOI: 10.1056/NEJMoa1310753.

Crowley, J., Santos, R., Peter, R., Puma, J. A., Schwab, S. J., Phillips, H. R., . . . Conlon, P. J. (1998). Progression of renal artery stenosis in patients undergoing cardiac catheterization. *American Heart Journal, 136*(5), 913–918.

Dworkin, L., & Cooper, C. (2009). Renal artery stenosis. *New England Journal of Medicine, 361*, 1972–1978.

Hackam, D. G., Duong-Hua, M., Mamdani, M., Li, P., Tobe, S. W., Spence, J. D., & Garg, A. X. (2008). Angiotensin inhibition in renovascular disease: A population-based cohort study. *American Heart Journal, 156*, 549–555.

Ives, N. J., Wheatley, K., Stowe, R. L., Krijnen, P., Plouin, P. F., van Jaarsveld, B. C., & Gray R. (2003). Continuing uncertainty about the value of percutaneous revascularization in atherosclerotic renovascular disease: A metaanalysis of randomized trials. *Nephrology, Dialysis, Transplantation, 18*, 298–304.

Mailloux, L., Napolitano, B., Bellucci, A., Vernace, M., Wilkes, B. M., & Mossey, R. T. (1994). Renal vascular disease causing end stage renal disease, incidence, clinical correlates, and outcomes. A 20 year clinical experience. *American Journal of Kidney Diseases, 24*(4), 622–629.

Pickering, T. G., Herman, L., Devereux, R. B., Sotelo, J. E., James, G. D., Sos, T. A., . . . Laragh, J. H. (1988). Recurrent pulmonary oedema in hypertension due to bilateralrenal artery stenosis: Treatment by angioplasty or surgical revascularisation. *Lancet, 2*(8610), 551.

Pillay, W. R., Kan, Y. M., Crinnion, J. N., Wolfe, J. H.; Joint Vascular Research Group, UK. (2002). Prospective multicentre study of the natural history of atheroscleroticrenal artery stenosis in patients with peripheral vascular disease. *British Journal of Surgery, 89*, 737–740.

Plouin, P., Chatellier, G., Darne, B., & Raynaud, A. (1998). Blood pressure outcome of angioplasty in atherosclerotic renal artery stenosis: A randomized trial. Essai Multicentrique Medicaments vs Angioplastie (EMMA) Study Group. *Hypertension, 31*, 823–829.

Radermacher, J., Chaven, A., Bleck, J., Vitzthum, A., Stoess, B., Gebel, M. J., . . . Haller, H. (2001). Use of Doppler ultrasonography to predict the outcome of therapy for renal artery stenosis. *New England Journal of Medicine, 344*, 410–417.

Safian, R., & Textor, S. (2001). Renal artery stenosis. *New England Journal of Medicine, 344*, 431–442.

Siddiqui, S., MacGregor, M., Glynn, C., Roditi, G., & Deighan, C. J. (2005). Factors predicting outcome in a cohort of patients with atheroscleroticrenal artery disease diagnose by magnetic resonance angiography. *American Journal of Kidney Diseases, 46*(6), 1065–1073.

Slovut, D., & Olin, J. (2004). Fibromuscular dysplasia. *New England Journal of Medicine, 350*, 1862–1871.

The ASTRAL investigators. (2009). Revascularization versus medical therapy for renal artery stenosis. *New England Journal of Medicine, 361*, 1953–1962.

Trinquart, L., Mounier-Vehier, C., Sapoval, M., Gagnon, N., & Plouin, P. F. (2010). Efficacy of revascularization for renal artery stenosis caused by fibromuscular dysplasia: A systematic review and meta-analysis. *Hypertension, 56*, 525–532.

Van Jaarsveld, B. C., Krijnen, P., Pieterman, H., Derkx, F. H., Deinum, J., Postma, C. T., . . . Schalekamp, M. A. (2000). The effect of balloon angioplasty on hypertension inatherosclerotic renal artery stenosis. *New England Journal of Medicine, 342*, 1007–1014.

Webster, J., Marshall, F., Abdalla, M., Dominiczak, A., Edwards, R., Isles, C. G., . . . Wilkinson, R. (1998). Randomized comparison of percutaneous angioplasty vs continued medical therapy for hypertensive patients with atheromatous renal artery stenosis. Scottish and Newcastle Renal Artery Stenosis Collaborative Group. *Journal of Human Hypertension, 12*, 329–335.

CHAPTER 65

ENDOCRINE HYPERTENSION

William J. Elliott

HYPERALDOSTERONISM

1. What is hyperaldosteronism?

   Hyperaldosteronism is a disorder with a characteristic set of signs and symptoms resulting from excessive effects of aldosterone or a similar mineralocorticoid agent, which typically include:
   - Hypertension: usually unresponsive to angiotensin converting-enzyme (ACE) inhibitors, angiotensin receptor blockers (ARBs), or direct renin inhibitors
   - Intravascular volume expansion
   - Hypokalemia

2. Describe the most common subtypes or causes of hyperaldosteronism.

   Hyperaldosteronism can be either primary or secondary. As a result of an autonomously functioning adrenal adenoma, it is called Conn syndrome, after Jerome William Conn (1907 to 1994). More common is bilateral adrenal hyperplasia (sometimes called idiopathic hyperaldosteronism), in which both glands oversecrete aldosterone. Glucocorticoid-remediable hyperaldosteronism results from a chimeric gene on chromosome 8 that crosses the regulatory sequence for corticotropin, 11β-hydroxylase, with the enzyme coding sequences for aldosterone synthase. Hyperaldosteronism from an adrenal carcinoma is rare (~30 cases worldwide) and usually presents as a large tumor.

   Secondary hyperaldosteronism includes obstructive sleep apnea (OSA). OSA is one of the more common causes of resistant hypertension. Renovascular hypertension is another example of secondary hyperaldosteronism causing hypertension.

3. How common is hyperaldosteronism?

   The prevalence of hyperaldosteronism depends on where and how one looks for it. Some referral centers report a prevalence of hyperaldosteronism related to sleep apnea at about 20%, similar to the original estimate for aldosterone-secreting adenomas proposed by Conn in 1954. Other population-based studies suggest that such a high prevalence is a result of a lack of specificity of the aldosterone-renin ratio that is often used to screen for the condition. In a consecutive series from the Mayo Clinic, about 10% of community-dwelling hypertensives had an "abnormal" ratio, but no tumors suggestive of adrenal adenomas were detected by computed tomography (CT) scanning. Small (often bilateral) tumors are occasionally seen in patients with bilateral hyperplasia but not with OSA.

4. What is the most appropriate test to screen for hyperaldosteronism?

   After total body potassium stores have been repleted, the ratio of plasma aldosterone to renin measured in (optimally, untreated) patients in the seated position at 8 AM is the most widely recommended test. A plasma aldosterone/renin activity ratio >20 ng/dL per ng/mL per hour and the plasma aldosterone level >15 ng/dL is a positive screen for primary hyperaldosteronism. Potential confounders of the test are listed in Box 65.1.

5. What additional tests may be useful in identifying patients with hyperaldosteronism?

   Many different tests have been proposed to distinguish between an aldosterone-producing adenoma and bilateral adrenal hyperplasia, including an assay of blood or urine for aldosterone (and/or other mineralocorticoids) before and after infusion of 2 L of saline, after a high-sodium diet, postural change, either an ACE inhibitor or an ARB, or an assay of serum 11- or 18-oxo-aldosterone. None of these are perfect discriminators, but the updated 2016 Endocrine Society guidelines suggest usually performing one of these confirmatory tests before imaging the adrenals. A CT scan of the abdomen, with thin (5 mm) cuts through the adrenals, is usually selected. If a unilateral hypodense mass >1 cm is found, particularly in a patient younger than 40 years, a surgeon is often consulted for laparoscopic removal (see later). Some physicians prefer a magnetic resonance imaging (MRI) scan, again with thin cuts through the adrenals, but this is less sensitive (because of the higher spatial resolution of CT scans).

   Although challenged by the results of a randomized trial, adrenal venous sampling is recommended by the updated 2016 Endocrine Society guidelines for all surgical candidates over age 40 years, because CT scans have only 78% sensitivity and 75% specificity for unilateral adrenal adenomas. The procedure

449

Box 65.1. Potential Confounders of the Aldosterone-Renin Ratio

Decrease ARR (higher likelihood of a false-negative test)
- Diuretics
- Angiotensin-converting enzyme inhibitors
- Angiotensin receptor antagonists
- Dihydropyridine calcium antagonists (smaller effect)
- Hypokalemia
- Pregnancy
- Renovascular hypertension
- Hypertensive emergency (formerly, "malignant hypertension")

Increase ARR (higher likelihood of a false-positive test)
- Beta-adrenergic antagonists
- Alpha-1 adrenergic agonists
- Nonsteroidal antiinflammatory drugs
- High-potassium diet (or "potassium loading")
- Older age
- Chronic kidney disease
- Pseudohypoaldosteronism, type 2

Changes in dietary sodium and potassium consumption can also affect the ARR, but the magnitude and direction of the changes depend on many other factors.
ARR, Aldosterone-renin ratio.

---

is complex and is typically done only at large, experienced centers, but it can help avoid removing an enlarged but nonfunctioning adrenal gland.

Glucocorticoid-remediable hyperaldosteronism can be detected by genetic testing of leukocyte DNA.

6. List of treatments for hyperaldosteronism.
   - **Conn adenoma:** Unilateral adrenalectomy, now often by laparoscopic surgery.
   - **Bilateral adrenal hyperplasia:** Chronic therapy with an aldosterone antagonist. Spironolactone had superior efficacy in lowering blood pressure compared to eplerenone in one international clinical trial, but the latter has fewer adverse effects.
   - **For hyperaldosteronism related to sleep apnea:** Spironolactone (or eplerenone) is effective in the vast majority of cases; continuous positive airway pressure is recommended for the signs and symptoms of sleep apnea.
   - **For glucocorticoid-suppressible hyperaldosteronism:** Low-dose glucocorticoid.

7. What are the short- and long-term challenges after surgery?
   Strict attention to eukalemia is important, particularly in the first few days after the operation. Most patients receive normal saline, without potassium, during the immediate postoperative period. A day after the procedure, a plasma aldosterone level is measured, potassium supplements and aldosterone antagonists are discontinued, and the patient is counseled to consume more dietary sodium than usual, to minimize the risk of hyperkalemia while the contralateral adrenal gland recovers function. Hyperkalemia is more common in patients with chronic kidney disease (albuminuria, increased serum creatinine, or both). Long-term resolution of hypokalemia is common, but about 50% of patients remain hypertensive (and require antihypertensive medications), even after a successful operation. Persistent hypertension is more common in older patients and those with a longer duration of hypertension before the diagnosis was made.

CUSHING SYNDROME AND CONGENITAL ADRENAL HYPERPLASIA

8. What is Cushing syndrome?
   Cushing syndrome is a characteristic set of signs and symptoms resulting from excessive effects of cortisol, initially attributed to a basophilic pituitary adenoma (Cushing disease) by Harvey Cushing in 1932.

9. Describe the most common clinical features of Cushing syndrome.
   Cushing syndrome is characterized by progressive physical changes, which are often best appreciated in serial photographs:
   - Central (truncal) obesity
   - Moon facies
   - Dorsocervical fat pad (buffalo hump)
   - Purple abdominal striae may be the most specific physical sign if >2.5 cm wide
   - Plethora

- Ecchymoses
- Hypertrichosis
- Muscle weakness and atrophy, which are typically noted when climbing stairs or arising from a chair.
    Other features of Cushing syndrome include emotional and cognitive changes, menstrual irregularity, glucose intolerance, and hypertension. Growth restriction is universal in children with Cushing syndrome.

10. **How common is hypertension in Cushing syndrome?**
    About 80% of patients with Cushing syndrome have hypertension.

11. **Explain the mechanism of hypertension in patients with Cushing syndrome.**
    Hypertension in patients with hypercortisolism is multifactorial:
    - Excessive cortisol exposure increases systemic vascular resistance by:
        - Enhancing the effects of catecholamines and angiotensin II
        - Suppressing synthesis of endogenous vasodilatory agents, including nitric oxide and prostaglandins
    - Cortisol also stimulates sodium reabsorption in the distal nephron, and to a lesser extent in the proximal nephron
    - Synthesis of certain mineralocorticoids are increased in corticotropin (formerly adrenocorticotropic hormone [ACTH])-dependent Cushing syndrome

12. **List the most common causes of Cushing syndrome.**
    Corticotropin-dependent:
    - Pituitary microadenoma (~68% of endogenous hypercortisolemia)
    - Ectopic corticotropin production (~12%, from other tumors, typically small-cell lung cancer)
    - Ectopic corticotropin-releasing hormone secretion (<1%)
    Corticotropin-independent:
    - Exogenous glucocorticoid administration (iatrogenic causes are the most common in the United States)
    - Adrenal adenoma (~10%)
    - Adrenal adenocarcinoma (~8%)
    - Primary pigmented nodular adrenal hyperplasia (<1%)
    - McCune-Albright syndrome (<1%)
    - Macronodular adrenal disease (<1%)
    - Hyperfunction of adrenal rest tissue (<1%)

13. **What is the difference between Cushing syndrome and Cushing disease?**
    Cushing syndrome includes all patients with hypercortisolism. Cushing disease refers to that subset of patients with Cushing syndrome due to a corticotropin-secreting pituitary microadenoma.

14. **What are the best tests to screen for Cushing syndrome?**
    Plasma cortisol levels >15 μg/dL in the afternoon or evening (in an unstressed patient) are suggestive of hypercortisolism; British endocrinologists prefer a midnight cortisol level, which can be measured noninvasively in saliva.
    Urinary free cortisol values >100 μg/day are abnormal, and values >400 μg/day (more than four times the upper limit of the reference range) are suggestive of Cushing syndrome.
    Many clinicians use the overnight dexamethasone suppression test (which is more convenient than the classical "low-dose" test) as a screen for Cushing syndrome. Morning (8 AM) plasma cortisol levels >5 μg/dL are suggestive of Cushing syndrome; patients with levels >1.8 μg/dL are candidates for further testing. Table 65.1 summarizes the usual test results for patients with Cushing syndrome.

15. **What additional tests may be useful in identifying the cause of Cushing syndrome?**
    Classically, the high-dose dexamethasone suppression test (2 mg every 6 hours for eight doses) suppresses the production of cortisol by >90% (and its urinary metabolites) in patients with Cushing disease, because pituitary microadenomas remain sensitive to high levels or activity of circulating corticosteroids. A more convenient "high-dose" test measures plasma cortisol at bedtime, followed by one 8 mg dose of dexamethasone and another cortisol level test 8 hours later; "suppression" is diagnosed if the cortisol level drops by 50% compared to baseline. This test does not distinguish between Cushing disease and the far less common ectopic corticotropin secretion, so a chest x-ray is usually scrutinized for evidence of a tumor that is secreting corticotropin.

Table 65.1. Summary of Typical Test Results in the Evaluation of Cushing Syndrome

PATHOLOGY	PLASMA/ URINARY CORTISOL LEVELS	CORTICOTROPIN LEVEL	CORTISOL LEVEL AFTER LOW-DOSE DEXAMETHA-SONE SUPPRESSION TEST	CORTISOL LEVEL AFTER HIGH-DOSE DEXAMETHA-SONE SUPPRESSION TEST
Pituitary microad-enoma (Cushing disease)	Elevated	Elevated	Not suppressed[a]	Suppressed[b]
Ectopic source of corticotropin	Elevated	Elevated	Not suppressed	Not suppressed
Ectopic source of corticotropin-releasing hormone	Elevated	Elevated	Not suppressed	Variable, but usually suppressed
Adrenal tumor or hyperplasia	Elevated	Suppressed	Not suppressed	Not suppressed
Pseudo-Cushing syndrome	Normal or slightly elevated, often with deranged circadian variation	Variable, but often suppressed	Usually suppressed; formerly used as an "objective" indicator of severity of depression	Suppressed

[a]Suppressed: <1.8 µg/dL. [b]Suppressed: <50% of baseline.

Head and abdominal CT scans may identify a pituitary or adrenal tumor; MRI is slightly less sensitive for adrenal tumors than a CT with thin cuts (5 mm) through the adrenals. Sometimes a chest x-ray and/or a chest CT is done because the most common source of ectopic corticotropin secretion is lung cancer, usually small cell.

16. List of treatment options for the various etiologies of Cushing syndrome.
   • Pituitary adenoma resection for Cushing disease
   • Adrenalectomy, particularly unilateral adrenalectomy, but occasionally bilateral adrenalectomy if the pituitary tumor cannot be resected
   • Resection of the corticotropin-secreting tumor

17. Is there a role for medical therapy for Cushing syndrome?
   Agents that modulate corticotropin release (cyproheptadine, bromocriptine, valproic acid) or inhibit cortisol synthesis and/or production (mitotane, trilostane, ketoconazole, aminoglutethimide, and metyrapone) may be useful preoperatively or for patients who are not surgical candidates.

18. Should all patients with hypertension who are obese be evaluated for Cushing syndrome?
   No. Testing should be considered for patients with hypertension who present with the characteristic clinical features of Cushing syndrome.

19. Define congenital adrenal hyperplasia (CAH).
   CAH is a diverse family of autosomal-recessive disorders characterized by deficient function of one of the enzymes necessary for cortisol synthesis (Fig. 65.1).
   The reduction in cortisol synthesis leads to a loss of feedback inhibition of the hypothalamic-pituitary-adrenal axis, with excessive production of corticotropin. Exposure to excessive corticotropin leads to adrenal hyperplasia, overproduction of adrenal steroids that do not require the deficient enzyme, and deficiency of steroids distal to the deficient enzyme.

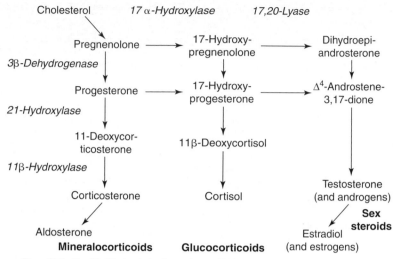

Figure 65.1. Simplified biochemical pathways for steroid biosynthesis (enzymes are given in italics).

20. List the typical clinical manifestations of CAH.
    The specific clinical features depend on the deficient enzyme involved:
    • Abnormal fetal genital development. Postnatal consequences of this include sex steroid imbalance, including abnormal patterns of growth and maturation, and impaired fertility.
    • Abnormal blood pressure regulation: disturbance in sodium and potassium homeostasis. Abnormal salt wasting or volume overload is important for blood pressure.

21. What is the most common cause of CAH?
    The most common cause of CAH is deficiency of 21-hydroxylase. This accounts for >90% of cases of CAH and represents 1:14,000 live births.

22. What are other causes of CAH?
    Deficiency of 11β-hydroxylase activity (5% to 8% of cases) is the second most common cause of CAH. Rare causes include 3β-hydroxysteroid dehydrogenase deficiency, 17α-hydroxylase deficiency, and lipoid CAH.

23. Which forms of CAH are associated with hypertension?
    11β-hydroxylase deficiency and 17α-hydroxylase deficiency are associated with hypertension.

24. What about 21 hydroxylase deficiency?
    Patients with classic 21-hydroxylase deficiency do not have hypertension, but instead have severe salt wasting with dehydration, hyponatremia, and hyperkalemia, which is related to aldosterone deficiency.

25. Describe the pathophysiology of 11β-hydroxylase deficiency.
    11β-hydroxylase (P450c11) is the mitochondrial enzyme responsible for the biosynthetic step immediately before cortisol production. More than 30 mutations have been identified in *CYP11B1*, the gene on chromosome 8, which encodes 11β-hydroxylase. Inadequate activity of 11β-hydroxylase leads to inadequate cortisol production, an excessive effect of corticotropin, and increased levels of the precursor deoxycorticosterone (DOC). Steroid biosynthesis is largely diverted to androgen production.

26. What are the important clinical features of 11β-hydroxylase deficiency (Bongiovanni syndrome)?
    • 11β-Hydroxylase deficiency occurs in about 1:100,000 births.
    • All affected females are born with some degree of masculinization of the external genitalia, including clitoromegaly and partial or complete fusion of the labioscrotal folds. Internal genitalia are normal.
    • Other symptoms of androgen excess that occur postnatally include rapid somatic growth with accelerated skeletal maturation, leading to premature closure of the epiphyses and short adult stature.
    • Mineralocorticoid excess leads to hypokalemic metabolic alkalosis in many patients.

- About 67% of these patients have low-renin hypertension beginning early in life (e.g., ages 1 to 2 years).

27. **Explain the pathophysiology of hypertension in patients with 11β-hydroxylase deficiency.**
    Hypertension is the result of volume expansion mediated by increased levels of DOC, a mineralocorticoid with weak activity, compared to aldosterone. High levels of circulating DOC produce significant sodium and water retention.

28. **Describe the pathophysiology of 17α-hydroxylase deficiency.**
    17α-Hydroxylase (P450c17) is the enzyme responsible for the biosynthetic step that converts mineralocorticoids to glucocorticoids (17α-hydroxylase activity) and glucocorticoids to sex steroids (17,20-lyase activity). More than 20 mutations have been identified on *CYP17*, the gene on chromosome 10 that encodes 17α-hydroxylase. Abnormal enzyme activity can be manifested as isolated 17α-hydroxylase deficiency, 17,20-lyase deficiency, or their combination. Inadequate 17α-hydroxylase activity leads to inadequate cortisol production, excessive effects of corticotropin, and increased levels of DOC. In contrast to 11β-hydroxylase deficiency, sex steroid production is decreased.

29. **What are the important clinical features of 17α-hydroxylase deficiency (Biglieri syndrome)?**
    - Because patients with 17α-hydroxylase deficiency do not have excessive androgen synthesis, they tend to present later than patients with 11β-hydroxylase deficiency.
    - Males may present with incomplete virilization, and females may present with primary amenorrhea and sexual infantilism at the time of puberty.
    - Occasionally, genetic males with a female phenotype may present for evaluation of a hernia or inguinal mass.
    - Mineralocorticoid excess leads to hypokalemic metabolic alkalosis and low-renin hypertension.

30. **Explain the pathophysiology of hypertension in patients with 17α-hydroxylase deficiency.**
    As in patients with 11β-hydroxylase deficiency, hypertension is the result of volume expansion mediated by increased levels of DOC.

31. **How is CAH diagnosed?**
    Patients with various forms of CAH are diagnosed by their clinical features and plasma and urine steroid profiles. In general, the corticotropin stimulation test results in marked elevation of precursor steroids proximal to the deficient enzyme. Neonatal screening for 21-hydroxylase deficiency is available across the United States and in many countries worldwide. There is currently no screening program for the hypertensive forms of CAH because of the low incidence of these disorders.

32. **In which patients with hypertension should CAH be considered in the differential diagnosis?**
    All patients with hypertension with the following:
    - Hypokalemic metabolic alkalosis
    - Abnormal external genitalia (virilized female, incompletely virilized male, or infantile female)
    - History of infertility

33. **Discuss the treatment options for CAH.**
    In general, CAH is treated with the long-term administration of hydrocortisone at a dose of 10 to 15 mg/m^2 per day. This provides negative feedback to the pituitary, decreases corticotropin release, and corrects excessive mineralocorticoid and sex steroid synthesis. In salt-wasting forms of CAH, such as 21-hydroxylase deficiency, the administration of fludrocortisone and sodium chloride is usually necessary. Virilized females with 11β-hydroxylase deficiency require surgical correction of the external genitalia. Sex steroids are necessary in patients with hypogonadotropic hypogonadism, such as in 17α-hydroxylase deficiency. Maternal treatment with dexamethasone during pregnancy has been successful in preventing abnormal fetal genital development. On the horizon is gene therapy, which works in adrenocortical cell lines and animal models.

34. **Which antihypertensive agents are most often used for patients with hypertension and CAH?**
    Potassium-sparing diuretics (spironolactone, possibly eplerenone, or amiloride) and calcium antagonists are used most often.

35. **Which antihypertensive agents should be avoided?**
    Because renin is suppressed, angiotensin-converting enzyme inhibitors, direct renin inhibitors, and ARBs are unlikely to be effective. Thiazide diuretics should be avoided because of the increased risk of hypokalemia.

PHEOCHROMOCYTOMA

36. **What is pheochromocytoma?**
Pheochromocytoma is a catecholamine-producing tumor arising from the chromaffin cells of the sympathetic nervous system derived embryonically from the primitive neural crest cells. Most pheochromocytomas are found in the adrenal gland; the second most common site is the organ of Zuckerkandl (ganglia at the bifurcation of the aorta), although paragangliomas (which have very similar presenting features, evaluation, and treatment) can arise anywhere along the parasympathetic chain.

37. **What is the incidence of pheochromocytoma?**
The annual incidence is about 1.5 to 2.1 cases per million population.

38. **What catecholamines are produced by pheochromocytoma?**
Most pheochromocytomas secrete primarily norepinephrine. Epinephrine-secreting tumors are more commonly malignant or extra-adrenal in location. Very rarely, a tumor is deficient in dopamine beta-hydroxylase; this causes secretion of large amounts of dopamine.
Pheochromocytomas also store and secrete many peptides: endogenous opioids, endothelin, erythropoietin, parathyroid hormone-related protein, neuropeptide-Y, and chromogranin-A; the latter has been used as a diagnostic marker.

39. **What are the clinical manifestations of pheochromocytoma?**
The most common finding is hypertension, which occurs in more than 90% of patients but it is paroxysmal in 25% to 33% of cases. Hypertension is often accompanied (especially in paroxysmal hypertension) by tachycardia, headache, tremor, sweating, and pupillary dilatation. Orthostatic hypotension may occur from decreased sympathetic reflexes, after downregulation of adrenergic receptors. Weight loss may result from chronic hypermetabolism. Hyperglycemia may occur as a consequence of the inhibitory effects of catecholamines on pancreatic beta cells.

40. **What are the five H's associated with pheochromocytoma?**
This mnemonic derives from five of the following clinical manifestations:
   • Hypertension
   • Headache
   • Hyperhidrosis
   • Hyperglycemia
   • Hypermetabolism
      A large French series suggested that hypertension, headache, and hyperhydrosis are present in 95% of cases diagnosed in that country.

41. **What is the "rule of ten (percent)"?**
Classically, each of the following accounts for about 10% of all pheochromocytomas:
   • Bilateral (in **both** adrenal glands)
   • Extra-adrenal
   • Malignant
   • Familial (associated with multiple endocrine neoplasia [MEN] syndromes)
   • Pediatric
      In reality, few large series show the expected 10% incidence; recent data suggest that about 20% of pheochromocytomas are heredofamilial (see next question).

42. **What conditions are associated with pheochromocytoma?**
   • von Recklinghausen disease (neurofibromatosis)
   • Tuberous sclerosis (de Bourneville or Pringle disease)
   • Sturge-Weber syndrome
   • von Hippel-Lindau disease
   • Ataxia telangiectasia
   • MEN syndromes:
      • MEN type 2 (or 2a): pheochromocytoma (usually bilateral, but seldom synchronous), parathyroid adenoma, medullary thyroid carcinoma (which is typically diagnosed first)
      • MEN type 3 (or 2b): pheochromocytoma, medullary carcinoma of thyroid, mucosal neuromas, abdominal gangliomas, Marfanoid body habitus (the prevalence of this syndrome is only about 5% of that of MEN 2 or 2a)
   • Familial paraganglioma (typically associated with mutations in the succinate dehydrogenase gene)

43. What are some clinical clues to the diagnosis of pheochromocytoma?
    - Sustained or paroxysmal hypertension associated with the triad of headache, palpitations, and diaphoresis
    - Hypertension and family history of pheochromocytoma
    - Refractory hypertension especially if associated with weight loss
    - Sinus tachycardia
    - Orthostatic hypotension
    - Recurrent cardiac dysrhythmias
    - Features of MEN type 2 (or 2a) or 3 (or 2b)
    - Hypertensive crises during surgery or anesthesia (typically during induction)
    - Pressor response to a beta-blocker
    - Incidentally discovered adrenal mass

44. What are the most common causes of death of patients with pheochromocytoma?
    - Myocardial infarction
    - Malignant cardiac dysrhythmias
    - Cerebrovascular accident
    - Renal failure
    - Dissecting aortic aneurysm

45. Elaborate on the biochemical screening for pheochromocytoma.
    Plasma metanephrines have the highest sensitivity (~96%), but a low specificity (~85%), so this test is most appropriate for patients at very high risk (e.g., those with family histories or strong histories and a positive scan). A 24-hour urine collection for fractionated metanephrines can be recommended for patients at low risk; vanillylmandelic acid (false-positive rate in patients at low risk ~15%) and total catecholamines can be added for those at higher risk. Collecting a 24-hour urine after a "spell" can increase the sensitivity of urinary tests.

46. What are the potential sources of error in chemical screening tests?
    Plasma levels of catecholamines and metabolites may be falsely elevated with any type of stress. In patients with paroxysmal hypertension, urinary concentration of catecholamines and their metabolites may be normal if the 24-hour urine is collected when the patient is normotensive and asymptomatic. Common drugs that affect catecholamine and metabolite levels are listed in Table 65.2.

47. What tests should be performed in equivocal cases?
    A number of pharmacologic tests can be performed but usually are not necessary (Table 65.3).

48. What studies are used to localize a pheochromocytoma?
    Imaging studies are generally indicated only after biochemical screening is positive. Using a scan as a screening test increases the risk of discovering an "incidentaloma" (i.e., a nonfunctioning tumor). CT scan or MRI of the abdomen is about 95% sensitive and 65% specific; the T2-weighted MRI has a higher specificity because chromaffin tumors usually "light up." ^{123}I-metaiodobenzylguanidine (MIBG) scintigraphy is about 80% sensitive and 99% specific for chromaffin tissue; it is usually used for large (>10 cm) tumors or to evaluate extra-adrenal tumors. When imaging studies are equivocal, somatostatin receptor imaging, positron emission scanning, or even selective venous sampling of the vena cava at various levels can help locate the tumor.

Table 65.2. Common Drugs That Affect Catecholamine and Metabolite Levels

INCREASE	DECREASE
Tricyclic antidepressants	Metyrosine
Amphetamine(s)	Methylglucamine
Beta-blockers (labetalol, sotalol)	Reserpine
Benzodiazepines	
L-dopa, methyldopa	
Ethanol	
Withdrawal from clonidine and other alpha-agonists	

Table 65.3. Tests for Pheochromocytoma

TEST	RATIONALE
Regitine® (phentolamine) test	Phentolamine is an alpha-blocker, and a reduction in blood pressure after its intravenous administration suggests a catecholamine excess. The test is neither sensitive nor specific
Histamine test	This old test is seldom performed today because it is neither sensitive nor specific and can be dangerous
Glucagon stimulation test	Glucagon stimulates catecholamine release and raises blood pressure and pulse rate in a patient with a pheochromocytoma. The risk of precipitating a hypertensive crisis can be blocked by prior administration of an alpha-adrenoceptor antagonist
Clonidine suppression test	Clonidine decreases central sympathetic outflow in normal or nervous subjects, but does not suppress autonomous catecholamine production by a tumor. Failure to suppress plasma norepinephrine by more than 50%, and into the normal range, within 2–3 h after administration of an appropriate dose (0.2–0.3 mg) of clonidine is highly suggestive of a pheochromocytoma

49. What is the treatment of choice for pheochromocytoma?

Surgical removal of the tumor is the treatment of choice and is curative in >90% of cases. Small, single tumors are now most often removed laparoscopically, but large tumors usually require the traditional midline incision, careful inspection of the paravertebral ganglionic chain, and longer recuperation. Medical therapy is used mainly for perioperative management. Chronic medical therapy in the form of α- and (sometimes) β-blockade or inhibition of catecholamine synthesis with α-methyl-paratyrosine can be used for patients with inoperable, recurrent, multicentric, or malignant pheochromocytoma.

50. Describe perioperative management.

The goal of preoperative medical therapy is to control blood pressure (for 1 to 4 weeks prior to surgery) and to block the cardiovascular consequences of increased catecholamine levels. Alpha-blockers should be given first; phenoxybenzamine, a long-acting, oral, noncompetitive alpha-blocker, is preferred. The more selective, competitive, postsynaptic alpha$_1$-blockers (prazosin, terazosin, doxazosin) have a shorter duration of action and provide incomplete α-blockade, so failures have been described. When tachycardia or cardiac dysrhythmias persist, a β-adrenergic blocker may be given, but only *after* achieving α-blockade to avoid unopposed α-receptor stimulation and further vasoconstriction.

51. What clinical parameters should be monitored in the postoperative period?

- Persistent hypertension reflects:
  - Fluid overload
  - Return of autonomic reflexes
  - Inadvertent ligation of renal artery
  - Presence of residual tumor
- Persistent hypotension often reflects:
  - Blood loss
  - Altered vascular compliance
  - Residual effect of preoperative α-blockade
  - Downregulation of adrenoceptors (left over from chronic stimulation preoperatively)
- Hypoglycemia
  - Removal of inhibitory effect of catecholamines on pancreatic beta cells
  - Increased sensitivity of the beta cells to glucose level after tumor removal
  - Cessation of enflurane anesthesia, which leads to reflexive increase in insulin
- Assess risk for familial syndromes and possible genetic testing
  - Serum calcium, calcitonin, and intact parathyroid hormone
  - Ophthalmologist examination for retinal angiomas; consider head CT for cerebellar hemangioblastomas
  - Consider mutation analysis for the *ret* proto-oncogene for familial and other high-risk cases

- Assess risk for residual tumor
  - A screening test that was positive preoperatively should be repeated 1 to 2 weeks after surgery and annually thereafter

52. **What about treatment for malignant pheochromocytoma?**
Malignant pheochromocytoma accounts for less than 10% of all pheochromocytomas. These are usually slow growing and are poorly responsive to radiotherapy or chemotherapy. Surgical debulking is occasionally necessary to decrease catecholamine synthesis. High-dose radioactive MIBG has been used with some success to ablate primary and metastatic sites.

53. **What is the prognosis of pheochromocytoma?**
- 5-year survival:
  - 95% in non-malignant pheochromocytoma
  - <50% in malignant pheochromocytoma
- Recurrence rate after surgery is <10% in non-malignant pheochromocytoma.
- Resection cures hypertension in 75% of affected patients. In the remaining 25%, hypertension persists but is easier to control with standard antihypertensive agents.

KEY POINTS

1. Hyperaldosteronism can be either primary (e.g., Conn adenoma, bilateral adrenal hyperplasia) or secondary (renovascular hypertension, sleep apnea). Primary hyperaldosteronism is distinguished by an elevated plasma aldosterone/renin ratio, although the test has frequent false positives.
2. Although exogenous administration of corticosteroids is the most common cause of Cushing syndrome, a basophilic adenoma of the pituitary gland (Cushing disease) is the most common non-iatrogenic cause. It is classically diagnosed by a non-suppressed serum cortisol level after low-dose dexamethasone, but a suppressed serum cortisol level after high-dose dexamethasone.
3. Although many treatments for Cushing syndrome exist, their success largely depends on accurate identification of the overproduced hormone and its source.
4. Congenital adrenal hyperplasia is rarely seen in adults because pediatricians are so efficient at recognizing affected babies and children. For most, low-dose glucocorticoid (and occasional mineralocorticoid) therapy provides effective long-term treatment.
5. Although very rare, patients with pheochromocytoma typically present with hypertension, headaches, and hyperhidrosis (excessive sweating). Patients can be diagnosed with either urinary or plasma catecholamine and/or metabolites. People with pheochromocytoma require pretreatment before surgery with alpha-blockers (and occasional beta-blockade) to prevent a hypertensive crisis. Other family members of patients with features of heredofamilial syndromes should be screened for these diseases.

BIBLIOGRAPHY

Hyperaldosteronism

Amar, L., Lorthioir, A., Azizi, M., & Plouin, P. F. (2015). Progress in primary aldosteronism. Mineralocorticoid antagonist treatment for aldosterone-secreting adenoma. *European Journal of Endocrinology, 172,* R125–R129.

Asbach, E., Williams, T. A., & Reincke, M. (2016). Recent developments in primary aldosteronism. *Experimental and Clinical Endocrinology and Diabetes, 124,* 335–341.

Funder, J. W., Carey, R. M., Mantero, F., Murad, M. H., Reincke, M., Shibata, H., . . . Young, W. F., Jr. (2016). The management of primary aldosteronism: Case detection, diagnosis, and treatment: An Endocrine Society Clinical Practice Guideline. *Journal of Clinical Endocrinology and Metabolism, 101,* 1889–1916.

Muth, A., Ragnarsson, O., Johannsson, G., & Wängberg, B. (2015). Systematic review of surgery and outcomes in patients with primary aldosteronism. *British Journal of Surgery, 102,* 307–317.

Cushing Syndrome and Congenital Adrenal Hyperplasia

Lacroix, A., Feelders, R. A., Stratakis, C. A., & Nieman, L. K. (2015). Cushing's syndrome. *Lancet, 386,* 913–927.

Lodish, M., & Stratakis, C. A. (2016). A genetic and molecular update on adrenocortical causes of Cushing syndrome. *Nature Reviews Endocrinology, 12,* 255–262.

Lonser, R. R., Nieman, L., & Oldfield, E. H. (2017). Cushing's disease: Pathobiology, diagnosis, and management. *Journal of Neurosurgery, 126,* 404–417.

Nieman, L. K, Biller, B. M., Findling, J. W., Murad, M. H., Newell-Price, J., Savage, M. O., . . . Endocrine Society. (2015). Treatment of Cushing's syndrome: An Endocrine Society clinical practice guideline. *Journal of Clinical Endocrinology and Metabolism, 100,* 2807–2831.

Nieman, L. K., Biller, B. M., Findling, J. W., Newell-Price, J., Savage, M. O., Stewart, P. M., & Montori, V. M. (2008). The diagnosis of Cushing's syndrome: An Endocrine Society clinical practice guideline. *Journal of Clinical Endocrinology and Metabolism*, *93*, 1526–1540.

Speiser, P. W., Azziz, R., Baskin, L. S., Ghizzoni, L., Hensle, T. W., Merke, D. P., . . . Endocrine Society. (2010). Congenital adrenal hyperplasia due to steroid 21-hydroxylase deficiency: An Endocrine Society clinical practice guideline. *Journal of Clinical Endocrinology Metabolism*, *95*, 4133–4160.

Pheochromocytoma

Fishbein, L. (2016). Pheochromocytoma and paraganglioma: Genetics, diagnosis and treatment. *Hematology/Oncology Clinics of North America*, *30*, 135–150.

Lenders, J. W., Duh, Q. Y., Eisenhofer, G., Gimenez-Roqueplo, A. P., Grebe, S. K., Murad, M. H., . . . Endocrine Society. (2014). Pheochromocytoma and paraganglioma: An Endocrine Society clinical practice guideline. *Journal of Clinical Endocrinology and Metabolism*, *99*, 1915–1942.

Martucci, V. L., & Pacak, K. (2014). Pheochromocytoma and paraganglioma: Diagnosis, genetics, management and treatment. *Current Problems in Cancer*, *38*, 7–41.

Pappachan, J. M., Raskauskiene, D., Sriraman, R., Edavalath, M., & Hanna, F. W. (2014). Diagnosis and management of pheochromocytoma: A practical guide to clinicians. *Current Hypertension Reports*, *16*, 442.

Pillai, S., Gopalan, V., Smith, R. A., & Lam, A. K. (2016). Updates on the genetics and the clinical impacts on phaeochromocytoma and paraganglioma in the new era. *Critical Reviews in Oncology and Hematology*, *100*, 190–208.

CHAPTER 66

OTHER FORMS OF SECONDARY HYPERTENSION

William J. Elliott

1. **Besides renovascular and the traditional endocrine causes of hypertension, what are eight uncommon, but important, causes of secondary hypertension?**
   - Obstructive sleep apnea (typically causing hyperaldosteronism)
   - Drug-induced hypertension (especially nonsteroidal antiinflammatory drugs, steroids, and/or other immunosuppressants)
   - Thyroid disorders (hypothyroidism more commonly than hyperthyroidism)
   - Coarctation of the aorta (typically manifested as different blood pressures in the arms or a lower blood pressure in the legs)
   - Hyperparathyroidism (hypertension is found in only 10% of patients with hyperparathyroidism in the general population and up to 60% of those with additional endocrinopathies, especially multiple endocrine neoplasia syndrome. Removal of the parathyroid adenoma does not always lower blood pressure
   - Acromegaly (18% to 60% [increasing with age at diagnosis] of patients with acromegaly have hypertension; many have left ventricular hypertrophy; most respond well to antihypertensive drugs; and some have blood pressures that revert to normal when the acromegaly is cured)
   - "Neurogenic" hypertension
   - Liddle syndrome (a rare genetic disorder that is also called pseudohyperaldosteronism)

2. **What is the usual sequence of diagnostic and therapeutic steps for patients with sleep apnea?**
   Most such patients are overweight or obese, and many have bed partners who note snoring and/or witness apneic episodes during sleep. The Berlin questionnaire may be useful in screening, but a polysomnographic sleep study is typically required for diagnosis. Cohort studies have shown a significant improvement in survival if continuous positive airway pressure (CPAP) is used during sleep; a meta-analysis of 18 randomized, clinical trials suggests that CPAP significantly lowers 24-hour ambulatory blood pressures (by about 2/2 mm Hg) but not cardiovascular events (odds ratio [OR] = 0.84, 95% confidence interval [CI]: 0.62 to 1.13) or death (OR = 0.85, 95% CI: 0.35 to 2.06). In patients with hyperaldosteronism and sleep apnea, CPAP is recommended primarily for its improvement in quality of life; blood pressure can typically be reduced even further by adding spironolactone or eplerenone; a serum aldosterone/renin ratio is often measured before starting such treatment.

3. **What are the most common drug-induced causes of hypertension?**
   Nonsteroidal antiinflammatory drugs (including agents that are more selective for the second isoform of cyclooxygenase, e.g., celecoxib) are probably the most common cause of drug-induced hypertension due to their widespread, unregulated use. The mechanism is not well worked out, although alteration in intrarenal prostaglandin metabolism, sodium retention, and edema formation is likely.

   Anabolic steroids, glucocorticoids, and mineralocorticoids all raise blood pressure, and the usual recommendation is to use the lowest possible dose for the shortest possible time to decrease the risk of long-term consequences (including hypertension and its sequelae).

   Patients with chronic kidney disease or transplant recipients often take drugs that raise blood pressure, including cyclosporine, erythropoietin, and tacrolimus. Elevated blood pressures after use of tyrosine kinase inhibitors (given for various cancers) are associated with a favorable tumor response. These drugs are so important for the patient's overall health that they are continued, and more antihypertensive agents are added.

   Many "street" drugs can raise blood pressure acutely; acute withdrawal from nicotine, heroin, or other opioids can have the same effect. The drugs most often causing hypertension in an Emergency Department setting are cocaine, methylphenidate (or other stimulants), gamma-hydroxybutyrate, ketamine, and ergotamine. Chronic ingestion of alcohol increases the risk of hypertension; a meta-analysis of 36 trials involving 2865 participants showed a dose-dependent, significant reduction in blood pressure (by 5.5/3.0 mm Hg, on average) in those who reduced their consumption from >2 drinks/day.

A large variety of other prescription drugs (e.g., phenylpropanolamines, oral contraceptive pills, venlafaxine) can raise blood pressure. A wide variety of other drugs can interfere with antihypertensive medications either directly or via inhibition of metabolic pathways (typically hepatic cytochrome P_{450} or CYP oxidoreductases). Stimulants used in the treatment of ADHD can cause hypertension. methylphenidate, dextroamphetamine, and lisdexamfetamine can cause hypertension.

4. What are the "usual and customary" antihypertensive treatment strategies for patients who have drug-induced hypertension?
   See Table 66.1.

5. What are three primary diseases of the thyroid that can affect blood pressure?
   - **Hypothyroidism** is the most common thyroid disease that is associated with hypertension (3% of newly diagnosed hypertensives), although the mechanism is unclear. After appropriate thyroid replacement, blood pressure typically falls without specific antihypertensive therapy. Because hypothyroidism is a rare cause of secondary hypertension, a serum-ultrasensitive thyroid-stimulating hormone was not generally recommended as an initial test for all patients newly diagnosed with hypertension until the 2017 American College of Cardiology/American Heart Association hypertension guidelines (although other historical and physical findings might justify it).
   - **Hyperthyroidism** typically presents in younger patients with tachycardia, hypertension, a wide pulse pressure, and other traditional signs, but older people sometimes lack one or more of these typical features. The now-standard initial test is a serum-ultrasensitive thyroid-stimulating hormone level. Therapy is usually propranolol, which treats the hypertension, tachycardia, and (at least according to traditional pharmacologic teachings, now widely challenged) inhibits the peripheral conversion of thyroxine (T_4) to triiodothyronine (T_3).

6. What is the usual anatomy of coarctation of the aorta, its typical signs, and diagnostic evaluation scheme?
   Although congenital localized narrowing of the aorta may occur anywhere between the aortic valve and the abdominal aorta, it most commonly occurs in adults near or at the location of the former ductus arteriosus (ligamentum arteriosum after regression). It is the fourth leading cause of congenital heart disease, but it is an uncommon cause of hypertension in children and is even less common in adults. Physical examination nearly always shows a lower blood pressure in the leg (measured supine, with a cuff over the thigh and auscultating in the popliteal fossa), radial-femoral delay, and diminished pulses in the lower extremities. Continuous cardiac murmurs are common in chronic untreated coarctation, as a result of development of collateral blood flow around the narrowing. The classic chest x-ray findings include rib notching (from dilated intercostal arteries on the inferior surfaces of ribs) and the "3 sign" (consisting of a dilated proximal aorta, the coarctation, and the poststenotic dilatation). An esophagram (obtained after swallowing barium or other contrast medium) often shows the "reverse 3" sign. The most useful diagnostic test for patients suspected of having a coarctation is an echocardiogram; some centers prefer magnetic resonance angiograms, although some surgeons still require traditional aortography and a full cardiac catheterization in adults to prove the absence of major coronary heart disease and/or other associated congenital anomalies.

Table 66.1. Antihypertensive Treatments for Drug-Induced Hypertension

DRUGS THAT INDUCE HYPERTENSION	ANTIHYPERTENSIVE DRUG TREATMENT(S)
Corticosteroids, mineralocorticoids	Angiotensin-converting enzyme inhibitor, diuretic
Nonsteroidal antiinflammatory drug	Diuretic, calcium antagonist, maybe alpha-1-blocker
Phenylpropanolamine(s)	Beta-blocker
Nasal decongestant(s)	Alpha-1-blocker or alpha-beta-blocker
Cocaine	Alpha-blocker (typically phentolamine)
Antidepressants (monoamine oxidase inhibitors, serotonin reuptake inhibitors, etc.)	Alpha-blocker, calcium antagonist (?)
Oral contraceptive pills	None; stop oral contraceptive pills instead

7. What are the recommended treatment options for patients with coarctation of the aorta and their effects on hypertension and mortality?
Multiple surgical procedures have been used, including resection of the involved aortic segment with end-to-end reanastomosis, grafting of an overlying aortic flap, and/or placement of a synthetic graft. More recently, balloon angioplasty has been successful in many infants and children, but the procedure can be technically challenging in adolescents and adults. If left untreated, about 50% of patients with coarctation die by age 30; the 30-year survival improves to 93% if successfully repaired before age 5 years. Hypertension is "cured" in about 50% of children who have successful repairs of coarctation. When the coarctation is discovered in an adult, the life expectancy is reduced, primarily because the hypertension is more difficult to control (and often does not disappear after repair), and more target organ damage has already occurred.

8. What is the relationship between hypertension and hyperparathyroidism?
Hypertension occurs in a variable proportion of patients with primary hyperparathyroidism, depending on the population surveyed; "cure" of hypertension is similarly unpredictable after resection of the parathyroid adenoma. Oddly enough, other chronic conditions that produce similar levels of hypercalcemia (e.g., sarcoidosis, myeloma, or other malignancies) are not associated with hypertension. This has led to increased attention to the serum parathyroid hypertensive factor, a unique 3000 to 4000 Da protein, which is normally released from parathyroid glands, and raises blood pressure when infused into rats or humans. Although its plasma concentration can now be measured by radioimmunoassay, it is not routinely measured in clinical laboratories.

9. What is the relationship between hypertension and acromegaly?
Although human growth hormone and insulin-like growth factor-1 (somatomedin C) may increase blood pressure a little (and treatment of normotensive people with acromegaly lowers blood pressure a little), most authorities attribute the higher-than-expected prevalence of hypertension in patients with acromegaly to their hypertrophied hearts and vascular systems; sleep apnea also plays a role. Octreotide and other antagonists of growth hormone have little antihypertensive effect. Treating hypertension in acromegaly probably improves their prognosis because most of them die of premature cardiovascular disease.

10. What is neurogenic hypertension? What are the most common forms? Are there any specific treatments?
Any pathologic process that acutely increases intracranial pressure can cause hypertension and bradycardia, which is known as the Cushing reflex. Thus, acute stroke, intracranial tumors, severe head injury, and occasionally patients with quadriplegia and other spinal cord pathology are often complicated by new-onset hypertension or worsened blood pressure control in those with a prior history of hypertension. In most cases, addressing the primary neurologic problem lowers blood pressure, often in as little as 24 hours. The presumed mechanism is neurovascular compression of the left ventrolateral medulla and associated sympathetic nervous system stimulation.

11. What are the common causes of, and the treatment options for, neurogenic orthostatic hypertension?
Neurogenic orthostatic hypotension is a distinctive and often treatable sign of cardiovascular autonomic dysfunction. It is caused by a failure of noradrenergic neurotransmission, and is most often associated with diabetic neuropathy, Parkinson disease, dementia with Lewy bodies, multiple system atrophy, or pure autonomic failure (in order of increasing risk). It has a prevalence of 5% to 30% in older, general US populations. The loss of homeostatic mechanisms to control blood pressure fluctuations raises blood pressure while supine, while causing orthostatic hypotension, typically within 6 seconds after assuming a seated or standing position. These changes are most easily demonstrated during a tilt-table test. Affected patients often need short-acting antihypertensive medications (e.g., clonidine) at bedtime and stimulants (e.g., midodrine, droxidopa) during the day.

12. What is the genetic defect in Liddle syndrome, and how are such patients treated?
Liddle syndrome is a rare (~30 pedigrees described through 2008) autosomal-dominant disorder caused by a gain of function mutation of the epithelial sodium channel (ENaC) in the cortical collecting tubule. The mutation causes increased sodium reabsorption, volume expansion, and blood pressure. The clinical presentation is distinguished from hyperaldosteronism by the low serum aldosterone, but hypokalemia, metabolic alkalosis, and hypertension are present in both. Treatment with amiloride or triamterene blocks the constitutively active ENaC in the collecting tubule, corrects the hypokalemia, and lowers blood pressure. Spironolactone or eplerenone is ineffective because aldosterone is not primarily involved in the pathogenesis of Liddle syndrome.

KEY POINTS

1. Obstructive sleep apnea is a recognized cause of hypertension because we have methods for efficient screening (with the Berlin questionnaire), diagnosis (with overnight polysomnographic testing, often in the home), and treatment (typically involving aldosterone antagonists), in addition to CPAP during sleep.
2. The most common cause of drug-induced hypertension is nonsteroidal antiinflammatory drugs. Other drugs that cause hypertension include steroids, cyclosporine, erythropoietin, tyrosine kinase inhibitors, or tacrolimus.
3. Hypothyroidism is a more common cause of hypertension than hyperthyroidism, but routine testing of serum thyroid-stimulating hormone was not warranted at diagnosis for all patients with hypertension until the 2017 ACC/AHA hypertension guidelines.
4. Coarctation of the aorta should be suspected if there is a lower blood pressure in an arm or a leg compared to the other arm or leg; an echocardiogram can confirm the diagnosis in most cases, and endoluminal therapies are available (and are especially useful in younger children).
5. The many single-gene mutations associated with hypertension have taught us a great deal about hypertension, but they account for a tiny fraction of the prevalence of the condition.

Bibliography

Cai, Y., Ren, Y., & Shi, J. (2011). Blood pressure levels in patients with subclinical thyroid dysfunction: A meta-analysis of cross-sectional data. *Hypertension Research, 34*, 1098–1105.
Calhoun, D. A., Jones, D., Textor, S., Goff, D. C., Murphy, T. P., Toto, R. D., . . . Carey, R. M. (2008). Resistant hypertension: Diagnosis, evaluation, and treatment: A scientific statement from the American Heart Association Professional Education Committee of the Council for High Blood Pressure Research. *Hypertension, 51*, 1403–1419.
Grossman, A., Messerli, F. H., & Grossman, E. (2015). Drug-induced hypertension: An underappreciated cause of secondary hypertension. *European Journal of Pharmacology, 763*, 15–22.
Guo, J., Sun, Y., Xue, L. J., Huang, Z. Y., Wang, Y. S., Zhang, L., . . . Yuan, L. X. (2016). Effect of CPAP therapy on cardiovascular events and mortality in patients with obstructive sleep apnea: A meta-analysis. *Sleep and Breathing, 20*, 965–974.
Marin, J. M., Carrizo, S. J., Vicente, E., & Agusti, A. G. (2005). Long-term cardiovascular outcomes in men with obstructive sleep apnoea-hypopnoea with or without treatment with continuous positive airway pressure: An observational study. *Lancet, 365*, 1046–1053.
Melmed, S., Casanueva, F. F., Klibanski, A., Bronstein, M. D., Chanson, P., Lamberts, S. W., . . . Giustina, A. (2013). A consensus on the diagnosis and treatment of acromegaly complications. *Pituitary, 16*, 294–302.
Metzler, M., Duerr, S., Granata, R., Krismer, F., Robertson, D., & Wenning, G. K. (2013). Neurogenic orthostatic hypotension: Pathophysiology, evaluation and management. *Journal of Neurology, 260*, 2212–2219.
Nakamura, K., & Stefanescu Schmidt, A. (2016). Treatment of hypertension in coarctation of the aorta. *Current Treatment Options in Cardiovascular Medicine, 18*, 40.
Padmanabhan, S., Caulfield, M., & Dominiczak, A. F. (2015). Genetic and molecular aspects of hypertension. *Circulation Research, 116*, 937–959.
Patrono, C. (2016). Cardiovascular effects of non-steroidal anti-inflammatory drugs. *Current Cardiology Reports, 18*, 25.
Roerecke, M., Kaczorowski, J., Tobe, S.W., Gmel, G., Hasan, O. S. M., & Rehm, J. (2017). The effect of reduction of alcohol consumption on blood pressure: A systematic review and meta-analysis. *Lancet Public Health, 2*, 108–120.
Sardella, C., Urbani, C., Lombardi, M., Nuzzo, A., Manetti, L., Lupi, I., . . . Bogazzi, F. (2014). The beneficial effects of acromegaly control on blood pressure values in normotensive patients. *Clinical Endocrinology (Oxf), 81*, 573–581.
Whelton, P.K., Carey, R.M., Aranow, W.S., et al. (2017). 2017 ACC/AHA/AAPA/ABC/ACPM/AGS/APhA/ASH/ASPC/NMA/PCNA guideline for the prevention, detection, evaluation, and management of high blood pressure in adults. A report of the American College of Cardiology/American Heart Association Task Force on Clinical Practice Guidelines. Hypertension, epub before print on 13 NOV 17; doi: 10.1161/HYP.0000000000000066; simultaneously published in *J Am Coll Cardiol*, doi: 10.1016/j.jacc.2017.11.006.

CHAPTER 67

RESISTANT HYPERTENSION

Susan Patricia Steigerwalt

1. **What is resistant hypertension (RH)? Is it the same as refractory hypertension?**
   Hypertension is considered resistant if the blood pressure (BP) cannot be reduced below target levels (Box 67.1) in patients who are compliant with an optimal triple-drug regimen that includes a diuretic typically with an angiotensin converting enzyme inhibitor (ACEI) or angiotensin receptor blocker (ARB) plus calcium channel blocker (CCB), or those who have controlled BP but are on four or more medications to achieve BP control. RH is increasing in frequency due to increased age and obesity. Most patients with hypertension respond favorably to 1 to 3 antihypertensive drugs. RH is present in about 21% of U.S. adults with hypertension, though a much smaller fraction, about 3%, are truly refractory. Refractory hypertension is an inability to control high BP with the use of five or more classes of antihypertensive agents, including a long-acting thiazide-type diuretic, such as chlorthalidone, and a mineralocorticoid receptor antagonist, such as spironolactone. As with the definition of RH, this diagnosis does not take into account out-of-office BP. Up to 37% of patients labeled as *resistant hypertension* are actually controlled when BP is measured by 24-hour ambulatory BP monitoring.

Box 67.1. Causes of Refractory Hypertension

- Pseudoresistance
  - White-coat hypertension (see measurement)
  - Pseudohypertension in older patients (rare)
  - Use of small cuff in patients who are obese
- Nonadherence to prescribed therapy; present to some degree in 50%
- Volume overload
- Drug-related causes
  - Doses too low
  - Wrong type of diuretic
  - Inappropriate combinations
  - Drug actions and interactions
  - Sympathomimetics
    - Nasal decongestants
    - Stimulants, particularly medications for attention deficit hyperactivity disorder (methylphenidate), narcolepsy (modafinil), and appetite suppressants
    - Cocaine
    - Oral contraceptives (rare)
    - Adrenal steroids
    - Licorice (as may be found in chewing tobacco)
    - Cyclosporine, tacrolimus
    - Erythropoietin
    - Antidepressants, particularly monoamine oxidase inhibitors and the selective serotonin reuptake inhibitors-SSNI venlafaxine
    - Nonsteroidal antiinflammatory drugs
- Concomitant conditions
  - Obesity
  - Sleep apnea (present in up to 90% of patients with RH)
  - Ethanol intake of more than 1 oz (30 mL) per day
  - Severe emotional trauma resulting in labile blood pressure surges (pseudopheochromocytoma)
  - Anxiety, hyperventilation
- **Secondary causes of hypertension** (e.g., primary aldosteronism, renovascular hypertension, adrenal causes, and kidney disease, etc.)

Both patients with RH, whether controlled (on four pills) or uncontrolled (on three), and refractory hypertension (uncontrolled on five) have increased cardiovascular risk. This is true for patients with and without chronic kidney disease (CKD). African Americans and patients with CKD are at elevated risk of resistant or refractory hypertension.

Although the definition of RH is currently "in-office BP greater than 140/90," the SPRINT trial has called into question that BP goal established by clinical practice guidelines, at least in high-risk patients, and the manner of BP measurement. This means that the definition of RH may change too.

If a patient's BP is uncontrolled on multiple antihypertensive drugs, but one of them is not a diuretic, a diagnosis of RH should be delayed until after a trial of a properly dosed diuretic. It is worthwhile remembering that an "optimal" dose may not necessarily equate to a "full" dose. An optimal dose is the highest dose tolerated by the patient, or a dose governed by concomitant conditions, such as CKD or congestive heart failure.

2. Discuss the epidemiology of RH.
Although not representing typical office practices, the data from the Anti-hypertensive and Lipid-Lowering Treatment to Prevent Heart Attack Trial (ALLHAT) provides an estimate of the prevalence of RH in the community setting. In ALLHAT, 34% of the study participants had BP >140/90 mostly on two medications, with 27% requiring three or more medications. Based on the 5-year observations in ALLHAT, the incidence of RH was approximately 15%. In the Controlled ONset Verapamil INvestigation of Cardiovascular End Points (CONVINCE) study, 18% of the patients had a BP level >140/90 mm Hg on three or more medications.

Patients with diabetes are more resistant to antihypertensive drugs than nondiabetic subjects are, so they will typically require more antihypertensive drugs to achieve goal BP.

3. What are the most common causes of RH?
When a patient with hypertension demonstrates RH, proper management requires the identification of possible etiologies (Table 67.1). Before making drastic therapeutic changes, certain questions should come to the physician's mind:
• **Does the patient truly have "resistant hypertension"?**
BP measurement is key to the diagnosis of RH. Evaluate BP appropriately with cuffs allowing unob-served automated BP: either the Omron 907 XL, which was used in the SPRINT trial (5-minute rest followed by three readings 1 minute apart), or the BPTru, which measures six readings after 1-minute rest, deletes the first reading, then averages the last five. These methods are accurate, validated, and correlate with target organ damage. On average, using either auto-mated cuff, the systolic BP (SBP) readings are 8 to 15 mm lower than casual office BP read-ings. There is considerable inter-individual variability in the degree of difference, so one can-not reliably adjust casual office readings to approximate automated readings. The solution is for offices to adopt automated BP machines.
In a large Spanish cohort of patients with RH, 24-hour ambulatory BP measurements showed that one-third of patients diagnosed with RH in the office have BPs that were well controlled out of office.
The BP cuff needs to circle 80% of the upper arm and needs to be greater than 40% of the length of the upper arm to be accurate. Accurate BP readings require that the patients have their feet on the floor, their back supported, their arm at the level of their heart, and their urinary bladder empty.

Table 67.1. JNC 7 Classifications

OFFICE BP CLASSIFICATION	SBP (mm HG)		DBP (mm HG)
Normal	<120	and	<80
Prehypertension	120–139	or	80–89
Stage I hypertension	140–159	or	90–99
Stage II hypertension	≥160	or	≥100

24-hour ABPM: average <130/80; daytime <135/85; nighttime <120/75
ABPM, Ambulatory blood pressure monitoring; BP, blood pressure; DBP, diastolic blood pressure; JNC 7, seventh report of the Joint National Committee on Prevention, Detection, Evaluation and Treatment of High Blood Pressure; SBP, systolic blood pressure.

- **Are there any patient/environmental factors?**
  - Nonadherence is common. When blood or urine drug testing is used to confirm adherence of hypertensive patients to their prescribed medication, up to 50% of patients are at least partially nonadherent. The most accurate method to assess adherence, which has not been tested widely in office practice, is high-performance liquid chromatography (HPLC)-mass spectroscopy of blood or urine, to look for prescribed medications. HPLC-mass spectroscopy is an analytical chemistry technique that identifies complex compounds, including antihypertensive medications. Its availability and cost varies. It is widely available in Europe but not in the United States.
  - Alternatives to biochemical testing of compliance include having patients bring pill bottles or calling the pharmacy about refills at each visit. The increase in cardiovascular risk noted in RH has been studied in populations where some nonadherence is very likely. So, although nonadherence may be present in RH, it is not a "cause" per se.
  - Common medications the patient may be taking that will increase BP. Methylphenidate, venlafaxine, and daily use of nonsteroidal antiinflammatory agents can all raise the BP. Vascular endothelial growth factor inhibitors, high-dose steroids, and calcineurin inhibitors all worsen BP. European black licorice, found in complementary alternative medications and chewing tobacco, plus traditional Chinese medicines and other supplements may have enough glycyrrhizic acid to cause pseudohyperaldosteronism. Many supplements do not accurately list their ingredients.
  - Many patients are inadequately diuresed. Hydrochlorothiazide and furosemide do not lower BP over a 24-hour period. Chlorthalidone is a thiazide-type diuretic that is superior to hydrochlorothiazide for controlling BP and preventing cardiovascular events. Its effectiveness is likely due to its long duration of action. Additionally, there are data showing effective BP control down to an estimated glomerular filtration rate of 20, and a larger, confirmatory trial is under way. In patients that require loop diuretics, torsemide is a better choice than furosemide due to its long half-life and predictable bioavailability.
  - Most patients with RH consume a high-sodium diet. The Dietary Approaches to Stopping Hypertension (DASH) diet, along with sodium restriction, can significantly improve BP. In the original study, BPs dropped 8 to 13 mm Hg systolic in the hypertensive sub-cohort. Sustained sodium restriction may result in profound improvements in SBP (13 to 17 mm Hg) in CKD stage 3 and 4 hypertensive patients.
  - Exercise for 30 minutes 5 days a week has been shown to be the equivalent of an additional drug in patients with RH.
  - It has been reported that cigarette smoking can interfere with BP control mechanisms. Smoking cessation should be encouraged to stabilize kidney function and decrease cardiovascular risk.
  - Excessive alcohol consumption (more than 2 oz or 60 mL daily) raises the SBP, sometimes to dangerously high levels.
  - Obesity is an important cause of a lot of hypertension. To date, no careful trials have been performed in RH, but the usual weight-appropriate recommendations for structured weight loss or bariatric surgery (which does reduce BP) may result in improvement in otherwise RH.
  - Pseudopheochromocytoma. Severe emotional stress in childhood or young adulthood, such as incest, witnessed suicide, or chronic severe unremitting stress, may be associated with labile hypertension without overt anxiety. It has been described as a calm panic attack. The preferred drugs include alpha blockers, antidepressants, and β-blockers.
- **Does the patient have a secondary form of hypertension, such as primary aldosteronism or renovascular disease?**
  Screen all patients with RH with an aldosterone renin ratio. An elevated aldosterone and suppressed renin is indicative of primary aldosteronism. Fully 20% of resistant hypertensives screen positive for primary aldosteronism. If the screen is positive (aldosterone at or near 15, renin less than 1), follow up with further evaluation. The Endocrine Society updated its guidelines on primary aldosteronism in 2016. If an adenoma is found on a computed tomography scan as part of the evaluation, the patient should also be screened for cortisol excess. Although pheochromocytoma is vanishingly rare, it is easily ruled out with a plasma metanephrine and normetanephrine assay.
  In older patients, if clinical suspicion is high due to diffuse vascular disease and recurrent bouts of pulmonary edema, or persistent azotemia with the use of an angiotensin-converting enzyme (ACE) inhibitor, further evaluation for renal artery stenosis is indicated, although careful selection of patients for renal revascularization is critical. A subset of patients in the Cardiovascular Outcomes in Renal Atherosclerotic Lesions (CORAL) study without proteinuria had good outcomes with stenting.
  Consider polycystic ovary syndrome in young women with refractory hypertension. Rare adrenal (11 and 17-hydroxylase deficiency) and mineralocorticoid receptor alterations (Liddles, 11 β-OH

SD deficiency), which usually manifests in childhood, may cause RH. It is also important to check thigh BP measurement in patients younger than age 30 to screen for coarctation of the aorta.
- **Does the patient have obstructive sleep apnea?**
  Always evaluate patients with RH for sleep apnea. Examine their mouth for a Mallampati score and perform a sleep apnea screen, such as the STOP-BANG or Epworth sleepiness scale. Refer appropriately for a positive screen. Large drops in BP with treatment are disappointingly rare; however, treatment of sleep apnea may improve diabetes and ease weight loss. Patients with excessive daytime sleepiness that improves following continuous positive airway pressure may have a greater drop in BP, which is otherwise typically only 2 to 3 mm Hg.

DRUG INTERACTIONS
Drug interactions can occur due to alterations in the drug pharmacokinetics or pharmacodynamics of concomitant drugs administered for different indications (Table 67.2).

4. Are there any particular recommended drug treatment add-ons or combination regimens for RH?
   The PATHWAY-2 trial showed spironolactone to be the best choice as the fourth-line drug, except in those whose renin level is extremely elevated. In patients with CKD, there is concern regarding hyperkalemia. In CKD stages 1 to 3, if the initial potassium is less than 4.5 when adding 25 mg of spironolactone, hyperkalemia is rare; nevertheless, it is mandatory to check the potassium at 1 and 4 weeks after the initiation of treatment. It is also important to forewarn patients that if they become ill or stop eating and drinking, to discontinue spironolactone and proceed to an emergency room for a potassium measurement. Although a small observational trial showed improved BP in CKD stage 4, the risk of hyperkalemia precludes further recommending it. There is currently interest in the use of novel oral potassium binders (e.g., patiromer in combination with spironolactone) to control hyperkalemia while offering the benefit of a mineralocorticoid antagonist. This is being studied in patients with RH in the AMBER trial.
   Combination calcium channel blocker regimens (from dihydropyridine and non-dihydropyridine groups) have been demonstrated to be synergistic for BP control in this population. Decreasing the total pill burden with combination therapy may improve adherence.
   In CKD, activation of the sympathetic nervous system is present, and clonidine twice daily or once daily guanfacine may be a helpful add-on after spironolactone. Somnolence and bradycardia can occur with these drugs, as well as rebound hypertension from abrupt cessation.

5. What is the role of volume regulation in RH? How does it interfere with the efficacy of antihypertensive agents?
   Volume overload from any underlying mechanism may not only increase the BP but may offset the effectiveness of antihypertensive drugs. Excessive salt intake and retention increases the plasma volume and causes resistance to antihypertensive drugs, and can actually raise the BP in some patients. Elderly and African American patients are particularly sensitive to fluid overload, as are patients with chronic kidney disease and congestive heart failure. Some antihypertensive drugs, such as direct vasodilators, antiadrenergic agents, and most of the non-diuretic antihypertensive drugs, cause plasma and extracellular fluid expansion, thus interfering with BP control. Of all the non-diuretic antihypertensive drugs, ACE inhibitors, angiotensin receptor blockers, and calcium antagonists are the least likely to cause fluid retention. Antihypertensive responsiveness can be regained by restricting the sodium intake; adding or increasing the dose of the diuretic; and, in some instances, switching

Table 67.2. Drug Interactions That May Lead to Resistant Hypertension

ANTIHYPERTENSIVE AGENTS	INTERACTING DRUGS
Chlorthalidone, indapamide	Cholestyramine
Propranolol	Rifampin
Angiotensin-converting enzyme inhibitors	Indomethacin
Diuretics	Indomethacin
All drugs	Cocaine Tricyclics Prescription stimulants

to a loop diuretic from thiazides. In patients with advanced CKD, dialysis might be required for the adequate control of BP. Hypertension may be seemingly refractory if the antihypertensive drugs are used in suboptimal doses, or when an inappropriate diuretic is used (e.g., using a thiazide-type diuretic as opposed to a loop diuretic in patients with chronic kidney disease, congestive heart failure, and in those who are taking potent vasodilators, such as minoxidil or hydralazine). Inappropriate combinations can also limit their therapeutic potential. Adverse drug–drug interactions can raise the BP in patients with and without hypertension.

6. What are the treatment options for RH—a philosophical approach?
Rational management of RH requires a systematic approach based on the direct causes of the RH (see above). It should be re-emphasized that because uncontrolled hypertension can cause significant morbidity and mortality, aggressive therapeutic management should be implemented. An overall management approach should be based on careful evaluation and rational medical therapy, which may be complex.
Doctors should try to reduce the pill burden with combination medications where possible.
Correction of volume overload is one of the key strategies in managing RH. Excessive salt intake must be curtailed. Adequate diuretic therapy should be implemented. The doses of antihypertensive drugs should be titrated systematically to determine whether the patient is responding to the treatment. Drug interactions should be considered and eliminated in the treatment of hypertension. Patients should be supplied with a complete list of drugs that can increase BP: steroids, oral contraceptives, sympathomimetics, nasal decongestants, cocaine, appetite suppressants, and so on. Patients should be counseled about alcohol consumption, weight control, salt intake, and regular physical activity. Conditions such as obstructive sleep apnea or chronic pain should be vigorously addressed.
Secondary causes of hypertension, such as those listed in Box 67.2, should be considered in the overall evaluation of patients with RH. Any underlying cause should be corrected, if possible, to permit better BP control. Patients with RH experience and suffer from a high degree of target organ damage.
Assuming that the hypertension has failed to respond to conventional therapies, consideration should be given to the use of hydralazine or minoxidil (in conjunction with a β-blocker and a diuretic). Because direct vasodilators cause significant reflex activation of sympathetic nervous system and fluid retention, their use should be accompanied by the co-administration of a β-blocker and a loop diuretic.
Aggressive cardiovascular risk management is mandatory in patients with RH due to their increased risk of events.
Another current consideration is referral to a center that performs clinical trials on renal denervation. The DenervHTN trial just reported from Europe shows an additive effect of renal denervation to maximum medical therapy in refractory hypertension patients, (average 5.1 medications) controlled for adherence. In the near future, clinical trials on carotid baroreceptors stimulation, and iliac arteriovenous fistulae may also be restarted.
Referral to a hypertension specialist (or becoming one through the American Society of Hypertension Program) may also be helpful. Shared decision making with the patient regarding outcomes and side effects is critically important.
The problem of RH can be treated successfully in a systematic fashion and on a rational basis.

Box 67.2. Some Examples of Secondary Forms of Hypertension

- Primary aldosteronism (present in 20% of resistant hypertensives)
- Kidney disease
- Renal artery stenosis-fibromuscular-young
- Atherosclerotic-old
- Pheochromocytoma (rare)
- Hypothyroidism
- Hyperthyroidism (systolic hypertension)
- Hyperparathyroidism
- Aortic coarctation (rare: do not forget to perform blood pressure measurement in the leg on the first visit)

KEY POINTS

1. Up to 20% of RH is associated with primary aldosteronism, so always screen for this.
2. Up to 50% of RH is associated with at least partial nonadherence to medications. The use of combinations to reduce the total pill burden may help.
3. RH is associated with increased morbidity and mortality.
4. Sodium restriction will assist in BP control.

BIBLIOGRAPHY

Epidemiology

Braam, B., Taler, S. J., Rahman, M., FIllaus, J. A., Greco, B. A., Forman, J. P., . . . Hedayati, S. S. (2017). Recognition and management of resistant hypertension. *Clin J Am Soc Nephrol, 12*(3), 524–535. doi:10.2215/CJN.06180616.
Calhoun, D. A., Jones, D., Textor, S., Goff, D. C., Murphy, T. P., Toto, R. D. . . . Carey, R. M. (2008). Resistant hypertension: Diagnosis, evaluation, and treatment. *Hypertension, 51*, 1403–1419.
Dudenbostel, T., Siddiqui, M., Oparil, S., & Calhoun, D. A. (2016). Refractory hypertension. *Hypertension, 67*, 1085–1092.
Muntner, P., Davis, B. R., Cushman, W. C., Bangalore, S., Calhoun, D. A., Pressel, S. L., . . . ALLHAT Collaborative Research Group. (2014). Treatment-resistant hypertension and the incidence of cardiovascular disease and end-stage renal disease: Results from the Antihypertensive and Lipid-Lowering Treatment to Prevent Heart Attack Trial (ALLHAT). *Hypertension, 64*(5), 1012–1021.
Thomas, G., Xie, D., Chen, H. Y., Anderson, A. H., Appel, L. J., Bodana, S., . . . CRIC Study Investigators. (2016). Prevalence and prognostic significance of apparent treatment resistant hypertension in chronic kidney disease. *Hypertension, 67*, 387–396.

Sprint and Blood Pressure Measurement

de la Sierra, A., Segura, J., Banegas, J. R., Gorostidi, M., de la Cruz, J. J., Armario, P., . . . Ruilope, L. M. (2011). Clinical features of 8295 patients with resistant hypertension classified on the basis of ambulatory blood pressure monitoring. *Hypertension, 57*(5), 898–902.
Kjeldsen, S. E., Lund-Johansen, P., Nilsson, P. M., & Mancia, G. (2016). Unattended blood pressure measurements in the systolic blood pressure intervention trial. *Hypertension, 67*, 808–812.
The Sprint Research Group. (2015). A randomized trial of intensive versus standard blood-pressure control. *NEJM, 373*(22), 2103–2116.

Drug Adherence

Jung, O., Gechter, J. L., Wunder, C., Paulke, A., Bartel, C., Geiger, H., & Toennes, S. W. (2013). Resistant hypertension? Assessment of adherence by toxicological urine analysis. *J Hypertens, 31*, 766–774.
Strauch, B., Petrák, O., Zelinka, T., Rosa, J., Somlóová, Z., Indra, T., . . . Widimský, J., Jr. (2013). Precise assessment of noncompliance with the antihypertensive therapy in patients with resistant hypertension using toxicological serum analysis. *J Hypertens, 31*, 2455–2461.

Chlorthalidone

Agarwal, R., Sinha, A. D., Pappas, M. K., & Ammous, F. (2014). Chlorthalidone for poorly controlled hypertension in chronic kidney disease: An interventional pilot study. *Am J Nephrol, 39*, 171–182.
Roush, G. C., Ernst, M. E., Kostis, J. B., Tandon, S., & Sica, D. A. (2015). Head-to-head comparisons of hydrochlorothiazide with indapamide and chlorthalidone. *Hypertension, 65*(5), 1041–1046. http://dx.doi.org/10.1161/HYPERTENSION.114.05021.

Bariatric Surgery and Resistant Hypertension

Blumenthal, J. A., Sherwood, A., Smith, P. J., Mabe, S., Watkins, L., Lin, P. H., . . . Hinderliter, A. (2015). Lifestyle modification for resistant hypertension: The TRIUMPH randomized clinical trial. *Am Heart J, 170*, 986–994.e5.
Schiavon, C. A., Drager, L. F., Bortolotto, L. A., Amodeo, C., Ikeoka, D., Berwanger, O., & Cohen, R. V. (2016). The role of metabolic surgery on blood pressure control. *Curr Atheroscler Rep, 18*, 50.
Zhang, H., Pu, Y., Chen, J., Tong, W., Cui, Y., Sun, F., . . . Zhu, Z. (2014). Gastrointestinal intervention ameliorates high blood pressure through antagonizing overdrive of the sympathetic nerve in hypertensive patients and rats. *J Am Heart Assoc, 3*, e000929. doi:10.1161/JAHA.114.000929.

Primary Aldosteronism and The Role of Spironolactone

Funder, J. W., Carey, R. M., Mantero, F., Murad, M. H., Reincke, M., Shibata, H., . . . Young, W. F., Jr. (2016). The management of primary aldosteronism: Case detection, diagnosis, and treatment: An endocrine society clinical practice guideline. *J Clin Endocrinol Metab, 101*(5), 1889–1916.
Khosla, N., Kalaitzidis, R., & Bakris, G. L. (2009). Predictors of hyperkalemia risk following hypertension control with aldosterone blockade. *Am J Nephrol, 30*(5), 418–424.
Williams, B., MacDonald, T. M., Morant, S., Webb, D. J., Sever, P., McInnes, G., . . . British Hypertension Society's PATHWAY Studies Group. (2015). Spironolactone versus placebo, bisoprolol, and doxazosin to determine the optimal treatment for drug-resistant hypertension (PATHWAY-2): A randomized, double-blind, crossover trial. *Lancet, 386*, 2059–2068.

Renal Denervation and Miscellaneous Secondary

Böhlke, M., & Barcellos, F. C. (2015). From the 1190s to CORAL (Cardiovascular Outcomes in Renal Atherosclerotic Lesions) trial results and beyond: does stenting have a role in ischemic nephropathy? *Am J Kidney Dis, 65*(4), 611–622.

Calhoun, D. A. (2016). Renal nerve denervation, adherence, and management of resistant hypertension. *Circulation, 134,* 858–860.

Grossman, A., Messerli, F. H., & Grossman, E. (2015). Drug induced hypertension—an unappreciated cause of secondary hypertension. *Eur J Pharmacol, 763*(Pt A), 15–22.

Malha, L., & Mann, S. J. (2016). Loop diuretics in the treatment of hypertension. *Curr Hypertens Rep, 18*(4), 27.

Oliveras, A., Marmario, P., Clarà, A., Sans-Atxer, L., Vázquez, S., Pascual, J., & De la Sierra, A. (2016). Spironolactone versus sympathetic renal denervation to treat true resistant hypertension: results from the DENERVHTA study—a randomized controlled trial. *J Hypertens, 34*(9), 1863–1871.

CHAPTER 68

HYPERTENSIVE EMERGENCIES
William J. Elliott

1. How does a "hypertensive emergency" differ from "hypertensive urgency"?
   A "hypertensive emergency" is a clinical situation in which severely elevated blood pressure is associated with acute, progressive target-organ damage that needs to be treated immediately with a safe and controlled reduction of blood pressure. "Hypertensive urgencies" (if they truly exist; see Question 15 below) are characterized by elevated blood pressures in a patient who has no acute, progressive target-organ damage; these are typically treated with oral antihypertensive medications and close follow-up thereafter. Typical scenarios that are hypertensive emergencies include the following:
   • Hypertensive encephalopathy: typically a diagnosis of exclusion (see later)
   • Acute left ventricular failure and/or pulmonary edema (see later)
   • Subarachnoid or intracerebral hemorrhage
   • Acute aortic dissection: Target blood pressure is <120/70 mm Hg, within 20 minutes (see later).
   • Acute myocardial infarction or acute coronary syndrome
   • Adrenergic crisis: for example, pheochromocytoma, phencyclidine, or cocaine overdose (see later)
   • Glomerulonephritis or acute kidney injury
   • Epistaxis, gross hematuria, or threatened suture lines after vascular surgery
   • Eclampsia (some authorities would include preeclampsia here, but most obstetricians hasten to deliver the baby and lower blood pressure BEFORE a seizure occurs)
      The absolute level of blood pressure does not distinguish between emergencies and urgencies. Patients who were previously normotensive can develop a hypertensive emergency with a blood pressure that is only 30 to 50 mm Hg higher than their usual and customary blood pressure (e.g., 160/100 in a woman with preeclampsia). Conversely, some patients with chronic hypertension remain asymptomatic and might qualify as only hypertensive urgencies, even with a blood pressure of 250/150 mm Hg. Seldom, if ever, does such a high blood pressure require hospitalization if there is no acute target-organ damage.

2. What is "malignant hypertension," and how does it differ from "accelerated hypertension"?
   Malignant hypertension is the term historically given when severely elevated blood pressure was accompanied by retinal hemorrhages, exudates, and originally papilledema. The term arose in the 1920s when no effective treatment was available, and the prognosis of patients with this condition was similar to cancer. Now that treatment is available and effective, the term is used predominantly by hospital-based coders. In the last millennium, "accelerated hypertension" was severely elevated blood pressure without papilledema; this term is now only rarely used outside its historical context.

3. What are the epidemiologic characteristics of patients who present with a hypertensive emergency?
   Most such patients have a history of stage 2 hypertension that has not been adequately treated. The most common cause of this is nonadherence to prescribed medication. In the last millennium, patients presenting with "malignant hypertension" typically had very high blood pressures (before treatment) and were often cigarette smokers. Secondary hypertension, especially renovascular hypertension, was often found in patients with Keith-Wagener-Barker Grade III (hemorrhages/exudates) or IV (frank papilledema) retinopathy; chronic kidney disease was also very common in such patients in the 1970s.

4. What is the pathophysiology of "malignant hypertension"?
   A rapid and sustained rise in blood pressure causes endothelial dysfunction and then frank arteritis, leading to platelet and fibrin deposition within the vessel and eventually fibrinoid necrosis. The juxtaglomerular apparatus of the kidney releases renin when it senses relative ischemia, which increases circulating angiotensin II levels and causes severe vasoconstriction. The kidney responds to the elevated blood pressure with natriuresis, causing relative volume depletion and further activating the renin-angiotensin-aldosterone system. These events typically reinforce each other and lead to the "vicious cycle" of increasing blood pressure and worsening vascular function.

5. **What were the typical pathologic findings in "malignant hypertension?"**
   The patient's blood vessels undergo myointimal proliferation (and medial thickening, leading to the "onion-skin" appearance) and fibrinoid necrosis. If the process is chronic, vascular smooth muscle hypertrophy occurs and collagen deposits in the small vessels and arterioles.

6. **Historically, what were the common clinical features of "malignant hypertension"?**
   Typically the blood pressure was very high (often diastolic >140 mm Hg). The optic fundi showed bilateral papilledema, often with hemorrhages and exudates in the periphery. Hypertensive encephalopathy was common, usually preceded by headache, somnolence, visual changes, and confusion. Microangiopathic hemolytic anemia, with schistocytes and helmet cells on peripheral smear, and increased serum lactate dehydrogenase often were associated with fibrinoid necrosis of arterioles. Normal kidney function was distinctly unusual; most patients had oliguria, azotemia, proteinuria, and (usually microscopic) hematuria. The major reason malignant hypertension is uncommon today is that, in early studies, even a single antihypertensive drug reduced the risk of malignant hypertension by more than 90%.

7. **How does one diagnose hypertensive encephalopathy?**
   Such patients typically present with very high blood pressures and altered mental status. Optic fundi may show Grade III (hemorrhages/exudates) or IV (papilledema) retinopathy. Usually other evidence of hypertensive target-organ damage is present, such as hematuria, elevated serum creatinine, or left ventricular hypertrophy. Although the differential diagnosis in such a patient is long and complex, consideration can be given to starting a short-acting, easily titratable, intravenous antihypertensive agent while transporting the patient to the computed tomographic scanner. It is rewarding to see an improvement in central nervous system function after the blood pressure is reduced even by 10%. However, other causes of stupor and coma have to be considered, appropriately evaluated, and eliminated before one can make the diagnosis of hypertensive encephalopathy.

8. **What are the major principles of treating a patient with a hypertensive emergency?**
   Normal autoregulation of vascular beds allows a tissue to receive relatively constant perfusion across a wide range of blood pressures. In hypertensive emergencies, the autoregulatory capacity of many vascular beds is reset, so that the autoregulatory zone is optimized for the much higher blood pressure in the days to weeks before the medical encounter. This allowed the vessels, over time, to constrict and continue to deliver an appropriate (if not quite normal) flow of blood and oxygen, despite the very high blood pressures. A primary treatment goal is to gradually reduce the blood pressure over a short but sufficient amount of time to allow vascular beds to adjust to the "new, lower" pressure without causing ischemia. A corollary is that lowering blood pressure into the "normal" range should be avoided, because prior to the patient's presentation, the threshold for ischemia has also been shifted to the right.
   Most authorities recommend admission to an intensive care unit, although a method to monitor blood pressure (intraarterial line versus automated oscillometric device), an intravenous line to deliver the antihypertensive agent, and an attentive physician can begin treatment in the emergency department.
   No trials have been done to establish a blood pressure target (Table 68.1), but most authorities recommend a decrease in mean arterial pressure by about 10% in the first hour and no more than 25% during the first 2 hours. Most patients tolerate a blood pressure of about 160 to 180/100 mm Hg well after the first 2 hours or so, but the antihypertensive medication dose should be individualized and should be reduced if deterioration occurs when the blood pressure is decreased "too fast" or "too far." After the blood pressure has been stabilized (usually for 6 to 24 hours) and after oral treatment is administered, intravenous antihypertensive therapy can be withdrawn.

9. **What drugs are used for treatment of hypertensive emergencies?**
   Fortunately, many drugs are available (Table 68.2), each with their own advantages and disadvantages. Nitroprusside is the most widely available, has the shortest time to effect, and can be easily titrated up or down as needed. It breaks down to cyanide and thiocyanate, which can cause metabolic acidosis, an anion gap, blurred vision, tinnitus, and/or confusion; the risk of these adverse effects increases with the dose and duration of infusion. The newer agents—esmolol, fenoldopam, and clevidipine—are reasonably short-acting agents that are a beta blocker, dopamine-1 agonist, and calcium antagonist, respectively; these attributes can be helpful in certain clinical scenarios (see Table 68.1).

10. **What is the long-term prognosis of patients with a hypertensive emergency?**
    Patients who experience a hypertensive emergency or urgency have worse outcomes than those whose blood pressure is chronically well controlled, but there are several confounders. With prompt

Table 68.1. Types of Hypertensive Emergencies, With Suggested Drug Therapy and Blood Pressure Targets

TYPE OF EMERGENCY	DRUG OF CHOICE	BLOOD PRESSURE TARGET
Aortic dissection	Beta blocker + nitroprusside[a]	120 mm Hg systolic in 20 min (if possible)
Cardiac Ischemia/infarction	Nitroglycerin, nitroprusside, nicardipine, or clevidipine	Cessation of ischemia
Heart failure (or pulmonary edema)	Nitroprusside[a] and/or nitroglycerin	Improvement in failure (typically only a 10%–15% decrease is required)
Hemorrhagic Epistaxis, gross hematuria, or threatened suture lines	Any (perhaps with anxiolytic agent)	To decrease bleeding rate (typically only 10%–15% reduction over 1–2 h is required)
Obstetric Eclampsia or preeclampsia	$MgSO_4$, hydralazine, methyldopa	Typically <90 mm Hg diastolic, but often lower
Catecholamine Excess States Pheochromocytoma	Phentolamine	To control paroxysms
Drug withdrawal	Drug withdrawn	Typically only one dose necessary
Cocaine (and similar drugs)	Phentolamine	Typically only 10%–15% reduction over 1–2 h
Renal Major hematuria or acute renal impairment	Fenoldopam	0%–25% reduction in mean arterial pressure over 1–12 h
Neurologic Hypertensive encephalopathy	Nitroprusside[a]	25% reduction over 2–3 h
Acute head injury/trauma	Nitroprusside[a]	0%–25% reduction over 2–3 h (controversial)

[a]Some physicians prefer an intravenous infusion of clevidipine, fenoldopam, or nicardipine, none of which has potentially toxic metabolites, over nitroprusside. Acute improvements in renal function occur during therapy with fenoldopam but not with nitroprusside.

Modified from Elliott, W. J. (2003). Management of hypertensive emergencies. *Current Hypertension Reports, 5,* 486–492.

and effective therapy, the prognosis in hypertensive emergencies depends more on kidney function at presentation (the higher the serum creatinine, the greater the risk of dialysis). The other important factor is the willingness/ability of the patient to take prescription antihypertensive drugs, as nonadherence is now the most common antecedent to hypertensive emergencies. Although the prognosis was dismal (~10% 1-year survival) before antihypertensive drug therapy was available, most recent series show higher than 95% 1-year survival rates. Although kidney function sometimes deteriorates acutely during and after blood pressure lowering (except, perhaps, with fenoldopam), some patients have recovered enough kidney function to discontinue dialysis after the blood pressure was well controlled on an outpatient basis.

11. **How does a hypertensive emergency with aortic dissection differ from others?**
    Such patients typically present with a characteristic history of chest or back pain, often described as "tearing" or "ripping," with radiation to the arms or upper abdomen. Typically blood pressures are

Table 68.2. Useful Drugs for Hypertensive Emergencies

DRUG	ONSET OF ACTION	ELIMINATION HALF-LIFE	USUAL DOSE (IV)	POSITIVE ATTRIBUTES	RISKS
Sodium nitroprusside	Seconds	~2 min	0.25–8.0 μg/kg per minute	Very effective; fast-acting, easily titrated, or stopped	Photosensitive; metabolized to cyanide and thiocyanate
Nitroglycerin	2–5 min	1–4 min	5–100 mcg/min	Useful for coronary ischemia	Methemoglobinemia; special tubing needed
Labetalol	5–10 min	5–6 h	20–80 mg bolus every 10–15 min, or 0.5–2.0 mg/min infusion	Useful for coronary ischemia; oral formulation available	Asthma, acute left ventricular dysfunction
Enalaprilat	15–30 min	11 h	1.25–5.0 mg every 6 h	Useful in left ventricular dysfunction	Avoid in acute myocardial infarction
Nicardipine	2–5 min	45 min, 14 h	5 mg/h, increased to 15 mg/h	Useful for cardiac ischemia	Interacts with cimetidine, cyclosporine; oral formulation available
Esmolol	5–10 min	9 min	250–500 mcg/kg per minute for 1 min, then 50–100 mcg/kg per minute	Useful for aortic dissection and perioperative state	Asthma, left ventricular dysfunction
Fenoldopam	2–5 min	5 min	0.1–0.3 mcg/kg per minute initially, increase 0.1–0.2 every 15 min	Improves several parameters of renal function	Raises intraocular pressure; may cause hypokalemia
Clevidipine	2–4 min	~1 min	1–2 mg/h, increased every 90 s	Useful for cardiac ischemia, perioperative state	Photosensitive; comes in lipid emulsion

lower in the legs than in the arms, and a murmur of acute aortic regurgitation may be present. A chest x-ray may show nothing, a widened aortic shadow, or a widened mediastinum; in appropriate patients, consideration should be given to initiating therapy before the imaging study (transesophageal echocardiogram, computed tomogram of the chest) is completed.

Therapy for aortic dissection differs in three important ways from other hypertensive emergencies. Therapy should include a beta blocker (unless otherwise contraindicated) to decrease the shear forces driving the dissection. Although not "evidence-based," the recommended blood pressure target is <120 mm Hg systolic, and it should be achieved within 20 minutes of starting therapy to minimize progression. A cardiothoracic surgeon should be consulted quickly; type A dissections (proximal to the aortic arch) nearly always require emergent surgery, sometimes including valve replacement.

12. How does a hypertensive emergency with acute left ventricular failure differ from other hypertensive emergencies?
These patients typically present with dyspnea, cough, frothy, pink-tinged sputum, and hypoxia. Physical examination nearly always shows distended neck veins, râles in most of the lung fields, and an S_3. Chest x-ray typically shows pulmonary vascular redistribution, hilar congestion, and diffuse infiltrates in most of the lung fields. Prompt therapy with oxygen, intravenous loop diuretics, morphine, and nitroglycerin are usually effective acutely, although nitroprusside may be added to help lower both preload and afterload if nitroglycerin is an insufficient hypotensive agent. Appropriate evaluation of the reason for the acute decompensated heart failure is appropriate during the intensive care unit stay. Intravenous enalaprilat has been shown in a small study to improve prognosis in these patients, but its hypotensive effect is variable and may lead to acute hypotension that is difficult to reverse.

13. How does an adrenergic crisis differ from other hypertensive emergencies?
These patients present with acutely increased alpha-adrenergic tone, typically because of:
• Excess catecholamines or their congeners
• Abrupt withdrawal of oral alpha-2 adrenergic agonists (e.g., clonidine, guanabenz, guanfacine)
• Ingestion of cocaine, amphetamines
• Ingestion of tyramine-rich foodstuffs during monoamine oxidase inhibitor therapy
    These patients are usually treated successfully with phentolamine (or the alpha-2 agonist that they stopped abruptly), although some physicians prefer labetalol, which also has beta-adrenergic inhibitory effects.

14. Are there some drugs that should not be used to treat hypertensive emergencies?
Generally drugs that can cause precipitous hypotension and cannot be recalled or stopped should be avoided. Nifedipine capsules once were widely used for hypertensive urgencies and even emergencies, but the US Food and Drug Administration did not grant this indication, because the blood pressure lowering was unpredictable and sometimes caused serious hypotension, shock, and death. Most physicians prefer to use drugs that have a short "time to effect," can be easily titrated, and have a short "off-time" just in case the blood pressure drops, and the medication has to be reduced in dosage or stopped altogether. Drugs with a long elimination half-life, even when given intravenously, are more likely to cause a problem in these conditions.

15. What is the evidence base supporting the acute pharmacologic treatment of hypertensive urgencies?
Prevailing expert opinion from about 1950 to 2008 often recommended acute drug treatment for patients with very elevated blood pressures, but research produced no evidence of acute, ongoing target organ damage. Courts ruled that physicians who evaluated but did not treat a patient with a hypertensive urgency were liable for any adverse outcome (e.g., stroke, myocardial infarction) shortly afterward. Some felt that the hypertensive urgency was a "teachable moment" that would impress the patient with the importance of controlling blood pressure. Then there were reports that acute hypotensive agents (especially nifedipine capsules) were temporally associated with ischemic events, perhaps because the blood pressure was lowered unpredictably and/or excessively. Recently two studies have compared long-term outcomes in patients presenting to either emergency departments ($n = 1016$) or outpatient centers ($n = 59,535$) with hypertensive urgencies; in neither report was acute drug treatment associated with improved prognosis. These data suggest that once acute, ongoing target organ damage is ruled out, the patient is best managed by timely referral to an appropriate source of outpatient care, where effective antihypertensive therapy can be prescribed and good follow-up assured.

KEY POINTS

1. Hypertensive emergencies are clinical scenarios in which acute target-organ damage is progressive and requires blood pressure to be reduced gradually and safely within minutes to hours.
2. The most common clinical scenarios that qualify as hypertensive emergencies include acute myocardial infarction, pulmonary edema, intracranial hemorrhage, glomerulonephritis, eclampsia, adrenergic crisis, uncontrolled bleeding, or hypertensive encephalopathy.
3. In hypertensive emergencies the treatment goal is to lower blood pressure by about 10% in the first hour and a further 10% to 15% in the next hour. Do not target a blood pressure of <140/90 mm Hg in the hours after presentation.
4. Although one of many intravenous antihypertensive drugs can be used for hypertensive emergencies, the pharmacokinetic advantages of sodium nitroprusside (very short onset of action, very short elimination half-life) usually outweigh the risk of cyanide or thiocyanate poisoning, which are more common with high doses or long durations of therapy.
5. Acute aortic dissection differs from all other hypertensive emergencies because the recommended systolic blood pressure target is <120 mm Hg within 20 minutes of diagnosis and an intravenous beta blocker is used to decrease the shear stress on the ruptured intimal flap.

BIBLIOGRAPHY

Adebayo, O., & Rogers, R. L. (2015). Hypertensive emergencies in the emergency department. *Emergency Medicine Clinics of North America, 33,* 539–551.

Cremer, A., Amraoui, F., Lip, G. Y., Morales, E., Rubin, S., Segura, J., . . . Gosse, P. (2016). From malignant hypertension to hypertension-MOD: A modern definition for an old but still dangerous emergency. *Journal of Human Hypertension, 30,* 463–466.

González, R., Morales, E., Segura, J., Ruilope, L. M., & Praga, M. (2010). Long-term renal survival in malignant hypertension. *Nephrology Dialysis Transplantation, 25,* 3266–3272.

Grassi, D., O'Flaherty, M., Pellizzari, M., Bendersky, M., Rodriguez, P., Turri, D., . . . Kotliar, C., for the REHASE Program Investigators. (2008). Hypertensive urgencies in the emergency department: Evaluating blood pressure response to rest and to antihypertensive drugs with different profiles. *Journal of Clinical Hypertension (Greenwich), 10,* 662–667.

Johnson, W., Nguyen, M. L., & Patel, R. (2012). Hypertension crisis in the emergency department. *Clinical Cardiology, 30,* 533–543.

Keating, G. M. (2014). Clevidipine: A review of its use for managing blood pressure in perioperative and intensive care settings. *Drugs, 74,* 1947–1960.

Levy, P. D., Mahn, J. J., Miller, J., Shelby, A., Brody, A., Davidson, R., . . . Welch, R. D. (2015). Blood pressure treatment and outcomes in hypertensive patients without acute target organ damage: A retrospective cohort. *American Journal of Emergency Medicine, 33,* 1219–1224.

Muiesan, M. L., Salvetti, M., Amadoro, V., di Somma, S., Perlini, S., Semplicini, A., . . . Pedrinelli, R. (2015). An update on hypertensive emergencies and urgencies. *Journal of Cardiovascular Medicine (Hagerstown), 16,* 372–382.

Padilla Ramos, A., & Varon, J. (2014). Current and newer agents for hypertensive emergencies. *Current Hypertension Reports, 16,* 450.

Patel, K. K., Young, L., Howell, E. H., Hu, B., Rutecki, G., Thomas, G., & Rothberg, M. B. (2016). Characteristics and outcomes of patients presenting with hypertensive urgency in the office setting. *JAMA Internal Medicine, 176,* 981–988.

Vlcek, M., Bur, A., Woisetschläger, C., Herkner, H., Laggner, A. N., & Hirschl, M. M. (2008). Association between hypertensive urgencies and subsequent cardiovascular events in patients with hypertension. *Journal of Hypertension, 26,* 657–662.

PHARMACOLOGIC TREATMENT OF HYPERTENSION

James Brian Byrd, C. Venkata S. Ram, and Edgar V. Lerma

CHAPTER 69

1. **When is pharmacologic treatment of hypertension indicated?**
   When an individual's blood pressure (BP) does not fall below goal after a suitable period of intensive lifestyle modifications, antihypertensive drug therapy is universally recommended. There is general agreement that antihypertensive drug therapy is one of the major reasons for the decline in stroke and coronary heart disease mortality over the past 50 years. Compared to placebo or no treatment, active drug treatment in clinical trials significantly reduced fatal or nonfatal stroke by ~35%, myocardial infarction by ~15% to 25%, heart failure by ~25%, and all-cause mortality by ~12%. Most meta-analyses suggest that the cardiovascular protective effects of most antihypertensive drug classes can be most easily attributed to their BP-lowering properties, despite the fact that they do so by different molecular mechanisms. However, a large meta-analysis showed that compared with other antihypertensive drug classes, beta blockers more effectively reduce risk of coronary heart disease events in the first several years after myocardial infarction. In addition, the same meta-analysis suggested that calcium channel blockers (CCBs) have less of a protective effect against heart failure compared with several other antihypertensive drug classes.

   Frequently updated guidelines are available from the Canadian Hypertension Education Program. Available at: http://guidelines.hypertension.ca/prevention-treatment/. Accessed October 10, 2016.

2. **What are the current recommended goals for treatment of hypertension?**
   BP treatment goals are controversial despite the recent publication of a trial intended to bring clarity to the issue. By way of background, although epidemiologic data indicate that a BP <115/75 mm Hg is associated with the lowest risk of cardiovascular morbidity and mortality, several studies have suggested that "lower BP" is not necessarily better to prevent cardiovascular events. The traditional BP target of <140/90 mm Hg for all patients with hypertension was lowered to a target of <130/80 mm Hg in patients with diabetes, people with chronic kidney disease (CKD), or those with established heart disease, but recent guidelines have not suggested special BP goal for these groups. Relatively few outcome-based clinical trials have been performed that randomized subjects with hypertension to different BP targets. One of the exceptions is the Action to Control Cardiovascular Risk in Diabetes Blood Pressure (ACCORD-BP) Trial, which showed no significant benefit in patients with hypertension and diabetes randomly assigned to a systolic BP target of <120 mm Hg except for the secondary endpoint of stroke.

   Another prominent trial that randomized patients to different BP goals was the Systolic Blood Pressure Intervention Trial (SPRINT). SPRINT enrolled over 9000 hypertensive patients at least 50 years of age and randomized them to intensive BP-lowering (goal systolic BP 120 mm Hg) or less intensive BP-lowering treatment (goal systolic BP 140 mm Hg). SPRINT excluded patients with diabetes or prior stroke. The trial was halted before scheduled completion after the Data Safety Monitoring Board revealed a 25% lower risk of fatal and nonfatal major cardiovascular events and death from any cause in the intensive BP-lowering arm. On the other hand, adverse events were more common with intensive treatment. SPRINT's generalizability has come into question because of the use of unattended automated office BPs in the trial to measure the achieved BP, which was the primary intervention in the trial. The precise correlation of BP measured this way with BP measured in others ways is unclear, although the findings should be applicable to patients who matched the enrollment criteria and whose BP is measured using a similar method.

   In November 2017 the American Heart Association (AHA) and American College of Cardiology published the Clinical Practice Guideline for Hypertension. This redefined hypertension as follows:
   - Normal: systolic BP (SBP) <120 mm Hg AND diastolic BP (DBP) <80 mm Hg
   - Elevated: SBP 120–129 mm Hg AND DBP <80 mm Hg
   - Stage 1 hypertension: SBP 130–139 mm Hg OR DBP 80–89 mm Hg
   - Stage 2 hypertension: SBP ≥140 mm Hg OR DBP ≥90 mm Hg

Treatment decisions are based on individual patients' cardiovascular risk. For patients with diabetes, known cardiovascular disease, or more than a 10% risk of an atherosclerotic event in the next 10 years the guideline recommends treating if the BP >130/80 with a treatment goal of a blood pressure below 130/80.

3. **What have we learned about monotherapy for hypertension?**
Only a minority of patients with hypertension reach their BP targets using only a single drug, so most patients require multiple drugs. Several influential hypertension treatment guidelines have converged on four drug classes as preferred initial therapy, with some exceptions for patients with certain characteristics. In order of their historical introduction, they are:
1. Thiazide or thiazide-like diuretics
2. Calcium channel antagonists
3. Angiotensin-converting enzyme (ACE) inhibitors
4. Angiotensin receptor blockers
    Most guideline committees agree that if a patient has a condition for which a specific type of antihypertensive drug improves prognosis, that medication can be used as initial therapy to lower BP. A hypertensive survivor of a recent myocardial infarction, for example, would benefit from a β-blocker to reduce the risk of death or recurrent infarction, so a β-blocker would be appropriate initial antihypertensive therapy in such a case. All guideline committees recognize the existence and importance of contraindications (including allergies), even for drugs that might otherwise be first-line choices. Recent guidelines have become more concordant with one another with respect to first-line choices of antihypertensive medications (Table 69.1).

4. **Is combination therapy better than monotherapy?**
Meta-analyses have suggested that, for most antihypertensive drug classes, combining two different classes of drugs at moderate doses is more likely to lower BP than pushing any one drug to its maximum dose. This also reduces adverse effects. Combining a CCB with an ACE inhibitor, or probably an angiotensin II receptor blocker (ARB), tends to reduce incidence and severity of pedal edema seen with higher-dose CCBs. In the Avoiding Cardiovascular events through COMbination therapy in Patients Living with Systolic Hypertension (ACCOMPLISH) trial, patients at high risk for cardiovascular events were randomized to a combination of benazepril and amlodipine or a combination of benazepril and hydrochlorothiazide (HCTZ). The combination of benazepril and amlodipine reduced cardiovascular events more than the combination of benazepril and HCTZ.

5. **What classes of antihypertensive agents are currently available?**
Diuretics, CCBs, ACE inhibitors, ARBs, direct renin inhibitors, β-blockers, and α-blockers are available. There are additional drug classes available, which have more profound adverse effects and which are not first-line or second-line or even third-line agents. These include mineralocorticoid receptor antagonists, α-adrenergic receptor agonists (e.g., clonidine, guanfacine, methyldopa), and direct-acting vasodilators (e.g., hydralazine, to be considered only in combination with a β-blocker due to reflex tachycardia).

6. **Discuss the use of diuretics.**
Diuretics were the first drug class to show benefits in patients with hypertension, although they were usually used in combination with other agents, even in the early trials. They primarily work by reducing extracellular sodium and volume, although some also have vasodilatory properties, perhaps at the calcium channel. Thiazide and thiazide-like diuretics act primarily in the distal convoluted tubule and are the most widely used, particularly in patients with normal renal function. Today, diuretic doses are much lower than those used in early clinical trials. The lower doses reduce the incidence and severity of adverse effects, particularly hypokalemia, which is blamed for some of the long-term metabolic effects (diabetes, increased cholesterol) of thiazides. The BP-lowering effects of diuretics can be overcome with dietary or other sources of sodium and with the use of nonsteroidal antiinflammatory drugs (NSAIDs). Most authorities agree that chlorthalidone is both more potent in lowering BP and has a longer duration of action than HCTZ.
    Diuretics that act primarily in the thick ascending limb of the loop of Henle, "loop diuretics," are usually required for patients with Stage 4 and higher CKD. They are also often used for patients with heart failure. If short-acting furosemide or bumetanide is given once daily, fluid accumulation can occur during the 12 to 18 hours before the next dose, particularly if the evening meal contains most of the day's dietary sodium. Most loop and thiazide diuretics are sulfonamides, so they are contraindicated in patients with true sulfa allergies. Oral ethacrynic acid is a sulfur-free loop diuretic.
    The two mineralocorticoid receptor blockers, spironolactone and eplerenone, have largely been used in patients with heart failure or primary aldosteronism. However, the recent PATHWAY-2 randomized, crossover trial provided evidence that spironolactone is an effective add-on therapy

Table 69.1. Effects of Different Classes of Antihypertensive Agents on Surrogate Markers of Cardiovascular Disease

	CENTRAL α-AGONISTS	α-BLOCKERS	α-, β-BLOCKER	VASODILATOR	β-BLOCKERS	ACE INHIBITORS	ATRAS	CCBS	DIURETICS
Metabolic									
LDL cholesterol	↑	↑	↑	↑	↓↑[a]	↑	↑	↑	↓↑
HDL cholesterol	↑	←	↑	↑	↓	↑	↑	↑	↑
Insulin resistance	↑	→	↓↑	↓↑	↓↑	→	→	↑	↓↑
Glucose control	↑	↑	↑	↑	↑	→↑	↑	↓→	↓↑
Cardiovascular									
Left ventricular hypertrophy	→	→	→	↓↑	→	→	→	→	↓↑
Renal									
Microalbuminuria	↑	↑	↓→	↓↑	↓↑	↓↓	↓↓	↓[b]	↓↑

[a]Only β-blockers with intrinsic sympathomimetic activity.

[b]Only nonhydropyridine calcium channel blockers (verapamil, diltiazem).

ACE, Angiotensin-converting enzyme; ATRAs, angiotensin II receptor antagonists; CCBs, calcium channel blockers; LDL, low-density lipoprotein; HDL, high-density lipoprotein; →, no effect; ↑, increase; ↓, decrease.

From Johnson, R. J., & Feehally, J. (2003). *Comprehensive clinical nephrology* (2nd ed.). Philadelphia: Mosby.

for treatment-resistant hypertension across a spectrum of plasma aldosterone concentrations. An important safety consideration in the use of spironolactone is the risk of potentially fatal hyperkalemia; monitoring of serum potassium is essential.

7. Discuss the use of CCBs.

The many available CCBs can be divided pharmacologically into two subgroups: dihydropyridines (e.g., nifedipine, amlodipine) and nondihydropyridines (e.g., verapamil, diltiazem). The latter typically have negative inotropic and chronotropic properties, whereas the former are more vasoselective and can increase heart rate, especially acutely if immediate-release preparations are given. All CCBs inhibit the flux of calcium into smooth muscle cells, resulting in vasodilation. Many CCDs are approved for patients with angina pectoris. Verapamil can cause dose-related constipation, and immediate-release dihydropyridine compounds can cause flushing, tachycardia, and dose-dependent pedal edema; only the latter is seen with long-acting preparations. The BP-lowering of CCBs is generally little affected by dietary sodium or NSAIDs. Although studies in the last millennium suggested that CCBs were associated with a significantly higher risk of cardiovascular events than other antihypertensive drug classes, recent meta-analyses of comparative clinical trials indicate that they are as effective in preventing both stroke and coronary heart disease as diuretics. The risk of heart failure is significantly increased (by about 44%) by CCBs, both dihydropyridine and nondihydropyridine. This may be due to diuretics' ability to treat CHF symptoms as well as CCBs' proclivity to cause congestive heart failure (CHF)-mimicking pedal edema. In addition, verapamil and diltiazem are able to reduce left ventricular ejection fraction.

8. Discuss the use of ACE inhibitors.

ACE inhibitors inhibit the conversion of angiotensin I to angiotensin II, thereby producing vasodilation and lowering BP. Because the hydrolysis of bradykinin is also inhibited by these drugs, cough (7% to 12%) can occur. Angioedema (0.7%) can also occur via pathobiology that remains obscure, and its occurrence can be life-threatening. Like any drug that inhibits the renin-angiotensin system, ACE inhibitors can cause acute renal failure in patients with renal artery stenosis, and they are teratogenic. These drugs cause birth defects, even if given during the first trimester of pregnancy.

ACE inhibitors are usually effective in lowering BP, but their efficacy is reduced by dietary or other sources of sodium, and renal function may be further threatened if given with NSAIDs. ACE inhibitors are also very useful for patients with heart failure or CKD (particularly type 1 diabetics and nondiabetic CKD).

9. Discuss the use of angiotensin receptor blockers.

ARBs inhibit the binding of angiotensin II to its subtype 1 receptor, which also results in vasodilation and BP lowering. They do not cause as much cough as ACE inhibitors, and whether they cause angioedema is unclear. Just like ACE inhibitors, ARBs should not be used in pregnancy and only cautiously in the presence of renal artery stenosis. Some ARBs have been approved for type 2 diabetic nephropathy and heart failure with diminished left ventricular function.

Several clinical trials of ARBs have provided disappointing results, either compared with CCBs Valsartan Antihypertensive Long-Term Use Evaluation trial [VALUE] or placebo (TRANSCEND, PRoFESS). The design of these trials has been criticized because either the dose was too low to cause equivalent BP lowering (e.g., VALUE), or the randomized agents were given in addition to other antihypertensive and other preventive therapies rather than as initial treatments (TRANSCEND, PRoFESS). There are no direct comparisons of diuretics with ARBs, because nearly all the ARB trials used a diuretic as second-line therapy. The major advantage of ARBs seems to be their relatively benign adverse effect profile; this probably accounts for why they have the highest persistence rates of all antihypertensive agents in general clinical practice. The combination of an ARB plus an ACE inhibitor was found to lower BP only a little more than either drug alone, not significantly improve clinical outcomes, and be associated with a much higher rate of adverse effects (especially renal) in the ONTARGET trial.

10. Discuss the use of (direct) renin inhibitors.

Initial enthusiasm for these drugs has been tempered by the findings of the ALTITUDE trial, which randomized patients with type 2 diabetes mellitus to:

- Aliskiren and an ACEi inhibitor or ARB; or
- Placebo and an ACEi inhibitor or ARB

ALTITUDE was stopped early, after there was a signal for increased stroke in the aliskiren group, as well as a trend to increased renal and cardiovascular events with aliskiren.

11. Discuss the use of β-blockers.

Although traditionally an acceptable first-line therapy for hypertension, β-blockers (particularly atenolol, which has 72% of the clinical trial data) are not recommended by contemporary guidelines as initial therapy for patients with uncomplicated hypertension. Four possible mechanisms have been invoked for how β-blockers reduce BP:
1. Inhibit renin release from the juxtaglomerular apparatus of the kidney.
2. Diminish tonic sympathetic outflow from the central nervous system.
3. Reduce myocardial contractility.
4. Reduce cardiac output, and vasodilate (some more than others).

Some β-blockers have ancillary properties, including greater selectivity for the β1-adrenoreceptor, water solubility, intrinsic sympathomimetic activity, membrane-stabilizing activity, or other properties (e.g., α1-blocking activity, enhancement of nitric oxide bioavailability). Several β-blockers are effective second-line therapy (after ACE inhibitors) for heart failure. Adverse effects include bradycardia, fatigue, bronchoconstriction, dyspnea on exertion, and impairment of recognition of hypoglycemia in brittle diabetics. Many β-blockers decrease high-density lipoprotein cholesterol levels, raise triglycerides, and may impair glucose tolerance. They are nonetheless very useful for reducing pulse rate and BP and are often used in patients with aortic dissection, coronary disease, cardiac arrhythmias, and other selective indications.

12. Discuss the use of α-blockers.

α-Blockers block neuromuscular transmission by occupying the postsynaptic α1-adrenoceptor on the smooth muscle cell, causing vasodilation. Their major adverse effects are dizziness, headache, orthostatic hypotension (particularly first-dose hypotension), and an increased risk of falls and hip fractures. Since the early termination of the doxazosin arm of Antihypertensive and Lipid-Lowering Treatment to Prevent Heart Attack trial (ALLHAT), resulting from a significantly increased risk of combined cardiovascular events (especially heart failure), α-blockers have been relegated to, at best, second-line therapy for uncomplicated hypertension; doxazosin was used successfully as the third therapy in ASCOT. α-Blockers are beneficial (in combination with other antihypertensive drugs) for men with symptoms of benign prostatic hyperplasia and have "favorable" effects on lipids and glucose metabolism.

13. Discuss the use of other antihypertensive drugs.

Clonidine and other centrally acting α2-agonists (e.g., methyldopa, guanfacine) work by decreasing sympathetic outflow from the central nervous system; in small doses, this causes vasodilation and BP lowering. In larger doses, sedation, dry mouth, drowsiness, and other symptomatic adverse effects occur, which are presumably the reason clonidine was the least well-tolerated drug in the Department of Veterans Affairs monotherapy trial. Sudden discontinuation of short-acting α2-agonists causes rebound hypertension, which is best treated by reinstituting therapy. Clonidine is the only transdermal antihypertensive available in the United States.

Direct vasodilators (hydralazine, minoxidil) are typically used with a diuretic and β-blocker to counteract their tendency to cause sodium and fluid retention and reflex tachycardia. Accordingly, these drugs are typically used third-line or higher, as was hydralazine in ALLHAT. Hydralazine is typically limited to ≤300 mg/day because of the risk of drug-induced lupus, and it should be combined with a β-blocker to decrease reflex tachycardia; minoxidil causes hair growth that is not well tolerated by most women.

KEY POINTS

1. Compared with placebo or no treatment, active drug treatment in clinical trials significantly reduced fatal or nonfatal stroke by ~35%, myocardial infarction by ~15% to 25%, heart failure by ~25%, and all-cause mortality by ~12%.
2. For most antihypertensive drug classes, combining two different classes of drugs at moderate doses is more likely to lower BP than pushing the dose of any one drug to its maximum.
3. Although traditionally an acceptable first-line therapy for hypertension, β-blockers (particularly atenolol, which has ~72% of the clinical trial data) are not currently recommended by either United States or United Kingdom guidelines as initial therapy for patients with uncomplicated hypertension.

BIBLIOGRAPHY

ACCORD Study Group, Cushman, W. C., Evans, G. W., Byington, R. P., Goff, D. C., Jr., Grimm, R. H., Jr., . . . Ismail-Beigi, F. (2010). Effects of intensive blood-pressure control in type 2 diabetes mellitus. *New England Journal of Medicine, 362*(17), 1575–1585.

ALLHAT Officers and Coordinators for the ALLHAT Collaborative Research Group. (2003). Diuretic versus alpha-blocker as first-step antihypertensive therapy: Final results from the Antihypertensive and Lipid-Lowering Treatment to Prevent Heart Attack Trial (ALLHAT). *Hypertension, 42,* 239–246.

Chobanian, A. V., Bakris, G. L., Black, H. R., Cushman, W. C., Green, L. A., Izzo, J. L., Jr., . . . Roccella, E. J. (2003). Seventh report of the joint national committee on prevention, detection, evaluation and treatment of high blood pressure National High Blood Pressure Education Program Coordinating Committee. *Hypertension, 42,* 1206–1252.

ESH/ESC Task Force for the Management of Arterial Hypertension. (2013). 2013 Practice guidelines for the management of arterial hypertension of the European Society of Hypertension (ESH) and the European Society of Cardiology (ESC): ESH/ESC Task Force for the Management of Arterial Hypertension. *Journal of Hypertension, 31*(10), 1925–1938.

Jamerson, K., Weber, M. A., Bakris, G. L., Dahlöf, B., Pitt, B., Shi, V., . . . Velazquez, E. J, for the ACCOMPLISH Trial Investigators. (2008). Benazepril plus amlodipine or hydrochlorothiazide for hypertension in high-risk patients. *New England Journal of Medicine, 359,* 2417–2428.

James, P. A., Oparil, S., Carter, B. L., Cushman, W. C., Dennison-Himmelfarb, C., Handler, J., . . . Ortiz E. (2014). 2014 evidence-based guideline for the management of high blood pressure in adults: Report from the panel members appointed to the Eighth Joint National Committee (JNC 8). *JAMA, 311*(5), 507–520.

Law, M. R., Morris, J. K., & Wald, N. J. (2009). Use of blood pressure lowering drugs in the prevention of cardiovascular disease: Meta-analysis of 147 randomised trials in the context of expectations from prospective epidemiological studies. *British Medical Journal, 338,* b1665.

The ONTARGET Investigators. (2008). Telmisartan, ramipril or both in patients at high risk for vascular events. ONTARGET Investigators. *New England Journal of Medicine, 358,* 1547–1559.

SPRINT Research Group, Wright, J. T., Jr, Williamson, J. D., Whelton, P. K., Snyder, J. K., Sink, K. M., . . . Ambrosius, W. T. (2015). A randomized trial of intensive versus standard blood-pressure control. *New England Journal of Medicine, 373*(22), 2103–2116.

Whelton, P.K., Carey, R.M., Aronow, W.S., et al. (2017). ACC/AHA/AAPA/ABC/ACPM/AGS/APhA/ASH/ASPC/NMA/PCNA guideline for the prevention, detection, evaluation, and management of high blood pressure in adults: Executive summary: A report of the American College of Cardiology/American Heart Association Task Force on Clinical Practice Guidelines. *Hypertension.*

Williams, B., MacDonald, T. M., Morant, S., Webb, D. J., Sever, P., McInnes, G., . . . Brown, M. J. (2015). British Hypertension Society's PATHWAY Studies Group. Spironolactone versus placebo, bisoprolol, and doxazosin to determine the optimal treatment for drug-resistant hypertension (PATHWAY-2): A randomised, double-blind, crossover trial. *Lancet, 386*(10008), 2059–2068.

NONPHARMACOLOGIC TREATMENT OF HYPERTENSION

Martin J. Andersen and Rajiv Agarwal

CHAPTER 70

1. **What nonpharmacologic strategies can be used to treat hypertension?**

   Several nonpharmacologic strategies are available to improve blood pressure control among essential hypertensive patients. By extension, similar strategies may be effective among patients with chronic kidney disease. These strategies include salt restriction, weight loss, exercise, moderation of alcohol intake, and treatment of obstructive sleep apnea (OSA).

2. **How effective is salt restriction?**

   Although some experts recommend caution in advocating for dietary sodium restriction, as some studies show an inverse relation between dietary sodium and mortality, we feel that it is an effective modality for hypertension management. Sodium restriction has been shown to reduce blood pressure, both in randomized trials and in meta-analyses. The Dietary Approaches to Stop Hypertension (DASH) trial revealed a −6.7/−3.5 mm Hg blood pressure reduction when dietary sodium was reduced from 3 to 1.5 g. A large meta-analysis found that a reduction of approximately 2.3 g in dietary sodium reduced systolic blood pressure by 3.7 mm Hg among hypertensive patients, an effect that was more pronounced among older patients. Sodium sensitive hypertensive patients who restrict dietary sodium convert from nondipping to dipping status (dipping refers to ≥10% decrease in blood pressure while asleep; nondipping, hypertensive patients are at increased cardiovascular risk compared to dipping patients). Dietary sodium restriction reduces left ventricular hypertrophy, improves the anti-proteinuric effects of angiotensin-converting enzyme (ACE) inhibitors and angiotensin receptor blockers for both diabetic and nondiabetic chronic kidney disease patients, and may reduce kidney disease progression. Long-term follow-up of patients enrolled in the Trials of Hypertension Prevention revealed that a reduction of dietary sodium of approximately 750 to 1000 mg daily reduced cardiovascular events (myocardial infarction, coronary bypass surgery, coronary angioplasty, stroke, or cardiovascular death) by 25%.

   A 24-hour urine collection that quantifies sodium excretion provides a reasonable estimate of dietary sodium intake, and a recently published analysis of patients enrolled in the Chronic Renal Insufficiency Cohort (CRIC) study revealed interesting results regarding dietary sodium intake and cardiovascular events. The CRIC study is a prospective cohort study of chronic kidney disease patients that evaluates the risk factors for kidney disease progression and cardiovascular disease. Among a group of nearly 3800 racially diverse patients, those patients whose dietary sodium (estimated from a mean of three 24-hour urine collections over the first 2 years of the study) resided in the highest quartile (≥4548 mg) experienced a 36% relative risk increase in nonfatal cardiovascular events (a composite of stroke, myocardial infarction, or congestive heart failure), a 34% relative risk increase in congestive heart failure, and an 81% relative risk increase for nonfatal stroke, compared to those patients whose dietary sodium was in the lowest quartile (<2894 mg). Every 1000 mg increase in daily dietary sodium increased the risk for the composite end-point 10%, the risk for congestive heart failure 9%, and the risk for nonfatal stroke 16%.

   The National Academy of Sciences and the American Heart Association recommend that dietary sodium be limited to 1.5 g daily—a goal that would need both government and industry cooperation. The U.S. Department of Health and Human Services also recommends dietary sodium restriction: no more than 1.5 g daily for adult African Americans, patients ≥51 years, or patients with diabetes mellitus, hypertension, or chronic kidney disease. The Kidney Disease Improving Global Outcomes guidelines also recommend low dietary sodium for chronic kidney disease patients, though only to a level of <2 g. While sodium restriction may initially be difficult, patients become acclimated to the diet over several weeks. A population-wide reduction of dietary sodium to 1200 mg may save approximately $10 billion to $24 billion annually in health care costs.

3. **How effective is the DASH diet?**
   Americans, besides consuming excess salt, eat foods high in saturated fats and low in fiber and potassium. Low dietary potassium predisposes to sodium retention, volume expansion, and hypertension. Potassium supplementation can decrease blood pressure in hypertensive patients. The mechanism by which fiber may prevent hypertension is not well delineated, although a meta-analysis showed that diets supplemented by fiber lower blood pressure (−1.13/−1.26 mm Hg). The DASH diet emphasizes fruits and vegetables and low-fat foods. During an 8-week trial, the DASH diet, in patients with and without hypertension, lowered blood pressures by 5.5/3 mm Hg. If the DASH diet is coupled with low sodium intake (1.5 g daily), blood pressures will decrease by −8.9/−4.5 mm Hg compared to an average American diet. Unfortunately, the National Health and Nutrition Examination Survey (NHANES) data reveal that nearly 91% of Americans consume more than 2300 mg of sodium daily. Only 1.2% patients who would benefit from reducing dietary sodium to ≤1.5 g (i.e., African Americans, patients ≥51 years, or patients with diabetes mellitus, hypertension, or chronic kidney disease) actually restrict dietary sodium appropriately. Over 60% of these patients consume more than 3 g of sodium daily. DASH dietary instructions have been published for easy reference.

   While the appropriateness of the DASH diet for chronic kidney disease patients has not been studied extensively, a small pilot study of 11 patients recently showed that the DASH diet is safe for patients with moderate kidney disease (i.e., an estimated glomerular filtration rate of 30 to 59 mL/min per 1.73 m^2). No significant hyperkalemia occurred during the 2-week study, and nighttime systolic blood pressure decreased by 5.3 mm Hg.

4. **How effective is the treatment of OSA?**
   Patients with OSA experience oxygen desaturation and sympathetic activation. Persistent, untreated OSA leads to hypertension. In the Wisconsin Sleep Cohort Study, 709 patients were followed for 4 years, and those patients with an apnea-hypopnea index of ≥5 had a more than twofold higher risk for hypertension, compared to patients with no apnea-hypopnea events. A meta-analysis of five randomized, controlled trials revealed that continuous positive airway pressure (CPAP) therapy improved the blood pressure control of OSA patients: 24-hour systolic and diastolic ambulatory blood pressures decreased 4.78 and 2.95 mm Hg, respectively, compared to no treatment. While nocturnal ambulatory systolic blood pressure did not change significantly with CPAP, nocturnal ambulatory diastolic blood pressure fell 1.53 mm Hg.

   OSA is common in chronic kidney disease—up to 60% of these patients may have OSA—and chronic kidney disease may increase sleep apnea severity. Severe OSA (apnea-hypopnea index ≥ 30), in conjunction with resistant hypertension, increases the odds of chronic kidney disease by more than 13-fold. It is possible that treatment of OSA in chronic kidney disease patients may improve blood pressure control and kidney outcomes.

5. **What is the role of alcohol in hypertension?**
   A morning blood pressure surge is a risk factor for cardiovascular mortality, and studies show that alcohol is a risk factor for stroke—primarily hemorrhagic stroke. A possible mechanism is related to alcohol's circadian effect on blood pressure. Acutely, alcohol ingestion will lower blood pressure through vasodilation. However, hours later, blood pressure rises, possibly as a result of sympathetic activation. A recent Japanese trial demonstrated that ambulatory blood pressures surged in drinkers shortly after awakening.

   The popular press has championed moderate alcohol intake as a treatment to reduce cardiovascular disease risk. Red wine, because of its antioxidant content, has been particularly noted. However, studies show that red wine's purported benefits result from the different drinking and dietary habits of red wine drinkers, compared to those who drink primarily beer or spirits. Moderate alcohol intake (one to two drinks daily for men and one drink daily for women) may be beneficial by increasing high-density lipoprotein levels and lowering platelet aggregation. These benefits are seen mostly in older patients. The benefits disappear with higher amounts of alcohol intake or binge drinking. The World Health Organization estimates that worldwide alcohol consumption contributes 16% to the risk of becoming hypertensive.

   Finally, while most studies do not find a direct correlation between alcohol consumption and kidney disease, some researchers note that drinking 30 g of alcohol daily (approximately three drinks) is associated with albuminuria.

6. **How effective are weight loss and exercise?**
   Weight loss and exercise are integral for hypertension control. Americans are increasingly becoming more sedentary and overweight. According to the latest NHANES data, 36.3% of adult American

aged ≥20 years are obese: 34.3% of men are obese, while 38.3% of women are obese. African American women are at particularly high risk, as nearly 57% are obese. Obesity predisposes patients to become hypertensive. Weight loss through exercise improves hypertension because exercise improves antioxidant effects and reduces systemic vascular resistance. The PREMIER trial showed that intensive lifestyle modification, entailing a low-sodium DASH diet, weight loss, and exercise, is successful in lowering blood pressure in patients with pressures 120 to 159/80 to 95 mm Hg. The average improvement, from baseline, was −4.3/−2.6 mm Hg. Two meta-analyses showed that approximately 1 kg in weight loss translates to approximately 1 mm Hg improvement in systolic blood pressure. Physicians should keep in mind that obesity itself is a risk factor for chronic kidney disease, as it can cause glomerular hyperfiltration and proteinuria. A recent meta-analysis found that weight loss reduces proteinuria and systolic blood pressure (~8 mm Hg for nonsurgical interventions [e.g., diet, exercise, or medications] and ~23 mm Hg for surgical interventions [e.g., gastric bypass]). Glomerular hyperfiltration improved, with the GFR decreasing ~25.6 mL/min, in those morbidly obese patients undergoing surgery, providing possible long-term kidney protection.

As the American population ages and more patients face chronic disease, expert opinion recognizes the importance of exercise to reduce cardiovascular events. Patients with chronic kidney disease are at high risk because this disease is an independent cardiovascular risk factor. Guidelines advocate that older patients perform moderate-intensity exercise (e.g., walking) for a minimum of 30 minutes 5 days weekly or vigorous activity (e.g., jogging) for a minimum of 20 minutes thrice weekly. In a small group of chronic kidney disease patients, regular exercise significantly reduced blood pressure. However, once these patients stopped their exercise training, their blood pressures promptly increased. A study of patients with chronic kidney disease undergoing cardiac rehabilitation showed improvements in weight, physical well-being, and lipid profiles. Finally, a study in which obese, chronic kidney disease patients underwent exercise training, dietary education, and orlistat therapy (a drug that reduces fat malabsorption) revealed that these patients can effectively lose weight. This is important because obesity is a barrier to transplantation, and transplantation provides a survival benefit to chronic kidney disease patients, as compared to dialysis, through reduction in cardiovascular risk.

KEY POINTS

1. Severe OSA with resistant hypertension increases the risk of chronic kidney disease by more than 13-fold.
2. OSA treatment can improve blood pressure control and/or simplify a blood pressure medication regimen.
3. Only moderate alcohol intake (i.e., one to two drinks daily for men and one drink daily for women) has shown possible benefits on cardiovascular risk; higher amounts of alcohol intake increase the risk for hypertension.
4. Weight loss can improve blood pressure: approximately 1 kg in weight loss can translate to an improvement in systolic blood pressure by 1 mm Hg.
5. A moderate exercise regimen (i.e., walking for 30 minutes 5 days weekly or jogging for 20 minutes thrice weekly) can improve blood pressure control for older patients and for chronic kidney disease patients.

BIBLIOGRAPHY

Appel, L. J., Champagne, C. M., Harsha, D. W., Cooper, L. S., Obarzanek, E., Elmer, P. J., . . . Writing Group of the PREMIER Collaborative Research Group. (2003). Effects of comprehensive lifestyle modification on blood pressure control: Main results of the PREMIER clinical trial. *Journal of the American Medical Association, 289*(16), 2083–2093.

Aucott, L., Rothnie, H., McIntyre, L., Thapa, M., Waweru, C., & Gray, D. (2009). Long-term weight loss from lifestyle intervention benefits blood pressure? A systematic review. *Hypertension, 54*(4), 756–762.

Cook, N. R., Cutler, J. A., Obarzanek, E., Buring, J. E., Rexrode, K. M., Kumanyika, S. K., . . . Whelton, P. K. (2007). Long term effects of dietary sodium reduction on cardiovascular disease outcomes: Observational follow-up of the trials of hypertension prevention (TOHP). *British Medical Journals, 334*(7599), 885–888. doi:10.1136/bmj.39147.604896.55.

Liu, L., Cao, Q., Guo, Z., & Dai, Q. (2016). Continuous positive airway pressure in patients with obstructive sleep apnea and resistant hypertension: A meta-analysis of randomized controlled trials. *Journal of Clinical Hypertension, 18*(2), 153–158.

Midgley, J. P., Matthew, A. G., Greenwood, C. M., & Logan, A. G. (1996). Effect of reduced dietary sodium on blood pressure: A meta-analysis of randomized controlled trials. *Journal of the American Medical Association, 275*(20), 1590–1597.

Mills, K. T., Chen, J., Yang, W., Appel, L. J., Kusek, J. W., Alper, A., . . . Chronic Renal Insufficiency Cohort (CRIC) Study Investigators. (2016). Sodium excretion and the risk of cardiovascular disease in patients with chronic kidney disease. *Journal of the American Medical Association, 315*(20), 2200–2210.

Navaneethan, S. D., Yehnert, H., Moustarah, F., Schreiber, M. J., Schauer, P. R., & Beddhu, S. (2009). Weight loss interventions in chronic kidney disease: A systematic review and meta-analysis. *Clinical Journal of the American Society of Nephrology, 4*(10), 1565–1574.

Neter, J. E., Stam, B. E., Kok, F. J., Grobbee, D. E., & Geleijnse, J. M. (2003). Influence of weight reduction on blood pressure: A meta-analysis of randomized controlled trials. *Hypertension, 42*(5), 878–884.

Sacks, F. M., Svetkey, L. P., Vollmer, W. M., Appel, L. J., Bray, G. A., Harsha, D., . . . DASH-Sodium Collaborative Research Group. (2001). Effects on blood pressure of reduced dietary sodium and the Dietary Approaches to Stop Hypertension (DASH) diet. *New England Journal of Medicine, 344*(1), 3–10.

Venkataraman, R., Sanderson, D., & Dittor, V. (2005). Outcomes in patients with chronic kidney disease undergoing cardiac rehabilitation. *American Heart Journal, 150*(6), 1140–1146.

XIII
ACID-BASE AND ELECTROLYTE DISORDERS

VOLUME DISORDERS AND ASSESSMENT

Nathaniel Reisinger and Michael Berkoben

CHAPTER 71

VOLUME

1. **What is meant by volume?**

   Physicians use the terms "volume" and "extracellular fluid volume" interchangeably. Because sodium is largely restricted to the extracellular fluid (ECF), total body sodium determines the ECF volume. Therefore changes in total body sodium lead to changes in ECF volume. A typical Westerner consumes about 150 mmol of sodium chloride per day. Let's consider the hypothetical case of adding 150 mmol of sodium chloride to the ECF of a normal human. The resultant rise in the plasma sodium concentration and plasma osmolality will stimulate thirst and antidiuretic hormone (ADH) secretion. Ingestion of water and reabsorption of water by the collecting ducts will restore the plasma sodium concentration and plasma osmolality to normal. The end result is that 1 L of an isosmotic solution has been added to the ECF compartment; an increase in total body sodium has led to an increase in ECF volume.

2. **How is ECF volume regulated?**

   If ECF volume is to remain constant, the amount of sodium ingested must be matched by the amount of sodium excreted by the kidneys. In the example above, expansion of the ECF volume must somehow be sensed. What is sensed is not ECF volume, but rather a portion of ECF called effective arterial volume. Effective arterial volume (also called effective circulating volume or sensed volume) is that portion of the ECF that is in the arterial tree and effectively perfusing tissues. An increase in effective arterial volume is sensed by baroreceptors in the aortic arch, carotid sinus, central veins, cardiac chambers, and afferent arterioles. In addition, an increase in effective arterial volume leads to an increase in renal tubular flow, which is sensed by the macula densa. Signals (suppression of renal sympathetic nerve activity and suppression of the renin angiotens in aldosterone system) are then sent to the kidneys, which lead to diminished sodium reabsorption by the renal tubules and increased sodium excretion by the kidneys. In the example above, 150 mmol of sodium will be excreted by the kidneys, returning ECF volume to normal.

HYPERVOLEMIA

3. **What is hypervolemia?**

   Hypervolemia is due to an excess of total body sodium and water, which leads to expansion of the ECF compartment. Hypervolemia is therefore synonymous with ECF volume overload. Hypervolemia is typically due to kidney retention of sodium and water. This kidney retention may be primary or secondary. Primary kidney sodium retention may be caused by kidney failure; in this setting the diseased kidneys may be unable to match sodium excretion with sodium intake. Drugs may also lead to primary kidney retention. The direct vasodilator minoxidil and the thiazolidinedioines commonly cause kidney sodium retention and edema. The dihydropyridine calcium channel blockers may cause edema; with these drugs, capillary leak plays an important role in the development of edema. Secondary kidney retention occurs when there is a reduction in effective arterial volume. The most common causes of reduced effective arterial volume are congestive heart failure (CHF) and cirrhosis. In these conditions, the reduction in sensed volume leads to enhanced kidney sympathetic nerve activity, enhanced activity of the renin-angiotensin-aldosterone system, and enhanced secretion of ADH. Avid kidney sodium and water reabsorption ensue. In the case of the nephrotic syndrome, both primary and secondary kidney sodium retention may contribute to varying degrees. The kidney disease itself may lead to primary sodium retention (overfill hypothesis). The low plasma oncotic pressure from hypoalbuminemia may lead to movement of fluid from the intravascular compartment to the interstitial compartment. The contraction of the intravascular volume leads to secondary kidney sodium retention (underfill hypothesis).

4. **What are the manifestations of hypervolemia?**
   The ECF compartment is composed of the vascular compartment (one-fourth of ECF volume) and the interstitial compartment (three-fourths of ECF volume). Patients with hypervolemia have expansion of the interstitial compartment; they may or may not have expansion of the vascular compartment.
   - Patients with primary kidney sodium retention may have elevated jugular venous pressure, pulmonary edema, and peripheral edema.
   - Patients with CHF may also have elevated jugular venous pressure, pulmonary edema, and peripheral edema.
   - Patients with cirrhosis may develop portal hypertension and splanchnic vasodilatation. Portal hypertension leads to an increase in hydraulic pressure in the hepatic sinusoids. Fluid in the sinusoids moves across the hepatic capsule into the peritoneum. Ascites formation and splanchnic vasodilatation lead to a state of low effective arterial volume, which in turn leads to avid reabsorption of ingested sodium and water. Kidney retention of sodium and water serves to increase effective arterial volume—but also augments ascites formation. Patients with cirrhosis may also have lower extremity edema. Jugular venous pressure, however, is usually not elevated, and patients with cirrhosis do not develop pulmonary edema.
   - Patients with the nephrotic syndrome typically have peripheral edema. If primary kidney sodium retention is predominant in an individual patient with the nephrotic syndrome, jugular venous pressure may be elevated. If vascular underfilling from movement of fluid from the intravascular to the interstitial compartment is predominant, the jugular venous pressure will not be elevated.

5. **Is the history and physical exam reliable for the detection of hypervolemia?**
   The history and physical exam is neither sensitive nor specific for diagnosing hypervolemia. No one exam finding or historical feature is 100% accurate in the determination of volume status. There may be false negatives. A patient with kidney disease or heart failure may not have crackles or edema on exam, yet have significant extracellular volume expansion. Moreover, a patient may have no dyspnea by history, yet still harbor significant pulmonary congestion. Nor are certain physical exam findings entirely specific for hypervolemia (false positives). For instance, a patient may have edema related to venous stasis or pulmonary crackles from atelectasis despite intravascular effective arterial volume depletion. Some physical exam signs are technically challenging and have variable interoperator reliability. Obesity, valvular heart disease, and impaired right heart function make interpretation of jugular venous distention contentious. These difficulties have led to the proliferation of innumerable techniques to aid in assessment of volume status.

6. **What are some adjuvant techniques to enhance the history and physical in assessing hypervolemia?**
   Given the association of volume overload with excess mortality and readmissions in heart failure and kidney disease, a variety of methods have been developed for noninvasively assessing volume overload. These methods take advantage of changes in physical properties as ECF volume increases. As with the history and physical exam, each method has limitations and their utility may be in the aggregate. This chapter will look at the noninvasive techniques with availability in inpatient or outpatient settings that have the best validation and most clinical utility:
   - Bioimpedance spectroscopy (BIS)
   - Lung-water ultrasound
   - Intradialytic blood volume monitoring (BVM) devices

7. **What is bioimpedance spectroscopy and how is it used?**
   Bioelectrical impedance analysis refers to several related techniques for determining body composition based on measuring electrical impedance or opposition to flow of a small alternating current applied to the body. Electrical impedance is the alternating current corollary to resistance in direct current circuits and is composed of resistance as well as reactance, which is made up itself of inductance (current induced by magnetic fields) and capacitance (the ability of circuit components to store charge). Body composition is determined by modeling the human body as an alternating current circuit using estimation equations derived from physical properties of the human body. Fat-free mass has lower impedance given its higher electrolyte-rich water content, whereas fat mass is relatively anhydrous and has higher impedance. In general, the greater the fluid content, the lower the impedance.
   Whole-body BIS is the most validated of these methods. In this method, electrodes are placed on a hand and foot and alternating currents over a broad band of frequencies are applied to the body to estimate impedance. BIS has been validated against deuterium, bromide, and radioactive potassium radioisotope dilution techniques for determination of total body water (TBW), ECF, and intracellular fluid (ICF), respectively. BIS appears to have value in detecting occult fluid overload patients with

end-stage kidney disease (ESKD) on HD. In retrospective cohort analysis, fluid overload as measured by BIS has been associated with increased all-cause mortality. In a large prospective cohort, fluid overload as measured by BIS was strongly and independently associated with all-cause mortality. Duration of exposure to fluid overload was associated with all-cause mortality in a dose-dependent fashion. These effects were durable across blood pressure tertiles. In two small clinical trials, estimation of dry weight enhanced by BIS showed improvement in all-cause mortality versus clinical evaluation alone. Similarly, in heart failure literature, one study validated transthoracic impedance to specifically measure ECF in the lung and found improvements in cardiovascular outcomes, all-cause mortality, and readmission. However, a multi-center randomized-controlled trial including 50 patients with fluid overload of 15% or more as demonstrated by BIS comparing three methods of dry weight reduction showed a high (31%) rate of dialysis-related complications across all groups demonstrating the difficulty of fluid removal in the dialysis population.

8. **What is the role of thoracic ultrasound?**
Formerly, ultrasound of the lung was thought to be valueless apart from the easy identification of pleural effusions. The lung is composed of numerous air-filled alveoli that represent multiple air-fluid interfaces. These interfaces reflect sound waves and generate reverberation artifacts that impair accurate tomographic visualization of normal lung parenchyma. These artifacts are termed A-lines and can be visualized as serial, equally spaced reflections of the pleural line (Fig. 71.1).

In patients with kidney disease or heart failure, fluid accumulates in the interlobular septa separating alveoli and the A-line pattern gives way to a B-line pattern (Fig. 71.2) with more B-lines corresponding with increasing fluid overload. The B-line pattern is visualized as radially oriented hyperechoic (bright) lines emanating perpendicularly from the pleural line running to the edge of the field. Counting B-lines serially over a predefined pattern of 28 intercostal spaces yields a B-line score.

B-line score has been validated using gravimetry in a post-mortem pig model and using invasive techniques available in the intensive care unit, such as transpulmonary thermodilution. B-line score correlates well with volume overload, outperforming the chest radiograph in detection of pulmonary edema, with higher score correlating with increased lung water. In patients with ESKD on HD, B-lines were demonstrated to disappear dynamically on dialysis correlating with ultrafiltration volume. In these patients, B-line score correlates with cardiovascular outcomes, death, and readmissions in retrospective data. A large, prospective, multi-center randomized controlled trial (Lung Water by Ultrasound Guided Treatment in Hemodialysis Patients or LUST Study) is ongoing to determine whether measurement of B-line score enhances estimation of dry weight and improves cardiovascular outcomes in patients with ESKD on HD and comorbid cardiac disease. Preliminary data from this trial has shown that the prevalence of asymptomatic pulmonary congestion is high and often goes undetected by the physical exam.

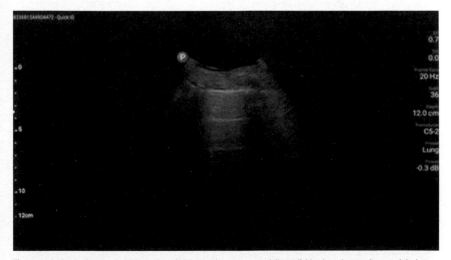

Figure 71.1. Lung ultrasound. A-line pattern. Obtained using a commercially available phased array ultrasound device paired with a tablet computer. Serial parallel hyperechoic lines parallel to the pleural line.

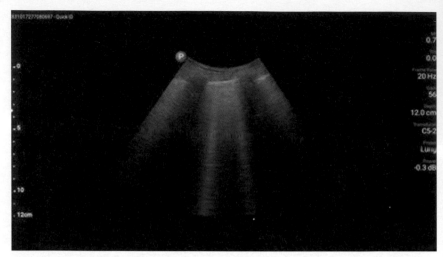

Figure 71.2. Lung ultrasound. B-line pattern. Obtained using a commercially available phased array ultrasound device paired with a tablet computer. Note the hyperechoic lines running perpendicular to the pleural line.

Lung ultrasound is easy to learn. Inter-observer reliability has been demonstrated using web-based tutorials and image review by expert trainers. There are limitations to lung ultrasound. A full 28-point exam takes about 5 minutes to perform and requires the patient to disrobe. Importantly, other disease processes can present as a diffuse B-line pattern, including the acute respiratory distress syndrome, diffuse interstitial lung diseases, and multifocal pneumonias.

9. What is the role of intradialytic BVM devices?

Patients undergoing ultrafiltration therapy have sodium and water removed from the intravascular compartment, leading to hemoconcentration as red cell mass is distributed in less volume. This is matched by mobilization of retained salt and water from the ECF compartment, termed capillary refill. The movement of water results in hemodilution, a fall in hematocrit. If the rate of ultrafiltration exceeds capillary refill, the patient develops effective arterial volume depletion. This can lead to intradialytic hypotension, decreased tissue perfusion, and myocardial and cerebral stunning.

The principle behind intradialytic BVM devices is to noninvasively estimate the hematocrit in real time during dialysis in order to avoid overaggressive ultrafiltration and prevent intradialytic hypotension.

Initial studies using intradialytic BVM devices showed improvement in intradialytic hypotension. However, a larger randomized controlled trial (the Crit-Line Intradialytic Monitoring Benefit or CLIMB Study) comparing these devices with standard of care demonstrated a significantly higher adverse event rate and mortality with intradialytic BVM. Further study is ongoing.

10. Why does edema develop?

Edema develops because of a perturbation in the Starling forces that govern the distribution of fluid between the vascular and the interstitial compartments.

- In primary kidney sodium retention, there is overfilling of the vascular compartment. This leads to increased venous pressure and increased capillary hydraulic pressure. Capillary hydraulic pressure is one of the Starling forces; increased capillary hydraulic pressure favors movement of fluid into the interstitium. Continued kidney retention of ingested sodium and water augments this process.
- In CHF, there is also overfilling of the vascular compartment, increased venous pressure, and increased capillary hydraulic pressure, which favors movement of fluid into the interstitium. Although there is overfilling of the vascular compartment, effective arterial volume is low. In other words, vascular underfilling is sensed. Avid kidney reabsorption of ingested sodium and water serves to increase effective arterial volume and increase effective tissue perfusion—but also augments edema formation.
- In cirrhosis, splanchnic vasodilatation is an early phenomenon. Sinusoidal obstruction in the cirrhotic liver leads to an increase in the hydraulic pressure in the sinusoids. Fluid in the sinusoids moves

across the hepatic capsule into the peritoneum. Ascites formation and splanchnic vasodilatation lead to a state of low effective arterial volume. Low effective arterial volume leads to avid reabsorption of ingested sodium and water, which augments ascites formation.

- In nephrotic syndrome, two mechanisms of edema formation (to varying degrees in individual patients) may be operative. Primary kidney sodium retention may lead to increased capillary hydraulic pressure and movement of fluid into the interstitium. Alternatively, low plasma oncotic pressure from hypoalbuminemia may lead to movement of fluid into the interstitium and vascular underfilling; secondary kidney retention of sodium and water augments edema formation.

11. **How is hypervolemia treated?**
Successful treatment of hypervolemia is accomplished by inducing negative sodium balance. A reduction in total body sodium will lead to a reduction in ECF volume. Output of sodium from the body may be increased by diuretic administration, by ultrafiltration (in patients with kidney failure), and by paracentesis (in patients with ascites). However, the goal of therapy is not merely to increase sodium output. The goal is to have sodium output exceed sodium intake. Therefore dietary sodium restriction is a cornerstone of therapy. Failure to adhere to dietary sodium restriction is a common cause of refractory edema.

12. **Is there a limit for volume removal?**
Diuretics cause fluid loss from the vascular space. This contraction of the vascular space leads to a fall in venous pressure and in capillary hydraulic pressure. The fall in capillary hydraulic pressure promotes movement of edema fluid from the interstitial space into the vascular space. The rate at which replenishment of the vascular space occurs varies. Overly rapid diuresis leads to a significant reduction in the vascular space, which will in turn lead to decreased venous return to the heart, decreased cardiac filling pressures, decreased stroke volume, decreased cardiac output, and ultimately hypotension. Impaired kidney perfusion may lead to prerenal azotemia. Most patients, however, can tolerate gradual correction of volume overload. In patients with substantial peripheral edema, edema fluid can be mobilized from most capillary beds. As a result, a negative fluid balance of 2 to 3 L/day can generally be accomplished without significant reduction in vascular volume. The case of the patient with cirrhosis and ascites but without peripheral edema is discussed below.

13. **How do diuretics work?**
All diuretics block sodium reabsorption by the kidney. Diuretics are classified according to the site in the nephron at which they block sodium reabsorption. There are four classes of diuretics.
- The thiazide diuretics (e.g., hydrochlorothiazide, chlorthalidone, and metolazone) inhibit the Na^+-Cl^- cotransporter in the luminal membrane of the distal tubule and connecting tubule.
- The loop diuretics (furosemide, bumetanide, torsemide, and ethacrynic acid) block the Na^+-K^+-$2Cl^-$ carrier in the luminal membrane of the thick ascending limb of the loop of Henle.
- The potassium-sparing diuretics (amiloride, triamterene, spironolactone, and eplerenone) block sodium reabsorption in the collecting tubule. Amiloride and triamterene inhibit Na^+ channels in the luminal membrane of the principal cell of the collecting tubule. Spironolactone and eplerenone are competitive inhibitors of aldosterone and indirectly block sodium reabsorption in the collecting tubule.
- The carbonic anhydrase inhibitor acetazolamide impairs proximal tubular Na^+, Cl^-, and HCO_3^- reabsorption.

14. **Should a thiazide diuretic or loop diuretic be used to treat hypervolemia?**
Approximately 25% of sodium filtered by the glomeruli is reabsorbed by the loop of Henle. Approximately 3% to 5% of filtered sodium is reabsorbed by the distal tubule and connecting segment. Because of their greater potency, loop diuretics are used to treat symptomatic hypervolemia. As described below, thiazide diuretics can be useful adjuncts to loop diuretics in refractory edema.

15. **Should a thiazide diuretic or loop diuretic be used to treat hypertension?**
In patients with normal kidney function, thiazide diuretics are preferred to loop diuretics. The thiazide diuretics have a longer duration of action than do loop diuretics. Furosemide, for example, has a duration of action of approximately 6 hours. After 6 hours, activation of the renin-angiotensin-aldosterone-system leads to renal sodium retention and limits the antihypertensive effect of the drug. The thiazide diuretics, especially chlorthalidone, have a much longer duration of action. However, the thiazide diuretics become much less effective when the glomerular filtration rate falls below about 30 mL/min. In patients with impaired kidney function, then, loop diuretics are more effective antihypertensive agents. It must be emphasized that a thiazide or loop diuretic is an essential component of an antihypertensive regimen for patients with resistant hypertension.

16. **How does one choose a loop diuretic dose for a patient with generalized edema?**
    The first order of business is to determine the effective dose. Loop diuretics have a dose-response curve. Loop diuretics are secreted into the tubular lumen and act on the luminal membrane. A threshold rate of diuretic excretion must be attained before natriuresis occurs. A typical initial intravenous dose of furosemide for a patient with generalized edema is 20 to 40 mg. If administration of 40 mg intravenous furosemide does not produce diuresis within a few hours, one can assume that the threshold rate of diuretic excretion has not been reached. Repeated administrations of 40 mg doses will not be effective. Instead, the dose should be increased to 80 mg. The dose may be increased in stepwise fashion to a maximum of 200 mg until the single effective dose is determined. This effective dose should then be administered at least twice daily in order to achieve effective diuresis. Because the bioavailability of oral furosemide averages about 50%, one must double the dose of furosemide when converting a patient from intravenous to oral therapy. This is not necessary for the other loop diuretics, which have greater oral bioavailability. On occasion, the maximum intravenous dose of a loop diuretic may not produce diuresis. The mechanisms of and approach to diuretic resistance are described in Tables 71.1 and 71.2.

17. **Are there special considerations when treating patients with the nephrotic syndrome?**
    Patients with the nephrotic syndrome may be resistant to diuretic therapy because of hypoalbuminemia and albuminuria. Because diuretics are highly protein-bound, they are confined to the vascular space and delivered rapidly to the kidney. The *hypoalbuminemia* in patients with the nephrotic syndrome expands the volume of distribution of the drug and slows the rate of delivery to the kidney. (In spite of this, administration of a solution of albumin to which a loop diuretic has been added does not substantially increase diuresis.) Except for the aldosterone antagonists, spironolactone and eplerenone, diuretics act on the luminal membrane. However, intraluminal binding of thiazide and loop diuretics by *albumin in the tubular fluid* makes them inactive. For these reasons, blocking sodium reabsorption at an additional site in the nephron may be necessary to achieve diuresis. A thiazide diuretic is typically chosen. The combination of a loop diuretic and a thiazide diuretic can precipitate severe hypokalemia; the plasma potassium concentration must be monitored carefully. Angiotensin inhibition by angiotensin-converting enzyme inhibitors or by angiotensin receptor blockers can be an important adjunct to diuretic therapy. These drugs may decrease albuminuria and increase the plasma albumin concentration, thereby enhancing the response to diuretics.

18. **Are there special considerations when treating patients with CHF?**
    Patients with CHF may be resistant to diuretic therapy. CHF leads to diminished kidney perfusion and consequently to diminished delivery of the diuretic to the kidney. In addition, increased activity of

Table 71.1. Intravenous Loop Diuretic Dose Equivalencies

DIURETIC	INITIAL DOSE	MAXIMUM DOSE[a]	CONTINUOUS INFUSION[a]
Furosemide	20–40 mg	200 mg	40–80 mg bolus, then 5–40 mg/h[b]
Bumetanide	0.5–1 mg	8–10 mg	1 mg bolus, then 0.5–2 mg/h[b]
Torsemide	10–20 mg	100 mg	20 mg bolus, then 5–20 mg/h[b]

[a]High doses of intravenous loop diuretic may be necessary in patients with resistance to diuretics (e.g., those with heart failure, nephrotic syndrome, or kidney failure). See text.
[b]Repeat loading dose before increasing the infusion rate.

Table 71.2. Thiazide Diuretic Doses in Refractory Edema[a]

DIURETIC	DOSE
Chlorothiazide	500–1000 mg IV daily or twice daily
Hydrochlorothiazide	25–50 mg by mouth twice daily[b]
Chlorthalidone	12.5–25 mg by mouth twice daily[b]
Metolazone	2.5–20 mg by mouth daily[b]

[a]When used in addition to loop diuretic.
[b]If the loop diuretic is given intravenously, administration of oral thiazide diuretic should precede administration of intravenous loop diuretic by a few hours.

the renin-angiotensin-aldosterone system leads to increased sodium reabsorption at other nephron sites. Finally, in patients treated with an oral loop diuretic, delayed intestinal absorption of the loop diuretic may prevent the threshold rate of diuretic excretion to be reached. Because of these phenomena, addition of a thiazide diuretic may be necessary. Chlorothiazide is the only thiazide diuretic that can be administered intravenously. However, oral hydrochlorothiazide, chlorthalidone, and metolazone are also effective. There are several other special considerations when treating patients with CHF:

- For patients treated with an oral loop diuretic, torsemide or bumetanide may be better choices than furosemide. The bioavailability of oral furosemide averages about 50%, but ranges from 10% to 100%. In addition, the bioavailability may vary greatly over time in an individual patient. The bioavailability of torsemide and bumetanide is more predictable.
- Spironolactone and eplerenone improve survival in patients with heart failure with reduced ejection fraction. This benefit is thought to be independent of the diuretic effect.
- Diuresis may lead to contraction of the vascular compartment, decreased venous return to the heart, decreased cardiac filling pressures, decreased cardiac output, decreased kidney perfusion, and prerenal azotemia. However, patients with elevated central venous pressure have elevated kidney venous pressure. Elevated kidney venous pressure impairs kidney perfusion. In such patients, diuresis may lead to improvement in kidney function.
- Patients with chronic obstructive pulmonary disease may have chronic respiratory acidosis and cor pulmonale. Diuresis can lead to contraction alkalosis. Contraction alkalosis can depress ventilation, thereby exacerbating the hypoxemia and hypercapnia. In this situation, correction of the contraction alkalosis can be achieved by the administration of the carbonic anhydrase inhibitor acetazolamide.

19. **Are there special considerations when treating patients with decompensated cirrhosis?**
    The initial diuretic regimen for a patient with cirrhosis and ascites typically consists of oral spironolactone 100 mg daily and oral furosemide 40 mg daily. The doses may be increased if necessary, maintaining the ratio of spironolactone to furosemide at 100 mg to 40 mg. In cirrhotic patients with generalized edema, diuresis can be rather rapid. In these patients, interstitial fluid can be mobilized rapidly through capillary beds, thereby maintaining vascular volume. In patients with ascites but without peripheral edema, one must be more cautious. In these patients, ascitic fluid can be mobilized only via the peritoneal capillaries. The maximum rate at which such mobilization can occur is approximately 500 mL/day. If negative fluid balance exceeds 500 mL/day, vascular volume may fall, leading to azotemia or even hepatorenal syndrome. If more rapid fluid removal is desired in a patient with ascites but without peripheral edema, large-volume paracentesis should be considered. Care must also be taken to avoid diuretic-induced hypokalemia in cirrhotic patients. Hypokalemia leads to exchange of potassium and hydrogen ions across cell membranes. Potassium moves out of cells, and protons move into cells. The resultant intracellular acidosis stimulates ammonia synthesis in the proximal tubular cells. Hyperammonemia may induce or exacerbate hepatic encephalopathy.

20. **Are there special considerations when treating patients with kidney failure?**
    Kidney failure leads to retention of anions, which competitively inhibit proximal tubular secretion of diuretic into the tubular lumen. This phenomenon leads to resistance to diuretics.

HYPOVOLEMIA

21. **What is hypovolemia? Is it different from dehydration?**
    Hypovolemia is generally synonymous with ECF volume contraction. Physicians should distinguish between ECF volume contraction and dehydration. ECF volume contraction implies a loss of sodium and water. Dehydration implies a loss of water. For example, a loss of 1 L of fluid containing 150 mmol sodium will cause the ECF volume to fall by 1 L. Because the lost fluid is isotonic, plasma osmolality will not change. A loss of 1 L water, however, will cause much less ECF volume contraction. Water will be lost proportionally from all body fluid compartments. Because two-thirds of total body water is intracellular and one-third is extracellular, a loss of 1 L water will cause the ECF volume to fall by only 0.33 L. Plasma osmolality will rise. A loss of 1 L water is more properly called dehydration. Losses of water, then, are less likely to cause manifestations of ECF contraction than are losses of sodium and water (Fig. 71.3). Losses of water, however, may cause manifestations of hypernatremia.

22. **What leads to ECF volume losses?**
    ECF volume losses may be due to losses of sodium and water through the gastrointestinal tract, through the kidneys, or through the skin. ECF may also be sequestered in a third space.

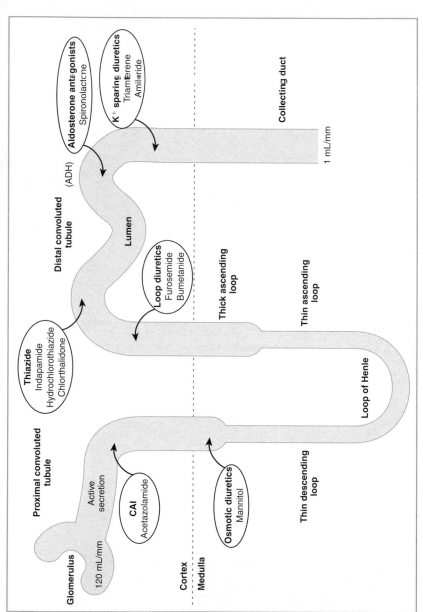

Figure 71.3. Site of diuretic action. ADH, Antidiuretic hormone; CAI, carbonic anhydrase inhibitors. (From Kester, M., Karpa, K. D., Quraishi, S., et al. (2007). Elsevier's integrated pharmacology. Philadelphia: Mosby.)

23. What are the common gastrointestinal causes of hypovolemia?
    - Gastrointestinal bleeding is a common cause of volume contraction.
    - Loss of fluid from the gastrointestinal tract can cause volume contraction. Secretions from the stomach, pancreas, gallbladder, and intestines total about 3 to 6 L/day, but almost all of this secreted fluid is reabsorbed. If reabsorption is prevented because of vomiting or external drainage of secretions (as with tube drainage or ostomies), volume contraction can ensue. If secretions increase (as with diarrhea), volume contraction can ensue.

24. What are the common kidney causes of hypovolemia?
    - Diuretics impair kidney sodium reabsorption. Overuse can cause volume contraction.
    - Osmotic diuresis can cause volume contraction. The presence of a nonreabsorbable solute in the tubular fluid inhibits sodium and water reabsorption. In uncontrolled diabetes mellitus, the rate at which glucose is filtered by the glomeruli exceeds the rate at which glucose can be reabsorbed by the renal tubules. Glucose in the tubular fluid acts as an osmotic agent and can produce large losses of sodium and water.
    - Adrenal insufficiency can cause volume depletion and hypotension. In this disorder, aldosterone deficiency leads to kidney sodium losses.
    - Diabetes insipidus is due to impaired ADH secretion (central diabetes insipidus) or impaired kidney response to ADH (nephrogenic diabetes insipidus). These disorders are characterized by decreased water reabsorption by the collecting tubules and by the excretion of large volumes of dilute urine. In well patients, this water loss will be matched by water intake. In patients with altered mental status or without easy access to water, however, ongoing water losses may produce hypernatremia and volume contraction.
    - Bilateral urinary tract obstruction can produce kidney failure and volume overload. Urine output often increases after relief of bilateral urinary tract obstruction. In almost all cases, however, this post-obstructive diuresis represents physiologic correction of volume overload. Attempts to match urine output with intravenous fluid intake will lead to persistently high urine output.

25. When do losses from the skin lead to hypovolemia?
    Evaporation of water from the skin and respiratory tract totals about 700 to 1000 mL/day. These losses are called insensible water losses. Sweat is hypotonic (sodium concentration 15 to 65 mmol/L), and production of sweat is low in day-to-day life. However, exercising in a hot environment will greatly increase sweat production and lead to deficits of sodium and water. Burns can lead to large losses of fluid from the interstitial compartment to the external environment. This fluid has electrolyte concentrations similar to those of plasma.

26. What conditions cause sequestration into a third space?
    A third space is a space that is not in equilibrium with the ECF space. The following conditions can cause sequestration of fluid into a third space.
    - Crush injuries. ECF is sequestered into the damaged skeletal muscle.
    - Severe pancreatitis. ECF is sequestered into the inflamed pancreas.
    - Intestinal obstruction. ECF is sequestered in the intestinal lumen.
    - Skeletal fractures. A large amount of blood may be sequestered in adjacent tissues.

27. How does one assess volume status?
    Assessment of volume status can be challenging. The wise clinician gathers evidence from the history, physical examination, and laboratory investigations. Each type of evidence has its limitations, and, in many cases, the evidence is conflicting. The following can be helpful in the assessment of volume status:
    - History. When assessing a patient with dyspnea, paroxysmal nocturnal dyspnea and orthopnea suggest that heart failure is the culprit.
    - Blood pressure. Patients with severe volume contraction may, of course, be hypotensive. However, if there is severe vasoconstriction, blood pressure may be normal even in patients with shock.
    - Postural vital signs. In patients with suspected blood loss, an increase in the pulse of at least 30 beats per minute or severe postural dizziness (preventing measurement of standing pulse and blood pressure) suggests a blood loss of at least 1 L.
    - Venous pressure. The external jugular vein may be examined. The normal venous pressure is 1 to 8 cm H_2O. Examination of the external jugular vein can be helpful both in the assessment of volume status and in the assessment of the response to volume replacement or diuresis. Venous pressure may also be measured by insertion of a catheter into the right atrium.

- Peripheral edema. Pitting edema occurs when the interstitial fluid is diluted with fluid with a low concentration of protein. Pitting edema indicates that there is an excess of interstitial fluid but not necessarily an excess of intravascular fluid.
- Skin turgor. The loss of interstitial fluid that occurs with ECF volume contraction causes the skin to recoil more slowly after pinching. Because elasticity of skin decreases with age, however, reduced skin turgor may not be a reliable sign of volume contraction in elderly patients.
- Dry axillae suggest the presence of volume depletion in the elderly. Moist mucous membranes suggest that volume depletion is not present.
- BUN: creatinine ratio. Proximal tubular reabsorption of filtered urea is passively linked to reabsorption of sodium and water. In hypovolemia *and in states of low effective arterial volume*, proximal tubular reabsorption of sodium, water, and urea will be enhanced. This may cause the BUN:creatinine ratio to exceed 20:1.
- Urine sodium concentration. The urine sodium concentration is typically less than 25 mmol/L in hypovolemia *and in states of low effective arterial volume*.
- Hematocrit and plasma albumin concentration. Acute loss of fluid from the vascular space can cause hemoconcentration.

28. When may the urine sodium concentration be misleading?
The urine sodium concentration may be misleading in the following circumstances.
- In metabolic alkalosis (as with nasogastric suction or vomiting), bicarbonaturia obligates excretion of a cation. Therefore, the urine sodium concentration may not be low in cases of volume contraction. In this circumstance, the urine chloride concentration should be measured. The urine chloride concentration will typically be less than 15 mEq/L in cases of volume contraction.
- In states of low effective arterial volume (heart failure and cirrhosis), there may be avid kidney tubular sodium reabsorption even in cases of severe hypervolemia. Physical findings of hypervolemia will usually suggest that such patients need to be diuresed.
- If a patient with acute kidney injury is being treated with diuretics, the urine sodium concentration may not be low, even in the presence of volume contraction. In this circumstance, the fractional excretion of urea should be calculated. A fractional excretion of urea of less than 35% suggests the presence of volume contraction and prerenal azotemia.
- If volume contraction and acute tubular necrosis coexist. Because kidney tubular function is impaired, the urine sodium concentration may not be low.

29. What acid-base and electrolyte changes are associated with hypovolemia?
- Gastric secretions contain high concentrations of H^+ and Cl^-. Therefore vomiting and nasogastric suction often cause metabolic alkalosis. The increased filtered load of bicarbonate leads to increased delivery of sodium and bicarbonate to the collecting tubule. Because of volume depletion, aldosterone secretion is enhanced. This hyperaldosteronism enhances sodium reabsorption and potassium secretion in the collecting tubule. Therefore vomiting and nasogastric suction may also be accompanied by hypokalemia.
- Secretions from the gallbladder, pancreas, and intestines have high concentrations of bicarbonate. Losses of these fluids, as from diarrhea or external drainage, may cause normal anion gap metabolic acidosis. Because these secretions contain potassium, hypokalemia may also be present.
- Overuse of diuretics is typically accompanied by hypokalemia and metabolic alkalosis. Diuretics lead to contraction of the ECF volume around a constant amount of bicarbonate, leading to contraction alkalosis. Loop and thiazide diuretics increase sodium delivery to the collecting tubule. Hyperaldosteronism secondary to volume contraction promotes sodium reabsorption and potassium secretion in the collecting tubule, leading to hypokalemia.
- Osmotic diuresis from uncontrolled diabetes mellitus can cause perturbations in plasma sodium and potassium concentrations. Hyperglycemia causes movement of water from the intracellular space to the extracellular space, depressing the plasma sodium concentration. However, the plasma sodium concentration is often higher than expected because of free water loss caused by the osmotic diuresis. Osmotic diuresis from uncontrolled diabetes mellitus generally causes a large total body potassium deficit because of urinary losses from the osmotic diuresis. Despite this potassium deficit, the plasma potassium concentration is usually normal or elevated. There are two reasons for this phenomenon. Because insulin promotes uptake of potassium by cells, insulin deficiency promotes hyperkalemia. In addition, the hyperosmolality caused by hyperglycemia causes water to move out of the cells into the ECF. Potassium will be "dragged" out of the cells in a process called solvent drag. Even if the initial plasma potassium concentration is normal, then,

one must monitor it closely. Insulin administration will reverse the processes described above and can lead to severe hypokalemia. Uncontrolled Type I diabetes mellitus may be accompanied by diabetic ketoacidosis.

- Diabetes insipidus leads to water losses and can cause severe hypernatremia in patients who do not have access to water.
- Any case of hypovolemia, if severe enough, can cause shock and lactic acidosis.

30. **Give some guidelines for the rate of volume replacement in hypovolemia.**
    In the absence of hypotension or shock, gradual volume repletion is preferred. The goal of therapy is to achieve positive fluid balance, not merely to administer a large volume of intravenous fluid. For example, a patient may have an ostomy output of 3 L/day. The patient's insensible losses are approximately 1 L/day. When one takes urine output into account, one can see that well more than 4 L of fluid must be administered per day if positive fluid balance is to be achieved and volume contraction is to be corrected.

    - In cases of hypovolemic shock, rapid volume repletion is preferred to restore tissue perfusion and to prevent shock from becoming irreversible. At least 1 to 2 L of isotonic saline should be given in the first hour. Blood should be given in cases of hemorrhagic shock. Blood pressure and mental status may be used to guide subsequent intravenous fluid administration. Central venous pressure measurement may be needed in patients who fail to respond to initial therapy, especially if there is substantial ongoing fluid loss.

31. **Are colloids better than crystalloids for volume replacement?**
    No. Fluid repletion with colloid-containing solutions (albumin solution or hyperoncotic starch solutions) would seem to have potential advantages over fluid repletion with crystalloids (0.9% saline or lactated Ringer's). Because the colloid remains in the vascular space, colloid-containing solutions should more effectively expand vascular volume. Also, because repletion with colloid-containing solutions increases plasma oncotic pressure and favors fluid movement from the interstitial space to the vascular space, repletion with colloid-containing solutions should lower the risk of pulmonary edema. However, studies have failed to demonstrate benefits from administration of colloid-containing solutions. In addition, administration of hyperoncotic starch solutions is associated with increased risk of acute kidney injury. Crystalloids are preferred to colloid-containing solutions, then, in the treatment of hypovolemia not due to bleeding. Because about three-fourths of administered isotonic saline will redistribute into the interstitial space, a much greater volume of crystalloid must be administered to achieve a similar degree of vascular volume expansion.

KEY POINTS

1. Hypervolemia is synonymous with ECF volume overload.
2. ECF volume overload is due to an excess of total body sodium.
3. To correct ECF volume overload, sodium output must exceed sodium intake. Sodium output is typically augmented by diuretics. Excessive dietary sodium intake can negate the effects of a diuretic regimen.
4. To correct ECF volume overload, an effective dose of diuretic must be determined, and, in some circumstances, more than one diuretic may need to be administered.
5. ECF volume contraction implies a deficit of sodium and water. Dehydration implies a deficit of water. A deficit of water is less likely to produce manifestations of ECF volume contraction than is a deficit of sodium and water.
6. To assess volume status, the clinician gathers evidence from the history, physical examination, and laboratory investigations. Each type of evidence has its limitations, and, in many cases, the evidence is conflicting.
7. A low urine sodium concentration does not necessarily imply the presence of volume contraction. A high urine sodium concentration does not necessarily imply the absence of volume contraction.
8. Immediate and rapid volume repletion is indicated in hypovolemic shock in order to prevent shock from becoming irreversible.
9. Crystalloids are preferred over colloid-containing solutions in the treatment of hypovolemia not due to hemorrhage.

BIBLIOGRAPHY

Andreoli, T. E. (1997). Edematous states: An overview. *Kidney Int, 51*(Suppl. 59), S2–S10.

Balter, P., Artemyev, M., & Zabetakis, P. (2015). Methods and challenges for the practical application of Crit-Line™ monitor utilization in patients on hemodialysis. *Blood Purif, 39*(1-3), 21–24.

Bleich, M., & Greger, R. (1997). Mechanism of action of diuretics. *Kidney Int, 51*, S11–S15.

Bock, H. A., & Stein, J. H. (1988). Diuretics and the control of extracellular fluid volume: Role of counterregulation. *Semin Nephrol, 8*, 264.

Chazot, C., Wabel, P., Chamney, P., Moissl, U., Wieskotten, S., & Wizemann, V. (2012). Importance of normohydration for the long-term survival of haemodialysis patients. *Nephrol Dial Transplant, 27*(6), 2404–2410.

Ellison, D. H. (1994). Diuretic drugs and the treatment of edema: From clinic to bench and back again. *Am J Kidney Dis, 23*, 623.

Enghard, P., Rademacher, S., Nee, J., Hasper, D., Engert, U., Jörres, A., & Kruse, J. M. (2015). Simplified lung ultrasound protocol shows excellent prediction of extravascular lung water in ventilated intensive care patients. *Crit Care, 19*, 36.

Ernst, M. E., & Moser, M. (2009). Use of diuretics in patients with hypertension. *N Engl J Med, 361*(22), 2153–2156.

Garro, R., Sutherland, S., Bayes, L., Alexander, S., & Wong, C. (2015). CRIT-LINE: A noninvasive tool to monitor hemoglobin levels in pediatric hemodialysis patients. *Pediatr Nephrol, 30*(6), 991–998.

Ginès, P., Cárdenas, A., Arroyo, V., & Rodés, J. (2004). Management of cirrhosis and ascites. *N Engl J Med, 350*, 1646–1654.

Humphreys, M. H. (1994). Mechanisms and management of nephrotic edema. *Kidney Int, 45*, 266.

Hur, E., Usta, M., Toz, H., Asci, G., Wabel, P., Kahvecioglu, S., . . . Ok, E. (2013). Effect of fluid management guided by bioimpedance spectroscopy on cardiovascular parameters in hemodialysis patients: A randomized controlled trial. *Am J Kidney Dis, 61*(6), 957–965.

Kraemer, M., Rode, C., & Wizemann, V. (2006). Detection limit of methods to assess fluid status changes in dialysis patients. *Kidney Int, 69*(9), 1609–1620.

Leypoldt, J. K., Cheung, A. K., Steuer, R. R., Harris, D. H., & Conis, J. M. (1995). Determination of circulating blood volume by continuously monitoring hematocrit during hemodialysis. *J Am Soc Nephrol, 6*(2), 214–219.

Martin, P. Y., & Schrier, R. W. (1997). Sodium and water retention in heart failure: Pathogenesis and treatment. Review. *Kidney Int, 51*(Suppl. 59), S57–S61.

Moissl, U. M., Wabel, P., Chamney, P. W., Bosaeus, I., Levin, N. W., Bosy-Westphal, A., ... Fuller, N. J. (2006). Body fluid volume determination via body composition spectroscopy in health and disease. *Physiol Meas, 27*(9), 921–933.

Moore, C. L., & Copel, J. A. (2011). Point-of-care ultrasonography. *N Engl J Med, 364*(8), 749–757.

Noble, V. E., Murray, A. F., Capp, R., Sylvia-Reardon, M. H., Steele, D. J. R., & Liteplo, A. (2009). Ultrasound assessment for extravascular lung water in patients undergoing hemodialysis. Time course for resolution. *Chest, 135*(6), 1433–1439.

Onofriescu, M., Hogas, S., Voroneanu, L., Apetrii, M., Nistor, I., Kanbay, M., & Covic, A. C. (2014). Bioimpedance-guided fluid management in maintenance hemodialysis: a pilot randomized controlled trial. *Am J Kidney Dis, 64*(1), 111–118.

Palmer, B. F., & Henrich, W. L. (2008). Recent advances in the prevention and management of intradialytic hypotension. *J Am Soc Nephrol, 19*(1), 8–11.

Picano, E., & Pellikka, P. A. (2016). Ultrasound of extravascular lung water: A new standard for pulmonary congestion. *Eur Heart J, 37*(27), 2097–2104.

Pitt, B., Zannad, F., Remme, W. J., Cody, R., Castaigne, A., Perez, A., . . . Wittes, J. (1999). The effect of spironolactone on morbidity and mortality in patients with severe heart failure. *N Engl J Med, 341*, 709.

Reddan, D. N., Szczech, L. A., Hasselblad, V., Lowrie, E. G., Lindsay, R. M., Himmelfarb, J., . . . Owen, W. F., Jr. (2005). Intradialytic blood volume monitoring in ambulatory hemodialysis patients: A randomized trial. *J Am Soc Nephrol, 16*(7), 2162–2169.

Rose, B. D., & Post, T. W. (2001). *Clinical physiology of acid-base and electrolyte disorders* (5th ed.). New York: McGraw-Hill.

Santoro, A., Mancini, E., Paolini, F., Cavicchioli, G., Bosetto, A., & Zucchelli, P. (1998). Blood volume regulation during hemodialysis. *Am J Kidney Dis, 32*(5), 739–748.

Schrier, R. W., Gurevich, A. K., & Cadnapaphornchai, M. A. (2001). Pathogenesis and management of sodium and water retention in cardiac failure and cirrhosis. *Semin Nephrol, 21*, 157–172.

Torino, C., Gargani, L., Sicari, R., Letachowicz, K., Ekart, R., Fliser, D., . . . Zoccali, C. (2016). The agreement between auscultation and lung ultrasound in hemodialysis patients: The LUST Study. *Clin J Am Soc Nephrol, 11*(11), 2005–2011.

Wilcox, C. S. (2002). New insights into diuretic use in patients with chronic renal disease. *J Am Soc Nephrol, 13*, 798.

Wilson, J. G., & Breyer, K. E. (2016). Critical care ultrasound: a review for practicing nephrologists. *Adv Chronic Kidney Dis, 23*(3), 141–145.

Wizemann, V., Wabel, P., Chamney, P., Zaluska, W., Moissl, U., Rode, C., . . . Marcelli, D. (2009). The mortality risk of overhydration in haemodialysis patients. *Nephrol Dial Transplant, 24*(5), 1574–1579.

Zannad, F., McMurray, J. J., Krum, H., van Veldhuisen, D. J., Swedberg, K., Shi, H., . . . EMPHASIS-HF Study Group. (2011). Eplerenone in patients with systolic heart failure and mild symptoms. *N Engl J Med, 364*, 11–21.

Zoccali, C. (2017). Lung ultrasound in the management of fluid volume in dialysis patients: potential usefulness. *Semin Dial, 30*(1), 6–9.

Zoccali, C., Torino, C., Tripepi, R., Tripepi, G., D'Arrigo, G., Postorino, M., . . . Lung US in CKD Working Group. (2013). Pulmonary congestion predicts cardiac events and mortality in ESRD. *J Am Soc Nephrol, 24*(4), 639–646.

GENETIC DISORDERS OF SODIUM TRANSPORT

Hakan R. Toka

1. **What is the difference between Mendelian (or monogenic) forms of hypertension and essential hypertension?**

   Essential hypertension has a multifactorial etiology, including demographic and environmental (dietary) factors, and genetic predisposition, which results from multiple gene–gene and gene–environment interactions. Large genome-wide association studies among various populations mapped many gene loci for essential hypertension; however these loci have been predicted to have a very small effect on individual blood pressure variation, often estimated to be less than 2%. In contrast, Mendelian (or monogenic) forms of hypertension have a large effect on blood pressure level, with identifiable and often effectively treatable causes. The most common mechanism involves activation of the mineralocorticoid pathway, leading to increased kidney sodium reabsorption and volume expansion. Up to 20% of cases with resistant hypertension have either aldosterone-producing adrenal adenomas (APA) or bilateral adrenal hyperplasia. Based on recent DNA sequencing studies from adrenal adenoma tissues, ~50% of APA cases are caused by somatic mutations in genes controlling adrenal zona glomerulosa cell proliferation and aldosterone production. APA is the most common form of secondary hypertension, estimated to affect up to ~10% of patients with hypertension. Nevertheless, most monogenic forms of hypertension are exceedingly rare and estimated to be less than 2% of newly diagnosed hypertension. They result from mutations in a single gene and are mostly inherited in a Mendelian pattern. Since the early 1990s, more than 20 genes have been implicated in the etiology of Mendelian hypertension (Table 72.1). Similarly, many Mendelian genes have been identified that lower blood pressure (Table 72.2), with renal salt wasting being the main mechanism.

2. **Which clinical characteristics support the diagnosis of monogenic hypertension?**

   Monogenic hypertension should be considered in patients below the age of 30 years, who present with severe or refractory hypertension and a family history of early-onset hypertension. In addition, associated biochemical abnormalities should raise suspicion. The presence of hypokalemia associated with metabolic alkalosis is suggestive of excess presence or activation of the mineralocorticoid pathway. Familial or spontaneous severe hypertension associated with hyperkalemia and metabolic acidosis (in setting of normal glomerular filtration rate) can be suggestive of pseudohypoaldosteronism type 2 (PHA 2; formerly known as Gordon syndrome).

   A low renin value is shared by most of these disorders. Aldosterone activity may be decreased or increased. A typical example of low renin and aldosterone levels is Liddle syndrome. In contrast, a higher level of aldosterone release is seen in glucocorticoid-remediable aldosteronism (GRA, familial hyperaldosteronism type I). Both familial and sporadic forms of primary hyperaldosteronism exhibit typically a serum aldosterone-renin ratio (ARR) greater than 30 and a serum aldosterone value ≥15 ng/dL. A positive ARR should be confirmed with a 24-hour urine aldosterone measurement of greater than 14 µg in the setting of high salt intake (urine sodium over 200 mEq/day).

3. **What is the genetic basis of unilateral aldosterone-producing adrenal adenomas (APA, familial hyperaldosteronism type 3)?**

   The etiology of APA is de novo, somatic mutations in adrenal zona glomerulosa cells. Exome sequencing from adrenal adenoma tissues identified that ~30% of APA are due to somatic mutations in one gene, the inwardly rectifying potassium channel KCNJ5, causing amino acid substitutions in one of two highly conserved residues (G151R and L168R). In vitro experiments suggest that these rare somatic mutations lead to chronic depolarization of adrenal cells, causing constitutive aldosterone production as well as adrenal cell proliferation and unilateral adenoma. Interestingly, KCNJ5 mutations occur approximately twice as often in female than male individuals with APA. Also of interest, one rare genomic KCNJ5 mutation (T158A), transmitted in autosomal-dominant fashion, was identified in one family with bilateral familial adrenal adenomas associated with severe hypertension.

501

Table 72.1. Monogenic Syndromes of Hypertension

SYNDROME	MAIN FEATURES	TREATMENT	LOCUS	INHERITANCE	DISEASE GENE
Liddle syndrome	• Salt-sensitive • Hypokalemia and metabolic alkalosis • Renin and aldosterone suppressed	ENaC inhibitors	16p12	AD	*ENaC* (Epithelial Na+ channel)
Glucocorticoid-remediable aldosteronism (GRA)	• Salt-sensitive • Hypokalemia and metabolic alkalosis • Renin suppressed • Aldosterone normal or elevated • "Unusual" urine steroid metabolites	Corticosteroid therapy	8q24	AD	*CYP11B1/CYP11B2* (chimeric gene)
Apparent mineralocorticoid excess (AME)	• Salt-sensitive • Hypokalemia and metabolic alkalosis • Renin and aldosterone suppressed • Nephrocalcinosis can be seen • Elevated urinary cortisol-to-cortisone ratio	Spironolactone and ENaC inhibitors	16q22	AR	*11 β-HSD 2*
Mineralocorticoid receptor (MR) activating mutation	• Salt-sensitive • Hypokalemia and metabolic alkalosis • Renin and aldosterone suppressed • Exacerbated in pregnancy • Spironolactone acts as agonist	ENaC inhibitors	4q31	AD	*NR3C2*
Aldosterone-producing adrenal adenomas (APA)	• Salt-sensitive • Hypokalemia and metabolic alkalosis • Renin suppressed • Aldosterone elevated • Imaging can show adrenal adenoma	Spironolactone or eplerenone adenomectomy	11q24 3p21 1p13 Xq28	De novo/AD de novo De novo De novo	*KCNJ5 CACNA1D* *ATP1A1* *ATP2B3*
Congenital adrenal hyperplasia (CAH)	• Salt-sensitive • Hypokalemia and metabolic alkalosis • Renin and aldosterone suppressed • ACTH elevated • Mineralocorticoids (e.g., DOC) elevated • Glucocorticoid deficiency and abnormal sex hormones	Corticosteroid therapy	10q24 8q24	AR AR	*17α-hydroxylase* *11β-hydroxylase*

Disorder	Features	Treatment	Location	Inheritance	Gene
Pseudohypoaldosteronism type 2 (PHA 2)	• Salt-sensitive • Hyperkalemia and metabolic acidosis • Renin suppressed • Aldosterone normal • Hypercalciuria can be seen	Thiazide diuretics	12p13 17q21 5q31 2q36	AD AD AR/ de novo	WNK1 WNK4 Kelch-like3 Cullin3
Pheochromocytoma	• Labile hypertension • Orthostatic hypotension • Renin and aldosterone elevated • Hypokalemia can be seen • Elevated metanephrines	Alphablocker Surgery	10q11 17q11 3p25 1p36 1q23 11q23 12q13 etc.	AD/ de novo de novo	Ret NF1 VHL SDHB SDHC SDHD KMT2D etc.
Hypertension-brachydactyly syndrome	• Not salt-sensitive • Renin and aldosterone suppressed • Baroreceptor dysfunction • Orthostatic hypertension • Short stature • Brachydactyly type E	Multidrug therapy	12p12	AD	PDE3A
Hypertension, hypomagnesemia, and hypercholesterolemia; mitochondrial	• Hypomagnesemia • Hyperlipidemia • Incomplete penetrance	Multidrug therapy	mDNA	Maternal	tRNAIle

AD, Autosomal-dominant; *AR*, autosomal-recessive; *ATP1A1*, Na+/K+ ATPase α-1 subunit; *ATP2B3*, ATPase, Ca++ transporting, plasma membrane3; *11β HSD*, 11β-hydroxysteroid dehydrogenase 2; *CACNA1D*, calcium channel, voltage-dependent, L type, α-1D subunit; *DOC*, Deoxycorticosterone; *KCNJ5*, K+ inwardly-rectifying channel, subfamily J, member 5; *KMT2D*, Histone-lysine N-methyltransferase 2D; *mDNA*, mitochondrial DNA; *NF1*, neurofibromatosis 1; *PDE3A*, phosphodiesterase 3A; *Ret*, rearranged during transfection; *SDHB/C/D*, succinate dehydrogenase subunit B, C or D; *PDE3A*, phosphodiesterase 3A; *tRNAIle*, tRNA Isoleucin; *Ret*, rearranged during transfection; *VHL*, von Hippel-Lindau; *WNK1*, With-No-Lysine(K) 1.

Table 72.2. Monogenic Syndromes of Renal Salt-Wasting Lowering Blood Pressure

SYNDROME	INHERITANCE	MAIN FEATURES	TREATMENT	LOCUS	DISEASE GENE
Bartter syndrome (TAL) Type 1 Type 2 Type 3 Type 4 Type 4b Type 5	AR AR AR AR AR AD	• Hypokalemia and metabolic alkalosis • Renin and Aldosterone elevated • Nephrocalcinosis (types 1 and 2) • Neonatal manifestation (types 1, 2, 4, and 4b) • Deafness (types 4 and 4b) • Hypercalciuria • Renal failure (rare)	• Increase salt intake • Potassium supplementation • NSAIDs • K+-sparing diuretic	15q21 11q24 1p36 1p32 1p36 3q13	SLC12A1 (NKCC2) KCNJ1 (ROMK) CLCNKB BSND (Barttin) CLCNKB/CLCNKA CASR
Gitelman syndrome (DCT)	AR	• Hypokalemia and metabolic alkalosis • Renin and Aldosterone elevated • Hypomagnesemia • Hypocalciuria • Increased bone density • Chondrocalcinosis (rare)	• Increase salt intake • Potassium supplementation • Magnesium supplementation • K+-sparing diuretic • NSAIDs	16q13	SLC12A3 (NCCT)
EAST syndrome (DCT, CNT, and CD)	AR	• Hypokalemia and metabolic alkalosis • Renin and Aldosterone elevated • Hypomagnesemia • Hypocalciuria • Seizures • Hearing loss	• Increase salt intake • Potassium supplementation • Magnesium supplementation • K-sparing diuretics	1q23	KCNJ10
Pseudohypo-aldosteronism Type 1 (PHA I) (CD)	AD AR AR	• Hyperkalemia and metabolic acidosis • Renin elevated • Failure to thrive • Resistance to steroid treatment	• Saline infusion • Bicarbonate supplementation • Dialysis	4q31 12p‾3 16p‾3 16p.3	NR3C2 SCNN1A SCNN1B SCNN1G

ACE, angiotensin-converting-enzyme; AD, Autosomal-dominant; AGT, angiotensinogen; AGT1R, angiotensin 2 type 1 receptor; AR, autosomal-recessive; BSND, Barttin; CD, collecting duct; CLCNKB, chloride channel, voltage-sensitive Kb; CNT, connecting tubule; DCT, distal convoluted tubule; EAST, Epilepsy, Ataxia, Sensorineural deafness, Tubulopathy; KCNJ1, potassium inwardly-rectifying channel, subfamily J, member 1; Kir 4.1, inward rectifier-type K+ channel, member 4.1; NR3C2, nuclear receptor subfamily 3, group C, member 2; NSAIDs, nonsteroidal antiinflammatory drugs; REN, renin; SCNN1A, 1B or 1C, sodium channel, non-voltage-gated 1, α-subunit, β-subunit or γ-subunit (genes encoding for ENaC subunits); SLC12A1, solute carrier family 12, member 1; TAL, thick ascending limb.

Less common APA-causing somatic mutations in other genes are more frequently seen in males, including ATP1A1 (Na/K ATPase α1 subunit) and ATP2B (Ca++ ATPase). The causes for these gender differences are unknown; hormonal differences could play a role. Another gene implicated in APA is CACNA1D (a voltage-gated calcium channel); affected individuals feature seizures and other neurological abnormalities. Additional, rarer APA genes have been recently identified.

4. **Which hypertension syndrome features unusual steroid metabolites in the urine that typically do not exist?**

GRA, familial hyperaldosteronism type 1, is an autosomal-dominant hypertensive disorder resulting from a hybrid gene located on chromosome 8. The defective gene consists of the regulatory gene of 11β-hydroxylase gene and the structural region of the aldosterone synthase gene. Normally, angiotensin-II (Ang-II) induces the production of aldosterone by stimulating the aldosterone gene, CYP11B2, whereas adrenocorticotropic hormone (ACTH) stimulation of the 11β-hydroxylase gene, CYP11B1, leads to cortisol production. A highly similar DNA sequence of these two genes and an unequal crossing over are the causes for GRA etiology. The ACTH-stimulated chimeric gene produces aldosterone in the zona fasciculata instead of the zona glomerulosa, and thus mineralocorticoid production is unresponsive to its traditional regulators Ang-II and potassium. Steroid analysis of urine in affected individuals shows the presence of unusual steroid metabolites of a chimeric protein normally not seen, 18-oxocortisol and 18-hydroxycortisol, which can be helpful to diagnose this condition.

In GRA, plasma renin is reduced, whereas aldosterone level can be increased. Hypokalemia is commonly seen. Given the severity of hypertension at presentation, patients suffer hemorrhagic strokes from ruptured aneurysms. Hence cerebral magnetic resonance angiography is a requisite in these patients at the time of diagnosis; repeat imaging every 5 years should be considered. Low-dose glucocorticoid therapy suppresses ACTH and aldosterone production, thereby serving an important therapeutic role. Both amiloride and spironolactone are also effective.

5. **Which syndrome features elevated cortisol-to-cortisone ratio in the urine despite normal serum cortisol levels?**

The syndrome of apparent mineralocorticoid excess (AME) is characterized by autosomal recessive hypertension and hypokalemia associated with metabolic alkalosis. In some cases, nephrocalcinosis and renal cysts are observed. The syndrome is caused by bi-allelic loss-of-function mutations in the kidney-specific isoform of 11β-hydroxysteroid dehydrogenase (11β-HSD 2), which allow concentrations of cortisol to rise in distal tubular cells and subsequent activation of the mineralocorticoid receptor (MR). Usually the 11β-HSD 2 enzymes "protect" MR from cortisol by oxidizing it to its inactive metabolite cortisone. The function of 11β-HSD 2 is important, since cortisol has the same affinity for the MR as aldosterone and typically a 10-fold greater level than aldosterone. An elevated urine (tetrahydro)cortisol-to-(tetrahydro)cortisone ratio greater than 0.5 establishes the diagnosis. The mainstay of therapy hinges on MR blockade with spironolactone. Adjunctive therapy includes potassium supplementation and low sodium diet.

6. **Which candy, additive to chewing tobacco, or liquor can cause a syndrome mimicking mineralocorticoid excess, and what is the mechanism?**

Individuals ingesting large amounts of high-quality licorice, which contains glycyrrhetinic acid, can develop hypertension associated with hypokalemia and metabolic alkalosis. This condition resembles an acquired form of AME. Glycyrrhetinic acid inhibits 11β-hydroxysteroid dehydrogenase 2 (11-β-HSD 2), thereby increasing cortisol in the distal tubule cells in the kidney, activating MR and increasing sodium reabsorption similar to that which occurs in AME syndrome. A frequently aggravating factor can be high salt content of certain licorice brands. Glycyrrhetinic acid can also be found in chewing tobacco, anise liquors (Ouzo, Arak, Raki, Sambuca), and carbenoxolone, a synthetic analog that is licensed in the United Kingdom for treatment of mucosal ulcerations.

7. **Which hypertension syndromes are characterized by low cortisol levels and abnormal sex hormones?**

Congenital adrenal hyperplasia (CAH) refers to several autosomal recessive conditions caused by mutations in genes mediating biochemical steroidogenesis in the adrenal gland. In CAH, the adrenal glands secrete excessive or deficient amounts of sex hormones and mineralocorticoids during prenatal development. Low cortisol production is characteristic of these conditions. CAH is often classified into the common "salt-wasting" forms, mostly due to 21-α-hydroxylase mutations, and the rare nonclassical forms (<10%), which are associated with hypertension due to increased ACTH production. Bi-allelic loss-of-function mutations in CYP11B1 (11-β-hydroxylase) or CYP17A1 (17-α-hydroxylase) can cause CAH associated with hypertension. In CAH, both cortisol and sex steroid levels are altered, leading to increased mineralocorticoid precursor production (mainly 11-deoxy-corticosterone, deoxycorticosterone [pDOC], and corticosterone) and activating the MR. Patients typically develop childhood hypertension caused by volume expansion associated hypokalemia and metabolic alkalosis. Treatment with glucocorticoids suppresses ACTH, thereby reducing mineralocorticoid precursor production and lowering the blood pressure. In 11-β-hydroxylase deficiency, female virilization is common, and in 17-α-hydroxylase deficiency, genetic males feature ambiguous genitalia and females can have failure to ovulate.

8. Describe a mechanism in which spironolactone and progesterone increase blood pressure.
   Geller syndrome is an autosomal-dominant form of hypertension resembling Liddle syndrome, associated with hypokalemia, metabolic alkalosis, and suppressed renin and aldosterone level. Affected individuals develop hypokalemia and early-onset hypertension, which in females, is exacerbated by pregnancy, often requiring premature delivery in the absence of preeclampsia. Candidate gene sequencing followed by structural protein analysis revealed that a mutated MR (S810L) allowed for activation by steroids lacking a 21-hydroxyl group, such as progesterone, which under normal conditions is not possible. At baseline, the mutated MR is constitutively active, explaining its features of increase distal sodium reabsorption via downstream activation of ENaC.
   In this disorder, a novel leucine residue (instead of serine) at position amino acid 810 lies within the MR ligand-binding domain, allowing activation of the receptor by spironolactone instead of inhibition. Amiloride and triamterene are used for treatment of this rare condition.

9. Why are amiloride or triamterene used to treat Liddle syndrome?
   First described by Grant W. Liddle in 1963, individuals with this autosomal-dominant form of hypertension feature hypokalemia and metabolic alkalosis, suggesting hyperaldosteronism; however, their aldosterone levels are completely suppressed. Interestingly, affected individuals do not respond to spironolactone treatment; however, they show significant improvement of blood pressure with any blockers of ENaC. Candidate gene analysis identified gain-of-function mutations in two of the three subunits that form the epithelial sodium channel ENaC as responsible cause for this syndrome. Missense mutations and deletions in the cytoplasmic tails of the β- or γ-subunits of ENaC lead to impaired deactivation of the channel from the luminal surface in the distal nephron, thereby causing upregulated sodium reabsorption.
   In vitro studies showed that the internalization of the mutated ENaC channels from the cell surface (either by ubiquitination or clathrin-mediated endocytosis) is impaired, and the ENaC channels remain active on the apical cell surface mediating unopposed sodium reabsorption. This mechanism explains the superb efficacy of ENaC blockers, such as amiloride, in the treatment of this disease.

10. Why is hydrochlorothiazide an effective treatment for PHA 2. familial hyperkalemic hypertension?
    PHA 2 is a heterogeneous condition that can be transmitted in autosomal-dominant, autosomal-recessive, or de novo fashion. In addition to hypertension and hyperkalemia, patients feature hyper-chloremic metabolic acidosis. Aldosterone levels are typically in the low normal range, reflecting the opposing effects of hyperkalemia, which normally stimulates aldosterone release, and extracellular fluid volume expansion, which normally inhibits it. Renin activity is typically suppressed. Hypercalciuria has been described.
    The molecular mechanisms of PHA 2 is defined by activation of the sodium-chloride-cotransporter (NCCT) in the distal convoluted tubule (DCT). In addition to salt-sensitive hypertension, blood pressure is chloride dependent; the exchange of sodium bicarbonate or citrate infusions for sodium chloride infusion ameliorates blood pressure elevation. These findings explain why thiazide diuretics represent a highly effective treatment for all features of this syndrome.

11. Name at least on gene defect that will lead to the clinical and biochemical profile of (PHA 2).
    Several genes have been identified for the etiology of PHA 2. The first ones were two (With-No-Lysine [K]) kinases, WNK1, and WNK4, identified by linkage analysis using (large) pedigrees of affected families. These WNK kinases have multiple functions in the distal nephron, including regulation of the NCCT in the DCT via cascade of various kinases, including WNK3. In part, they are regulated by intracellular chloride concentration. When these kinases are mutated (WNK1: intronic gain-of-function deletions, WNK4: loss-of-function mutations), distal sodium reabsorption via NCCT is increased regardless of volume status, resulting in salt-sensitive hypertension. Mutations in the WNKs are believed to cause increased NCCT plasma membrane abundance and therefore increased activity. Another hallmark of PHA 2 is hyperkalemia; the mechanisms leading to decreased potassium excretion are complex and can be explained by WNK participation in determining the nature of aldosterone

action, which has distinct functions in the setting of hypovolemia (sodium retention) and hyperkalemia (potassium excretion). The inhibition of potassium excretion despite marked hyperkalemia occurs likely by both, direct inhibition of the potassium channel renal outer medullary K (ROMK) (increased endocytosis) in the DCT and decreased potassium excretion in the collecting duct (CD; lower sodium concentration in the lumen leads to decreased diffusion gradient for movement of cellular potassium into the urine). The role of NCCT activation in the pathophysiology of PHA 2 explains why this condition is so responsive to treatment with thiazide diuretics.

Two more gene defects for PHA 2 have been identified by exome sequencing; Kelch-like 3 (KLHL3) and Cullin 3 (CUL3). These genes are expressed in the DCT and co-localize with WNK1, WNK4, and the NCCT. They form a complex, a KLHL3-CUL3 E3 ubiquitin ligase, which regulates WNK1 and WNK4 activity in the DCT in complex fashion and ubiquitination (deactivation) of NCCT from cell surface.

The phenotype of individuals affected by these different gene defects in PHA 2 differs. Patients with KLHL3 and CUL3 mutations appear more severely affected as they develop PHA 2 at younger age and present with more severe hyperkalemia and also a failure to thrive. Patients with WNK1 mutations have a milder phenotype, whereas patient with WNK4 mutations can feature hypercalciuria. However, thiazide diuretics are a very effective treatment of choice in all forms of PHA 2.

12. **Which monogenic form of hypertension can feature both elevated renin and aldosterone level?**
Pheochromocytoma (PCC) is caused by catecholamine-producing adrenal tumors and is associated with various symptoms depending on the type and secretory pattern of the produced catecholamine(s). Hypertension can present as paroxysmal and labile hypertension, complicated by orthostatic hypotension and persistent hypertension. Hypokalemia is often seen, and renin and aldosterone levels are elevated due to volume depletion and catecholamine-mediated renin release from the juxtaglomerular cells. Familial forms of PCC are common. The majority are associated with multiple endocrine neoplasia type 2 (MEN type 2) and caused by gain-of-function mutations in the RET protooncogene. In addition to RET, more than 10 genes have been associated with familial PCC (including genes causing the phakomatoses von Hippel-Lindau disease and Neurofibromatosis type 1; Table 72.1). Overall, known genetic mutations may account for the pathogenesis of up to ~60% of PCC and paragangliomas. A recent exome sequencing study from nonsyndromic adrenal PCC tissue identified de novo somatic mutations in genes associated with apoptosis-related pathways. Particularly, mutations in the "cancer" gene KMT2D (lysine [K]-specific methyltransferase 2D) were more frequent (~14% of tissues).

The treatment of choice is surgical resection of the affected adrenal gland(s) or paraganglioma, respectively. Treatment with irreversible alpha-blockade prior to surgery is mandatory to prevent life-threatening hypertensive complications.

13. **Which salt-wasting tubulopathy represents the mirror image of (PHA 2)?**
Individuals affected by Gitelman syndrome present with symptoms identical to those who are on thiazide diuretics; the features of this condition mirror the findings in PHA 2 with the exception of hypomagnesemia and include hypochloremic metabolic alkalosis, hypokalemia, and hypocalciuria. Affected individuals are typically asymptomatic; however, muscular cramps, weakness/fatigue, and irritability have been described. More severe symptoms, such as tetany and paralysis, are rare.

The condition is caused by homozygous or compound heterozygous loss-of-function mutations in SLC12A3 encoding the NCCT, inactivating NCCT expression in the apical membrane of DCT epithelia, thereby causing urinary sodium wasting. Individuals with heterozygous loss-of-function mutations in NCCT may have a survival benefit due to a lower blood pressure level and increased bone mineral density.

14. **Which salt-wasting tubulopathy represents the mirror image of Liddle syndrome?**
Pseudohypoaldosteronism type 1 (PHA 1) is characterized by salt-wasting resulting from renal unresponsiveness to aldosterone. Affected individuals present with neonatal renal salt wasting associated with hyperkalemic acidosis, despite high aldosterone levels. There are two genetic subtypes, which can be distinguished by severity of symptoms: the milder type 1A is inherited in an autosomal-dominant fashion, and the more severe type 1B is transmitted in an autosomal recessive pattern.

The recessive form, PHA type 1B, is caused by biallelic loss-of-function mutations in any one of the three genes encoding the α-, β-, and γ-subunits of ENaC, leading to decreased channel activity and severe renal salt wasting. This condition is the mirror image of Liddle syndrome. Patients with this form can feature a severe systemic disorder, starting in infancy and persisting into adulthood, and require lifelong follow-up.

PHA type 1 A is caused by loss-of-function mutations in the MR gene and could be considered as mirror image of Geller syndrome (hypertension exacerbated in pregnancy by activating mutation of the MR). Affected individuals improve with aging and usually become asymptomatic without treatment by adulthood. Nevertheless, elevated aldosterone levels can be found. Affected individuals are at higher risk with intercurrent illness associated with volume depletion.

15. **Explain the various types of Bartter syndrome.**

In Bartter syndrome, renal salt wasting occurs in the thick ascending limb of Henle (TAL). It is a heterogeneous, autosomal-recessive renal-tubular disorder characterized by hypokalemia, hypochloremia, metabolic alkalosis, and hyperreninemia with low-normal blood pressure. The primary defect is an impaired transepithelial transport of sodium chloride across the TAL, resulting in excessive urinary losses of sodium, chloride, and potassium. The combination of secondary hyperaldosteronism and increased distal sodium delivery enhances potassium (and hydrogen) secretion at the secretory sites in the distal nephron, leading to hypokalemia. In addition to volume depletion, increased renal release of vasodilating prostaglandins PGE2 contributes to the features of Bartter syndrome.

Failure to thrive is a typical occurrence in children with neonatal Bartter syndrome, caused by loss-of-function mutations in the Na-K-2Cl cotransporter (NKCC2, Bartter type 1) and the kidney outer medullary potassium channel (ROMK, Bartter type 2), both of which are expressed at the apical membrane of TAL epithelia.

In comparison, the classic Bartter syndrome (type 3) is caused by loss-of-function mutations in the basolateral chloride channel Kb (CLCNKB), often diagnosed at school age or later in adulthood. Increased urinary calcium excretion is significantly milder in classic Bartter; however, kidney stones can develop. Kidney function is typically normal; however, progression to end-stage kidney disease has been reported. Since CLCNKB is also expressed in the DCT, type 3 Bartter syndrome is classified by some authors as a mixed disorder of the TAL and DCT or as a disorder of the thiazide–furosemide pharmacotype; therefore hypomagnesemia can be present in classic Bartter syndrome.

Type 4 Bartter syndrome is caused by mutations in Barttin (BSND), an accessory β-subunit of the CLCNKB, and associated with sensorineural deafness. Hearing loss in Bartter type 4 is explained by loss-of-function of Barttin, which is also expressed in the inner, serving also as a subunit to the chloride channel CLCNKA. The recently described Bartter type 4b is caused by simultaneous homozygous mutations in both CLCNKB and CLCNKA and is also associated with deafness. Both type 4 and 4b can manifest in early childhood and can be associated with kidney failure.

Autosomal-dominant gain-of-function mutations in the calcium-sensing receptor gene (CASR) can also cause renal salt wasting in a subset of affected individuals. Although parathyroid hormone levels are severely suppressed in this syndrome, this condition is classified by some as a variant or phenocopy of Bartter (type 5) due to the expression of CASR on the basolateral membrane of TAL epithelia. Hypomagnesemia can be seen.

16. **What distinguishes Bartter from Gitelman syndrome?**

Urinary calcium excretion is increased in Bartter syndrome, in contrast with the hypocalciuria found in patients with Gitelman syndrome. Hypomagnesemia is a hallmark findings in Gitelman syndrome and uncommon in Bartter. Another distinguishing feature is the lack of change in urinary chloride in Gitelman patients with thiazide administration.

Interestingly, the Gitelman variant has a relatively high allele frequency of up to 1 in 100 to 400 individuals. Lower blood pressure and increased bone mineral density may be a survival benefit in Gitelman variant carriers. Regardless, both Gitelman and Bartter syndromes have autosomal recessive transmission and are therefore uncommon; when suspected in adults, it is important to exclude surreptitious vomiting and diuretic use.

17. **Which salt wasting nephropathy resembling Gitelman syndrome is associated with seizure and ataxia?**

EAST syndrome (epilepsy, ataxia, sensorineural deafness, and tubulopathy) features renal salt wasting and electrolyte imbalance. The mode of inheritance is autosomal recessive and consanguinity has been described in some families. The responsible gene, *KCNJ10*, is expressed in the basolateral membranes of the DCT, connecting tubule (CNT) and CD epithelia. The identified electrolyte and acid–base abnormalities are similar to those seen in Gitelman syndrome and include hypokalemia, hypomagnesemia, and metabolic alkalosis (see Table 72.2). Renin and aldosterone levels are both elevated. Patients typically crave salt, suggesting that they compensate for renal salt losses with an increased consumption of salt to maintain normal blood pressure values. In vitro studies suggest that loss-of-function mutations in *KCNJ10* impair the activity of the Na-K-ATPase in the DCT (by decreased potassium "recycling"), located at the basolateral membrane of epithelia. The additional features seen in this syndrome are due to the expression of KCNJ10 in neuronal tissues and in cells of the inner ear.

KEY POINTS

1. Monogenic hypertension results from a mutation in a single gene, typically one that affects electrolyte transport in the distal nephron.
2. Patients with monogenic hypertension present at a young age with severe or refractory hypertension, have a strong family history of hypertension, and have typical changes in serum electrolytes.
3. Excess sodium absorption is characteristic of most genetic mutations that cause hypertension with low renin. Whereas metabolic alkalosis and hypokalemia are most common, a phenotypic variant with hyperkalemia and hyperchloremic metabolic acidosis can also be observed.
4. Mutations of sodium transport also lead to renal salt wasting. Patients with Bartter or Gitelman syndrome present typically with hypokalemia and metabolic alkalosis. Patients with PHA 1 develop salt wasting with hyperkalemia and non-gap metabolic acidosis.

BIBLIOGRAPHY

Choi, M., Scholl, U. I., Yue, P., Björklund, P., Zhao, B., Nelson-Williams, C., . . . Lifton, R. P. (2011). K+ channel mutations in adrenal aldosterone-producing adenomas and hereditary hypertension. *Science, 331*(6018), 768–772.

Hoorn, E. J., Nelson, J. H., McCormick, J. A., & Ellison, D. H. (2011). The WNK kinase network regulating sodium, potassium, and blood pressure. *Journal of the American Society of Nephrology, 22*(4), 605–614.

Ji, W., Foo, J. N., O'Roak, B. J., Zhao, H., Larson, M. G., Simon, D. B., . . . Lifton, R. P. (2008). Rare independent mutations in renal salt handling genes contribute to blood pressure variation. *Nature Genetics, 40*(5), 592–599.

Lifton, R. P., Dluhy, R. G., Powers, M., Rich, G. M., Cook, S., Ulick, S., & Lalouel, J. M. (1992). A chimaeric 11 beta-hydroxylase/aldosterone synthase gene causes glucocorticoid-remediable aldosteronism and human hypertension. *Nature, 355*(6357), 262–265.

Mune, T., Rogerson, F. M., Nikkilä, H., Agarwal, A. K., & White, P. C. (1995). Human hypertension caused by mutations in the kidney isozyme of 11 beta-hydroxysteroid dehydrogenase. *Nature Genetics, 10*(4), 394–399.

Seyberth, H. W., & Schlingmann, K. P. (2011). Bartter- and Gitelman-like syndromes: Salt-losing tubulopathies with loop or DCT defects. *Pediatric Nephrology, 26*(10), 1789–1802.

Shimkets, R. A., Warnock, D. G., Bositis, C. M., Nelson-Williams, C., Hansson, J. H., Schambelan, M., . . . Findling, J. W. (1994). Liddle's syndrome: Heritable human hypertension caused by mutations in the beta subunit of the epithelial sodium channel. *Cell, 79*(3), 407–414.

Speiser, P. W., & White, P. C. (2003). Congenital adrenal hyperplasia. *New England Journal of Medicine, 349*(8), 776–788.

CHAPTER 73

DYSNATREMIAS

N. Winn Seay and Arthur Greenberg

1. **What are dysnatremias?**
   The term *dysnatremia* applies when an aberration in plasma sodium concentration is present. Changes in plasma sodium concentration can result in fluid shifts between the intra- and extracellular compartments of the body. In the healthy state, the body's osmoregulatory system maintains the plasma sodium concentration between 135 and 145 mEq/L. Failure of this system begets an imbalance of free water intake and excretion. When free water intake exceeds excretion, the plasma sodium concentration decreases below 135 mEq/L, a condition known as hyponatremia. In contrast, hypernatremia, defined as a serum sodium concentration >145 mEq/L, occurs when electrolyte-free water excretion exceeds intake. Less commonly, pure loss or addition of sodium without a primary disturbance in water balance may also lead to hypo- or hypernatremia.

2. **How is plasma osmolality determined?**
   Plasma osmolality can be calculated with the following equation:

$$(2 \times [Na^+] \, (mEq/L) + blood \; urea \; nitrogen \; (mg/dL)/2.8 + glucose \, (mg/dL)/18 \; =$$
$$Plasma \; osmolality \; (mOsm/kg \, H_2O)$$

   As the equation implies, serum sodium concentration is by far the main determinant of plasma osmolality. Plasma osmolality can be directly measured with an osmometer. An osmolar gap exists if there is greater than a 10 mOsm/kg H_2O discrepancy between the calculated and measured osmolality, indicative of the presence of a solute not routinely measured in plasma.

3. **Can osmolality be normal despite an abnormal serum sodium concentration?**
   Yes! Serum sodium concentration is usually measured using indirect ion-selective electrodes with specimen dilution and depends on the assumption that water comprises approximately 93% of plasma. The presence of high concentrations of plasma lipid or protein, however, will reduce the aqueous contribution to plasma volume. As a result, the measured serum sodium concentration will be falsely low. This condition is known as pseudohyponatremia. Ultracentrifugation and separation of the lipid layer can correct for lab artifact due to hyperlipidemia. Direct ion-selective electrodes are not confounded by hyperlipidemia or hyperproteinemia, but only about a third of chemical analyzers use this technique. Blood gas laboratories use ion-selective electrodes and thus are not susceptible to this artifact.

4. **Is plasma osmolality the same as plasma tonicity?**
   No! While plasma hypertonicity implies hyperosmolality, hyperosmolar plasma is not necessarily hypertonic. The effective osmolality, often termed plasma tonicity, denotes the concentration of osmoles in plasma that do not move freely across the cell membrane. Such osmoles can generate concentration gradients across cell membranes and in turn drive shifts in water between the extra- and intracellular compartments. While sodium and glucose as effective osmoles contribute to tonicity, urea and ethanol are ineffective osmoles as they freely cross cell membranes. High concentrations of these latter molecules confer hyperosmolality without affecting tonicity. In the absence of ethanol or other unexpected solutes, the effective osmolality is simply the measured osmolality minus blood urea nitrogen (BUN) (mg/dL)/2.8.

5. **In what states of tonicity and osmolality can dysnatremias occur?**
   Because sodium is an effective osmole, hypernatremia by definition indicates both a hyperosmolar and hypertonic state. Hyponatremia, however, can arise in various states of osmolality and tonicity.

6. **In what hyponatremic states can a patient be hyperosmolar or hypertonic?**
   The two most clinically relevant occurrences of hyperosmolar hyponatremia are azotemia and hyperglycemia. Buildup of nitrogenous waste, that is, urea, in the setting of impaired kidney function increases plasma osmolality. If present alone, kidney dysfunction does not lead to a change in serum

sodium concentration. However, if a simultaneous disorder in water balance leading to hyponatremia is present, hyponatremia with normal or elevated serum osmolality may result. Such patients are truly *hypotonic*, because the decreased sodium, an effective osmole, leads to a decrease in tonicity while urea, an ineffective osmole, does not increase tonicity.

In hyperglycemia, increased serum glucose increases both the total and effective plasma osmolality, leading to a hypertonic state. The hypertonic plasma draws water from the cells into the extracellular compartment, lowering the serum sodium concentration. For every 100 mg/dL increase in glucose above normal, the serum sodium falls by approximately 1.6 mEq/L even as tonicity rises due to the hyperglycemia. In cases of more severe hyperglycemia (i.e., serum glucose >400 mg/dL), the ratio approximates a 2.4 mEq/L drop in serum sodium for every 100 mg/dL rise in serum glucose. A similar process occurs with administration of mannitol. Any such correction factor is an approximation, and osmolality should be measured directly when clinically relevant.

7. What causes hypotonic hyponatremia?
   While there are many discrete etiologies of hypotonic hyponatremia, there are three general processes:
   1. Inadequate solute intake
   2. Excess electrolyte-free water intake
   3. Retention of electrolyte-free water
      Not infrequently, the latter two are present simultaneously.

8. What are the clinical manifestations of hyponatremia?
   Not all patients with hyponatremia will be symptomatic. While neurons are especially sensitive to osmotic stress, astrocyte-mediated expulsion of electrolytes into the extracellular fluid (ECF) over several hours followed by organic osmolytes (e.g., taurine and glutamate) over the ensuing 24 to 48 hours prevents intracellular swelling. Thus, patients who develop a serum sodium concentration between 125 and 135 mEq/L over greater than 48 hours will often have minimal or no symptoms. Observational studies, however, have demonstrated an association between even mild hyponatremia (serum sodium concentration 130 to 134 mEq/L) and increased in-hospital mortality, falls, and reduced bone density. Other studies have noted impaired motor function and gait even with modest reductions in serum sodium concentration. The combination of cognitive impairment, unsteady gait, increased falls, and osteoporosis constitute a "perfect storm" for development of bone fractures. An increase in fracture risk has indeed been documented. Rapid decreases in plasma sodium concentration (from >134 to <125 mEq/L within 48 hours) are faster than compensatory loss of intracellular solute, so the relatively hypertonic intracellular compartment osmotically absorbs water. This cellular swelling particularly affects the brain given the limit to expansion within a tightly encasing cranium. Thus, the manifestations of hyponatremia are predominantly neurologic and include nausea, vomiting, malaise, headache, lethargy, confusion, and muscle cramps. In severe cases, seizures, coma, tentorial herniation, and neurogenic pulmonary edema can occur.

9. What is the initial diagnostic approach to hypotonic hyponatremia?
   Once hypotonicity is confirmed with an effective osmolality <275 mOsm/kg H_2O, the urine osmolality is instrumental in assessing whether or not the kidneys are reabsorbing electrolyte-free water. In the absence of chronic kidney disease, a urine osmolality <100 mOsm/kg indicates an intact diluting mechanism and a state of maximal electrolyte-free water excretion. Conversely, a urine osmolality >100 mOsm/kg suggests that electrolyte-free water reabsorption is occurring, which would be inappropriate from the point of view of tonicity alone. Patients with chronic kidney disease may have an impairment in maximal ability to dilute the urine. In such cases a urine osmolality of <200 mOsm/kg reflects maximal free-water excretion. The diagnostic approach to hyponatremia is further outlined the Fig. 73.1.

10. How is hypotonic hyponatremia with dilute urine further assessed?
    If the urine is maximally dilute, the pituitary-kidney axis is doing what it is supposed to be doing, and hypotonic hyponatremia is arising from electrolyte-free water ingestion in excess of what the kidneys can excrete. In the typical Western diet, approximately 800 mOsm of solute derived from ingested electrolytes and protein is consumed or generated and excreted in the urine on a daily basis. Assuming a maximal urine diluting capacity of 50 mOsm/kg H_2O, such a solute load is sufficient to permit excretion of up to 16 L of urine (800 mOsm solute/50 mOsm/kg = 16 L). If electrolyte-free water intake exceeds this limit, the kidneys' electrolyte-free water excretory capacity is overwhelmed, and hypotonic hyponatremia ensues. This condition, known as primary polydipsia, typically occurs among psychiatric patients. Inadequate solute intake impairs free water clearance. If solute intake decreases to 200 mOsm/day and intake of protein that would lead to urea production is reduced—as occurs

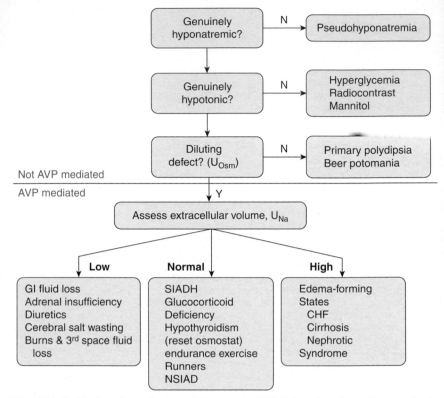

Figure 73.1. Algorithm for evaluation of patients with hyponatremia. *NSIAD*, Nephrogenic syndrome of inappropriate anti-diuresis, a rare-heritable disorder characterized by constitutive activation of the collecting duct vasopressin receptor with normal pituitary function and suppressed vasopressin release. *SIADH*, syndrome of inappropriate anti-diuretic hormone secretion. *AVP*, Arginine vasopressin; *CHF*, congestive heart failure; *GI*, gastrointestinal.

with a "tea and toast diet" or beer potomania—the volume of maximally dilute urine the kidneys can excrete may be as little as 4 L. Water ingestion above this amount can more easily be achieved and will also result in hyponatremia.

11. What causes hyponatremia with concentrated (less than maximally dilute) urine?
    Electrolyte-free water reabsorption. Water reabsorption is mediated by binding of vasopressin, or antidiuretic hormone (ADH—same stuff, 2 names), to vasopressin 2 (V2) receptors on the basolateral membranes of principal cells in the collecting ducts of nephrons. Vasopressin binding in turn stimulates insertion of aquaporin water channels into the luminal membrane. Water then flows through these aquaporin channels into cells and onward to the hypertonic medullary interstitium via constitutively active basolateral aquaporin channels. ADH release is regulated by osmoreceptors in the hypothalamus. Normally, vasopressin release is inhibited when the serum sodium concentration falls below 135 mEq/L. However, poor effective circulating volume—as sensed by carotid baroreceptors as a decrease in arterial pressure—serves as a potent stimulus for ADH secretion despite osmoregulatory inhibition. Hyponatremia in the setting of hypovolemia arises from hemodynamically driven ADH release and should improve with volume repletion. ADH secretion in the setting of arterial underfilling, due either to a low output state in the case of heart failure or to splanchnic vasodilation in cirrhosis, occurs by the same hemodynamic mechanism. These patients, conversely, will appear hypervolemic on exam. They are hyponatremic and hypotonic despite a clear excess in total body sodium content.

12. How is hypervolemic hyponatremia managed?
    Unlike hypovolemic hyponatremia, the mainstay of therapy for hypervolemic hyponatremia arising from either heart failure or cirrhosis is water restriction. Loop diuretics can also be effective in

hyponatremia associated with heart failure. By inhibiting sodium reabsorption in the ascending limb of the Loop of Henle, loop diuretics decrease the tonicity of the medulla and thereby diminish the driving force for ADH-mediated water reabsorption in the collecting duct. (By acting in the distal tubule of the cortex, *thiazide* diuretics block sodium reabsorption only at a site where sodium is reabsorbed without water. Moreover, generation of a hypertonic medullary interstitium is unaffected, leaving conditions persistently favorable for electrolyte-free water reabsorption. Thus, thiazide diuretics tend to induce *hyponatremia*.) When water restriction and loop diuretics fail, a vasopressin receptor antagonist (vaptan) may be useful. Conivaptan (a non-selective V1/V2 antagonist) and tolvaptan (a pure V2 antagonist) can be used to promote aquaresis in volume-overloaded heart failure patients with mild-to-moderate symptomatic hyponatremia. Conivaptan should be used with caution in patients with cirrhosis due to a theoretically increased risk for hypotension or variceal bleeding via antagonism of the V1 pressor receptor. Tolvaptan is relatively contraindicated in patients with cirrhosis as well due to the possibility of hepatotoxicity. More common side effects associated with these medications include thirst and dry mouth.

13. **What etiologies give rise to euvolemic hyponatremia with less than maximally dilute urine?**
Most commonly, euvolemic hyponatremia with less than maximally dilute urine arises from the syndrome of inappropriate antidiuretic hormone secretion (SIADH, discussed below). Other potential causes include exercise-associated hyponatremia (EAH), methylenedioxy-*N*-methamphetamine (MDMA or ecstasy) ingestion, hypothyroidism, and glucocorticoid insufficiency. EAH is classically observed among marathon runners, who become overhydrated in the face of excessive water ingestion coupled with impaired water excretion from non-osmotically driven ADH release. By stimulating both ADH secretion and polydipsia via activation of serotonergic pathways, MDMA ingestion can lead to acute, severe hyponatremia and death if not promptly addressed. Although the mechanism is not definitively clear, the negative systemic effects of profound thyroid hormone deficiency on cardiac output and peripheral vascular resistance appear to trigger nonosmotic ADH secretion and hyponatremia. Since cortisol suppresses ADH release, isolated glucocorticoid deficiency can result in hyponatremia from uninhibited vasopressin secretion. This entity is distinct from Addison disease or other causes of adrenal gland destruction where mineralocorticoid deficiency and consequent volume depletion are present along with glucocorticoid lack.

14. **What is the SIADH?**
SIADH refers to ADH secretion that persists in the absence of an osmotic or hemodynamic stimulus. Other potential etiologies of hyponatremia including adrenal or glucocorticoid insufficiency, heart failure, liver failure, hypothyroidism, advanced kidney disease, or diuretics (usually thiazide) should be ruled out. Although CHF and cirrhosis patients can have persistent ADH secretion despite hypotonicity, such patients as well as individuals with advanced kidney failure (due to intrinsic defects in urinary dilution) are excluded by convention from the diagnosis of SIADH. Patients with SIADH classically present with hypotonic, *euvolemic* hyponatremia and U_{osm} >100 mOsm/kg H_2O. The urine osmolality need not be higher than plasma osmolality; it only need be greater than maximally dilute. The modest intravascular volume expansion that results from ADH-induced water retention results in decreased renin angiotensin aldosterone system (RAAS) activity and sodium reabsorption. Assuming a normal dietary sodium intake, the urine sodium concentration is consequently >30 mmol/L. Likewise, an associated serum uric acid level of less than 4 mg/dL reflects increased urinary urate excretion. BUN and creatinine tend to be low normal or normal; a high normal or elevated BUN should make clinicians consider volume depletion or diminished effective arterial volume as the cause of hyponatremia. Directly measuring vasopressin levels is in general of very limited utility, as urine osmolality is an adequate surrogate measure of ADH activity. Furthermore, ADH levels will be elevated in patients with hypervolemic or hypovolemic hyponatremia, so levels do not help distinguish among these disorders. SIADH can arise in a variety of malignancies, pulmonary disorders, and central nervous system (CNS) disease. Many medications, most notably selective serotonin reuptake inhibitors, narcotics, and antipsychotics, can also cause SIADH.

15. **How is SIADH managed?**
SIADH should resolve if the underlying cause is eliminated—something often easier said than done. Discontinuation of culprit medications, antimicrobial therapy for pulmonary or CNS infections, and treatment of an underlying malignancy will be helpful. Treatment is otherwise dictated by chronicity and severity of symptoms of the hyponatremia. Asymptomatic or minimally symptomatic patients with chronic SIADH should be water restricted initially. The degree of fluid restriction can be estimated by calculating the ratio of the sum of urinary potassium and sodium concentrations to plasma sodium concentration. A ratio less than 1 allows for more liberal water restriction (i.e., 1 L/day); a ratio greater

than 1 requires stricter (and often impractical) measures (<500 mL/day). Unsurprisingly, the effectiveness of water restriction is limited by patient compliance. Alternatively, increased protein and salt consumption may be helpful. Oral urea supplementation (30 g/day), by increasing solute intake and hence urine volume, is effective but has been poorly tolerated historically, though newer formulations have proven to be more palatable. When these interventions fail, the vaptans can be used for euvolemic, mild-to-moderate hyponatremia with mild attributable symptoms. The vaptans do not reliably increase the serum sodium in a rapid fashion. Meta-analyses of randomized controlled trials have demonstrated a mean rise in the plasma sodium concentration of approximately 5 mEq/L occurring over several days in the case of tolvaptan. Thus, these medications should *not* be given for hyponatremia with severe neurologic symptoms, which would otherwise merit more rapid correction. In such cases, hypertonic saline should be administered.

16. **When and how fast should hypertonic saline be given?**
    If the ratio of the sum of urine potassium and sodium to plasma sodium is greater than 1 in a patient with SIADH, infusion of normal saline will likely lead to worsening hyponatremia as the NaCl is excreted in a smaller, more concentrated volume of urine and the remaining electrolyte-free water is then retained. Administration of hypertonic (3%) saline, however, can quickly raise the serum sodium concentration irrespective of etiology of hyponatremia. Rapid correction is warranted in severely symptomatic patients, particularly if the hyponatremia developed over less than 48 hours, since these patients are at highest risk for seizures and tentorial herniation. Even very small increases in serum sodium concentration can reduce the amount of cerebral edema present and markedly lower the risk of these life-threatening events. Elevation of the serum sodium concentration by 4 to 6 mEq/L acutely is sufficient to prevent these complications. This can be accomplished with up to three 100 mL boluses of hypertonic saline given over 10 minutes at a time. If emergent correction is not required, hypertonic saline can be administered by continuous infusion without initial boluses. A number of formulas have been proposed to model the rate of serum sodium concentration rise. However, they ignore factors such as ongoing water and electrolyte excretion that may influence the rate of rise of serum sodium concentration. Consequently, we favor use of a simple prediction formula: infusion of 1 mL/kg per hour of hypertonic saline with the expectation that it will raise the serum sodium concentration by approximately 1 mEq/L per hour. How much the serum sodium concentration should be increased depends on the rate of development of hyponatremia. With chronic hyponatremia, strict limits for overall rate of correction should be observed to avoid complications from overly rapid correction itself (see below). Any formula is only a crude estimation, so it is essential to measure serum sodium concentration frequently during the initial stages of treatment to assure that the rate of rise matches the goal.

17. **What complications of treatment can occur?**
    As discussed in Question 8, neurons, in response to hypotonic hyponatremia, expel electrolytes and organic osmolytes to reduce intracellular tonicity and limit brain swelling. When the serum sodium concentration rises too fast for the cells to reverse the prior compensation by regaining or regenerating osmolytes, water flows down its osmotic gradient and out of the cells into the newly relatively hypertonic interstitium causing cell shrinkage and, potentially, demyelination of neurons. This condition, termed osmotic demyelination syndrome (ODS), is characterized by an array of often irreversible neurologic manifestations including dysarthria, dysphagia, movement disorders (particularly spasticity), quadriparesis, behavioral abnormalities, seizures, delirium, and coma. In more severe cases, patients can become "locked in"—that is, conscious but unable to move, speak, or swallow. This complication occurs several days after the rapid correction, and the findings may be permanent. The classic presentation is a patient who initially becomes more alert as serum sodium concentration is corrected, then deteriorates a few days later.

18. **Who is at risk for ODS?**
    Patients with acute hyponatremia developing over less than 24 to 48 hours are at low risk for ODS, and there is accordingly no potential for harm in rapid correction of hyponatremia in this group. ODS is also unlikely to arise as a complication of treatment in patients presenting with a serum sodium >125 mEq/L. Conversely, an initial serum sodium <105 mEq/L, hypokalemia, alcoholism, malnutrition, and advanced liver disease are risk factors for ODS in patients with chronic hyponatremia. Strategies for sodium correction aimed at preventing ODS are outlined in the Table 73.1. Notably, hyponatremia should be assumed to be chronic and managed as such unless its onset is clearly known to be <48 hours.

Table 73.1. Goals and Limits for Treatment of Hyponatremia Stratified by Duration and Risk of Osmotic Demyelination Syndrome

PRESENTATION	RISK FOR ODS	GOAL INCREASE IN [Na+]	LIMIT TO INCREASE IN [Na+]	TREATMENT STRATEGY
Acute Hypotonic Hyponatremia (duration verified to be <48 h)				
Severe symptoms	Negligible	Rapid increase by 4–6 mEq/L, then gradual increase to normalization	None	Rapidly increase serum Na by 4–6 mEq/L with up to three 100 mL boluses of hypertonic saline given over 10 min at a time, followed by hypertonic saline at 1 mL/kg/h until substantial normalization
Mild or moderate symptoms	Negligible	Normalization	None	Fluid restriction alone if etiology rapidly reversible. Otherwise, hypertonic saline at 1 mL/kg/h until substantial normalization
Chronic Hypotonic Hyponatremia (duration known to be >48 h or duration uncertain)				
Severe, moderate, or mild symptoms	High[a]	4–6 mEq/L in 24 h	8 mEq/L in any 24 h period	Treatment according to etiology (e.g., volume repletion for hypovolemic hyponatremia, water restriction with SIADH or hypervolemic hyponatremia) and severity of symptoms. Can consider hypertonic saline for severely symptomatic euvolemic hyponatremia with risk of seizures or herniation or a vaptan for mild-to-moderate, refractory euvolemic or hypervolemic hypernatremia. Closely monitor [Na+] every 2–4 h and urine output. Re-lower [Na+] with IV 5% dextrose or enteral water ± desmopressin 1–2 mcg Q6 h if overly rapid correction
Severe, moderate, or mild symptoms	Intermediate	4–8 mEq/L in 24 h	10–12 mEq/L in any 24 h and no more than 18 mEq/L in any 48 h period	Same strategy as high-risk ODS patients, except with less strict [Na+] correction goals and limits
Moderate or mild symptoms	Low (initial [Na+] > 125 mEq/L)	Normalization	Normalization	Treatment according to etiology. Can consider vaptan for mild-to-moderate, refractory euvolemic or hypervolemic hypernatremia

[a][Na+] ≤105 mEq/L, hypokalemia, alcoholism, malnutrition, advanced liver disease.

In patients with significant risk of ODS, especially those with starting [Na+] <120 mEq/L, who experience a rise in [Na+] exceeding recommended limit, consider re-lowering [Na+] to a value below target by administration of electrolyte-free water. Urine output and/or osmolality should also be followed to detect onset of a spontaneous water diuresis (volume depletion, thiazide-associated) that can lead to overly rapid correction. Desmopressin may be useful in this setting to limit ongoing urinary water loss.

IV, Intravenous; [Na+], serum sodium concentration; ODS, osmotic demyelination syndrome; SIADH, syndrome of inappropriate antidiuretic hormone secretion.

19. **How should correction be monitored?**

    The serum sodium should be monitored every 2 to 4 hours during hypertonic saline infusion. Urine volume should also be closely watched during this period. Patients with hypovolemic or thiazide-induced hyponatremia may experience a spontaneous water diuresis once volume depletion has been corrected, sometimes after only a modest amount of normal saline given for volume repletion. The occurrence of such a water diuresis will put the patient at risk for ODS. In some patients, spontaneous correction is so rapid that the major therapeutic consideration is how to limit the rise in serum sodium concentration. Although initiation of hypertonic saline infusion in patients with severe symptoms should not be delayed until intensive care unit (ICU) transfer, monitoring urine output on an hourly basis and serum sodium concentration every 2 hours is most readily accomplished in the IOU.

20. **What should be done if correction is too rapid?**

    As the onset of symptoms of osmotic demyelination occurs days after over-rapid correction, preemptive administration of electrolyte-free water with or without desmopressin (synthetic vasopressin) to block further urinary electrolyte-free water loss is warranted to re-lower the serum sodium to the target increase level even in the absence of ODS symptoms.

21. **What are the clinical manifestations of hypernatremia?**

    In an otherwise healthy individual, hypernatremia manifests as thirst, which prompts increased electrolyte-free water intake and serum sodium concentration normalization. Thirst can dissipate, however, as hypernatremia worsens. Thirst aside, patients otherwise are typically asymptomatic until the serum sodium rises to near 160 mEq/L. In more severe cases, hypernatremia-induced brain shrinkage can lead to vascular tension and rupture with intracranial hemorrhage. Infants and children are at particular risk for this devastating complication. While lethargy, coma, and muscle weakness are associated with hypernatremia, such symptoms are often manifestations of other comorbidities as opposed to the hypernatremia itself. Note that while clinicians oftentimes refer to hypovolemic patients as being "dehydrated," when used rigorously, the term "dehydration" is reserved for hypernatremic patients, who demonstrate a true deficit of electrolyte-free water relative to sodium.

22. **What causes hypernatremia?**

    Rapid administration of hypertonic fluid—as often occurs with administration of ampules of sodium bicarbonate during cardiopulmonary resuscitation—and baby formula mixing errors can result in hypernatremia from pure solute gain. The overwhelming majority of cases, however, arise because thirst perception or access to water is impaired. Outside of the hospital, hypernatremia occurs most commonly among the institutionalized elderly and infants, who at baseline depend on others for access to water. Increased insensible water losses in the setting of febrile illness can incite hypernatremia among the elderly. In other instances, urine-concentrating defects resulting from loop diuretics or diabetes insipidus (DI) (see below) contribute to hypernatremia. Among hospitalized patients, iatrogenic hypernatremia is common and found among all age groups, particularly intubated patients and patients with increased enteral fluid losses from either diarrhea or nasogastric drainage whose fluid prescription contains an insufficient amount of hypotonic fluid. Loop diuretics, by reducing the tonicity of the medulla, diminish ADH-mediated water reabsorption and predispose to hypernatremia.

23. **What is DI?**

    DI is a disorder characterized by a deficiency in vasopressin-mediated electrolyte-free water reabsorption. DI can denote a defect either in pituitary vasopressin secretion (neurogenic or central DI) or vasopressin action (nephrogenic DI). It manifests as polyuria—defined as more than 3 L of daily urine output. The urine is dilute due to excessive urinary electrolyte-free water loss. In most patients, an intact thirst perception and ready access to electrolyte-free water prevent a rise in the serum sodium concentration. However, hypernatremia will ensue if free water access is limited. Note that polyuria with polydipsia are also characteristic of primary polydipsia, but the polyuria is secondary, not primary; serum sodium concentration is normal or low, and water restriction does not lead to hypernatremia.

    Neurogenic DI can result from a number of etiologies including trauma, granulomatous disease, tumors, infection, or aneurysm affecting the hypothalamus or pituitary. Nephrogenic DI can be either congenital or acquired, the latter being associated with intrinsic kidney disease, hypercalcemia, hypokalemia, and drugs including lithium and demeclocycline. Unlike nephrogenic DI, patients with the neurogenic form will exhibit a robust response to administration of a vasopressin agonist by producing concentrated urine.

24. **How is hypernatremia managed?**
Treatment of hypernatremia first requires addressing the underlying cause. This includes discontinuation of culprit medications (e.g., laxatives, lithium, demeclocycline, and loop diuretics), correction of hypokalemia and hypercalcemia, and treatment of fever. In addition, the patient should be repleted with electrolyte-free water either enterally or intravenously with hypotonic fluids. While central DI can be managed with desmopressin (a vasopressin analogue), management of nephrogenic DI is more difficult and begins with removal of offending agents. By inducing volume contraction, thiazide diuretics can be helpful in stimulating more proximal reabsorption of sodium and water and, in turn, decreased water delivery to the pathologically ADH-insensitive collecting duct.

25. **Are there complications of treatment?**
To prevent hypernatremia-induced brain shrinkage, neurons accumulate electrolytes in a matter of hours followed by organic osmolytes over several days to increase intracellular tonicity. Due to this adaptation, rapid correction of chronic hypernatremia can, in theory, result in cerebral edema. This phenomenon has been characterized in children but is not usually observed in adults.

26. **How rapidly should electrolyte-free water be administered for hypernatremia?**
Most cases of hypernatremia develop slowly over several days. Recommendations for treatment of chronic hypernatremia are not as well established as for chronic hyponatremia. Some authorities recommend that for hypernatremia developing over an interval longer than 48 hours, the rate of serum sodium concentration reduction should be limited to 10 mEq/L per day to minimize the theoretical risk for cerebral edema. A common strategy entails replenishing half of a patient's electrolyte-free water deficit in the first 24 hours and the remaining half in the following 24 to 48 hours. If hypernatremia developed in less than 48 hours, it can be corrected faster. A patient's free water deficit can be estimated with the following equation:

$$\text{Electrolyte-free water deficit} = \text{Total body water} \times [1 - (\text{Desired serum Na} \div \text{Current serum Na})]$$

Total body water can be estimated by multiplying the patient's weight in kilograms by 0.5 in the case of women or 0.6 in men. These fractions are further reduced in the obese and elderly. Using this equation, the electrolyte-free water deficit in an intubated 60 kg woman with a serum sodium of 167 mEq/L is approximately 4.8 L of water ($60 \times 0.5 \times [1 - 140/167] = 4.8$ L). Half of this deficit can be replaced in the first 24 hours by administering 300 mL of water via orogastric tube every 3 hours, followed by 150 mL of water every 3 hours in the subsequent 48 hours. Of note, if her electrolyte-free water deficit is corrected with intravenous 0.45% saline, she would require double this volume, as this fluid is only half electrolyte-free water by volume. This formula is only an approximation, so careful monitoring of the serum sodium concentration during the correction period is required. Finally, the formula does not take into account electrolyte-free water losses that are still ongoing. The fluid prescription should be augmented to match any such losses. Returning to our example above, if we assume our patient produces 1600 mL of urine daily, half of which is electrolyte-free water, 400 mL of water via orogastric tube every 3 hours in the first 24 hours (3200 mL) would match the ongoing urinary loss of electrolyte-free water (800 mL) and replenish half (2400 mL) of her free water deficit. In the ensuing 48 hours, 250 mL of water every 3 hours should be given to correct for ongoing urinary water excretion and address the remainder of her free water deficit. If the patient has 3 L/day urine output, an additional 700 mL of water administration would be required each day if the assumption that electrolyte-free water output is half of urine output remains valid. Particularly at high urine output rates and in patients with DI, the urine sodium and potassium should be measured to allow a more precise estimate of urinary electrolyte-free water loss. Since diarrheal fluid is hypotonic, additional electrolyte-free water will also be needed in patients with copious ongoing diarrhea, as with *Clostridium difficile* colitis.

KEY POINTS

1. When hypernatremia is present, a hypertonic state must be present as well; hyponatremia can occur in various states of tonicity.
2. Hypotonic hyponatremia arises from inadequate solute intake, excess intake of electrolyte-free water, or reduced excretion of electrolyte-free water. Urine osmolality can distinguish the latter mechanism from the first two.

3. The classic presentation for syndrome of inappropriate anti-diuretic hormone secretion is euvolemic, hypotonic hyponatremia with $U_{Osm} > 100$ mOsm/kg H_2O and urine sodium concentration >30 mmol/L in the absence of adrenal or glucocorticoid insufficiency, heart failure, liver failure, hypothyroidism, advanced kidney disease, or diuretics.
4. Hypotonic hyponatremia that developed acutely can be rapidly corrected without risk. Since over-rapid correction of chronic hyponatremia may result in the osmotic demyelination syndrome, correction should be targeted to defined limits. If it occurs, over-rapid correction may require reversal by administration of hypotonic fluids with or without a vasopressin agonist.
5. The vast majority of cases of hypernatremia occur when thirst perception or access to water are impaired. If the urine is not maximally or near maximally concentrated, the presence of an osmotic diuresis or central or nephrogenic diabetes insipidus should be suspected

BIBLIOGRAPHY

Adrogue, H. J., & Madias, N. E. (2000). Hypernatremia. *New England Journal of Medicine, 342*, 1493–1499.
Adrogue, H. J., & Madias, N. E. (2000). Hyponatremia. *New England Journal of Medicine, 342*, 1581–1589.
Berl, T. (2015). Vasopressin antagonists. *New England Journal of Medicine, 372*, 2207–2216.
Berl, T., Quittnat-Pelletier, F., Verbalis, J. G., Schrier, R. W., Bichet, D., Ouyang, J., . . . for the SALTWATER Investigators. (2010). Oral tolvaptan is safe and effective in chronic hyponatremia. *Journal of the American Society of Nephrology, 21*(4), 705–712.
Ellison, D. H., & Berl, T. (2007). Clinical practice. The syndrome of inappropriate antidiuresis. *New England Journal of Medicine, 356*, 2064–2072.
Hillier, T. A., Abbott, R. D., & Barrett, E. J. (1999). Hyponatremia: Evaluating the correction factor for hyperglycemia. *American Journal of Medicine, 106*, 399–403.
Lehrich, R. W., Ortiz-Melo, D. I., Patel, M. B., & Greenberg, A. (2013). Role of vaptans in the management of hyponatremia. *American Journal of Kidney Diseases, 62*, 364–376.
Palevsky, P. M., Bhagrath, R., & Greenberg, A. (1996). Hypernatremia in hospitalized patients. *Annals of Internal Medicine, 124*, 197–203.
Perianayagam, A., Sterns, R. H., Silver, S. M., Grieff, M., Mayo, R., Hix, J., & Kouides, R. (2008). DDAVP is effective in preventing and reversing inadvertent overcorrection of hyponatremia. *Clinical Journal of the American Society of Nephrology, 3*, 331–336.
Renneboog, B., Musch, W., Vandemergel, X., Manto, M. U., & Decaux, G. (2006). Mild chronic hyponatremia is associated with falls, unsteadiness, and attention deficits. *American Journal of Medicine, 119*, 71–78.
Schrier, R. W., Gross, P., Gheorghiade, M., Berl, T., Verbalis, J. G., Czerwiec, F. S., & Orlandi C. (2006). Tolvaptan, a selective oral vasopressin V2-receptor antagonist, for hyponatremia. *New England Journal of Medicine, 355*, 2099–2112.
Sterns, R. H. (2015). Disorders of plasma sodium—causes, consequences, and correction. *New England Journal of Medicine, 372*, 55–65.
Verbalis, J. G., Goldsmith, S. R., Greenberg, A., Korzelius, C., Schrier, R. W., Sterns, R. H., & Thompson, C. J. (2013). Diagnosis, evaluation, and treatment of hyponatremia: Expert panel recommendations. *American Journal of Medicine, 126*, S1–S42.
Wald, R., Jaber, B. L., Price, L. L., Upadhyay, A., & Madias, N. E. (2010). Impact of hospital-associated hyponatremia on selected outcomes. *Archives of Internal Medicine, 170*, 294–302.

CHAPTER 74

HYPOKALEMIA AND HYPERKALEMIA

Vikram Patney and Adam Whaley-Connell

1. **Describe normal potassium balance.**
   Approximately 98% of total body potassium resides inside cells, making it the most abundant cation in the intracellular fluid (ICF). The total body stores approximately 3000 mEq or more (approximately 50 to 70 mEq/kg body weight) of K^+, with the skeletal muscle cells providing the biggest storage site for intracellular K^+. ICF concentration of potassium is approximately 140 mEq/L compared to only 4 to 5 mEq/L in the extracellular fluid (ECF).

2. **Why is potassium balance important?**
   Since most of the total body potassium is intracellular, a large gradient exists between the ICF and ECF. This potassium gradient across the cell membrane is partially responsible for maintaining the potential difference across the cell membrane. This potential difference is critical for the function of cells, particularly excitable tissues like nerves and muscles.

3. **What is the primary cellular mechanism that maintains potassium balance?**
   Most cells contain Na^+-K^+-ATPase pump on the cellular membrane which pumps 2 molecules of K^+ in and 3 molecules of Na^+ out of the cell. This pump is regulated by catecholamines, insulin, and the potassium level itself. The ability to rapidly shift potassium from the extracellular to the intracellular compartment is vital to prevent severe increases in the serum potassium from routine dietary ingestion.

4. **What are the mechanisms for maintaining the internal potassium balance?**
   A typical Western diet ingests approximately 70 to 80 mEq of K^+ per day. Almost all the ingested potassium is absorbed by the intestine. Adjustments in the kidney potassium excretion to match potassium intake is the principal mechanism for maintaining potassium balance. Because the changes in the kidney excretion of potassium occur over several hours, the initial buffering of an increase in ECF potassium occurs by movement of potassium into skeletal muscle. With intact kidney function, only about 10% of dietary potassium is excreted in the feces.

5. **Why don't serum potassium levels go up when we eat a dietary potassium load (such as hamburger or soda)?**
   The ingestion of food causes release of insulin, which binds to its receptor on the cell membrane leading to the insertion of GLUT4 into the cell membrane (a glucose transporter). Similarly, insulin causes the membrane insertion and stimulation of Na^+-K^+-ATPase pump, leading to movement of potassium into the cell, preventing a rise in the serum potassium.

6. **What are the "feedback control" and "feed-forward" effects in potassium balance?**
   Elevation of plasma potassium causes the activation of mechanisms (insulin and aldosterone effects) that lower plasma potassium. This is an example of a negative feedback system where potassium excretion increases in response to increases in the plasma potassium level.
   On the other hand, a feed-forward system responds to potassium intake in a manner that is independent of changes in the systemic plasma potassium level. In sheep, intake of potassium-rich foods triggers a significant increase in urinary potassium excretion without an increase in the serum potassium. The signal between the gastrointestinal (GI) tract and the kidney potassium handling that is responsible for this feed-forward control is unknown.

7. **How do catecholamines affect internal potassium balance?**
   β2 adrenergic stimulation by catecholamines leads to increased Na^+-K^+-ATPase pump activity through a cyclic adenosine monophosphate (AMP) and protein kinase A dependent pathway primarily in the skeletal muscle leading to increased cellular uptake. This physiological effect is the basis for using β2 agonists like albuterol in the treatment of hyperkalemia.

8. **What role do skeletal muscle cells play in internal balance of potassium during exercise?**
   In addition to taking part in cellular uptake of potassium under the influence of insulin, skeletal muscle cells also participate in the changes of ECF potassium that occur with exercise. Exercise increases ECF potassium, which limits muscle excitability and contractility leading to fatigue. Increased ECF potassium also causes vasodilation, increasing blood flow to exercising muscle. Exercise causes β2 adrenergic mediated stimulation of Na^+-K^+-ATPase pump that shifts potassium back into the cells.

9. **What factors can cause hypokalemia by shifting potassium into cells?**
   Hypokalemia due to intracellular shift of K^+ primarily occurs due to insulin, β2 adrenergic stimulation, α-adrenergic antagonists, and metabolic alkalosis.

10. **What factors can cause hyperkalemia by shifting potassium out of cells?**
    Hyperkalemia due to shift of potassium from the cells can occur in metabolic acidosis, exercise, insulin deficiency, β-adrenergic blockade, and α-adrenergic stimulation, as well as conditions like hyperglycemia that increase serum osmolality. Hyperglycemia, which pulls water from the cells, can lead to a solvent drag that also shifts potassium from cells.

11. **Describe kidney potassium handling?**
    Two-thirds of the potassium that is filtered by the glomerulus is passively reabsorbed with sodium and water in the proximal tubule. After further reabsorption in the ascending limb of loop of Henle via the Na^+-K^+-$2Cl^-$ cotransporter, only about 10% of the filtered load reaches the distal nephron. The ability to secrete potassium begins in the early distal convoluted tubule and progressively increases along the distal nephron into the cortical collecting duct. The rate of potassium secretion by the distal nephron depends on the physiological need. The principal cells in the initial collecting duct and the cortical collecting duct are responsible for potassium secretion through the renal outer medullary potassium (ROMK) and large conductance potassium (BK) channels. In states of potassium depletion, reabsorption of potassium occurs in the collecting duct via the apical H^+-K^+ ATPase on α-intercalated cells.

12. **What factors determine kidney potassium excretion?**
    The two principal factors that determine the potassium secretion in the distal nephron are mineralocorticoid activity (aldosterone) and distal delivery of sodium and water (urine flow).

13. **How does distal delivery of sodium and volume increase potassium excretion?**
    Increased distal delivery of sodium allows reabsorption via the epithelial sodium channel (ENaC) in the late distal convoluted tubule, the connecting tubule, and the cortical collecting duct. Reabsorption of sodium generates a negative charge in the lumen, which enhances potassium secretion through the ROMK channels. With higher urine flow, the secreted potassium is diluted and washed away, maintaining a diffusion gradient leading to continued potassium secretion. While ROMK channels are activated under physiological conditions, the BK channels are activated by increased urine flow.

14. **How does aldosterone effect kidney potassium excretion?**
    Aldosterone stimulates sodium reabsorption in the distal nephron through activation of the ENaC and also increases the intracellular potassium concentration by stimulating the Na^+-K^+-ATPase in the basolateral membrane of these cells. Sodium reabsorption via ENaC increases electronegativity in the lumen, leading to an electrical gradient favoring potassium secretion.

15. **What conditions stimulate release of aldosterone in a normal person?**
    Aldosterone is produced by the Zona Glomerulosa of the adrenal gland in response to hyperkalemia and angiotensin II released due to the activation of the renin-angiotensin-aldosterone system in response to hypotension or hypovolemia.

16. **What is the aldosterone paradox?**
    The ability of aldosterone to cause kidney retention of sodium without potassium secretion in states of volume depletion and stimulate kidney potassium secretion without sodium retention in hyperkalemia is called the aldosterone paradox.
    During hypovolemia, angiotensin II and aldosterone have a synergistic effect on the sodium chloride cotransporter (NCC) and the ENaCs in the distal nephron, resulting in maximal sodium reabsorption. The resulting decreased distal delivery of sodium, as well as urine flow, reduces the secretion of potassium. In addition, angiotensin II has an inhibitory effect on ROMK, thereby reducing potassium secretion.

Hyperkalemia causes a renin and angiotensin II–independent increase in aldosterone secretion. In the absence of increased angiotensin II levels, NCC inhibition leads to increased sodium delivery to the ENaC. This leads to electrochemical absorption of sodium through ENaC coupled with secretion of potassium through the uninhibited ROMK channels.

17. **How does chronic kidney disease affect kidney and colonic potassium excretion?**
The loss of nephron mass in patients with progressive chronic kidney disease (CKD) is counterbalanced by an adaptive increase in potassium secretion by the functioning nephrons. This adaptation results in preserved potassium homeostasis until the glomerular filtration rate falls below 15 to 20 mL/min when hyperkalemia may ensue due to the inability to excrete daily dietary potassium load. In addition to kidney clearance, colonic potassium secretion is upregulated in advanced CKD as BK channels in the colonic mucosa increase several fold under the influence of aldosterone.

18. **What are some common causes of hypokalemia?**
Hypokalemia can occur from one of four mechanisms:
1. Pseudo-hypokalemia: Artifactual decrease in potassium level after phlebotomy, most commonly due acute leukemia where white blood cells take up the potassium from blood sample.
2. Redistribution: Shifts from ECF to ICF due to insulin, aldosterone and β2 adrenergic agonists, hypokalemic period paralysis.
3. Increased GI losses: chronic diarrhea, vomiting, nasogastric suction, laxative abuse.
4. Kidney potassium loss: Drugs (diuretics and others), primary and secondary hyperaldosteronism, hypomagnesemia, Bartter, Gitelman, and Liddle syndrome, bicarbonaturia from metabolic alkalosis, and renal tubular acidosis. Reduced effective arterial blood volume due to GI fluid losses or diuretics stimulates aldosterone secretion increasing potassium secretion.

19. **How do loop or thiazide diuretics cause kidney potassium loss?**
Diuretics increase distal delivery of sodium and water:
- Loop diuretics inhibit Na^+-K^+-$2Cl^-$ cotransporters in the thick ascending limb of loop of Henle
- Thiazide and thiazide-like diuretics inhibit Na^+-Cl^- cotransporter in the distal convoluted tubule
This leads to increased potassium secretion in the principal cells of the distal nephron. In addition, the volume depletion caused by diuretics stimulates increased aldosterone production resulting in increased potassium secretion.

20. **What urine studies can help in the evaluation of hypokalemia?**
A spot urine potassium-to-creatinine ratio of more than 13 mEq/g of creatinine in the presence of hypokalemia suggests kidney potassium wasting. Similarly, a 24-hour urine potassium excretion of more than 25 to 30 mEq/day in the setting of hypokalemia may suggest kidney potassium wasting.

21. **What are some of the signs and symptoms of hypokalemia?**
Hypokalemia may be asymptomatic until the potassium level is below 3.0 mEq/L. Patients may present with muscle weakness, cramps, rhabdomyolysis, and myoglobinuria. Neuromuscular weakness can also manifest as gastric dilatation, adynamic ileus, and respiratory muscle weakness leading to respiratory failure. Hypokalemia may present as cardiac arrhythmias including premature atrial and ventricular beats, sinus bradycardia, atrial and junctional tachycardia, atrioventricular block, ventricular tachycardia, and fibrillation. Hypokalemia can increase blood pressure by 5 to 10 mm Hg. Chronic hypokalemia can result in kidney tubulointerstitial fibrosis, kidney cyst formation, metabolic alkalosis, CKD, and impaired kidney concentrating ability causing polyuria.

22. **What are the cardiac effects and electrocardiogram (EKG) changes that may occur due to hypokalemia?**
Cardiac arrhythmias due to hypokalemia include premature atrial and ventricular beats, sinus bradycardia, paroxysmal atrial or junctional tachycardia, arteriovenous (AV) block, and ventricular tachycardia, or fibrillation. Hypokalemia-induced EKG changes include: prolonged QT interval, depression of the ST segment, decreased amplitude of the T wave, and increased amplitude of U waves that occur at the end of the T wave. EKG changes may not correlate well with the degree of hypokalemia, so consideration of continuous telemetry monitoring is warranted in patients with prolonged QT interval, arrhythmias due to hypokalemia, presence of conditions that predispose to arrhythmias (acute myocardial infarction, digitalis toxicity), intravenous (IV) replacement at a rate greater than 10 mEq/h, and patients at risk for rebound hyperkalemia (patients with thyrotoxic periodic paralysis).

23. When should hypokalemia be corrected by oral supplementation?

   Even though widely variable, in the absence of transcellular potassium shifts, the average serum potassium decreases by 0.3 mEq/L for each 100 mEq reduction in total body potassium stores. Oral or enteral administration is preferred when GI function is intact; the patient has mild ($K^+ > 3$ mEq/L) to moderate (K^+ 2.5 to 3 mEq/L) asymptomatic hypokalemia with normal kidney function. Oral KCl can be given at 10 to 20 mEq PO thrice daily for mild and 40 to 60 mEq PO thrice daily for moderate hypokalemia. If ongoing losses are present, these doses can be scheduled. The serum K^+ should be checked frequently and supplementation stopped or adjusted.

24. When should IV potassium supplementation be used to treat hypokalemia?

   This may be necessary emergently in hypokalemic periodic paralysis, severe hypokalemia prior to urgent surgery, acute myocardial infarction (MI), and significant ventricular ectopy, or other situations where the gut cannot be used. KCl should not be diluted in dextrose containing IV fluids, because insulin release can stimulate potassium to shift intracellularly. IV potassium supplementation should be accompanied by continuous EKG monitoring. The recommended maximum rate of IV potassium replacement in most patients should not be more than 10 to 20 mEq of KCl per hour to prevent acute hyperkalemia and sudden death. Initial rapid rate of replacement of 20 to 40 mEq/h can be given cautiously through a central venous catheter with continuous EKG monitoring in patients with life-threatening hypokalemia.

25. What are the common causes of hyperkalemia?

   Pseudohyperkalemia may be due to hemolysis-related potassium release after phlebotomy, ischemia from increased tourniquet time, increased red cell fragility due to rheumatoid arthritis, infectious mononucleosis, red cell membrane disorders, chronic lymphocytic leukemia, and thrombocytosis. Redistribution of potassium from ICF to ECF may occur with hyperosmolarity seen with severe hyperglycemia, severe nonorganic acidosis, and also with medications like β-blockers and digoxin that prevent cellular potassium uptake. Increased potassium intake as food, supplementation, or salt substitutes in the setting of impaired kidney function. Decreased kidney potassium excretion due to acute kidney injury, CKD, medications, or rare genetic disorders like Gordon syndrome.

26. What are the mechanisms by which commonly used medications cause hyperkalemia?

   See Table 74.1.

27. How can you differentiate true from pseudohyperkalemia?

   Pseudohyperkalemia is suspected when the laboratory value of the measured potassium is high but the patient does not manifest signs of hyperkalemia such as an abnormal EKG. Some authors have defined pseudohyperkalemia as a difference between serum and plasma potassium concentrations of more than 0.4 mmol/L when samples remain at room temperature and are tested within one hour of collection.

   Pseudohyperkalemia due to mechanical cell lysis can be identified by keeping the tourniquet time less than 1 minute and avoiding fist clenching to obtain an atraumatic sample. Serum is the supernatant obtained by centrifuging a blood sample that has been allowed to clot after collection in a red top tube (no anticoagulant). Plasma is the supernatant obtained after removing cells by centrifuging a sample of blood collected in tube with an anticoagulant (lavender top or light blue top). The process of clotting causes cell lysis and thus release of intracellular potassium. In pseudohyperkalemia, the plasma potassium will be normal in the face of an elevated serum potassium.

28. Does inhibiting the renin-angiotensin aldosterone system (RAAS) with angiotensin-converting enzyme inhibitors, angiotensin receptor blockers, and mineralocorticoid receptor antagonists (MRA) cause hyperkalemia in patients on dialysis?

   End-stage kidney disease (ESKD) patients on dialysis may be oliguric or anuric and hence do not depend on kidney excretion of potassium. These patients depend on dialysis and restriction of oral intake of potassium to maintain acceptable levels. Recent evidence from small-sized studies has shown that administration of low-dose MRA provides cardioprotective effects in both hemodialysis and peritoneal dialysis patients without significantly increasing the risk of hyperkalemia. MRA may improve mortality in ESKD dialysis patients, but larger studies are needed to establish safe protocols for their use in dialysis patients.

29. How does hyperkalemia present?

   Hyperkalemia may be asymptomatic or present with mild symptoms like muscular weakness. Severe hyperkalemia can produce life-threatening conditions like respiratory failure due to paralysis of the

Table 74.1. Mechanisms by Which Commonly Used Medications Cause Hyperkalemia

CLASS	MECHANISM
Potassium containing drugs like KCl, penicillin G, potassium citrate	Increased intake of potassium usually in the setting of decreased GFR
β-blockers	Inhibit renin release and cellular uptake of potassium
ACE inhibitors like lisinopril, captopril, enalapril, ramipril	Inhibit conversion of angiotensin I to angiotensin II, leading to ↓ aldosterone effect
Angiotensin receptor blockers like losartan, valsartan	Inhibit activation of angiotensin II receptors by angiotensin II and thus ↓ aldosterone synthesis and secretion
Direct renin inhibitors	↓ renin activity leading to ↓ angiotensin II production
Heparin	Inhibits enzyme aldosterone synthase in adrenals
Mineralocorticoid receptor antagonists like spironolactone	Block aldosterone receptor activation
Potassium-sparing diuretics like amiloride, triamterene (trimethoprim and pentamidine have similar structure)	Block apical ENaC in collecting duct, thus ↓ the electrical gradient needed for potassium secretion
NSAIDs and COX-2 inhibitors	Inhibit prostaglandin stimulation of collecting duct secretion; inhibit renin release
Digoxin	Inhibit Na^+-K^+-ATPase pump on collecting duct necessary for providing potassium for secretion
Calcineurin inhibitors (tacrolimus, cyclosporine)	Activates WNK3 and WNK4 which upregulate sodium chloride cotransporter (thiazide sensitive transporter). This decreases sodium delivery to the ENaC needed for potassium secretion

ACE, Angiotensin converting enzyme; *COX-2,* cyclooxygenase-2; *ENaC,* epithelial sodium channel; *GFR,* glomerular filtration rate; *NSAIDs,* nonsteroidal anti-inflammatory drugs.
Modified from Weiner, D. I., Linas, S. L., & Wingo C. S. (2015). Disorders of potassium metabolism. In *Comprehensive clinical nephrology.* Philadelphia: Elsevier Saunders.

diaphragm, or ventricular fibrillation. The serum potassium concentration may not correlate with the progression of EKG changes.

30. What EKG changes are seen in patients with hyperkalemia?
    - Early, peaked T waves, initially in precordial and then in all leads
    - Followed by increased PR interval and QRS complex widening
    - This is followed by progressive flattening and then disappearance of P waves.
    - Merging of the widened QRS and peaked T waves leads to a sine-wave pattern.
    - This may be followed by ventricular fibrillation.

31. Are hemodialysis patients more tolerant of mild hyperkalemia as compared to the general population?
    The lower susceptibility of ESKD patients to the cardiac toxicity of hyperkalemia may be attributable to its chronic nature. ESKD or advanced CKD patients may not demonstrate symptoms or EKG changes with serum potassium levels more than 6 mEq/L. In these patients, it is thought that membrane potentials of excitable cardiac tissues can adapt to the chronic elevation of potassium. In contrast, acute hyperkalemia can cause a rapid reduction in resting membrane potential, depolarization, muscle excitability, and EKG changes.

32. What is transtubular potassium gradient (TTKG) and how can it be used in diagnosis of hyperkalemia?
    TTKG is a measurement of the potassium gradient between urine in the distal nephron (cortical collecting tubule) and the peritubular capillaries after correcting for changes in urine osmolality.
    TTKG = Urine K^+ / Serum K^+ × Serum Osmolality/Urine Osmolality

It was originally proposed that a TTKG >10 suggests normal aldosterone secretion and action and a TTKG <5 to 7 was thought to suggest aldosterone deficiency or resistance. Use of TTKG in the evaluation of patients with hyperkalemia is no longer recommended.

33. **Why has the utility of TTKG as an assessment of aldosterone secretion and action been questioned?**
TTKG was thought to represent the activity of aldosterone on the basis of an assumption that there is no appreciable reabsorption of osmoles downstream from the cortical collecting duct. This assumption has been found to be invalid after the discovery of the fact that urea is actively absorbed in the medullary collecting duct, a process that is regulated by vasopressin and aids in the secretion of potassium. Thus, TTKG represents potassium excretion due to both aldosterone and vasopressin action, and its utility in the diagnosis of hyperkalemia has been questioned.

34. **What is the acute treatment for life-threatening hyperkalemia?**
Calcium gluconate or calcium chloride, 10% solution, 10 mL IV over 10 minutes can help antagonize the membrane effects of hyperkalemia on the myocardial conducting system. This effect lasts for 30 to 60 minutes. Calcium chloride is preferred in patients with cardiac arrest due to hyperkalemia because it releases active calcium immediately upon infusion, unlike calcium gluconate, which requires hepatic metabolism to release calcium. Calcium gluconate can be administered IV via a peripheral vein but calcium chloride requires a central line because extravasation can cause tissue necrosis.

35. **What are other acute treatments that can be used for management of severe hyperkalemia?**
Shift potassium into the cells by using:
1. Regular insulin 10 units IV with 50% dextrose 50 mL. Dextrose is not needed if the plasma glucose is above 250 mg/dL. Always recheck the blood glucose after giving insulin.
2. Nebulized albuterol 10 mg can also be used with similar lowering of potassium. These effects last 2 to 6 hours and must be followed by strategies to definitively remove potassium from the body.

36. **How can one definitively remove potassium from the body in an acute situation?**
- Diuretics can increase kidney excretion of potassium in patients that make urine.
- Dialysis can be used acutely in patients with acute kidney injury or ESKD with hyperkalemia.

37. **What are some treatment strategies in patients who have persistent hyperkalemia, especially in patients who may need to be on medications that cause elevation of potassium as a side effect (example: ACE inhibitors in diabetic kidney disease)?**
- Dietary reduction of potassium is beneficial in all patients but may not be enough.
- Review of all medications and supplements to consider stopping agents that can raise serum potassium.
- Increase excretion of potassium in the stool by using potassium binders.

38. **Describe the various K⁺-binding agents for the management of hyperkalemia.**
See Table 74.2.

Table 74.2. K⁺-Binding Agents for the Management of Hyperkalemia

	SODIUM POLYSTYRENE SULFONATE	PATIROMER	SODIUM ZIRCONIUM CYCLOSILICATE (ZS-9)
Status	In use for past 60 years	Introduced in 2016	Approval pending
Characteristic	Resin	Resin/polymer	Crystal
Mechanism of action and specificity	Exchanges sodium for calcium, magnesium, K⁺, and ammonium in the colon/rectum	Exchanges calcium for K⁺, magnesium, and ammonium in the distal colon	Exchanges sodium and hydrogen ions for K⁺ throughout the GI tract; selective for K⁺ and ammonium
Dose and routes of administration	Oral: 15 g orally q6h Rectal: 30–50 g q6h	Oral: 8.4–25.2 g/day	Oral: pending FDA approval; 5–10 g/day

Table 74.2. K$^+$-Binding Agents for the Management of Hyperkalemia—cont'd

	SODIUM POLYSTYRENE SULFONATE	PATIROMER	SODIUM ZIRCONIUM CYCLOSILICATE (ZS-9)
Onset of action	1–2 h	7 h	1 h
Adverse events	Nausea, vomiting, constipation, diarrhea, gastric irritation, colonic necrosis; sodium retention, hypokalemia, hypomagnesemia, hypocalcemia, metabolic alkalosis	Constipation, diarrhea, nausea, vomiting, flatulence; hypokalemia, hypomagnesemia, and possible calcium load.	Constipation, diarrhea, nausea, vomiting; hypokalemia, sodium retention, edema

FDA, U.S. Food and Drug Administration.
Modified from Chaitman, M., Dixit, D., & Bridgeman, M. B. (2016). Potassium-binding agents for the clinical management of hyperkalemia. *P & T, 41*, 43–50.

KEY POINTS

1. Ninety-eight percent of potassium is intracellular, making it the most abundant intracellular cation.
2. The large potassium gradient between the intracellular and extracellular compartments is partially responsible for maintaining the potential difference across the cell membrane, which is critical for the function of cells, particularly excitable tissues like nerves and muscles.
3. Adjustments in the kidney excretion of potassium is the principal mechanism for maintaining potassium balance by matching potassium intake with excretion.
4. The principal factors that determine the potassium secretion in the distal nephron are mineralocorticoid activity (aldosterone) and distal delivery of sodium and water (urine flow).
5. Potassium-binding agents may be useful in situations where the use of RAAS inhibitors or MRA is limited due to the occurrence of hyperkalemia.

BIBLIOGRAPHY

Bomback, A. S. (2016). Mineralocorticoid receptor antagonists in end-stage renal disease: Efficacy and safety. *Blood Purification, 41*, 166–170.
Bomback, A. S., & Klemmer, P. J. (2007). The incidence and implications of aldosterone breakthrough. *Nature Clinical Practice Nephrology, 3*, 486–492.
Chaitman, M., Dixit, D., & Bridgeman, M. B. (2016). Potassium-binding agents for the clinical management of hyperkalemia. *P & T, 41*, 43–50.
Einhorn, L. M., Zhan, M., Hsu, V. D., Walker, L. D., Moen, M. F., Seliger, S. L., . . . Fink, J. C. (2009). The frequency of hyperkalemia and its significance in chronic kidney disease. *Archives of Internal Medicine, 169*, 1156–1162.
Epstein, M., & Lifschitz, M. D. (2016). Potassium homeostasis and dyskalemias: The respective roles or renal, extrarenal, and gut sensors in potassium handling. *Kidney International Supplements, 6*(1), 7–15.
Gennari, F. G. (1998). Hypokalemia. *New England Journal of Medicine, 339*, 451–458.
Gumz, M. L., Rabinowitz, L., & Winso, C. S. (2015). An integrated view of potassium homeostasis. *New England Journal of Medicine, 373*, 60–72.
Kamel, K. S., & Halperin, M. L. (2011). Intrarenal urea recycling leads to a higher rate of renal excretion of potassium: An hypothesis with clinical implications. *Current Opinion in Nephrology and Hypertension, 20*, 547–554.
Mount, D. B. (2017). *Clinical manifestations and treatment of hypokalemia in adults.* Uptodate. Retrieved from https://www.upto date.com/contents/clinical-manifestations-and-treatment-of-hypokalemia-in-adults?source=history_widget#H169061725.
Mount, D. B., Sterns, R. H., Emmett, M., & Forman, J. P. (2016). *Clinical manifestations and treatment of hypokalemia in adults.* Retrieved June 20, 2016, from http://www.uptodate.com.
Mount, D. B., Sterns, R. H., & Forman, J. P. (2014). *Causes and evaluation of hyperkalemia in adults.* Retrieved June 20, 2016, from http://www.uptodate.com.
Palmer, B. F. (2015). Regulation of potassium homeostasis. *Clinical Journal of American Society of Nephrology, 10*, 1050–1060. doi:10.2215/CJN.08580813.
Sterns, R. H., Grieff, M., & Bernstein, P. L. (2016). Treatment of hyperkalemia: Something old, something new. *Kidney International, 89*, 546–554.
Tawada, M., Suzuki, Y., Sakata, F., Mizuno, M., & Ito, Y. (2016). Mineralocorticoid receptor antagonists in dialysis patients. *Renal Replacement Therapy*, 2–9.
Weiner, D. I., Linas, S. L., & Wingo C. S. (2015). Disorders of potassium metabolism. In *Comprehensive clinical nephrology.* Philadelphia: Elsevier Saunders.
Weir, M. R. (2016). Current and future treatment options for managing hyperkalemia. *Kidney International Supplements, 6*, 29–34.

CHAPTER 75

HYPOCALCEMIA AND HYPERCALCEMIA

Lavinia Aura Negrea

1. **What is calcium homeostasis?**
   Calcium homeostasis refers to the regulation of the calcium concentration in the extracellular fluid. Normal serum calcium concentration varies between laboratories, but is usually 8.5 to 10.5 mg/dL (2.1 to 2.6 mmol/L) and it represents the sum of the three circulating fractions: 45% protein bound (albumin ~80%, globulins ~20%), 15% complexed to anions (citrate, bicarbonate, lactate, phosphate), and 40% free, or ionized. The ionized calcium is the physiologically active form, which is recognized by the calcium-sensing receptor (CaSR). The main hormonal regulators of ionized calcium are parathyroid hormone (PTH) and 1,25 dihydroxyvitamin D (1,25D).

2. **Which are the units of measurements for serum calcium and what is the conversion between them?**
   Serum calcium is expressed in conventional units, as mg/dL, in SI (Système International) units, as mmoles/L, and sometimes as mEq/L. Calcium has a molecular weight of 40 and its valence is 2. Therefore:

   Calcium (mg/dL) $\times$ 0.25 = Ca (mmol/L)
   Calcium (mg/dL) $\times$ 0.5 = Ca (mEq/L)
   Calcium (mEq/L) $\times$ 0.5 = Ca (mmol/L)

3. **Describe the normal calcium balance.**
   Calcium balance represents the net difference between calcium intake and output in the body in steady state. This balance is positive during skeletal growth in children, zero in adults, and negative in the elderly. In a healthy adult on an average Western diet of 1000 mg elemental calcium per day, the net intestinal calcium absorption is ~200 mg; bone mineral accretion (~500 mg) equals bone resorption (~500 mg). The kidneys, under hormonal control, will excrete ~200 mg calcium in the final urine, rendering a neutral calcium balance. Calcium homeostasis and balance become altered in advanced chronic kidney disease (CKD). A positive calcium balance has been demonstrated in patients with CKD stage 3 and 4 placed either on a 2000 mg calcium diet or on 1500 mg calcium carbonate supplements. Thus calcium supplementation in this population should be used with caution, to avoid calcium overload.

4. **What causes spurious hypocalcemia?**
   Total serum calcium is routinely measured with colorimetric assays. The commonly used arsenazo–III reagent complexes with certain gadolinium compounds (like gadodiamide and gadoversetamide), blocking the detection of calcium. The artifact can be as large as 6 mg/dL and persists until the gadolinium is excreted from the body. The ionized calcium is unchanged in this situation and can confirm the spurious hypocalcemia.

5. **What causes pseudohypocalcemia?**
   Unlike true hypocalcemia (low ionized calcium), pseudohypocalcemia is defined as a normal ionized calcium, with low total serum calcium. This usually occurs in conditions associated with low serum albumin (malnutrition, nephrotic syndrome, cirrhosis, etc.). In general, the concentration of calcium falls by 0.8 mg/dL for every 1 g/dL decrease in serum albumin concentration. One of the formulas to correct serum calcium for low albumin, derived from studies in cirrhotic patients with low albumin, is:

   Ca corrected = Ca measured + [(4.0 - serum albumin measured) $\times$ 0.8)]

   A study of CKD patients not yet on dialysis showed that total calcium and albumin-corrected calcium failed to identify true hypocalcemia or hypercalcemia in 20% of the patients. Directly measuring the ionized calcium is preferred in this population.

6. How does the acid-base status affect the ionized calcium?

   Serum pH is inversely related to the ionized calcium. An increase in pH causes an increased binding of calcium to albumin, resulting in a drop in ionized calcium, while the opposite occurs when the pH drops. Total calcium remains unchanged in these situations. In patients with CKD with metabolic acidosis, measurement of total calcium underestimates the ionized calcium.

7. What are some common causes of hypocalcemia?

   Here is a list of the various causes; each is discussed in more detail in further questions:
   - Hypoparathyroidism: genetic and acquired (post-surgical)
   - PTH resistance (pseudohypoparathyroidism)
   - Vitamin D deficiency or resistance
   - Kidney disease
   - Hypomagnesemia
   - Hyperphosphatemia
   - Hungry bone syndrome
   - Medications
   - Human immunodeficiency virus
   - Acute pancreatitis
   - Sepsis and critical illness

8. What are some causes of hypoparathyroidism?

   Idiopathic hypoparathyroidism may be the result of the absence of parathyroid glands, brachial dysembriogenesis (DiGeorge syndrome), or polyglandular autoimmune disorder. Acquired forms can result from surgery, neck irradiation, or infiltrative diseases like hemochromatosis, amyloidosis, and thalassemia. The most common cause is hypomagnesemia.

9. What is pseudohypoparathyroidism?

   In contrast to hypoparathyroidism, in which the synthesis or secretion of PTH is impaired or absent, in pseudohypoparathyroidism, target tissues are unresponsiveness to the actions of PTH. Chronic hypocalcemia in this disorder leads to hyperplastic parathyroid glands and increased levels of PTH.

10. Briefly discuss the vitamin D–related causes of hypocalcemia.
    - Vitamin D deficiency: associated with inadequate exposure to ultraviolet light, poor dietary intake, or malabsorption. Also, vitamin D deficiency may occur in patients with nephrotic syndrome as a result of losses of vitamin D–binding protein in the urine.
    - Abnormalities of vitamin D metabolism: either reduced hydroxylation of vitamin D to 25-hydroxyvitamin D (25D) in chronic liver diseases or reduced hydroxylation of 25D to 1,25D in kidney failure or vitamin D–dependent rickets type I (deficiency of 1α-hydroxylase).
    - Resistance to the actions of vitamin D: vitamin D–dependent rickets type II (molecular defects in the vitamin D receptor).

11. What factors contribute to hypocalcemia in CKD?
    - Hyperphosphatemia
    - Decreased levels of 1,25D
      - Decreased kidney mass as kidney disease progresses
      - Accumulation of bone-derived hormone fibroblast growth factor 23 (FGF-23). FGF-23 reduces the activity of the 1-hydroxylase enzyme in the kidney.
    - Skeletal resistance to the calcemic action of PTH.

12. How does abnormal serum magnesium cause hypocalcemia?
    - Magnesium levels below 1 mg/dL produce PTH resistance. With more severe hypomagnesemia, the secretion of PTH can also be impaired. Correction of the hypocalcemia requires first restoring magnesium.
    - Magnesium levels over 6 mg/dL can suppress PTH secretion causing hypocalcemia.

13. Explain how hypocalcemia can result from hyperphosphatemia.

    Hyperphosphatemia can induce hypocalcemia through an increase in calcium $\times$ phosphorus product with subsequent precipitation of calcium phosphate salts in soft tissues. This commonly occurs with excessive enteral or parenteral phosphate administration (during treatment of hypophosphatemia) or with massive release of intracellular phosphate in patients with tumor lysis syndrome, severe hemolysis, or rhabdomyolysis. It can also occur in acute kidney injury or advanced CKD due to decreased renal phosphorus excretion.

14. **What is "hungry bone syndrome"?**
Also known as recalcification tetany, this condition can occur immediately after parathyroidectomy for hyperparathyroidism (primary or secondary) and consists of rapid skeletal uptake of calcium and phosphate by the bones, causing hypocalcemia. It is usually more severe in parathyroidectomy following the secondary hyperparathyroidism of renal failure and may require high doses of calcium and calcitriol for weeks.

15. **What other diseases commonly encountered in clinical practice are associated with hypocalcemia and how?**
HIV disease. Hypocalcemia in HIV is about 6 times more common than in the general population and recognized multiple causes: antiretroviral therapy, vitamin D deficiency, hypomagnesemia, etc. PTH hyporesponsiveness to hypocalcemia has also been reported.
   Acute pancreatitis. Hypocalcemia is due to deposition of "calcium soaps" consisting of calcium and fatty acids. Calcitonin-mediated hypocalcemia was reported in some but not all studies.
   Sepsis. Hypocalcemia in patients with sepsis is usually accompanied by hypophosphatemia, high levels of PTH and calcitonin. The mechanism of hypocalcemia in these patients is likely heterogeneous and has not been rigorously studied.

16. **What are some of the medications that cause hypocalcemia and how?**
Many medications can cause hypocalcemia through a variety of mechanisms:
   • Calcium chelators: citrate, ethylenediaminetetraacetic acid (EDTA)
   • Complex formation: foscarnet
   • Inhibition of bone resorption: bisphosphonates, denosumab, etc.
   • Drug-induced hypoparathyroidism: cinacalcet
   • Altered vitamin D metabolism: phenytoin, 5 fluorouracil/leucovorin

17. **What laboratory tests are helpful in the evaluation of hypocalcemia?**
Ionized calcium will confirm true hypocalcemia. Serum PTH is the most helpful test in evaluating hypocalcemia and should assist in differentiating between conditions associated with low or elevated PTH levels. Further, serum magnesium, phosphorus, and creatinine, 25D, and 1,25D can be obtained, as suggested by the patient's clinical and medication history.

18. **What are the clinical manifestations of hypocalcemia?**
The manifestations of hypocalcemia depend as much on the rate of its occurrence as on the degree of the reduction in plasma calcium. Symptoms include neuromuscular manifestations such as tetany, muscle spasm, cramps, carpopedal spasm, irritability, and seizures. Cardiovascular manifestations include hypotension, and congestive heart failure.
   Electrocardiographic abnormalities: prolonged QT intervals, QRS complex and ST-segment changes that resemble acute myocardial infarction, conduction abnormalities.

19. **What is the treatment for acute symptomatic hypocalcemia?**
Acute symptomatic hypocalcemia requires therapy with intravenous calcium. This can be given as 10 to 20 mL of calcium gluconate (90 mg of Ca^{++} per 10-mL ampule) infused at no more than 2 mL/min. This should be repeated as needed to keep the patient free of symptoms. In hypocalcemia associated with hypomagnesemia, magnesium replacement also is required.

20. **What is pseudohypercalcemia?**
In pseudohypercalcemia the ionized calcium is normal, but the total serum calcium is elevated due to increased calcium binding to serum proteins. This can be seen in patients with hyperalbuminemia due to dehydration. Also, in certain multiple myeloma cases, the abnormal paraprotein can bind excessively to calcium, resulting in elevated total serum calcium.

21. **What are some common causes of hypercalcemia?**
Hyperparathyroidism and malignancy represent about 90% of all cases of hypercalcemia. Other etiologies include:
   • Granulomatous diseases
   • Immobilization
   • Medications: excessive vitamin D, vitamin A, lithium, Tamoxifen, etc.
   • Milk-alkali (or calcium alkali) syndrome
   • Endocrine: thyrotoxicosis, etc.

22. **Describe the mechanism of hypercalcemia and its consequences in primary hyperparathyroidism.**
PTH causes hypercalcemia by stimulating osteoclastic bone resorption and by increasing kidney calcium reabsorption in the distal nephron. PTH also stimulates 1,25D synthesis, which leads to

increased intestinal calcium absorption and increased calcium reabsorption in the distal nephron. Hypercalcemia will increase the filter load of calcium, exceeding the tubular reabsorption capability and causing hypercalciuria and increased kidney stones.

23. How do malignancies cause hypercalcemia?
    - Humoral hypercalcemia of malignancy refers to hypercalcemia from secretion of PTH-related peptide (PTH-rP) by tumors including squamous cell carcinomas of the lung, head, or neck and renal cell carcinoma. PTH-rP mimics the actions of PTH by binding to the same receptor ($\sim$80% of cases).
    - Local osteolytic hypercalcemia. Secretion of bone-resorbing cytokines (such as interleukin-1, interleukin-6, and macrophage inflammatory protein-α) has been reported with some solid tumors metastatic to the bone and multiple myeloma ($\sim$20% of cases).
    - Extra-renal 1,25D production. Certain lymphomas, ovarian dysgerminoma, will convert 25 OH vitamin D to the active 1,25 form (less than 1% of cases).
    - Authentic ectopic hyperparathyroidism. Rare occurrence with ovarian, lung, thyroid carcinomas, etc.

24. What conditions, other than malignancy, can present with elevated 1,25D levels?
    - Increased production of 1,25D by non-renal tissues has been reported with sarcoidosis, certain infections (tuberculosis, invasive histoplasmosis, etc.), and other granulomatous disorders (granulomatosis with polyangiitis, Crohn disease, giant cell polymyositis, foreign–body granulomas from silicone, paraffin, polymethyl methacrylate, etc.).
    - Reduced catabolism of 1,25D (loss of function mutation of the 24-hydroxylase encoding gene, CYP24A1) can present as unexplained hypercalcemia. The adult phenotype includes varying degrees of hypercalcemia, hypercalciuria, nephrolithiasis/nephrocalcinosis, low PTH, higher than expected 1,25D levels, and CKD. Pregnancy associated hypercalcemia in women without prior hypercalcemia or nephrocalcinosis has been reported, and can be complicated by maternal hypertension, acute pancreatitis, and fetal demise.

25. How does hypercalcemia occur during immobilization?
    Immobilization regularly leads to accelerated bone resorption and hypercalcemia primarily in individuals with high rates of bone turnover (e.g., adolescents on bed rest or patients with Paget disease). Hypercalcemia is preceded by hypercalciuria, which may lead to kidney stones. Hypercalcemia promptly reverses with the resumption of normal weight bearing.

26. What commonly used medications cause hypercalcemia and how?
    Vitamin D toxicity, which usually develops in vitamin faddists, manifests clinically with hypercalcemia. In general, serum 25D levels above 80 ng/mL are necessary for vitamin D toxicity, though much higher levels are typically seen in symptomatic hypercalcemia.

    Hypercalcemia also occurs in CKD patients treated for secondary hyperparathyroidism with pharmacologic doses of active vitamin D, like calcitriol (1,25D) or synthetic analogs (paricalcitol, doxercalciferol, etc.). Hypercalcemia is dose-dependent and transient, resolving within a few days of the drug being discontinued.

    Vitamin A intoxication, more commonly seen today with dermatologic or oncologic use of vitamin A analogues, causes hypercalcemia via osteoclast-mediated bone resorption.

    Thiazide diuretics reduce urinary calcium excretion via the sodium-calcium exchanger in the distal tubule. However, hypercalcemia from thiazide diuretics occurs mainly in patients with underlying mild primary hyperparathyroidism.

    Lithium interferes with CaSR, resulting in an increase in the set point at which calcium is suppressed. Patients on chronic lithium therapy can develop mild hypercalcemia, which subsides when medication is stopped in most cases.

27. What is the milk-alkali syndrome?
    The milk-alkali syndrome consists of hypercalcemia, hyperphosphatemia (although with use of calcium supplements such as calcium carbonate, phosphate binding in the gastrointestinal tract may produce hypophosphatemia), metabolic alkalosis, and kidney failure. It was most commonly observed years ago in patients who were treated for peptic ulcer disease with large doses of sodium bicarbonate or calcium carbonate antacids and milk. Kidney failure was mediated by metastatic calcification of the kidney resulting from excessive calcium and phosphorus absorption. Kidney failure accounted for impairment of bicarbonate excretion. Currently it results from the use of calcium supplements in patients seeking to enhance bone formation, such as postmenopausal women with osteoporosis.

28. **What are the clinical manifestations of hypercalcemia? Why does polyuria occur?**
Clinical manifestations vary with acuity and severity of hypercalcemia. In the more acute settings, these include fatigue, weakness, lethargy, confusion, anorexia, nausea, abdominal pain, constipation, polyuria, and polydipsia. Cardiac abnormalities like electrocardiographic changes (short QT, ST segment elevation), arrhythmias (bradyarrhythmias or heart block), and potentiation of digitalis toxicity have been reported.
    Polyuria is a manifestation of nephrogenic diabetes insipidus that occurs in hypercalcemia by the following proposed mechanisms:
    • Inhibition of salt reabsorption in the medullary thick ascending limb with resultant "washing out" of the medullary interstitium and reduction of the countercurrent gradient.
    • Inhibitory effect of the CaSR on vasopressin-stimulated water reabsorption in the inner medullary collecting duct.

29. **Which laboratory tests are helpful in the evaluation of hypercalcemia?**
Serum PTH level will help distinguish a PTH-mediated from a non-PTH–mediated hypercalcemia. In patients with normal kidney function, an elevated serum-intact PTH level will diagnose primary hyperparathyroidism in more than 90% of cases. If serum PTH is low (usually <20 pg/mL or so), evaluation of PTH-rP, 25D and 1,25D, phosphorus, creatinine, vitamin A level, serum, and urine protein electrophoresis should be pursued based on the patient's clinical and medication history.

30. **How can urinary calcium help in the diagnosis of hypercalcemia?**
Evaluation of urine calcium (spot studies, or preferably a 24-hour collection) is helpful in distinguishing primary hyperparathyroidism from familial hypocalciuric hypercalcemia (FHH), an inactivating mutation of CaSR with autosomal-dominant transmission, presenting sometimes in adulthood. FHH is manifested as mild hypercalcemia, slightly elevated PTH, and increased kidney reabsorption of calcium causing hypocalciuria. The urinary calcium/creatinine ratio is below 0.01 (mg/mg) in FHH, while a ratio over 0.2 (mg/mg) is seen in primary hyperparathyroidism; ratios between 0.01 and 0.2 are indeterminate.

31. **What are the general therapeutic interventions in the management of hypercalcemia?**
In symptomatic patients, general measures that facilitate urinary calcium excretion include administration of intravenous saline, followed by furosemide once volume expansion has been achieved. Loop diuretics are calciuric and help prevent pulmonary congestion. Patients with impaired kidney function who are unable to excrete the sodium load may require hemodialysis against a low calcium bath.

32. **What specific treatment can be used in the management of hypercalcemia?**
Glucocorticoids are the first line of therapy for hypercalcemia-associated elevated 1,25D levels in sarcoidosis and have been successfully used in other cases of granulomatous hypercalcemia like tuberculosis, silicone-induced granulomas, etc. Oral calcium intake as low as 400 mg/day is also recommended in these cases (to limit its intestinal absorption).
    For hypercalcemia of malignancy associated with bone resorption, bisphosphonates (pamidronate, zoledronic acid), which induce osteoclast apoptosis, are considered first line of therapy. The clinical response is apparent in a few days. Calcitonin inhibits osteoclast bone resorption within hours, but its use is limited by the modest effect and rapid development of tachyphylaxis. Denosumab, a monoclonal antibody that blocks osteoclast activation by targeting the receptor activator of NF-kB ligand, has been used in some case series of bisphosphonates-resistant hypercalcemia.
    Cinacalcet activates the CaSR in the parathyroid gland, thus inhibiting PTH secretion; it may be used in patients with parathyroid cancer in whom surgical parathyroid resection is not curative.

KEY POINTS

1. A positive calcium balance has been demonstrated in patients with CKD stages 3 and 4 consuming a diet containing 2000 mg of calcium per day, or calcium carbonate supplements of 1500 mg/day. Calcium supplementation in this population should be used cautiously.
2. Correcting the total serum calcium for albumin in patients with advanced kidney failure may lead to errors in estimating ionized serum calcium. Therefore ionized serum calcium should be directly measured if hypocalcemia or hypercalcemia is suspected.
3. Elevated 1,25D levels due to mutations of the 24-hydroxylase gene have been reported recently in adults. This possibility should be considered in the differential diagnosis of adults with unexplained hypercalcemia associated with high 1,25D levels, low PTH, nephrolithiasis/nephrocalcinosis, and CKD.

ACKNOWLEDGMENT

The author would like to thank Dr. Stanley Goldfarb for his contribution to this chapter.

BIBLIOGRAPHY

Bazari, H., Palmer, W. E., Baron, J. M., & Armstrong, K. (2016). Case records of the Massachusetts General Hospital. Case 24-2016. A 66-year-old man with malaise, weakness, and hypercalcemia. *New England Journal of Medicine, 375*(6), 567–574.

Cooper, M. S., & Gittoes, N. J. (2008). Diagnosis and management of hypocalcaemia. *British Medical Journal, 336,* 1298–1302.

Evenepoel, P., & Wolf, M. (2013). A balanced view of calcium and phosphate homeostasis in chronic kidney disease. *Kidney International, 83*(5), 789–791.

Fraser, W. D. (2009). Hyperparathyroidism. *Lancet, 374,* 145–158.

Hill, K. M., Martin, B. R., Wastney, M. E., McCabe, G. P., Moe, S. M., Weaver, C. M., & Peacock M. (2013). Oral calcium carbonate affects calcium but not phosphorus balance in stage 3-4 chronic kidney disease. *Kidney International, 83*(5), 959–966.

Medarov, B. I. (2009). Milk-alkali syndrome. *Mayo Clinic Proceedings, 84,* 261–267.

Reagan, P., Pani, A., & Rosner, M. H. (2014). Approach to diagnosis and treatment of hypercalcemia in a patient with malignancy. *American Journal of Kidney Diseases, 63*(1), 141–147.

Schafer, A. L., & Shoback, D. (2013). Hypocalcemia: Definition, etiology, pathogenesis, diagnosis, and management. In C. J. Rosen (Ed.), *Primer on the metabolic bone diseases and disorders of mineral metabolism* (8th ed.). Ames, IA: John Wiley & Sons, Inc.

Shoback, D. (2008). Clinical practice. Hypoparathyroidism. *New England Journal of Medicine, 359,* 391–403.

Spiegel, D. M., & Brady, K. (2012). Calcium balance in normal individuals and in patients with chronic kidney disease on low- and high-calcium diets. *Kidney International, 81*(11), 1116–1122.

Tebben, P. J., Singh, R. J., & Kumar, R. (2016). Vitamin D mediated hypercalcemia: Mechanisms, diagnosis and treatment. *Endocrine Reviews, 37*(5), 521–547.

Woods, G. N., Saitman, A., Gao, H., Clarke, N. J., Fitzgerald, R. L., & Chi, N. W. (2016). A young woman with recurrent gestational hypercalcemia and acute pancreatitis due to CYP24A1 deficiency. *Journal of Bone and Mineral Research, 31*(10), 1841–1844. doi:10.1002/jbmr.2859.

CHAPTER 76

DISORDERS OF PHOSPHORUS METABOLISM

Mina El Kateb and Joel M. Topf

NORMAL PHOSPHORUS PHYSIOLOGY

1. **What is the difference between phosphate and phosphorus and how are they measured in clinical medicine?**
   Phosphorus is a critical element in physiology. Phosphorus is an essential component of bone (hydroxyapatite), DNA, lipid membranes (phospholipids), signal molecules (phosphorylation activates numerous enzymes), and chemical energy storage (adenosine triphosphate and creatine phosphate). In the serum, phosphorus circulates as phosphate, PO_4^{-3} usually with one or two protons, $H_2PO_4^-$ or HPO_4^{2-} (Fig. 76.1).
   The atomic weight of phosphorus is 31 g/mole and the average valence (pH 7.4) is 1.8. Normal serum phosphorus is 2.5 to 4.5 mg/dL. This converts to 0.8 to 1.45 mmol/L or 1.45 to 2.61 mEq/L.

2. **Where is phosphorus found in the body?**
   There is 780 mg in a typical 70 kg man. Almost all of it (80% to 85%) is found in teeth and bones as hydroxyapatite. Only 0.1% is found in the extracellular fluid.

3. **Tell me about dietary phosphorus intake.**
   Organic phosphorus is found in meat, fish, dairy, whole grains, and nuts. However, most of the phosphorus we encounter in our diet is in the form of inorganic phosphorus added during food processing to enhance flavor and to improve color, and it serves as a preservative. Between 40% and 80% of dietary phosphorus is absorbed. The variability is largely due to the type of phosphorus consumed. Organic phosphorus is typically bound to proteins and must be metabolized to phosphate prior to absorption. Only about 40% to 60% of organic phosphorus is absorbed. Phosphate from animal protein is better absorbed than plant phosphate (phytate). Inorganic phosphate is more bioavailable, with as high as 90% absorption. The institute of medicine recommends 750 mg of phosphorus per day, with larger requirements (1250 mg/day) for children and pregnant women.
   Food tables that list the phosphorus content do not include the phosphorus used as preservatives and so tend to underestimate daily phosphorus intake by as much as 272 to 350 mg.
   Phosphate absorption in the gastrointestinal (GI) tract is largely unregulated, so increased dietary phosphate ingestion increases phosphate absorption. Active (1,25-OH) vitamin D also increases phosphate absorption.

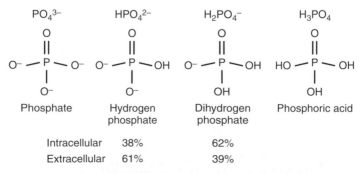

Figure 76.1. There are four forms of phosphate, with two found in the body. Hydrogen phosphate is the dominant form in the extracellular compartment, while dihydrogen phosphate is more common in the intracellular compartment. The other forms are essentially nonexistent in the body.

$$\text{Tubular reaborption of phosphorus} = \left(1 - \frac{Cr_{serum} \times Phos_{urine}}{Cr_{urine} \times Phos_{serum}}\right) \times 100$$

Equation 76.1. The tubular reabsorption of phosphorus is the percentage of filtered phosphorus, which is subsequently reabsorbed. It is one minus the fractional excretion of phosphorus. It is generally between 75% and 85%.

4. **How is phosphorus handled by the kidney?**
   The kidney filters between 3700 and 6100 mg of phosphate a day. Phosphate excretion is about 600 to 1500 mg/day, so about 75% to 85% of filtered phosphate is reabsorbed by the kidney. The proximal tubule reabsorbs about 85% of the filtered load via a triad of sodium-phosphate cotransporters (NaPi-2a, NaPi-2c, PiT-2). Phosphate reabsorption is regulated by numerous dietary, metabolic, and hormonal factors. Calculating the tubular reabsorption of phosphorous (TRphos) can provide insight into renal phosphorus handling. See Equation 76.1.
   Factors that lead to increased renal phosphate absorption include a low phosphate diet, 1,25-OH vitamin D, and thyroid hormone. On the other hand, parathyroid hormone (PTH), fibroblast growth factor (FGF)23, a high phosphate diet, metabolic acidosis, potassium deficiency, glucocorticoids, dopamine, hypertension, and estrogen lower phosphate absorption.

5. **What is FGF-23?**
   FGF-23 is classified as a phosphotonin—a hormone that increases urinary phosphorus. It is produced and released by osteocytes in response to increased serum phosphorus. When FGF-23 binds its receptor and the receptor's co-factor, Klotho, it decreases phosphorus reabsorption in the proximal tubule. It also decreases 1-alpha hydroxylase, lowering 1,25-OH D levels. FGF-23 also can directly suppress PTH. Increases in FGF-23 are found early in chronic kidney disease (CKD) and is responsible for the decreased 1,25-OH D levels found in CKD. It helps maintain normal phosphate levels despite compromised glomerular filtration rate (GFR).

HYPOPHOSPHATEMIA

6. **What is the difference between phosphate depletion and hypophosphatemia?**
   Phosphate depletion is a decrease in the total body soluble phosphate. Hypophosphatemia is a low serum phosphate level. Hypophosphatemia can be due to a decreased total phosphate level or to altered transcellular distribution of phosphorus into the intracellular compartment. Often, patients with phosphate depletion can maintain normal phosphate levels for a while, but are predisposed to sudden and acute drops in phosphate levels from events that shift phosphate into cells.

7. **What is the definition of hypophosphatemia and how common is it?**
   Hypophosphatemia is defined as serum phosphate level less than 2.5 mg/dL (0.8 mmol/L). In unselected hospitalized patients, hypophosphatemia has a prevalence of 2% to 3%. However, that increases dramatically in selected populations: 34% for intensive care unit patients, 65% to 80% for patients with sepsis.

8. **What are the causes of hypophosphatemia?**
   The causes of hypophosphatemia should be organized by decreased intake and GI losses, transcellular shift, and increased renal phosphate wasting. Since phosphorus is a common constituent of food, decreased dietary intake is a rare cause of hypophosphatemia. However, malabsorption or increased colonic secretion from diarrhea can result in hypophosphatemia. Some cases of hypophosphatemia occur with chronic overuse of phosphorus binders or calcium-, magnesium-, or aluminum-containing antacids that block phosphorus absorption. Pharmaceutical niacin causes a modest reduction in serum phosphorus (0.3 mg/dL, 0.1 mmol/L), which is thought to be due to decreased GI absorption.
   Increased renal phosphate excretion is a common cause of hypophosphatemia. Since PTH decreases renal phosphorus absorption by decreasing sodium-phosphate cotransporter activity in the proximal tubule, primary hyperparathyroidism is the prototypical example of renal phosphorous wasting. A unique form of hyperparathyroidism can occur after a kidney transplant. Patients with significant secondary hyperparathyroidism prior to transplant often have prolonged hypophosphatemia because they are unable to adequately suppress PTH following the transplant. In others, the hypophosphatemia persists despite normal PTH. In a series of 27 living donor transplants, FGF-23 was found to correlate best with post-transplant phosphorus levels.

Vitamin D deficiency can lead to hypocalcemia. This causes secondary hyperparathyroidism, which decreases serum phosphorus. This is made worse by decreased dietary phosphorus absorption from the lack of vitamin D.

Generalized dysfunction in the proximal tubule, Fanconi syndrome, is characterized by hypophosphatemia, in addition to glucosuria, proximal renal tubular acidosis, hypokalemia, and aminoaciduria.

Autosomal dominant hypophosphatemic rickets causes renal wasting of phosphorus. Patients are unable to mineralize bones so they end up with soft bones. It is due to an inability to inactivate FGF-23, which results in increased renal phosphorus wasting. A similar phenotype is seen in *X-linked hypophosphatemic rickets*; however, in this condition, there is an inactivating mutation of PHEX, which normally decreases the expression of FGF-23.

The last major cause of hypophosphatemia is transcellular shift, where phosphorus is either shifted into cells or taken up by bones. The former occurs with increases in insulin. Refeeding syndrome occurs in patients with total body phosphorus depletion, who then undergo a fast of 2 to 3 days. When they resume eating, the sudden increase in carbohydrates causes a release of insulin which shifts glucose, potassium, and phosphorus into cells. Phosphorus, which is already somewhat depleted, is rapidly consumed with the conversion of glucose to glucose 6-phosphate.

Respiratory alkalosis reliably causes a shift of phosphorus into cells.

The other sudden cause of hypophosphatemia is hungry bone syndrome, which occurs in patients with significant secondary or tertiary hyperparathyroidism, which is then corrected by surgical removal of the parathyroid glands. This triggers a sudden drop in PTH and rapid remineralization of osteoid throughout the skeleton, causing sudden drops in serum calcium, phosphorus, magnesium, and potassium.

9. How does hypophosphatemia present?

Since phosphorus is a key ingredient to the cellular energy molecule, adenosine triphosphate (ATP), hypophosphatemia causes symptoms related to the lack of ATP. Symptoms are rare until the phosphorus falls below 1 mg/dL (0.32 mmol/L). The most severe hypophosphatemia can cause hemolysis from decreased red blood cell deformability due to ATP depletion. Hypophosphatemia can also cause rhabdomyolysis. Hemolysis and rhabdomyolysis both release intracellular phosphorus covering the tracks of the inciting hypophosphatemia.

A number of studies have associated hypophosphatemia with increased hospital mortality; however, the lack of randomized, interventional trials keeps the question open of whether the hypophosphatemia causes or is associated with the increased mortality.

Hypophosphatemia has been associated with decreased respiratory muscle strength resulting in increased duration of mechanical ventilation. Others have reported decreased myocardial contractility, and improved left ventricular performance was documented with the correction of severe (<1 mg/dL or 0.3 mmol/L) but not moderate hypophosphatemia. Decreased phosphorus can result in central nervous system (CNS) symptoms ranging from paresthesias (perioral numbness) to irritability, delirium, seizures, and coma.

10. How should one approach evaluating the cause of hypophosphatemia?

Generally, the cause of the hypophosphatemia can be elucidated from the patient's history, focusing on diet, nutritional status, social habits, and medication use. In situations where it is not clear, a 24-hour urinary phosphate or calculating the TRphos can distinguish renal wasting from GI loss or cellular redistribution. A 24-hour urinary phosphate excretion <100 mg or TRphos >95% is indicative of appropriate renal phosphate retention in the setting of hypophosphatemia.

11. How should hypophosphatemia be treated?

Moderate hypophosphatemia (phosphorus >1 mg/dL, 0.32 mmol/L) and asymptomatic patients can be treated with oral phosphate. Cow's milk is a good source of phosphate. Typical oral dosing is 40 to 80 mmol (124 to 248 mg) divided into four doses over 24 hours. Severe hypophosphatemia (<1 mg/dL, 0.32 mmol/L) and patients who cannot tolerate oral replacement need intravenous (IV) replacement. IV phosphorus can cause hypocalcemia, kidney failure, hypotension, hyperphosphatemia, and electrocardiogram (ECG) abnormalities. These complications can be avoided with moderate doses. A safe dose is considered to be 15 mmol over 2 hours; however, doses graded by weight and phosphorus level were shown to be more effective and just as safe in a prospective trial.

This protocol (Table 76.1) corrected 78% of patients with hypophosphatemia with a single dose administered over 6 hours (compared to 47% prior to the protocol) and resulted in no cases of hyperphosphatemia (compared to 16 episodes prior to the protocol).

Table 76.1. Phosphorus Treatment Protocol

PHOSPHORUS LEVEL		WEIGHT		
mmol/l	mg/dl	40–60 kg	61–80 kg	81–120 kg
<0.32	1.0	30 mmol Phos	40 mmol Phos	50 mmol Phos
0.32–0.54	1.0–1.7	20 mmol Phos	30 mmol Phos	40 mmol Phos
0.55–0.70	1.7–2.2	10 mmol Phos	15 mmol Phos	20 mmol Phos

From Taylor, B. E., Huey, W. Y., Buchman, T. G., Boyle, W. A., & Coopersmith, C. M. (2004). Treatment of hypophosphatemia using a protocol based on patient weight and serum phosphorus level in a surgical intensive care unit. *Journal of the American College of Surgeons*, 198(2), 198–204.

HYPERPHOSPHATEMIA

12. What is the definition of hyperphosphatemia?
   Hyperphosphatemia is defined by a serum phosphate level greater than 1.45 mmol/L or 4.5 mg/dL. In patients on dialysis, a looser standard of 5.5 mg/dL (1.77 mmol/L) is sometimes adopted.

13. What is the incidence of hyperphosphatemia?
   The incidence of hyperphosphatemia is largely determined by kidney function. In unselected hospitalized patients, the rate is about 9%. The patients with hyperphosphatemia had an average estimated GFR (eGFR) of 22 mL/min/1.73 m^2, while the patients with normal phosphorus were 93 mL/min/ 1.73 m^2. Among patients on dialysis, the rate is 47%, despite using a looser definition for hyperphosphatemia (1.77 instead of 1.45 mmol/L).

14. What is pseudohyperphosphatemia?
   Elevated phosphorus levels, often mildly elevated (but have been as high as 31 mg/dL), have been encountered in the setting of normal kidney function, calcium, parathyroid hormone, and vitamin D level, suggesting spurious elevation or lab errors: this is pseudohypophosphatemia. It is often a result of a lab assay interference, which can be seen in cases of paraproteinemia, and with the use of liposomal amphotericin B, recombinant tissue plasminogen activator, and heparin sulfate. It is important to be aware of this problem in order to prevent unnecessary and potentially harmful treatments geared at lowering serum phosphorus levels.

15. What are the causes of hyperphosphatemia?
   Hyperphosphatemia can be due to increased intake, transcellular distribution, and decreased kidney clearance.
   Cathartics may contain sodium phosphate. When used as the principal bowel prep for colonoscopies and GI procedures, the recommended dose is 11.5 g of phosphorus in 90 mL of solution. Patients routinely become hyperphosphatemic, though usually only transiently. Increased age, abnormal bowel motility, and decreased kidney function are all risk factors for persistent and significant hyperphosphatemia. Similar results have been reported with sodium phosphate enemas.
   In advanced CKD, increased dietary phosphorus is associated with hyperphosphatemia. Foods with high phosphorus need to be avoided in order to keep dietary phosphorus below 1200 mg for pre-dialysis CKD patients, and 800 mg for dialysis patients.
   The anti-seizure medication, fosphenytoin, is metabolized to phenytoin, formaldehyde, and phosphorus. Acute episodes of hyperphosphatemia have been reported in patients with kidney failure.
   Cell breakdown in the setting of tumor lysis syndrome, rhabdomyolysis, or hemolysis releases intracellular phosphate. Breakdown of these cells also releases uric acid, myoglobin, and hemoglobin, respectively, resulting in acute kidney injury. This compromises the excretion of phosphate. With tumor lysis syndrome in particular, calcium phosphate, uric acid, and xanthine can precipitate in the tubules, resulting in inflammation and obstruction. Increased urine pH predisposes to the crystallization of calcium phosphate. Chemotherapy protocols that call for alkalinization of the urine to prevent uric acid nephropathy may unwittingly predispose to calcium phosphate precipitation.
   Hyperphosphatemia is common in diabetic patients presenting with ketoacidosis. However, the phosphorus rapidly falls with treatment, and by 12 hours the phosphorus may be below normal. The increased phosphorus is due to transcellular shift and a lack of insulin. After treatment is initiated, phosphorus shifts back in the cells and reveals underlying total body phosphorus depletion.

PTH decreases kidney reabsorption of phosphorus, so decreases in PTH result in hyperphosphatemia. Hypoparathyroidism is most commonly seen as a complication of parathyroid, thyroid, or neck surgery. Both hypo- and hypermagnesemia can cause functional hypoparathyroidism. DiGeorge, or velocardiofacial syndrome due to a micro deletion of 22q11, is a congenital cause of hypoparathyroidism. Acromegaly is thought to cause hyperphosphatemia through the action of an insulin-like growth factor, which stimulates phosphorus reabsorption in the proximal tubule. Vitamin D toxicity increases both calcium and phosphorus absorption. The increased calcium suppresses PTH, which further compromises phosphorus excretion. Bisphosphonates induce a mild hyperphosphatemia by stimulating phosphorus reabsorption. Primary hyperphosphatemic tumoral calcinosis is a condition characterized by multiple calcified, painless masses. Patients have normal calcium levels but elevated phosphorus levels with normal kidney function. This is due to an inactivating mutation to FGF-23, Klotho, or GALNT3, resulting in decreased renal phosphorus excretion.

As mentioned earlier, decreased renal clearance is arguably the most important cause of hyperphosphatemia. In acute kidney injury, as kidney dysfunction resolves, so does the hyperphosphatemia. In early CKD, increases in FGF-23 and PTH are able to maintain the phosphorous balance, but as the GFR falls below 20 mL/min, the frequency of hyperphosphatemia begins to increase.

16. What are the symptoms of hyperphosphatemia?
Acute hyperphosphatemia is usually asymptomatic, but when there are symptoms, they are typically consistent with the concurrent hypocalcemia seen with hyperphosphatemia. Hypocalcemia primarily causes cardiac and CNS toxicity. The primary ECG changes are QTc prolongation and it can also cause myocardial depression leading to hemodynamic instability. The neurologic effects include perioral numbness, Chvostek and Trousseau signs, lethargy, laryngospasm, seizure, and coma.

Chronic hyperphosphatemia is generally asymptomatic; however, there are a few complications that are significant. Increased phosphorus is associated with poor patient outcomes. In a study of inpatients, those with hyperphosphatemia had a longer length of stay (6 compared to 3 days) and higher mortality. The CARE study was a randomized, controlled trial of pravastatin in patients with a previous myocardial infarction and hypercholesterolemia. The average GFR was 70 mL/min. The investigators found a 27% increase in the risk of death for every 1 mg/dL (0.32 mmol/L) increase in phosphorus. In patients on dialysis, multiple studies from all over the world have found an association with high phosphorus and mortality.

Another complication of hyperphosphatemia is calcific uremic arteriolopathy (formerly known as calciphylaxis). This disease is usually seen in dialysis patients and affects the arterioles. Histologically, it is characterized by apoptosis, differentiation of smooth muscle cells into bone forming osteoblast-like cells, and increased inflammation. Patients develop painful, deep soft-tissue plaques that progress to black eschars and necrotic ulcers. Sodium thiosulfate administered with dialysis has emerged as a promising treatment strategy.

17. How do you treat acute hyperphosphatemia?
The best treatment is avoiding acute hyperphosphatemia in the first place. Sodium phosphate bowel cleanses should be avoided, especially in patients with CKD and abnormal gut motility. Once the patient has hyperphosphatemia, the focus should be on maintaining kidney function to prevent accumulation. IV fluids should be started if the patient can tolerate them. Insulin can shift phosphorus into the cells, though it is unclear if this is beneficial. If the patient has kidney failure, consideration should be given to dialysis.

18. How do you treat chronic hyperphosphatemia?
Chronic hyperphosphatemia as seen with end-stage kidney disease should be treated with phosphorus binders. Binders are cationic compounds that bind phosphate anions in the gut and prevent absorption. One of the first phosphorus binders used was aluminum hydroxide. The use of aluminum hydroxide was associated with adynamic bone disease and dementia. Aluminum gave way to calcium-based binders, primarily calcium acetate and calcium carbonate. Additional binders include sevelamer, lanthanum carbonate, and two iron-based binders: sucroferric oxyhydroxide and ferric citrate. All of these have shown efficacy in lowering serum phosphorus. In multiple meta-analyses sevelamer has demonstrated a survival advantage over calcium-based binders. However, this finding is largely dependent on the positive results of a single large trial, Di Lori's open-label INDEPENDENT Trial. INDEPENDENT showed a huge reduction in cardiovascular mortality with sevelamer (hazard ratio [HR] 0.09; total mortality HR 0.23) that other studies were unable to detect.

The use of phosphate binders in CKD is less clear. The drugs appear to be effective and reduce both serum phosphorus and 24-hour urine phosphorus; however, vascular calcification, an important surrogate endpoint, actually increased rather than decreased. No randomized trials have demonstrated survival or improved kidney function through the use of phosphorus binders in CKD.

19. **What is the *calcium-phosphorus product* and what is its significance?**
The term *calcium-phosphorus product* (Ca x P) was first coined in 1922 by Howland and Kramer, attempting to explain risk factors for children who developed rickets. A few years later, this concept was tied to ectopic calcification—calcification that happens outside of bone. It was presumed that this simple second-order relationship was representative of intravascular calcification and, consequently, could be tied to outcomes, especially in dialysis patients. Despite ectopic calcification being an established risk factor for outcomes in dialysis patients, the calcium-phosphorus product could not be established as a risk factor for ectopic calcification, and altering this product did not impact outcomes. Consequently, this concept has fallen out of favor.

20. **Can IV calcium be given if the phosphorus is high?**
While the calcium phosphorus product does not represent the relationship of intravascular calcification, adding calcium to a patient with hyperphosphatemia does induce ectopic calcification. That being said, the risks of acute hypocalcemia including arrhythmia, laryngospasm, and hemodynamic compromise outweigh the long-term risks of vascular calcification. So calcium can be given for symptomatic hypocalcemia even in the presence of hyperphosphatemia.

21. **Do sodium phosphate (Fleet brand) enemas cause kidney failure?**
Sodium phosphate enemas (SPE), often referred to by the brand name "Fleet," have been rarely associated with acute phosphate nephropathy. In a 2012 case series highlighting the negative impact of SPE, Ori et al showed acute kidney injury in 11 elderly patients receiving Fleet enemas for constipation. These patients presented with severe hyperphosphatemia, hypocalcemia, and hypotension, with one patient presenting with a phosphorus level of 45 mg/dL (14.5 mmol/L) and calcium of 2 mg/dL (0.5 mmol/L). In a retrospective cohort from the VA system, 70,499 patients receiving either SPE alone, SPE with polyethylene glycol (PEG), or PEG alone for colonoscopy prep were analyzed for estimated glomerular filtration rate (eGFR) decline. The authors, after an adjusted analysis, indicated that there was a greater portion of long-term (>6 months) decline in eGFR in the SPE group over the PEG group, without a higher risk of acute drop in eGFR. The pathologic feature of phosphate toxicity is calcium phosphate deposition within the tubular cells, the tubular lumen, and the interstitium, leading to obstruction and inflammation. The glomeruli are left relatively intact. This has been termed acute phosphate nephropathy.

22. **What about aluminum-based binders?**
In the early 1970s, aluminum hydroxide was one of the major binders used in the treatment of hyperphosphatemia in dialysis patients. It was assumed that most of the aluminum would bind to phosphorus and would be excreted in feces; however, aluminum accumulated in the CNS causes dementia, and aluminum accumulated in the bone results in osteomalacia and anemia. A more aggressive form of this dementia, called dialysis encephalopathy, presents as acute encephalopathy, with seizures and sometimes respiratory failure. Currently, the National Kidney Foundation guidelines recommend the use of aluminum only in patients who have an elevated phosphorus >7 mg/dL (2.3 mmol/L), refractory to other binders, and only for a limited time period (<4 weeks).

KEY POINTS

1. Phosphorus is the main component of ATP, the basic energy molecule of all human cells.
2. Hypophosphatemia is common, but clinically significant hypophosphatemia (<1 mg/dL) is rare, manifesting as muscle breakdown, decreased cardiac contractility, CNS dysfunction, lethargy, seizures, and death.
3. There is an increasing amount of inorganic phosphorus in our diets, mostly from preservatives; however, intact kidneys maintain phosphate balance.
4. Patients with acute or chronic kidney disease are highly susceptible to hyperphosphatemia.
5. Rarely, excessive ingestion overwhelms the kidney's ability to handle phosphorus; this can be seen with sodium phosphate cathartics and enemas.

BIBLIOGRAPHY

Beloosesky, Y., Grinblat, J., Weiss, A., Grosman, B., Gafter, U., & Chagnac, A. (2003). Electrolyte disorders following oral sodium phosphate administration for bowel cleansing in elderly patients. *Archives of Internal Medicine, 163*(7), 803–808.

Bhan, I., Shah, A., Holmes, J., Isakova, T., Gutierrez, O., Burnett, S. M., . . . Wolf, M. (2006). Post-transplant hypophosphatemia: Tertiary 'Hyper-Phosphatoninism'? *Kidney International, 70*(8), 1486–1494.

Block, G. A., Wheeler, D. C., Persky, M. S., Kestenbaum, B., Ketteler, M., Spiegel, D. M., . . . Chertow, G. M. (2012). Effects of phosphate binders in moderate CKD. *Journal of the American Society of Nephrology, 23*(8), 1407–1415.

Howland, J., & Benjamin, K. (1922). Factors concerned in the calcification of bone. *Tractates of the American Pediatric Society, 34*, 204.

Izzedine, H., Oamouo, L., Bourry, F. Azar, N., Leblond, V., & Deray, G. (2007). Make your diagnosis. Multiple myeloma-associated with spurious hyperphosphatemia. *Kidney International, 72*(0), 1025–1036.

Kalantar-Zadeh, K., Gutekunst, L., Mehrotra, R., Kovesdy, C. P., Bross, R., Shinaberger, C. S., . . . Kopple, J. D. (2010). Understanding sources of dietary phosphorus in the treatment of patients with chronic kidney disease. *Clinical Journal of the American Society of Nephrology, 5*(3), 519–530.

Kidney Disease: Improving Global Outcomes (KDIGO) CKD-MBD Work Group. (2009). KDIGO clinical practice guideline for the diagnosis, evaluation, prevention, and treatment of Chronic Kidney Disease-Mineral and Bone Disorder (CKD-MBD). *Kidney International Supplement, 76*(113), S1–130.

Kraft, M. D., Btaiche, I. F., Sacks, G. S., & Kudsk, K. A. (2005). Treatment of electrolyte disorders in adult patients in the intensive care unit. *American Journal of Health System Pharmacy, 62*(16), 1663–1682.

Levin, A., Bakris, G. L., Molitch, M., Smulders, M., Tian, J., Williams, L. A., & Andress, D. L. (2007). Prevalence of abnormal serum vitamin D, PTH, calcium, and phosphorus in patients with chronic kidney disease: Results of the study to evaluate early kidney disease. *Kidney International, 71*(1), 31–38.

Liamis, G., Liberopoulos, E., Barkas, F., & Elisaf, M. (2013). Spurious electrolyte disorders: A diagnostic challenge for clinicians. *American Journal of Nephrology, 38*(1), 50–57.

Maccubbin, D., Tipping, D., Kuznetsova, O., Hanlon, W. A., & Bostom, A. G. (2010). Hypophosphatemic effect of niacin in patients without renal failure: A randomized trial. *Clinical Journal of the American Society of Nephrology, 5*(4), 582–589.

Marik, P. E., & Bedigian, M. K. (1996). Refeeding hypophosphatemia in critically ill patients in an intensive care unit. A prospective study. *Arch Surg, 131*(10), 1043–1047.

Nigwekar, S. U., Brunelli, S. M., Meade, D., Wang, W., Hymes, J., & Lacson, E. (2013). Sodium thiosulfate therapy for calcific uremic arteriolopathy. *Clinical Journal of the American Society of Nephrology, 8*(7), 1162–1170.

O'Neill, W. C. (2007). The fallacy of the calcium-phosphorus product. *Kidney international, 72*(7), 792–796.

Ori, Y., Rozen-Zvi, B., Chagnac, A., Herman, M., Zingerman, B., Atar, E., . . . Korzets, A. (2012). Fatalities and severe metabolic disorders associated with the use of sodium phosphate enemas: A single center's experience. *Archives of Internal Medicine, 172*(3), 263–265.

Palmer, S. C., Gardner, S., Tonelli, M., Mavridis, D., Johnson, D. W., Craig, J. C., . . . Strippoli, G. F. (2016). Phosphate-binding agents in adults with CKD: A network meta-analysis of randomized trials. *American Journal of Kidney Disease, 68*(5), 691–702.

Parkinson, I. S., Ward, M. K., & Kerr, D. N. (1981). Dialysis encephalopathy, bone disease and anaemia: The aluminum intoxication syndrome during regular haemodialysis. *Journal of Clinical Pathology, 34*(11), 1285–1294.

Port, F. K., Pisoni, R. L., Bommer, J., Locatelli, F., Jadoul, M., Eknoyan, G., . . . Young, E. W. (2006). Improving outcomes for dialysis patients in the international Dialysis Outcomes and Practice Patterns Study. *Clinical Journal of the American Soceity of Nephrology, 1*(2), 246–255.

Prié D., & Friedlander G. (2010). Genetic disorders of renal phosphate transport. *New England Journal of Medicine, 362*(25), 2399–2409.

Schaefer, M., Littrell, E., Khan, A., & Patterson, M. E. (2016). Estimated GFR decline following sodium phosphate enemas versus polyethylene glycol for screening colonoscopy: A retrospective cohort study. *American Journal of Kidney Diseases, 67*(4), 609–616.

Taylor, B. E., Huey, W. Y., Buchman, T. G., Boyle, W. A., & Coopersmith, C. M. (2004). Treatment of hypophosphatemia using a protocol based on patient weight and serum phosphorus level in a surgical intensive care unit. *Journal of American Colonoscopy and Surgery, 198*(2), 198–204.

Zazzo, J. F., Troché, G., Ruel, P., & Maintenant, J. (1995). High incidence of hypophosphatemia in surgical intensive care patients: Efficacy of phosphorus therapy on myocardial function. *Intensive Care Medicine, 21*(10), 826–831.

CHAPTER 77

DISORDERS OF MAGNESIUM METABOLISM

Mina El Kateb and Joel M. Topf

NORMAL MAGNESIUM PHYSIOLOGY

1. How is magnesium measured?
   The molecular weight of magnesium is 24.3 g/mol, with a 2+ valence (Mg2+). The normal serum magnesium level is 0.7 to 0.85 mmol/L, but it is often expressed as equivalents per liter, 1.4 to 1.7 mEq/L (mEq/L = mmol/L × valence), or in conventional units, 1.7 to 2.1 mg/dL (mg/dL = mmol/L × molecular weight divided by 10). Normal reference levels vary from laboratory to laboratory (Table 77.1).

2. Where is magnesium found in the body?
   The average human body contains a total of 25 g of magnesium, which is roughly equivalent to 2000 mEq or 1 mole of magnesium. Nearly 99% of this magnesium is intracellular, with just over half trapped in bone. Only 1% is extracellular, a third of which (2.6 mmol) is present in plasma (Fig. 77.1). Like calcium, only the ionized fraction of magnesium is metabolically active, and represents 55% to 70% of serum magnesium.
   The intracellular magnesium concentration is 10 to 20 mM/L; however, the majority of this magnesium is bound to adenosine triphosphate (ATP), while a smaller potion is bound to nucleotides and proteins. Only 5% of the cytosolic magnesium (0.5 to 1 mM/L) is unbound.

Table 77.1. Normal Magnesium Levels in Various Units

UNITS	NORMAL MAGNESIUM CONCENTRATION
mmol/L	0.7–0.85 mmol/L
mEq/L	1.4–1.7 mEq/L
mg/dL	1.7–2.1 mg/dL
mg/L	17–21 mg/L

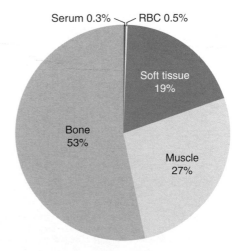

Figure 77.1. The distribution of magnesium in the body. *RBC,* Red blood cell.

3. **What are the roles of magnesium?**
   Magnesium is a critical cofactor for over 600 enzymatic reactions. It maintains the stability of ATP as well as the tertiary structure of DNA. Given magnesium's central role in ATP generation, it should not be a surprise that magnesium is important for muscle contraction, relaxation, normal neurological function, and release of neurotransmitters. Magnesium also has a role in DNA replication and repair, RNA transcription, amino acid synthesis, protein formation, and glucose metabolism.
       There is evidence that magnesium has a role in insulin secretion, and some clinical trials have shown improved metabolic profiles in diabetics given magnesium supplementation.

4. **What are the primary nutritional sources of magnesium?**
   Dietary sources of magnesium are primarily dark leafy vegetables, whole grains, nuts, beans, and seafood. A typical Western diet contains less than the FDA recommended 420 mg for males and 320 mg for women, because the soil in which fruits and vegetables are grown is depleted of magnesium. Also, Western diets are rich in refined grains, and as much as 90% of the Mg is lost in processing. Hard water is a source of dietary magnesium. Globally, magnesium intake has dropped due to increased consumption of processed (refined) grains and increased water softening.

5. **How does the gastrointestinal (GI) tract absorb and excrete magnesium?**
   Only about a quarter, or 100 mg, of the ingested magnesium is absorbed by the GI tract and the rest is excreted. Much of the absorption takes place through passive paracellular transport, driven by an electrochemical gradient and solvent drag. There is a second active transport system mediated by TPRM 6 and 7 channels (TRPM stands for "transmembrane receptor potential subfamily melastatin"). The active magnesium transport becomes more active with low magnesium status and is downregulated with magnesium excess. This active transport system is more active in the terminal ileum and proximal colon (Fig. 77.2).

6. **What is different about kidney magnesium handling from other electrolytes?**
   Unlike most other electrolytes, where absorption takes place in the proximal tubule, magnesium reabsorption occurs predominantly at the thick ascending limb of the loop of Henle (TAH). That being said, roughly 20% of filtered magnesium is reabsorbed in the proximal tubule. About 70% of the filtered magnesium is absorbed in the thick ascending loop of Henle. This occurs through paracellular tight junctions down the electrical gradient. The electrical gradient is established by the renal outer medullary potassium (ROMK) channel, which allows intracellular potassium to flow into the tubule. Potassium is the rate-limiting reagent for the sodium, potassium, two chloride (NK2Cl) channel (Fig. 77.3).

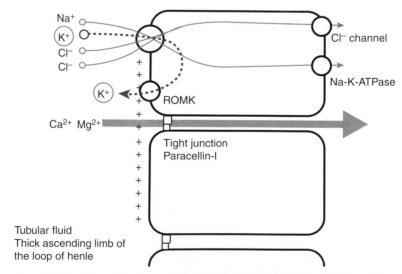

Figure 77.2. Potassium reabsorbed by the NaK2Cl channel flows back out through the renal outer medullary potassium channel, so the net movement of charge is two anions and one cation into the cell leaving the tubular fluid with a net positive charge. This charge drives the paracellular reabsorption of magnesium and calcium.

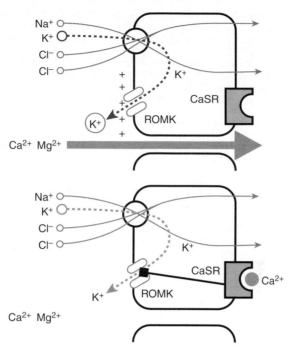

Figure 77.3. When calcium binds the calcium sensing receptor it slows potassium efflux form the thick ascending limb of the loop of Henle cell, lowering the positive tubular charge that drives magnesium and calcium reabsorption, which antagonizes the renal outer medullary potassium.

The kidneys are able to dynamically adjust the reabsorption of magnesium to respond to changes in magnesium levels. In the presence of low magnesium, fractional reabsorption of magnesium can rise to 99.5%. With magnesium excess, the fractional excretion of magnesium can fall to 30%.

7. What hormones regulate magnesium levels?
   No known hormone has any appreciable effect on renal magnesium handling.

HYPOMAGNESAEMIA

8. What is the difference between hypomagnesemia and magnesium deficiency?
   Hypomagnesemia is defined as serum magnesium level less than 1.7 mg/dL (1.4 mEq/L or 0.7 mmol/L). However, since serum magnesium represents on 0.3% of total body magnesium, serum magnesium may not correspond with total body magnesium. Some patients with normal serum magnesium may have signs or symptoms of low magnesium. This is referred to as normomagnesemic magnesium depletion and should be considered in patients with risk factors for hypomagnesemia (alcoholics, patients with poorly controlled diabetes, or diarrhea), and refractory hypokalemia or unexplained hypocalcemia.

9. How common is hypomagnesemia and who is at risk for hypomagnesemia?
   Hypomagnesemia is found in 10% of hospitalized patients. In the intensive care unit (ICU) this may be as high as 60%. Patients at risk include chronically malnourished, alcoholic, and patients with diabetes.

10. What type of GI disorders lead to hypomagnesemia?
    GI losses occur with diarrhea and vomiting. Lower GI losses cause more hypomagnesemia due to a higher magnesium content in the secretions (up to 15 mEq/L with lower GI compared with 1 mEq/L with upper GI losses). This is particularly important in malabsorptive syndromes.

In acute pancreatitis, lipase metabolizes triglycerides to free fatty acids. The fatty acids are capped by carboxyl group with a charge of −1. The carboxyl group binds cations, specifically calcium and magnesium. The carboxyl complex precipitates out of solution lowering the calcium and magnesium. This process is called *saponification*.

Proton pump inhibitors can cause severe hypomagnesemia. The mechanism has not been fully worked out, but it appears that renal magnesium handling is intact and most attention is focused on active magnesium absorption by TRPMP6 channels in the terminal ileum and colon. It is hypothesized that the higher pH of intestinal secretions with proton pump inhibitor (PPI) decreases TPRM6/7 affinity for magnesium. It resolves with discontinuation of the drug but returns with rechallenge.

Primary intestinal hypomagnesemia is a rare congenital hypomagnesemic condition. Patients will typically also have renal magnesium wasting, because the molecular defect in the apical magnesium channel, TRPMC, is also found in the kidney. The condition has variable inheritance. It typically presents in infancy and early childhood but can present in young adults.

11. **What type of kidney disorders lead to hypomagnesemia?**
Kidney magnesium losses are increased with increased urine output. This occurs with diuretics, osmotic diuresis (as seen in diabetes), excessive intravenous saline, postobstructive diuresis, the recovery phase of acute tubular necrosis (ATN), and following a kidney transplant.

Loop diuretics specifically disrupt the NaK2Cl channel needed to generate the positive tubular lumen charge that drives magnesium and calcium reabsorption in the TAH. Thiazide diuretics induce hypomagnesemia by preventing the distal absorption of magnesium.

Hypercalcemia increases kidney magnesium wasting through a mechanism similar to that of loop diuretics. The cells of the TAH have a calcium-sensing receptor (CaSR) on the basolateral membrane. When activated, the CaSR antagonizes the ROMK channel, preventing the generation of the positive luminal charge that drives magnesium reabsorption (Fig. 77.3).

A number of other drugs can cause hypomagnesemia through increased kidney loss of magnesium, including:
a. Aminoglycosides
b. Amphotericin B
c. Pentamidine
d. Cisplatin
e. Epidermal growth factor (EGF) monoclonal antibodies
f. Calcineurin inhibitors

Chronic ethanol abuse causes a kidney magnesium leak. It can take weeks of abstinence to reverse this injury. In addition to the kidney leak, these patients often have poor dietary magnesium and increased GI losses, which contributes to the hypomagnesemia.

There are numerous inherited magnesium wasting nephropathies; none of them are common. The two most well known are Gitelman syndrome and Bartter syndrome.

Gitelman syndrome is an autosomal recessive disorder resulting from an inactivating mutation of the thiazide-sensitive sodium chloride cotransporter gene (NCCT) of the distal convoluted tubules. These patients present with signs and symptoms of chronic thiazide ingestion, including mild salt wasting, volume depletion, hypokalemia, metabolic alkalosis, and hypomagnesemia.

Bartter syndrome is a kidney sodium wasting nephropathy that mimics chronic loop diuretic use. It is typically autosomal recessive, though there is an autosomal-dominant form. Patients typically have low blood pressure, hypokalemia, metabolic alkalosis, hypocalcemia, and hypomagnesemia. The hypomagnesemia tends to be less severe than that seen in Gitelman syndrome.

The congenital kidney magnesium wasting syndromes are summarized in Table 77.2.

12. **What other conditions lead to hypomagnesemia?**
Decreased oral intake by itself is a rare cause of hypomagnesemia, but it can occur, more so in combination with other additional risk factors.

Hungry bone syndrome is an uncommon cause of hypomagnesemia. Following prolonged hyperparathyroidism, if a patient goes for a parathyroidectomy, it can result in sudden remineralization of the demineralized osteoid. This can result in sudden and prolonged consumption of serum electrolytes, including calcium, potassium, and magnesium.

13. **What electrolyte abnormalities occur with hypomagnesemia?**
Hypomagnesemia causes modest hypocalcemia. This is presumed to be due to bone resistance to parathyroid hormone.

Table 77.2. Congenital Renal Magnesium Wasting Syndromes

SYNDROME	INHERITANCE	DEFECT	PRESENTATION
Gitelman (most common)	AR	Thiazide-sensitive sodium chloride cotransporter (SLC12A3)	Children/adolescents/ adults with salt wasting, hypokalemic metabolic alkalosis, and **hypocalciuria**
Bartter syndrome	AR	Loop-sensitive sodium, potassium, 2Chloride channel (Na-K-2Cl)	Neonate/Infancy with salt wasting, hypokalemic metabolic alkalosis, and **hypercalciuria**
Familial hypomagnesemia with hypercalciuria and nephrocalcinosis (FHHNC)	AR	Caludin-16 gene	Children/adolescent with **hypercalciuria**, recurrent nephrocalcinosis, and progressive renal failure
Isolated dominant hypomagnesemia with hypocalciuria	AD	Gamma subunit of Na-K-ATPase pump resulting in misrouting	Children with hypomagnesemia and **hypocalciuria** and no stones
Voltage-gated potassium channel	AD	Voltage-gated potassium channel (KCNA1), which interacts with TMRP6	Isolated hypomagnesemia and renal magnesium wasting

AD, Autosomal dominant; AR, autosomal recessive.

Hypomagnesemia causes treatment-resistant hypokalemia. Of note, many causes of hypomagnesemia also independently cause hypokalemia (diuretics, alcoholism, and chronic diarrhea, etc.), so some hypokalemia is not due to the hypomagnesemia, but rather due to the process causing hypomagnesemia. It is estimated that 50% of patients with hypokalemia also have a magnesium deficiency, and replacing potassium alone will not correct the hypokalemia. Magnesium binds the inner surface of the ROMK channel of the cortical collecting duct, limiting potassium efflux. With magnesium depletion, this inhibition of potassium efflux is lost, causing increased kidney potassium loss (Fig. 77.4).

14. What are the signs, symptoms, and consequences of hypomagnesemia?
    Since hypomagnesemia causes hypokalemia and hypocalcemia, all three electrolyte abnormalities commonly occur simultaneously. Because of this it is difficult to know if specific manifestations of hypomagnesemia are due strictly to the magnesium deficiency or to low calcium, potassium, or a mixture. Given that warning, here are the commonly reported manifestations of hypomagnesemia.
    Neurologic manifestations are primarily hyperexcitability, which can present as muscle spasms, cramps, Trousseau and Chvostek signs, and tremors. Other symptoms include weakness, apathy, delirium, convulsions, and coma.

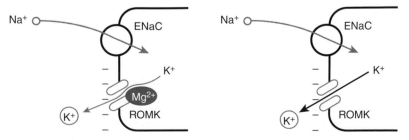

Figure 77.4. In the distal convoluted tubule and cortical collecting duct, intracellular magnesium decreases the activity of the ROMK channel slowing potassium efflux. Hypomagnesemia can lower intracellular magnesium levels enough that this inhibition is lost, increasing renal potassium loss.

Cardiovascular manifestations begin with widened QRS and peaked T-waves, and then progress to prolonged PR interval, further widening of the QRS, and loss of the T-waves with worsening hypomagnesemia. Atrial and ventricular arrhythmias including torsades de pointes are possible.

In retrospective analysis, low magnesium has been associated with increased mortality in multiple clinical scenarios, including ICU, general medicine wards, and in dialysis patients. Though this signal is seen even with controlling for severity of illness, prospective studies have not been done to show a decrease in mortality with replacing magnesium.

15. **How should one approach the diagnosis of hypomagnesemia?**
For most cases of hypomagnesaemia, the etiology can be elicited from a thorough history—focusing on diet, bowel habits, medications, comorbidities, diabetic control, and alcohol intake.

Additional testing includes the fractional excretion of Mg (FeMg; Equation 77.1). The serum magnesium is multiplied by 0.7 to account for the 30% of serum magnesium that is protein bound and not filtered at the glomerulus.

$$\text{Fractional excretion of magnesium} = \frac{Cr_{serum} \times Mg_{urine}}{Cr_{urine} \times 0.7 \times Mg_{serum}} \times 100 \qquad \text{[Equation 77.1]}$$

Normal values were established in patients with preserved kidney function in the setting of normal and low serum magnesium levels. Typical levels of FEMg were provided by Elisaf in a study of 216 patients (142 with normal magnesium and 74 with low magnesium of mixed etiologies). There was good separation of kidney wasting from extrarenal wasting in the study (Table 77.3).

A fractional excretion of magnesium over 4% is typical for kidney magnesium wasting, though some references say 3% and others 2%.

Twenty-four-hour urine for magnesium can also be done. Urine magnesium should be less than 24 mg in the absence of treatment and extrarenal magnesium loss. If there is a magnesium kidney loss, the urinary magnesium will be greater than 24 mg.

16. **How should hypomagnesemia be treated?**
Patients with severe symptomatic hypomagnesemia (i.e., seizures, tetany, or arrhythmia) need intravenous (IV) magnesium. One to 2 g of magnesium sulfate (8 to 17 mEq of magnesium) can be given by rapid IV push in patients in cardiac arrest or over an hour in patients with a pulse. This should be followed by a longer, slow infusion of another 4 to 8 g (33 to 66 mEq) of magnesium over 24 hours. This continuous infusion can be repeated safely for up to 3 consecutive days in order to ensure adequate repletion of intracellular and bone stores. Doses should be lowered in chronic kidney disease. Intravenous magnesium inhibits magnesium reabsorption in the loop of Henle, so patients will have increased kidney magnesium wasting during treatment. Up to 50% of infused magnesium will be excreted within a day of the infusion.

Magnesium sulfate increases kidney losses of potassium. This can exacerbate hypokalemia, so concomitant therapy with potassium should be considered. In addition, magnesium sulfate can lower ionized calcium.

Patients with asymptomatic or mildly symptomatic hypomagnesemia can be treated with oral magnesium replacement. Patients should be prescribed 240 to 1000 mg of elemental magnesium daily, in divided doses. Oral magnesium can cause diarrhea, worsening the hypomagnesemia, so the dose needs to be adjusted to avoid this side effect. See Table 77.4 for a list of oral magnesium preparations.

Patients who cannot tolerate oral magnesium can be replaced with intravenous magnesium. Doses range from 1 to 8 g over 12 to 24 hours, depending on the severity of hypomagnesemia (Table 77.5).

Table 77.3. Fractional Excretion of Magnesium, Interpretation

CONDITION	AVERAGE	RANGE
Normal magnesium level	1.8%	0.5%–4%
Renal magnesium wasting	15%	4%–48%
Extrarenal magnesium wasting	1.4%	0.5%–2.7%

Table 77.4. Oral Magnesium Preparations

DRUG	ELEMENTAL MAGNESIUM
Magnesium oxide (Uro-Mag)	84.5 mg I 7.0 mEq I 3.5 mmol
Magnesium chloride (Slow-Mag)	71.0 mg I 6.0 mEq I 3.0 mmol
Magnesium l-lactate (MAG-TAB SR)	84.0 mg I 7.0 mEq I 3.5 mmol
Magnesium aspartate	65.0 mg I 5.4 mEq I 2.7 mmol

Table 77.5. Empirical Treatment of Hypomagnesemia

SEVERITY	SERUM MAGNESIUM CONCENTRATION (MG/DL)	IV MAGNESIUM REPLACEMENT DOSE[a,b]
Mild to moderate	1.0–1.5	8–32 meq magnesium (1–4 g magnesium sulfate), up to 1.0 meq/kg
Severe	<1.0	32–64 meq magnesium (4–8 g magnesium sulfate), up to 1.5 meq/kg

[a]In patients with normal renal function; patients with renal insufficiency should receive ≤50% of the initial empirical dose. Maximum rate of infusion = 8 meq magnesium per hour (1 g magnesium sulfate per hour), up to 100 meq magnesium (approximately 12 g magnesium sulfate) over 12 hours if asymptomatic; up to 32 meq magnesium (4 g magnesium sulfate) over 4–5 minutes in severe symptomatic hypomagnesemia. 1 g magnesium sulfate = 8.1 meq magnesium.

[b]The authors suggest using adjusted body weight (AdjBW) in patients who are significantly obese (weight of >130% of ideal body weight [IBW] or have a body mass index of ≥30 kg/m2): AdjBW (men) = ([wt (kg) – IBW (kg)] × 0.3) + IBW; AdjBW (women) = ([wt (kg) – IBW (kg)] × 0.25) + IBW.

Originally published in Kraft, M. D., Btaiche, I. F., Sacks, G. S., et al. (2005). Treatment of electrolyte disorders in adult patients in the intensive care unit. *American Journal of Health-System Pharmacy, Inc.* 62(16), 1663-1682. All rights reserved. Reprinted with permission. (R1707).

HYPERMAGNESEMIA

17. **What is the definition and prevalence of hypermagnesemia?**
Hypermagnesemia occurs when serum magnesium rises over 2.1 mg/dL (1.75 mEq/L or 0.86 mmol/L). Hypermagnesemia is less common than hypomagnesemia. Nearly all hypermagnesemia goes undiagnosed. In a study of magnesium levels in 1179 consecutive blood samples sent for electrolytes among hospitalized patients, 59 (5.7%) had a magnesium level over 2.4 mg/dL (0.99 mmol/L), but a magnesium was requested in only 7 of those 59. Studies of outpatients in the community have shown rates from 3% to 10%, depending on the population and magnesium level used to define hypermagnesemia.
Hypermagnesemia is more common in patients with ESRD. In a screening of 101 asymptomatic dialysis patients, ingestion of as little as 281 mg of magnesium resulted in hypermagnesemia.
Though biochemical hypermagnesemia is rare, it is generally well tolerated, and symptomatic hypermagnesemia is quite unusual.

18. **What condition is either the sole cause or an important contributor to hypermagnesemia?**
Almost all cases of hypermagnesemia have kidney failure as the primary or contributing etiology. The kidney is able to ramp up excretion of magnesium by minimizing magnesium reabsorption, so in most cases of clinically significant hypermagnesemia, there is a component of chronic kidney disease (CKD). In addition to CKD, there is usually another inciting event: increased GI intake, IV infusion, or cell destruction.

19. **Explain how increased magnesium intake can be a cause of hypermagnesemia.**
Magnesium is an active ingredient in multiple laxatives and antacids. Epsom salt is magnesium sulfate. It can be taken as an enema or orally. Epsom salts are a folk remedy for a variety of ailments from abdominal pain (it is an effective cathartic) to cerebral edema (ineffective) to halitosis (unable to find convincing blinded analysis). One tablespoon of Epsom salt contains approximately 35 g of magnesium sulfate, which is 3.4 g of elemental magnesium.

IV magnesium leads to hypermagnesemia. Magnesium is the most common agent used to treat eclampsia and preeclampsia. Patients are typically loaded with 4 g of IV magnesium sulfate, followed by an infusion of 1 to 2 g/h. This typically produces stable magnesium levels of 6 to 8.5 mg/dL (2.5 to 3.5 mmol/L). Most clinicians do not follow biochemical levels, but screen for toxicity by checking the patellar reflex. Loss of the reflex occurs at magnesium levels above 8.5 mg/dL (3.5 mmol/L). Magnesium for eclampsia and preeclampsia can occasionally cause a solute diuresis.

The intracellular concentration of magnesium is roughly 10 to 20 times as high as the extracellular concentration. Cell lysis due to rhabdomyolysis, infarction, or hemolysis releases intracellular magnesium, causing hypermagnesemia.

20. What types of kidney conditions cause hypermagnesemia?

Since the kidney is responsible for clearing magnesium absorbed from the GI track, and the body has limited ability to regulate GI absorption, decreased kidney function (either acute or chronic) is an important cause of hypermagnesemia. Among hemodialysis patients, hypermagnesemia was associated with a daily magnesium intake greater than 281 mg (less than the RDA of magnesium: 420 mg for men, 320 mg for women).

In addition to generalized decreases in glomerular filtration rate (GFR), familial hypocalciuric hypercalcemia is a tubular disorder associate with modest hypermagnesemia. Hypocalciuric hypercalcemia is an autosomal dominant loss-of-function mutation of the CaSR. The abnormal CaSR is less responsive to serum calcium, so higher calcium concentrations are needed to suppress PTH and shut down calcium and magnesium reabsorption in the TAL (see Fig. 77.3).

21. How does hypermagnesemia present?

Hypermagnesemia decreases neuromuscular transmission. The first sign will typically be diminished deep-tendon reflexes (DTR), followed eventually by complete loss of DTR. As the magnesium level rises, patients develop progressive somnolence, paralysis, and ultimately apnea.

Cardiovascular effects occur due to magnesium acting as both a calcium and potassium channel antagonist. This leads to PR, QRS, and QT prolongation presenting as bradycardia and hypotension. Ultimately, hypermagnesemia can cause complete heart block and cardiac arrest.

Magnesium is tightly linked to calcium metabolism. Hypermagnesemia inhibits parathyroid hormone (PTH) release, leading to mild hypocalcemia; this may be of little consequence but can worsen QT prolongation and compound cardiac arrhythmia.

Table 77.6 has a summary of signs and symptoms according to severity of hypermagnesemia.

22. How is hypermagnesemia treated?

The best way to treat hypermagnesemia is preventing it from happening in the first place. Avoid magnesium-containing products in patients with CKD or those with AKI. Also, patients receiving magnesium infusions should be monitored regularly.

Treatment in patients with preserved kidney function or only mild CKD is primarily stopping all magnesium-containing medications and initiating intravenous fluids with normal saline. The addition of loop diuretics can further assist with kidney magnesium clearance.

Table 77.6. Symptoms of Hypomagnesemia Based on Serum Magnesium Level

MAGNESIUM LEVEL	NEUROMUSCULAR	CARDIOVASCULAR	ELECTROLYTE	OTHER
4–6 mEq/L 4.8–7.2 mg/dL	Diminished DTR	Flushing from vasomotor dilation, PR interval prolongation and QRS interval prolongation		Nausea, vomiting
6–10 mEq/L 7.2–12 mg/dL	Loss of DTR	Hypotension, bradycardia,	Hypocalcemia, suppression of PTH	Somnolence
>10 mEq/L >12 mg/dL	Paralysis, respiratory depression, apnea	AV dissociation, complete heart block, cardiac arrest		Coma

DTR, Deep-tendon reflexes.

If the patient has severe CKD and significant symptomatic hypermagnesemia, the primary therapy is hemodialysis. IV calcium can be given to reverse the neuromuscular and cardiovascular effects of magnesium while preparing for hemodialysis.

23. **What is the relationship between multifocal atrial tachycardia (MAT) and magnesium?**
MAT is a type of atrial tachycardia where the P-wave originates from multiple foci in the atrium, outside of the sinoatrial node. This results in multiple morphologies of the P-wave. IV magnesium is considered an effective therapy for MAT, especially when associated with hypomagnesemia.

24. **Is there an association between hypomagnesemia and diabetes?**
Magnesium has been linked to glycemic control in diabetic patients. Hypomagnesemia is common in patients with diabetes, occurring in 13% to 47% of diabetic, nonhospitalized patients. Magnesium tends to go down as glycemic control worsens. Hypomagnesemia has been linked to reduced insulin sensitivity, and supplementing magnesium in type 2 diabetic patients has been shown to improve insulin sensitivity and metabolic control. No major diabetic institutions have made any recommendations for chronic or routine magnesium supplementation in diabetic patients.

25. **What is the role of magnesium is asthma?**
There is a role for IV magnesium in status asthmaticus. A Cochrane meta-analysis revealed that magnesium is beneficial in patients with severe asthma exacerbations, resulting in reduced admissions and improved lung function. Typical protocols call for a rapid infusion of 1.2 to 2 g over a 15 to 30 minutes period.

26. **Is magnesium useful in myocardial infarction?**
Magnesium causes systemic and coronary vasodilation, platelet inhibition, and has antiarrhythmic effects. Consequently, it seems like an ideal agent in the setting of acute myocardial infarction (AMI). The LIMIT-2 trial, published in the *Lancet* in 1992, randomized more than 2000 patients suspected to have AMI to either placebo or IV magnesium infusion. This randomized, double-blind, controlled trial demonstrated a mortality benefit, with 24% relative risk reduction when magnesium was used over a placebo. Magnesium supplementation consisted of 8 mmol over 5 minutes followed by 65 mmol over 24 hours. In the angioplasty era, the data seems less promising. In 2002, the MAGIC trial, published in the Lancet randomized over 6000 patients with ST elevation myocardial infarct (STEMI) to either placebo or a rapid (2 g over 15 minutes) followed by a slow (17 g of 24 hours) magnesium infusion. Both groups underwent percutaneous coronary intervention. There was no significant difference in the 30-day all-cause mortality between the two groups.

KEY POINTS

1. Unlike other electrolytes that are primarily reabsorbed in the proximal tubule, magnesium is primarily reabsorbed in the thick ascending limb of the loop of Henle.
2. Conditions associated with increased urine output predispose to low magnesium. This includes diuretics, IV fluids, and poorly controlled diabetes.
3. Low magnesium causes other electrolytes to fall. Hypomagnesemia can cause hypokalemia and hypocalcemia.
4. Hypermagnesemia is usually only found with renal failure, either acute or chronic.
5. Increased magnesium causes decreased deep tendon reflexes and can ultimately cause muscle weakness and respiratory arrest.

BIBLIOGRAPHY

Agus, Z. S. (1999). Hypomagnesemia. *Journal of the American Society of Nephrology, 10*(7), 1616–1622.
Antman, E. M., Magnesium in Coronaries (MAGIC) Trial Investigators. (2002). Early administration of intravenous magnesium to high-risk patients with acute myocardial infarction in the Magnesium in Coronaries (MAGIC) Trial: A randomised controlled trial. *Lancet, 360*(9341), 1189–1196.
Barbagallo, M., & Dominguez, L. J. (2015). Magnesium and Type 2 Diabetes. *World Journal of Diabetes, 6*(10), 1152–1157.
Blaine J., Chonchol, M., & Levi, M. (2015). Renal control of calcium, phosphate, and magnesium homeostasis. *Clinical Journal of the American Society of Nephrology, 10*(7), 1257–1272.
Danziger, J., William, J. H., Scott, D. J., Lee, J., Lehman, L. W., Mark, R. G., . . . Mukamal, K. J. (2013). Proton-pump inhibitor use is associated with low serum magnesium concentrations. *Kidney International, 83*(4), 692–699.
de Baaij, J. H., Hoenderop, J. G., & Bindels, R. J. (2015). Magnesium in man: Implications for health and disease. *Physiological Reviews, 95*(1), 1–46.

De Marchi, S., Cecchin, E., Basile, A., Bertotti, A., Nardini, R., & Bartoli, E. (1993). Renal tubular dysfunction in chronic alcohol abuse–effects of abstinence. *New England Journal of Medicine, 329*(26), 1927–1934.

Elisaf, M., Panteli, K., Theodorou, J., & Siamopoulos, K. C. (1997). Fractional excretion of magnesium in normal subjects and in patients with hypomagnesemia. *Magnesium Research, 10*(4), 315–320.

Freitag, J. J., Martin, K. J., Conrades, M. B., Bellorin-Font, E., Teitelbaum, S., Klahr, S., & Slatopolsky, E. (1979). Evidence for skeletal resistance to parathyroid hormone in magnesium deficiency: Studies in isolated perfused bone. *Journal of Clinical Investigation, 64*(5), 1238–1244.

Kew K. M., Kirtchuk, L., & Michell, C. I. (2014). Intravenous magnesium sulfate for treating adults with acute asthma in the emergency department. *Cochrane Database System Review*, (5), CD010909. doi:10.1002/14651858.CD010909.pub2.

Lu, J. F., & Nightingale, C. H. (2000). Magnesium sulfate in eclampsia and pre-eclampsia: Pharmacokinetic principles. *Clinical Pharmacokinetics, 38*(4), 305–314.

McCord, J. K., Borzak, S., Davis, T., & Gheorghiade, M. (1998). Usefulness of intravenous magnesium for multifocal atrial tachycardia in patients with chronic obstructive pulmonary disease. *American Journal of Cardiology, 81*(1), 91–93.

Rodríguez-Morán, M., & Guerrero-Romero, F. (2003). Oral magnesium supplementation improves insulin sensitivity and metabolic control in type 2 diabetic subjects: A randomized double-blind controlled trial. *Diabetes Care, 26*(4), 1147–1152.

Ryzen, E., Wagers, P. W., Singer, F. R., & Rude, R. K. (1985). Magnesium deficiency in a medical ICU population. *Critical Care Medicine, 13*(1), 19–21.

Whang, R., & Ryder, K. W. (1990). Frequency of hypomagnesemia and hypermagnesemia. Requested vs routine. *JAMA, 263*(22), 3063–3064.

Wolf, F., & Hilewitz, A. (2014). Hypomagnesaemia in patients hospitalised in internal medicine is associated with increased mortality. *International Journal of Clinical Practice, 68*(1), 111–116.

Wong, E. T., Rude, R. K., Singer, F. R., & Shaw, S. T., Jr. (1983). A high prevalence of hypomagnesemia and hypermagnesemia in hospitalized patients. *American Journal of Clinical Pathology, 79*(3), 348–352.

Woods, K. L., Fletcher, S., Roffe, C., & Haider, Y. (1992). Intravenous magnesium sulphate in suspected acute myocardial infarction: Results of the second Leicester Intravenous Magnesium Intervention Trial (LIMIT-2). *Lancet, 339*(8809), 1553–1558.

Wyskida, K., Witkowicz, J., Chudek, J., & Więcek, A. (2012). Daily magnesium intake and hypermagnesemia in hemodialysis patients with chronic kidney disease. *Journal of Renal Nutrition, 22*(1), 19–26.

CHAPTER 78

METABOLIC ACIDOSIS

David S. Goldfarb and Jon-Emile S. Kenny

METABOLIC ACIDOSIS

The "secrets" of metabolic acidosis will be the emphasis of this chapter, given the breadth of this topic. This chapter is parsed into, first, a brief overview of relevant physiology and, second, an algorithmic, clinically relevant approach to the metabolic acidosis. The final section of the chapter will discuss, in more detail, specific examples of this diverse group of metabolic abnormalities.

BACKGROUND AND KEY PHYSIOLOGY

1. The difference between acidemia and acidosis.
   Acid*emia* describes the concentration of hydrogen ions ($[H^+]$) in plasma; thus it includes all conditions where $[H^+]$ in plasma is higher than the values observed in normal subjects (40 $\pm$ 2 nmol/L, or a pH less than 7.38). Acid*emia* has two general causes, and this leads to the concept of acid*osis*. An acid*osis* is any *process* by which there is increased $[H^+]$ and a decrease in the concentration and/or the content of bicarbonate (HCO_3^-) in the extracellular fluid (ECF) compartment. As noted previously, there are two general processes whereby $[H^+]$ is increased in plasma. First, there may be a high carbon dioxide tension in arterial blood (i.e., the $PaCO_2$—called a respiratory acidosis) or, second, a high $[H^+]$ in plasma from a low bicarbonate (called metabolic acidosis). Notably, an acidosis does not necessarily mean there is an acidemia. This is because there may be multiple processes—of metabolic or respiratory origin—that cause $[H^+]$ in plasma to fall despite there being an identified metabolic acidosis.

2. What is metabolic acidosis?
   A metabolic acidosis is a metabolic process resulting in increased $[H^+]$; there are two main etiologies:
   A. The addition of an acid (Fig. 78.1, shift in equation 1 from left to right)
   B. The loss of HCO_3, usually with sodium (Na^+) ($NaHCO_3$), or potassium (K^+), or both (see Fig. 78.1, shift in equation 3 from right to left).

3. What risks does metabolic acidosis entail for the patient?
   The risks that metabolic acidosis pose to the patient arise from multiple mechanisms:
   • There is risk engendered by the underlying disorder responsible for the metabolic acidosis (e.g., shock).
   • There are the adverse effects of high $[H^+]$ (binding of H^+ to intracellular proteins in vital organs (e.g., brain and heart; see equation 2 in Fig. 78.1), as well as possible dangers associated with the anions that accompany the H^+ load (e.g., chelation of ionized calcium during citric acidosis).
   • There are risks from toxins produced in the metabolic process that lead to the production of these acids (e.g., formaldehyde produced during the metabolism of methanol to formic acid or glycoaldehyde produced during metabolism of ethylene glycol to glycolic acid) or as a marker of a serious

$$(1) \quad \text{Acid} \longrightarrow \boxed{H^+} + \text{Anion}$$

$$(2) \quad \boxed{H^+} + \text{Protein}^0 \longrightarrow \boxed{\text{PTH-H}^+}$$

$$(3) \quad \boxed{H^+} + HCO_3^- \longleftrightarrow \boxed{CO_2} + H_2O$$

Figure 78.1. Buffer systems to remove a H^+ load. Although equations 2 and 3 describe buffer systems to remove H^+ in terms of chemistry of this process, there is a different emphasis in physiologic terms. In this context, flux through equation 2 must be minimized. This occurs if these added H^+ are forced to bind to bicarbonate (HCO_3^-) by lowering the PCO_2 in capillaries of skeletal muscles (equation 3) where this buffer system is most abundant, thereby pulling equation 3 to the right, which lowers the concentration of H^+ in plasma and minimizes binding of H^+ to intracellular proteins in vital organs (e.g., brain and heart).

metabolic threat (e.g., production of pyroglutamic acid after overdoses of acetaminophen, as this indicates depletion of the reduced form of glutathione—the protein that scavenges reactive oxygen species).

4. **What are the benefits of metabolic acidosis?**
   It should also be recognized that there may be benefits from metabolic acidosis. Most importantly, the Bohr effect leads to a shift of the hemoglobin-O_2 dissociation curve to the right, leading to more unloading of O_2 to tissues. Whatever adverse effects occur as the result of acidosis, treatment of metabolic acidosis is not necessarily beneficial, particularly when acute. Administration of sodium bicarbonate may not lead to the expected benefit and can itself lead to adverse effects.

5. **What is the bicarbonate buffer system (BBS)?**
   To minimize binding of H^+ to intracellular proteins, another process must prevent $[H^+]$ from rising, despite the H^+ load. This occurs if added H^+ are forced to bind to bicarbonate (HCO_3^-), the predominant extracellular buffer (see Fig. 78.1, equation 3), and this illustrates the BBS. The vast majority of HCO_3^- is in skeletal muscle. If the BBS in skeletal muscle is not appropriately titrating, and therefore removing H^+ in a patient with metabolic acidosis, acidemia will be more pronounced, and more of the H^+ load will be titrated in vital organs (e.g., brain and heart; Fig. 78.2). Critically, for the BBS to function there

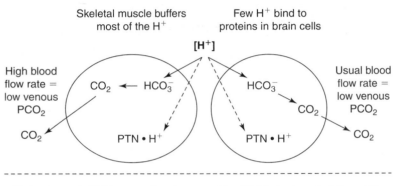

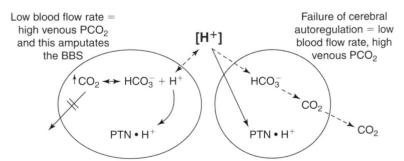

Figure 78.2. Physiology of the bicarbonate buffer system *(BBS)*. Skeletal muscle cells are shown to the left and brain cells to the right; because the brain is one-twentieth the size of muscle, it has far less intracellular fluid (ICF) and therefore less HCO_3^-. When the extracellular fluid (ECF) volume is low, the PCO_2 in the venous blood draining muscle is high. This minimizes the removal buffering of H^+ by the BBS in its ECF and ICF. As a result, the $[H^+]_{plasma}$ rises and more H^+ will be removed in brain cells. As the cerebral blood flow rate is autoregulated, the PCO_2 in the jugular venous blood draining the brain will change minimally, and hence the BBS in the brain will still function to titrate the H^+ load. Furthermore, if the degree of ECF volume contraction is severe, cerebral autoregulation fails and the blood flow to the brain falls. Hence the PCO_2 in brain cells will rise and more H^+ will bind to proteins in brain cells. In contrast, when intravenous saline is administered, blood flow to skeletal muscle rises, its venous PCO_2 should fall, and more H^+ are removed by its BBS. As a result, the $[H^+]_{plasma}$ falls and H^+ will be released from proteins in brain cells.

must be a low concentration of carbon dioxide (CO_2) in capillaries around skeletal muscle; in other words, equation 3 *must maintain its rightward direction* (i.e., Fig. 78.1, equation 3).

6. How do you assess the adequacy of the BBS?
   A high tension of capillary CO_2 within skeletal muscle will lead to a failure to maintain rightward shift (equation 3 in Fig. 78.1), thus extinguishing the BBS. CO_2 tension within muscle capillaries can be assessed with a venous blood gas (VBG). This is because the PCO_2 in capillaries of skeletal muscle reflects the PCO_2 in its cells and interstitial space; further, there is no CO_2 added once the blood leaves the capillaries and enters the veins. The secret here is that if the partial pressure of carbon dioxide in the venous effluent ($PvCO_2$) is high, the BBS in skeletal muscle is less effective (i.e., the rightward direction of equation 3 is blunted). Acidemia will be more pronounced, as more of the H^+ load will be titrated in vital organs.

7. What are the major reasons for a high $PvCO_2$?
   The $PvCO_2$ is essentially the summation of the arterial PCO_2 ($PaCO_2$) entering the capillaries and the CO_2 added by cellular metabolism. At the usual blood flow rate at rest, this results in a brachial $PvCO_2$ of 46 mm Hg, assuming a normal input arterial $PaCO_2$ of 40 mm Hg. Accordingly, the reasons for a high $PvCO_2$ are due to either a high $PaCO_2$ (i.e., respiratory suppression/failure), which raises the lowest possible value for $PvCO_2$, and/or a slow blood flow rate to muscle (e.g., poor perfusion states such as evolving shock). The reason that diminished tissue perfusion raises $PvCO_2$ is outlined as follows:
   1. When capillary blood flow falls, tissue oxygen consumption remains constant.
   2. Constant oxygen consumption leads to constant CO_2 production (as related by the respiratory quotient; i.e., 0.7 to 1.0 mmol of CO_2 will be formed per mmol of O_2 consumed).
   3. Despite constant CO_2 production, in the context of low flow, there is relatively more CO_2 added to each liter of blood volume; consequently, $PvCO_2$ rises.

CLINICALLY RELEVANT APPROACH TO A PATIENT WITH METABOLIC ACIDOSIS

8. What is the general approach to metabolic acidosis evaluation?
   Metabolic acidosis can be thought of as comprising two major subgroups: one underpinned by the addition of [H^+] and the other driven by the loss of $NaHCO_3$. The distinction here is generally guided by the calculation of the anion gap. Prior to this, however, it is prudent to identify and manage underlying threats to the patient's life consequent to the acidosis. In addition, therapy for the acidosis may unmask adverse effects that should be anticipated. Examples will be considered later on in this chapter, during the discussion of specific disorders. Lastly, when able, assess the adequacy of the BBS by comparing the arterial and venous tensions of CO_2. Therapy directed at lowering arterial $PaCO_2$ should be instituted if there is concomitant respiratory failure, and tissue perfusion should be enhanced if there is a gradient (i.e., more than 10 mm Hg) between the $PaCO_2$ and $PvCO_2$. As noted previously, lowering the venous and therefore capillary CO_2 shifts equation 3 rightward. In this way, bicarbonate rather than tissue proteins buffer the excess protons. The initial steps in our clinical approach to the patient with metabolic acidosis are illustrated in Fig. 78.3.

9. How do you calculate the anion gap?
   The presence of new anions in plasma can be detected with the calculation of the $P_{Anion\ gap}$.
   Electroneutrality requires that Na^+ + unmeasured cations (UC) = Cl^- + HCO_3^- + unmeasured anions (UA). Actually, almost everything *is* measured, but for simplicity's sake we pretend that the potassium, calcium, phosphate, and others are not.
   Then, rearranging, $Na^+ - Cl^- - HCO_3^-$ = UA – UC = anion gap. Assuming some usual normal values, $140 - 104 - 24 = 12$ (normal range 6 to 12). The major UA is albumin—about 3 mEq negative charge for each g/dL. So with normal albumin concentration of 4.0 g/dL, it contributes 12 mEq/L, roughly equal to the anion gap. From that equation, it can be seen that an increase in the anion gap is due to an increase in the UA (e.g., lactate) and/or a decrease in the UC (e.g., globulins).
   Accordingly, the baseline value of the $P_{Anion\ gap}$ must be adjusted for the $P_{Albumin}$. A rough guide for correcting the baseline value of $P_{Anion\ gap}$ for $P_{Albumin}$ is that at $P_{Albumin}$ of 4.0 g/dL (40 g/L), the $P_{Anion\ gap}$ is 12 mEq/L; hence for every 1.0 g/dL (10 g/L) decrease in $P_{Albumin}$, the $P_{Anion\ gap}$ will be lower by ~3 mEq/L. The converse is true for a rise in the $P_{Albumin}$ (Box 78.1).

10. In a patient with an increased anion-gap metabolic acidosis, what is the cause of overproduction of acids?
    A list of the causes of metabolic acidosis is provided in Box 78.2, and a clinical approach to the diagnosis of the cause of metabolic acidosis is summarized in Fig. 78.4.

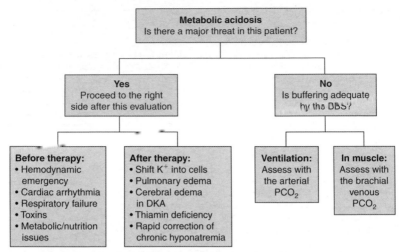

Figure 78.3. Initial steps in the clinical approach to a patient with metabolic acidosis. When the extracellular fluid (ECF) volume is significantly contracted, one must use a definition of metabolic acidosis that is based not only on the P_{HCO_3} but also on the content of HCO_3^- in the ECF compartment. Our initial step is to determine threats for the patient that may be present and anticipate those that may develop during therapy *(left side of the flow chart)*. The next step is to assess buffering by the bicarbonate buffer system *(BBS)* in both the ECF and intracellular fluid of skeletal muscle by measuring brachial or femoral venous PCO_2. *DKA,* Diabetic ketoacidosis.

Box 78.1. Abbreviations and Normal Values in Plasma

pH: 7.40 ± 0.02
[H+]: 40 ± 2 nmol/L
[HCO₃⁻] in plasma (P_{HCO_3}): 25 ± 2 mmol/L
Arterial PCO₂: 40 ± 2 mm Hg
Brachial venous PCO₂: <10 mm Hg higher than the arterial PCO₂.
Albumin in plasma ($P_{Albumin}$): 4.0 g/dL or 40 g/L.
Accounts for ~ 12 mEq/L of the anionic charge in plasma.

Anion gap in plasma ($P_{Anion\ gap}$): 12 ± 2 mEq/L (must adjust for the valence from the PAlbumin)
Henderson equation: $[H^+]$ (nmol/L) $= PCO_2$ (mm Hg) $\times$ (25 or 24)/ P_{HCO_3}
To make the mathematics easier at the bedside, one can use 25 or 24 as the constant.

Box 78.2. Causes of Metabolic Acidosis

Acid Gain

With retention of anions in plasma:
1. L-lactic acidosis
   A. Due predominantly to overproduction of L-lactic acid
      Hypoxic lactic acidosis
      Inadequate delivery of O_2 (cardiogenic shock, shunting of blood past organs [e.g., sepsis], or excessive demand for oxygen [e.g., seizures])
      Increased production of L-lactic acid in absence of hypoxia
      Overproduction of NADH and accumulation of pyruvate in the liver (e.g., metabolism of ethanol plus a deficiency of thiamin)
      Decreased pyruvate dehydrogenase activity (e.g., thiamin deficiency, inborn errors of metabolism)

   Compromised mitochondrial electron transport system (e.g., cyanide, riboflavin deficiency, inborn errors affecting the electron transport system)
   Excessive degree of uncoupling of oxidative phosphorylation (e.g., phenformin)
   B. Due predominantly to reduced removal of L-lactate: liver failure (e.g., severe acute viral hepatitis, shock liver, drugs)
   C. Due to a combination of reduced removal and overproduction of L-lactic acid
      Antiretroviral drugs (inhibition of mitochondrial electron transport plus hepatic steatosis)
      Metastatic tumors (especially large tumors with hypoxic areas plus liver involvement)
2. Ketoacidosis (diabetic ketoacidosis, alcoholic ketoacidosis, hypoglycemic ketoacidosis including starvation, ketoacidosis due to a large supply of

Box 78.2. Causes of Metabolic Acidosis *(Continued)*

short-chain fatty acids [i.e., acetic acid from fermentation of poorly absorbed carbohydrate plus inhibition of acetyl-coenzyme A carboxylase])
3. Kidney insufficiency (metabolism of dietary sulfur-containing amino acids and decreased kidney excretion of NH_4^+)
4. Metabolism of toxic alcohols (e.g., formic acid from metabolism of methanol, glycolic acid, and oxalic acid from metabolism of ethylene glycol)
5. D-lactic acidosis (and other organic acids produced by gastrointestinal bacteria)
6. Pyroglutamic acidosis

With a high rate of excretion of anions in urine:
1. Glue sniffing (hippuric acid overproduction)
2. Diabetic ketoacidosis with excessive ketonuria

NaHCO₃ Loss

Direct loss of NaHCO₃:
1. Via the GI tract (e.g., diarrhea, ileus, fistula)
2. Via the urine (proximal renal tubular acidosis or low carbonic anhydrase II or IV activity)

Indirect loss of NaHCO₃ (low urinary NH_4^+ secretion):
1. Low glomerular filtration rate

2. Renal tubular acidosis
   A. Low availability of NH_3 (urine pH $\sim$5) = problem in PCT ammoniagenesis: hyperkalemia, alkaline pH in PCT cells
   B. Defect in net distal H^+ secretion (urine pH often $\sim$7):
      H^+ ATPase defect or alkaline α-intercalated cells (a number of autoimmune disorders or disorders with hypergammaglobulinemia; e.g., Sjögren syndrome)
      H^+ back leak (e.g., amphotericin B)
      HCO_3 secretion in the collecting ducts (e.g., a molecular defect in the Cl^-/HCO_3^- anion exchanger leading to its mistargeting to the luminal membrane of α-intercalated cells, as in some patients with Southeast Asian ovalocytosis)
   C. Problem with both distal H^+ secretion and medullary NH_3 (urine pH <6): Diseases involving the kidney interstitial compartment (e.g., sickle cell disease)

PCT, Proximal convoluted tubule.

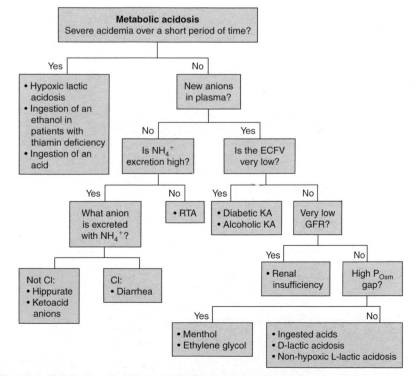

Figure 78.4. Clinical approach to the diagnosis of the cause of metabolic acidosis. *ECFV*, Extracellular fluid volume; *GFR*, glomerular filtration rate; *KA*, ketoacid anions; *RTA*, renal tubular acidosis.

A secret heuristic for the causes of an elevated anion gap is "KULT":

- Ketones (diabetic, fasting and alcoholic ketoacidosis)
- Uremia (with retained phosphate and sulfate and others)
- Lactate (e.g., with hypoxia and septic shock)
- Toxic ingestions (especially ethylene glycol and methanol)

While ketones are typically detected from the clinical history, a secret is that ketonuria may not be detected on a standard urinalysis if there is a high NADH/NAD ratio (e.g., contaminant, ethanol intake). The reason is that beta-hydroxybutyrate (BHB) is favored when NADH is abundant, and BHB is not detected by the nitroprusside test, which is the urinalysis based assay. The next test to be sought is the venous lactate measurement. When a VBG is available, also take note of the $PvCO_2$, as noted previously. Lastly, consider assessing for toxic ingestions by calculating a serum osmolal gap ($P_{Osmolal\ gap}$). This will determine whether new uncharged particles are present in plasma:

$$P_{Osmolal\ gap} = \text{measured } P_{osm} - (P_{Glucose} + P_{Urea} + 2\,P_{Na}), \text{ all in mmol/L units.}$$

However, as the toxic alcohols ethylene glycol and methanol are metabolized to oxalate and formic acid, the osmolal gap falls as the anion gap rises. Early after ingestion, before metabolism has occurred, the osmolal gap is present. Subsequently, metabolism leads to a rising anion gap such that the time of the peak for both anion and osmolal gaps may not coincide (Table 78.1).

11. Is there a reproducible quantitative relationship between the fall in [HCO_3^-] and the rise in the $P_{Anion\ gap}$ in all patients with metabolic acidosis?

    The relationship between the rise in the $P_{Anion\ gap}$ and the fall in the concentration of bicarbonate [HCO_3^-] is used to detect the presence of coexisting metabolic alkalosis in a patient with metabolic acidosis (i.e., the rise in $P_{Anion\ gap}$ is larger than the fall in [HCO_3^-]) and/or the presence of both an acid overproduction type and a $NaHCO_3$ loss type of metabolic acidosis (i.e., the rise in $P_{Anion\ gap}$ is smaller than the fall in [HCO_3^-]). It must be recognized, however, that this relationship uses *concentration* rather than *content* terms and therefore will underestimate the magnitude of the HCO_3^- deficit if there is significant contraction of the ECF. That is, diminished ECF volume will suggest an underlying alkalosis (i.e., a process that is *increasing* the *content* of bicarbonate), when in fact there is none. This carries clinical relevance in bicarbonate-wasting metabolic acidosis, because the provision of bicarbonate-free fluid resuscitation may lead to a rapid, unexpectedly large fall in [HCO_3^-] and unmask a severe metabolic acidosis, described as follows under specific disorders (e.g., diarrhea; see Table 78.1).

Table 78.1. Laboratory Tests in the Diagnosis of Metabolic Acidosis

QUESTION	PARAMETER ASSESSED	TOOLS TO USE
Is the content of HCO_3^- low in the ECF?	ECF volume	Hematocrit or total plasma proteins
Have new acids accumulated?	Appearance of new anions in the body or the urine	$P_{Anion\ gap}$ Urine anion gap
Are toxic alcohols present?	Detect alcohols as unmeasured osmoles	$P_{Osmolal\ gap}$
Is the renal response to acidemia adequate?	Examine the rate of excretion of NH_4^+	Urine osmolal gap
If NH_4^+ excretion is high, which anion was excreted?	GI loss of $NaHCO_3$ Acid added, but its new anions are excreted	Urine Cl^- is high Urine anion gap
What is the basis for a low rate or excretion of NH_4^+?	Low net distal H^+ secretion Low NH_3 availability Both defects	Urine pH >6.5 Urine pH ~5.0 Urine pH ~6.0
Where is the defect in H^+ secretion?	Distal H^+ secretion Proximal H^+ secretion	PCO_2 in alkaline urine FE_{HCO3}, $U_{Citrate}$

ECF, Extracellular fluid; *GI*, gastrointestinal.

12. Estimate the "corrected" bicarbonate concentration when there is significant ECF volume contraction.

The hematocrit or total protein levels in plasma may be used to obtain a quantitative estimate of the ECF volume.

Sample calculation: If the patient does not have preexisting anemia or polycythemia, use the hematocrit (though the concentration of albumin or total proteins in plasma may also be used) to obtain a quantitative estimate of the ECF volume and calculate its *content* of HCO_3^-. In a normal adult, the usual hematocrit is 0.40 (40%); this represents a blood volume of 5 L (2 L of red blood cells [RBC] and 3 L of plasma):

Hematocrit (0.40) = 2 L RBC/Blood volume (5 L total volume), (2 L RBC + 3 L plasma)

Therefore when the hematocrit is 0.50, the plasma volume equals the of RBC volume (i.e., 2 L):

Hematocrit (0.50) = (4 L total volume, 2 L RBC L blood volume)

The present blood volume is 4 L, and thus the plasma volume is 2 L. Hence the plasma volume is reduced by 1 L from its normal value of 3 L. Ignoring changes in Starling forces for simplicity, the ECF volume is diminished by $\sim$33%; this implies that rapid restoration of ECF volume would lead to a $[HCO_3^-]$ that is 33% of its measured value.

13. In a patient without an elevated anion gap, with a hyperchloremic metabolic acidosis, estimate the urinary excretion of NH_4^+.

If increased protons are added to the circulation with the "unmeasured" anions discussed previously, an increase in the anion gap occurs. But if such anions are not present, added protons will appear to have been added as hydrochloric acid, HCl. This is because when protons accumulate and serum bicarbonate falls, the kidney will have to reabsorb Na^+ with Cl^-, out of proportion to normal $[Cl^-]$. The result is that the anion gap does not change and hyperchloremic acidosis ensues. A major example is renal tubular acidosis (RTA), where the kidney fails to excrete protons. The loss of HCO_3^- in the stool, with diarrhea, is another example. Again, Na^+ is reabsorbed in the kidney with Cl^-, and hyperchloremic acidosis occurs. For practical purposes, hyperchloremic metabolic acidosis is due either to diarrhea or RTA. Other disorders that lead to hyperchloremic metabolic acidosis generally fall into one of these categories.

In the context of a *chronic* hyperchloremic metabolic acidosis and normal renal function, the urinary excretion NH_4^+ of should rise, and can exceed 200 mmol/day. Most laboratories do not measure U_{NH_4} (without good reason); therefore one way to indirectly estimate U_{NH_4} is the urine osmolal gap ($U_{Osmolal\ gap}$). Because NH_4^+ is excreted with an anion, U_{NH_4} is half the calculated value of $U_{Osmolal\ gap}$.

$$U_{Osmolal\ gap} = Measured\ U_{Osm} - Calculated\ U_{Osm}$$

$$Calculated\ U_{Osm} = 2\,(U_{Na} + U_K) + U_{Urea}\ all\ in\ mmol/L$$

$\left(\text{The concentration of glusoce in the urine} \left(U_{Glucose}\right) \text{ should be added in patients with hyperglycemia}\right)$.

To convert U_{NH_4} into an excretion rate, divide it by the concentration of creatinine in the urine ($U_{Creatinine}$). If the ratio of $U_{NH_4}/U_{Creatinine}$ is considerably <40 mmol/g creatinine (or <4, in mmol/mmol terms), a low rate of excretion of NH_4^+ is likely to be an important cause of the acidemia; such pathophysiology is a hallmark of RTA.

14. In a patient without an elevated anion gap (with hyperchloremic metabolic acidosis) and a low rate of excretion of NH_4^+, what is the basis for a low NH_4^+ excretion rate (Fig. 78.5)?

The urine pH is most valuable to identify the pathophysiology of the low rate of excretion of NH_4^+. If the urine pH is greater than 6.5, the low rate of excretion of NH_4^+ is likely the result of a reduced net rate of distal H^+ secretion. In contrast, if the urine pH $\sim$5, the low rate of excretion of NH_4^+ is usually the result of a disease, leading to a diminished production of NH_4^+ in the proximal convoluted tubule (PCT). However, if urine pH is $\sim$6, there will be a defect that lowers the availability of both H^+ and NH_3 in the lumen of the medullary collecting duct.

15. In a patient with hyperchloremic metabolic acidosis and a low rate of excretion of NH_4^+, is there a defect in H^+ secretion in the PCT?

Patients with defective reabsorption of $NaHCO_3$ in the PCT have proximal RTA (also called Type 2 RTA). Since the distal tubule secretes protons normally, such patients will usually have an acidic urine pH (less than 6) as long as they are not administered alkali. While not readily available in most clinical labs, urinary bicarbonate measurement can help detect a proximal defect. A fractional excretion of

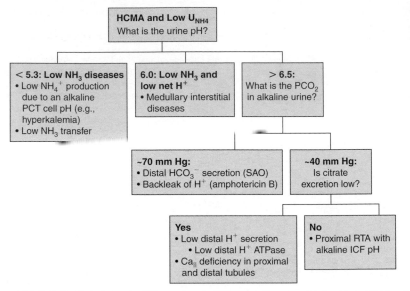

Figure 78.5. Evaluating the basis for a low NH_4^+ excretion rate. *HCMA*, Hyperchloremic metabolic acidosis; *ICF*, intracellular fluid; *PCT*, proximal convoluted tubule; *RTA*, renal tubular acidosis; *SAO*, Southeast Asian ovalocytosis.

HCO_3^- that is more than 15% of the filtered load after giving a $NaHCO_3$ load that increases the $[HCO_3]$ to $\sim$24 mmol/L indicates a defect in H^+ secretion (via the sodium-hydrogen exchanger [NHE3]) in the PCT. Only when given alkali will these patients experience an alkaline urine pH. This test, however, should not be performed in a patient with hypokalemia until the P_K has been raised to the normal range, because of the risk of worsening hypokalemia and inducing a cardiac arrhythmia.

One secret for detecting the presence of reduced PCT function in patients with an alkaline PCT is the finding of a high rate of urinary citrate excretion. High urinary citrate excretion may result from isolated or generalized (e.g., Fanconi syndrome) PCT dysfunction. Other causes of metabolic acidosis (hyperchloremic metabolic acidosis or distal RTA) are expected to stimulate PCT reabsorption of citrate via a sodium-dicarboxylate cotransporter that is pH sensitive. Citrate, like other organic anions, represents a potential base, and should be reclaimed in states of metabolic acidosis.

16. What is the basis of hyperchloremic metabolic acidosis in a patient with a low rate of excretion of NH_4^+ and a urine pH >6.5?
    If the urine pH is >6.5, the low rate of excretion of NH_4^+ is a result of a reduced net rate of distal H^+ secretion. Such patients have distal RTA (also called Type I RTA). Again, while not readily available in most clinical laboratories, the basis of the distal lesion can be elucidated by measurement of the PCO_2 in alkaline urine (see Fig. 78.5); one group has reported the use of blood gas analysis machines to measure urinary pH and carbon dioxide with calculation of urinary bicarbonate via the Henderson-Hasselbalch equation. Patients with H^+ pump defect (a congenital or an acquired defect resulting from a number of autoimmune or disorders with hypergammaglobulinemia; e.g., Sjögren syndrome) have a PCO_2 in their alkaline urine that approaches its value in their arterial blood. Conversely, in disorders whereby HCO_3^- is secreted in the distal nephron (some patients with Southeast Asian ovalocytosis, with mutations in a Cl/HCO_3 anion exchanger, AE1, present in RBC and in the nephron) or if H^+ back-diffuse in the distal nephron (e.g., due to effects of drugs such as amphotericin B), the PCO_2 in alkaline urine will be elevated. A high rate of urinary citrate excretion in these patients indicates that the underlying lesion also involves the proximal tubule cells (e.g., carbonic anhydrase II deficiency). These patients fail to excrete their daily proton load and are in positive acid balance.

17. In a patient with hyperchloremic metabolic acidosis and a high rate of excretion of NH_4^+, what anion accompanied NH_4^+ in the urine?
    In a patient with hyperchloremic metabolic acidosis and a high rate of excretion of NH_4^+, if the urine anion is Cl^-, the cause of the hyperchloremic metabolic acidosis is usually loss of $NaHCO_3$ via the GI

tract or, potentially, hyperchloremia from the infusion of normal saline, which has a higher $[Cl^-]$ than plasma. By contrast, if the anion is not Cl^-, suspect that the cause of metabolic acidosis is overproduction of an organic acid, the anion of which is excreted in the urine at a very rapid rate (e.g., secreted hippuric acid in the patient with glue sniffing). The presence of a high rate of excretion of organic anions or HCO_3^- (very high urine pH) in the urine can be detected with the calculation of the urine anion gap ($U_{Na} + U_K + U_{NH_4} - U_{Cl}$, all in mEq/L terms); for this calculation, the concentration of NH_4^+ in the urine (U_{NH_4}) can be estimated using the urine osmolal gap as described previously (see Table 78.1).

18. Does the strong ion difference provide an improved way to determine the cause of an acid–base disorder?

    The calculation of the strong ion difference (the Stewart approach) and the $P_{Anion\ gap}$ are used by clinicians to detect the addition of new acids in a patient with metabolic acidosis. Although the strong ion difference is popular with some specialists, the authors do not use it. The advantage of the strong ion difference approach is that its calculation takes into account the net negative charge on $P_{Albumin}$. The calculation of the strong ion difference is complex; this advantage over the calculation of the $P_{Anion\ gap}$ is easily negated if one were to adjust the baseline value of the $P_{Anion\ gap}$ for the $P_{Albumin}$ routinely. Of note, both the strong ion difference and the $P_{Anion\ gap}$ approaches rely on the concentration of HCO_3^- and ignore the content of HCO_3^- in the ECF compartment. Furthermore, as pointed out earlier, an important initial step in the clinical approach in patients with metabolic acidosis is to determine if the BBS in skeletal muscle is functioning effectively to remove the bulk of the added new H^+ and minimize the rise in the concentration of H^+ and thereby the binding of H^+ to intracellular proteins in vital organs such as the brain and the heart; this information can be only obtained by measuring the brachial or the femoral venous PCO_2. This is, however, not part of the usual clinical approach whether clinicians use the strong anion difference or the $P_{Anion\ gap}$, because both approaches rely *solely* on the arterial PCO_2 to assess buffering of H^+ by the BBS.

SPECIFIC DISORDERS: THE ANION GAP ACIDOSES

19. Does the presence of elevated serum lactate indicate the presence of cellular hypoxia?

    The secret here is that lactate elevation, even during severe sepsis and septic shock, often occurs in cells that are *not* hypoxic. *Both* glycolysis *and* lactate formation are "anaerobic," because oxygen is not required for these reactions to occur; it is *anaerobic chemistry* regardless of the status of the mitochondria and function of oxidative phosphorylation. The reason for lactate elevation under physiological stress is the activity of epinephrine on muscle and increased glycolysis (discussed later); lactate concentration falls with provision of volume, not because hypoxic tissue is reperfused, but because the stress response is mitigated, just as the heart rate falls in response to volume.

    The formation of lactate does not generate an intracellular proton load (discussed later). Nevertheless, when oxygen consumption in tissue falls (e.g., in ischemic gut or arterial thromboses), true tissue-hypoxic physiology will take hold. In this situation, the protons generated by intracellular adenosine triphosphate (ATP) hydrolysis can no longer be recycled by oxidative phosphorylation. Lactate rises because oxidative phosphorylation has ceased, but it is not the lactate that is causing the acidosis; the elevation of lactate is coincident to the cessation of oxidative phosphorylation, which itself is the reason for the elaboration of intracellular protons.

20. What is the biomedical basis for very rapid rates of production of L-lactate?

    The secret to understanding this pathophysiology is that there are two substrates for glycolysis (glucose and adenosine diphosphate [ADP]). In addition, the availability of ADP controls the rate of conversion of glucose to pyruvate and, consequently, L-lactate:
    1. Work + ATP $\rightarrow$ ADP + Pi + H^+
    2. Glucose + 2Pi + 2ADP + 2NAD$^+$ $\rightarrow$ 2Pyruvate + 2ATP + 2NADH + 2 H^+ + 2H_2O
    3. 2Pyruvate + 2NADH + 2 H^+ $\rightarrow$ 2Lactate + 2NAD$^+$

    First, note that the conversion of glucose to pyruvate *produces 2 protons*, while metabolism of pyruvate to lactate *consumes 2 protons* (compare equations 2 and 3). Thus it is not the generation of lactate per se that causes acidosis. Second, L-lactate production from glucose also depends on having high levels of ADP as a substrate (equation 2).

    Fast production of L-lactate occurs under states of increased biochemical/cellular work and high glycolytic flux. Increased work can be the result of physiological stress and epinephrine release, for example with strenuous exercise, seizure, and sepsis. Notably, the increase in cellular $[H^+]$ is not from a malfunctioning electron transport chain. Rather, increased ATP hydrolysis releases protons and increased glycolysis raises lactate—even under fully aerobic conditions. This reiterates the following important—and often clinically confusing—distinction: lactate production is "anaerobic" only in that oxygen is not chemically required for its synthesis; *however, "anaerobic" chemistry does not necessitate cellular hypoxia!*

Nevertheless, in states of *severe* organ hypoperfusion, L-lactate will rise rapidly if tissue oxygen delivery becomes so critical that tissue oxygen consumption falls (e.g., when systemic hemodynamics is severely compromised); this usually requires a cardiac output of less than 2 L/min. Lactate elevation in this situation is consequent to true tissue hypoxia.

Slower forms of L-lactate elevation occurs when the usual rate of lactate removal is diminished. The major reason for this pathophysiology is a marked decrease in liver mass or a compromised metabolism of pyruvate resulting from lower activities of the major enzymes that catalyze pyruvate metabolism: pyruvate dehydrogenase (PDH) or pyruvate carboxylase. A diminished activity of PDH may result from lesser amounts of the enzyme, the absence of one of its essential cofactors (e.g., vitamin B_1 or thiamine), or the presence of inhibitors of PDH activity such as the products of oxidation of fat-derived fuels (e.g., high ATP or low ADP, high acetyl-coenzyme A [CoA] or low CoASH, or high NADH or low NAD^+). Similarly, low activity of pyruvate carboxylase or the availability of its cofactor, biotin, can lead to the need for higher levels of pyruvate (and hence L-lactate) in liver cells to permit the conversion of pyruvate to glucose or glycogen.

21. Under what circumstances will the ingestion of ethanol cause a serious degree of L-lactate elevation? As shown in this equation, NADH is the other substrate for L-lactate dehydrogenase:

$$Pyruvate + NADH \rightarrow L\text{-Lactate} + NAD^+.$$

A means by which NADH rises within the cytosol is the metabolism of ethanol:

$$Ethanol + NAD^+ \rightarrow Acetate + NADH.$$

Hence the combination of a high concentration of pyruvate *and* a high concentration of NADH will result in a very large accumulation of L-lactate. In other words, when the *only* lesion is thiamine deficiency, the result will be a modest increase in the $P_{L\text{-lactate}}$. Similarly, high rates of oxidation of ethanol will result in a high concentration of NADH but only a modest rise in the rate of L-lactate production and $P_{L\text{-lactate}}$ of ~4 to 5 mmol/L. Accordingly, should a patient—who is thiamine deficient—consume a large amount of ethanol, plasma L-lactate may rise to a greater degree than expected.

22. What is the basis of chronic L-lactate elevation in patients who are malnourished?
   • Thiamine deficiency: Thiamine (vitamin B_1) deficiency is reasonably common in chronic alcoholics. Absence of this cofactor retards the conversion of pyruvate into acetyl-CoA because thiamine is a component of the active form of PDH. Importantly, because the oxidation of glucose via PDH must occur in the brain, these patients need therapy with thiamine at the outset to prevent the development of Wernicke-Korsakoff encephalopathy.
   • Riboflavin deficiency: Deficiency of riboflavin (vitamin B_2) impairs oxidative phosphorylation because vitamin B_2 is a necessary cofactor for the conversion of ADP to ATP in mitochondria. This is more likely if the patient is taking a tricyclic antidepressant drug, because this class of drugs prevents the formation of the active form of riboflavin.

23. Discuss lactate elevation and acidosis in metformin toxicity.
   Metformin—and its predecessor phenformin—provide another opportunity to distinguish between *lactate elevation* and *acidosis*. The mechanism of the acidosis is the inability of oxidative phosphorylation to function properly. These antidiabetic medications act as uncoupling agents (i.e., poisons that carry H^+ across the inner mitochondrial membrane, which decreases the rate of regeneration of ATP by mitochondria). Thus the proton load, which needs to be dealt with by the BBS, comes from dysfunctional mitochondria. The lactate elevation is coincident to impaired oxidative phosphorylation, but is not, in and of itself, the etiology of the proton bolus.
   • Metformin is not very soluble in lipids and is therefore a weak uncoupler; it rarely (in the absence of an acute overdose) is the sole cause of lactate elevation and acidosis. In contradistinction, phenformin is a much stronger uncoupler because it is much more soluble in the lipid in the inner membranes of hepatic mitochondria. Consequently, to a much greater degree, it prevents the conversion of ADP + Pi + H+ → ATP when oxygen is consumed. Because ADP + Pi are the

other substrates for glycolysis, there is much more L-lactate formed than can be removed by metabolic means:

$$Work + ATP^{4-} \rightarrow ADP^{3-} + PI^{2-} + H^+$$

$$Glucose + 2Pi + 2ADP + 2NAD^+ \rightarrow 2Pyruvate + 2ATP + 2NADH + 2H^+ + 2H_2O$$

$$2Pyruvate + 2NADH + 2H^+ \rightarrow 2Lactate + 2NAD^+$$

As noted previously, the secret here is that instead of oxygen acting as the terminal electron/proton *consumer* (converted to water), pyruvate acts as the electron and proton *consumer* and is converted to lactate. The result of uncoupling, therefore, is metabolic acidosis *with coincident lactate elevation*.

The current recommendation is to initiate metformin in patients only when their estimated glomerular filtration rate (eGFR) is above 45 mL/min/1.73 m^2; consider the risks and benefits of continuation when eGFR is between 30 and 45 mL/min/1.73 m^2 and discontinue when eGFR is less than 30 mL/min/1.73 m^2. Notably, lactic acidosis associated with metformin use, though rare, is more likely at lower levels of glomerular filtration rate (GFR). The fact that the incidence of metformin-associated lactic acidosis remains extremely low, and that the drug is associated with significant benefit for hyperglycemia, has led to some controversy and debate about these recommendations.

24. Discuss D-lactate elevation.

There are multiple putative mechanisms for D-lactate elevation and its clinical consequences. First, there is a functional separation between glucose absorption in the jejunum and bacteria, which are located primarily in the colon. If this functional segregation is disturbed, the risk of D-lactate elevation is increased because it is gut bacteria, which elaborate D-lactate. Disruption of normal bacterial flora (e.g., from antibiotic therapy) may result in their abnormal migration and proliferation in the small intestine. Further, certain sugars (e.g., fructose) that are poorly absorbed in the small intestine may be delivered to the colon when their intake is high. In addition, decreased bowel motility (e.g., blind loops, drugs) increases the contact time for bacteria and sugar, and as a result, more organic acids may be produced. Lastly, antacids or drugs that inhibit gastric H$^+$ secretion may lead to a higher pH that is more favorable for bacterial growth and metabolism.

Organic acids, noxious alcohols, aldehydes, amines, and mercaptans produced during fermentation may lead to many of the central nervous system symptoms that are observed in this disorder.

Humans metabolize D-lactate more slowly than L-lactate. D-lactate may also be excreted in the urine, and hence the rise in the P$_{Anion\ gap}$ may be lower than expected, as judged from the fall in bicarbonate concentration.

The usual laboratory test for "lactate" detects L-lactate but not D-lactate. Hence a specific assay for D-lactate must be performed to confirm the diagnosis. An anion gap will be present, but the lactate measurement will be falsely low.

Treatment should be directed at the gastrointestinal (GI) problem. The oral intake of fructose and complex carbohydrates should be decreased. Antacids should be avoided, and drugs that diminish GI motility should be stopped. Poorly absorbed antibiotics (e.g., vancomycin) could be used to change the bacterial flora. Insulin may be helpful by lowering the rate of oxidation of fatty acids and hence permitting a higher rate of oxidation of organic acids.

25. Discuss alcoholic ketoacidosis as a cause of metabolic acidosis.

One substrate of acetyl-CoA production is ethanol: both contain two carbon atoms. In starvation, a substrate for acetyl-CoA are the fatty acids. Acetyl-CoA has multiple fates, one of which is the genesis of ketoacids. For high levels of ketoacids to accumulate, however, the conversion of acetyl-CoA to fatty acids (lipogenesis) must cease. Acetyl-CoA carboxylase is the key enzyme that transforms acetyl-CoA into fatty acids, and it is inhibited by epinephrine, which may be present in alcoholics due to subtle volume depletion from deficient solute intake. In addition, hypoglycemia (described later) stimulates epinephrine release.

There is an important difference, however, between ketoacid formation from fatty acids (e.g., starvation) versus ethanol as a major substrate. When long-chain fatty acids are the foundation for ketogenesis, there is a lag period before ketoacids are produced at a rapid rate; there is no lag when ethanol is the substrate. Thus, in alcoholic ketoacidosis, there tends to be a "rapid ketosis." Nevertheless, the degree of acidemia may be blunted by the presence of metabolic alkalosis (e.g., from vomiting) or respiratory alkalosis (e.g., hyperventilation from aspiration pneumonia or alcohol withdrawal).

Patients with alcoholic ketoacidosis can be classified into two groups with regard to their clinical presentation. The first group consists of normal subjects who consumed a large amount of ethanol, and the second group consists primarily of chronic alcoholics who had a binge intake of ethanol. The $P_{Glucose}$ on admission may help identify each group because patients in the latter group who are malnourished will usually have hypoglycemia. This point is emphasized because these patients are likely to have other nutritional deficiencies (e.g., thiamine deficiency). It is critical to administer thiamine (and probably riboflavin) early in therapy in these patients; this will permit aerobic oxidation of glucose in the brain once ketoacids disappear and prevent the development of Wernicke's encephalopathy.

These patients are likely also to be potassium depleted (especially if there is a prolonged history of vomiting), despite normokalemia and perhaps hyperkalemia on presentation, because the α-adrenergic surge inhibits the release of insulin and causes potassium to shift out of cells. Once the effective arterial blood volume is expanded, the α-adrenergic surge disappears, insulin is released, and potassium moves back into the cells. Do not wait for hypokalemia to develop before administering KCl.

No specific therapy is needed for ketoacidosis because excessive production of ketoacids ceases once the alcohol disappears. Furthermore, utilization of ketoacids by the brain (as the ethanol level falls) and the kidney (as GFR improves) increases. Therapy with $NaHCO_3$ is not needed in most cases (and may be dangerous if the patient is potassium depleted).

26. **What is the basis of hypoglycemia in alcohol dependence?**
When ethanol is oxidized in the liver, there is a rise in the $NADH:NAD^+$ ratio in hepatocytes. This leads to the conversion of pyruvate to lactate, because these two metabolic intermediates can be interconverted by a NAD^+-like dehydrogenase with a very large catalytic capacity. This reduces the rate of formation of glucose from pyruvate (i.e., hepatic gluconeogenesis) and leads to hypoglycemia in the malnourished alcoholic. This high $NADH:NAD^+$ ratio also leads to conversion of acetoacetic acid to β-hydroxybutyric acid, which becomes the major form of ketoacids released from the liver. This leads to less formation of acetone, and hence its odor may not be detected in exhaled air at the bedside. Furthermore, the nitroprusside test result, which is used as a quick assay for ketones, may be falsely negative because it detects acetone and acetoacetate but not β-hydroxybutyrate.

27. **Discuss starvation ketoacidosis as a cause of metabolic acidosis.**
The brain needs biochemical fuel to oxidize the regeneration of the ATP consumed when work is performed in this organ. Its major fuels are glucose in the fed state and ketoacid anions during starvation.

When there is hypoglycemia, insulin levels decline because the major stimulus to release insulin from β cells of the pancreas is glucose. Further, when glucose is low, more epinephrine is released, which augments lipolysis in adipose tissue and promotes hepatic ketogenesis by inhibiting acetyl-CoA carboxylase, the key enzyme in the conversion of acetyl-CoA to fatty acids (described previously). As the concentration of acetyl-CoA rises in hepatocytes, the synthesis of ketoacids increases.

The degree of acidemia in pure starvation is usually modest (P_{HCO_3} ~19 mmol/L, with a normal ECF volume so there is a very modest decrease in the content of HCO_3^- in the ECF compartment), although the rate of production of ketoacids may be as high as in a patient with diabetic ketoacidosis (DKA). This is because there is a relatively rapid rate of removal of ketoacids in the brain (the $P_{Glucose}$ is low, which permits a higher rate of ketoacid oxidation in the brain) and in the kidneys (GFR is not low, so the kidneys will oxidize more fuel [ketoacid anions] to provide the ATP needed to reabsorb the filtered Na^+).

Treatment of starvation ketoacidosis is simply the provision of glucose.

28. **Discuss DKA as a cause of metabolic acidosis.**
DKA is a very broad topic. A few secrets to consider are cerebral edema (CE), gastric emptying, and the notion of 1:1 change in the anion gap to fall in venous bicarbonate.

CE occurs in very young patients and is responsible for mortality or significant morbidity in ~1 of 150 children treated for DKA, even in the best pediatric medical centers. CE occurs more commonly during the first episode of DKA, which is often more severe, possibly because of the long delay in making the diagnosis. CE usually becomes evident, with little warning, 5 to 15 hours after therapy is instituted.

CE is a clinical diagnosis—it should be suspected if a headache or vomiting develops, if there is unexpected deterioration in neurologic status, or if there is an unexpected rise in blood pressure and a fall in heart rate. Therefore these patients should be admitted to a unit where they can be observed closely, because therapy must be instituted without delay to minimize the risk of permanent brain damage.

The secret here is that because serum $[Na^+]$ tends to fall in the setting of hyperglycemia, one may be tempted to think that rapid correction of serum glucose, with consequent *rise* in serum $[Na^+]$, would place the patient at risk for osmotic demyelination syndrome. The risk, however, is *cerebral*

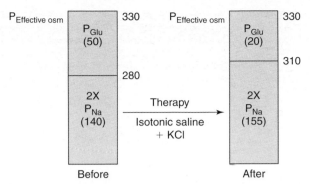

Figure 78.6. Defense of the effective osmolality of plasma. A rise in the P_{Na} is needed to prevent a fall in the $P_{Effective\ Osm}$ when there is a fall in the $P_{Glucose}$. If the P_{Na} on admission is close to 140 mmol/L, the P_{Na} should rise to 155 mmol/L when the $P_{Glucose}$ falls from 50 mmol/L (900 mg/dL) to 20 mmol/L (360 mg/dL) to maintain a constant $P_{Effective\ Osm}$.

edema. The intracellular volume is the largest intracranial compartment; the shift of glucose into cells will be accompanied by water with subsequent cell swelling. Therefore it is imperative that one prevent a fall in the effective osmolality in plasma ($P_{Effective\ osm}$). Because the most common cause for a large fall in the $P_{Effective\ osm}$ is the large decrease in the $P_{Glucose}$ early during therapy, the P_{Na} must rise by one half of the fall in the $P_{Glucose}$ (glucose in mmol/L) to prevent a fall in the $P_{Effective\ osm}$; Fig. 78.6).

There may be an "occult" factor that contributes to the development of a rapid infusion of free water into the vascular compartment. Although stomach emptying is usually slow in the patient with a high $P_{Glucose}$, it is a source of an infusion of water with or without glucose but with few electrolytes. Although this is more likely to occur once the $P_{Glucose}$ has decreased, it may also occur at other times.

29. What are the clues to suggest that there was an occult stomach emptying?
When a subject drinks a beverage that contains sugar to quench his or her thirst, some of this glucose (and water) will remain in the stomach because hyperglycemia slows stomach emptying. This will represent a gain of water after this fluid is absorbed and its glucose is removed by metabolic means. The following observations, however, are clues that stomach emptying and absorption of a sugar-containing solution occurred in a patient with hyperglycemia. However, a fall in $P_{Effective\ osm}$ may suggest that stomach emptying and absorption of water has occurred.
- A rise in $P_{Glucose}$ in the absence of an infusion of solutions containing glucose or a precursor of glucose, such as L-lactate
- A sudden large rise in the urine output as a result of a glucose-induced osmotic diuresis
- Absence of a sufficient fall in $P_{Glucose}$ despite the excretion of glucose in the urine

30. What therapy should be given if CE is suspected?
Because there is such a high mortality and morbidity rate once CE develops as a result of brain herniation, one must draw water out of the brain. This means that the patient must be given a rapid intravenous infusion of hypertonic saline, using the clinical response as the guide to further therapy. The goal is for an increase in $[Na^+]$ to oppose the decrease in $P_{Glucose}$. Do not send the patient for imaging studies, because the CE can worsen very quickly. Be aware because the stomach may contain fluid that will become hypotonic after it is absorbed and the glucose is removed by metabolic means.

31. Will the venous bicarbonate fall to the same degree as the rise in anion gap?
Consider a 50-kg patient with DKA, a P_{HCO_3} of 10 mmol/L and the "expected" 1:1 relationship between the rise in the plasma anion gap ($P_{Anion\ gap}$) and the fall in the plasma bicarbonate concentration $[HCO_3^-]$. The patient had a normal ECF volume of 10 L before DKA developed, but as a result of the glucose-induced osmotic diuresis, his current ECF volume is 8 L. Examine the *contents* of bicarbonate and ketoacids (Table 78.2), when the fall in the bicarbonate *concentration* and the rise in the ketoacid *concentration* are equal. The deficit of HCO_3^- is 170 mmol, but the quantity of new anions in the ECF is only 120 mEq; in other words, more bicarbonate is lost than one would predict using only concentrations, not contents, as a guide (see Table 78.1).

But why is more bicarbonate lost? There was an indirect loss of HCO_3^- when ketoacids were added; some of the ketoacid anions were excreted in the urine with Na^+, an indirect form of $NaHCO_3$

Table 78.2. Changes in the Content of HCO_3^- and New Anions in the Extracellular Fluid Compartment

CONDITION	ECF VOLUME	HCO_3^- CONCENTRATION (Mmol/L)	HCO_3^- CONTENT (Mmol)	KA^- CONCENTRATION (Mmol/L)	KA^- CONTENT (Mmol)
Normal	10 L	25	250	0	0
DKA	8 L	10	80	15	120
Balance	-2 L	—	170	—	-120

DKA, Diabetic ketoacidosis; ECF, extracellular fluid; KA^-, ketoacid anions.
In these calculations, we ignored changes in the $P_{Albumin}$ for simplicity.

loss. This loss of HCO_3^- is not reflected by an increase in $P_{Anion\ gap}$. Hence the rise in $P_{Anion\ gap}$ did not reveal the actual quantity of ketoacids that were added, and the fall in bicarbonate concentration did not reflect the actual magnitude of the deficit of HCO_3^-. With re-expansion of the ECF volume with the administration of saline, the true deficit of HCO_3^- will become evident because the fall in the $P_{Anion\ gap}$ will not be matched by an equal rise in the $[HCO_3^-]$. In addition, the anion gap will fall to a greater degree, as more ketoacid anions will be lost in urine. This is because their filtered load is increased with the increase in GFR as a result of re-expansion of effective arterial blood volume.

32. Discuss toxin-induced metabolic acidosis.
    Ingestion of methanol, propanediol, or ethylene glycol should be suspected in a patient with metabolic acidosis, an elevated $P_{Anion\ gap}$, and no obvious cause for these findings, especially if the ECF volume is not significantly contracted. Failure to make this diagnosis can be devastating. If ingestion of these alcohols is suspected, one must calculate the $P_{Osmolal\ gap}$; be suspicious if this value is considerably greater than 20 mOsm/kg H_2O. As discussed previously, the $P_{Osmolal\ gap}$ may be present early in the presentation and the $P_{Anion\ gap}$ only later. As the former disappears, the latter increases. It is not the ingested parent compound that is toxic, but rather the downstream metabolites. Because of this, the metabolism must be stopped with fomepizole, an alcohol dehydrogenase inhibitor. Fomepizole is preferred in the treatment of patients with methanol or ethylene glycol poisoning instead of ethanol, which itself leads to reduced levels of consciousness and other adverse effects. Fomepizole is easy to dose and administer, and side effects are rare; its main disadvantage is its high cost. It may not be available in all locations. Administering fomepizole or ethanol to prevent metabolism of the alcohols to their toxic metabolites (oxalate for ethylene glycol and formaldehyde and formic acid for methanol) is appropriate when these ingestions are suspected, even before the facts are made clear by direct assays for toxic alcohols.

33. What type of metabolic acidosis develops in patients who receive propane 1,2-diol?
    Propane 1,2-diol (propylene glycol) is commonly used as a diluent for many intravenous (or intramuscular) drug preparations (e.g., lorazepam, which may be used in large doses as a sedative in the intensive care unit and to treat delirium tremens). It is also used as a solvent for other drugs like cough medicine and, at times, without proper labeling. When given in large quantities, this alcohol can be detected by finding a large $P_{Osmolal\ gap}$. The danger associated with its use is that one of its metabolites is an aldehyde, which is in general very toxic.
    Propane 1,2-diol is a 50:50 mixture of D and L isoforms. Approximately 40% of the administered dose is excreted unchanged in the urine, whereas 60% is metabolized in the liver by alcohol dehydrogenase to lactaldehyde. L-lactaldehyde is then metabolized by aldehyde dehydrogenase to L-lactic acid (Fig. 78.7). D-lactaldehyde, however, is not a good substrate for aldehyde dehydrogenase. Therefore it accumulates and leads to many of the toxic effects observed in this setting. D-lactaldehyde can be metabolized in the liver via an alternate pathway that uses reduced glutathione (GSH) as a cofactor to D-lactic acid. Because D-lactic acid is metabolized much slower than L-lactic acid, the acid that accumulates is principally D-lactic acid. The most important step in therapy is to stop the formation of D-lactaldehyde by giving ethanol or fomepizole. This must be followed up by removal of propane 1,2-diol by hemodialysis.

34. What are considerations in patients who ingest rubbing alcohol?
    The principal use of isopropanol (commonly known as "rubbing alcohol") is as a topical antiseptic. This three-carbon alcohol has the β-OH group on the middle carbon. When oxidized by hepatic

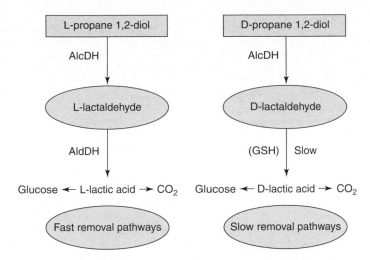

Figure 78.7. Metabolism of propane 1,2-diol to L-lactic acid and D-lactic acid. When a large quantity of propane 1,2-diol is ingested, the body is presented with a racemic mixture. Both the L-form *(shown to the left of the vertical dashed line)* and the D-form *(shown to the right of the vertical dashed line)* are substrates for alcohol dehydrogenase *(AlcDH)*; hence their metabolism occurs in the liver. The products are L-lactaldehyde and D-lactaldehyde, which are substrates for aldehyde dehydrogenase *(AldDH)*, but the D-form is a much poorer substrate, and the D-lactaldehyde accumulates and is responsible for most of the toxicity. The cofactors, NAD^+ and NADH, are not shown for simplicity. *GSH*, Glutathione.

NAD^+-linked alcohol dehydrogenase, the alcohol group is converted to a keto group forming acetone:

$$\text{Isopropyl alcohol} + NAD^+ \rightarrow \text{Acetone} + NADH$$

Thus there is no accumulation of H^+ in this metabolic process. The acetone is volatile and has a characteristic fruity odor; it reacts with the Ketostix reagent, yielding a positive test for ketones, which in the absence of metabolic acidosis and a high value for the plasma osmolal gap should lead the clinician to the correct diagnosis.

No toxic effects can be attributed to acetone. Patients may appear intoxicated and should be managed in a similar fashion to patients with ethanol overdose. Hemodialysis is rarely indicated, except in patients with massive ingestion who are hemodynamically unstable despite aggressive supportive measures.

35. What is the danger in patients who have high levels of pyroglutamic acid?

    In this situation, with acetaminophen overdoses, the metabolic acidosis is a marker of a more serious underlying disorder; the threat to life results from depletion of glutathione and hence compromised ability to detoxify reactive oxygen species. The metabolic acidosis warns the clinician of this pathophysiology; the treatment is not directed at the acidosis, but rather at the repletion of glutathione. The clinician should consider administering N-acetyl cysteine to prevent potentially lethal hepatic toxicity. Riboflavin should also be given because flavin nucleotides are cofactors for glutathione reductase.

SPECIFIC DISORDERS: THE NON-ANION GAP ACIDOSES

36. Discuss diarrhea as a cause of metabolic acidosis.

    Contemplating a case of severe diarrhea can help reveal some of the physiological secrets of the non-anion gap metabolic acidoses.

    Case: A previously healthy 25-year-old man develops massive diarrhea over 24 hours (stool volume was estimated ~5 L) after he drank contaminated water. His blood pressure is 90/60 mm Hg with a pulse of 110 beats/min, and his jugular venous pressure is low. He has no urine output since arrival. Acid–base measurements in arterial blood reveal a pH of 7.39, P_{HCO_3} 12 mmol/L, and a $PaCO_2$ of 21 mm Hg; his $P_{Anion\ gap}$ is 20 mEq/L, his hematocrit is 0.60 and total protein is 11 g/dL.

37. Does this patient have a metabolic acidosis?
   Recall from the previous discussion the difference between acidosis and acidemia. An acidosis is a process that contributes to a low serum pH (i.e., addition of protons or loss of bicarbonate), yet this does not guarantee an acidemia, which is a measured proton excess in the blood. One can have an acidosis without an acidemia if there is a compensatory or competing alkalosis. Therefore the patient does not have an acidemia, but certainly has an underlying, severe acidosis, as evidenced by the low serum bicarbonate.

38. What are the concurrent/competing alkaloses?
   Importantly, because the bicarbonate concentration reflects the content of HCO_3^- in the ECF compartment divided by the ECF volume, the measured concentration is elevated by a very large decrease in the ECF volume. Notably the hematocrit of 0.60 provides a quantitative, minimum estimate that his plasma volume was reduced from 3.0 L to ~1.3 L (i.e., >50%).
   Furthermore, the patient has a mild respiratory alkalosis potentially triggered by anxiety or volume depletion itself. Using Winter's formula ($[1.5 \times \{HCO_3^-\}] + 8 \pm 2$), the expected $PaCO_2$ is 24 to 28 mm Hg; his is measured at 21 mm Hg. Accordingly, there is a mild respiratory alkalosis.
   Thus he has multiple, concurrent acid–base disorders: metabolic acidosis secondary to bicarbonate/potential bicarbonate loss from the gut and metabolic alkalosis from the very low ECF volume. In addition, there is a mild respiratory alkalosis. The competing processes resulted in a normal proton concentration (pH).

39. What is the basis for the high $P_{Anion\ gap}$?
   One must distinguish between a process leading to a deficit of HCO_3^-, for example (as suggested by a history of diarrhea, and a process that caused the addition of acids [as suggested by the rise in $P_{Anion\ gap}$]) because of different implications for therapy. The high $P_{Anion\ gap}$ resulted mainly from a very high $P_{Albumin}$ (as evidenced by the high total protein) rather than the addition of new acids. This was confirmed because the concentrations of lactate and ketoacid anions in plasma were less than 2 mmol/L. An increase in the anion gap secondary to hyperproteinemia in cholera has been well described and may be considered an important secret.

40. What dangers should be anticipated when this patient is given a large infusion of isotonic saline?
   - **A very severe degree of acidemia:** There will be a fall in the bicarbonate concentration when a large volume of saline without $NaHCO_3$ is given to a patient who has a very severe degree of ECF volume contraction, because this infused solution will lower the bicarbonate concentration by dilution. In fact, it is reported that when saline was infused very rapidly, a subset of these patients developed pulmonary edema before the ECF volume was totally re-expanded. Putatively, this is the result of a severe acidemia and consequent redistribution of blood from the peripheral to the central circulating blood volume. It is important to recognize this complication, because pulmonary edema can be prevented and treated successfully with an infusion of fluid that contains $NaHCO_3$ (or an anion that can be metabolized quickly to produce HCO_3^-; e.g., L-lactate in Ringer lactate solution). In addition to dilution, two other mechanisms may lead to an unanticipated severe acidemia with the infusion of a large amount of saline in these patients.
   - **Loss of more $NaHCO_3$ in diarrhea fluid:** Re-expansion of the arterial blood volume will increase splanchnic blood flow if the heart is fluid responsive. This will permit a much larger volume of Na^+ and Cl^- to be secreted in the small intestine. When a large volume of luminal fluid containing Na^+ and Cl^- reaches the colon, more Cl^- will be reabsorbed in exchange for HCO_3^-, as compared with the reabsorption of Na^+ in exchange for secreted H^+; hence the loss of $NaHCO_3$ in diarrhea fluid might rise markedly.
   - **Back titration of HCO_3^- by H^+ that were bound to intracellular proteins in muscle:** With increased flow through the muscles, *less* CO_2 will be added to each liter of blood, as carbon dioxide production will remain the same. Hence the tissue PCO_2 and the venous PCO_2 will decline. As a result of the fall in tissue PCO_2, equation 3 (see Fig. 78.1) will shift rightward and bicarbonate will be consumed in the ICF and ECF compartments of muscle. The protons that combine with the bicarbonate are unbound from intracellular proteins; hence the concentration HCO_3^- of in the ECF compartment will decline (see Fig. 78.2).
   - **Hypokalemia:** Despite an important degree of K^+ depletion from loss of K^+ in diarrhea fluid, hypokalemia may not be present on admission, presumably because K^+ shifts out of cells. The mechanism for K^+ shift can be a stress-induced (i.e., adrenergic-related) insulin deficiency. The stimulus for epinephrine release is the contracted arterial blood volume. Hence one should anticipate a significant drop in the P_K with re-expansion of the ECF volume, because this will lead to a fall in

circulating α-adrenergic hormone levels and a rise in plasma insulin levels. One should also be aware that the degree of hypokalemia may become more severe with the infusion of $NaHCO_3$, and more aggressive therapy with KCl will likely be needed. If a severe degree of K^+ depletion with hypokalemia develops, bowel motility may diminish to a degree such that intestinal secretions are pooled in the gut and diarrhea is no longer observed.

41. Does this patient have respiratory acidosis?
Because the pH and $PaCO_2$ (39 mm Hg) in arterial blood were in the normal range, he does not have a hypoventilation form of respiratory acidosis. His brachial venous $PvCO_2$, however, was much higher (i.e., 55 mm Hg) than the usual value of ~6 mm Hg step-up from the $PaCO_2$. This is because the blood flow rate to muscle was very low as a result of the significant degree of effective circulating blood volume contraction. Hence more O_2 was extracted from each liter of blood, and almost an identical amount of CO_2 was added to capillary blood, raising the muscle venous $PvCO_2$. The higher concentration of CO_2 in interstitial space and in cells of muscles abrogates the BBS.

42. Discuss RTA as a cause of metabolic acidosis.
As considered previously, there are essentially two types of RTA: proximal RTA (type II) and distal RTA (type I). Although *both* types have a low rate of excretion of NH_4^+, in type II RTA there is also decreased capacity for the reabsorption of HCO_3^- in the PCT.

Proximal, or type II, RTA may present as an *isolated* defect in reabsorption of HCO_3^- in the PCT or as a component of a *generalized* PCT dysfunction—that is, Fanconi syndrome. When there is generalized reduction of PCT function, there will also be glucosuria, aminoaciduria, and increased excretion of urate, phosphate, and citrate, in addition to the loss of HCO_3^-. The most common cause of Fanconi syndrome in the pediatric population is cystinosis, whereas common causes in adult population are paraproteinemias and autoimmune disorders. The steps in the clinical approach and differential diagnosis in patients with RTA were outlined in Fig. 78.5.

In patients with proximal RTA, treatment with $NaHCO_3$ does not maintain the P_{HCO_3} near the normal range, because bicarbonaturia ensues as the distal capacity for the reabsorption of HCO_3^- is exceeded. Do not be aggressive with the administration of $NaHCO_3$, because bicarbonaturia may lead to the development of hypokalemia and the alkaline urine pH may increase the risk of formation of calcium phosphate stones. Conversely, $NaHCO_3$ seems to be beneficial in still-growing pediatric patients with proximal RTA and growth retardation.

In patients with distal, or type I, RTA from a defect in net distal H^+ secretion, the major threat to the patient on presentation is cardiac arrhythmia resulting from hypokalemia. Hypokalemia may also cause respiratory muscle weakness and severe acidemia from superimposed respiratory acidosis. $NaHCO_3$ should not be given until enough potassium is given to raise plasma potassium to a safe level (~3 mmol/L). After the plasma bicarbonate concentration (P_{HCO_3}) is corrected, the dose of $NaHCO_3$ needed to maintain P_{HCO_3} in the normal range is usually less than 30 or 40 mmol/day (i.e., enough to titrate the acid load produced from the metabolism of sulfur-containing amino acids).

Patients with distal RTA, unlike those with proximal RTA, are in net positive proton balance, as they cannot secrete their daily proton load, assuming a "Western," acid-producing diet. Some of these protons are titrated by bone, leading to release of some calcium from bone, causing decreased bone mineral density and hypercalciuria. Hypocitraturia results as absorption of citrate in the PCT is stimulated. Citrate binds calcium and keeps it soluble, while in its absence, calcium can bind to oxalate or phosphate and form stones. With the alkaline urine pH of distal RTA, calcium phosphate deposition is favored over calcium oxalate. The result is that patients may have diminished GFR due to nephrocalcinosis and may have frequent stones. Administration of potassium citrate, sometimes with thiazides to reduce urine calcium excretion, is often appropriate.

The diagnostic category of type III RTA was never clearly defined and did not stand the test of time; most of these patients probably had a combination of proximal and distal RTA, with findings similar to that of patients administered carbonic anhydrase inhibitors. The term "type IV RTA" is usually used to describe the constellation of findings of hyperkalemia and metabolic acidosis resulting from a low rate of excretion of NH_4^+. These patients are usually said to have hyporenin, hypoaldosteronism, though the actual endocrine findings are highly variable when they are assessed. While the syndrome is often noted in diabetics, the most common cause today is the use of angiotensin-converting enzyme inhibitors and angiotensin receptor blockers.

It is important to realize that there are two ways that hyperkalemia and a low rate of excretion of NH_4^+ may coexist. In one, hyperkalemia, attributed to reduced aldosterone secretion, is responsible for the low rate of excretion of NH_4^+ because hyperkalemia is associated with an alkaline PCT cell pH, which leads to inhibition of ammoniagenesis. The urine pH is then invariably acid, given the lack of buffer, with distal proton secretion intact. In these patients, if the plasma potassium is corrected, the metabolic acidosis should also resolve. Since these patients often have hypertension and reduced GFR, administration of furosemide or thiazides may be appropriate. However, in a second subset of patients, hyperkalemia is not the major reason for the low rate of excretion of NH_4^+; rather, these patients have medullary interstitial disease, causing the low rate of excretion of NH_4^+, which also involves the cortical distal nephron, leading to hyperkalemia. Distinguishing these two etiologies may not always be possible. In both groups, the administration of $NaHCO_3$ or sodium citrate is appropriate, as it will ameliorate hyperkalemia, both by causing shift of potassium into cells and by increasing distal tubular sodium delivery. In addition, recent evidence suggests that alkali may be beneficial for reducing the progression of chronic kidney disease in diabetic nephropathy and possible other causes of chronic kidney disease.

43. Can you summarize the approach to the diagnosis of metabolic acidosis?
- Initial steps in the diagnostic approach in a patient with metabolic acidosis include the following:
    1. Identify and deal with emergencies; at times one may need to know the etiology to institute therapy.
    2. Anticipate and prevent risks that are likely to develop during therapy.
- Two major amendments are needed to the traditional approach to the patient with metabolic acidosis:
    1. **One should not rely solely on concentration terms to determine if metabolic acidosis is present when the ECF volume is contracted.** Rather, a quantitative estimate of the ECF volume is needed to calculate the *content* of HCO_3^- in this setting. Use the hematocrit to calculate the plasma volume and thereby to calculate the content of HCO_3^- in the ECF compartment, especially if this latter volume may be contracted.
    2. **One may assess the effectiveness of the BBS.** When the BBS is compromised in skeletal muscle, more H^+ will bind to proteins in cells of vital organs (e.g., brain, heart), and this may compromise their essential functions. One should not rely solely on the arterial $PaCO_2$ for this assessment. Rather, the brachial or femoral venous $PvCO_2$ reflects the capillary CO_2 tension in that drainage bed. This is required to evaluate the effectiveness of the vast bulk of this buffer system to remove added H^+.
- **Determine whether the basis of the metabolic acidosis is a result of added acids and/or a deficit of $NaHCO_3$:** Look for new anions in plasma (high $P_{Anion\ gap}$ adjusted for the $P_{Albumin}$) and urine (high urine anion gap) and assess the rate of excretion of NH_4^+. At times the new anions may cause serious other problems (e.g., chelation of ionized calcium by citrate anions).
- **Assess the rate of excretion of NH_4^+:** The major renal response in chronic metabolic acidosis is a high rate of excretion of NH_4^+. The urine osmolal gap provides the best indirect test to detect very high urinary NH_4^+ concentration.

44. How is acute metabolic acidosis treated?
The treatment of metabolic acidosis must focus on the underlying disorder. Treatment of diarrhea with antibiotics, oral rehydration solutions, or antimotility medications might be appropriate. Treating the acidosis per se, in order to increase the arterial pH, requires the administration of bicarbonate or potential base, such as citrate. However, administration of alkali for acute metabolic acidosis is not clearly beneficial and constitutes a topic of some long-standing controversy.

Acute metabolic acidosis is especially controversial, since few data demonstrate that administration of sodium bicarbonate in acute lactic acidosis leads to the changes in outcomes one would hope for. There are various etiologies that may explain this failure of administration of alkali in such circumstances. Most importantly, the evidence does not show that intracellular pH changes in the desired manner. Bicarbonate may fail to have the desired effect on what is ultimately most important to cellular and protein function. In some settings, especially in the face of cardiac arrest and cardiopulmonary resuscitation, intravenous bicarbonate is titrated by protons and forms CO_2 that can enter cells readily, faster than HCO_3, and lower intracellular pH. Acute administration of sodium bicarbonate has other adverse effects. It leads to an increase in extracellular volume and a risk of pulmonary edema. It is hypertonic and can lead to hypernatremia. The titration of protons off albumin exposes negative charges that can bind calcium and cause a fall in extracellular ionized calcium, leading to a risk for arrhythmia, reduced cardiac contractility, and hypotension; perhaps administering intravenous calcium when bicarbonate is administered would be appropriate, but this strategy has not been tested adequately. The current "Surviving Sepsis" guidelines recommend against administration of sodium bicarbonate for arterial pH of 7.15 or more, and express uncertainty about whether giving it when pH is lower has any utility.

In DKA, administration of insulin will lead to metabolism of acetoacetate and BHB, consuming a proton and, in effect, generating bicarbonate. Administration of bicarbonate is generally not needed unless the pH is extremely low, and can lead to metabolic alkalosis once the ketosis is terminated.

Alternative therapies for metabolic acidosis have been studied and thus far are not in common use. Tris-hydroxymethyl aminomethane (THAM) is a base that can neutralize protons without producing CO_2, but has not found widespread use. Carbicarb is a preparation of sodium bicarbonate and sodium carbonate, which similarly also produces less CO_2 when neutralizing protons. Currently there are studies attempting to show that blockade of sodium/hydrogen exchange may protect from an effect of bicarbonate that increases intracellular calcium driving cellular injury.

45. **How is chronic metabolic acidosis treated?**
Chronic metabolic acidosis, the result of chronic kidney disease (CKD) or RTA, more clearly benefits from treatment. Recent data suggest that the treatment of acidosis, even if relatively mild with serum bicarbonate concentrations less than 24 mEq/L, is associated with a decrease in the progression of CKD. Perhaps even patients with normal serum bicarbonate concentrations benefit from the administration of alkali, either in the form of sodium citrate or sodium bicarbonate. Some people tolerate sodium citrate better than they do sodium bicarbonate because the latter is associated with some production of CO_2 in the stomach, with the base titrated by gastric HCl. Most preparations of sodium citrate include citric acid, which increases palatability but has no net effect on acid–base balance. This is because all organic acids, such as citric acid, malic acid, and acetic acid (vinegar), will be metabolized, yielding bicarbonate that is titrated by the accompanying proton, so that the effect on acid–base balance is nil. This accounts for the fact that citrus juices have an acidic pH but increase (rather than decrease) urine pH. This is due to the fact that some of the carboxyl anions are accompanied by potassium, yielding bicarbonate, and some are accompanied by protons, yielding no net change in acid–base balance.

The benefit may be the result of the ensuing decline in ammoniagenesis, with some evidence that ammonia is capable of activating complement in the kidney. Another possibility is that alkali antagonizes the effects of endothelin, which both increases blood pressure and stimulates inflammation. In any case, the administration of alkali to patients with CKD appears to be safe and not linked to the increases in blood pressure associated with increased intake of NaCl. In addition, the treatment of metabolic acidosis appears to decrease muscle wasting in CKD.

The treatment of the acidosis resulting from RTA has other benefits. First, it is associated with preservation of bone mineral density. Second, the administration of citrate is useful to prevent kidney stones, and may also reduce the progression of nephrocalcinosis, a cause of reduced GFR. Citrate is an antagonist of calcium crystallization, inhibiting both calcium oxalate and calcium phosphate precipitation. Some of the citrate will be metabolized, chiefly in the liver, and consume protons, the equivalent of generating bicarbonate. Though in the case of stone prevention the goal is to increase urinary citrate, there will inevitably also be an increase in urine pH. While it is suggested that the increase in urine pH may promote calcium phosphate precipitation, the increase in citrate appears to largely overcome this effect, as the anecdotal evidence shows that stones are inhibited by citrate administration in RTA.

For RTA, citrate administration is usually achieved by giving potassium citrate, rather than sodium citrate, since the patients are often hypokalemic. Some people have dyspepsia from the preparation, in which case potassium bicarbonate may be better tolerated. Another reason that sodium citrate is to be avoided is because the sodium load will be accompanied by an increase in urinary calcium excretion, which is undesirable when kidney stone prevention and improved bone mineral density are the goals.

LABORATORY DATA

pH = 7.20 (64 [H+] nmol/L)
PCO$_2$ (arterial) = 25 mm Hg
HCO$_3^-$ = 11 mmol/L
Glucose = 180 mg/dL (10 mmol/L)
Creatinine = 1.8 mg/dL (160 μmol/L)
Calcium (total) = 10 mg/dL (2.5 mmol/L)

Na$^+$ = 143 mmol/L
K$^+$ = 6.3 mmol/L
Cl$^-$ = 99 mmol/L
Albumin = 4.5 g/dL (45 g/L)
Blood urea nitrogen (urea) = 8.4 mg/dL (3.0 mmol/L)
L-lactate = 2.0 mmol/L

Acknowledgments

This chapter was originally authored by Dr. Kamel Kamel and Dr. Mitch Halperin. Rather than start from scratch, we have simply updated and revised this chapter. We acknowledge their outstanding contribution to the understanding of the relevant physiology and medicine. Our work must pay tribute to their many contributions.

KEY POINTS

1. The diagnostic category of metabolic acidosis is made up of two major subgroups: one where the basis of the disorder is the addition of acids, and the other where the basis is a major loss of $NaHCO_3$.
2. When the extracellular fluid (ECF) volume is significantly contracted, one must use a definition of metabolic acidosis that is based not only on the plasma HCO_3 but also on the content HCO_3 of in the ECF compartment.
3. In patients with proximal renal tubular acidosis (RTA), one should not be too aggressive with the administration of $NaHCO_3$, because bicarbonaturia may lead to the development of hypokalemia and the alkaline urine pH may increase the risk of formation of calcium phosphate stones. In patients with distal RTA from a defect in net distal H^+ secretion, the major threat to the patient on presentation is cardiac arrhythmia from hypokalemia. Osteoporosis, nephrocalcinosis with chronic kidney disease, and kidney stones are also risks.
4. The elaboration of lactate *consumes* protons when pyruvate becomes the terminal electron acceptor under states of either increased physiological stress/work or when there is true tissue hypoxia/impaired oxidative phosphorylation. Under either condition, glycolysis and lactate production are "anaerobic" only in that their chemistry is *independent of* tissue oxygen. Thus the finding of lactate elevation does not necessarily mean true tissue hypoxia is present. The underlying etiology of hyperlactatemia must be sought and treated rationally.

BIBLIOGRAPHY

Dyck, R. F., Asthana, S., Kalra, J., West, M. L., & Massey, L. (1990). A modification of the urine osmolal gap: An improved method for estimating urine ammonium. *American Journal of Nephrology, 10,* 359–362.

Goraya, N., & Wesson, D. E. (2014). Is dietary acid a modifiable risk factor for nephropathy progression? *American Journal of Nephrology 39,* 142–144.

Gowrishankar, M., Kamel, K. S., & Halperin, M. L. (2007). Buffering of a H1 load: A 'brain-protein-centered' view. *Journal of the American Society of Nephrology, 18,* 2278–2280.

Kamel, K. S., Briceno, L. F., Santos, M. I., Brenes, L., Yorgin, P., Kooh, S. W., & Halperin, M. L. (1997). A new classification for kidney defects in net acid excretion. *American Journal of Kidney Diseases, 29,* 126–136.

Kamel, K. S., & Halperin, M. L. (2006). An improved approach to the patient with metabolic acidosis: A need for four amendments. *Clinical Nephrology, 65,* S76–S85.

Levy, B. (2006). Lactate and shock state: The metabolic view. *Current Opinion in Critical Care, 12*(4), 315–321.

Preminger, G. M., Sakhaee, K., Skurla, C., & Pak, C. Y. (1985). Prevention of recurrent calcium stone formation with potassium citrate therapy in patients with distal renal tubular acidosis. *Journal of Urology, 134,* 20–23.

Rastegar, A. (2009). Clinical utility of Stewart's method in diagnosis and management of acid-base disorders. *Clinical Journal of the American Society of Nephrology, 4,* 1267–1274.

Rhodes, A., Evans, L. E., Alhazzani, W., Levy, M. M., Antonelli, M., Ferrer, R., . . . Dellinger, R. P. (2017). Surviving sepsis campaign: International guidelines for management of sepsis and septic shock: 2016. *Intensive Care Medicine, 43*(3), 304–377.

Shull, P. D., & Rapoport, J. (2010). Life-threatening metabolic acidosis caused by alcohol abuse. *Nature Reviews Nephrology, 6,* 555–558.

Sousa, A. G., Cabral, J. V., El-Feghaly, W. B., de Sousa, L. S., & Nunes, A. B. (2016). Hyporeninemic hypoaldosteronism and diabetes mellitus: Pathophysiology assumptions, clinical aspects and implications for management. *World Journal of Diabetes, 7,* 101–111.

METABOLIC ALKALOSIS

David S. Goldfarb and Jon-Emile S. Kenny

CHAPTER 79

INTRODUCTION AND PHYSIOLOGY

1. What is metabolic alkalosis?

   The metabolic alkaloses represent a heterogeneous group of disorders that have in common a high concentration of plasma bicarbonate [HCO_3^-] and a low concentration of H^+ in plasma. This constellation of findings can be seen in a number of different pathophysiologic entities. Hence metabolic alkalosis is a syndrome of metabolic findings and not a final diagnosis.

   As addressed in the chapter on metabolic acidosis, an alkalosis is a process that favors an alkaline blood pH or alkalemia. However, an alkalosis does not guarantee alkalemia, and other processes, such as acidosis, may be concurrent.

2. What are the mechanisms by which metabolic alkaloses develop and persist?

   Traditionally, the factors responsible for a rise in [HCO_3^-] have been classified as those that directly raise [HCO_3^-] and those that account for the failure of the kidneys to excrete the excess bicarbonate anions (Fig. 79.1). Six broad mechanisms are recognized. A and B are processes that generate metabolic alkalosis; C to E are contributors to the maintenance of metabolic alkalosis.

   Generation:
   A. The loss of a nonvolatile acid from the extracellular fluid (ECF) compartment (e.g., vomiting)
   B. Addition of exogenous alkali (e.g., ingestion of $NaHCO_3$)
   C. Loss of NaCl-rich fluid, leading to reabsorption of $NaHCO_3$ (e.g., loop and thiazide diuretics)

   Maintenance:
   D. Increased reabsorption of bicarbonate within the proximal tubule
   E. Increased regeneration of bicarbonate at the distal nephron
   F. Increased bicarbonate produced from the bicarbonate buffer system

   With respect to A, the most common clinical example is vomiting or nasogastric suction causing loss of HCl (Fig. 79.2). These are common generators of metabolic alkalosis. Addition of base (B) is also a possible underlying mechanism but a relatively infrequent event, such as ingestion of $NaHCO_3$. A large input of $NaHCO_3$ cannot maintain metabolic alkalosis because the kidneys will readily excrete sodium (Na^+) and HCO_3^- or potential HCO_3^- (citrate) very quickly, unless reduced kidney function is present. Milk-alkali syndrome is an example in which base administration occurs, and reduced glomerular filtration rate (GFR) accounts for a reduction in the kidney's ability to excrete the excess base.

   The secrets surrounding direct HCl loss are elaborated in much more detail later.

   In the metabolic alkalosis frequently seen with the use of both loop and thiazide diuretics, the urine produced contains mostly NaCl and KCl, removing a portion of plasma that will lead to a higher [HCO_3]. This initial generating phase is termed "contraction" alkalosis. The failure of the kidney to correct the [HCO_3] is due to the ensuing deficiency of both Cl and K, leading to maintenance of the contraction-initiated alkalosis.

   Augmentation of proximal bicarbonate reabsorption (D) is considered a perpetuator of alkalosis rather than a trigger. Bicarbonate reabsorption at the proximal convoluted tubule (PCT) is driven largely by angiotensin II and hypokalemia, both of which favor PCT proton excretion, which captures filtered bicarbonate for reabsorption. These processes, which help maintain metabolic alkalosis, are important mediators in states of extracellular volume depletion, or reduced effective arterial blood volume, which stimulate renin and angiotensin II production. When there is a reduction in effective arterial blood volume, reabsorption of sodium predominates over the kidney's ability to maintain acid-base balance. Angiotensin directly stimulates proximal Na^+/H^+ exchange (NHE3), leading to reabsorption of $NaHCO_3$ regardless of [HCO_3^-]. Because loss of gastric acid, or the action of diuretics, causes loss of Cl, the reabsorption of Na^+ in the PCT must be accompanied by HCO_3. Potassium depletion with both vomiting and diuretic effects also contribute to the maintenance process.

   Distal bicarbonate regeneration (E) occurs in response to distal sodium delivery and the action of aldosterone. These two prerequisites allow for sodium-proton exchange; the excreted proton leaves

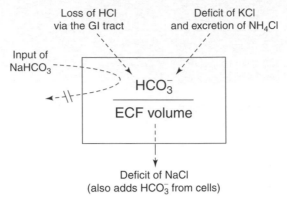

Figure 79.1. Mechanisms that may lead to a rise in the P_{HCO3}. *ECF,* extracellular fluid; *GI,* gastrointestinal.

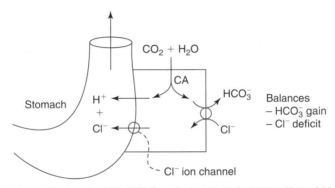

Figure 79.2. Electroneutrality during the deficit of HCl. The stylized structure is the stomach with a parietal cell on its right-hand border. In this cell, $CO_2 + H_2O$ are converted to H^+ and HCO_3^- by a reaction catalyzed by carbonic anhydrase *(CA).* H^+ are secreted into the lumen of the stomach by the H^+/K^+-ATPase, whereas K^+ recycle back into the parietal cell (not shown for simplicity). Cl^- from the extracellular fluid compartment enter parietal cells on the basolateral Cl^-/HCO_3^- anion exchanger; Cl^- enter the lumen of the stomach via Cl^- ion channels. Overall, there is a loss of Cl^- and a gain of HCO_3^- in the body. Thus there is also electroneutrality in all compartments.

the urine as ammonium chloride. Thus hyperaldosteronism is a potential generator of alkalosis. A secret here is that aldosterone promotes the action of the distal proton-ATPase (H^+-ATPase); this protein lies on the luminal side of the distal convoluted tubule and excretes hydrogen ions into the lumen such that bicarbonate is reclaimed. In addition, hypokalemia enhances distal proton-potassium-ATPase (H^+/K^+-ATPase)—a luminal facing hydrogen ion, potassium antiporter—which also leads to bicarbonate absorption. Thus hypokalemia and hyperaldosteronism *independently* potentiate the magnitude of renal proton excretion (or distal bicarbonate regeneration). Another secret is that chronic elevations of arterial carbon dioxide tension ($PaCO_2$) up-regulate the expression of distal H^+-ATPase and H^+/K^+-ATPase—the basis for metabolic compensation for chronic respiratory acidosis; note that these processes most appropriately are considered "compensation" rather than "primary metabolic alkalosis." Stimulation of both distal H^+-ATPase and H^+/K^+-ATPase are associated with enhanced appearance of bicarbonate in the blood as long as the generated protons appear in the urine.

Lastly, bicarbonate can come from underperfused muscle (F). In states with a low effective arterial blood volume and diminished blood flow to muscles, PCO_2 in capillary blood rises. Because CO_2 must diffuse from cells to capillaries, it follows that the intracellular PCO_2 must also be high. As shown in Fig. 79.3, this high PCO_2 will drive its conversion to H^+ and HCO_3^- within skeletal muscle. The H^+ binds to proteins in cells while the HCO_3^-. exits via the Cl^-/HCO_3^- anion exchanger. This condition will persist as long as the blood flow rate to muscles remains low.

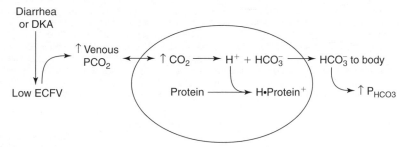

Figure 79.3. Generation of new HCO_3^- in skeletal muscle when there is a deficit of NaCl. The oval represents a cell membrane containing HCO_3^- and protein buffer systems. When the effective arterial blood volume is contracted, the rate of blood flow is reduced. The subsequent extraction of most of the O_2 from each liter of blood flowing through the capillaries raises both the capillary and the intracellular fluid PCO_2 *(left portion of the figure)*. The higher PCO_2 in the interstitial fluid and in these cells drives the synthesis of H^+ and HCO_3^-; the H^+ bind to intracellular proteins while the HCO_3^- is exported to the extracellular fluid *(right portion of the figure)*. The net result is a rise in the P_{HCO3}. After the infusion of enough saline, there is a decline in capillary and, thereby, the PCO_2 in cells. When these events are reversed, there will be a fall in the P_{HCO3}. *DKA,* Diabetic ketoacidosis; *ECFV,* extracellular fluid volume.

3. **How does hypokalemia affect the excretion of HCO_3^-?**
   Loss of potassium from the extracellular space is associated with movement of potassium from the intracellular space to the extracellular space, necessitating movement of protons into cells. The result is *lower intracellular pH* in cells of the PCT causing activation of the NHE3 in the luminal membrane of this nephron segment. Consequently, there is augmented secretion of H^+, leading to more reabsorption of $NaHCO_3$ during hypokalemia, frequently contributing to the maintenance of metabolic alkalosis. Hypokalemia and the associated fall in PCT intracellular pH also stimulate ammoniagenesis, increasing ammonium ion (NH_4^+) production and excretion:

$$Glutamine^0 \rightarrow 2\ NH_4^+\ 2\ HCO_3^-.$$

   Each ammonium appearing in the urine represents the addition of an HCO_3^- to the plasma.

4. **Is there a tubular maximum for the renal reabsorption of filtered HCO_3^-?**
   Under normal conditions, the kidneys reabsorb greater than 90% of filtered HCO_3^- in the PCT. As stated earlier, the stimuli for this process are the ambient level of angiotensin II and the usual intracellular pH in cells of the PCT. Consequently, to inhibit this reabsorption of HCO_3^-, the effective arterial blood volume must be corrected (e.g., create a positive Na^+ balance in cases of reduced total body Na^+ content or improve cardiac output in cases of congestive heart failure) to diminish the release of angiotensin II, or the pH in the cells of the PCT must rise. In addition, low GFR is often invoked as a perpetuator of alkalosis because low GFR prevents the high $[HCO_3^-]$ present during alkalosis from exceeding the maximum reabsorption (Tm) of bicarbonate. That is, the low GFR prevents greater HCO_3^- filtration from occurring so that Tm is not reached. In that case, there is no bicarbonaturia and systemic alkalosis is maintained. Bearing this in mind, we shall examine the conditions that were present in experimental studies that were interpreted to indicate that there is a renal threshold (Tm) for the reabsorption of HCO_3^- by the kidneys.
   • **Data to suggest that there is a renal threshold for the reabsorption of HCO_3^- by the kidneys:** In the seminal experiments by Pitts et al. in the late 1940s, the infusion of $NaHCO_3$ was large enough to expand the ECF volume sufficiently to diminish circulating levels of angiotensin II and to raise the pH in cells of the PCT. Hence the two physiologic stimuli for the proximal reabsorption of HCO_3^- were removed. Rather than relate these findings to the changes in physiologic variables, the conclusion was that there is a tubular maximum for the renal reabsorption of HCO_3^-.
   • **Data to suggest that there is not a renal threshold for the reabsorption of HCO_3^-:** The design of these experiments (e.g., Purkerson et al.) was to avoid a large expansion of the ECF volume while creating a positive balance of $NaHCO_3$. Even though the HCO_3^- rose, there was little bicarbonaturia, and hence a tubular maximum for the renal reabsorption of $NaHCO_3$ was not observed. In support of this view, the range for the $[HCO_3^-]$ is from 22 to 31 mmol/L in normal subjects consuming a typical Western diet, and there is no appreciable bicarbonaturia at the upper range values for the $[HCO_3^-]$, despite much higher filtered loads for HCO_3^-, because the GFR is relatively constant throughout the day.

In summary, the enthusiasm for a T_m for HCO_3^- reabsorption in the PCT is based on data from experimental conditions that removed the usual stimuli for the reabsorption of filtered HCO_3^-. Furthermore, an infusion of $NaHCO_3$ does not represent a normal physiologic occurrence.

Two other points merit emphasis. First, a steady state with metabolic alkalosis can be achieved and maintained when the blood pH rises sufficiently to overcome the stimulatory actions of angiotensin II of the reabsorption of HCO_3^- in cells of the PCT. Second, the excretion of *potential* HCO_3^- in the form of organic anions such as citrate is augmented by a *high pH* in cells of the PCT. Higher intracellular pH inhibits the action of the sodium-dicarboxylate cotransporter in the PCT, leading to excretion of citrate.

5. What other mechanism may lead to a rise in the plasma bicarbonate concentration?

Because concentrations have numerators and denominators, the $[HCO_3^-]$ will rise when there is a net addition of HCO_3 to the ECF compartment and/or when the volume of the ECF compartment declines (see Fig. 79.1):

$$P_{HCO3} = \text{Content of } HCO_3^- \text{ / ECF volume}$$

The secret here is that the deficit of Na^+ and Cl^- raises $[HCO_3^-]$ for two reasons. As noted earlier, the first reason is a fall in the denominator of the ratio of HCO_3^- to ECF volume (see equation in Question 4); this is because the major function of Na^+ is to retain water in the ECF compartment. Second—as in part 2D earlier—there is generation of new HCO_3^- in skeletal muscle because the blood flow declines appreciably to this organ for hemodynamic reasons. To maintain steady oxygen consumption, more oxygen is extracted per liter of blood flow. This oxygen is converted to CO_2, which leads to a high capillary PCO_2 and thereby a higher intracellular PCO_2 (see Fig. 79.3). As protons are buffered by proteins, bicarbonate leaves the cell in exchange for chloride.

6. What is the most reliable way to perform a quantitative analysis of the ECF volume in patients with metabolic alkalosis?

Accurate quantitative data about the ECF volume are not reliably obtained by the physical examination; instead, the hematocrit or total protein level in plasma can often be used to obtain this information. The hematocrit or the concentration of hemoglobin in blood will rise when there are more red blood cells (RBCs) or fewer liters of plasma. If one ignores the Starling forces across capillaries, the changes in the plasma volume will reflect alterations in the ECF volume. The hematocrit on admission provides helpful information to guide initial decisions about intravenous fluid therapy and to decide when to slow down this infusion rate.

For example, assume that the hematocrit is 0.40 and the blood volume is 5 L. Therefore the plasma volume will be 3 L and volume of RBCs is 2 L:

$$\text{Hematocrit (0.4)} = \text{RBC volume (2L)/plasma vloume (3 L)} + \text{RBC volume (2 L)}$$

If the hematocrit on admission is 0.60 in a patient who does not have polycythemia, the new plasma volume can be calculated as follows:

$$\text{Hematocrit of (0.6)} = \text{RBC volume (2L)/Blood volume (XL)}$$

On rearranging this equation, 0.6 X = 2.0 L and X is 3.3 L. Because 2 of these liters are red blood cells, the remaining volume is the plasma volume (3.3 L − 2.0 L = 1.33 L). Thus the plasma volume has fallen from 3 to 1.33 L, and, by inference, the ECF volume is reduced to 44% of its normal volume (i.e., 100 × 1.33 L/3.0 L = 44%). Because hematocrit values of 0.6 can be seen in patients with diabetic ketoacidosis or in states with severe diarrhea (e.g., cholera), the measured $[HCO_3^-]$ will be more than twofold higher than in a similar patient who did not have such a contracted ECF volume.

7. What causes the contraction of the ECF volume?

When there is a *deficit of NaCl* without a simultaneous loss of $NaHCO_3$, the content of HCO_3^- in the ECF compartment does not change, but the $[HCO_3^-]$ rises because the denominator of the content of HCO_3^-/ECF volume (see equation in Question 4) is diminished. This contraction type of metabolic alkalosis is particularly important when there is a large decrease in the ECF volume (e.g., in patients with massive diarrhea or when diuretics are given to patients with congestive heart failure).

8. Are the abnormalities in metabolic alkalosis restricted to the ECF compartment?

No. There are abnormalities in both the ECF and intracellular fluid (ICF) compartments in patients with metabolic alkalosis. The primary stimulus for these changes largely arises secondary to deficits of compounds that contain Cl^-. In a small number of patients, there will be a positive balance for $NaHCO_3$, but in these patients, hypokalemia plays a central role. To understand the pathophysiology, one must examine how electroneutrality and balance were achieved in the ECF and ICF compartments and in the urine, as highlighted in the following clinical example.

CLINICAL EXAMPLES OF METABOLIC ALKALOSIS

9. Loss of gastric contents: what is the impact of a deficit of H^+ and Cl^-?
   Removal of HCl from the stomach was first studied in seminal experiments performed by Schwartz and Kassirer. The initial loss of gastric contents is considered the generation phase for metabolic alkalosis. A deficit of Cl^- without a deficit of Na^+ or K^+ occurs. Based on electroneutrality, this must represent a deficit of an equimolar amount of H^+. Hence there is a net gain of an equimolar amount of HCO_3^- in the body, causing alkalemia and a higher $[HCO_3^-]$. Because gastric fluid contains relatively little Na^+ and K^+, there are no important changes in Na^+ or K^+ balance. Hence there are no important changes in the ICF compartment, merely a loss of Cl^- and an equivalent gain of HCO_3^- in the ECF compartment.
   When the deficit is purely HCl, one could, in theory, give HCl to the patient. This choice is rarely made, because the administration of HCl via intravenous infusion is somewhat inconvenient. Alternatively, one could give NaCl, because the expanded ECF volume will result in the excretion of the administered Na^+ with the extra HCO_3^- that was present in the ECF compartment. The administered Cl^- will be retained.
   However, as this initial period of gastric acid loss persists, additional events occur before the steady state develops. The rise in serum $[HCO_3^-]$ leads to an increase in filtered $[HCO_3^-]$. This is because sodium is not yet lost and there is not a significant stimulus for renin and angiotensin II; consequently, there is little bicarbonate reabsorption in the PCT. Bicarbonaturia ensues, demonstrated by an increase in the urine pH, and obligating loss of Na^+ and K^+. The loss of extracellular fluid volume (ECFV) and the development of hypokalemia are therefore the result of renal, not gastric, losses. Increased renin and angiotensin II then follow.
   Untreated, even were the vomiting and loss of gastric fluid to stop, a maintenance period would follow. The deficiency of both Cl^- and K^+ will prevent the excretion of the excess generated $[HCO_3^-]$. During this phase, as the filtered HCO_3^- is reabsorbed in the PCT, there is no further bicarbonaturia, and the urine pH is acidic. This observation is the paradoxical aciduria of metabolic alkalosis, representing the failure of the kidneys to excrete the excess generated bicarbonate. Further urinary losses of Na^+ and K^+ do not occur. Because the deficit is now mostly of KCl, the administration of KCl is most important. Giving NaCl alone will not correct the deficit of KCl acutely. To the extent that the ECFV is contracted, administration of NaCl is appropriate and will allow suppression of renin and angiotensin II. Repletion of Cl^- allows the kidneys to reabsorb Na^+ with Cl^- instead of HCO_3^-, and repletion of K^+ suppresses other mechanisms associated with bicarbonate reabsorption discussed previously.

10. What are the diagnostic hallmarks of metabolic alkalosis resulting from depletion of HCl?
    Because of the deficit of Cl^-, the urine should be virtually free of Cl^-. Despite a contracted ECF volume, Na^+ may be excreted if the urine contains bicarbonate, or anions other than Cl^-. This is particularly the case in the generation phase when bicarbonaturia occurs, urine pH is higher than 6.0, and urinary Na^+ and K^+ losses are occurring. The secret here is that the fractional excretion of sodium *may be high* in the context of volume depletion secondary to loss of gastric acid. In addition, the urine may contain K^+ even though the patient has chronic hypokalemia.

11. What is the pathophysiology of metabolic alkalosis in patients with primary high mineralocorticoid activity?
    In patients with primary hyperaldosteronism, caused by either benign adrenal adenomas or bilateral adrenal hyperplasia, metabolic alkalosis and hypertension are expected. H^+-ATPase activity is directly stimulated. There is an initial positive balance of NaCl as a result of actions of mineralocorticoids. Distal tubular and collecting duct epithelial sodium channel (ENaC) activity are increased and hypertension results. Renin and angiotensin II secretion are suppressed. Secondly, there is excretion of K^+. Mineralocorticoids facilitate kaliuresis through several mechanisms. Stimulation of ENaC activity makes the luminal potential difference more negative, facilitating K^+ secretion by the renal outer medullary K^+ channel, ROMK. ROMK channel open activity also is increased. In addition, this negative luminal potential difference facilitates the activity of H^+-ATPase, further stimulating distal proton secretion.

The resulting deficit of K^+ and hypokalemia acidifies proximal convoluted tubular cells, stimulates proximal $NaHCO_3$ reabsorption, and stimulates sodium/citrate reabsorption, causing retention of dietary alkali and lowering excretion of citrate. However, this process is opposed by suppression of renin and angiotensin II by the volume-expanding effect of aldosterone, suppressing NHE3 activity. An increased rate of excretion of NH_4^+ due to hypokalemia also follows.

In total body terms, there is net gain of $NaHCO_3$. When plasma bicarbonate rises sufficiently to return the ICF pH toward normal, these patients can achieve acid-base balance by excreting appropriate amounts of NH_4^+ and organic anions in the urine, as dictated by their dietary intake but at a higher $[HCO_3^-]$. Note that these patients are not Cl^- depleted and urine Cl^- is not low. As H^+-ATPase activity is stimulated, urine pH is generally 6.0 or less.

OLINIOAL APPROACH

12. What is the optimal clinical approach to the patient with metabolic alkalosis?
    A concise and clinically relevant approach to the patient with metabolic alkalosis is provided in Fig. 79.4. The first step is to rule out the common causes of metabolic alkalosis: vomiting and use of diuretics. Although this may be evident from the clinical history, some patients may deny the intake of diuretics or previous vomiting. Examining the urine electrolytes is particularly helpful for this diagnosis. The traditional classification distinguishes those with Cl^--responsive alkalosis from those with Cl^--unresponsive alkalosis, so begin with the concentration of Cl^- in the urine (U_{Cl}). A very low U_{Cl} is expected when there is a deficit of HCl and/or NaCl as in vomiting. The recent intake of diuretics will cause the urinary excretion of Na^+ and Cl^- to be elevated. However, note that after diuretic action wears off, U_{Cl} will be low, so that diuretics should be seen as causing Cl^--responsive alkalosis. The U_{Na} may be high if there is a recent episode of vomiting, representing further generation of metabolic alkalosis, in which case bicarbonaturia and higher urine pH are expected. This increase in U_{Na} during

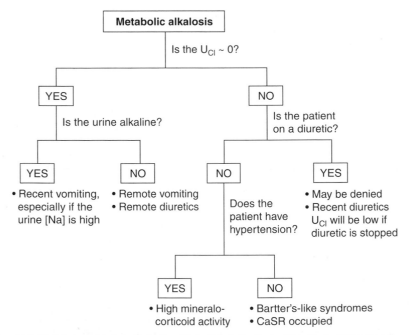

Figure 79.4. Clinical approach to the patient with metabolic alkalosis. The U_{Cl} should be close to nil if the cause of metabolic alkalosis is vomiting or the remote use of diuretics. If the U_{Cl} is not low, an assessment of "effective" arterial blood volume and blood pressure helps separate patients with disorders of high primary mineralocorticoid activity from those with Bartter's-like syndromes. *CaSR*, Calcium sensing receptor in thick ascending limb of the loop of Henle; U_{Cl}, concentration of Cl^- in the urine.

the generation of metabolic alkalosis is why the U_{Cl} is considered the best test because it is low whether the patient is in the generation or maintenance phases.

Another state of Cl^--responsive metabolic alkalosis is posthypercapneic metabolic alkalosis. This occurs in patients with chronic respiratory acidosis whose metabolic compensation in response to increases in PCO_2 leads to increases in serum $[HCO_3^-]$. If exacerbation of pulmonary disease leads to sudden intubation and some degree of hyperventilation with a decrease in PCO_2, the bicarbonate is now high, the PCO_2 is near normal, and metabolic alkalosis is present. This posthypercapneic alkalosis is a state of Cl^- depletion as the kidneys were responding to the respiratory acidosis by preferentially reabsorbing Na^+ in the PCT with HCO_3^- and excreting Cl^-. Correction of the serum $[HCO_3^-]$ will occur only when Cl^- is administered. Because giving Na^+ is often undesirable in such situations, when heart failure may be present and the goal is to keep the alveoli dry, KCl is usually the preferred therapy.

Cl^--unresponsive metabolic alkalosis is generally associated with syndromes that have increased mineralocorticoid activity. If the U_{Cl} is not low, assessment of effective arterial blood volume and blood pressure will help diagnose patients with disorders of high primary mineralocorticoid activity (effective arterial blood volume is not low, hypertension is present). These patients may be separated from those with syndromes causing tubular dysfunction of normal Na^+-reabsorptive processes. These patients resemble those taking diuretics because they have mutations in genes coding for Na^+ transporters. Patients with mutations in genes that lead to changes in the activity of the K-dependent sodium chloride transporter in the thick ascending limb of the loop of Henle have Bartter syndrome and have a phenotype similar to those taking loop diuretics. Those with mutations causing dysfunction in the sodium chloride cotransporter expressed in the distal tubule have Gitelman syndrome and appear as though they are taking thiazides. Both have low effective arterial blood volume with the absence of hypertension. Both have hypokalemia and metabolic alkalosis. However, the patients with Gitelman have low urine calcium, consistent with the effects of thiazides, whereas those with Bartter have increased urine calcium, consistent with the effect of loop diuretics. Another secret for distinguishing genetic abnormalities from surreptitious diuretic use is serial measurements of U_{Cl} in spot urine samples. Patients with Bartter or Gitelman syndromes should have *persistently* high U_{Cl}, whereas those with diuretic abuse will have *intermittently* high U_{Cl}.

13. **What is the major differential diagnosis in a patient who has metabolic alkalosis, a urine Cl^- concentration that is not low, and a contracted ECF volume?**
In this setting, one must look for the basis for a deficit of HCl, KCl, and/or NaCl. The most common cause is the chronic use of diuretics; to reiterate, the U_{Cl} is low when the diuretics are not working. There is also one other group of causes to exclude—the presence of a drug, cation, or cationic protein that binds to the calcium-sensing receptor (Ca-SR) in the basolateral membrane of the thick ascending limb of the loop of Henle. The major ligands for the Ca-SR are a high concentration of ionized calcium in plasma, cationic antibiotics such as gentamicin, and circulating cationic proteins as seen in immunologic disorders or with disorders such as multiple myeloma. A clue for the latter condition is a lower-than-expected value for the anion gap in plasma adjusted for the concentration of albumin in plasma.

14. **When is base administration associated with persistent metabolic alkalosis?**
Base administration may be a generation phase of metabolic alkalosis when kidney function is reduced and the kidneys do not excrete the bicarbonate as rapidly as usual. Occasionally patients with kidney failure may take $NaHCO_3$ as an antacid and with very low GFR develop metabolic alkalosis. They may have correction of the high $[HCO_3]$ at the time of their next dialysis treatment, at which time they should undergo hemodialysis with a lower dialysate $[HCO_3]$. Eventually, normal metabolism and diet will lead to production of protons that will also reduce the $[HCO_3]$.

Another cause is the milk-alkali syndrome. Administration of calcium-containing antacids, mostly calcium carbonate, cause reduced GFR, hypercalcemia, and hypercalciuria. Deposition of calcium phosphate in the kidney parenchyma is a cause of nephrocalcinosis and chronic kidney disease, which also reduces GFR. The carbonate is potential base, titrating protons, and vomiting is sometimes present as well. Metabolic alkalosis contributes to perpetuating the hypercalcemia as it stimulates distal tubular reabsorption of calcium. Hypercalcemia worsens GFR by causing renal vasoconstriction and stimulating the Ca-SR, leading to natriuresis and diuresis and volume depletion. Suppression of PTH leads to reduced bone turnover, which suppressed the ability of bone to take up calcium.

ACKNOWLEDGMENTS

This chapter was original authored by Dr. Kamel Kamel and Dr. Mitch Halperin. Rather than start from scratch, we have simply updated and revised this chapter. We acknowledge their outstanding contribution to the understanding of the relevant physiology and medicine. Our work must pay tribute to their many contributions.

KEY POINTS

1. Concentrations have numerators and denominators. Thus the $[HCO_3^-]$ will rise when the content of HCO_3^- increases and/or when the volume of the extracellular fluid (ECF) compartment declines. Hence metabolic alkalosis represents a heterogeneous group of disorders
2. Support for a T_m for HCO_3^- reabsorption in the proximal convoluted tubule is derived from data from the infusion of $Na^+ + HCO_3^-$, but this is not a physiologically relevant setting.
3. Classification of the common forms of metabolic alkalosis should be based on deficits of HCl, KCl, and/or NaCl (i.e., do not focus only on Cl^- deficiency because this is a partial description of the pathophysiology).
4. Measuring the concentration of Cl^- in the urine is an excellent first step in the clinical approach to patients with metabolic acidosis.
5. A quantitative estimate of the degree of contraction of the ECF volume is helpful because it will indicate the magnitude of the deficit or surplus of HCO_3^- in the ECF compartment.

BIBLIOGRAPHY

Cogan, M. G. (1990). Angiotensin II: A powerful controller of sodium transport in the early proximal tubule. *Hypertension, 15,* 451–458.

Felsenfeld, A. J., & Levine, B. S. (2006). Milk alkali syndrome and the dynamics of calcium homeostasis. *Clinical Journal of the American Society of Nephrology, 1,* 641–654.

Gennari, F. J. (2011). Pathophysiology of metabolic alkalosis: A new classification based on the centrality of stimulated collecting duction transport. *American Journal of Kidney Diseases, 58,* 626–636.

Gowrishankar, M., Kamel, K. S., & Halperin, M. L. (2007). Buffering of a H^+ load: A "brain-protein-centered" view. *Journal of the American Society of Nephrology, 18,* 2278–2280.

Hebert, S. C. (1996). Extracellular calcium-sensing receptor: Implications for calcium and magnesium handling in the kidney. *Kidney International, 50,* 2129–2139.

Kassirer, J. P., & Schwartz, W. B. (1996). The response of normal man to selective depletion of hydrochloric acid. *American Journal of Medicine, 40,* 10–18.

Pitts, R. F., Ayer, J. L., Schiess, W. A., & Miner, P. (1949). The renal regulation of acid-base balance in man. III. The reabsorption and excretion of bicarbonate. *Journal of Clinical Investigation, 28*(1), 35–44.

Purkerson, M. L., Lubowitz, H., White, R. W., & Bricker, N. S. (1969). On the influence of extracellular fluid volume expansion on bicarbonate reabsorption in the rat. *Journal of Clinical Investigation, 48,* 1754–1760.

Scheich, A., Donnelly, S., Cheema-Dhadli, S., Schweigert, M., Vasuvattakul, S., & Halperin, M. L. (1994). Does saline 'correct' the abnormal mass balance in metabolic alkalosis associated with chloride-depletion in the rat? *Clinical & Investigative Medicine, 17,* 448–460.

Simpson, D. (1983). Citrate excretion: A window on renal metabolism. American *Journal of Physiology, 244,* F223–F234.

Zalunardo, N., Lemaire, M., Davids, M. R., & Halperin, M. L. (2004). Acidosis in a patient with cholera: A need to redefine concepts. *Quarterly Journal of Medicine, 97,* 681–696.

XIV
PALLIATIVE CARE IN NEPHROLOGY

PALLIATIVE CARE IN NEPHROLOGY

Amar D. Bansal and Jane O. Schell

CHAPTER 80

OVERVIEW OF PALLIATIVE CARE AND ROLE IN NEPHROLOGY CARE

1. **What is palliative care?**
   Palliative care is specialized care that treats the symptoms and burdens associated with serious illness. Palliative care is delivered by an interdisciplinary team that includes physicians, nurses, social workers, and chaplains.
       Palliative care is not synonymous with hospice care (see later).

2. **What are the domains of palliative care?**
   Palliative care collaboratively addresses multiple domains for patients with serious illness. These domains include:
   - treatment of distressing physical and psychological symptoms
   - help outline goals and preferences for treatment decision making and end of life
   - support spiritual needs and beliefs
   - address caregiver needs

3. **How does palliative care differ from hospice?**
   Palliative care is appropriate at any stage of serious illness. Hospice care is a Medicare benefit provided to patients with terminal illness or when prognosis is likely less than 6 months and the goals of care have shifted toward symptom management rather than life-prolonging therapies. The broad domains of palliative care are still used, but the structure of care is focused on symptom relief and bereavement needs as patients' approach end of life.
       A helpful schematic (Fig. 80.1) shows the gradual shift from curative to palliative care and eventual hospice care over the illness course.

4. **What age group of the chronic kidney disease (CKD) population has the highest rates of dialysis initiation?**
   Based on data from the US Renal Data Service (USRDS), adults older than 75 years have the highest rates for dialysis initiation. This subset of patients presents an important challenge to nephrologists due to their limited prognosis, high symptom burden, and increased need for palliative care.

5. **How can palliative care be helpful in nephrology practice?**
   Nephrologists care for a medically complex population who are at risk for having untreated symptoms, medical setbacks, and limited survival. Palliative care domains that specifically address nephrology needs fall into three domains:
   - Symptom management
   - Shared decision making
   - Advance care planning

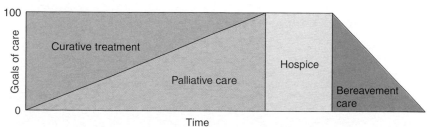

Figure 80.1. Focus of care through chronic disease. The spectrum of curative treatment, palliative care, and hospice through chronic disease. *(Modified from Ferris, F. D., Balfour, H. M., Bowen, K., Farley, J., Hardwick, M., Lamontagne, C., . . . West, P. J. (2002). A model to guide patient and family care: Based on nationally accepted principles and norms of practice. Journal of Pain and Symptom Management, 24, 115. Elsevier.)*

SYMPTOM MANAGEMENT

6. What is the prevalence of symptoms in end stage kidney disease (ESKD)?
   Studies from patients with ESKD have shown that physical symptoms such as pain, fatigue, and pruritus are present in a majority of hemodialysis patients. The severity of symptom burden correlated with decreased health-related quality of life. Dialysis patients are at increased risk for depressive symptoms, with a prevalence of approximately 20%.

7. Is there a substantial difference in the symptoms reported by patients with CKD versus those who have started dialysis?
   The prevalence of patient-reported symptoms, quality of life, and presence of depression are not substantially different between patients with CKD and those who have started dialysis.

8. What are the most common symptoms reported by patients with advanced CKD or ESKD?
   Fatigue, worrying, pruritus, dry skin, dry mouth, feelings of sadness, sleep disturbances, irritability, loss of libido, and muscle cramps were reported by at least 40% of patients in either the CKD or ESKD group in a study of 177 patients.
   From the same study, at least 20% of patients in either the CKD or ESKD group reported having pain or soreness, shortness of breath, anxiety, constipation, edema, restless legs, diarrhea, anorexia, headache, cough, nausea, lightheadedness or dizziness, and lower extremity paresthesias.

9. How aware are nephrologists of symptoms reported by patients?
   Symptom management is a top priority for patients. Despite this, these symptoms are not commonly identified or known by their treating nephrologists. Based on a study of dialysis patients and their providers, at least 25% of providers answered "Don't know" for the 10 most commonly reported symptoms by patients. Current evidence suggests that nephrology providers' unawareness of symptoms is one of the main barriers to improving quality of life for patients with renal disease.

10. What screening tools are available to help nephrologists uncover symptoms?
    Four commonly used tools are the Palliative Care Outcome Scale, Dialysis Symptom Index, Kidney Disease Quality of Life, and Edmonton Symptom Assessment System.

11. What are the treatment options for these common symptoms?
    A variety of treatment options exist with a wide spectrum in the quality of the underlying evidence. See Table 80.1 for a summary of the general approach to three common symptoms that affect nephrology patients.

Table 80.1. Approaches to Address Symptoms Associated With Kidney Disease

SYMPTOM	GENERAL APPROACH
Fatigue	Evaluate for common conditions such as anemia, hypothyroidism, severe hyperparathyroidism, depression, malnutrition, sleep disturbances, or hypotension. Perform a careful medication review 　Adverse drug reactions (especially from antihypertensives) are common. Consider adjustments to the dialysis prescription. 　This may include changes to shift timing, treatment duration, and treatment frequency.
Pruritus	Evaluate for common conditions such as uremia, hyperphosphatemia, hypercalcemia, hyperparathyroidism, dry skin, contact dermatitis, anemia, or drug sensitivity/allergies. Skin care measures include 　Minimizing use of harsh soaps and fragrances 　Use of topical emollients 　Avoidance of hot water during bathing or showering 　Use of humidifiers in winter seasons Potential pharmacologic therapies include: 　Low-dose gabapentin 　Phototherapy 　Topical camphor or menthol Dermatologic consultation may be needed for select patients

Table 80.1. Approaches to Address Symptoms Associated With Kidney Disease *(Continued)*

SYMPTOM	GENERAL APPROACH

Pain	Assess for description of pain; whether the pain is episodic or constant; and whether the duration is expected to be acute or chronic
	Distinguish pain from dialysis associated cramping
	Determine whether pain is thought to be nociceptive or somatic (or both)
	    Analgesics should target appropriate pain type
	    Individualized plan for analgesic selection based on age and comorbidities
	Inquire about ongoing psychosocial distress, depression, anxiety, sleep complaints, or labile mood
	    If present, addressing these first may be beneficial
	    Consideration can be given to nonopioid treatments and nonpharmacologic
	      measures such as mild to moderate exercise or cognitive behavioral therapy
	Use of opioids should be used if other measures fail
	    With proper assessment of risk for misuse, opioids can be safely used in dialysis
	      patients
	    Opioids safe in dialysis patients include fentanyl and methadone. Hydromorphone
	      and oxycodone can be used though doses should start low with longer time
	      intervals between doses (e.g., every 6–8 h as needed instead of every 4 h).

SUPPORT SHARED DECISION MAKING

12. What is shared decision making?

    Shared decision making is a collaborative process through which the clinician and patient arrive at a decision that is mutually agreeable to both of them and informed by the patient's values and preferences. A shared expertise is necessary to develop a patient-centered plan of care—the clinician as the expert in current evidence and best practice, with the patient as the expert in his or her own values and preferences.

13. What characteristics of patients with kidney disease underscore the importance for shared decision making in this population?

    - Limited life expectancy: Survival among patients with ESKD is comparable to many common malignancies, and 1-year mortality for nursing home patients initiated on dialysis is more than 50%. Shared decision making is therefore an essential mechanism to deliver care that is consistent with patients' values and preferences.
    - Unmet symptom and end-of-life needs: Nephrology patients report substantial unmet needs in palliative care, and hospice use remains low for ESKD patients. Shared decision making encourages providers and patients to discuss and plan for future burdens and setbacks related to a given treatment path.
    - Modality selection: For those initiating renal replacement therapy, modality selection is fundamentally based on the process of shared decision making.

14. How can prognostication facilitate shared decision making?

    Most patients want to hear prognostic information. Knowing their prognosis may help patients make decisions that are consistent with their values and preferences and be more engaged in their care, not just with nephrology providers, but with their family and/or surrogate decision makers.

15. Are there tools to help estimate prognosis?

    Validated prognostication tools have been described in the literature. It is important to emphasize that these tools share the same limitations as any prediction algorithm; the accuracy of their results tends to be highest at an aggregate, population level. Their accuracy is limited in evaluating individual patients. Table 80.2 describes some of these prediction models.

16. Do patients want to know their prognosis?

    Based on data from a Canadian study involving 584 patients with advanced CKD, more than 90% reported that it was somewhat or extremely important for them to be informed about their prognosis.

Table 80.2. Studies Examining Survival Prediction in Kidney Disease

PROGNOSTIC MODEL	VALIDATION COHORT	USEFUL FOR	DESCRIPTION
Cohen LM et al.[a]	Patients on maintenance hemodialysis at outpatient centers in the northeastern United States	Estimating chance of survival at 6 months	An integrated model that uses five components: 1. Advanced age 2. Dementia 3. Peripheral vascular disease 4. Decreased albumin 5. Positive "surprise question" ("Would I be surprised if the patient died within the next 6 months?")
Moss AH et al. "Surprise question"	Patients on maintenance hemodialysis at outpatient centers in West Virginia	Identifying patients who may benefit from palliative care intervention	Nurse practitioners were asked if they would be surprised if the patient died in the next 12 months. The odds ratio for death in 12 months in the "no" group versus the "yes" group was 3.5 (95% CI, 1.4–9.1)[b]
Thamer M et al.	Retrospective observational cohort study of 69,441 patients who started dialysis in the United States with an analysis of pre-ESKD Medicare claims to build a prediction model	Estimating risk of 3- and 6-month mortality for incident dialysis patients	A simple risk score is computed from common clinical characteristics. Scores range from 0 to 9, with higher scores correlating with shortened survival.
Couchoud CG et al.[a]	Retrospective observational cohort study of 24,348 patients who started dialysis in France	Estimating risk of 3-month mortality for incident dialysis patients	A risk score is computed from common clinical characteristics. Scores range from 0 to 25, with higher scores correlating with shortened survival.

[a]Denotes that an online calculator is available at https://www.qxmd.com/calculate/.
[b]Denotes confidence interval.

Data from Cohen, L. M., Ruthazer, R., Moss, A. H. & Germain, M. J. (2010.) Predicting six-month mortality for patients who are on maintenance hemodialysis. *Clin J Am Soc Nephrol 5*, 72–79; Moss, A. H. et al. (2008.) Utility of the 'surprise' question to identify dialysis patients with high mortality. *Clin J Am Soc Nephrol 3*, 1379–1384; Thamer, M. et al. (2015.) Predicting Early Death Among Elderly Dialysis Patients: Development and Validation of a Risk Score to Assist Shared Decision Making for Dialysis Initiation. *Am. J. Kidney Dis. 66*, 1024–1032; Couchoud, C. G. G., Beuscart, J.-B. R. B., Aldigier, J.-C. C., Brunet, P. J. & Moranne, O. P. (2015). Development of a risk stratification algorithm to improve patient-centered care and decision making for incident elderly patients with end-stage renal disease. *Kidney Int. 88*, 1178–1186.

17. **Aside from renal replacement therapy and transplantation, what treatment options are available to patients with advanced CKD?**
    Although an individualized approach is essential, there are two main options:
    • Comprehensive conservative care (CCC): a multidisciplinary approach using the principles of nephrology, palliative care (and hospice when necessary), to manage CKD without dialysis.
    • Time-limited trial of dialysis: initiation of dialysis for the purpose of achieving predetermined goals within a specified timeframe.

18. **What is the philosophy of comprehensive conservative care?**
    To use medical therapies such as blood pressure and volume control, anemia management, nutritional interventions, and palliative care assessments to maximize quality of life. There is a shift in focus from biochemical optimization to aggressive symptom management.

19. **Are there subsets of patients for whom the benefit of initiating dialysis is unclear?**
There are two broad categories of patients for whom dialysis may be of unclear benefit. The first category is in the *outpatient setting,* where patients with advanced CKD and other comorbidities may be candidates for CCC. CCC is ideal for patients for whom dialysis is unlikely to add benefit and may cause substantial burdens. These characteristics include but are not limited to:
    - Advanced age (>75 years) with frailty or ischemic heart disease with reduced ejection fraction
    - Patients who have limited prognosis due to advanced coexisting conditions
    - Patient goals that are consistent with maximizing quality of life and for whom dialysis would negatively impact quality of life
    - Presence of geriatric syndromes such as cognitive or functional impairment.
    The second category is in the *inpatient setting,* where critically ill patients with acute kidney injury prompt dialysis discussions. In these situations, in which the chances for meaningful recovery are very small or the burdens of the dialysis treatment itself are great, withholding dialysis or a time-limited trial may be suitable. These decisions often depend on the patient's goals and preferences.

ADVANCE CARE PLANNING (ACP)

20. **What is advance care planning?**
Advance care planning is the process through which healthcare providers engage patients and their caregivers about their preferences for current and future care with emphasis on facilitating future choices. This process typically includes a discussion about advanced therapies (such as dialysis or chemotherapy) and end-of-life preferences.

21. **What is an "illness trajectory"?**
Illness trajectories describe the time-related decline of functional status across a spectrum of illnesses (Fig. 80.2). The concept is useful at an epidemiologic scale and may help clinicians predict future care needs and care preferences. Variability and uncertainty among illness trajectories, including sudden declines in functional ability, highlight the importance of timely discussions of patients' preferences and identification of surrogate decision makers.

22. **Is there an ideal time to discuss advance care planning?**
ACP is appropriate for all patients with kidney disease and not merely reserved for the elderly, frail, or those suffering from a terminal illness. It is not necessarily limited to the end-of-life context, but includes decision making about curative, invasive, or advanced therapies throughout the illness course. When dealing with a CKD population, a discussion of ACP topics should therefore be woven throughout longitudinal interactions with patients.

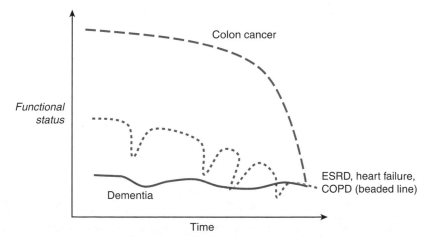

Figure 80.2. Illness trajectories in serious illness. *COPD,* Chronic obstructive pulmonary disease. *ESRD,* End stage renal disease. *(Data from Holley, J.L. (2012). Advance care planning in CKD/ESRD: an evolving process.* Clin J Am Soc Nephrol, *7:1033–1038, and Murtagh, F.E.M., Addington-Hall, J.M. (2007). Symptoms in advanced renal disease: a cross-sectional survey of symptom prevalence in stage 5 chronic kidney disease managed without dialysis.* J Palliat Med. *10:1266–1276.)*

Table 80.3. Advance Directives

TYPE	DESCRIPTION OR PURPOSE
Generic advance directive or "living will"	A document of variable length, specificity, and interpretability that aims to clarify a patient's preferences about medical therapies and/or end-of-life care.
Declaration of surrogate decision-maker	Identifies an adult individual who can make healthcare decisions for the patient when he/she is unable to do so.
Physician Orders for Life Sustaining Treatment (POLST)	An actual physician signed order that outlines a patient's care goals, including code status and preferences for life-sustaining treatments. Because POLST forms are a translation of a patient's goals and preferences into an order, they are less ambiguous than some typical advance directive documents. POLST forms are available in most states and document names will differ by state.
Do not resuscitate (DNR)	A physician order (sometimes with patient co-signature) that prohibits initiation of cardiopulmonary resuscitation in the event of cardiac arrest. A patient who elects a DNR plan of care is still able to receive curative therapies such as invasive procedures, intensive care unit care, chemotherapy, mechanical ventilation, or dialysis.

To maintain broad applicability, general terminology is used. There is state-level variability in terminology and legal differences exist throughout the United States.

23. **Who should be involved in ACP?**
   Evidence suggests that patients think communication about ACP topics is important. Specifically, stronger involvement of the nephrologist is something that patients may desire when it comes to discussing their values and preferences. This process should also involve family and caregivers who often serve as surrogate decision makers when a patient no longer has capacity or is too medically ill to participate in end-of-life decision making.

24. **What are some of the documents used in ACP?**
   There are many documents beyond the Do Not Resuscitate form that may be useful for ACP. Some of these include physician orders for life-sustaining treatment, Five Wishes, and state- or institution-specific advance healthcare directives. Table 80.3 provides an overview of the purpose of many of these forms. Reviews of useful advance directives, as well as their limitations, are available in the literature (Holley JL, *Clin J Am Soc Nephro*, 2012).

25. **How can ACP help patients?**
   The ACP process results in delivery of care that aligns with patients' preferences and therefore results in increased patient satisfaction. In addition, because identification of a surrogate decision maker is an important part of ACP, involvement of family and caregivers results in an improvement in bereavement outcomes, such as depression and anxiety among surviving family members.

26. **What is known about end-of-life preferences for dialysis patients?**
   There are limited data on this issue, but survey results suggest patients want to know more about hospice services and withdrawal from dialysis. Furthermore, results from a single study suggest that patients may prefer to die at home or in hospice rather than in a hospital.

27. **What is the end-of-life experience in ESKD?**
   A study examining the last month of life for ESKD Medicare recipients older than 65 years in the United States found that 76% were hospitalized, approximately half were admitted to an intensive care unit (ICU), and 29% received at least one intensive procedure (defined as cardiopulmonary resuscitation, mechanical ventilation, or insertion of a feeding tube). In addition, approximately 45% died in a hospital. Only 20% of ESKD patients used hospice services in the last month of life, whereas those with cancer or heart failure had hospice use rates at least twofold higher than dialysis patients.

28. **What is known about the dialysis withdrawal?**

There is heterogeneity in the literature in how to define deaths *due to* dialysis withdrawal. However, estimates from USRDS suggest that approximately 20% of patients with ESKD die due to withdrawal from dialysis.

Based on a retrospective analysis, patients who discontinued dialysis had a mean survival of 7 days after enrollment into hospice. This is significantly shorter than patients who enroll for reasons unrelated to renal failure. Clinical characteristics that predicted shortened survival include male sex, low functional status, referral from a hospital, and the presence of peripheral edema.

29. **Are there guidelines about dialysis initiation and withdrawal from dialysis that nephrology providers can use?**

A multidisciplinary clinical practice guideline including input from the Renal Physicians Association and the American Society of Nephrology has been published and makes recommendations focusing on many concepts covered in this chapter.

KEY POINTS

1. Palliative care focuses on treating or alleviating the symptoms and burdens associated with any serious illness.
2. Palliative care can be provided at any time during the course of a serious illness and is not synonymous with hospice, which is a Medicare benefit for patients with a terminal illness or a prognosis less than 6 months.
3. Incorporating palliative care principles into nephrology can help improve symptom management, shared decision making, and advanced care planning for patients with CKD or ESKD.
4. Hemodialysis patients have very high symptom burden and low health-related quality of life. A majority of them report pain, fatigue, and pruritus.
5. Shared decision making is a collaborative process through which the clinician and patient attempt to align goals in order to arrive at a decision that is mutually agreeable to both of them.
6. In situations in which dialysis is thought to have minimal benefit, other treatment options include comprehensive conservative management or a time-limited trial of dialysis.

BIBLIOGRAPHY

Abdel-Kader, K., Unruh, M., & Weisbord, S. (2009). Symptom burden, depression, and quality of life in chronic and end-stage kidney disease. *Clinical Journal of the American Society of Nephrology, 4,* 1057–1064.

Davison, S. N. (2010). End-of-life care preferences and needs: Perceptions of patients with chronic kidney disease. *Clinical Journal of the American Society of Nephrology, 2,* 195–204.

Davison, S. N., & Jassal, S. V. (2016). Supportive care: Integration of patient-centered kidney care to manage symptoms and geriatric syndromes. *Clinical Journal of the American Society of Nephrology, 10,* 1882–1891.

Galla, J. H. (2000). Clinical practice guideline on shared decision-making in the appropriate initiation of and withdrawal from dialysis. *Journal of the American Society of Nephrology 11,* 1340–1342.

Holley, J. L. (2012). Advance care planning in CKD/ESRD: An evolving process. *Clinical Journal of the American Society of Nephrology, 7,* 1033–1038.

Murtagh, F. E. M., & Addington-Hall, J. M. (2007). Symptoms in advanced renal disease: A cross-sectional survey of symptom prevalence in stage 5 chronic kidney disease managed without dialysis. *Journal of Palliative Medicine, 10,* 1266–1276.

O'Connor, N. R., Dougherty, M., Harris, P. S., & Casarett, D. J. (2013). Survival after dialysis discontinuation and hospice enrollment for ESRD. *Clinical Journal of the American Society of Nephrology, 8,* 2117–2122.

Weisbord, S., Fried, L., Mor, M., Resnick, A. L., Unruh, M. L., Palevsky, P. M., . . . Arnold, R. M. (2007). Renal provider recognition of symptoms in patients on maintenance hemodialysis. *Clinical Journal of the American Society of Nephrology, 2,* 960–967.

Wong, S., Kreuter, W., & O'Hare, A. (2012). Treatment intensity at the end of life in older adults receiving long-term dialysis. *Archives of Internal Medicine, 172,* 661–663.

Wright, A. A., Zhang, B., Ray, A., Mack, J. W., Trice, E., Balboni, T., . . . Prigerson, H. G. (2008). Associations between end-of-life discussions, patient mental health, medical care near death, and caregiver bereavement adjustment. *JAMA, 300,* 1665–1673.

XV
NEPHROLOGY
BEGINNINGS

CHAPTER 81

NEPHROLOGY BEGINNINGS

Garabed Eknoyan

1. Why the history of nephrology?

"To understand a science it is necessary to know its history," said August Comte (1798–1857), founder of modern sociology. Rooted in sociology, this saying evolved into what is now known as the theory of path dependence, which explains how decisions made in any given new circumstance are determined and limited by decisions made in the past, even though past circumstances may no longer be directly relevant to present ones. This almost intuitively self-evident truth of social behavior applies to the science of decision making in general and has led to three Nobel Prizes. This is why the history of any science, and that of nephrology in particular, does matter.

Broadly defined, one can argue that the history of diseases of the kidney can be traced to antiquity. On the other hand, strictly defined, the specialty dedicated to the study of the kidney and its diseases, nephrology, is a relatively new discipline that emerged in the latter half of the 20th century. Although the term *nephrology* appears in medical dictionaries of the 1840s, and most nephrologists trace their origins to Richard Bright's description of the association of proteinuria with kidney disease in 1827, the term did not enter medical parlance until the 1960s (see the following section of this chapter). As such, nephrology has a rather short albeit rapidly expanding history.

Why then the history of nephrology? From the outset, it is important to admit that historical knowledge is not necessary to the practice of good medicine by any well-rounded nephrologist, or to doing solid nephrology research by any well-trained investigator. The once lofty answer that, as a learned profession, medicine has interests that transcend its utilitarian purpose is no longer tenable. However, the fact remains that most notable leaders and contributors to the medical sciences are well versed in the humanities and knowledgeable of the history of their discipline as any reading of the acceptance lectures of past Nobel laureates in chemistry or physiology or medicine will clearly reveal (see: nobelprize.org). And as stated by a founder of scientific medicine, William Osler (1849–1919), *"History and the knowledge of men are as much part of medicine as the latest technical devices and the knowledge of science."*

That may sound as a tenuous argument, particularly by those enamored with the rapid pace of nephrologic advances, who in their quest for new truths reject the past as obsolescent. In this regard, it is worth noting that current research can be appreciated best when considered in its historical context. This should be evident to all medical investigators, no matter how narrow their field of research and whether or not they realize it, and not only because they are part of a grand historical tradition. More importantly, however limited their care for the history of nephrology, their ultimate research motivation is to discover some new truth to change the course of their very research topic. Stated otherwise, they are actually doing research in a quest for a place in history. As such, the realization of their own rich professional heritage and the very raison d'être of research can only enrich their intellectual satisfaction and will provide them with reassurance when facing the trials and tribulations of research. In essence, belittling the past is detrimental only to their own full appreciation of the very work they are engaged in.

By the same token, one may ask whether the practice of nephrology deprived of its history makes one an inferior clinician. Surely not. However, as a first consideration, it is worth noting that history is engrained in the very practice of medicine. Any good clinician—even those with no interest in history—must be a good historian who can dig up and record the facts of the "past medical history" of every patient encountered. That is the aim of every aspiring clinician so well promulgated by one considered the ultimate clinical scholar, William Osler, whose statement on the importance of the history of medicine has been quoted earlier. Osler's statement can be taken with a grain of salt in current rapidly evolving science of medicine, but familiarity with the work of one's predecessors does add to the appreciation and enjoyment of one's daily practice of medicine.

To sum up, why history in general, and that of nephrology in particular, is important may have been answered best by the English historian, Thomas Fuller (1608–1661):

History maketh a young man to be old, without either wrinkles or grey hairs; privileging him with the experiences of age, without either the infirmities or inconveniences thereof. Yea, it not only maketh things past, present; but enableth one to make a rational conjecture of things to come.

August Comte may have been right after all. Knowing the history of nephrology will not only make it easier to understand the science of nephrology but will also enrich its daily practice by those pursuing it as an avocation.

2. When did nephrology emerge as a medical specialty?

Words involving the Greek root *nephros* for the kidney have been used for centuries. The word "nephrology" as a discipline for the study of the kidney in health and disease came into use in the opening decades of the 19th century but did not actually enter the parlance of medicine until the middle of the 20th century, at which time several events contributed to the emergence of nephrology as a medical specialty. First was the continued and increasing number of published articles on kidney function that had been prompted by the World War II medical effort to study shock, climatic adaptation, renal clearance of drugs, and hemodynamics. Second was technological advances that were of direct clinical relevance to kidney disease, specifically dialysis, kidney transplantation, and kidney biopsy.

The first physician to call himself a "nephrologist," as one who specialized in diseases of the kidney, was Arthur Arnold Osman (1893–1972) in 1945, who went on to help found the U.K. Renal Association in 1950 and served as its first president for the next 6 years. The Italian Società Italiana di Nefrologia was founded thereafter in 1957, and the French Société de Nephrologie in 1959. The first medical publication devoted to the discipline, Minerva Nefrologica, appeared in Italy in 1957. As the number of physiologists, pathologists, and clinicians interested in the kidney increased, the membership of these societies increased and new national organizations were established. In 1960 the first international meeting of nephrologists was held in Evian, leading to the establishment of the International Society of Nephrology in 1961 and the launching of its first official journal, *Nephron,* in 1964. The American Society of Nephrology was founded in 1966, and its official journal, the *Journal of the American Society of Nephrology,* was published in 1990.

As a result, all the "nephrophiles" of the past and the budding "nephrologists" thereafter now had a discipline to rally around.

3. When was the first artificial kidney used in humans?

Thomas Graham (1805–1869), a physical chemist whose seminal work on osmotic forces of fluids paved the way to hemodialysis, has been dubbed the father of modern dialysis. His studies on the behavior of biological fluids across a semipermeable membrane presaged the development of an artificial kidney and formulated the scientific basis of clinical dialysis, specifically that blood flowing in a semipermeable membrane that is in contact with an electrolyte solution (dialysate) allowed for the diffusion of small molecules from blood into the dialysate.

The first use of dialysis in vivo, so called vividiffusion, was in rabbits and dogs by John Jacob Abel (1857–1928) and his associates at Johns Hopkins in 1912 and 1913. His primitive attempts at dialyzing a few patients were utter failures, but it was his machine that was first dubbed an "artificial kidney" by a correspondent of the *London Times.* Tentative attempts at dialysis of humans were undertaken by Georg Haas (1886–1971) in Giessen in the 1920s, using collodion membranes and hirudin as anticoagulant that had also been used by Abel. Collodion and hirudin had to be prepared fresh, were not standardized, were difficult to sterilize, and soon led to the abandonment of clinical dialysis.

Practical dialysis became possible in the early 1940s as a result of two new substances: a cellulose acetate (cellophane) membrane and a new anticoagulant heparin. Three early pioneers to use the new membrane and anticoagulant in clinical dialysis were Gordon Murray (1884–1972) in Canada, Niels Alwall (1906–1986) in Sweden, and Willem Kolff (1911–2009) in the Netherlands; but it was Kolff working in Kampen under the tensions and difficult conditions of war-torn Holland who achieved the first clinically successful hemodialysis in humans. Kolff's "rotating drum hemodialyzer" was a wooden, pumpless drum, wrapped 30 times with 130 feet of cellophane tubing (connected to the circulation) immersed in a ceramic bathtub containing a saline solution. Beginning in 1942, Kolff experimented with his artificial kidney. His first 16 patients never recovered and went on to succumb to kidney failure. Only 2.5 years later did his first patient, Sofia Maria Schafstadt, survive. Ironically, she had been a Nazi collaborator who was actually imprisoned. She had cholecystitis, developed septicemia, and was treated with one of the recently available sulfonamides. Her acute kidney injury was a result of sulfonamide crystal precipitation in the tubules, a common side effect of these early wonder antibacterial drugs then in use.

4. Who was the first patient to benefit from chronic maintenance hemodialysis?

The artificial kidney introduced after World War II remained experimental and was used mainly in exploratory attempts to sustain the lives of selected patients with acute kidney injury through the 1950s. The need for repeated access to the circulation limited the use of hemodialysis to the short term only in patients with acute kidney injury. Even in patients with acute kidney injury with delayed recovery, prolonged dialysis presented insurmountable problems that led to its abandonment before kidney function had recovered. The breakthrough came in March 1960, when Belding Scribner (1921–2003), a nephrologist, and Wayne Quinton (1921–2015), an engineer, working in Seattle, developed the so-called Quinton-Scribner shunt using Teflon, which had become available recently and was being used to coat implantable cardiac pacemakers. Shortly thereafter, the shunt was modified to be made from more flexible silicone tubing with Teflon tips inserted into the radial vasculature. The first patient to benefit from this new device was Clyde Shields (1921–1971), a 39-year-old Boeing machinist. In April 1960 Scribner took Clyde to the annual meeting of the American Society for Artificial Internal Organs in Atlantic City, New Jersey for a private demonstration of the shunt. The news traveled with lightning speed, and suddenly long-term maintenance hemodialysis became possible. For the first time in medicine, technology and creativity allowed the replacement of the functions of a vital body organ. Literally overnight, repeated hemodialysis allowed survival from the otherwise fatal disease described by Richard Bright (1789–1858) some 150 years earlier.

That was when dialysis moved from its rudimentary beginnings in the 1950s to a chronic life-sustaining modality of treatment, for which Kolff and Scribner were to share the Lasker Award in 2002. Unfortunately, the extremely limited resources then available in Seattle necessitated the creation of a committee to select who received maintenance dialysis (later dubbed "Life and Death Committee"). Even when restricted funds were made available, dialysis remained limited and choices of who was dialyzed continued to be made, albeit based on "medical criteria" and "first come, first served" basis imposed by the limited means and available dialysis machines. It was not until 1973, when Public Law 92-603 amendment to the 1972 Social Security Act went into effect, that dialysis care became accessible to almost everyone.

In response to mounting needs for maintenance dialysis, hospital-based dialysis centers moved into for-profit outpatient facilities and proliferated. The rush to save the life of otherwise dying patients outpaced the science of dialysis, resulting in the delivery of a treatment that was primarily empiric. Over the decades that followed, the complications of dialysis and the significant morbidity and mortality associated with it emerged as serious concerns of all stakeholders. Some of the early complications of dialysis (aluminum toxicity, water purity, hepatitis, anemia) were soon resolved; others (mineral bone disease, cardiovascular disease) linger on, while that of adequacy of dialysis still awaits resolution.

All those problems and concerns notwithstanding, Clyde Shields survived 11 years on dialysis, succumbing to a myocardial infarction in 1971.

5. When were the first kidney biopsies performed?
   Biopsies of the kidney on the operating table were performed by surgeons through the first decades of the 20th century for various reasons. Relevant to the history of nephrology was an open biopsy performed in 1896 by a British urologist, Reginald Harrison (1837–1908), as part of a kidney decapsulation procedure for the treatment of Bright disease. The first open kidney biopsy for a diagnostic purpose was performed in 1923 in Toronto by Norman B. Gwyn (1875–1952), a nephew and student of William Osler. The first report of systematically studied kidney biopsies was in subjects undergoing dorsolumbar sympathectomy for hypertension published in 1943 by a Boston surgeon, Reginald Smithwick (1899–1987), and a pathologist, Benjamin Castleman (1906–1982), better known for his long editorship of the clinicopathologic case reports in the *New England Journal of Medicine*.

   Percutaneous needle biopsy of the kidney was introduced after the successful use of cutting needles in liver biopsy. Nils Alwall (1904–1986) of Lund, also a pioneer of hemodialysis, performed the first systematic needle kidney biopsies in 1944. An early death of a patient after a biopsy led him to abandon the technique. He did not publish his results until 1952. In the meantime, Poul Iversen (1889–1966) and Claus Brun (1914–2014) of Copenhagen began using the technique in 1949. The initial needles, known as Vim-Silverman needles, were a modification of the liver biopsy cutting-edge needles. Apart from the skill needed in handling these needles, positioning of the kidney presented a major challenge in those early days. Credit for improvements and for popularizing the clinical utility of kidney biopsies is due to Robert M. Kark (1911–2002), Robert C. Muehrcke (1921–2003), and Conrad L. Pirani (1915–2005) from Chicago. The first international meeting on kidney biopsies was held in 1961, and meetings to discuss kidney pathology were precursors of the kidney pathology societies that emerged thereafter.

   Subsequent improved imaging and kidney ultrasound, together with new disposable gun biopsy needles, have literally revolutionized the procedure, which has evolved increasingly into another procedure undertaken by invasive radiologists.

6. How did the concept of acid-base balance emerge?
   Variable notions of acid and alkali have been part of medicine since antiquity. The concept of acidity and alkalinity were well known from their sensory perception, either gustatory from their taste or

visual from the color changes they produced in certain dyes. Their taste is what provided their initial nomenclature. Acids tasted sour, hence the origin of the term "acid" from the Latin *acere* (sour), and its prototype the taste of acetic acid in vinegar, still known in Italian as *aceto*. Alkali, referring to that of the ash of charred wood or plants, whose principal constituent is potassium carbonate, is derived from the Arabic, *al-qali,* the word for roasting. Its taste is harder to describe, but, as the opposite of acid, it lacks tartness but leaves a distinctive sleek, somewhat soapy aftertaste in the mouth.

The changes in color they produce were first explored by the Catalan scholar Arnaldus de Villa Nova (1240–1311) using litmus, a dye extract from lichen, to test acidity. They were expanded and systematized by Robert Boyle (1622–1691), who described plant extracts that changed color in the presence of acids and bases. One such was an extract of violets that is blue but turns green in solutions that are basic and red when acid.

Early chemical studies in the 17th century by Johann Glauber (1607–1673) working in Amsterdam identified salts that resulted from the union of various acids and bases and attributed disease to disturbances in their balance in the body. A German chemist, Justin Liebig (1803–1873), ascribed acidity to the presence of hydrogen ions. With methodologic advances in chemical measurement, it was then recognized that blood is alkaline and the urine is acidic. One of the earliest studies on urinary acid and base constituents was published in 1812 by the Swedish chemist, John Jacob Brezilius (1770–1843), considered one of the founding fathers of chemistry. Interest in acid-base balance grew thereafter but remained descriptive in the main. The theory of electrolyte dissociation in aqueous solutions and the presence of hydrogen ions in acids and hydroxyl ions in bases proposed by the Swedish physicist Svante Arrhenius (1859–1927) in 1887 were instrumental in the subsequent development of concepts of acid-base solutions and buffers. For his contributions, Arrhenius was awarded the 1903 Nobel Prize for Chemistry *"in recognition of the extraordinary services he has rendered to the advancement of chemistry by electrolytic theory of dissociation."* His concept was expanded by the Danish chemist Johannes N, Brønsted (1879–1947) and the Englishman Thomas M. Lowry (1874–1936), working independently, into the present Brønsted-Lowry theory characterizing acids by their affinity as proton donors and of alkali as proton acceptors.

Subsequent refinements in the instrumentation to measure the concentration of hydrogen and hydroxyl ions provided much of the advances in acid-base balance that followed. Research was stimulated by epidemics of cholera and subsequently diabetic ketoacidosis by such early pioneers in kidney physiology as Bernhard Naunyn (1839–1925), Lawrence Henderson (1878–1942), and Donald Van Slyke (1883–1971).

In 1911 Henderson introduced an equation for evaluating the buffering properties of weak acids and bases from their dissociation constant. The logarithmic transformation of Henderson's equation by Karl Hasselbach (1874–1962) in 1917 yielded what is known now as the Henderson-Hasselbach equation. The fundamental importance of this mathematic equation in the subsequent elucidation of acid-base disorders notwithstanding, its complexity remains the principal cause of the difficulty encountered by most in understanding acid-base disorders. The use of hydrogen ion concentration expressed in nanomoles would resolve much of the difficulty associated with the continued, but unnecessary, use of the negative logarithmic expression of pH, which is just understood by a select few but is confusing to everyone else.

Structured studies in acid-base homeostasis and the role of the kidney in maintaining acid-base balance were undertaken during the period between the two world wars. The role of the kidney in the process was elucidated in the 1940s to a great extent by the studies of Robert F. Pitts (1908–1977) and his associates at Cornell University.

7. When was the first successful kidney transplant performed?
Experimental allotransplants and xenotransplants of the kidney in animals were begun in the latter half of the 19th century. By the opening decades of the 20th century, unsuccessful attempts at xenotransplantation in humans were undertaken in Vienna by Emerich Ullman (1861–1937), who transplanted a pig kidney in the elbow of a young woman with uremia, and in Lyon by Mathieu Jaboulay (1860–1913), who transplanted a sheep kidney in one patient and a pig kidney in another. The first cadaveric kidney transplant was performed on April 3, 1933 in Kiev by Yuri Voronoy (1895–1961), who transplanted the kidney from a 60-year-old woman who had died from head injury to a 26-year-old woman with acute kidney injury from mercury poisoning, a common cause of kidney injury at the time. The patient died 48 hours later.

Technical difficulties and lack of an understanding of the immunologic basis of organ rejection hampered early efforts at organ transplantation. Their respective study and partial resolution resulted in two Nobel Awards in Physiology or Medicine: the first in 1912 to the French surgeon Alexis Carrel

(1873–1944) *"in recognition of his work on vascular suture and transplantation of blood vessels and organs,"* and the second in 1960 to the British biologist Peter Medawar (1915–1987) and the Australian virologist Frank Macfarlane Burnet (1899–1985) *"for discovery of acquired immunological tolerance."* The first documented kidney transplant in the United States was performed on June 17, 1950 on a 44-year-old woman with polycystic kidney disease in Evergreen Park, Illinois. The kidney was rejected. The first successful kidney transplant was performed in Boston by a team led by the nephrologist John P. Merrill (1917–1984) and the plastic surgeon Joseph Murray (1919–2012), who on December 23, 1954 transplanted a kidney from one identical twin, Ronald Herrick, to his brother, Richard. This was before chronic maintenance hemodialysis became feasible, and it generated considerable interest and excitement in the future treatment of kidney failure.

Richard Herrick recovered kidney function, married the recovery room nurse who had cared for him after the transplant, had two children, and enjoyed good health until his death in March 1963. In 1990 Joseph Murray received the Nobel Prize in Physiology or Medicine, shared with another American physician E. Donnall Thomas (1920–2012), for their contribution to *"organ and cell transplantation in the treatment of human disease,"* the third Nobel prize to be granted for work on transplantation.

8. What is the origin of the term "uremia"?
Much of our understanding of the pathophysiology of diseases comes from the analysis of body fluids that were being introduced into medicine in the 19th century. These early biochemical studies were instrumental in shaping much of the subsequent nomenclature and progress in the study of diseases in general and that of the end-stage kidney disease described by Richard Bright (1789–1858) at about that time.

Large volumes were necessary for the rather crude analytic methods available then, and it was generally easier to use the readily accessible and substantial quantities of urine rather than blood. Of the various chemical substances that were identified in the urine, it was probably that of urea which contributed most to what followed. First characterized as a *"urinary salt"* in 1662 and an *"unusual saponaceous salt residue of urine that tasted different than sea salt"* in 1732, urea was finally isolated as a pure salt by the Frenchmen François Fourcroy (1755–1809) and Nicolas Vaquelin (1763–1829) in 1799. By 1817 the properties, appearance, and chemical reactions of urea were described by the Englishman William Prout (1785–1850), who alluded to its presence in the blood. Shortly thereafter, in 1828 the German Friederich Wöhler (1800–1882) synthesized urea from two inorganic molecules, ammonia and cyanic acid, which prompted him to write triumphantly to his mentor Jöns Jacob Berzelius (1779–1848): *"I can make urea without the use of kidney, either man or dog."* This was a major breakthrough and turning point in the history of science that placed the notion of vitalism, which had dominated medical concepts theretofore, to rest and validated the chemical approach to biology that was to launch the new basic sciences of organic chemistry and biochemistry. Wöhler's discovery literally coincided with the description of Bright disease. Within a year, Robert Christison (1797–1882) reported increased urea levels in the serum of patients with Bright disease, which by 1847 led to the introduction by Pierre Piorry (1794–1879) of the term *urémie* (uremia), literally urine in the blood, to describe patients with high blood urea levels.

Over the years, the term *uremia* has come to encompass all the clinical manifestations of the failing kidneys. The sole role of urea to account for the symptom complex of uremic patients with advanced kidney disease was questioned from the outset. George Johnson (1818–1896), a contemporary of Richard Bright and a prominent authority on kidney disease who described the microscopic changes of Bright disease, wrote in 1852, *"It is in the highest degree probable that urea is a poisonous agent, but we have no proof that it is more so than other urinary constituents which must be retained or accumulated in the blood, when the kidneys are so much disorganized as they are often found to be."* A truth that still holds, notwithstanding which the uremia of Piorry remains in use to this day as a rather vague and catch-all medical term used to refer to abnormalities of kidney failure that remain unexplained and presumed to result from the still elusive chemical product(s) that should have been excreted by the kidneys.

Of note, it was the continued studies of urea that were to provide much of the experimental and theoretic concepts that led to the discovery of the artificial kidney. It was the studies of Thomas Graham (1805–1869) on the diffusion and osmotic properties of urea that laid the very conceptual foundations of hemodialysis, and it is the proportional clearance of urea from the body by dialysis (urea reduction ratio) that now provides a measure of the adequacy of dialysis in treating patients with kidney failure.

It was also studies on the clearance of urea that paved the way to the study of kidney function, introduced the concept of *renal efficiency,* and provided for the classification of kidney disease. Early studies of progressive ablation of kidney mass to produce uremia were refined by measurement of blood levels of urea and its renal clearance in patients with kidney disease by George Widal (1862–1929) in France and Hermann Strauss (1864–1944) in Germany. Widal meticulously evaluated the gradual retention of nitrogenous end products (*azotémie*), which he went on to classify as azotemia that is alarming, grave, and fatal, the first classification of kidney diseases based on the severity of lost kidney function.

9. What is the origin of the term *nephrotic syndrome*?

Nephrotic syndrome as a diagnostic term came into use in the 1920s to describe the triad of heavy proteinuria, hypoalbuminemia, and edema, usually with associated dyslipidemia and lipiduria. The common presenting symptom of edema, once called dropsy, has an ancient history. It was the association of dropsy with proteinuria that established the link of edema with kidney disease and launched the discipline that was to become nephrology. Dropsy, or the accumulation of fluid, was regarded as an entity of its own until the end of the 18th century. Its association with cirrhosis of the liver was well known in antiquity, its association with kidney disease was also described, particularly in patients with oliguria, but its association with diseases of the heart was indirect and generally ascribed to the broader concept of diseases of the chest, when fluid was detected in the lungs or pleural space of some patients with dropsy. Two landmark publications laid the foundations that were to clarify the role of the kidneys and the heart in dropsy, their interrelationships in health and disease, and ultimately the identification of edema as a symptom of underlying diseases rather than a disease itself.

First was the publication in 1785 of *An Account of the Foxglove and Some of Its Medical Uses* by William Withering (1741–1799), who showed that the administration of an infusion of the leaves of foxglove *(digitalis purpurea)* produced a diuresis and an amelioration of dropsical symptoms. However, it was obvious from the outset, including a third of the cases reported by Withering, that not all patients with dropsy responded to the infusion and that some of the nonresponders who died while taking the infusion were suffering from cirrhosis of the liver with ascites. No comment was made on the kidney of these nonresponders. The determination of the kidney as a principal cause of dropsy had to await a second landmark publication in 1827 of the *Reports of Medical Cases* by Richard Bright (1789–1858), which contained his description of end-stage kidneys and led to the distinction of dropsy as a result of kidney disease by the presence of heat-coagulable albuminous material in the urine.

The link of dropsy with hypoalbuminemia was suspected shortly thereafter from the low specific gravity of the serum of patients with Bright disease who had the heaviest albuminuria reported by Robert Christison (1799–1882) of Edinburgh in 1829 but had to await improved chemical methods to define it as due to hypoalbuminemia.

Although it was clear from the outset that kidney disease is not always associated with dropsy or albuminuria, Bright disease soon came to be accepted as a diagnostic term for albuminuric kidney disease. It was studies to differentiate the various kidney lesions of Bright disease and the evaluation of their possible association with proteinuria that determined the course of subsequent events in the emergence of nephrology. Richard Bright had described three principal types of the gross appearance of the kidneys he reported: (1) a hard, small (one-half normal size) kidney with cysts; (2) a soft, mottled, yellowish-grey kidney of normal size; and (3) a swollen, large (twice normal size), soft, pale kidney. It was the latter, which was associated with anasarca and heavier proteinuria, that ultimately came to be associated with nephrotic syndrome. The descriptive morphologic term *nephrosis,* derived from the German *nephrotische,* was introduced in 1905 by Friedrich von Müller (1858–1941), a pathologist working in Munich, to differentiate the morphologic features of these large kidneys from those of the small kidneys due to the inflammatory lesions of *nephritis.* The subsequent grouping of the common clinical manifestations of the various lesions of nephrosis under the term *syndrome of nephrosis*, *nephrosis syndrome*, and *nephrotic syndrome* were introduced between 1924 and 1929 in the writings of Henry A. Christian (1876–1951) of Boston. Of those, nephrotic syndrome received the better acceptance and entered medical parlance thereafter.

10. When did clinical nephrology begin its transformation into a science?

Thomas Addis (1881–1949), a pioneer in nephrology, was one of the first clinicians to systematize the study of kidney disease, quantify the cellular (especially red blood cells) constituents of the urine sediment, use the recently developed clearance technique to determine kidney function, and introduce dietary treatment for those with kidney failure. His book, titled *Glomerular Nephritis: Diagnosis and Treatment,* published in 1948, remains a reference worth perusal by anyone seriously interested in the beginnings of clinical nephrology. His most famous patient was the double Nobel laureate for

Chemistry and Peace, Linus Pauling (1901–1994), whom Addis treated with a protein-restricted diet. Relevant to the current debate on healthcare, it is of special interest that shortly before his death, Addis resigned from the American Medical Association in objection to its campaign against President Truman's national plan for health insurance.

The heritage of Addis is best summed in one of his sayings, *"When the patient dies the kidneys go to the pathologist, but when he lives the urine is ours. It can provide us day by day, month by month, and year by year, with a serial story of the major events going on within the kidney,"* a statement that deserves to be remembered and propagated daily by every nephrologist.

KEY POINTS

1. Richard Bright discovered the connection of proteinuria to kidney disease.
2. Willem Kolff conducted the first successful dialysis for acute kidney injury in a human (1944).
3. Clyde Shields was the first person to receive chronic dialysis via the newly invented Scribner shunt.
4. Joseph Murray performed the first successful kidney transplant by taking the organ from one twin brother (Ronald Herrick) and placing it in to the other (Richard Herrick), who had ESKD (1919–2012), on December 23, 1954.

BIBLIOGRAPHY

Astrup, P., & Severinghaus, W. (1986). *The history of blood gases, acids and bases.* Copenhagen: Munksgaard.
Cameron, J. S. (2002). *History of the treatment of renal failure by dialysis.* Oxford: Oxford University Press.
Cameron, J. S., & Hicks, J. (1999). The introduction of renal biopsy into nephrology from 1901–1961. A paradigm of the forming of nephrology by technology. *American Journal of Nephrology, 17,* 347–358.
Cameron, J. S., & Hicks, J. (2002). The origin and development of the concept of a "nephrotic syndrome." *American Journal of Nephrology, 22,* 240–247.
Eknoyan, G. (2016). Why the history of nephrology. *Giornale Italiano Di Nefrologia, 33*(1), 1–7.
Lemley, K. V., & Pauling, L. (1994). Thomas Addis: July 27, 1881–June 4, 1949. *Biographical Memoirs. National Academy of Sciences, 63,* 3–46.
Morris, P. J. (2004). Transplantation: A medical miracle of the 20th century. *New England Journal of Medicine, 351,* 2678–2680.
Peitzman, S. J. (2008). *Dropsy, dialysis, transplant: A short history of failing kidneys.* Baltimore: Johns Hopkins University Press.
Richet, G. (1988). Early history of uremia. *Kidney International, 33,* 1013–1015.
Schreiner, G. (1999). Evolution of nephrology. The caldron of its organizations. *American Journal of Nephrology, 19,* 295–303.

INDEX

Note: Page numbers followed by "f" refer to illustrations; page numbers followed by "t" refer to tables; page numbers followed by "b" refer to boxes.

608 INDEX

Elderly patients
  chronic kidney disease in, 123
    mortality, 345
  dialysis in, 345
  glomerular diseases in, 345
  hypertension in, 344, 441
  immunosuppression in, 346
  kidney clearance in, 344
  kidney diseases in, 342–347, 346b
  kidney transplant graft loss in, 346
  peritoneal dialysis in, 371
  prevalence of, 342
  simple cyst in, 346
  urinary tract infection in, 323
Electrocardiogram (EKG), hypokalemia-related
  changes in, 521, 523
Electrolyte abnormalities
  in cancer, 257
  in tumor lysis syndrome, 265
Electrolyte disorders, rhabdomyolysis caused by, 90t
Electrolyte-free water, in hypernatremia, 517–518
Electron microscopy, for immunoglobulin A
  nephropathy, 198
Elevated 1, 25D level, 529
Elimination, of drugs, in chronic kidney disease,
  169–170
Embolism
  air, hemodialysis-related, 362
  cholesterol, 146
Emphysematous pyelonephritis, 326
Empiric antimicrobial therapy, for complicated
  urinary tract infection, 325
Enalaprilat, 474t
Encephalopathy, hypertensive, 472
End-stage kidney disease (ESKD)
  in ADPKD, 299
  in African Americans
    incidence of, 348
    mortality rate of, 350
    recombinant human erythropoietin in, 350
    risk factors for, 348
  in elderly patients, 345
  home hemodialysis for, 363
  in living kidney donors, 401, 402
  membranoproliferative glomerulonephritis
    and, 205
  renal artery stenosis and, 444
  risk for, hypertension and, 441
End-stage renal disease (ESRD)
  chronic kidney disease, 580
  diabetic neuropathy progression to, 211–212
  end of life experience in, 584
  from lupus nephritis, extrarenal flares in, 221–222
  in membranous nephropathy, 194
  prevalence of, 580
  treatment options for, 580, 580–581t
Endocrine hypertension, 449–459, 458b
  congenital adrenal hyperplasia and, 450–454,
    453f
  Cushing syndrome and, 450–454
  hyperaldosteronism and, 449–450
  pheochromocytoma and, 455–458

Endothelin-1, in sickle cell nephropathy, 336
Endothelin A receptor antagonists, for diabetic
  kidney disease, 214
Enoxaparin, for chronic kidney disease, 176, 176t
Entecavir, for HBV glomerular disease, 239
Enteric hyperoxaluria, 318
Enzyme replacement therapy (ERT), for Fabry
  disease, 291
Eosinophilic granulomatosis with polyangiitis, 224
Eosinophiluria
  acute kidney injury and, 50
  in acute tubulointerstitial nephritis, 313
Ephedrine, kidney stone caused by, 118h
Epithelial sodium channel (ENaC), 520
Eplerenone, 478–480
Epoetin, 132
Epsilon-aminocaproic acid (EACA), for
  hematuria, 339
Epstein-Barr virus (EBV) infection
  post-transplant lymphoproliferative disorder
    and, 416
  posttransplant, 421
Equilibrated Kt/Vurea (eKt/Vurea), 358
Ergocalciferol, 137t
Ergotamine, secondary hypertension from, 460
Erlotinib, 259t
Erythromycin, drug interaction of, 406t
Erythropoiesis-stimulating agents (ESAs)
  administration of, 132
  for African Americans, with end-stage kidney
    disease, 350
  newer, 133
  during pregnancy, 333
  for sickle cell anemia, 339
  toxic, 133
Erythropoietin, deficiency of, 130
Escherichia coli
  posttransplant, 418
  in urinary tract infection, 321–322
Esmolol, 474t
Essential hypertension, 501
Estimated Post Transplant Survival Score (EPTS), 395
Ethanol, effect on catecholamine and metabolite
  levels, 456t
Ethylene glycol, metabolic acidosis and, 562
European Vasculitis Study, 103–104
Everolimus, 281
Exercise
  excessive, rhabdomyolysis and, 89–90
  for hypertension control, 484–485
  resistant hypertension and, 466
Exit site infection, peritoneal dialysis and, 381
Extended daily dialysis (EDD), 54
Extracellular fluid (ECF)
  bicarbonate in, 549, 562t, 564
  volume
    contraction of, 572
    losses of, 495
    quantitative analysis of, 572
    regulation of, 489
Extracorporeal albumin dialysis, for acute kidney
  injury-hepatorenal syndrome, 66

Hypertension *(Continued)*
  antihypertensive regimen for, 441–442
  blood pressure measurement technique for, 439–440
  as cardiovascular disease risk factor, 424t, 438–439
  classification of, 431, 432t
  congenital adrenal hyperplasia and, 453
  in Cushing syndrome, 451
    mechanism of, 451
  definition of, 431
  diabetes mellitus and, 439
  drug-induced, 460–461
  in elderly patients, 344
  end-stage kidney disease risk and, 441
  endocrine, 449–459, 458b
  epidemiology of, 438
  evaluation for, 432
  familial hyperkalemic, 506
  gestational, 332
    living kidney donation and, 402
  in 11β-hydroxylase deficiency, 454
  in 17α-hydroxylase deficiency, 454
  imaging work-up for, 33
  kidney disease causing, 441
  kidney parenchymal, 438–443, 442b
  low cortisol levels, 505–506
  malignant, 471
  Mendelian (or monogenic) *versus* essential, 501
  in minimal change disease, 182
  monogenic, 501, 507
  neurogenic, 460, 462
    orthostatic, 462
  in pregnancy, 332, 442
  prevalence of, 431–432
  primary, 429–437, 436b
    pathophysiology of, 433
  refractory, 464
  renal transplantation and, 397, 425
  renovascular, 444
  resistant, 464–470, 469b
  salt-sensitive, 433–434, 441
  secondary, 460–463, 463b, 468b
  secondary cause of, 434
  treatment of, 440–441
    in chronic kidney disease, 145
    combination therapy, 478
    diastolic, systolic, or pulse pressure, 439
    goals, 477–478
    initial, 432–433
    monotherapy, 478
    non-pharmacologic, 483–486, 485b
    pharmacologic, 477, 481b
    in renal transplant recipients, 425
  uncontrolled, 441
    revascularization for, 447
Hypertension-brachydactyly syndrome, 502t
Hypertension syndrome, 505
Hypertensive emergencies, 471–476, 476b
  with acute left ventricular failure, 475
  adrenergic crisis as, 475

Hypertensive emergencies *(Continued)*
  with aortic dissection, 473–475
  epidemiologic characteristics of, 471
  hypertensive urgency *versus,* 471
  long-term prognosis of, 472–473
  treatment of
    acute pharmacologic, 475–476
    drugs for, 472, 474t
    major principles in, 472
  types of, 473t
Hypertensive encephalopathy, 472
Hypertensive urgency, hypertensive emergencies *versus,* 471
Hyperthyroidism, secondary hypertension from, 461
Hypertonic saline, 514
Hyperuricemia, tumor lysis syndrome and, 263
Hypervolemia, 489–495
  adjuvant techniques to enhance history and physical in, 490
  definition of, 489
  manifestations of, 490
  physical exam reliable for, 490
  treatment of, 493
Hypoalbuminemia
  nephrotic syndrome and, 494
  peritoneal dialysis-related, 385–386
Hypocalcemia, 526–531, 530b
  acute symptomatic, treatment for, 528
  causes of, 527
  clinical manifestations of, 528
  diseases associated with, 528
  laboratory tests of, 528
  medications causing, 528
  rhabdomyolysis caused by, 90t
  spurious, causes of, 526
Hypocomplementemia, in membranoproliferative glomerulonephritis, 205–206
Hypogammaglobulinemia, in minimal change disease, 183
Hypoglycemia, in alcohol dependence, 560
Hypokalemia, 519–525, 525b
  causes of, 521
  in chronic tubulointerstitial nephritis, 318
  cortisol levels in, 505
  diarrhea and, 564–565
  evaluation of, 521
  factors of, shifting potassium into cells, 520
  IV potassium supplementation for, 522
  by oral supplementation, 522
  peritoneal dialysis-related, 385
  rhabdomyolysis caused by, 90t
  signs and symptoms of, 521
Hypomagnesemia, 502t, 541–544
  diabetes and, 547
  diagnosis of, 544, 544t
  electrolyte abnormalities and, 542–543
  hypocalcemia caused by, 527
  kidney disorders leading to, 542, 543f
  signs, symptoms, and consequences of, 543–544, 546t
  treatment for, 544, 545t